Child Abuse

MEDICAL DIAGNOSIS AND MANAGEMENT

4th Edition

Editors

Antoinette Laskey, MD, MPH, MBA, FAAP
Professor of Pediatrics
Division Chief and Medical Director
Center for Safe and Health Families
University of Utah School of Medicine
Salt Lake City, UT

Andrew Sirotnak, MD, FAAP
Professor and Vice Chair for Faculty Affairs
Department of Pediatrics
University of Colorado School of Medicine
Director, Child Protection Team
Children's Hospital Colorado
Aurora, CO

American Academy of Pediatrics
DEDICATED TO THE HEALTH OF ALL CHILDREN®

Mary Lou White, *Chief Product and Services Officer/SVP, Membership, Marketing, and Publishing*

Mark Grimes, *Vice President, Publishing*

Chris Wiberg, *Senior Editor, Professional/Clinical Publishing*

Theresa Wiener, *Production Manager, Clinical and Professional Publications*

Jason Crase, *Manager, Editorial Services*

Mary Louise Carr, MBA, *Marketing Manager, Clinical Publications*

Published by the American Academy of Pediatrics

345 Park Blvd
Itasca, IL 60143
Telephone: 630/626-6000
Facsimile: 847/434-8000
www.aap.org

The American Academy of Pediatrics is an organization of 67,000 primary care pediatricians, pediatric medical subspecialists, and pediatric surgical specialists dedicated to the health, safety, and well-being of infants, children, adolescents, and young adults.

The recommendations in this publication do not indicate an exclusive course of treatment or serve as a standard of care. Variations, taking into account individual circumstances, may be appropriate.

Any websites, brand names, products, or manufacturers are mentioned for informational and identification purposes only and do not imply an endorsement by the American Academy of Pediatrics (AAP). The AAP is not responsible for the content of external resources. Information was current at the time of publication.

The publishers have made every effort to trace the copyright holders for borrowed material. If they have inadvertently overlooked any, they will be pleased to make the necessary arrangements at the first opportunity.

This publication has been developed by the American Academy of Pediatrics. The authors, editors, and contributors are expert authorities in the field of pediatrics. No commercial involvement of any kind has been solicited or accepted in the development of the content of this publication. Disclosures: Dr Dias disclosed a safety monitoring board relationship with Allergan. Dr Dubowitz disclosed consulting relationship with Total Child Health and with Advanced Metrics. Dr Forkey disclosed family stock ownership with Precision C Corporation. Dr Greenbaum disclosed a family safety monitoring board relationship with Retrophin and with Relypsa and a family consu relationship with Vifor and with Bristol-Myers Squibb. Dr McTavish disclosed a consulting relationship with the World Health Organiza Dr Metz disclosed stock ownership in Vertex, Biogen, and Medtronic. The editors and many of the contributors to this book often provide witness testimony in court cases involving alleged child abuse and may be reimbursed for these services.

Every effort has been made to ensure that the drug selection and dosages set forth in this text are in accordance with the current recommendations and practice at the time of publication. It is the responsibility of the health care professional to check the package insert of each drug for any change in indications and dosages and for added warnings and precautions.

Every effort is made to keep *Child Abuse: Medical Diagnosis and Management* consistent with the most recent advice and information available from the American Academy of Pediatrics.

Special discounts are available for bulk purchases of this publication. Email Special Sales at aapsales@aap.org for more information

Printed in the United States of America

9-426/rep0925

2 3 4 5 6 7 8 9 10
MA0938
ISBN: 978-1-61002-358-0
eBook: 978-1-61002-359-7
Cover and publication design by Peg Mulcahy
Library of Congress Control Number: 2018967251

Contributors

Amy R. Beck, PhD
Weight Management Program
Center for Children's Healthy Lifestyles and Nutrition
Children's Mercy Kansas City
Associate Professor of Pediatrics
UMKC School of Medicine
Kansas City, MO

Elizabeth Benzinger, PhD
Ohio Bureau of Criminal Investigation
London, OH

Molly Curtin Berkoff, MD, FAAP
Associate Professor of Pediatrics
Division of General Pediatrics and Adolescent Medicine
Department of Pediatrics
University of North Carolina at Chapel Hill
Chapel Hill, NC

Stephen C. Boos, MD, FAAP
Associate Professor of Pediatrics
University of Massachusetts Medical School–Baystate
Springfield, MA
Adjunct Associate Professor of Pediatrics
Tufts University School of Medicine
Boston, MA

Ryan Brown, MD, FAAP
Clinical Associate Professor
Department of Pediatrics
The University of Oklahoma College of Medicine
Medical Director, Child Protection Team
The Children's Hospital at OU Medical Center
Oklahoma City, OK

Kara Byrne, PhD
Assistant Research Professor
College of Social Work
University of Utah
Salt Lake City, UT

Kristine Campbell, MD, MSc, FAAP
Associate Professor
Division of Child Protection and Family Health
Department of Pediatrics
University of Utah School of Medicine
Primary Children's Hospital Center for Safe and Healthy Families
Salt Lake City, UT

Mary Case, MD
Professor
Department of Pathology
St Louis University Health Sciences Center
St Louis, MO

Antonia Chiesa, MD
Associate Professor of Pediatrics
University of Colorado School of Medicine
Kempe Center for the Prevention and Treatment of Child Abuse and Neglect
Children's Hospital Colorado
Aurora, CO

Theresa M. Covington, MPH
Director, Within Our Reach
Alliance for Strong Families and Communities
Washington, DC

Paige Culotta, MD, FAAP
Child Abuse Pediatrician
Children's Hospital of New Orleans
Audrey Hepburn CARE Center
New Orleans, LA

Allan R. De Jong, MD, FAAP
Medical Director
Children at Risk Evaluation (CARE) Program
Nemours/Alfred I. duPont Hospital for Children
Wilmington, DE

Stephanie A. Deutsch, MD, FAAP
Co-Medical Director
Children at Risk Evaluation (CARE) Program

Nemours/Alfred I. duPont Hospital for Children
Wilmington, DE

Mark S. Dias, MD, FAAP, FAANS
Professor of Neurosurgery and Pediatrics
Penn State College of Medicine
Penn State Health Children's Hospital
Hershey, PA

Howard Dubowitz, MD, MS, FAAP
Professor
Department of Pediatrics
University of Maryland School of Medicine
Baltimore, MD

Karen Farst, MD, MPH, FAAP
Associate Professor and Section Chief for Children at Risk
Department of Pediatrics
University of Arkansas for Medical Sciences
Little Rock, AR

Kenneth Feldman, MD, FAAP
Clinical Professor of Pediatrics
University of Washington
Children's Protection Program
Seattle Children's Hospital
Seattle, WA

Amanda K. Fingarson, DO, FAAP
Child Abuse Pediatrics Program
Ann and Robert H. Lurie Children's Hospital of Chicago
Assistant Professor of Pediatrics
Northwestern University Feinberg School of Medicine
Chicago, IL

Martin A. Finkel, DO, FACOP, FAAP
Professor of Pediatrics
Institute Codirector
Child Abuse Research Education & Service (CARES) Institute
School of Osteopathic Medicine
Rowan University
Stratford, NJ

Diana H. Fishbein, PhD
Director, Program for Translational Research on Adversity and Neurodevelopment
Edna Bennett Pierce Prevention Research Center
Professor, Department of Human Development and Family Studies
The Pennsylvania State University
University Park, PA

Heather Forkey, MD, FAAP
Associate Professor
Department of Pediatrics
University of Massachusetts Medical School
Worcester, MA

Jordan Greenbaum, MD
Institute on Healthcare and Human Trafficking at the Stephanie V. Blank Center for Safe and Healthy Children
Children's Healthcare of Atlanta
Atlanta, GA
International Centre for Missing and Exploited Children
Alexandria, VA

Sarah E. Hampl, MD, FAAP
General Pediatrics and Weight Management
Center for Children's Healthy Lifestyles and Nutrition
Children's Mercy Kansas City
Professor of Pediatrics
UMKC School of Medicine
Kansas City, MO

Suzanne B. Haney, MD, FAAP
Assistant Professor of Pediatrics
University of Nebraska Medical Center
Children's Hospital and Medical Center
Omaha, NE

Tara L. Harris, MD, MS, FAAP
Assistant Professor of Clinical Pediatrics
Division of Child Protection Programs
Department of Pediatrics
Indiana University School of Medicine
Riley Hospital for Children
Indianapolis, IN

M. Katherine Henry, MD, MSCE, FAAP
Fellow
Department of Pediatrics
Perelman School of Medicine at the University of Pennsylvania
Safe Place: The Center for Child Protection and Health
Division of General Pediatrics
Children's Hospital of Philadelphia
Philadelphia, PA

Larissa Hines, MD, FAAP
Clinical Assistant Professor
Department of Pediatrics
The University of Oklahoma College of Medicine
Child Abuse Pediatrician
Child Protection Team
The Children's Hospital at OU Medical Center
Oklahoma City, OK

Brooks Keeshin, MD, FAAP
Assistant Professor
Department of Pediatrics
University of Utah
Center for Safe and Healthy Families
Primary Children's Hospital
Salt Lake City, UT

Emily Killough, MD, FAAP
Child Abuse Pediatrician
Division of Child Adversity and Resilience
Children's Mercy Kansas City
Assistant Professor of Pediatrics
Division of Child Abuse and Neglect
UMKC School of Medicine
Kansas City, MO

Barbara L. Knox, MD, FAAP
Professor of Pediatrics
University of Wisconsin School of Medicine and Public Health
Medical Director, University of Wisconsin Child Protection Program
University of Wisconsin American Family Children's Hospital
Madison, WI

Wendy G. Lane, MD, MPH, FAAP
Clinical Associate Professor
Department of Epidemiology and Public Health
Department of Pediatrics
University of Maryland School of Medicine
Baltimore, MD

Alex V. Levin, MD, MHSc, FRCSC, FAAP, FAAO
Chief, Pediatric Ophthalmology and Ocular Genetics
Wills Eye Hospital
Philadelphia, PA

Daniel M. Lindberg, MD
Associate Professor
Department of Emergency Medicine
Department of Pediatrics
University of Colorado School of Medicine
Attending Physician
Kempe Center for the Prevention and Treatment of Child Abuse and Neglect
Children's Hospital Colorado
Aurora, CO

Deborah Lowen, MD, FAAP
Associate Professor of Pediatrics
Vanderbilt University School of Medicine
Director, Center for Child Protection & Well-Being
Vanderbilt University Medical Center
Nashville, TN

François M. Luyet, MD
Clinical Assistant Professor of Pediatrics
University of Wisconsin School of Medicine and Public Health
University of Wisconsin Child Protection Program
University of Wisconsin American Family Children's Hospital
Madison, WI

Harriet MacMillan, CM, MD, MSc, FRCPC, FAAP
Distinguished University Professor
Department of Psychiatry and Behavioural Neurosciences

Department of Pediatrics
Chedoke Health Chair in Child Psychiatry
Offord Centre for Child Studies
McMaster University
McMaster Children's Hospital/ Hamilton Health Sciences
Hamilton, Ontario, Canada

Kathi Makoroff, MD, MEd, FAAP
Mayerson Center for Safe and Healthy Children
Cincinnati Children's Hospital Medical Center
Associate Professor
University of Cincinnati College of Medicine
Cincinnati, OH

Shelly D. Martin, MD
Child Abuse Pediatrician
Brooke Army Medical Center
San Antonio, TX
Associate Clinical Professor of Pediatrics
Uniformed Services University of the Health Sciences
Bethesda, MD

Jill McTavish, PhD
Postdoctoral Fellow
Department of Psychiatry and Behavioural Neurosciences
McMaster University
Hamilton, Ontario, Canada

John D. Melville, MD, MS, FAAP
Associate Professor of Pediatrics
Medical University of South Carolina
Charleston, SC

James Metz, MD, MPH, FAAP
Assistant Professor
Department of Pediatrics
University of Vermont
Larner College of Medicine
Division of General Pediatrics, ChildSafe Program
University of Vermont Children's Hospital
Burlington, VT

Mary E. Moffatt, MD, FAAP
Professor of Pediatrics
University of Missouri Kansas City School of Medicine
Director, Child Abuse Pediatrics Fellowship
Division of Child Adversity and Resilience
Division of Emergency Medicine
Children's Mercy Hospital, Kansas City
Kansas City, MO

Yair Morad, MD
Department of Ophthalmology
Assaf Harofeh Medical Center
Tel Aviv University
Tel Aviv, Israel

Wynne Morgan, MD
Assistant Professor
Department of Psychiatry
University of Massachusetts Medical School
Worcester, MA

Sandeep K. Narang, MD, JD, FAAP
Associate Professor of Pediatrics
Northwestern University Feinberg School of Medicine
Division Head, Child Abuse Pediatrics
Ann and Robert H. Lurie Children's Hospital of Chicago
Chicago, IL

Shalon M. Nienow, MD, FAAP
Medical Clinic Director
Chadwick Center for Children and Families
Rady Children's Hospital—San Diego
Clinical Assistant Professor
Division of Pediatric Emergency Medicine
University of California San Diego
San Diego, CA

Sarah A. W. Northrop, MD, FAAP
Department of Pediatrics
Brenner Children's Hospital
Assistant Professor of Pediatrics
Wake Forest School of Medicine
Wake Forest Baptist Health
Winston-Salem, NC

Vincent J. Palusci, MD, MS, FAAP
Professor of Pediatrics
New York University School of Medicine
New York, NY

Sarah Passmore, DO, FAAP
Department of Pediatrics
University of Oklahoma
Tulsa, OK

James G. Pawelski, MS
Director, State Advocacy
American Academy of Pediatrics
Itasca, IL

Hillary W. Petska, MD, MPH, FAAP
Assistant Professor
Department of Pediatrics
Medical College of Wisconsin
Child Abuse Pediatrician
Child Advocacy and Protection Services
Children's Hospital of Wisconsin
Milwaukee, WI

Mary Clyde Pierce, MD, FAAP
Child Abuse Pediatrics Program, Pediatric Emergency Medicine
Ann and Robert H. Lurie Children's Hospital of Chicago
Professor of Pediatrics
Northwestern University Feinberg School of Medicine
Chicago, IL

Corey J. Rood, MD, FAAP
Child Abuse Pediatrician
Assistant Professor of Pediatrics
Medical Director, Child Abuse Pediatrics
University of California Irvine
Orange, CA
Medical Director, Child Abuse and Prevention Team
Miller Children's and Women's Hospital
Long Beach, CA

Emma Jane Rose, PhD
Assistant Research Professor
Associate Director, Program for Translational Research on Adversity and Neurodevelopment
Edna Bennett Pierce Prevention Research Center
The Center for Healthy Children
The Pennsylvania State University
University Park, PA

Brooke D. Saffren, OMS-IV
Philadelphia College of Osteopathic Medicine
Philadelphia, PA

Susan A. Scherl, MD, FAAP
Professor
Department of Orthopaedics
University of Nebraska Medical Center
Attending Physician
Section of Pediatric Orthopaedics
Children's Hospital and Medical Center
Omaha, NE

Patricia G. Schnitzer, MS, PhD
National Center for Fatality Review and Prevention
Washington, DC

Lynn K. Sheets, MD, FAAP
Professor
Department of Pediatrics
Medical College of Wisconsin
Medical Director
Child Advocacy and Protection Services
Children's Hospital of Wisconsin
Milwaukee, WI

Lindsay Dianne Shepard, LCSW, MSW, MSC
Program Manager
Department of Pediatrics
University of Utah
Therapist
Center for Safe and Healthy Families
Primary Children's Hospital
Salt Lake City, UT

Kirsten Simonton, MD, FAAP
Assistant Professor of Pediatrics
Northwestern University Feinberg School of Medicine
Attending Physician

Division of Child Abuse Pediatrics
Ann and Robert H. Lurie Children's Hospital of Chicago
Chicago, IL

Katherine Snyder, MD, MPH, FAAP
Department of Pediatrics
Dell Medical School
University of Texas at Austin
Austin, TX

Jenna Spagnuolo, DCFI
Forensic Interviewer Supervisor
Child Abuse Program
Children's Hospital of The King's Daughters
Norfolk, VA

Lisa Spector, MD, FAAP
Professor of Pediatrics
University of Central Florida
Division Chief of Developmental and Behavioral Pediatrics
Nemours Children's Hospital
Orlando, FL

Suzanne P. Starling, MD, FAAP
Medical Director, Chadwick Center for Children & Families
Rady Children's Hospital of San Diego
Clinical Professor of Pediatrics, University of California San Diego
San Diego, CA

Sasha Svendsen, MD, FAAP
UMass Memorial Children's Medical Center
Westborough, MA
University of Massachusetts Medical School
Worcester, MA

Brooke Sweeney, MD, FAAP
Medical Director, Weight Management Services
Children's Mercy Kansas City
Clinical Assistant Professor of Pediatrics
UMKC School of Medicine
Kansas City, MO

Jonathan Thackeray, MD, FAAP
Chief Medical Community Health Officer
Department of Medical Affairs
Dayton Children's Hospital
Professor and Vice Chair
Department of Pediatrics
Wright State University Boonshoft School of Medicine
Dayton, OH

Kathryn Wells, MD, FAAP
Associate Professor and Section Head for Child Abuse and Neglect
Department of Pediatrics
University of Colorado School of Medicine
Aurora, CO

With enduring gratitude to those who came before and laid the foundation on which we were able to build and grow and from whom we have learned so much

To my professional rocks APS, SPS, and TPH, who have helped me grow into the professional I am

To ZWS, who has been there through it all and has turned into an amazing professional in his own right

And to JGL, AGL, and DEL, without whom I could not achieve all that I have set out to do

—ALL

To my colleagues, mentors, and peers, who have supported my professional growth and leadership journey

To JWW and my family, who have provided encouragement and sustained my resilience

And to all the students, fellows, and early career professionals who inspire me as we learn together and care for children

—APS

Contents

Part 3: Neglect

Part 4: Other Forms of Maltreatment

Part 5: Pathology of Child Maltreatment

Part 6: Professional Issues in Child Maltreatment

Part 7: Outcomes

Part 8: Prevention

Foreword

"To study the phenomena of disease without books is to sail an uncharted sea, while to study books without patients is not to go to sea at all."

Sir William Osler

Clinicians who evaluate patients to determine whether they have been harmed by neglect or sexual or physical maltreatment heed Olser's advice and use books along with peer-reviewed literature to complement their direct contact with these patients. It is, therefore, essential that authoritative books in the field of child abuse and neglect are available, current, and evidence based. This fourth edition of *Child Abuse: Medical Diagnosis and Management* continues its mission to present the best research available synthesized by leading experts.

The preface in the first edition, published in 1994, stated the "accumulation of understanding has appeared in such a diverse range of clinical and research journals that it requires constant vigilance to stay informed of recent advances. The practitioner needs an integrated resource for the strictly medical information when confronting a new case of child abuse." This is true to an even greater extent 25 years and more than 3,000 peer-reviewed articles published since Caffey's seminal article in 1946[1] and Kempe et al's article in 1962.[2] The relatively recent recognition of child maltreatment as a major contributor to morbidity and mortality in infancy, childhood, and adolescence has spawned the subspecialty of child abuse pediatrics. This new edition of *Child Abuse: Medical Diagnosis and Management* opens with a discussion of this evolving workforce.

In addition to the traditional core curriculum, comprehensively presented in the first 26 chapters, appropriate attention is also given to vicarious trauma and burnout, caring for the child in out-of-home care, and the medical and psychological sequelae of child abuse and neglect. The authors of the chapter on neurobiological consequences of child maltreatment address the central importance of adverse childhood experiences as critically significant in numerous adult pathologies. Finally, the concluding section discusses prevention and advocacy, persistently necessary approaches to the protection of children in a world fraught with challenges from all quarters of our social order.

Thanks are due to those who contributed chapters, the editors who selected them, and the American Academy of Pediatrics for publishing this book.

Robert M. Reece, MD, FAAP

References

1. Caffey J. Multiple fractures in the long bones of infants suffering from chronic subdural hematoma. *Am J Roentgenol Radium Ther.* 1946;56(2):163–173 PMID: 20995763
2. Kempe CH, Silverman FN, Steele BF, Droegemueller W, Silver HK. The battered-child syndrome. *JAMA*. 1962;181(1):17–24 PMID: 14455086 https://doi.org/10.1001/jama.1962.03050270019004

Acknowledgment

With this fourth edition, the editors and authors of the current edition wish to express their deep gratitude for the hard work and expertise of the previous editions' authors in creating a solid foundation on which we could build. Without their knowledge, effort, and mentorship, we would not be able to successfully advance this field of medicine.

Introduction

The Evolving Workforce

Antoinette Laskey, MD, MPH, MBA, FAAP
Andrew Sirotnak, MD, FAAP

Child maltreatment has affected children since long before medical professionals recognized the manifestations medically and psychologically in their patients. Over the years since the early publications identifying the specific findings that indicated a child had experienced sexual abuse, physical abuse, or neglect, there has been an increase in interest among certain medical professionals to care for these patients, to learn more about the conditions, and, importantly, to try to prevent the harm that can be done at the hands of a caregiver. The medical field has evolved from professionals without specific training but with a committed interest to this population to those who choose to obtain accredited fellowship training in child abuse pediatrics and to a growing interdisciplinary research community with a focus on the problem of child maltreatment.

There have also been important changes in how cases are handled among the multitude of professionals who are involved in the evaluation and management of the child who has potentially experienced abuse. What used to be a strictly siloed approach of each professional agency handling a case as it evolved is now an integrated, child-centered, ideally trauma-informed approach to caring for a child who has potentially experienced abuse. This is often accomplished through children's advocacy centers that bring together multidisciplinary teams committed to best practices and collaboration in working with children affected by violence. Partnerships between pediatricians and children's hospitals have been crucial in the development of a diverse range of programs, often associated or integrated within trauma, emergency, or pediatric medicine divisions. Building systems of care into communities, these programs often struggle to meet every need, ranging from medical evaluation, diagnosis, and management to follow-up care and trauma-informed behavioral therapy.

While some of us are attracted to pediatrics because we enjoy working with children, other medical professionals may think that child maltreatment is an issue that is irrelevant to them because they specifically chose *not* to go into the specialty of pediatrics. The truth is quite the opposite. As Robert Block, MD, one of the fathers of child abuse pediatrics and a former president of the American Academy of Pediatrics, once said, "All adults once were children, and who we are as adults is in many ways affected by our childhood experiences, environments, and relationships."

No matter the medical specialty, all medical professionals need to be aware of the prevalence, findings, and medical and psychological consequences of child maltreatment. It is important for all medical professionals to know what to do for current and past children who have experienced maltreatment to mitigate the potential negative health outcomes.

Since the first board certification examination offered in 2009, more than 400 pediatricians have obtained board certification from the American Board of Pediatrics in the subspecialty of child abuse pediatrics. Despite having these trained individuals who choose to focus on this aspect of pediatric medicine, there will always be a need for the frontline medical professionals around the country in community-based practices, community hospitals, and medical settings ranging from rural to urban, who see most of the children who have been maltreated. Some of these medical professionals have been informally and affectionately dubbed "Gen-CAPS" because they have a special interest in this population and are willing to work closely with their community partners such as law enforcement and child welfare agencies.

This new edition of *Child Abuse: Medical Diagnosis and Management* was developed with all these professionals in mind: the subspecialist trained in child abuse pediatrics, the Gen-CAP, the medical professional who sees children in his or her practice, and the medical learners who have yet to choose their clinical area of specialization. We hope that this edition will be a trusted education and clinical resource. We recognize that to effectively care for children who may have experienced maltreatment, there are many who must recognize maltreatment, respond, report when appropriate, and partner to provide ongoing medical and psychological care for the damage to be mitigated and the healing to begin.

Part 1

Physical Abuse

CHAPTER 1

Sentinel Injuries

Hillary W. Petska, MD, MPH, FAAP
Assistant Professor
Department of Pediatrics
Medical College of Wisconsin
Child Abuse Pediatrician
Child Advocacy and Protection Services
Children's Hospital of Wisconsin
Milwaukee, WI

Lynn K. Sheets, MD, FAAP
Professor
Department of Pediatrics
Medical College of Wisconsin
Medical Director
Child Advocacy and Protection Services
Children's Hospital of Wisconsin
Milwaukee, WI

Many children evaluated in a medical setting have incidental findings on physical examination of minor skin or intraoral injuries. Children who can walk, run, and jump often have bruises over bony prominences, such as the shins, knees, or forehead. Bruises in these locations are expected in active children and are not usually concerning for abuse. However, young infants who are not yet mobile typically have no bruises.[1–7] Any bruise in an infant who is not yet mobile should raise concerns for physical abuse or, much more rarely, a bleeding disorder. It is not until infants start to pull to a stand and take a few steps while holding onto something, or *cruise,* that an occasional bruise is expected. Similarly, intraoral injuries are common unintentional injuries in walking children but should raise concerns for physical abuse in young pre-cruising infants. Pediatricians, other physicians, and nonphysician clinicians must remain vigilant for these subtle signs of abuse, or *sentinel injuries,* in infants because a missed diagnosis may have fatal consequences.

Definition

A *sentinel injury* is a relatively minor injury in a pre-cruising infant that is poorly explained and therefore concerning for child physical abuse. Sentinel injuries are visible to a caregiver and may include bruising or intraoral injury (eg, torn frenum) (figures 1.1 and 1.2). Burns, radial head subluxation (ie, pulled [nursemaid] elbow), and subconjunctival hemorrhages have also been identified as possible sentinel injuries requiring careful evaluation (Figure 1.3).[8–10]

Superficial abrasions or transient reddening of the skin are not sentinel injuries because they are nonspecific and may occur in the normal care or activity of an infant (eg, infant unintentionally scratches her face with her fingernails).[6,11] Injuries such as rib fractures are also not sentinel injuries because they are often occult and not easily detectable by a caregiver.

Sentinel injuries typically heal quickly and completely without the need for medical intervention. However, these apparently trivial injuries are clinically significant because they are unexpected and because of

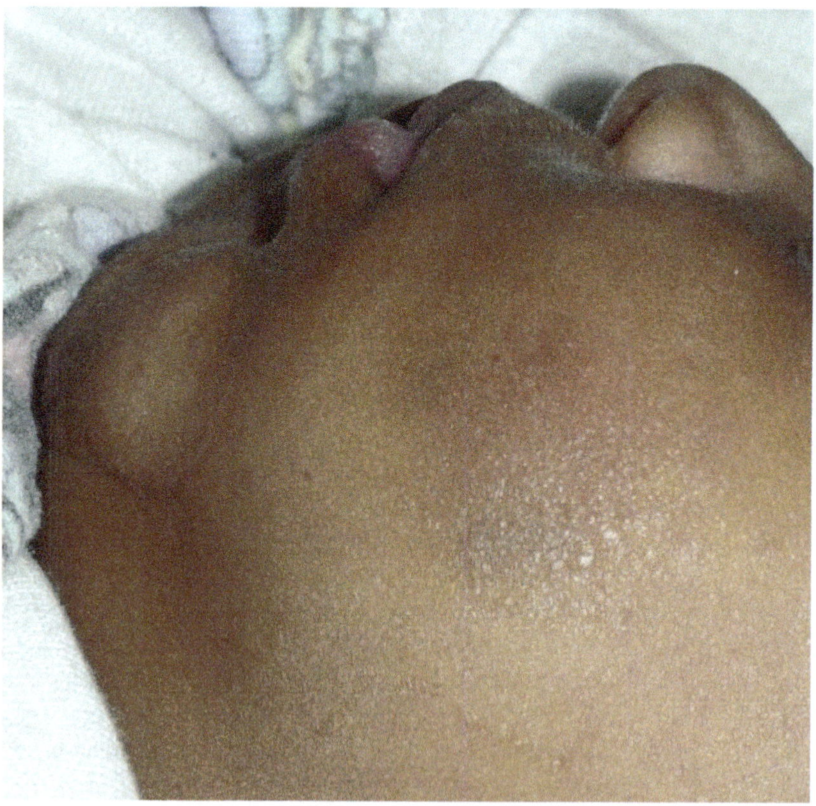

FIGURE 1.1
7-week-old presenting for constipation and fussiness with an unexplained cheek bruise noted on examination.

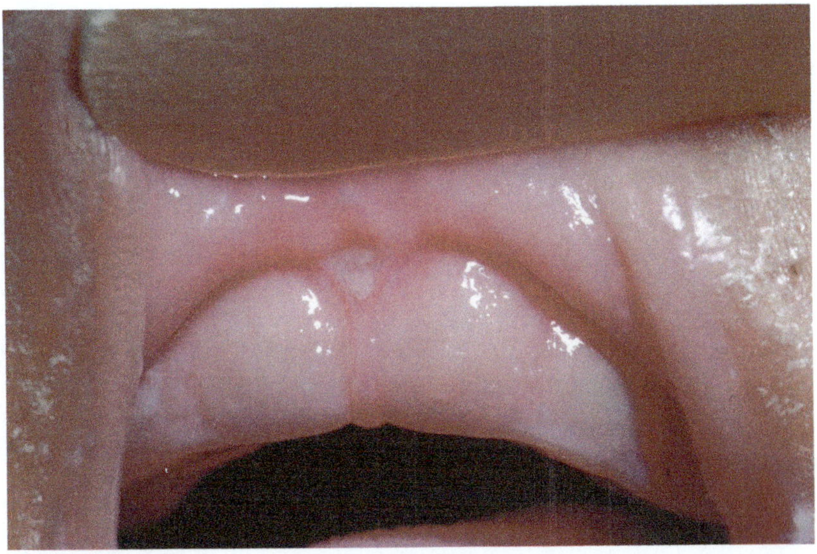

FIGURE 1.2
3-month-old with unexplained upper labial frenum injury and fractures.

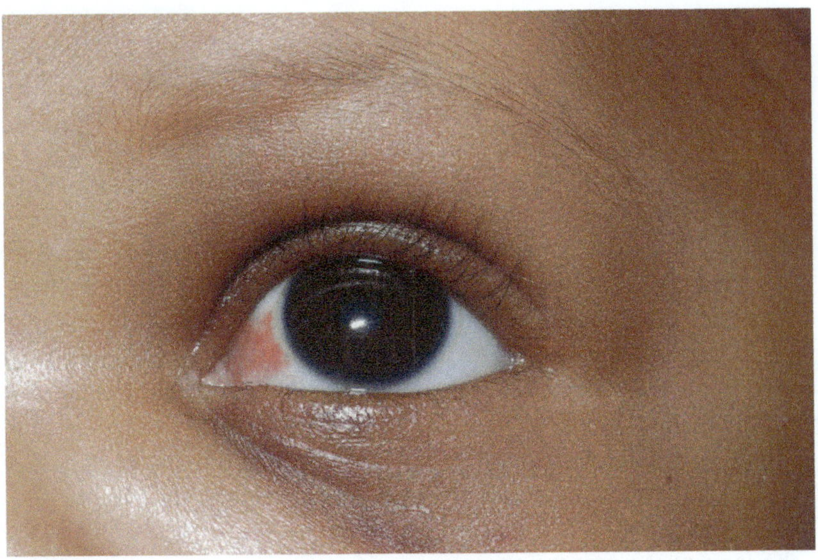

FIGURE 1.3
3-month-old with unexplained subconjunctival hemorrhage and fractures.

the concern they raise for physical abuse or, rarely, a bleeding disorder.[12] Bruising and intraoral injury are uncommon and unexpected in healthy infants and often precede more severe injury or death in infants who experience child abuse (Figure 1.4).[1–8,13–21]

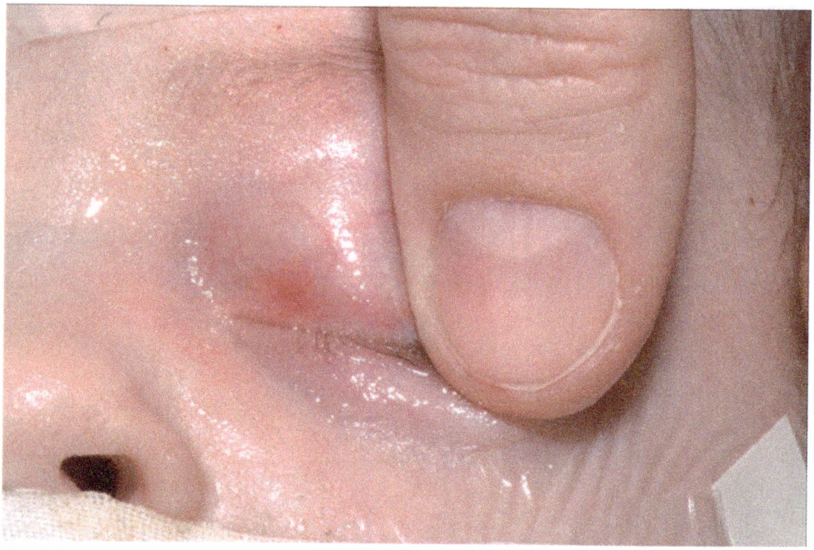

FIGURE 1.4
1-month-old with a non-blanching red eyelid bruise noted 1 day prior to admission for abusive head trauma.

The exact prevalence of sentinel injuries is unknown. Caregivers may not seek medical attention for injuries, and medical professionals may not document sentinel injuries if they are perceived as minor or unimportant. However, in the seminal study of infants who were evaluated for abuse by a hospital-based child protection team, 27.5% of children with a diagnosis of physical abuse had a previous history of a sentinel injury described by a parent. None of the children with no or low concern for abuse had a history of sentinel injury.[8] More recent studies have continued to show the association between sentinel injuries and subsequent more severe abuse, although some included mobile children and/or occult injuries in their definition.[22–24] The power of the term *sentinel injury* is in its ability to help medical and other professionals involved in protecting infants think about these seemingly minor injuries as severe injuries when they occur in pre-cruising infants.[25] Imprecise use should be avoided because it poses a risk to the value of the concept as a prevention strategy.

Clinical Presentation

Sentinel injuries are typically identified in 1 of 2 ways: during medical history from a caregiver or incidentally on examination, after which a history is sought. Given the risk of harm, pre-cruising infants should be screened routinely for sentinel injuries during every medical evaluation, including health supervision (well-child), urgent care, and emergency department visits. Regardless of the presenting chief complaint, specific questions about sentinel injuries and a naked skin examination are critical in young infants.

History

While many injuries concerning for abuse are evaluated in emergency departments, infants with sentinel injuries often present to primary care clinicians with unrelated concerns.[26] Soft tissue injury, such as bruising, is the most common presentation of child physical abuse as well as the most common sentinel injury.[6,8,27,28] Bruises are unusual and unexpected in infants younger than 6 months and in children who do not yet cruise (Table 1.1).[1–7,28] Therefore, any history of bruising, even a single bruise, in a young, pre-cruising infant should raise concern for physical abuse. In fact, in one study, the most serious subsequent injuries were seen in infants with a single, subtle bruise.[23]

During medical evaluation, caregivers should be asked specifically about any history of a sentinel injury, such as bruising, "red spots" on the whites of the eyes, or bleeding from the nose or mouth (eg, frenum injury), since minor injuries may not otherwise be remembered or concerning to a caregiver. In order to consider alternative causes for a sentinel injury, the medical history also should include birth, medical, developmental, family,

TABLE 1.1
Studies of Bruising in Typical Children by Age or Stage of Motor Development

Study	Age or Stage of Motor Development	% With Bruises
Roberton et al[1] (1982) N = 400	2 wk–2 mo 3–9 mo	3.3[a] 0.1
Mortimer and Freeman[2] (1983) N = 620	<1 y	0.9
Wedgwood[3] (1990) N = 24	Pre-cruisers	0
Carpenter[4] (1999) N = 177	Pre-crawlers	3.9
Sugar et al[5] (1999) N = 930	Pre-cruisers 0–2 mo 3–5 mo 6–8 mo	2.2 0.04 0.7 5.6
Labbé and Caouette[6] (2001) N = 1,467	0–8 mo	1.2[a]
Kemp et al[7] (2015) N = 328	Pre-mobile • Not rolling • Rolling	6.7 1.3 10.9

[a] Included abrasions.

and social history. When a sentinel injury is identified, further history regarding the injury should be elicited, including a detailed timeline of when the injury was first noticed, what it looked like, when it resolved, and any known history of trauma. The medical professional must then carefully consider whether the history provided adequately explains the injury.

A plausible unintentional injury event should include a mechanism consistent with the injury and developmental stage, such as a 6-month-old with a forehead bruise and a distinct, clear history of a witnessed fall from a sitting position onto a hard toy. Without this history, the bruise should prompt consideration of child physical abuse. A bruise over soft parts of the body without an underlying bony prominence or in a protected location should also heighten the level of concern for abuse.[7,29] Whereas a history of a fall with an object in the mouth may explain an intraoral injury in a mobile child, normal care, activity, or handling of a pre-cruising infant would not. Instead, this type of injury is typically caused by a direct blow or forceful insertion of a foreign object (eg, bottle, spoon, finger) into the mouth. Similarly, while a mobile child may sustain a pulled elbow from a caregiver grabbing his arm, picking up a young infant by one arm would not be considered appropriate care or handling. Finally, while subconjunctival hemorrhages may be caused by straining with constipation, coughing, or vomiting in an older child, they are unexpected in a young infant and should raise concern for abuse such as a direct blow or asphyxiation.[30]

A changing history, lack of a plausible history, inappropriate delay in seeking care, and history that is inconsistent with developmental stage or type or severity of injury are often associated with abuse.[31,32] In a series of pre-cruising infants with unexplained bruises, child abuse was the most common cause.[23] A common implausible history is self-inflicted injury,[33] because young infants are not able to generate the force required to cause sentinel injuries themselves.[23] Uncomplicated short household falls are also often reported. While a history of a fall is the most common true and false history in pediatric injury, short falls usually result in no injury.[34] Even with a history of trauma, bruising is rare in infants.[35] Bruising also does not occur during the typical care or handling of a healthy infant in the absence of abusive forces.

Clinicians must maintain a high level of suspicion when a caregiver offers a history to explain a sentinel injury in a pre-cruising infant (Table 1.2). Sometimes an implausible history is offered because the protective caregiver does not know how the injury occurred but assumes that it was caused through unintentional events or believes a false story provided by another caregiver. The medical professional should explore the history provided to better understand the source of information and why it is being attributed to a certain event (eg, did the caregiver witness a discrete event that caused injury, or is the caregiver speculating?).

Table 1.2
Common Suspicious Stories for Bruising in Pre-cruising Infants

Mechanism	Examples
Unknown/no history	• Injury not known until noted during examination. • Infant just woke up with injury.
Easy bruising/bleeding	• Infant has pale and/or sensitive skin that bruises easily. • Infant has a history of bruises that come and go.
Normal care and handling	• Infant injured when picked up or diaper changed. • Contact with caregiver jewelry or bony prominences while being held.
Short household fall	• Infant fell from a low height (<4 ft [1.2 m]) such as a couch, crib, bed, or chair. • Infant dropped from caregiver's arms.
Injury inflicted by another child or pet	• Slightly older sibling dropped a toy on the infant. • Pet was by the infant before injury noted.
Self-inflicted injury	• Infant poked self in the face or mouth. • Infant hit self with a toy. • Infant slept on a toy or pacifier (Figure 1.5). • Infant rolled into furniture (Figure 1.6).

Modified from Kirschner RH, Wilson H. Pathology of fatal abuse. In: Reece R, Ludwig S, eds. *Child Abuse: Medical Diagnosis and Management.* 2nd ed. Philadelphia, PA: Lippincott Williams & Wilkins; 2001:467–516.

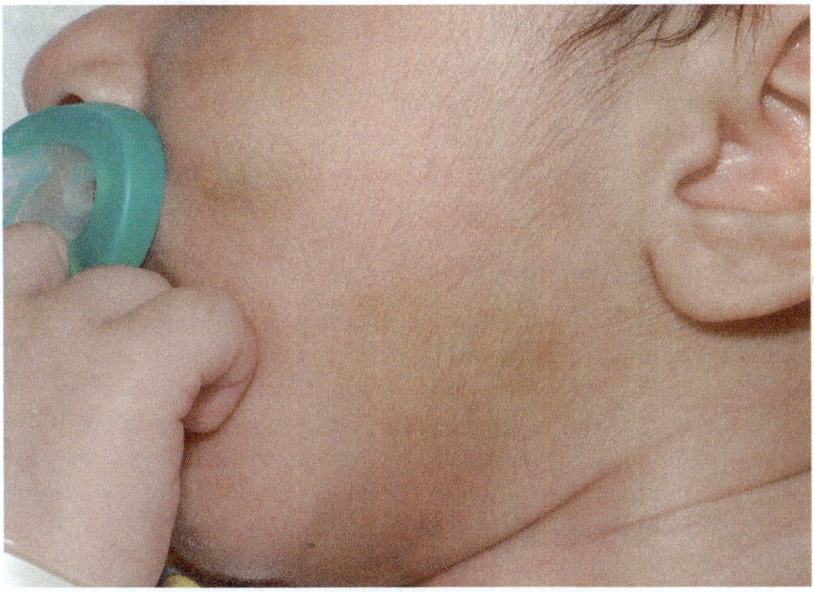

FIGURE 1.5
5-month-old who experienced abuse with facial bruising suggestive of bite injury reportedly caused by sleeping on a toy.

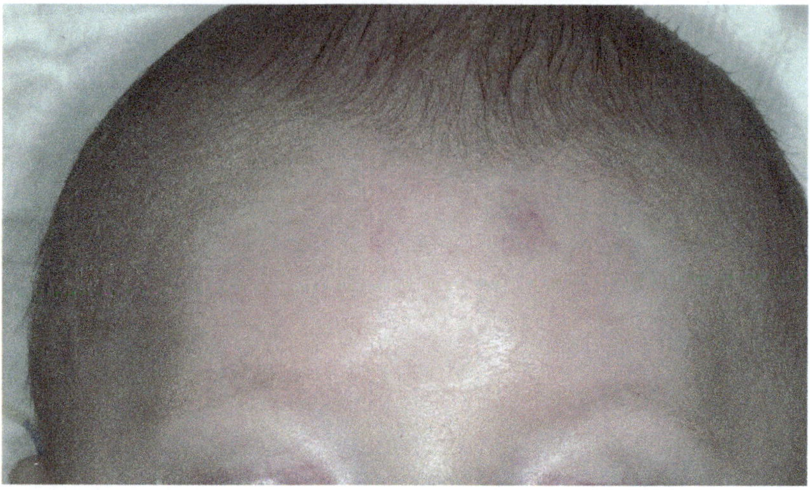

FIGURE 1.6
6-week-old who experienced abuse with forehead bruising reportedly caused by rolling into crib slats.

Certain historical elements have been identified as risk factors for child physical abuse and should be considered in the context of the entire evaluation. Infants have the highest rate of maltreatment, more than twice that of other children: 24.2 per 1,000 versus 9.2 per 1,000, respectively.[36] This may be related to the increased needs of young infants as well as their dependence on caregivers.[37] Crying also peaks during early infancy and is a commonly identified inciting infant behavior, or *trigger,* among perpetrators.[8,38–40] Other risk factors include young parental age, mental health disorders, substance abuse, domestic violence, and lower socioeconomic status.[31] It is important to note, however, that child physical abuse occurs in all geographic, ethnic, and socioeconomic settings. The presence of risk factors does not confirm the diagnosis of abuse; nor does their absence rule it out.

Physical Examination

Sentinel injuries may be subtle and are often missed on examination. Given the risk of subsequent harm in children with sentinel injuries, a complete physical examination should be performed for all young infants at every medical evaluation. The infant should be examined fully undressed with removal of the diaper for anogenital examination. An infant's skin and oral mucosa should then be carefully examined for signs of injury. While sentinel injuries are often located on the head or face,[8] injuries to the labial and sublingual frena, anterior and posterior ears, scalp, anogenital area, hands, and feet can be missed if not thoroughly inspected (figures 1.7 and 1.8).

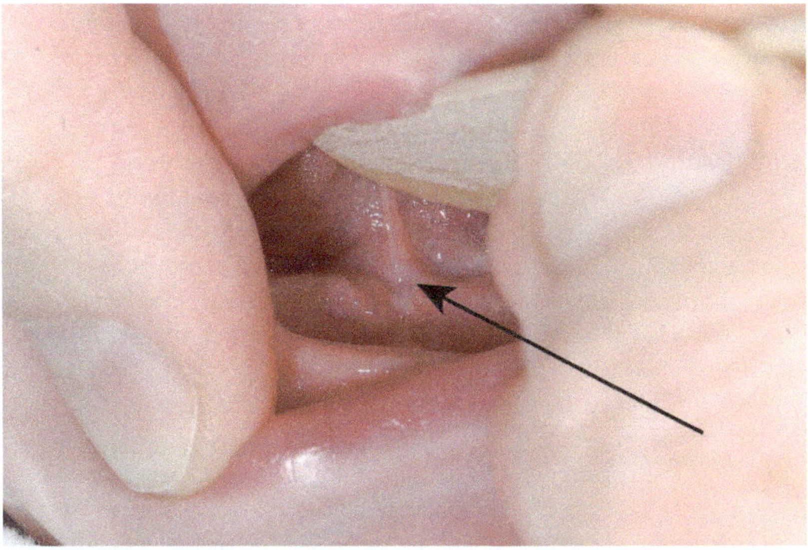

FIGURE 1.7
1-month-old with multiple fractures and bruising as well as injury at the base of the lingual frenum reportedly self-inflicted due to "tongue-tie."

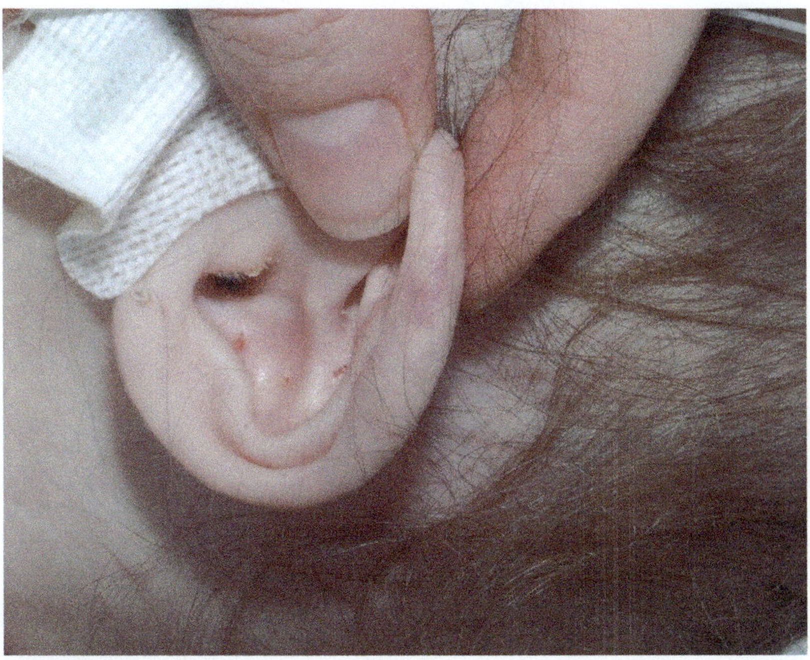

FIGURE 1.8
5-month-old with ear bruising reportedly caused by a 3-year-old sibling 1 week prior to admission for abusive head trauma.

Head circumference should also be measured routinely, even at sick visits; crossing of percentiles is often missed during medical evaluations and may be a sign of abuse.[14,21]

Any injury should be documented with a description of the location, size, and pattern and photographed if possible. Nonspecific words such as "mark" or "lesion" should be avoided if the precise type of injury, such as a bruise, is known. Bruising may appear red and/or linear and can be mistaken for abrasions (Figure 1.9). Bruises, unlike abrasions and minor skin irritation, will not blanch with application of pressure (see Figure 1.4). If unable to distinguish bruising from other skin findings, repeat or serial examinations may be necessary.

Even when injuries are noted on examination, an accurate diagnosis of abuse may be missed. In one study on sentinel injuries, a medical professional was reportedly aware of the injury in 41.9% of cases in which children were abused again. In more than half of these cases, abuse was not even considered in the differential diagnosis.[8] Injuries such as bruises that might not raise concerns in an ambulatory child have increased specificity for abuse in pre-cruising infants.[32] Abuse should be included on the differential diagnosis of any young infant presenting with bruising.

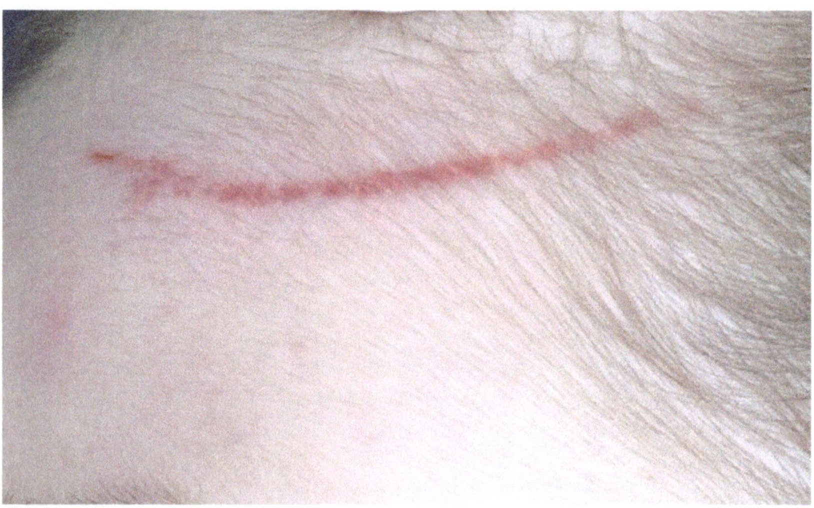

FIGURE 1.9
Linear bruise without overlying abrasion mistakenly documented as a "scratch" at the initial medical evaluation.

Management

Recognition of sentinel injuries and appropriate response can prevent further abuse. Numerous studies have shown an association between sentinel injuries and subsequent, more severe physical abuse.[8,13–21] Sentinel injuries must be recognized and responded to quickly since the interval between sentinel injury and subsequent abuse can be as little as 1 day (see Figure 1.4).[8] Despite increasing awareness, in a recent study on bruising in infants evaluated in the emergency department, only 50% of infants younger than 6 months with bruises underwent an evaluation for abuse.[24]

Infants with a sentinel injury identified on history or examination should undergo an urgent, protocol-based evaluation for occult injuries as well as predisposing medical conditions, when appropriate (Figure 1.10).[32,41] In one study of young infants presenting with unexplained bruising, 50% had an additional injury identified following evaluation. None of the infants evaluated for a bleeding disorder had a predisposing bleeding disorder.[12] Evaluation may be performed in the emergency department or primary care setting if laboratory and imaging services are available. Surveillance for other occult injuries should include

- Head computed tomography in infants younger than 6 months or with abnormal neurologic findings
- Initial skeletal survey in children younger than 2 years with follow-up skeletal survey 2 to 3 weeks later
- Laboratory studies to screen for abdominal injury[32]

Screening for occult drug exposure and underlying medical conditions such as a bleeding disorder should also be considered.[42,43] However, the workup for a medical condition should not delay appropriate management. In addition, the presence of a bleeding disorder does not rule out the possibility of abuse. The absence of additional injury on head computed tomography or skeletal survey should not diminish the level of concern for abuse because the sentinel injury may be the first or only abusive injury.

A sentinel injury on history or examination should be reported to authorities as mandated by law. Reporting only requires a reasonable suspicion of abuse, and abuse can be missed without a child protective services or law enforcement investigation.[23] A decision to report a sentinel injury can be distressing for medical professionals who perceive the injury as insignificant or who have an established relationship with a family. However, the safety of the infant must be prioritized; reporting

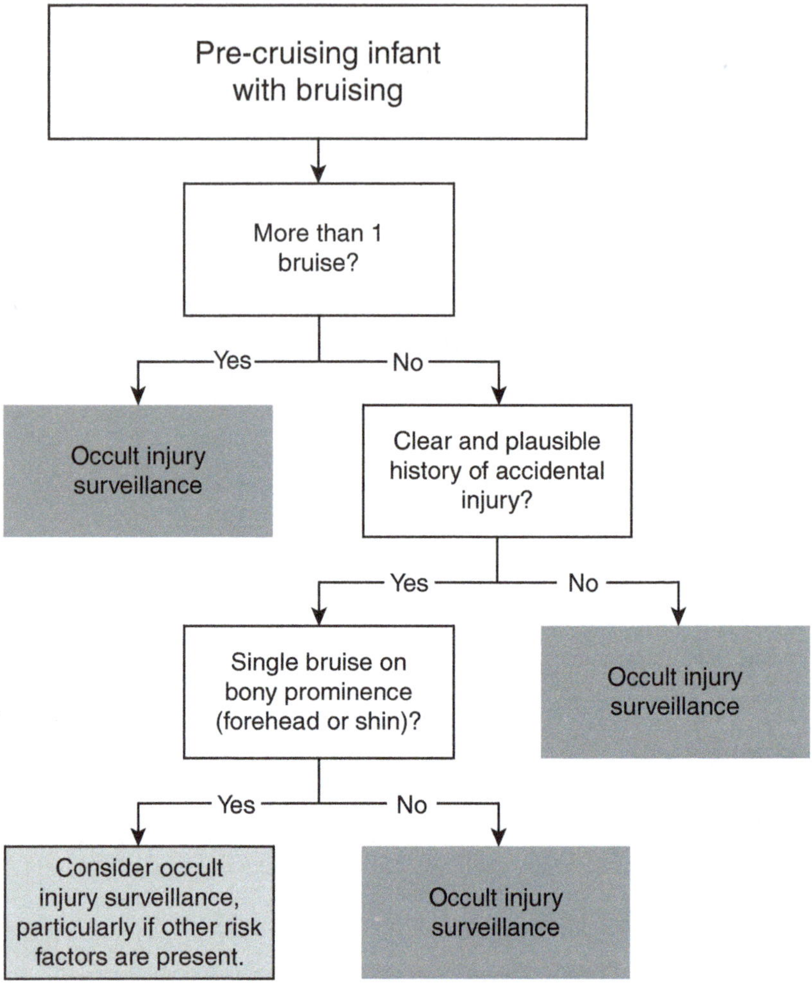

FIGURE 1.10
Algorithm to guide management of a pre-cruising infant (generally ≤ 6 months) with bruising.

may be the only opportunity to prevent further injury and/or death. When informing the family of the required reports, it is important to remain nonjudgmental because the infant may have been injured by someone other than the parents. If medical professionals are unsure about reporting or performing further workup, a pediatrician who specializes in child abuse can be contacted for guidance.

Regardless of the outcome of reporting, the occult injury surveillance and reports to investigators may serve as a deterrent to further abuse. Following a report, ongoing medical care for the child should include careful observation for subsequent injuries and anticipatory guidance and resources for the family, which may include screening for other types of violence in the home, such as intimate partner violence. Identification of sentinel injuries and intervention prior to escalation of abuse have significant potential to prevent further abuse.

References

1. Roberton DM, Barbor P, Hull D. Unusual injury? Recent injury in normal children and children with suspected non-accidental injury. *Br Med J (Clin Res Ed)*. 1982;285(6352):1399–1401 PMID: 6814575 https://doi.org/10.1136/bmj.285.6352.1399
2. Mortimer PE, Freeman M. Are facial bruises in babies ever accidental? *Arch Dis Child*. 1983;58(1):75–76 PMID: 6830281 https://doi.org/10.1136/adc.58.1.75-b
3. Wedgwood J. Childhood bruising. *Practitioner*. 1990;234(1490):598–601 PMID: 2392410
4. Carpenter RF. The prevalence and distribution of bruising in babies. *Arch Dis Child*. 1999;80(4):363–366 PMID: 10086945 https://doi.org/10.1136/adc.80.4.363
5. Sugar NF, Taylor JA, Feldman KW; Puget Sound Pediatric Research Network. Bruises in infants and toddlers: those who don't cruise rarely bruise. *Arch Pediatr Adolesc Med*. 1999;153(4):399–403 PMID: 10201724 https://doi.org/10.1001/archpedi.153.4.399
6. Labbé J, Caouette G. Recent skin injuries in normal children. *Pediatrics*. 2001;108(2): 271–276 PMID: 11483787 https://doi.org/10.1542/peds.108.2.271
7. Kemp AM, Dunstan F, Nuttall D, Hamilton M, Collins P, Maguire S. Patterns of bruising in preschool children—a longitudinal study. *Arch Dis Child*. 2015;100(5):426–431 PMID: 25589561 https://doi.org/10.1136/archdischild-2014-307120
8. Sheets LK, Leach ME, Koszewski IJ, Lessmeier AM, Nugent M, Simpson P. Sentinel injuries in infants evaluated for child physical abuse. *Pediatrics*. 2013;131(4):701–707 PMID: 23478861 https://doi.org/10.1542/peds.2012-2780
9. Browner EA. Nursemaid's elbow (annular ligament displacement). *Pediatr Rev*. 2013;34(8):366–367 PMID: 23908364 https://doi.org/10.1542/pir.34-8-366
10. Betts T, Ahmed S, Maguire S, Watts P. Characteristics of non-vitreoretinal ocular injury in child maltreatment: a systematic review. *Eye (Lond)*. 2017;31(8):1146–1154 PMID: 28338664 https://doi.org/10.1038/eye.2017.25
11. American Academy of Pediatrics Committee on Child Abuse and Neglect. When inflicted skin injuries constitute child abuse. *Pediatrics*. 2002;110(3):644–645 PMID: 12205272 https://doi.org/10.1542/peds.110.3.644
12. Harper NS, Feldman KW, Sugar NF, Anderst JD, Lindberg DM; Examining Siblings to Recognize Abuse Investigators. Additional injuries in young infants with concern for abuse and apparently isolated bruises. *J Pediatr*. 2014;165(2):383–388.e1 PMID: 24840754 https://doi.org/10.1016/j.jpeds.2014.04.004
13. Maguire S, Hunter B, Hunter L, Sibert JR, Mann M, Kemp AM; Welsh Child Protection Systematic Review Group. Diagnosing abuse: a systematic review of torn frenum and other intra-oral injuries. *Arch Dis Child*. 2007;92(12):1113–1117 PMID: 17468129 https://doi.org/10.1136/adc.2006.113001
14. Jenny C, Hymel KP, Ritzen A, Reinert SE, Hay TC. Analysis of missed cases of abusive head trauma. *JAMA*. 1999;281(7):621–626 PMID: 10029123 https://doi.org/10.1001/jama.281.7.621
15. Thackeray JD. Frena tears and abusive head injury: a cautionary tale. *Pediatr Emerg Care*. 2007;23(10):735–737 PMID: 18090110 https://doi.org/10.1097/PEC.0b013e3181568039

16. Oral R, Yagmur F, Nashelsky M, Turkmen M, Kirby P. Fatal abusive head trauma cases: consequence of medical staff missing milder forms of physical abuse. *Pediatr Emerg Care*. 2008;24(12):816–821 PMID: 19050665 https://doi.org/10.1097/PEC.0b013e31818e9f5d
17. Feldman KW. The bruised premobile infant: should you evaluate further? *Pediatr Emerg Care*. 2009;25(1):37–39 PMID: 19148012 https://doi.org/10.1097/PEC.0b013e318191db15
18. Pierce MC, Smith S, Kaczor K. Bruising in infants: those with a bruise may be abused. *Pediatr Emerg Care*. 2009;25(12):845–847 PMID: 20016354 https://doi.org/10.1097/PEC.0b013e3181c06217
19. Petska HW, Sheets LK, Knox BL. Facial bruising as a precursor to abusive head trauma. *Clin Pediatr (Phila)*. 2013;52(1):86–88 PMID: 22511190 https://doi.org/10.1177/0009922812441675
20. Thorpe EL, Zuckerbraun NS, Wolford JE, Berger RP. Missed opportunities to diagnose child physical abuse. *Pediatr Emerg Care*. 2014;30(11):771–776 PMID: 25343739 https://doi.org/10.1097/PEC.0000000000000257
21. Letson MM, Cooper JN, Deans KJ, et al. Prior opportunities to identify abuse in children with abusive head trauma. *Child Abuse Negl*. 2016;60:36–45 PMID: 27680755 https://doi.org/10.1016/j.chiabu.2016.09.001
22. Lindberg DM, Beaty B, Juarez-Colunga E, Wood JN, Runyan DK. Testing for abuse in children with sentinel injuries. *Pediatrics*. 2015;136(5):831–838 PMID: 26438705 https://doi.org/10.1542/peds.2015-1487
23. Feldman KW, Tayama TM, Strickler LE, et al. A prospective study of the causes of bruises in premobile infants. *Pediatr Emerg Care*. 2017 PMID: 29040244 https://doi.org/10.1097/PEC.0000000000001311
24. Pierce MC, Kaczor K, Acker D, et al. History, injury, and psychosocial risk factor commonalities among cases of fatal and near-fatal physical child abuse. *Child Abuse Negl*. 2017;69:263–277 PMID: 28500923 https://doi.org/10.1016/j.chiabu.2017.04.033
25. Laskey AL. Cognitive errors: thinking clearly when it could be child maltreatment. *Pediatr Clin North Am*. 2014;61(5):997–1005 PMID: 25242711 https://doi.org/10.1016/j.pcl.2014.06.012
26. Tiyyagura G, Beucher M, Bechtel K. Nonaccidental injury in pediatric patients: detection, evaluation, and treatment. *Pediatr Emerg Med Pract*. 2017;14(7):1–32 PMID: 28665574
27. Ellerstein NS. The cutaneous manifestations of child abuse and neglect. *Am J Dis Child*. 1979;133(9):906–909 PMID: 474541 https://doi.org/10.1001/archpedi.1979.02130090034005
28. Maguire S, Mann MK, Sibert J, Kemp A. Are there patterns of bruising in childhood which are diagnostic or suggestive of abuse? A systematic review. *Arch Dis Child*. 2005;90(2):182–186 PMID: 15665178 https://doi.org/10.1136/adc.2003.044065
29. Hibberd O, Nuttall D, Watson RE, Watkins WJ, Kemp AM, Maguire S. Childhood bruising distribution observed from eight mechanisms of unintentional injury. *Arch Dis Child*. 2017;102(12):1103–1109 PMID: 28847881 https://doi.org/10.1136/archdischild-2017-312847
30. DeRidder CA, Berkowitz CD, Hicks RA, Laskey AL. Subconjunctival hemorrhages in infants and children: a sign of nonaccidental trauma. *Pediatr Emerg Care*. 2013;29(2):222–226 PMID: 23546430 https://doi.org/10.1097/PEC.0b013e318280d663
31. Jenny C, ed. *Child Abuse and Neglect: Diagnosis, Treatment and Evidence*. St. Louis, MO: Saunders; 2011
32. Christian CW; American Academy of Pediatrics Committee on Child Abuse and Neglect. The evaluation of suspected child physical abuse. *Pediatrics*. 2015;135(5):e1337–e1354 PMID: 25917988 https://doi.org/10.1542/peds.2015-0356

33. Kirschner RH, Wilson H. Pathology of fatal abuse. In: Reece R, Ludwig S, eds. *Child Abuse: Medical Diagnosis and Management*. 2nd ed. Philadelphia, PA: Lippincott Williams & Wilkins; 2001:467–516
34. Haney SB, Starling SP, Heisler KW, Okwara L. Characteristics of falls and risk of injury in children younger than 2 years. *Pediatr Emerg Care*. 2010;26(12):914–918 PMID: 21088634 https://doi.org/10.1097/PEC.0b013e3181fe9139
35. Pierce MC, Magana JN, Kaczor K, et al. The prevalence of bruising among infants in pediatric emergency departments. *Ann Emerg Med*. 2016;67(1):1–8 PMID: 26233923 https://doi.org/10.1016/j.annemergmed.2015.06.021
36. US Department of Health and Human Services, Administration for Children and Families, Administration on Children, Youth and Families, Children's Bureau. *Child Maltreatment 2015*. Washington, DC: US Dept of Health and Human Services; 2017. https://www.acf.hhs.gov/programs/cb/research-data-technology/statistics-research/child-maltreatment. Reviewed November 16, 2018. Accessed January 15, 2019
37. Johnson CF, Showers J. Injury variables in child abuse. *Child Abuse Negl*. 1985;9(2):207–215 PMID: 4005661 https://doi.org/10.1016/0145-2134(85)90013-4
38. Flaherty EG. Analysis of caretaker histories in abuse: comparing initial histories with subsequent confessions. *Child Abuse Negl*. 2006;30(7):789–798 PMID: 16844217 https://doi.org/10.1016/j.chiabu.2005.12.008
39. Lee C, Barr RG, Catherine N, Wicks A. Age-related incidence of publicly reported shaken baby syndrome cases: is crying a trigger for shaking? *J Dev Behav Pediatr*. 2007;28(4):288–293 PMID: 17700080 https://doi.org/10.1097/DBP.0b013e3180327b55
40. Barr RG. Preventing abusive head trauma resulting from a failure of normal interaction between infants and their caregivers. *Proc Natl Acad Sci USA*. 2012;109(suppl 2):17294–17301 PMID: 23045677 https://doi.org/10.1073/pnas.1121267109
41. Livingston N. Bruising in infancy: when is it an emergency? *Pediatr Ann*. 2010;39(10):646–654 PMID: 20954611 https://doi.org/10.3928/00904481-20100922-09
42. Oral R, Bayman L, Assad A, et al. Illicit drug exposure in patients evaluated for alleged child abuse and neglect. *Pediatr Emerg Care*. 2011;27(6):490–495 PMID: 21629147 https://doi.org/10.1097/PEC.0b013e31821d860f
43. Anderst JD, Carpenter SL, Abshire TC; American Academy of Pediatrics Section on Hematology/Oncology and Committee on Child Abuse and Neglect. Evaluation for bleeding disorders in suspected child abuse. *Pediatrics*. 2013;131(4):e1314–e1322 PMID: 23530182 https://doi.org/10.1542/peds.2013-0195

CHAPTER 2

Cutaneous Manifestations of Child Abuse

Amanda K. Fingarson, DO, FAAP
Child Abuse Pediatrics Program
Ann and Robert H. Lurie Children's Hospital of Chicago
Assistant Professor of Pediatrics
Northwestern University Feinberg School of Medicine
Chicago, IL

Mary Clyde Pierce, MD, FAAP
Child Abuse Pediatrics Program, Pediatric Emergency Medicine
Ann and Robert H. Lurie Children's Hospital of Chicago
Professor of Pediatrics
Northwestern University Feinberg School of Medicine
Chicago, IL

Evaluation

When assessing children for possible abuse, a meticulous examination of the entire skin surface is essential. Any concerning injuries should be measured and described in medical documentation. Given that skin injuries can evolve and resolve quickly, photographs of the injuries should be obtained whenever feasible. Photography provides important information for investigators if a report to child protective services is made; it also allows for review by colleagues with expertise in child abuse. Photographs of bruises and other skin injuries should be taken with an adequate light source, and multiple photographs taken from different perspectives, angles, and levels of magnification should be obtained. Ideally, a ruler should be included in the photograph, and the camera should be perpendicular to the plane of the skin that is being photographed. If a measurement device is unavailable, an item with a known measurement, such as a coin or dollar bill, should be included in the photograph to assist with scale.

Plausibility Assessment

When evaluating children with cutaneous injuries, it is critical to obtain a detailed history accounting for the features of the injury. It is important to ask caregivers about any episodes of trauma that may account for skin findings and to interview a child in a private, developmentally appropriate way when feasible. Given that the potential for accidental injury increases as developmental capabilities increase, knowing about a child's developmental history is critical in assessing plausibility. Time between the injury and seeking care should also be taken into account, while acknowledging that some injuries (including many mild skin injuries) may not prompt reasonable caregivers to seek immediate medical care. Any other injuries noted on physical examination should also be evaluated and assessed. Caregivers and the child should also be asked about previous injuries that the child sustained. While the history provided to account for the child's current injury may be plausible, a pattern of previous injuries, particularly in a very young child, may raise concern for physical abuse or a neglectful environment.

In addition to raising concern for prior maltreatment, prior bruising may also suggest the possibility of a hematologic disorder. A careful history about any prior bruising (including bruising at birth) should be elicited. In addition, excessive bleeding with heel sticks, injections, circumcisions, and other procedures should be inquired about. Hematologic laboratory workup may be prudent in some cases, but this should be guided by the history and physical examination findings and should not delay involving child protective services when there is concern for possible maltreatment.[1]

Family history is another important part of the medical history, particularly in cases of isolated bruising. It is important to ask about a family history of known hematologic disorders in addition to asking about symptoms in family members, such as abnormal or excessive bruising, abnormal bleeding with dental or surgical procedures, recurrent epistaxis, or menorrhagia.

Children younger than 2 years with cutaneous injuries concerning for abuse should undergo a complete skeletal survey.[2] With infants, particularly very young infants and those with head or face bruising, consideration should be given to neuroimaging to assess for occult head injury.[3,4]

Incidence of Abusive Cutaneous Injuries

Cutaneous injuries include bruises, petechiae, burns, bite marks, lacerations, and abrasions. In 2016, data from the National Child Abuse and Neglect Data System of the US Department of Health and Human Services indicated that physical abuse constituted 18.2% of the 676,000 substantiated reports for child maltreatment.[5] Cutaneous injuries are the single most common presentation of physical child abuse. While the injuries may be minor and resolve without intervention, they may be the first indication that a child is being maltreated and may be the only indication of serious internal injury.[4,6]

Skin: An Overview

Human skin is an extraordinary organ, accounting for 16% of the weight of the human body.[7] It serves many important functions, including thermoregulation, regulation of blood pressure, protection from microorganisms and toxins, and maintenance of hydration.

Skin varies in thickness, depending on the location on the body. On the eyelid, it is 0.5 mm thick. On the soles of the feet, it can be up to 4 mm thick and can tolerate constant abrasion.[7] Skin consists of 2 basic layers, the epidermis and dermis.

Epidermis

The *epidermis* is the outer protective layer of the skin. It is made up of 5 cellular layers, all of which gradually migrate to the surface from the most basilar layer impinging on the basement membrane.

In addition to epithelial cells and their main product, keratin, the epidermis contains melanocytes, providing melanin to protect and color the skin. The epidermis is replaced every 2 to 4 weeks.[8]

Dermis

The underlying *dermis* provides the skin's elasticity and strength. The dermis itself is composed of 2 layers containing the proteins collagen, elastin, and reticulin and permeated by a mucopolysaccharide ground substance. Blood vessels, lymph vessels, and nerve fibers traverse the dermis. Fibroblasts, macrophages, and mast cells reside in the dermis. Hair follicles, sweat glands, and sebaceous glands protrude from the dermis to the epidermis and skin surface, providing regenerative potential after loss of the epidermis through illness or injury. Below the dermis, a subcutaneous layer attaches to fascia. This layer contains immune cells, blood and lymph vessels, nerves, and adipose tissue and protects the body (Figure 2.1).

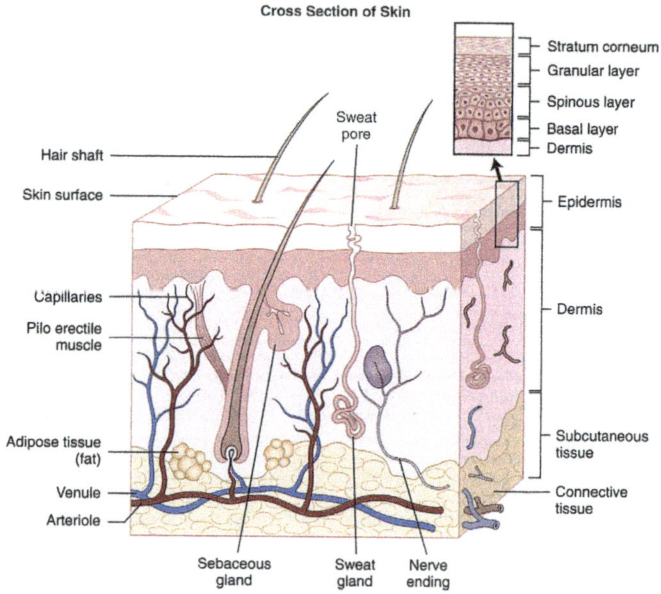

FIGURE 2.1

Anatomy of the skin.

Reprinted from Harris TL, Flaherty EG. Bruises and skin lesions. In: Jenny CJ, ed. *Child Abuse and Neglect: Diagnosis, Treatment and Evidence.* St. Louis, MO: Elsevier Saunders; 2011:239–251, with permission from Elsevier.

Properties of Skin

Skin has biomechanical properties that affect its function and healing. Temperature, humidity, and pH affect the biomechanical properties of skin. Skin is thinner but denser on the extremities. It increases in stiffness from the head to the foot.[9]

Dermal fibers in children are tortuous, unbranched, and loosely arranged. The lack of connection among fibers gives young skin greater mobility and elastic properties. When skin is strained, dermal fibers reorient to the direction of the load, becoming straightened and compact to minimize strain. With excess stress, the fibers fail and rupture, causing tissue failure. Young skin is less protected against large strains than is older skin. It is more viscous and less elastic.[10]

Injuries of the Skin

When sufficient force is delivered to skin, deformation and injury result. The injury experienced depends on the nature of the insult, the amount of force or energy applied, and the extent of surface area experiencing the force.[11] Injuries are categorized by the nature of disruption to the tissues.

- *Abrasions* result from friction removing superficial layers of skin. They are also called scrapes. Skinned knees are a typical example of abrasions.
- *Contusions* cause discoloration of the skin because of hemorrhage into the skin after blunt trauma.
- *Lacerations* are tears into the skin caused by shearing or crushing forces. Sharp or blunt objects can lacerate the skin, depending on the amount of force applied.

Healing of Injured Skin

Once skin is injured, the complex process of wound healing begins. There are 3 phases in this process, with overlap between phases.

The first phase is the *inflammatory phase,* which occurs when a platelet plug forms that limits bleeding and begins cytokine signaling.[12]

The second stage is the *proliferative phase,* which occurs from days 4 to 21. During the proliferative phase, granulation tissue made up of collagen and extracellular matrix is laid down and angiogenesis occurs.

The third stage, known as the *maturation stage,* involves a period of remodeling that lasts from 3 weeks until 1 year.[13] Maximum strength occurs around 42 to 60 days, which is the reason for the traditional recommendation of limiting activity for 6 weeks after major injury or surgery.[14] When a wound is fully healed, the skin is only 70% as strong as uninjured skin.[15]

Many factors can slow the rate of healing, including hypoxia, ischemia, chronic shear forces, hyperthermia, infection, foreign bodies in the wound, use of anti-inflammatory medications, use of tobacco, poor nutrition (including deficiencies of vitamins A, B, C, and E; zinc; copper; calcium; methionine; proteins; and essential fatty acids), and metabolic diseases (eg, diabetes) and other systemic disease.[16]

The central nervous system and the cutaneous sensory nerves play a role in healing. Denervated tissue heals more slowly than enervated tissue.[17] Better blood supply facilitates more rapid healing. The mouth, anus, and genitals heal most quickly, followed by the head and trunk. Healing of the extremities is slowest.[18]

Healing of skin injuries is faster in children than in adults. Larger wounds require longer healing time than smaller, less deep wounds, and crush injuries cause more devitalization of tissue than do shear injuries, thus delaying healing. The compressive force of crush injuries delivers more energy to larger amounts of tissue, causing more tissue disruption and greater risk of infection.[19] A scar (cicatrix) results from the deposition of fibrous tissue in the healed wound. A hypertrophic scar is limited to the original wound margin. A keloid, conversely, results from collagen deposited beyond the margins of the original wound. Keloids result from an imbalance in collagen production versus collagen degradation during wound healing.[20] Keloids are more likely to form on children whose skin is darkly pigmented and on certain areas of the body, including the earlobes, sternum, back, shoulder, and upper arm.[21]

Resolution of Bruises

Bruises differ from other wounds because the skin itself remains intact. Bruises are the result of the rupture of blood vessels and seepage of blood into interstitial spaces. In addition, local inflammation and capillary dilation may add to the bright red color of a fresh bruise. As the blood cells and hemoglobin break down, the bruise exhibits a succession of colors, including red, violet, black, blue, yellow, green, and/or brown. However, there does not seem to be a predictable order or chronology of color progression.

One study of visible bruises concluded that a bruise with any yellow coloration must be older than 18 hours.[22] Other bruise colors could occur at any time. This study was limited, however, in that only children and adults older than 10 years were included. Furthermore, studies have found that the ability to differentiate colors is variable and diminishes with age.[23] A study on the accuracy of forensic examiners in dating bruises in adults found that estimates were accurate to within 24 hours only 48% of the time.[24]

Bruises of identical age and cause on the same person may not appear the same and may change colors at different rates.[25] Many factors affect the rate of bruise resolution, including the amount of blood extravasated after the injury, the distance of the leakage of the blood from the skin surface, the amount of force applied and the amount of tissue damage incurred, the vascularity of the underlying tissue, the age of the person injured, and the underlying color of the injured person's skin.[25] Bruises are often less obviously noted on the skin of children whose skin is more darkly pigmented.[26] The location of the bruise also can be a factor. Loosely attached skin, such as the skin around the eyes or genitals, will bruise more readily than skin that is under more tension. Drugs (eg, corticosteroids) can alter the rate of bruise resolution. Aspirin or other anti-inflammatory drugs can increase susceptibility to bruising by platelet inhibition, and the bruised person's underlying clotting mechanisms can increase or decrease the size of the initial bruise that must be cleared.[27] In a recent review of peer-reviewed articles on the accuracy of dating bruises, Maguire and Mann concluded that the use of color to determine the age of a bruise is not based on science and should be avoided.[28]

Bruising in Children Who Have Experienced Abuse Versus Those Who Have Not Experienced Abuse

Overall, bruising is a common finding in children who have and have not experienced abuse, and features of the bruising and the child's age and development provide important information about the likelihood of abuse.

Bruising and Child Age and Development

Bruising in children is related to developmental stage (Table 2.1).[3,26,31–34] Studies have shown that infants who do not yet cruise holding onto furniture are unlikely to be bruised; therefore, bruises are very rare in infants younger than 6 months.[26,28,30,33,35,36] Feldman et al found that more than half of infants younger than 6 months who had initially unexplained bruises at presentation were ultimately found to have been abused.[37] The amount of bruising in toddlers increases as their motor skills increase.[28] Sugar et al found lower leg bruising to be common in children who could pull to standing or walk.[26] Head and face injuries were more common in 10- to 18-month-olds (when children are learning to cruise and walk) and uncommon in children older than 4 years. Whereas fewer than 1% of children younger than 3 years had lumbar bruises, the lumbar areas of 14% of school-aged children were bruised, again highlighting differences in activity based on development.[29]

Bruising and Accidental Injuries

The distribution of bruises in children who have been injured accidentally tends to be different from children who have experienced abuse. Bruises to "exploratory surfaces" such as the lower legs are common once children are mobile, and bruises to the trunk are less common. In their systematic review of 181 published articles, Maguire and Mann concluded that most bruises in walking children are small and occur over bony prominences and on the front of the body.[28]

Bruising is rare on the hands, buttocks, cheek, nose, forearms, or chest of children who have not experienced abuse.[26] Hibberd et al found no bruises to the ears, neck, or genitalia in 372 children with accidental injuries who had not experienced abuse. Bruising to the buttocks, upper arm, and back of the legs or feet was also rare.[38]

A study of accidentally injured children found that a single episode of trauma usually resulted in only 1 bruise (81.7%). Multiple bruises were rare with the exception of motor vehicle collisions and falls down more than 10 stairs.[38] Children with siblings have also been found to have an increased number of bruises.[39]

TABLE 2.1
Studies of Location of Skin Trauma in Children by Developmental Stage or Age

Location	Study	Population	Location of Injury	Age/Motor Development Stage	% With Lesions
Health clinics (United Kingdom)	Roberton et al[29] (1982)	Normal children (N = 400)	Lower leg	18 mo–3 y	> 40.0
				3–11 y	34.3
			Thigh/buttocks	< 18 mo	2.4
				> 18 mo	17.0
			Arms	< 18 mo	2.4
				> 18 mo	15.4
			Face and head	18 mo–3 y	16.6
				> 3 y	< 5.0
Health clinics (United Kingdom)	Mortimer and Freeman[30] (1983)	Normal children (N = 620)	Face	< 1 y	0.6
Forensic pathology (United Kingdom)	Atwal et al[31] (1998)	Fatal abusive head trauma cases (N = 18)		< 1 y	72.0
Physician offices (United States)	Sugar et al[26] (1999)	Health supervision (well-child) visits (N = 930)	Lower leg	Pre-cruiser	0.6
				Cruiser	11.9
				Walker	44.7
			Forehead	Pre-cruiser	0.6
				Cruiser	3.0
				Walker	5.7
			Scalp	Pre-cruiser	0.6
				Cruiser	5.0
				Walker	0.6
			Upper leg	Pre-cruiser	0.2
				Cruiser	1.0
				Walker	4.4
Hearing test clinics and child health clinics (United Kingdom)	Carpenter[32] (1999)	Assessments of children 6–12 mo (N = 177)	Face, head, and shins	Pre-cruiser	8.5
				Walker	37.5
Outpatient clinic and ED (Canada)	Labbé and Caouette[33] (2001)	Medical visits not related to trauma (N = 246)		< 9 mo	1.2
Child abuse teams in United States (20 teams)	Harper et al[3] (2014)	Physical child abuse consultations (N = 980)	Face/head	< 6 mo	75.3
			Trunk		31.5
			Extremities		26.7
Pediatric EDs in United States (3 EDs)	Pierce et al[34] (2016)	Pediatric ED visits (N = 2,488)		< 6 mo	1.3
				6–12 mo	6.4

Abbreviation: ED, emergency department.

Bruising and Physical Abuse

Certain bruising features and locations are more common in children who have experienced abuse. Abusive bruises tend to be away from bony prominences and involve the face, neck, ear, head, trunk, buttocks, and arms. Abusive bruises tend to be larger and multiple and often occur in clusters.[28,40]

Pierce et al compared children who had accidents versus children who experienced abuse and found that bruising to the torso, ear, or neck in a child younger than 4 years predicted abuse with 97% sensitivity and 84% specificity.[35] Harper et al found that bruising to the face, head, trunk, and extremities and patterned bruises were associated with abuse. They also found an association between bruising location and positive neuroimaging findings. Of those with positive neuroimaging findings, 90% had face or head bruising, suggesting that special consideration for screening neuroimaging for intracranial injury should be given for infants with bruising in this region.[3]

The number of bruises in children who have experienced abuse can vary widely, but these children tend to have a greater number of bruises identified at the time of diagnosis.[39] Pierce et al studied 95 patients in pediatric intensive care units with injuries from accident or abuse and found that those patients who had experienced abuse had more bruises than those who had been accidentally injured (median of 6 bruises vs 1.5 bruises).[35]

Children With Disabilities

Studies have found that children with disabilities have unique bruising features. As in typically developing children, knees were frequently bruised, but unlike typically developing children, feet, thighs, hands, arms, and the abdomen were also commonly bruised. Some of the unusual areas of bruising were attributable to mobility devices.[41] Goldberg et al found that overall, children with disabilities were more likely to have at least 1 bruise than typically developing children (18% vs 3.3%, respectively).[42]

Bruising as a Sentinel Injury

While many bruises are accidental, bruising is a common *sentinel injury,* defined as a previous injury reported in the medical history that raises suspicion for abuse.[43–47] (See Chapter 1, Sentinel Injuries.) Sheets et al found that of 200 infants who had experienced abuse, 27.5% had a sentinel injury, with 80% of these sentinel injuries being bruises.[6] A study of children with abusive head trauma found that for 25%, there had been prior opportunity to identify abuse in a medical setting; of this 25%, 11.7% involved bruising.[48] Thus, sentinel injuries may represent missed opportunities to prevent ongoing abuse and repeat injuries; improved recognition and correct interpretation of the significance of "atypical" bruising is paramount to improving outcomes for children who have experienced abuse.

Variations of Bruises in Children Who Have Experienced Abuse

Although many children who have not experienced abuse will manifest injuries, certain patterns of injury have been recognized to be frequently caused by inflicted rather than accidental or incidental trauma in children.

Pattern Marks

Injury inflicted with an object will often leave marks that reflect the outline of that object. Some of the more common patterned cutaneous injuries are noted herein.

Slap, Grab, and Closed-Fist Punch Marks

The hand can leave a negative imprint, particularly on the face, when capillaries break between the fingers as blood is pushed away from the point of impact. This creates a tramline appearance (Figure 2.2). Grab marks can result from a child being forcefully gripped by an extremity. The

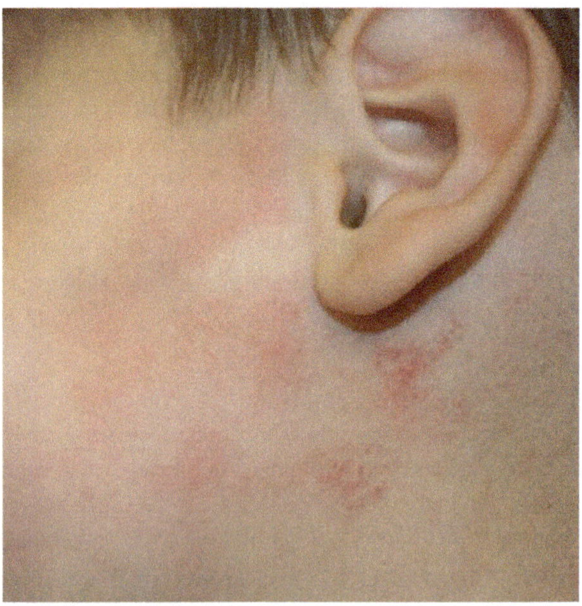

FIGURE 2.2
Inflicted handprint on the face of a child, leaving an outline of the fingers.

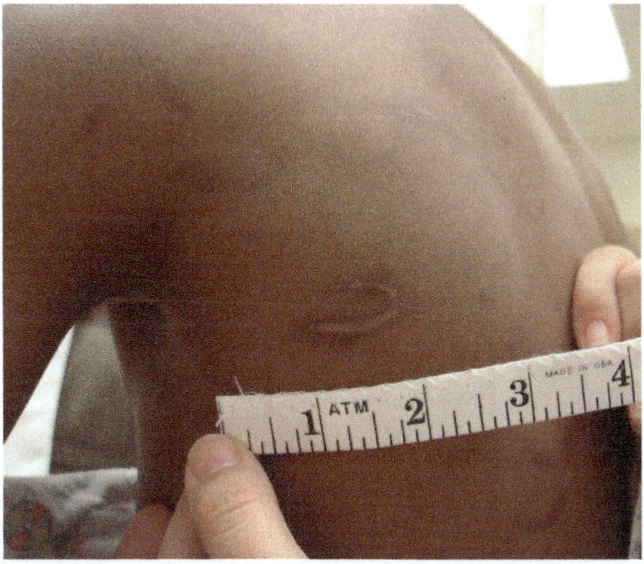

FIGURE 2.3
Inflicted patterned marks on a child's back.

bruises are often circular and correspond to the fingertips of an assailant.[49] Closed-fist punches usually result in 2 to 3 circular bruises that correspond to a knuckle on the hand of an assailant.

Marks From Implements

Cords, ropes, shoes, kitchen implements, and belt buckles can leave notable outlines on the skin.[50] Loop marks are generally worse at their extreme ends because the far end of the flexible cord travels at a faster rate of speed around the hand of the person inflicting the injuries[28] (Figure 2.3). Clothing that a child is wearing can also be imprinted on the skin during an assault.[51]

Vertical Bruises of the Gluteal Cleft

Blows to the buttocks can leave vertical marks at the junction where the buttocks curve into the gluteal cleft.[52,53] Such bruising can even be seen in infants because some caregivers begin the practice of "spanking" in early infancy (Figure 2.4).

Bite Marks

Bite marks are sometimes an abusive injury, and they can be inflicted by adults, children, or animals or self-inflicted by the patient. Bite marks

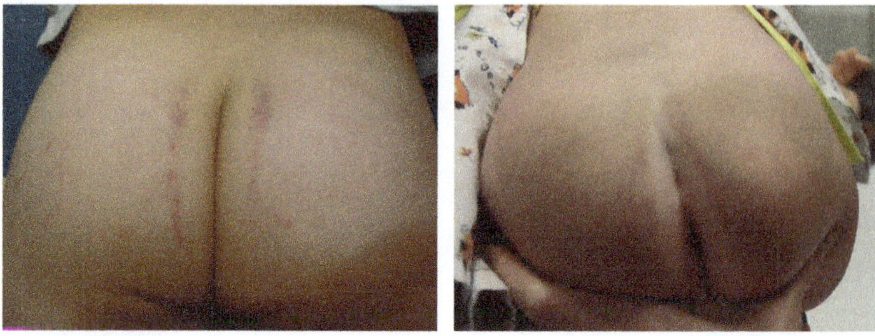

FIGURE 2.4
Buttock bruising from spanking/paddling.

are a unique form of cutaneous injury due to the possibility of obtaining the forensic identification of the perpetrator either through scientifically linking the dentition of a potential biter with a bite mark or by examining DNA left on the skin's surface. Human bite marks should be considered when bruising or abrasions are found in an elliptical, horseshoe-shaped, or ovoid pattern.[54] Central bruising is often present from compression of soft tissues between the teeth or from suction.[55] Traditionally, inter-canine distance was used to distinguish bites originating from a child versus an adult, with the distance being less than 2.5 cm in children, 2.5 to 3.0 cm in children or small adults, and 3.0 to 4.5 cm in adults. It has been found that adult dentition is reached by 12 years, and there is significant variation based on sex and race that should lead to caution in interpreting bite marks based purely on inter-canine distance.[56,57] A forensic dentist should be consulted when available, and bite marks should be carefully photographed with and without a size standard and swabbed with sterile water or saline to recover genetic markers left behind from saliva.

Tattooing

Purposely disfiguring a child's skin by tattooing the skin with an ink-filled needle has been reported.[58] While many cultures view tattooing as an acceptable practice that might reach children and teens (eg, Samoan, Polynesian, Māori tribe of New Zealand), this permanent disfigurement can lead to child abuse charges in many US jurisdictions. Tattooing is also common in human trafficking victims. In this scenario, the tattoos may be sexually explicit, indicate a gang affiliation, or show a name (indicating ownership).[59]

Subgaleal Hematomas

Violently pulling on a child's hair can cause subgaleal hematomas (hemorrhage under the scalp).[60] The scalp is lifted off the calvarium at the aponeurotic junction. This finding has also been reported in case reports of Afro-Caribbean hair braiding.[61] In addition to scalp swelling, traumatic alopecia (traumatic hair loss) can occur.[62] The hair loss is usually seen on the top of the head, is patchy, and may be confused with tinea capitis. The underlying scalp can appear normal, or petechial bruising can be seen.[28]

Petechiae

Petechiae are uncommon in accidental injuries. One study found petechiae in only 1 of 293 children presenting to an emergency department with bruising from accidental trauma.[38] Similarly, another study found that 21.9% of 128 children with abusive injuries had petechiae, while only 2.3% of the 250 children who were accidentally injured did. The location of the petechiae also differed. The petechiae in children who did not experience abuse tended to be on limbs and trunks. Petechiae in children who experienced abuse tended to be located on the head and neck.[63] Conjunctival hemorrhages and facial and neck petechiae (masque ecchymotique) can result from compression of the chest and neck, causing increased venous pressure. Strangulation or suffocation by occlusion of the airway can cause similar lesions (Figure 2.5).

Bruising of the External Ear

Blows to the side of the head can cause purpuric or petechial hemorrhages to occur on the external ear, often in the interior folds of the ears.[64] Pulling

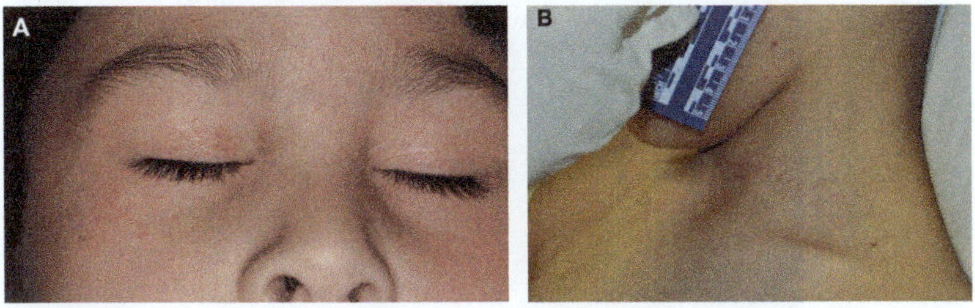

FIGURE 2.5

A, Facial petechiae caused by strangulation. B, Petechiae around neck and clavicles from physical abuse.

or pinching the top of the ear leaves bruises on the helix or behind the pinna. If a blow sharply folds and crimps the pinna at the apex of the helix, petechiae can result.[52] Certain regions of the ear are more predictive of abusive trauma than other areas; for example, the top of the ear/helical rim is more susceptible to simple falls against an object such as a coffee-table edge, whereas the inner folds of the ear are not easily bruised and most often indicate a substantial blow to the side of the head (figures 2.6 and 2.7).

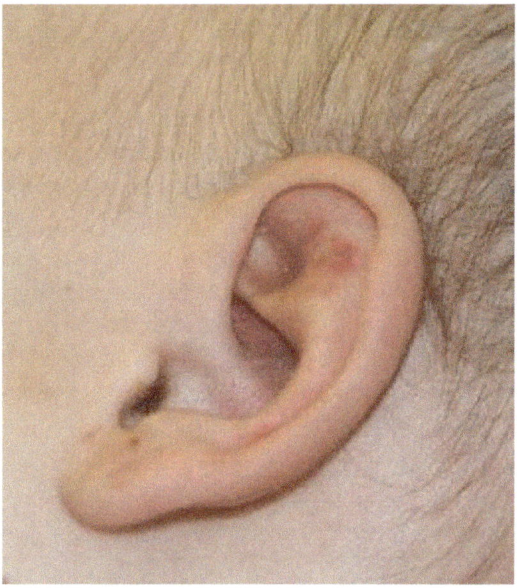

FIGURE 2.6
Child with abusive ear bruising.

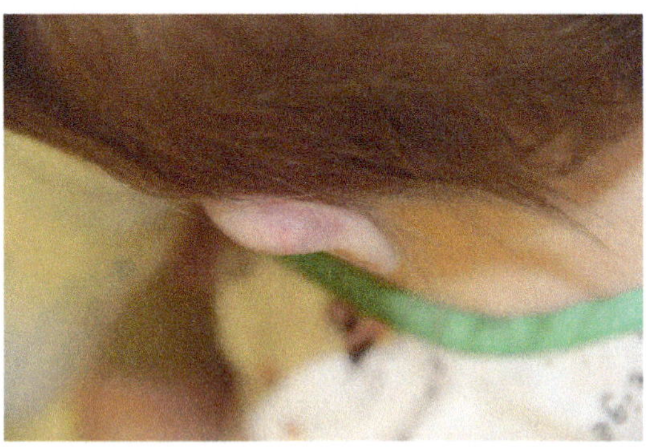

FIGURE 2.7
Child with accidental ear bruising.

Subungual Hematomas

Abusive biting of a child's fingers can cause chronic subungual hematomas. Leukonychia and swelling of the hands and feet also can be seen.[65] Hitting a child's fingers with an object might leave subungual hemorrhages as well.

Factitious Dermatitis (Dermatitis Artefacta)

Many different types of skin injuries can be purposefully inflicted on children by their caregivers to gain medical attention.[66,67] This factitious disorder by proxy often presents with chronic dermatitis or skin ulcers that heal poorly. They are more likely found on the face, chest, anterior surfaces of the legs, and dorsal surfaces of the arms. The condition resolves when the child is removed from the abuser.

Children who have experienced abuse (especially sexual abuse) are more likely to inflict injuries on themselves, cutting or burning themselves to distract themselves from emotional pain.[68,69]

Conditions in Differential Diagnosis for Inflicted Cutaneous Injuries

Many different pathologic conditions have been reported to be confused with inflicted injury.[53] Some of the more common conditions are described in the following sections:

Dermal Melanocytosis (Mongolian Spots, Slate Gray Nevi)

These slate-blue or blue-green patches with indistinct borders are commonly seen in newborns. From 80% to 90% of black infants, 75% of Asian infants, and 10% of white infants have dermal melanosis. They are most often found on the lumbosacral region but can occur anywhere on the body. Most fade by age 5 years.[70] These lesions are uniformly the same blue-gray color from one side of the lesion to the other, and the absence of swelling and erythema helps differentiate dermal melanocytosis from bruising. Whereas bruises fade over a few weeks, Mongolian spots remain unchanged during that time. Moreover, when asking parents when they first noticed these lesions, they will usually say that they were there at birth, and some will know the name Mongolian spots. Newborn records can help corroborate their presence at birth, although this finding is inconsistently documented by medical professionals (figures 2.8 and 2.9).

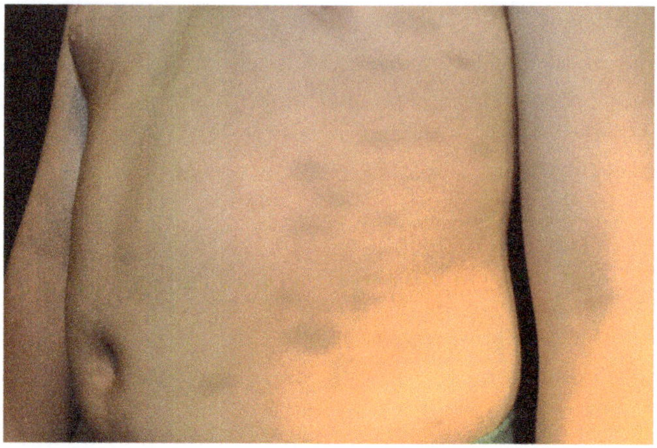

FIGURE 2.8
Older child with extensive, dark Mongolian spots (dermal melanosis).

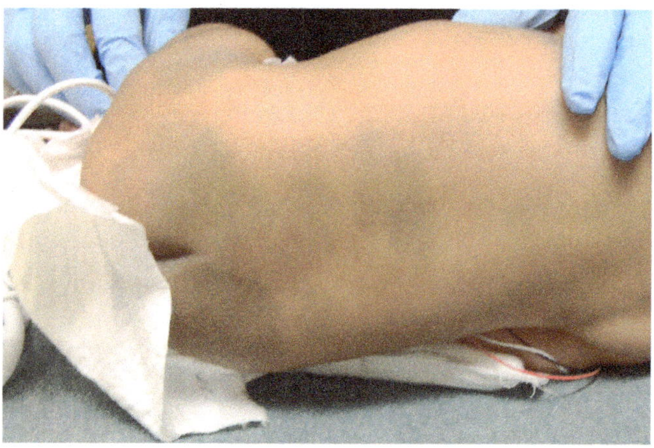

FIGURE 2.9
Mongolian spots (dermal melanosis) in an infant.

Chilblain (Pernio)

Chilblain occurs when tissues are exposed to wet, cold weather.[71] Bluish discoloration, erythema, and swelling occur, especially on the hands, feet, and face. Blistering or ulceration also can develop. Vasospasm induced by the cold leads to hypoxemia and localized inflammation of the tissues. "Popsicle pernio" occurs in some children secondary to holding popsicles in the corner of the mouth.

Bleeding Disorders

One study found that 16% of children evaluated for child abuse because of excessive bruising had a bleeding disorder.[72] Bruises in children with bleeding disorders differ from bruises in unaffected children in some important ways. Children with bleeding disorders have been found to have more and larger bruises at all ages. After becoming mobile, children with bleeding disorders are more likely to have bruises of the trunk, buttocks, limbs, hands, and feet than children without bleeding disorders.[73] The most common inherited bleeding disorder is von Willebrand disease, with up to 1% of the population having low von Willebrand factor levels (although far fewer having symptoms). The severity of symptoms in patients with von Willebrand disease varies. Some patients are completely asymptomatic, whereas others experience epistaxis, gingival bleeding, severe postoperative bleeding, menorrhagia, and easy ability to bruise. Immune thrombocytopenic purpura, hemophilia, and other bleeding disorders also have been confused with child abuse.[74]

When extensive unexplained bruising occurs, particularly in the absence of associated injuries, bleeding disorders should be considered. A complete blood cell count with platelet count, an activated partial thromboplastin time, a prothrombin time, factor VIII level, factor IX level, von Willebrand factor antigen, and von Willebrand activity (ristocetin cofactor) are useful in screening for unrecognized bleeding disorders.[1] Of note, patients with bleeding disorders should exhibit ongoing problems with bruising, rather than an isolated episode, although the severity of von Willebrand disease is known to wax and wane over time.

Henoch-Schönlein Purpura

Henoch-Schönlein purpura causes a nonthrombocytopenic purpuric rash that can be complicated by abdominal pain and bleeding, nephritis, and/or arthritis that can be confused with abusive injury.[75] The symmetrical rash tends to be more common over the buttocks and lower extremities but can be found in other places as well, including the face or ears. The lesions can look like multiple bruises, especially early in the course of the disease. Patients often have a thrombocytosis and an elevated erythrocyte sedimentation rate. Lesions occur in crops over time.[76]

Phytophotodermatitis

Phytophotodermatitis is an acute phototoxic skin eruption occurring after contact with certain fruits or plants followed by sun exposure.

The lesions often have bizarre configurations, making them appear to be inflicted burns or contusions.[77,78] As the lesions heal, they often become hyperpigmented and can mimic bruises. Citrus fruits and fruit juices, bergamot oil, figs, angelica, cow parsley, scurf pea, celery, wild parsnips, and rue are among the plants that can photosensitize the skin. Furocoumarins (psoralens) are the agents in the plants that cause the reaction[79] (Figure 2.10).

Hemangiomas

Hemangiomas can look like bruises and can ulcerate. They are not always obvious at birth and can become obvious later in infancy. On the genitals, they can mimic sexual abuse–related trauma.[80]

Maculae Ceruleae

Flat, purpuric macules can be associated with pediculosis. They occur distant from the actual site of the lice infestation. The exact cause of the lesions is unknown. Although maculae ceruleae are more commonly seen on the body as a complication of pubic crab lice, they have been associated with head lice as well.[81]

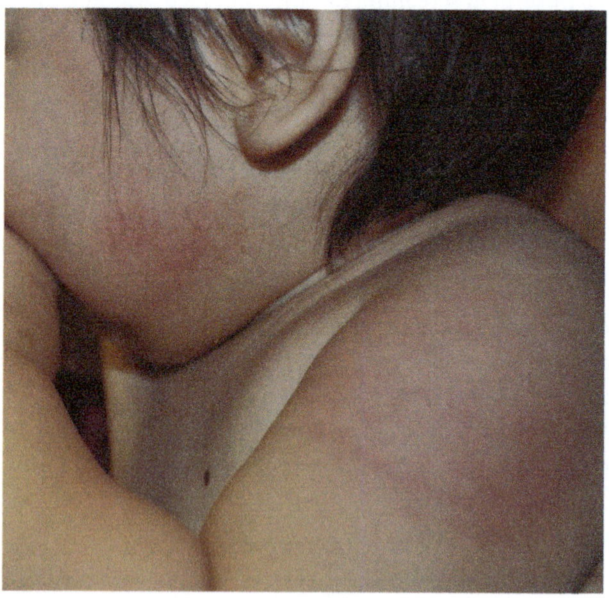

FIGURE 2.10
Phytophotodermatitis on a child's shoulder, mimicking inflicted injury.

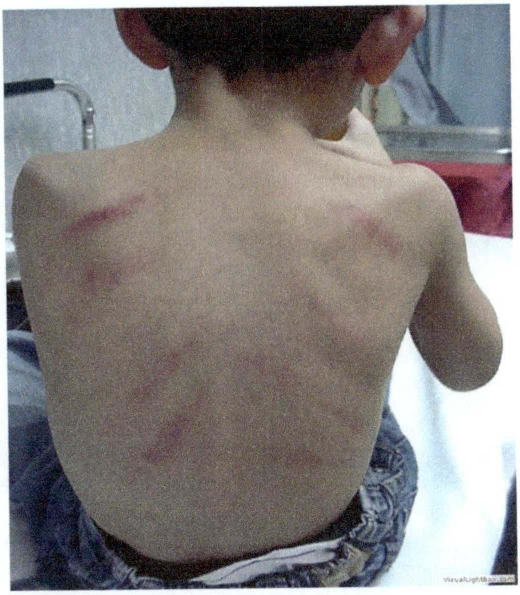

FIGURE 2.11
Coin rubbing, or cao gio, in which a coin, or the back of a spoon, is rubbed repeatedly over the skin. From Larson A, Hoffman-Rosenfield J, Tayama T. Bruises and other skin findings. In: Anderst JD, ed. *Visual Diagnosis of Child Abuse.* 4th ed. Elk Grove Village, IL: American Academy of Pediatrics; 2016.

Folk Remedies

Cao gio (coin rubbing; Figure 2.11) is a Southeast Asian remedy for fever, chills, and headache. The back or chest is massaged with mentholated oil and then vigorously rubbed with the edge of a coin until petechiae or purpura appear. *Cupping* (glass leaching; Figure 2.12) is used to treat a variety of ailments and involves a heated cup being applied to the skin, which results in patterned bruising from negative pressure. *Quat sha* (spooning) is a Chinese remedy used to relieve pain and headaches. Skin is scratched with a porcelain spoon until ecchymotic lesions appear. Studies have found that significant portions of the world use complementary and integrative medicine practices that may incorporate these elements, so medical professionals should be aware of these practices regardless of the ethnic backgrounds of their patients.[82]

Erythema Multiforme

Erythema multiforme often presents with red skin blotches that then darken. The lesions resemble traumatic contusions and bruises. The lesions evolve into the classic target lesions with central clearing associated with the disease.[83]

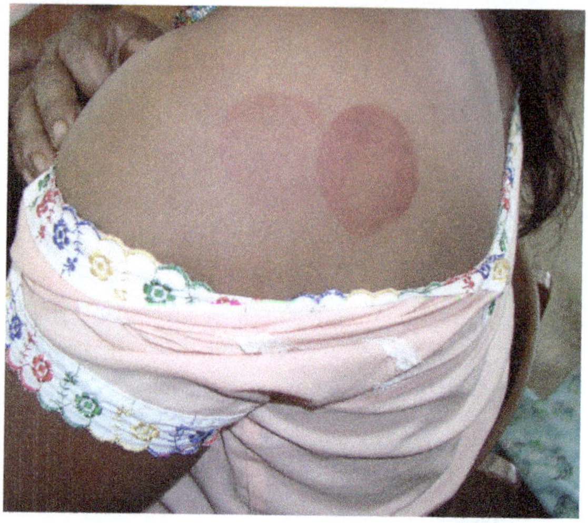

FIGURE 2.12
Cupping marks induced by suction from a heated cup placed on the skin.
Courtesy of Dale P. Woolridge, MD, PhD, University of Arizona.

Erythema Nodosum

Erythema nodosum presents as tender erythematous nodules that can evolve to bruise-like marks. It occurs most commonly on the lower limbs, and lesions can mimic trauma.[84]

Angioedema/Hypersensitivity Reactions

Recurrent angioedema limited to the scalp and face has been described in one case report as an atypical presentation mimicking trauma to the head; a diagnosis of trauma to the head and face was initially considered.[85] Hypersensitivity reactions limited to certain body parts, such as the lips or the penis, have the potential to also be confused with trauma.[86,87]

Striae

Physiological striae (stretch marks) are common and are sometimes found in adolescents who are growing rapidly. Striae in the lumbar area can occur horizontally across the back and hips, appearing to be linear inflicted pattern marks. Over time, they fade and take on a sclerotic appearance.[88,89]

Ehlers-Danlos Syndrome

Ehlers-Danlos syndrome is an inherited disease caused by the production of defective collagen. It is a clinically heterogeneous condition that includes joint hypermobility, frequent joint dislocations, increased skin elasticity, and poor blood vessel integrity. The defective collagen causes skin to be soft, friable, and easily traumatized. Injured skin heals with wide scars, appearing to have healed by secondary intention.[90] Although all currently recognized types of Ehlers-Danlos syndrome cause cutaneous manifestations, the vascular type (formerly type IV) is most notable for severe bruising.[91]

Loose Anagen Hair Syndrome

Loose anagen hair syndrome is a genetic disease frequently causing abrupt, patchy hair loss.[62] There is a lack of cohesion between the hair root sheaths and the cuticle during the growth phase of the hair-growth cycle (anagen). Anagen hairs can be pulled out easily and painlessly. The affected hair has a characteristic microscopic appearance, with dystrophic roots, longitudinal groove, lack of root sheaths, and a ruffled cuticle.[92]

Postmortem Insect Bites

Insect bites can be confused with burns or abrasions. Cockroaches (*Dictyoptera blattaria*) are notorious for scavenging bodies, particularly after death. They bite hands, toes, eyelashes, and areas of the skin with thin epidermis such as the face and ears. The bites are small and well circumscribed but irregular. They can sometimes be inflicted in a row and can have the appearance of abrasions or burns. Smaller bites can coalesce into larger lesions.[93]

Management

The management of cutaneous injuries caused by child abuse is related to the extent and severity of the wounds. Cutaneous injuries often do not require medical intervention. However, the medical professional must not equate the severity of the injury with the severity of the risk to a child. A seemingly mild skin injury may be a harbinger of an abusive environment.

Prevention

Prevention of inflicted skin injuries is related to prevention of child physical abuse in general. Primary prevention efforts aimed at reducing child physical abuse are important in reducing cutaneous injuries from child abuse.

Secondary prevention plays a large role in cutaneous injuries from abuse. If inflicted bruises are recognized when they first present, rather than bruises being overlooked sentinel injuries, further harm can be avoided. For abuse to be recognized before physical abuse recurs and escalates, education is necessary. Medical professionals, caregivers, and others interacting with children need to be aware of what constitutes concerning bruises by age and development and must understand the importance in reporting their concerns to state child protective services. Only when this gap is filled will children in unsafe environments be identified early and protected from further harm.

Prognosis

The prognosis of cutaneous injuries from child abuse is related to depth and extent of the skin injury. Although most non-burn cutaneous injuries do not cause permanent disability, complications can arise. Rhabdomyolysis can occur in cases with extensive injury and muscle involvement, particularly injuries to the buttocks and legs. Muscle damage from cutaneous trauma can also result in hyperkalemia, which can compromise renal function.[94]

Conclusion

The cutaneous manifestations of abuse are varied and often nonspecific. Careful consideration by the medical professional, including the medical history, physical examination, and psychosocial context, is necessary to diagnose child abuse accurately.

References

1. Anderst JD, Carpenter SL, Abshire TC; American Academy of Pediatrics Section on Hematology/Oncology and Committee on Child Abuse and Neglect. Evaluation for bleeding disorders in suspected child abuse. *Pediatrics*. 2013;131(4):e1314–e1322 PMID: 23530182 https://doi.org/10.1542/peds.2013-0195
2. Christian CW; American Academy of Pediatrics Committee on Child Abuse and Neglect. The evaluation of suspected child physical abuse. *Pediatrics*. 2015;135(5):e1337–e1354 PMID: 25917988 https://doi.org/10.1542/peds.2015-0356
3. Harper NS, Feldman KW, Sugar NF, Anderst JD, Lindberg DM; Examining Siblings to Recognize Abuse Investigators. Additional injuries in young infants with concern for abuse and apparently isolated bruises. *J Pediatr*. 2014;165(2):383–388.e81 PMID: 24840754
4. Rubin DM, Christian CW, Bilaniuk LT, Zazyczny KA, Durbin DR. Occult head injury in high-risk abused children. *Pediatrics*. 2003;111(6 Pt 1):1382–1386 PMID:12777556 https://doi.org/10.1542/peds.111.6.1382
5. US Department of Health and Human Services Administration for Children and Families, Administration on Children, Youth, and Families, and Children's Bureau. *Child Maltreatment 2016*. Washington, DC: US Dept of Health and Human Services; 2018. https://www.acf.hhs.gov/programs/cb/research-data-technology/statistics-research/child-maltreatment. Reviewed November 16, 2018. Accessed January 16, 2019

6. Sheets LK, Leach ME, Koszewski IJ, Lessmeier AM, Nugent M, Simpson P. Sentinel injuries in infants evaluated for child physical abuse. *Pediatrics*. 2013;131(4):701–707 PMID: 23478861 https://doi.org/10.1542/peds.2012-2780
7. Wilkes GL, Brown IA, Wildnauer RH. The biomechanical properties of skin. *CRC Crit Rev Bioeng*. 1973;1(4):453–495 PMID: 4581809
8. Fuchs E. Keratins and the skin. *Annu Rev Cell Dev Biol*. 1995;11(1):123–154 PMID: 8689554 https://doi.org/10.1146/annurev.cb.11.110195.001011
9. Ryan TJ. Mechanical resilience of skin: a function of blood supply and lymphatic drainage. *Clin Dermatol*. 1995;13(5):429–432 PMID: 8665453 https://doi.org/10.1016/0738-081X(95)00088-W
10. Edwards C, Marks R. Evaluation of biomechanical properties of human skin. *Clin Dermatol*. 1995;13(4):375–380 PMID: 8665446 https://doi.org/10.1016/0738-081X(95)00078-T
11. DiMaio DJ. *Forensic Pathology*. New York, NY: Elsevier; 1989
12. Periayah MH, Halim AS, Mat Saad AZ. Mechanism action of platelets and crucial blood coagulation pathways in hemostasis. *Int J Hematol Oncol Stem Cell Res*. 2017;11(4):319–327 PMID: 29340130
13. Mahdavian Delavary B, van der Veer WM, van Egmond M, Niessen FB, Beelen RH. Macrophages in skin injury and repair. *Immunobiology*. 2011;216(7):753–762 PMID: 21281986 https://doi.org/10.1016/j.imbio.2011.01.001
14. Childs DR, Murthy AS. Overview of wound healing and management. *Surg Clin North Am*. 2017;97(1):189–207 PMID: 27894427 https://doi.org/10.1016/j.suc.2016.08.013
15. Bernstein G. Healing by secondary intention. *Dermatol Clin*. 1989;7(4):645–660 PMID: 2676283 https://doi.org/10.1016/S0733-8635(18)30559-X
16. Stadelmann WK, Digenis AG, Tobin GR. Impediments to wound healing. *Am J Surg*. 1998;176(Suppl 2A):39S–47S PMID: 9777971
17. Ansel JC, Kaynard AH, Armstrong CA, Olerud J, Bunnett N, Payan D. Skin-nervous system interactions. *J Invest Dermatol*. 1996;106(1):198–204 PMID: 8592075 https://doi.org/10.1111/1523-1747.ep12330326
18. Rowell LB. Reflex control of the cutaneous vasculature. *J Invest Dermatol*. 1977;69(1):154–166 PMID: 326990 https://doi.org/10.1111/1523-1747.ep12497938
19. Jagodzinski NA, Weerasinghe C, Porter K. Crush injuries and crush syndrome—a review. Part 2: the local injury. *Trauma*. 2010;12(3):133–148 https://doi.org/10.1177/1460408610372441
20. Mari W, Alsabri SG, Tabal N, Younes S, Sherif A, Simman R. Novel insights on understanding of keloid scar: article review. *J Am Coll Clin Wound Spec*. 2016;7(1-3):1–7 PMID: 28053861
21. Laude TA. Approach to dermatologic disorders in black children. *Semin Dermatol*. 1995;14(1):15–20 PMID: 7742234 https://doi.org/10.1016/S1085-5629(05)80034-3
22. Langlois NE, Gresham GA. The ageing of bruises: a review and study of the colour changes with time. *Forensic Sci Int*. 1991;50(2):227–238 PMID: 1748358 https://doi.org/10.1016/0379-0738(91)90154-B
23. Munang LA, Leonard PA, Mok JY. Lack of agreement on colour description between clinicians examining childhood bruising. *J Clin Forensic Med*. 2002;9(4):171–174 PMID: 15274931 https://doi.org/10.1016/S1353-1131(02)00097-4
24. Pilling ML, Vanezis P, Perrett D, Johnston A. Visual assessment of the timing of bruising by forensic experts. *J Forensic Leg Med*. 2010;17(3):143–149 PMID: 20211455 https://doi.org/10.1016/j.jflm.2009.10.002

25. Langlois NE. The science behind the quest to determine the age of bruises-a review of the English language literature. *Forensic Sci Med Pathol.* 2007;3(4):241–251 PMID: 25869263 https://doi.org/10.1007/s12024-007-9019-3
26. Sugar NF, Taylor JA, Feldman KW; Puget Sound Pediatric Research Network. Bruises in infants and toddlers: those who don't cruise rarely bruise. *Arch Pediatr Adolesc Med.* 1999;153(4):399–403 PMID: 10201724 https://doi.org/10.1001/archpedi.153.4.399
27. Stephenson T. Ageing of bruising in children. *J R Soc Med.* 1997;90(6):312–314 PMID: 9227377 https://doi.org/10.1177/014107689709000605
28. Maguire S, Mann M. Systematic reviews of bruising in relation to child abuse—what have we learnt: an overview of review updates. *Evid Based Child Health.* 2013;8(2):255–263 PMID: 23877882 https://doi.org/10.1002/ebch.1909
29. Roberton DM, Barbor P, Hull D. Unusual injury? Recent injury in normal children and children with suspected non-accidental injury. *Br Med J (Clin Res Ed).* 1982;285(6352):1399–1401 PMID: 6814575 https://doi.org/10.1136/bmj.285.6352.1399
30. Mortimer PE, Freeman M. Are facial bruises in babies ever accidental? *Arch Dis Child.* 1983;58(1):75–76 PMID: 6830281 https://doi.org/10.1136/adc.58.1.75-b
31. Atwal GS, Rutty GN, Carter N, Green MA. Bruising in non-accidental head injured children; a retrospective study of the prevalence, distribution and pathological associations in 24 cases. *Forensic Sci Int.* 1998;96(2-3):215–230 PMID: 9854835 https://doi.org/10.1016/S0379-0738(98)00126-1
32. Carpenter RF. The prevalence and distribution of bruising in babies. *Arch Dis Child.* 1999;80(4):363–366 PMID: 10086945 https://doi.org/10.1136/adc.80.4.363
33. Labbé J, Caouette G. Recent skin injuries in normal children. *Pediatrics.* 2001;108(2): 271–276 PMID: 11483787 https://doi.org/10.1542/peds.108.2.271
34. Pierce MC, Magana JN, Kaczor K, et al. The prevalence of bruising among infants in pediatric emergency departments. *Ann Emerg Med.* 2016;67(1):1–8 PMID: 26233923 https://doi.org/10.1016/j.annemergmed.2015.06.021
35. Pierce MC, Kaczor K, Aldridge S, O'Flynn J, Lorenz DJ. Bruising characteristics discriminating physical child abuse from accidental trauma. *Pediatrics.* 2010;125(1):67–74 PMID: 19969620 https://doi.org/10.1542/peds.2008-3632
36. Wedgwood J. Childhood bruising. *Practitioner.* 1990;234(1490):598–601 PMID: 2392410
37. Feldman KW, Tayama TM, Strickler LE, et al. A prospective study of the causes of bruises in premobile infants. *Pediatr Emerg Care.* 2017;1 PMID: 29040244 https://doi.org/10.1097/PEC.0000000000001311
38. Hibberd O, Nuttall D, Watson RE, Watkins WJ, Kemp AM, Maguire S. Childhood bruising distribution observed from eight mechanisms of unintentional injury. *Arch Dis Child.* 2017;102(12):1103–1109 PMID: 28847881 https://doi.org/10.1136/archdischild-2017-312847
39. Kemp AM, Dunstan F, Nuttall D, Hamilton M, Collins P, Maguire S. Patterns of bruising in preschool children—a longitudinal study. *Arch Dis Child.* 2015;100(5):426–431 PMID: 25589561 https://doi.org/10.1136/archdischild-2014-307120
40. Dunstan FD, Guildea ZE, Kontos K, Kemp AM, Sibert JR. A scoring system for bruise patterns: a tool for identifying abuse. *Arch Dis Child.* 2002;86(5):330–333 PMID: 11970921 https://doi.org/10.1136/adc.86.5.330
41. Newman CJ, Holenweg-Gross C, Vuillerot C, Jeannet PY, Roulet-Perez E. Recent skin injuries in children with motor disabilities. *Arch Dis Child.* 2010;95(5):387–390 PMID: 20457703 https://doi.org/10.1136/adc.2009.163691
42. Goldberg AP, Tobin J, Daigneau J, Griffith RT, Reinert SE, Jenny C. Bruising frequency and patterns in children with physical disabilities. *Pediatrics.* 2009;124(2):604–609 PMID: 19620196 https://doi.org/10.1542/peds.2008-2900

43. Jenny C, Hymel KP, Ritzen A, Reinert SE, Hay TC. Analysis of missed cases of abusive head trauma. *JAMA*. 1999;281(7):621–626 PMID: 10029123 https://doi.org/10.1001/jama.281.7.621
44. Petska HW, Sheets LK. Sentinel injuries: subtle findings of physical abuse. *Pediatr Clin North Am*. 2014;61(5):923–935 PMID: 25242706 https://doi.org/10.1016/j.pcl.2014.06.007
45. Pierce MC, Smith S, Kaczor K. Bruising in infants: those with a bruise may be abused. *Pediatr Emerg Care*. 2009;25(12):845–847 PMID: 20016354 https://doi.org/10.1097/PEC.0b013e3181c06217
46. Feldman KW. The bruised premobile infant: should you evaluate further? *Pediatr Emerg Care*. 2009;25(1):37–39 PMID: 19148012 https://doi.org/10.1097/PEC.0b013e318191db15
47. Pierce MC, Kaczor K, Acker D, et al. History, injury, and psychosocial risk factor commonalities among cases of fatal and near-fatal physical child abuse. *Child Abuse Negl*. 2017;69:263–277 PMID: 28500923 https://doi.org/10.1016/j.chiabu.2017.04.033
48. Letson MM, Cooper JN, Deans KJ, et al. Prior opportunities to identify abuse in children with abusive head trauma. *Child Abuse Negl*. 2016;60:36–45 PMID: 27680755 https://doi.org/10.1016/j.chiabu.2016.09.001
49. Raimer BG, Raimer SS, Hebeler JR. Cutaneous signs of child abuse. *J Am Acad Dermatol*. 1981;5(2):203–212 PMID: 7263965 https://doi.org/10.1016/S0190-9622(81)80059-X
50. Showers J, Bandman RL. Scarring for life: abuse with electric cords. *Child Abuse Negl*. 1986;10(1):25–31 PMID: 3955425 https://doi.org/10.1016/0145-2134(86)90028-1
51. Kaczor K, Clyde Pierce M, Makoroff K, Corey TS. Bruising and physical child abuse. *Clin Pediatr Emerg Med*. 2006;7(3):153–160 https://doi.org/10.1016/j.cpem.2006.06.007
52. Feldman KW. Patterned abusive bruises of the buttocks and the pinnae. *Pediatrics*. 1992;90(4):633–636 PMID: 1408524
53. Jinna S, Livingston N, Moles R. Cutaneous sign of abuse: kids are not just little people. *Clin Dermatol*. 2017;35(6):504–511 PMID: 29191342 https://doi.org/10.1016/j.clindermatol.2017.08.002
54. Fisher-Owens SA, Lukefahr JL, Tate AR; American Academy of Pediatrics Section on Oral Health, Committee on Child Abuse and Neglect; American Academy of Pediatric Dentistry Council on Clinical Affairs, Council on Scientific Affairs; Ad Hoc Work Group on Child Abuse and Neglect. Oral and dental aspects of child abuse and neglect. *Pediatrics*. 2017;140(2):e20171487 PMID: 28771417 https://doi.org/10.1542/peds.2017-1487
55. Hinchliffe J. Forensic odontology, part 4. Human bite marks. *Br Dent J*. 2011;210(8):363–368 PMID: 21509016 https://doi.org/10.1038/sj.bdj.2011.285
56. Freeman AJ, Senn DR, Arendt DM. Seven hundred seventy eight bite marks: analysis by anatomic location, victim and biter demographics, type of crime, and legal disposition. *J Forensic Sci*. 2005;50(6):1436–1443 PMID: 16382842 https://doi.org/10.1520/JFS2005178
57. Maguire S. Which injuries may indicate child abuse? *Arch Dis Child Educ Pract Ed*. 2010;95(6):170–177 PMID: 20926622 https://doi.org/10.1136/adc.2009.170431
58. Johnson CF. Symbolic scarring and tattooing. Unusual manifestations of child abuse. *Clin Pediatr (Phila)*. 1994;33(1):46–49 PMID: 8156727 https://doi.org/10.1177/000992289403300108
59. Greenbaum VJ, Dodd M, McCracken C. A short screening tool to identify victims of child sex trafficking in the health care setting. *Pediatr Emerg Care*. 2018;34(1):33–37 PMID: 26599463 https://doi.org/10.1097/PEC.0000000000000602
60. Seifert D, Püschel K. Subgaleal hematoma in child abuse. *Forensic Sci Int*. 2006;157(2-3):131–133 PMID: 16191474 https://doi.org/10.1016/j.forsciint.2005.03.023
61. Onyeama CO, Lotke M, Edelstein B. Subgaleal hematoma secondary to hair braiding in a 31-month-old child. *Pediatr Emerg Care*. 2009;25(1):40–41 PMID: 19148013 https://doi.org/10.1097/PEC.0b013e318191db98

62. Whiting DA. Traumatic alopecia. *Int J Dermatol*. 1999;38(suppl 1):34–44 PMID: 10369538 https://doi.org/10.1046/j.1365-4362.1999.00006.x
63. Nayak K, Spencer N, Shenoy M, Rubithon J, Coad N, Logan S. How useful is the presence of petechiae in distinguishing non-accidental from accidental injury? *Child Abuse Negl*. 2006;30(5):549–555 PMID: 16698081 https://doi.org/10.1016/j.chiabu.2005.09.005
64. Hanigan WC, Peterson RA, Njus G. Tin ear syndrome: rotational acceleration in pediatric head injuries. *Pediatrics*. 1987;80(5):618–622 PMID: 3670962
65. Gavin LA, Lanz MJ, Leung DY, Roesler TA. Chronic subungual hematomas: a presumed immunologic puzzle resolved with a diagnosis of child abuse. *Arch Pediatr Adolesc Med*. 1997;151(1):103–105 PMID: 9006541 https://doi.org/10.1001/archpedi.1997.02170380107021
66. Jones DP. Dermatitis artefacta in mother and baby as child abuse. *Br J Psychiatry*. 1983;143(2):199–200 PMID: 6616121 https://doi.org/10.1192/bjp.143.2.199
67. Stankler L. Factitious skin lesions in a mother and two sons. *Br J Dermatol*. 1977;97(2):217–219 PMID: 911684 https://doi.org/10.1111/j.1365-2133.1977.tb15069.x
68. Gupta MA, Gupta AK. Dermatitis artefacta and sexual abuse. *Int J Dermatol*. 1993;32(11):825–826 PMID: 8270346 https://doi.org/10.1111/j.1365-4362.1993.tb02776.x
69. Wright J, Friedrich W, Cinq-Mars C, Cyr M, McDuff P. Self-destructive and delinquent behaviors of adolescent female victims of child sexual abuse: rates and covariates in clinical and nonclinical samples. *Violence Vict*. 2004;19(6):627–643 PMID: 16004066 https://doi.org/10.1891/vivi.19.6.627.66343
70. Cordova A. The Mongolian spot: a study of ethnic differences and a literature review. *Clin Pediatr (Phila)*. 1981;20(11):714–719 PMID: 7028354 https://doi.org/10.1177/000992288102001105
71. Giusti R, Tunnessen WW Jr. Picture of the month. Chilblains (pernio). *Arch Pediatr Adolesc Med*. 1997;151(10):1055–1056 PMID: 9343021 https://doi.org/10.1001/archpedi.1997.02170470089018
72. O'Hare AE, Eden OB. Bleeding disorders and non-accidental injury. *Arch Dis Child*. 1984;59(9):860–864 PMID: 6486863 https://doi.org/10.1136/adc.59.9.860
73. Collins PW, Hamilton M, Dunstan FD, et al. Patterns of bruising in preschool children with inherited bleeding disorders: a longitudinal study. *Arch Dis Child*. 2017;102(12):1110–1117 PMID: 27449675
74. Carpenter SL, Abshire TC, Anderst JD; American Academy of Pediatrics Section on Hematology/Oncology and Committee on Child Abuse and Neglect. Evaluating for suspected child abuse: conditions that predispose to bleeding. *Pediatrics*. 2013;131(4):e1357–e1373 PMID: 23530171 https://doi.org/10.1542/peds.2013-0196
75. Brown J, Melinkovich P. Schönlein-Henoch purpura misdiagnosed as suspected child abuse. A case report and literature review. *JAMA*. 1986;256(5):617–618 PMID: 3723759 https://doi.org/10.1001/jama.1986.03380050085026
76. Lanzkowsky S, Lanzkowsky L, Lanzkowsky P. Henoch-Schoenlein purpura. *Pediatr Rev*. 1992;13(4):130–137 PMID: 1626007 https://doi.org/10.1542/pir.13-4-130
77. Pfurtscheller K, Trop M. Phototoxic plant burns: report of a case and review of topical wound treatment in children. *Pediatr Dermatol*. 2014;31(6):e156–e159 PMID: 25424227 https://doi.org/10.1111/pde.12396
78. Goskowicz MO, Friedlander SF, Eichenfield LF. Endemic "lime" disease: phytophotodermatitis in San Diego County. *Pediatrics*. 1994;93(5):828–830 PMID: 8165090
79. Hill PF, Pickford M, Parkhouse N. Phytophotodermatitis mimicking child abuse. *J R Soc Med*. 1997;90(10):560–561 PMID: 9488014 https://doi.org/10.1177/014107689709001008

80. Greig AV, Harris DL. A study of perceptions of facial hemangiomas in professionals involved in child abuse surveillance. *Pediatr Dermatol*. 2003;20(1):1–4 PMID: 12558837 https://doi.org/10.1046/j.1525-1470.2003.03001.x
81. Ragosta K. Pediculosis masquerades as child abuse. *Pediatr Emerg Care*. 1989;5(4):253–254 PMID: 2602204 https://doi.org/10.1097/00006565-198912000-00016
82. Lilly E, Kundu RV. Dermatoses secondary to Asian cultural practices. *Int J Dermatol*. 2012;51(4):372–379 PMID: 22435423 https://doi.org/10.1111/j.1365-4632.2011.05170.x
83. Adler R, Kane-Nussen B. Erythema multiforme: confusion with child battering syndrome. *Pediatrics*. 1983;72(5):718–720 PMID: 6634277
84. Labbé L, Perel Y, Maleville J, Taïeb A. Erythema nodosum in children: a study of 27 patients. *Pediatr Dermatol*. 1996;13(6):447–450 PMID: 8987051 https://doi.org/10.1111/j.1525-1470.1996.tb00722.x
85. Thakur BK, Kaplan AP. Recurrent "unexplained" scalp swelling in an eighteen-month-old child: an atypical presentation of angioedema causing confusion with child abuse. *J Pediatr*. 1996;129(1):163–165 PMID: 8757580 https://doi.org/10.1016/S0022-3476(96)70207-X
86. Leung AK, Robson WL. Penile and oral angioedema associated with peanut ingestion. *J Natl Med Assoc*. 2006;98(12):2011–2012 PMID: 17225851
87. Smith GA, Sharma V, Knapp JF, Shields BJ. The summer penile syndrome: seasonal acute hypersensitivity reaction caused by chigger bites on the penis. *Pediatr Emerg Care*. 1998;14(2):116–118 PMID: 9583392 https://doi.org/10.1097/00006565-199804000-00007
88. Cohen HA, Matalon A, Mezger A, Ben Amitai D, Barzilai A. Striae in adolescents mistaken for physical abuse. *J Fam Pract*. 1997;45(1):84–85 PMID: 9228918
89. Heller D. Lumbar physiological striae in adolescence suspected to be non-accidental injury. *BMJ*. 1995;311(7007):738 PMID: 7549692 https://doi.org/10.1136/bmj.311.7007.738
90. Abtahi-Naeini B, Shapouri J, Masjedi M, Saffaei A, Pourazizi M. Unexplained facial scar: child abuse or Ehlers-Danlos syndrome? *N Am J Med Sci*. 2014;6(11):595–598 PMID: 25535610 https://doi.org/10.4103/1947-2714.145482
91. Patel B, Butterfield R. Common skin and bleeding disorders that can potentially masquerade as child abuse. *Am J Med Genet C Semin Med Genet*. 2015;169(4):328–336 PMID: 26502028 https://doi.org/10.1002/ajmg.c.31462
92. Dhurat RP, Deshpande DJ. Loose anagen hair syndrome. *Int J Trichology*. 2010;2(2):96–100 PMID: 21712911 https://doi.org/10.4103/0974-7753.77513
93. Denic N, Huyer DW, Sinal SH, Lantz PE, Smith CR, Silver MM. Cockroach: the omnivorous scavenger. Potential misinterpretation of postmortem injuries. *Am J Forensic Med Pathol*. 1997;18(2):177–180 PMID: 9185937 https://doi.org/10.1097/00000433-199706000-00014
94. Peebles J, Losek JD. Child physical abuse and rhabdomyolysis: case report and literature review. *Pediatr Emerg Care*. 2007;23(7):474–477 PMID: 17666931 https://doi.org/10.1097/01.pec.0000280514.05913.23

CHAPTER 3

Burns

Kenneth Feldman, MD, FAAP
Clinical Professor of Pediatrics
University of Washington
Children's Protection Program
Seattle Children's Hospital
Seattle, WA

James Metz, MD, MPH, FAAP
Assistant Professor
Department of Pediatrics
University of Vermont
Larner College of Medicine
Division of General Pediatrics, ChildSafe Program
University of Vermont Children's Hospital
Burlington, VT

Burn injuries, whether accidental or abusive, are some of the most visible signs of trauma. They can be relatively benign or result in severe disfigurement depending on the extent, depth, and location of the burn. Worldwide, burns are a leading cause of morbidity and lead to an estimated 180,000 death every year.[1] Burns disproportionally affect younger children and low-income populations.[1,2] The heavy economic effect of burns results from prolonged hospital recovery as well as disability-adjusted life years lost. For the United States in 2000, the direct costs associated with childhood burns exceeded $211 million.[1]

While most childhood burns are accidental, a significant number of burn injuries result from child abuse and neglect. Of children who have experienced physical abuse, 6% to 20% have sustained burns.[3] Medical professionals caring for children may have infrequent exposure to burns, but familiarity with the basic concepts and epidemiology of burns is important for recognizing when a burn may have been the result of abuse or neglect. As opposed to the frustrated, impulsive caregiver acts that cause most physical abuse, many burns require greater intent and planned effort to cause pain.

In the simplest terms, burn injuries require the transfer of destructive energy to tissue. Most often this energy is in the form of heat, but other types of energy are relevant, including cold, dry hot air, steam, radiant energy, microwave energy, x-rays, and chemical energy. The most common childhood burns, abusive and accidental, are caused by heated fluids or solids.

General Epidemiology

Burns affect people of all ages, although the burden of disease tends to favor younger children. The Web-based Injury Statistics Query and Reporting Systems (WISQARS)[4] of the Centers for Disease Control and Prevention, National Electronic Injury Surveillance System (NEISS)[5] of the US Consumer Product Safety Commission, and the National Safety Council[6] provide regularly updated burn incidence and fatality rates (Table 3.1).

A prospective emergency department (ED) and inpatient accidental burn study in the United Kingdom, excluding house fires, identified 1,215 burn victims.[7] Seventy-eight percent of 709 scald injuries were in children younger than 5 years. Children's development abilities modify their risk of experiencing or causing burn injuries. The youngest infant to pull fluid onto himself was 8 months old, the youngest to have hot water spilled on him by someone else was 4 months old, and the youngest to climb into a bathtub was 15 months old. The front of the body was injured in 96%, with younger children sustaining more face, arm, and upper trunk burns and older children more leg, hand, or lower trunk injuries. Contact burns

TABLE 3.1
National Burn Incidence Statistics

	0–14 y		0–4 y		5–9 y		10–14 y	
	No.	Rate[a]	No.	Rate[a]	No.	Rate[a]	No.	Rate[a]
WISQARS fire/burn nonfatal	93,688	152.79	56,476	284.13	20,941	102.06	15,275	73.89
WISQARS fire/burn nonfatal violence	995	1.63	641	3.22	118	0.57	237	1.15
WISQARS fire/burn deaths unintentional	235	0.39	138	0.69	83	0.41	51	0.25
WISQARS fire/burn deaths violence	23	0.04						
WISQARS house fire deaths all intent	215	0.35						
			0–1 y		1–4 y		5–14 y	
NSC fire/smoke/flame deaths[6]			17	0.4	128	0.8	135	0.3

Abbreviations: NSC, National Safety Council; WISQARS, Web-based Injury Statistics Query and Reporting System.
[a] Per 100,000.

were next in frequency at 32%, but more often they only required ED care. Children younger than 5 years accounted for 73% of contact burns. Most young children (83%) were injured when they touched a hot object, with 67% sustaining hand burns, including 82% of them having palmar injuries only. Of the 11% with multiple burns, 35 children had bilateral injuries. Other burn causes were flames (5.5%); radiation, including solar (1.6%); chemicals (1%); friction (1%); and electrical (0.4%).

While accidental burns are by far most common, abusive burns are particularly problematic. In a review of nearly 16,000 pediatric burn admissions in the American Burn Association registry, 5.8% were judged abusive.[8] The age of children with abusive burns was younger (mean 2.4 years old) than that of children with accidental burns (mean 3.9 years old). The adjusted mortality risk of children who experienced abuse was 4.9 times that of children who did not experience abuse; their absolute mortality rate was 2.5%. Also, hospital length of stay and the need for intensive care was greater in abusive burns. The most common areas for abusive burns were the buttock, perineum, and bilateral lower extremities. Abuse was less common among children who had head, neck, and torso injuries. Inhalation injuries and fire or flame sources were more common among children who were unintentionally injured. Rates of contact and scald injuries did not differ between abuse and unintentional injury.

In infants and children, scalds were the most common burn source among outpatient and inpatient burn case series (43%–65%)[7,9–20] (Table 3.2). Different study sites had unique burn cause distributions.

Abuse, including scalding, accounts for many childhood burns. In a Chicago, IL, study, 7.8% of childhood burns were abusive, 64% accidental, and 53% negligent. Of the abusive burns, 62% were due to scalds. Tap water was involved in 20% of accidental, 56% of neglectful, and 70% of abusive scalds, emphasizing tap water's importance among abusive and neglectful injuries.[13] Among 344 infants seen in the ED for a burn injury in Washington, DC, 13.4% resulted from abuse.[14] At Shriners Hospitals for Children—Boston, 18.5% of burn admissions were abusive.[15] Addition of a forensic scientist to an inpatient burn team in Turkey increased the number of cases of maltreatment burns from 59% to 72%.[16] Most of the maltreatment injuries in this study were attributed to neglect. From Parkland Hospital in Dallas, TX, 5.3% of burn admissions were abusive.[17] Scalds accounted for 45% and flames 29% overall. However, for children who had experienced abuse, scalds accounted for 90% of injuries and contact injuries 5%. Eighty-seven percent of 218 immersion scalds were caused by abuse. Unilateral or bilateral foot, buttock, and perineal distributions were associated with abuse, while arm, chest, and head and neck injuries were more often unintentional. Electrical, flame, and grease burns were more frequent with unintentional injury. Child abuse was a major contributor to burn mortality; the mortality rate for children who had experienced abuse was 5.7% versus 0.5% for children who were injured unintentionally.

TABLE 3.2
Selected Burn Studies, Causes/Sources of Burns

No. of Children/ Age Range	Setting	Scalds	Contact	Flame	Chemical/ Electrical	Other/Notes
106 <1 y	OP Finland[9]	61% 86% beverage 23% food 5% humidifier	38% 68% stove fireplace 12.5% radiator 10% kettles 7.5% irons 2.5% light bulbs			
29 0–6 mo	IP, ED Australia[10]	43%	39%			11% sunburn 7% IV extravasation
104 <1 y	IP United Kingdom[11]	65%	30% radiators/hot pipes	5%		
2,109 with scalds <15 y	IP, ED India[12]	42% (of all age)				
1,372 <10 y	ICU, IP South Africa[21]	76.5%		21.8%		1.8% electrical/ contact/other fluid
208 <17 y	ED, IP England[19]	51%	36%	11%		3% were assault or NAT
1,215 <17 y	IP, ED United Kingdom[7]	58% 50% beverage 37% tap water 13% food	32% (40% fixed objects, 60% mobile objects)	5.5%	0.9%	0.9% sunburn 0.9% friction 0.6% radiation

Abbreviations: ED, emergency department; ICU, intensive care unit; IP, inpatient; IV, intravenous; NAT, non-accidental trauma; OP, outpatient.

A study from a Seattle, WA, inpatient burn unit, from 1996 to 2000, found unintentional burn injuries were caused by hot fluid spills (82%), tap water spills (6%), other immersions (5%), tap water immersions (4%), and steam (3%).[18] Causes of abusive injuries included 6 tap water immersions (67%), 1 tap water spill (11%), and 2 other spills (22%). Abuse was the cause of 0.5% of scalds, but 46% of tap water immersions were abusive. Yet, only 1.3% of hot fluid spills resulted from abuse. The mean age of immersion victims was 18 months.

A British general practice study of 3.9 million children showed that risk factors for those who had experienced abuse compared with case controls were male sex, birth order later than third, single parent home, and teen or depressed mother.[20] Neither postpartum depression nor drug or alcohol problems were associated risk factors.

These are by no means exhaustive examples of the proportions and rates of childhood burn agents. These studies are mostly burn service studies that discuss children who have been seen primarily for burn injuries. As such, they underemphasize children who have been seen primarily for other injuries who happen to have associated burn injuries. This is not an unusual situation for children who have been beaten but also have associated punitive contact burns.

Burn rates change over time and between societies based on local customs and changes in regional technology.[22–27] For example, the US Flammable Fabrics Act dramatically reduced the incidence of childhood clothing ignition burns.[22] A law was passed in Washington (RCW 19.27A.060) limiting new water heater initial settings to 49°C (120°F) in 1983. By 2000, the rate of tap water burn admissions in King County, WA, was cut from 5.5 per year before the law to 1.6 per year.[18] Local culture and changing technology modify each area's burn incidence patterns.

Burn Mechanics

Fundamental to thermal burns is the relationship of substance temperature to time in defining burn risk. Among burn causes, the simplest energy transfer situation is from hot water to skin. Water has a heat content of 1 cal/mL/°C in 1 mL.[28] If hot water from a constant temperature reservoir is flowing over skin, it maintains a constantly replenished supply of similar temperature fluid on the skin's surface. Other fluids differ from water; most have higher heat content, and most are more viscous. Downhill flow of more viscous fluids is slowed. These attributes of fluids other than water produce more prolonged and intense thermal damage to the exposed skin.[29] For example, olive oil has a heat content of 7 cal/°C in 1 mL.[28] While water has a viscosity of 0.65 cP at 40°C (104°F), olive oil is 36 cP. Likewise, solids have variable heat content, heat conductance within the object, and surface emissivity by contact or radiation. As examples, heat conductivity, which is required to refresh the surface temperature of a solid object, in copper is 0.98 mW/cm/°C, while in concrete it is 0.002 mW/cm/°C. Copper has a heat content of 0.09 kcal/kg/°C, while concrete content is 0.18 kcal/kg/°C. Surface properties are also important. To prevent burns from steam transmission pipes, the insulation must limit the external pipe temperature to below 45°C (113°F) if the surface of the pipe is shiny metal.[30] If it is covered in white matte fabric, temperatures up to 60°C (140°F) are safe. Also, a solid's heat transfer may occur through intervening or coupling substances; consider walking on a sun-heated pool deck, with or without wet feet. These variables lead to much more complex predictions of the time and temperature thresholds for burns from substances other than water.

Initial Burn Assessment

The American Burn Association provides guidance on the initial assessment of burn size and depth.[31]

Scalds

Among burns of children, scalds are extremely common. Most arise from unintentional spills of food or drink. Several basic principles underlie analysis of scald burns: the hotter the liquid, the faster the burn; flowing water runs downhill; and standing water seeks a level.

Time–Temperature Relationships in Scalds

Our understanding of the time–temperature relationships for hot water burns stems from the 1940s research of Moritz and Henriques[32] (Figure 3.1). Using pigs exposed to constant temperature hot water, they defined the temperatures required to cause superficial epidermal and full-thickness epidermal burns. They termed these *threshold burns*. This threshold burn is consistent with the prior nomenclature of *superficial second-degree burns* or the current *superficial partial-thickness injury*. Pigs were used in the research because they have similar dermal and epidermal anatomy to humans but lack the ability to sweat. The researchers confirmed their findings using a limited number of adult human volunteers. They noted that skin compression, resulting in lack of blood flow during the burn event, did not modify burn times. The time–temperature burn curves were doubly asymptotic. Below 52.7°C (127°F), at which point adults sustain threshold burns in 1 minute, the time to burn increases dramatically with each degree lower of temperature. At 48.8°C (120°F) it takes 10 minutes to cause the same injury. At the other end of the burn curve, above 60°C (140°F), burn times rapidly fall with each degree of temperature rise, becoming almost instantaneous.

Henriques also described how burn injury rates are proportionate to the skin depth of interest. He used a rearrangement of the "error function."[28,34] Using his equation, one can define how burn times vary with or at different skin depths. At lower temperatures, deeper dermal tissues require a more prolonged time at the target temperature to sustain burn necrosis, but at higher temperatures necrosis is nearly instantaneous once the target temperature is reached. As a result, at low temperatures, the time to necrosis is determined by the total time at the target temperature, which is much longer than the time for heat penetration. Thus, at temperatures below 54.4°C (130°F), the time for penetration of heat to the target depth of the skin is insignificant and drops out of Henriques' equation. However, at high temperatures, with instantaneous skin necrosis, it is the heat penetration time that determines the time to burn. This means that children, who have thinner skin, will sustain superficial burns in nearly the same time as adults at lower temperatures but will burn more rapidly at higher temperatures. This disparity between adult and child burn times is magnified the deeper the level of interest is into the skin. At the extreme, burn times have been experimentally derived for preterm neonates who have very thin skin and little subcutaneous fat to develop safe standards for the use of heated oximetry probes. The probes can remain in place for 6 hours at 44.4°C (112°F) before causing dermal burns.[35]

Examples of experimental and calculated burn rates for children and adults for superficial epidermal injuries and the Moritz and Henriques threshold burns (epidermal/dermal junction) can be seen in Table 3.3. These rates were based on their experiments and also were calculated from Henriques' equation,[34,36,37] using pathologically described child and adult skin thickness. More recent papers have used ultrasound-derived skin thickness[38] to describe thresholds for deep dermal burns (second-degree/deep partial-thickness skin burns) (Table 3.3).[33]

Clothing can either be a barrier to hot liquids or cause prolonged contact, attenuating or increasing the burn severity. At the extremes, a close-fitting diaper can almost completely shield the perineum, while water spilled onto an absorbent and porous shirt increases burn time.

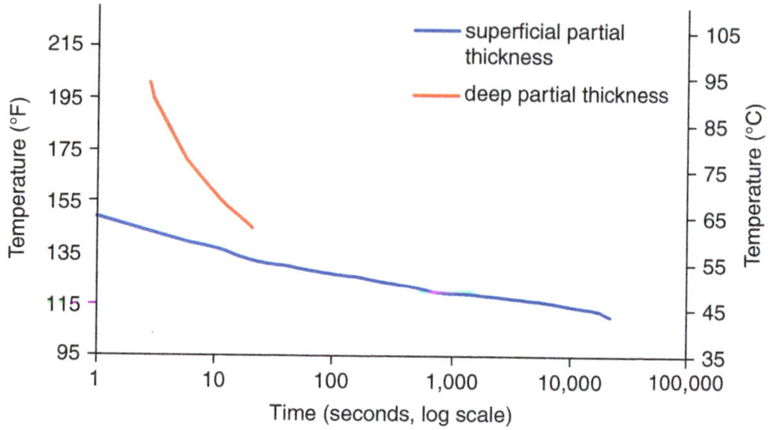

FIGURE 3.1
Burn time versus temperature. Superficial partial-thickness burn thresholds are derived from Moritz and Henriques for adult skin.[32] The deep partial-thickness values for children are after Abraham et al.[33]

TABLE 3.3
Selected Burn Injury Thresholds: Burn Times at Different Temperatures

Temperature °C (°F)	Burn Threshold[a] Onset Epidermal/First Degree (s)			Superficial Epidermal/Superficial Second Degree[a] (s)			Deep Partial-Thickness/Deep Dermal[b] (s)	
	Adult Calcu-lated	Adult Experi-mental	Child Calcu-lated	Adult Calcu-lated	Adult Experi-mental	Child Calcu-lated	Adult Calculated	Child Calcu-lated
49 (120)								
54 (129)	19.0	18	6.0	31.0	35	10.0		
56 (133)	8.1	8.3	–	13.0	16			
57 (135)	–	–	2.0	–	–	4.0		
60 (140)	2.3	2.6	0.5	3.0	5	1.0		
63 (145)							31	21
65 (149)	1.0	0.7	0.3	1.0	2	0.5		
66 (151)							23	15
68 (154)							17	12
70 (158)	0.4	–	–	0.5	1	–		
71 (160)							14	9.2
77 (171)							10	6.0

[a] After Moritz and Henriques[32] and Feldman.[36]
[b] After Abraham et al[33] (no postburn cooling).

Flow/Splash Pattern Scalds

If free to flow, the influence of gravity on the flow pattern of scalds should be apparent. This is most easily seen in unintentional coffee or tea burns (figures 3.2–3.4). One should be able to identify the point of initial fluid contact, the child's position in relation to vertical, and the flow pattern down the child's body. The "arrow down" scald pattern is typically seen with such unintentional incidents. Spilled, splashing, or thrown water tends to separate into smaller boluses that may still have sufficient heat content to burn but only if the water is still quite hot when it hits the skin. Water temperatures in the range of 60°C (140°F) to 65.6°C (150°F) are required. In Figure 3.2, separate splash marks can be seen. The corollary is that at lower

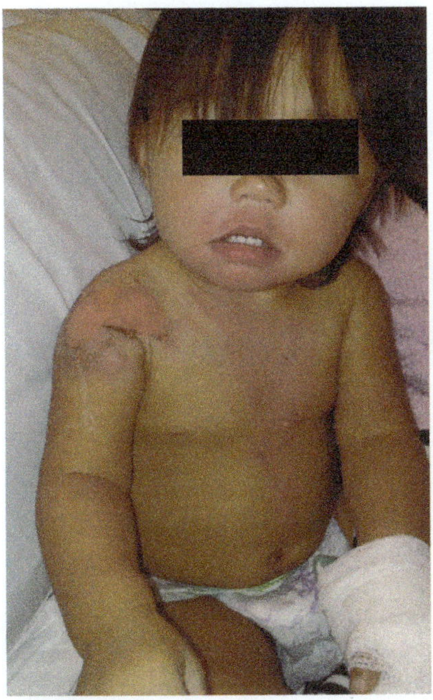

FIGURE 3.2

A 17-month-old girl pulled a cup of hot tea off a table at her child care. She sustained burns under her left chin and on her left chest and shoulder. Note the "arrow down" chest pattern and the splash burn below the main shoulder burn. Tea and coffee are often served at 71°C to 77°C (160°F–170°F). This is not abusive but poor child care safety practice.

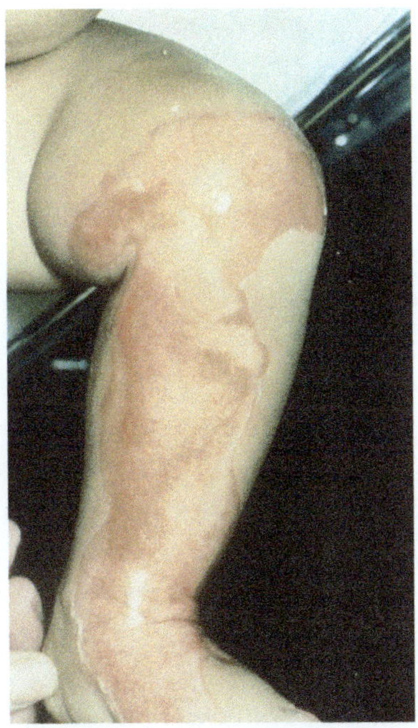

FIGURE 3.3

This toddler's family lived in rental housing with water supplied by a small tank water heater. They had set it at 77°C (170°F) to have sufficient hot water. They left the toddler bathing in shallow lukewarm water. He turned on the hot water handle alone and was found still holding the handle. The hot water flow pattern down and around his leg is apparent. The burn pattern is consistent with the accident as described, but it was negligent to leave so young a toddler bathing unsupervised.

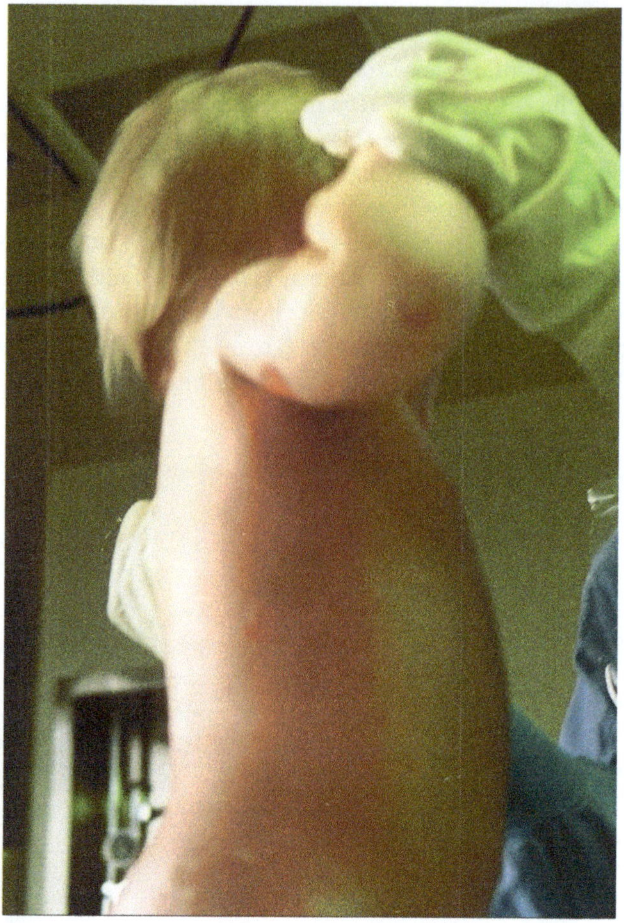

FIGURE 3.4

This child's babysitter burned her while cleaning off soil with a kitchen sink sprayer. The event was punishment for the soiling.

temperatures, the absence of splash marks is meaningless when thinking about burn mechanism. Likewise, because flow patterns are not uniform, the burn depth of the primary injury in flow scalds will be variegate.

Immersion Scalds

If a child's body part is forcibly immersed in a basin of standing hot water, body contour lines will define a sharp margin between burned and unburned skin. The burns themselves are mostly of uniform depth because of the similar exposure times of all the skin. This will, however, be modified if the immersed skin is of different thicknesses. As such, thicker palmar and plantar skin may have relative sparing compared with dorsal hand and foot scalds, if the burn times are short. The prototypical examples of such immersions are the abusive glove (Figure 3.5) or stocking (Figure 3.6) burns. More complex examples involve buttock and lower body immersions, often occurring in toddlers due to caregivers' toilet training frustrations (Figure 3.7). These injuries involve perineal and bilateral foot and/or leg injuries. Lower extremity symmetry is often present. If the child attempts to resist being held in the hot water, his or her hands may be burned as he or she attempts to "tripod" his or her perineum out of the water. Skin areas protected by skin-to-skin apposition in flexural creases can be spared if the child is immobile, as with restraint. If perineal burning is present, a doughnut hole of buttock sparing may be present where the child was forcibly held against the cooler tub bottom. Some of these burns have biphasic patterns because of superposition of the pattern of the initial immersion onto that of the child's defensive attempts.

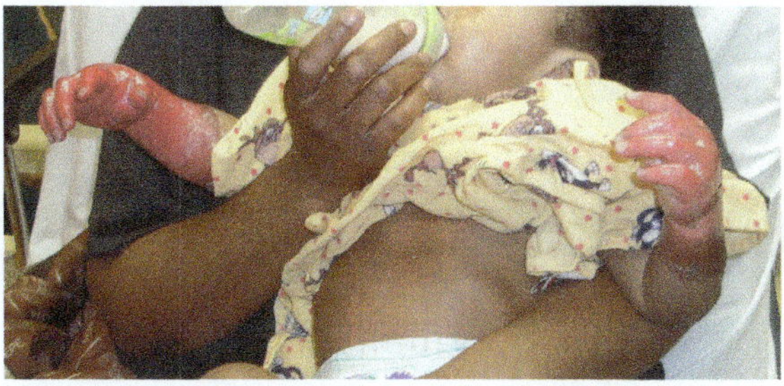

FIGURE 3.5
This 11-month-old's babysitter reported that he had sustained the burns when he tipped over a hot steam humidifier. However, he had typical glove burns of forced hand immersion, and not flow burns.

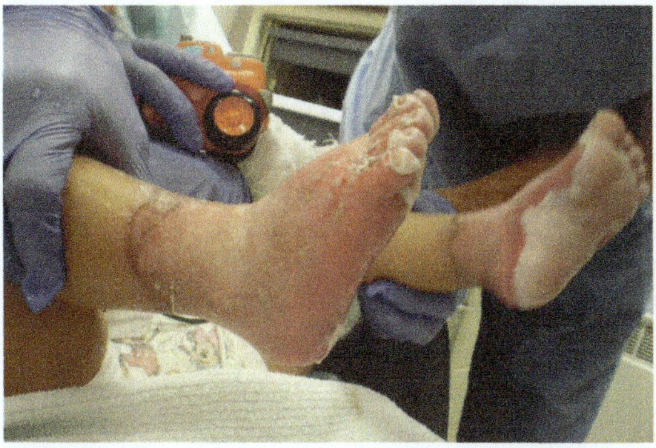

FIGURE 3.6
The mother's boyfriend reported that this 18-month-old boy had pulled over a pot of boiling macaroni, which caused his injuries. However, the child sustained bilateral stocking immersion burns caused by a forced immersion. The soles were partially spared because of their thicker skin.

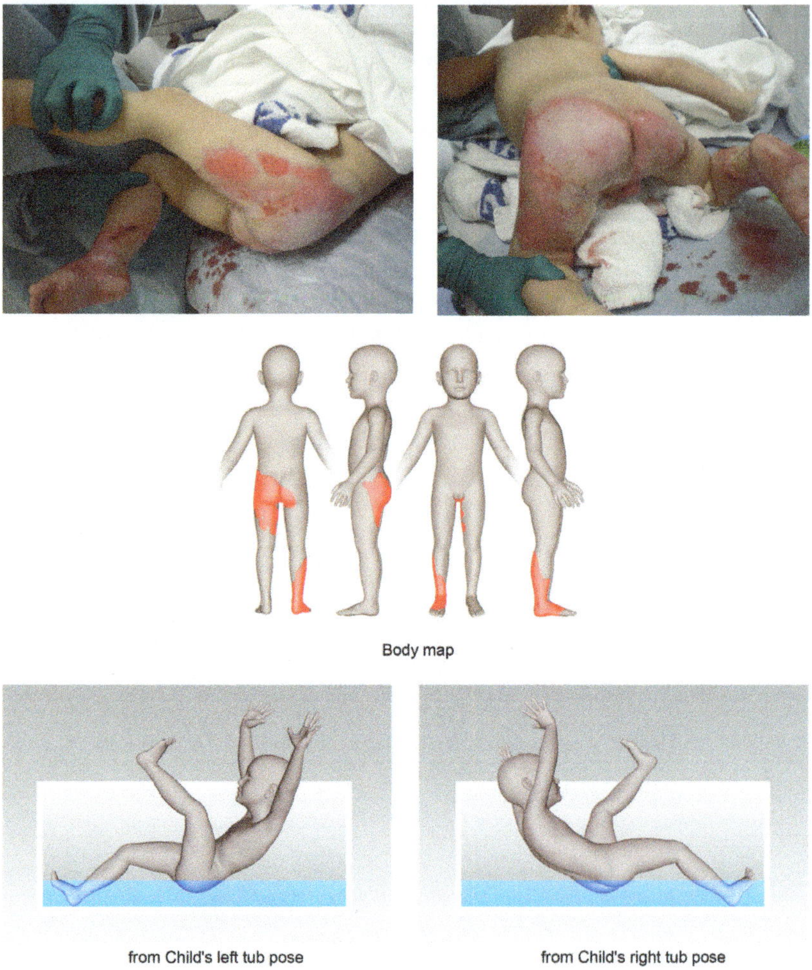

FIGURE 3.7
This 3-year-old boy's stepmother reported she had drawn his bath and checked the water temperature. Then she had left the water running while she went to check on her own 2-year-old. She reported the 3-year-old undressed, got in the tub, and then began yelling, "Owie." She found him thrashing about in the tub. The burn pattern indicates he was held in the water in a position he would be unable to sustain by himself. Except for the left hip, no splash areas are present. The burn distribution diagram and illustrated scene reconstruction assisted the jury in returning a guilty verdict.
Photos courtesy of Dr Rebecca Wiester. Medical illustration by Kate Sweeney.

Relationship of Pain to Burn Injuries

Adult pain thresholds for hot water have been reported to be 42.8°C to 45°C (109°F–113°F).[39] Children tend to be even more averse to hotter water temperatures, yet these temperatures are less than or equal to the 6-hour time required to cause superficial dermal burns. Young children comfortably bathe at 38.3°C (101°F). The general rule should be that *if it doesn't hurt, it doesn't burn.* Stories that the child was left comfortably bathing in the bathtub, but her skin was burned and was peeling when the caregiver returned, are patently false. However, children who are insensate in their lower body, lack the ability to perceive pain due to congenital pain insensitivity, are unconscious due to seizures occurring while in hot water, or lack cognitive or motor skills sufficient to escape injury are subject to burns that typical children could have avoided[40] (figures 3.8 and 3.9). Lagunju and colleagues reported that 57 of 125 children with epilepsy experienced seizure-related injuries, 3 of whom sustained burns.[41]

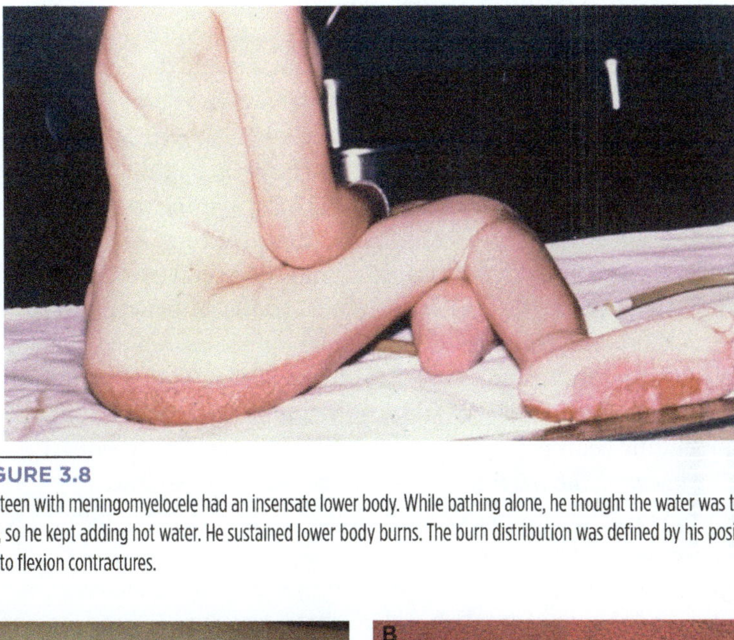

FIGURE 3.8

This teen with meningomyelocele had an insensate lower body. While bathing alone, he thought the water was too cool, so he kept adding hot water. He sustained lower body burns. The burn distribution was defined by his position due to flexion contractures.

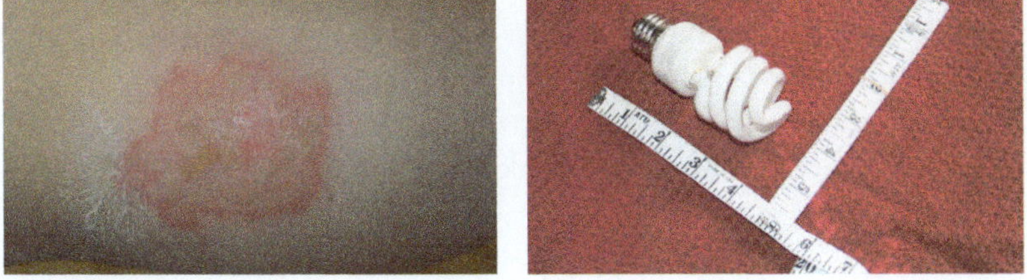

FIGURE 3.9

During a sleepover, an 8-year-old boy (A) and a friend found and drank a bottle of diphenhydramine. The next morning, on awakening, a compact fluorescent light had tipped over and was in contact with the boy's leg. The bulb's coil pattern (B) can be seen at the margin of the burn.
Photos courtesy of Dr Rebecca Wiester.

Child Behavior and Scalding Scenarios

Children can sustain unintentional immersion burns when they unknowingly enter a basin of drawn hot water or a peer or older sibling places them in already drawn hot water. However, attribution of burns to the child or siblings can be false histories to hide abuse.[42] Nine percent of infants as young as 10 months are capable of climbing into a 14-inch bathtub; by 12 to 15 months of age, 30% can do so.[43] Observations show that half enter feetfirst and half enter headfirst. It could be assumed that the corollary is that toddlers who can get into a tub should have the cognitive and motor skills to be able to get out if they experience pain.

Often, immersion injuries are accompanied by a parental history of drawing a shallow level of appropriate-temperature bathwater, putting the child in the tub, and leaving the room briefly to answer the phone or do a similar outside task. However, we should understand the dynamics of added hot water. The usual 125-L (33-gal) bathtub has 22.9 cm (9") between tub bottom and the overflow drain. If the child is left in 7.6 cm (3") of comfortable 38.3°C (101°F) bathwater and then turns on only the hot water at full flow, at an average faucet flow rate of 19 L (5 gal)/min, it would take 2 minutes to add an additional 7.6 cm or 42 L (11 gal) of hot water. If that added water were at 65.6°C (150°F) and fully mixed with the previously drawn, comfortable 38.3°C (101°F) water, 52.7°C (127°F) water would result. It takes an additional 2 minutes at that temperature to cause a threshold dermal burn, for a total time required to cause a burn of 4 minutes. It is hardly plausible that a toddler would not attempt to extricate himself as the temperature became painfully hot and before frank injury occurred. Likewise, knowing the water temperature and time–temperature relationship for child burning, one can often recognize that the child would have had to be kept in obviously painfully hot water for a prolonged duration. In abusive scald injuries with incomplete restraint and very hot water, a mixed picture with splash and immersion patterns may be present because the child struggles to escape. This speaks to the caregiver continuing to immerse the child long after the child's pain is clearly evident. This property indicates the caregiver's intention to inflict prolonged pain, even if the eventual injury is not intended. Burn infliction can be more sadistic than more impulsive modes of abuse, like shaking an infant.

Patterns and Locations of Inflicted Scalds

The incidence of abusive immersion burns peaks in the toddler years. Lower body immersions are often accompanied by a soiling history or other caregiver frustrations with typical toddler behavior as a trigger event.[44] If a child is forcibly held in a fixed flexion position, skin-to-skin contact (as in the groin creases) will prevent hot water entry within the flexion creases, resulting in burn-spared areas (Figure 3.10). Likewise, if the child's buttocks are forcibly held against the cooler tub bottom, a doughnut hole of sparing may be present on the child's buttocks (Figure 3.11). Intentional headfirst or face-first immersion burns have also been described (Figure 3.12).[17] Another abuse variation is the "up body" flowing burn pattern that implies that either the child was held in a nonphysiological position when fluid was poured on the child or the fluid was thrown upward. In a New Jersey study, 8.3% of burn injuries involved

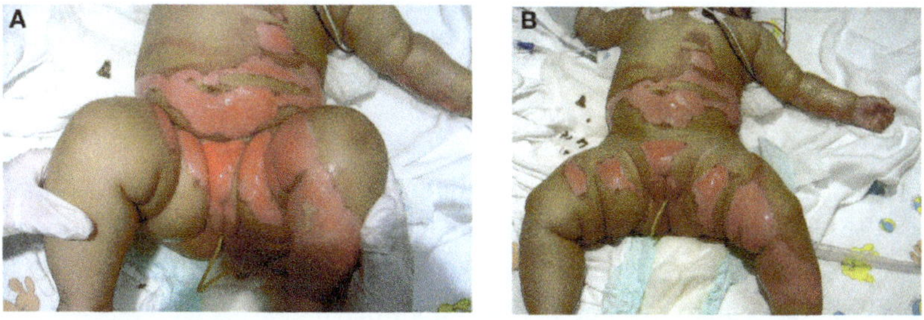

FIGURE 3.10
The mother initially reported that this infant had diaper rash from lotion but later admitted that the father might have poured hot water on the infant when the infant was in an infant car seat. The flexed photo (A) shows how skin-to-skin contact in the car seat caused flexion crease sparing, while the extended photo (B) shows the separate areas of burning. Note the lesser burn depth at the injury's upper margin. Such varied burn depths are typical of hot liquid flows or spills.

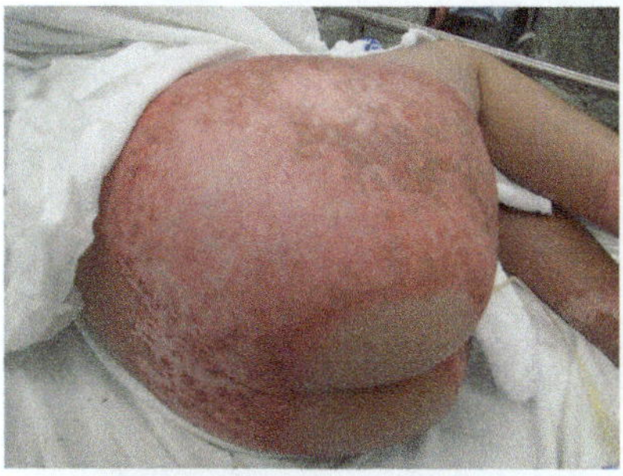

FIGURE 3.11
A 15-year-old girl with autism spectrum disorder, who had severe motor impairments, had 3 diarrheal stools in her diaper during the day. The third time, her caregiver drew a tub of hot water and placed her in it. The doughnut-hole sparing of her buttocks speaks to her immobility and restraint in the hot water; the tub's bottom remains cooler than the tub water. She would have been unable to enter the tub herself.

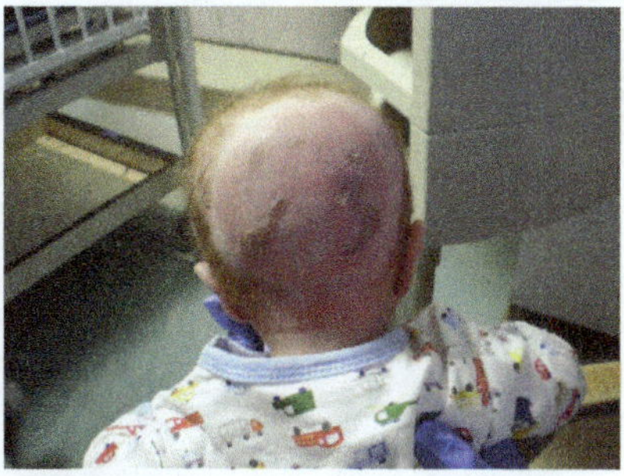

FIGURE 3.12
This 5-week-old's father reported he had run an infant bathing basin of comfortable water for the baby's bath, but he must have forgotten to turn off the hot water. He dipped the baby's occiput in the water, only then realizing it must have been too hot. No splash or flow marks are present. There was a prior history of a choking episode while the father was bathing the baby. The scenario indicates abuse.

children's genitals.[45] Scalds were a more common cause of genital burns in children younger than 5 years than older children (95% vs 78%), while flame burns caused more genital injuries (13% vs 2%) among older children. Abuse was the cause of 23% of younger children's and 5% of older children's genital injuries. Eighty-nine percent of unintentional and abusive genital injuries of all ages were caused by scalds.

Sink bathing has been found to be a risk for scald injury.[46] A New York, NY, study found that scalds occurred most often with impoverished families in substandard housing without other bathing facilities. Tap water accounted for 17% of all scalds, and sink bathing accounted for 46% of bathing scalds. Protective services referrals for concerns of abuse or neglect were common (27%) for children who had experienced scalds from sink bathing.

Accidental Scalds

Most flowing water burns result from childhood accidents in which hot drinks or food substances are spilled or pulled down on the victim. Injuries occur in toddlers who can reach and tip over food or drink containers, while older children tend to spill hot food or drink when preparing it themselves. Occasionally, abusive burns occur when hot liquids are intentionally run from the faucet, thrown, or spilled on the victim (Figure 3.13). Burns of the chest and forearms are most common with unintentional injuries. In abusive cases, burn patterns may suggest the fluid was coming from a direction opposite

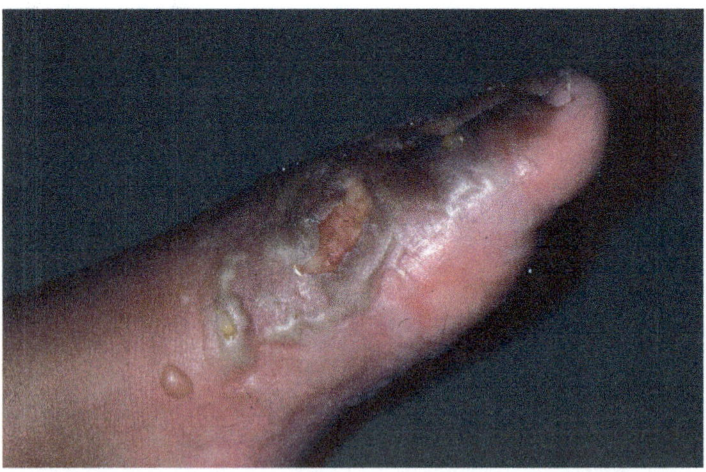

FIGURE 3.13

The mother's boyfriend reported he rescued this 2½-year-old girl from the bathtub after she had turned on only the hot water, sustaining flowing water scalds of the dorsum of both feet. Several years later, the girl told her physician she wouldn't have done anything that stupid; the boyfriend had turned on the hot water and held her feet under the flow as a punishment.

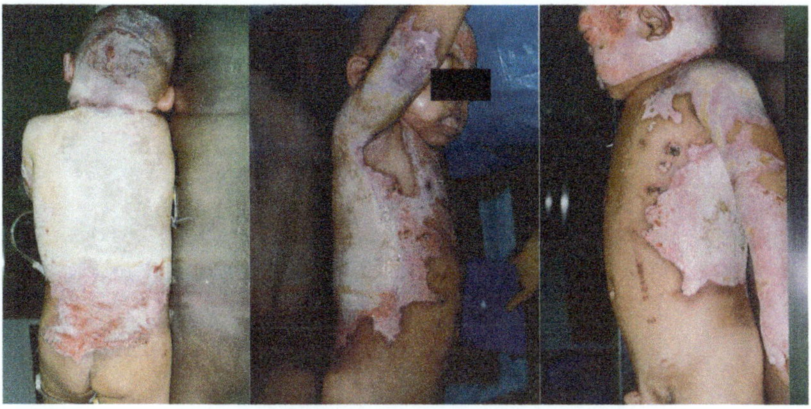

FIGURE 3.14

This 2½-year-old boy was reported to have, unwitnessed, pulled a pot of boiling water off the back burner of the stove. His mother heard him crying and found him in front of the stove, burned, with the spilled pot on the floor. In spite of his 53% body surface area scald, he wasn't brought to care until 2½ hours after the reported accident. He died of brain death and acute respiratory distress syndrome about 3 weeks after his injury. Note that his burn arose from flowing water from the left and behind his head. The water was hot enough to cause splash marks on the margins of the chest burns. There also were small groin splashes. The sparing of both anterior axillae suggests that his arms were at his sides at the time of injury, not reaching up. Most spills from pots pulled off a stove will involve the front of the child's body. It is unlikely he could have reached to the back burner. The burns seem most consistent with a seated child leaning forward, tripoding with his arms, as if he was restrained while hot water was poured over him. At the least, delay in seeking burn care was negligent and likely contributed to his fatal course.

of how the described "accidental spill" would have occurred; for example, the caregiver describes a "child pull down" accident, but the burn primarily affects the child's back (Figure 3.14). Flow or spill burns that are caused by more viscous liquids with higher heat content are likely to have more discrete tendrils of drip flow, causing deeper burn injuries.[29] Burn exposure times and temperatures have been found to depend on fluid viscosity and the angle of the burn surface relative to gravity.[47] Baby walker use remains a risk factor for accidental childhood pull-down scalds.[48] Sheridan has described abusive forced aspiration of hot liquids as a cause of some pharyngeal and airway burns.[49] Palatal and perioral injuries may also occur.

Contact Burns

Contact burn injuries are common with abusive and unintentional trauma. If occurring unintentionally, they happen when the child touches, brushes against, pulls down, or steps onto a hot object. Such events most often result in single, glancing injuries of normally unclothed skin. The site of the initial contact may look like a "comet head," while the child's attempts to withdraw or twist away result in its "tail." The standing or running child who sustains a glancing face burn while brushing against a cigarette held at her parent's side is a good example. Contact burns that are multiple, involve clothed or protected body parts, and are clearly, directly, and deeply imprinted are more likely to be abusive (Figure 3.15). Such injuries can result from contact with hot solids or smoldering objects, like cigarettes.[50] Cigarettes, if pressed directly into skin, cause deep, punched-out, 5- to 10-mm burns. They heal with heaped-up margins and eschar formation (Figure 3.16). However, these eschars, if small and circular, could be confused with deep-seated staphylococcal pyoderma. Toddlers are most vulnerable to contact burns from heaters (Figure 3.17) and stove or fireplace glass.[51–53] If they toddle up and touch hot surfaces, they may be unable

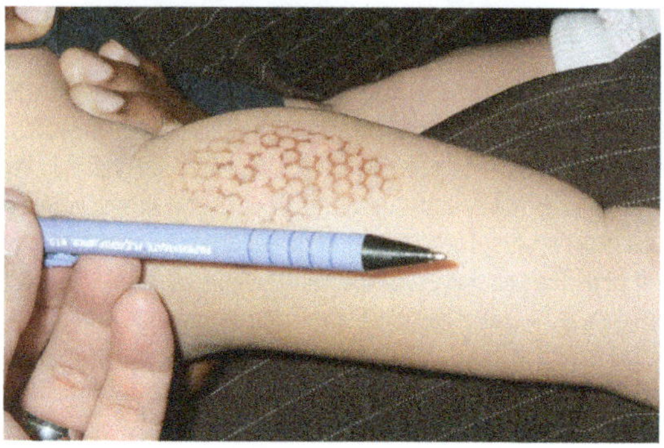

FIGURE 3.15

This infant sustained a burn from a metal grid. Note how clearly imprinted the burn is. A brushing, unintentional contact clearly is not an adequate explanation.

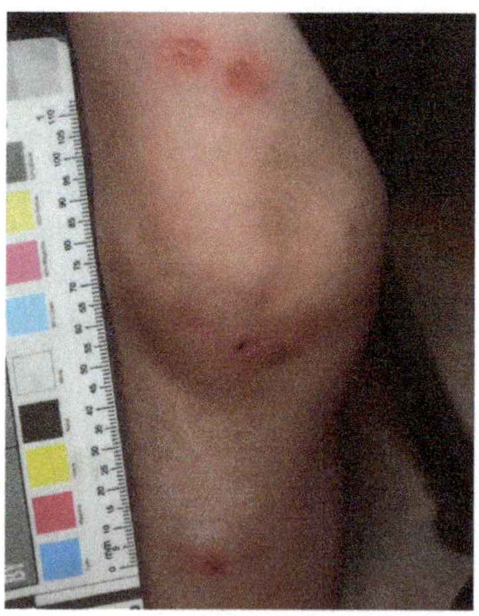

FIGURE 3.16

A 3-year-old girl came to child care with burns above and below her right knee. They were attributed to her 5-year-old brother running over her with his bicycle. A week before, she had had unexplained finger burns. Her mother attributed them to the child getting her hand under a door her brother had opened. The family had a past history of child protective services involvement and domestic violence. The lesions on her leg represented directly imprinted cigarette burns.

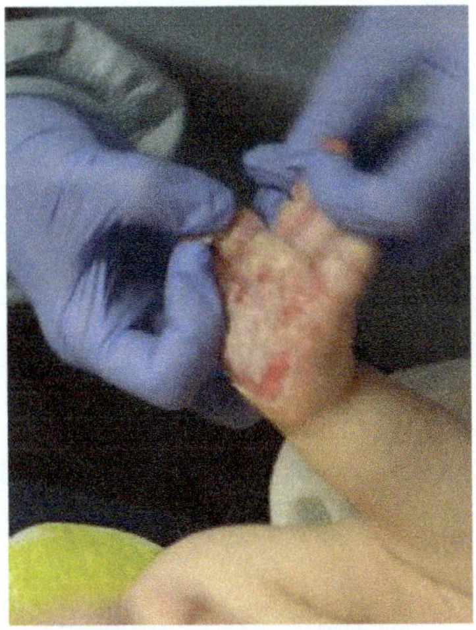

FIGURE 3.17
A toddler sustained bilateral, similar-appearing palmar burns when he walked to and touched a gas-powered room heater.

to remove their hands quickly. Hot curling or clothes irons that remain hot, firepits, and sun-heated pavement are other common unintentional contact burn sources. However, children also can be forcibly held against or touched by these objects. With heated oven or fireplace doors and hot pavement events, bilateral symmetrical injuries of the palms or soles, if accompanied by an appropriate scenario, are less concerning for abuse than other burn injury types (Figure 3.18). Clothes and hair styling irons are a common source of childhood burns, because they can retain their heat after they are shut off. If left within reach of an exploring toddler, they can cause unintentional burns. Irons are also a common implement for inflicting burns; inflicted iron burns show a different pattern than unintentional ones (Figure 3.19).[54] Unintentional styling iron burns usually result from glancing, falling irons or from a toddler grasping an iron, resulting in palmar and finger flexor surface injuries (Figure 3.20). Unintentional heated surface burns normally involved palmar surfaces, while 63% of intentional burns involved the back of the hand.[54–56] Three-fourths of unintentional burns from hot irons involve the hands. They occur when the child touches the iron or pulls the cord of a still heated or cooling iron.[54] The median injury age for this type of burn is 17 months old. It is important to look at the direction and body site of the burn in the context of how the object was left or would have fallen (Figure 3.20). Electric heaters in house floors reach an average temperature of 63.2°C (146°F). Gratings of these heaters leave distinctive patterns and have been the source of unintentional and abusive burns[56] (Figure 3.21). The tops of disposable cigarette lighters are commonly used to burn children (Figure 3.22).

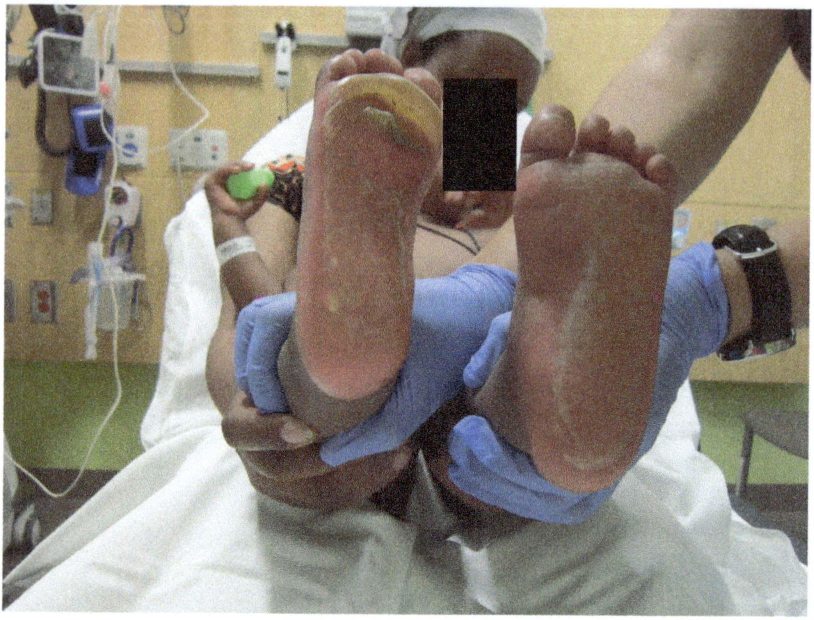

FIGURE 3.18
This 2½-year-old girl walked barefoot outside on a sunny July day. She sustained bilateral partial-thickness sole burns but no other injuries. In spite of the symmetry, this pattern is typical for sun-heated surface foot burns.

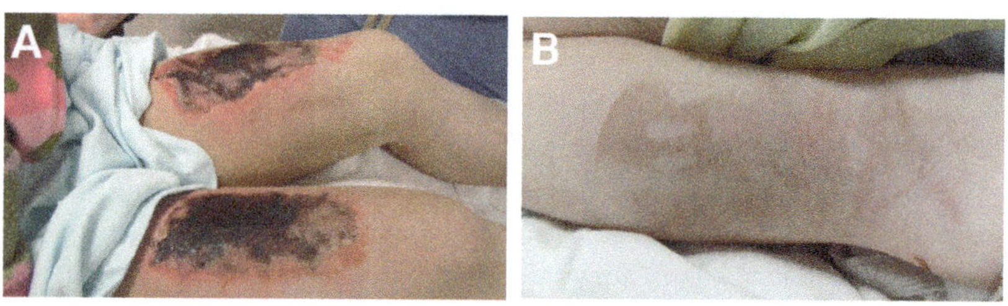

FIGURE 3.19
This 6-year-old girl and her 8-year-old brother experienced torture over the course of several weeks at the hands of their mother's boyfriend. The mother, who had experienced domestic violence, eventually sought help. The girl had deep eschars of both anterior thighs (A), both buttocks, and her right inner thigh. She had also been severely beaten and deprived of fluids. She was in myoglobin-uric renal failure at presentation. A less severe burn of her right arm (B) had a patterned injury suggesting a clothes iron burn; police were informed of this. During the police investigators' interviews, the children spoke of the boyfriend threatening and burning them with an iron. The police retrieved the iron, which matched the girl's burn pattern.

It takes 50 seconds of continuous flame with the lighter held upright for the metal top to reach 60°C (140°F), at which temperature contact burns can occur.[57] After the lighter has been burning for 180 seconds, it takes 60 seconds to cool below 60°C (140°F). These heating times imply that significant caregiver intent is required for such brandings to occur.

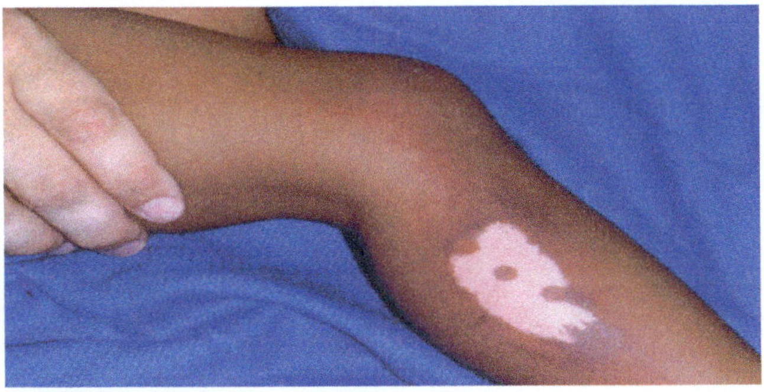

FIGURE 3.20
This toddler had sustained a clothes iron burn of her lateral right calf. If she had accidentally brushed against an iron left cooling on its heel, the burn should not have been pointed downward and it should not have been so clearly inscribed.
Photo courtesy of Dr Seth Asser.

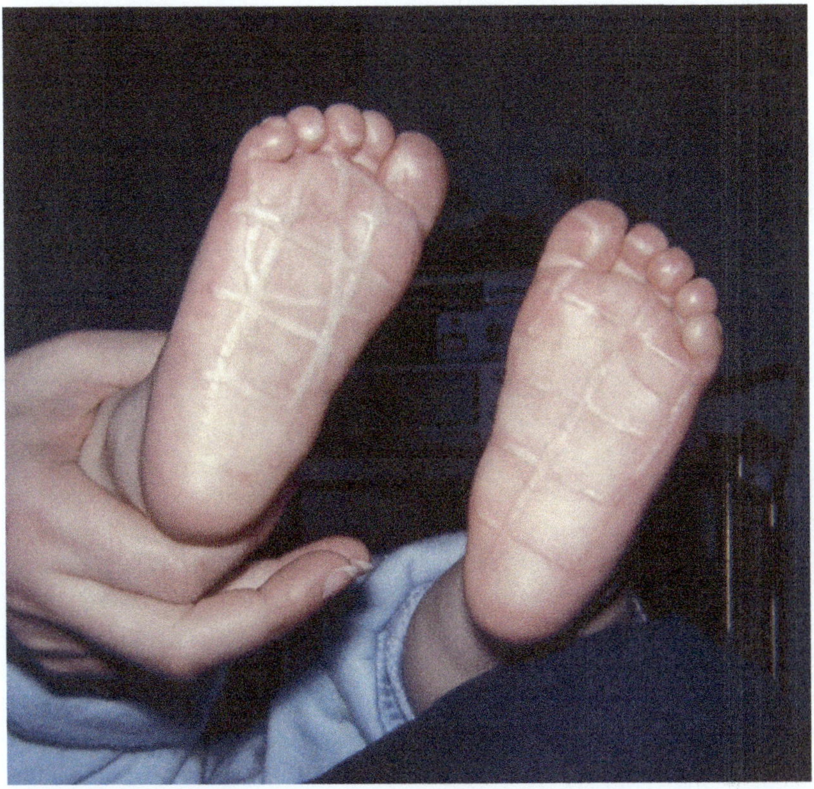

FIGURE 3.21
This toddler sustained hot metal floor heating grate grid burns. Note that the burns are clearly inscribed, but his right foot also has 2 overlapping burn images. In cool-enough home conditions to have the grate this hot, his soles would usually have been protected by socks and/or shoes.

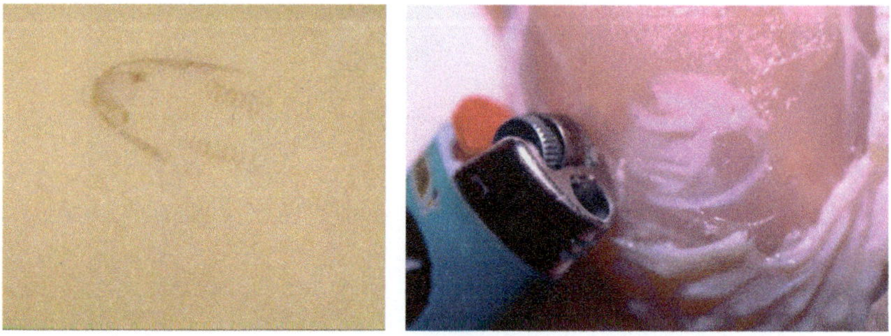

FIGURE 3.22
A police officer brought this burn injury photo, inquiring what object could have caused it. When told it was the top of a heated cigarette lighter, she confiscated the lighter from the mother's purse. She then executed the "poultry proof" by duplicating the burn pattern on a grocery store chicken breast.

Contact burns are often smaller injuries than scalds, so they may be underrepresented in inpatient burn studies. Also, the extent and severity of smaller contact burns might not mandate immediate medical care. Smaller injuries concerning for abuse often come to medical attention when observed and referred in by outside laypersons or when observed during the evaluation of other, more severe abusive injuries. Abusive contact burns are commonly in locations that are hidden or not easily visible, such as a cigarette burn on the dorsum of the foot or a hot iron burn on the buttocks. They may not present until concerns for secondary infection develop, or they may be incidentally found during the investigation of more serious abuse. Of note, 43% of children who had experienced torture in one study had contact burns and 18% had scalds[58] (Figure 3.23).

Accidental contact foot burns can result from stepping on hot coals or sun-heated surfaces.[59–61] While contact foot burns affect all ages, more than half of the foot scalds happened among infants younger than 1 year, and two-thirds happened to children younger than 4 years.[59] Although treadmills cause frictional foot burns, upper limb, especially hand, injuries are the predominant treadmill injury (91%).[62] Children with accidental foot burns from sun-heated surfaces commonly have bilateral plantar burns caused by walking onto hot pavement (82%) (see Figure 3.18).[60] However, crawling infants may have bilateral hand or knee, shin, and dorsal foot burns. Sun-heated asphalt can rise rapidly to 71°C (160°F).

A systematic review of the literature on contact, cigarette, and flame burns caused by abuse identified only 73 children from 2 series and additional case reports.[63] Among these children, non-scald burns accounted for 27% of all burns and 47% of abusive burns. Males (73%) were disproportionately injured. Although, in the Hicks and Stolfi study[64] in this systematic review, the mean age of the children without scalds was 2.9 years for the 2 combined case series, two-thirds were older than 3 years.[63] Forty-seven percent of children who had experienced abuse sustained multiple burns and 32% sustained additional abusive injuries. Contact burns with sharp, shape-defining margins caused 85% of abusive injuries. Included were 25% from cigarettes, 12% from clothes irons, 10% from hair dryers, and 14% from radiators, stoves, or heaters. Less common causes were hot grease, curling irons, a car hood, molten plastic, a light bulb, a stun gun, cigarette lighters, a heated knife, and a heated spatula. The cigarette injuries, in particular, included multiple deep, circular cigarette-diameter lesions. In addition, 10% of the children who had experienced abuse had flame burns, 4% had caustic injuries, and 3% had microwave oven burns. If medical professionals are concerned for abuse, the likelihood of hospital admission is 5.5 times higher.[13]

Other Burn Sources

A variety of other energy sources cause burn or burn-like injuries. Steam has a higher heat content than hot, dry air, so it is more prone to cause burn injuries. A shower steamer, designed to cause a sauna-like effect, has been reported as a cause of an unintentional toddler burn.[65] Steam or hot air can be the source of inflicted burns from sources like hair dryers and hot steam humidifiers. Unintentional scalding has resulted from breathing steaming air as a home remedy, both from commercially available vaporizers and from containers of boiling water.[66,67] Children can be burned by the hot air coming from a hair dryer if they are not able to get away from it (Figure 3.24). Hair dryers have also caused inflicted contact burns when their heated exit grating is pressed directly against skin (see Figure 3.23).[68] Likewise, electric hair straighteners can reach 145°C (293°F) within 2 minutes and take 7 minutes to cool below a 1-second adult burn threshold[69] (Figure 3.25). They have been implicated in abusive and unintentional contact burns. Outdoor cooking grills are estimated to cause more than 15,000 US childhood burns per year.[70] Upper-extremity injuries are the most common site of unintentional injury, but younger children may also sustain head and neck injuries. Most injuries result from the child running into the grill. Inflicted flame burns can occur when children's hands are held over open flames as punishment. Inflicted flame burns also occasionally include the use of accelerants and clothing ignition (figures 3.26 and 3.27). Microwave ovens most often cause burns when the food heated inside them spills on a child from heated baby bottles or

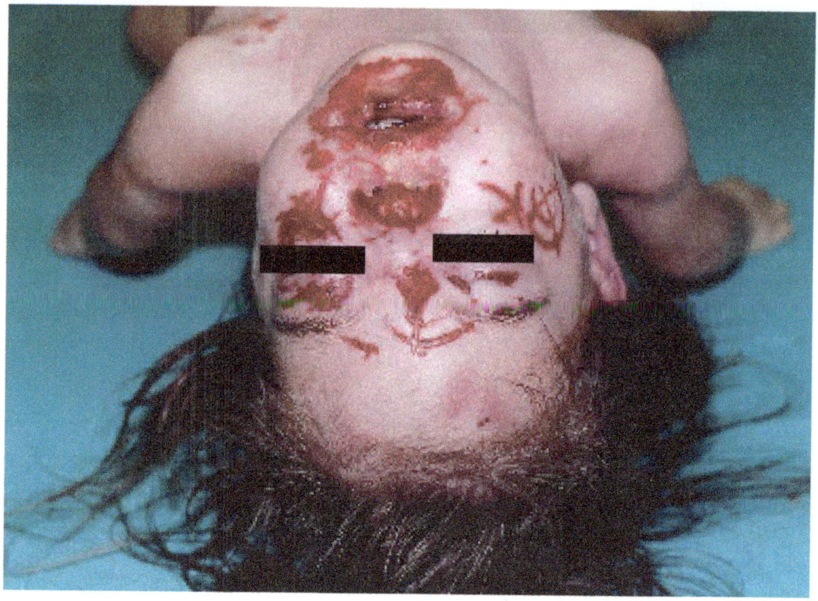

FIGURE 3.23

This 2-year-old girl's foster mother reported she had drowned in the bathtub, but the responding emergency medical services found both her and the bathtub dry. She had sustained perioral burns a few days earlier from being force-fed soup. Multiple directly impressed contact burns of her face were caused by a hair dryer grid (note low brow and left malar). Her upper brow and scalp had multiple bruises accompanying fatal abusive head trauma. Her overall injuries constituted torture.

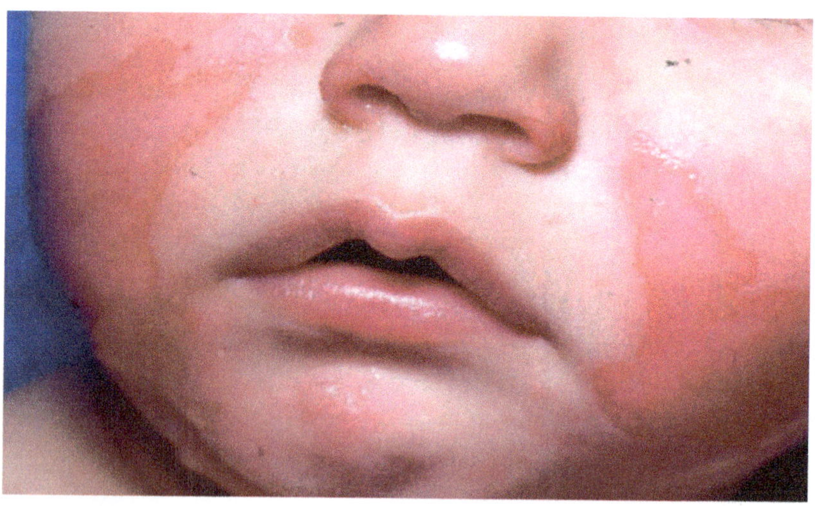

FIGURE 3.24

This infant's face was dried by blowing with a hot-air hair dryer. It was directed from below her chin. As a result, her chin and cheeks shadowed her perioral skin and protected them from burning.

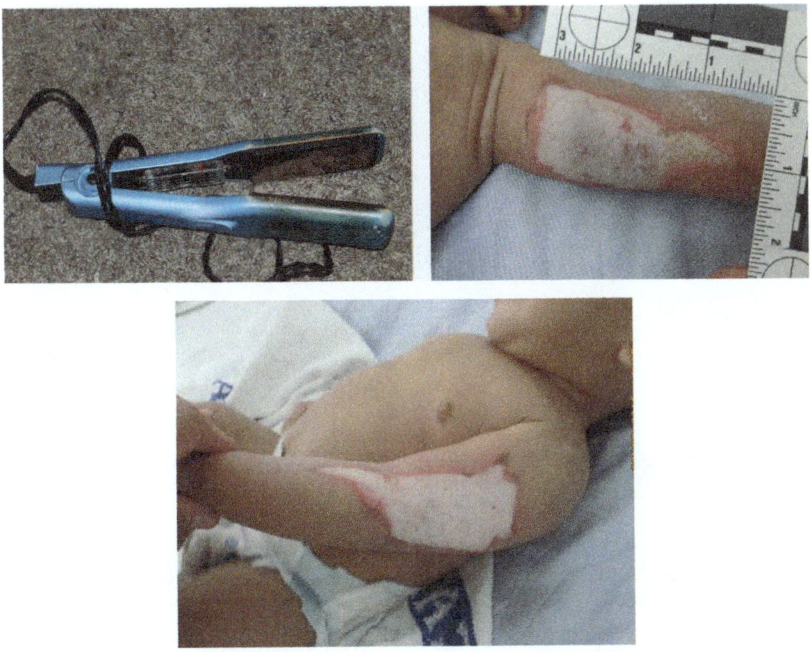

FIGURE 3.25
This toddler sustained deep contact burns on the inside and outside of his left arm. The burn pattern can be seen to slide downward, but it would have been unlikely for the jaws of the falling iron to have so perfectly and intensely affected both the inside and outside of his arm.

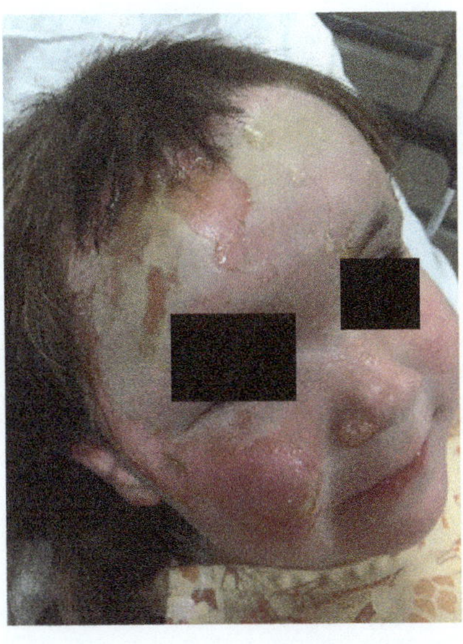

FIGURE 3.26
This 4-year-old girl caught her own hair on fire while playing with a cigarette lighter. She sustained significant burns to the face. Note the patchy distribution.

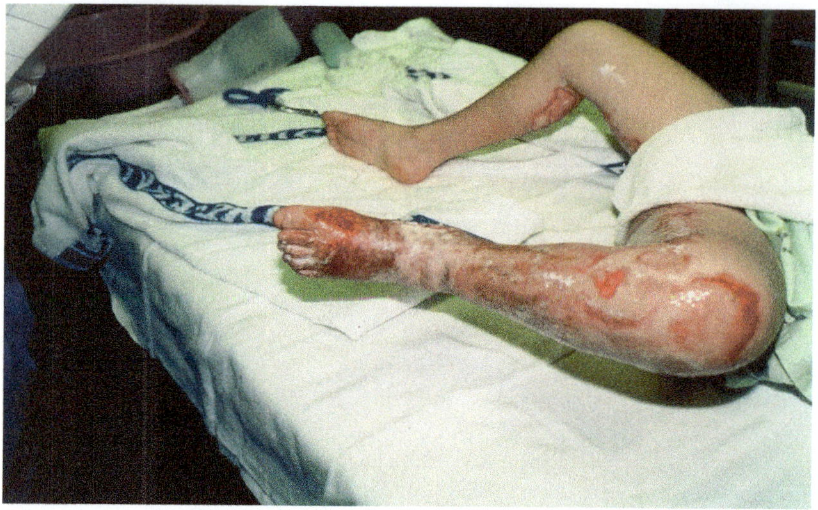

FIGURE 3.27
A 3½-year-old boy's uncle reported the child had accidentally spilled some gasoline into his rubber boot. The gasoline then ignited when he ran past a pile of burning leaves. However, both the boy and his older brother reported his uncle had poured the gasoline in his boot and then ignited it with a cigarette lighter. He also reported his uncle had shot him with a BB gun. The uncle had previously abused a different child. This child's boot was melted, and his burn pattern indicated he had been in a seated position, not running, when burned.

when solids, likes eggs or potatoes, explode.[71–74] Alexander et al reported an infant who had been "cooked" in a microwave.[75] Their further experiments demonstrated that microwave burns are uneven, with deeper water-containing tissues more affected than the superficial fatty layers that underlie the skin. This uneven heating in microwaves also leads to pockets of overheated formula in microwave-heated baby bottles. Inadequate subsequent formula mixing and temperature testing of infant bottles can cause unintentional oral burns.[76,77]

Caustic chemicals can cause inflicted burns. These most often occur in the course of adolescent or young adult interpersonal violence.[78] However, young children can be abusively or negligently exposed to caustics (Figure 3.28). These substances usually cause facial and/or intraoral injuries. In one study, caustics accounted for 35% of pediatric oral burns.[79,80] A variety of other less intensely caustic chemicals can also cause burn injuries, including bleach,[81] vinegar, nonindustrial cleaning strength acetic acid, ammonia (Figure 3.29), saturated salt solutions, and camphor.[82] They are generally small.[83] Two peaks in age distribution occurred at 2 and 15 years, but 70% occurred before 10 years. The main body regions injured included limbs (57%), trunk (34%), and head and neck (9%). Household cleaners caused most injuries, with lack of supervision playing a major role. The study's authors noted only 2 injuries

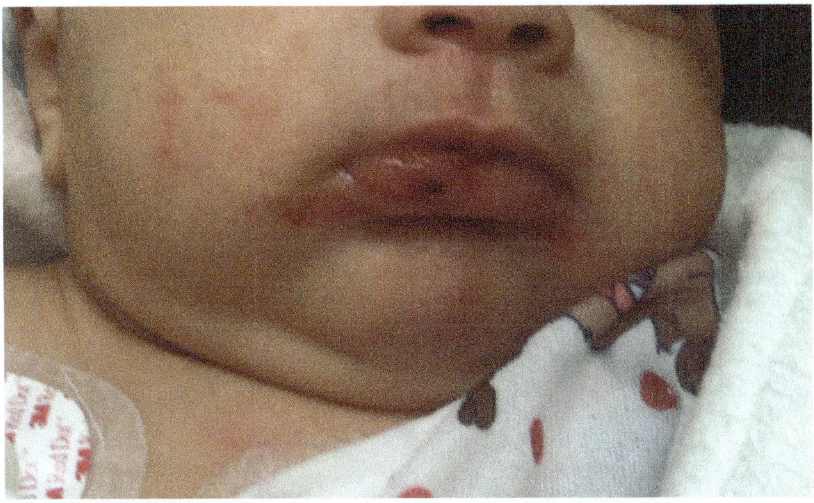

FIGURE 3.28
A 6-week-old was found by police, having been abandoned. She had white powder on her face. A container of LAs Totally Awesome Power Oxygen Base Cleaner was found nearby. She was hypothermic and had caustic burns scattered over her face.

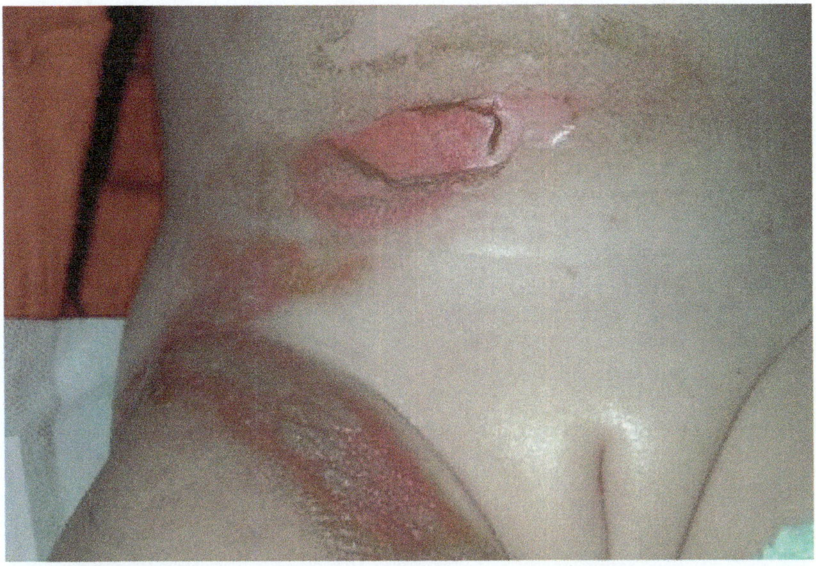

FIGURE 3.29
This toddler had normal-strength home ammonia accidentally spilled onto her lower abdomen and upper legs. Her diaper was protective, but the surrounding affected skin sustained chemical burns.

of questionable intent in young children. Hair straightening and braiding practices (ie, use of hot water and/or chemicals) can cause hot water burns and/or contact burns or contact allergy blistering, primarily in children of African ancestry (Figure 3.30).[84,85]

Electrical burns cause deep coagulation necrosis (Figure 3.31). They usually result from accidental childhood exploration. Typical is the crawling child who chews on an electrical cord, sustaining an angle-

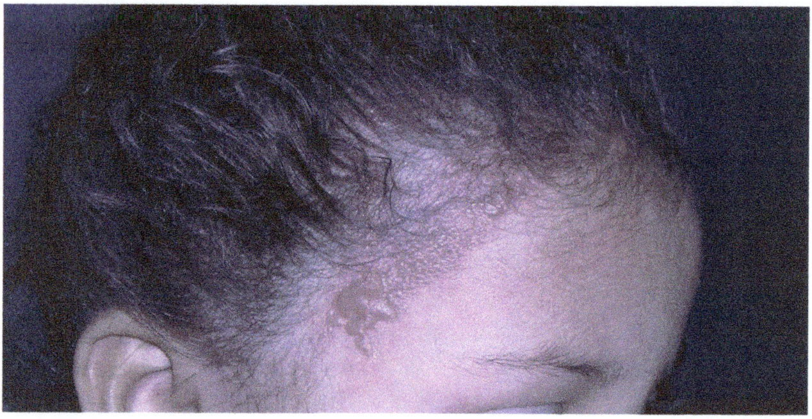

FIGURE 3.30

This 2½-year-old girl sustained an erythematous and vesiculating margin of the scalp rash, suggestive of a contact reaction to hair straighteners or other chemical treatments.

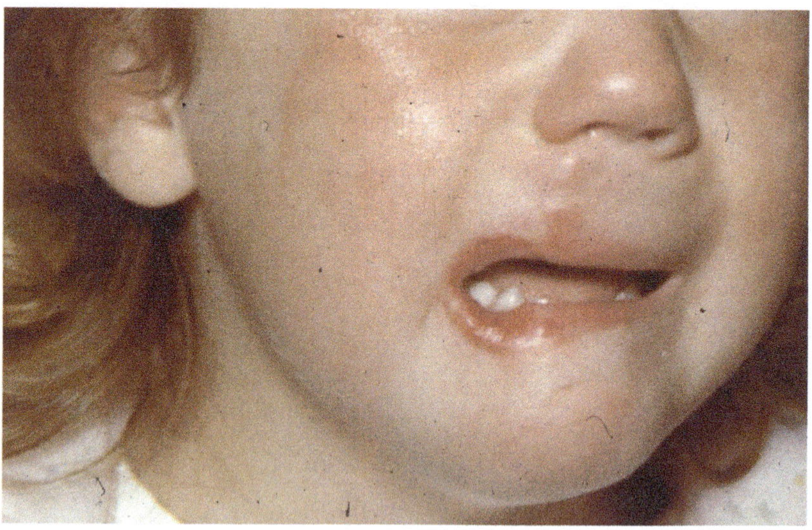

FIGURE 3.31

An angle-of-mouth electrical burn resulted from chewing on an electrical cord. It has deep coagulation necrosis. There is a risk for arterial bleeding when the eschar separates.

of-mouth burn. In one study, electrical injuries accounted for 12% of childhood oral burns.[80] Angle-of-mouth burns are prone to late arterial hemorrhage. In an Australian study, 82% of ED injuries were the result of low-power (< 1,000 W) exposures.[86] Myoglobinuria and permanent cardiac conduction problems were seen in some children, generally with higher-voltage injuries.[87]

Sunburns usually result from unintentional excess exposure, but they can result from intentional prolonged, unprotected exposure. Burns from infrared heat have been experimentally evaluated in a rat model.[88] Some negligent childhood injuries are caused by infrared heaters (Figure 3.32). Likewise, cold exposures usually cause frostbite through unintentional exposures,[89] but they can be caused by intentional exposure, including in torture cases. The youngest subject in the study was 8 months old, but the number of children was not specified. Ionizing radiation, although a source of burns, is unlikely to be available as a tool of abuse.

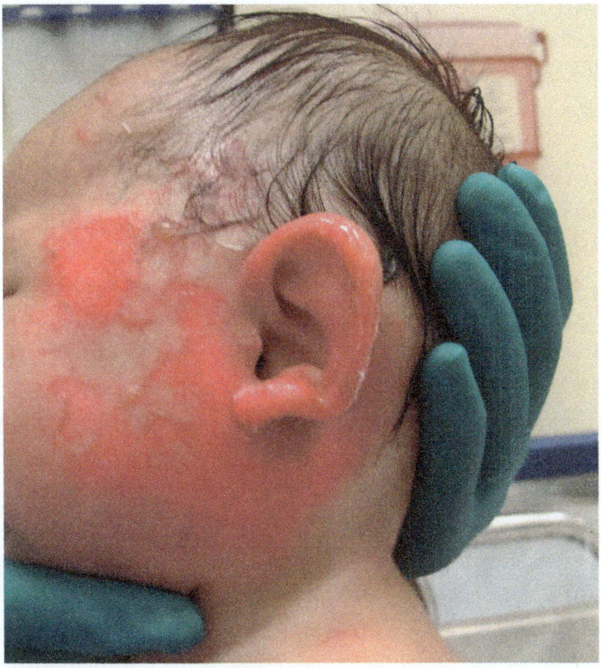

FIGURE 3.32
After her bath, this 6-month-old was left on a bed, near a small radiant heater. When found, she had face burns. Police referral was made to confirm the plausibility of an unintentional injury at the scene.

Neglect in Childhood Burns

Childhood burn injuries can involve caregiver neglect. In common with many preschool accidents, lapses in supervision allow child exploration and injury. Although it is normal to gradually allow preschool-aged children to have greater independence, lack of supervision becomes more problematic when it is developmentally premature, part of a pervasive parental pattern, or accompanied or caused by parental impairments, such as drug or alcohol dependence.[90] The role of negligence in burn injury has been best studied by Collier et al.[13] Negligent injuries were more likely to have a delayed presentation to medical care. Tap water burn injuries were more common, but stove and microwave scalds were less common than with children who were injured unintentionally. Overall and subtype rates of contact burns did not differ. However, hand and thigh contact burns were more common with negligence than with unintentional injury. Children with negligent injuries are no less likely than others to receive appropriate postburn cooling for 10 to 20 minutes, but it only occurs in about 45% of negligent, unintentional, and abusive injury cases. Topical ointments are used more often (53% vs 31%) for home treatment of negligent injuries than unintentional injuries.

In Iowa, 40% of children with confirmed burn abuse or neglect had positive urine or hair toxicology screen results.[91] Sixteen percent also had a positive skeletal survey result. Methamphetamine was detected in urine drug screens in 10% of the 62% of children screened at hospital admission.[92] Children with positive screening results had a combination of negligent, unintentional, and abusive injuries. Compared with children with negative screening results, these children sustained larger burns, more inhalation injuries, and more additional injuries.

From suburban Chicago, 22.5% of children admitted to the burn unit had been referred for child protective services (CPS) investigation.[93] Neglect concerns were most common. Single-parent homes, nonwhite families, primary caregivers who were unemployed, and a past history of CPS involvement were all risk factors for abuse or neglect confirmation.

When a hot hazard is present in children's environment, boys exhibit more hazard-directed behavior than girls, even when their mother is present.[94] Children who were observed to have more risk-taking behavior approached hazards more often. Only 34% of mothers who were present within line-of-sight view of their child showed proactive protective injury prevention behavior, but 98% were reactively defensive.

House fire deaths have been associated with acute parental intoxication.[95] The fire's ignition is often related to caregiver smoking.[95–97] In Birmingham, UK, 42% of childhood burn injuries were felt to warrant scene or social service investigation. Single-parent homes, prior CPS referrals, parental drug use, delayed care, lack of first aid, and deeper injuries were all risk factors.[98]

Anderst et al have developed a screen for supervisory neglect in general for use by protective services agencies, which could be applied to burns.[99]

Burn injuries are predictive of subsequent risk of abuse or neglect.[100] Among Australian children younger than 15 years, those hospitalized with abusive burns had odds of mortality of 1.6 times that of controls. Among those deaths, 38% were related to the burn injury and the rest to subsequent all-cause mortality. Their data suggest that the child's milieu is detrimental and predictive of acute and subsequent early mortality.[101]

Domestic Violence in Childhood Burn Injuries

Childhood burn injuries may occur when children are bystanders in domestic violence assaults.[102,103] Children can sustain burn injuries, usually from house fires, when parents attempt suicide with the intent that the children accompany them in death.

Abusive Burns: Statistical Associations

A variety of scald burn patterns have been statistically associated with abusive burns in a systematic literature review.[104] Included were contour line burns with clear upper margins, uniform burn depth or immersion pattern, buttock "doughnut-hole" sparing, and symmetrical perineal and/or lower extremity injuries. Just short of statistical significance were skip areas from forced flexion, stocking or glove injuries, a trigger event, and an unrelated adult bringing the child to care.

Unlike in other cases of physical abuse, in the aforementioned systematic literature review, delay in care did not reach statistical significance. The challenge with determining delay in care is that no one has defined or analyzed which burns are so significant that a "reasonable caregiver" should have sought expeditious care, instead of attempting home treatment. Moreover, burns evolve over time, making it difficult to determine when a burn was serious enough for a reasonable caregiver to be aware he or she should seek care. One study on tap water burns found 70% of the time when care was delayed more than 2 hours after injury or someone other than the caregiver at the time of injury brought the child to care, the injury was caused by abuse.[105] Abuse was felt to be the cause of 28% of these scalds. Due to negligent lack of supervision, 45% of the time the child or a sibling turned on the hot water. Having a mean of 19% and median of 12% body surface area (BSA) burns, the injuries were large and severe enough that they should have caused the reasonable caregiver to seek help.

In a subsequent study of 215 children with burns of all types, lack of an adequate history, a past history of abuse, immersion injuries, bilateral or symmetrical burns, more than 10% total BSA burns, full-thickness burns, and coexistent injuries were all associated with abusive burns.[44] A case control study also found patients with inflicted injuries had more groin, buttock, thigh, lower leg, and foot injuries.[13] Children with abusive (50%) and negligent (40%) injuries more often had a prior family history of CPS involvement than children who were unintentionally injured (8%). Immersion patterns were statistically more likely, in descending order, with abusive than negligent or unintentional burns. Chest injuries were more common with unintentional burns but back injuries more so with either abuse or neglect. Unintentional burns were smaller than abusive or negligent injuries. Flame burns were more common with negligence. Concomitant injuries were more common with negligent and abusive burn injuries. Children with negligent and abusive burn injuries had more injury complications. Large burns, tap water burns, immersion lines, young child age, delay in seeking care, non–2-parent family, young parents, inconsistent history, and injury patterns have all been associated with maltreatment.[53]

Screening for Abusive Burns and Associated Abusive Injuries

A screening tool was proposed for ED evaluation to assist in determining which burn injuries warrant further scrutiny.[106] It was effective in improving the frequency and appropriateness of CPS referral. The Dutch reviewed the utility of their general ED abuse screen, the SPUTOVAMO, for burn injuries.[107] The SPUTOVAMO was 73% sensitive and 95% specific for maltreatment with a positive predictive value of 58% and negative predictive value of 97%. Recently, an 8-factor screening tool for abusive burns was published.[108] Included were child age younger than 5 years, previous CPS involvement, full-thickness burn severity, concerning history, uncommon body location, supervision concerns, bilateral scald pattern, multiple burn sites for contact burns, use of first aid before seeking care, and longer than 24 hours to presentation. If 3 factors were positive, the tool was 87.5% sensitive and 81.5% specific for the need to evaluate for abuse.

Burn injuries have been felt to have fewer associated occult injuries, in particular skeletal injuries, than other forms of serious abuse, such as abusive head injury. However, studies by Hicks, DeGraw, Fagen, and Belfer indicate that skeletal survey results are positive in 6% to 33% of children whose burns were imaged.[64,109–111] A study of nearly 3,000 children referred to child abuse pediatricians for abuse evaluation found 41% of the cases to be concerning for abuse, with burns present in 7.6%.[44] For 87%, the burn was the primary reason for the referral. Of the 186 children with burns as the primary child abuse concern, 65% had at least 1 additional injury. Seventeen percent of the children had fractures, 10% oropharyngeal injury, 8% abusive head trauma, 3% retinal hemorrhage, 2% abdominal trauma, and 1% other abusive injury. These are likely minimum estimates, because occult injury testing was incomplete. A German clinical forensic medicine survey also found that 71% of those who had experienced abusive burn injuries had additional evidence of abuse or neglect.[112] As a result, regular age guidelines should be used for screening for occult injuries in children who have possibly experienced physically abusive burn injuries.

Burn Care

Sheridan provides a summary of outpatient and inpatient burn management for pediatricians.[113] Criteria for transfer to a burn center are provided in Box 3.1, and suggestions for outpatient management are given in Box 3.2.

BOX 3.1
American Burn Association Burn Center Transfer Criteria

- Second- and third-degree burns >10% TBSA in patients <10 or >50 years of age.
- Second- and third-degree burns >20% TBSA in other age groups.
- Second- and third-degree burns that involve the face, hands, feet, genitalia, perineum, and major joints.
- Third-degree burns >5% TBSA in any age group.
- Electrical burns, including lightning injury.
- Chemical burns.
- Inhalation injury.
- Burn injury in patients with preexisting medical disorders that could complicate management, prolong recovery, or affect mortality.

(continued)

BOX 3.1 (*continued*)

- Any patients with burns and concomitant trauma (eg, fractures) in which the burn injury poses the greatest risk of morbidity or mortality. In such cases, if the trauma poses the greater immediate risk, the patient may be treated initially in a trauma center until stable before being transferred to a burn center. Physician judgment will be necessary in such situations and should be in concert with the regional medical control plan and triage protocols.
- Hospitals without qualified personnel or equipment for the care of children should transfer children with burns to a burn center with these capabilities.
- Burn injury in patients who will require special social/emotional and/or long-term rehabilitative support, including cases involving suspected child abuse, substance abuse.

Abbreviation: TBSA, total body surface area.

Based on American Burn Association burn center referral criteria (http://ameriburn.org/wp-content/uploads/2017/05/burncenterreferralcriteria.pdf). From Sheridan RL. Burn care for children. *Pediatr Rev*. 2018;39(6):273–286.

BOX 3.2
Suggestions for Outpatient Burn Management

Patient Selection Suggestions

- Airway is clear.
- Burn small enough that fluid resuscitation not needed.
- Child can eat and drink.
- Family support adequate to meet monitoring, wound care, and transportation needs.
- Family clearly understands care plan and follow-up recommendations.
- No concern for abuse or neglect.

Wound Care Suggestions

- Debride loose tissue and debris.
- Gently debride leaking, loose, or thin blisters.
- Apply antibiotic ointment or silver-releasing membrane based on local experience and protocols.
- Schedule periodic inspections of the wound at 24 to 72 hours; consider a pain control plan that minimizes opioid use.
- Describe specific reasons for early return to family.
- Schedule and track clinic visits.
- Consult liberally with supporting inpatient burn facility.
- Use local visiting nurse and outpatient medical support resources.

From Sheridan RL. Burn care for children. *Pediatr Rev*. 2018;39(6):273–286.

Burn Documentation and Investigation

Excellent photodocumentation is critical to burn evaluation and management. Although burn injuries also should be diagrammed[31,113] (Figure 3.33), photographs provide more reliable data about burn distribution. For patterned injuries, photos taken at a right angle to the injury plane and with a ruler in the same plane and adjacent to the injury are needed to identify objects from the child's environment that could have caused the injury. Additionally, photos of the burns should be taken at a distance to allow for determination of the exact location and laterality of the injury.

For scald burns and immersions particularly, special attention should be paid to ensure that enough photos are taken to clearly define all of the burn's margins and skip areas. It is much easier to mentally reconstruct flow patterns or the child's immersion position in water if there are a full series of photos, as opposed to trying to reconstruct while the child is being painfully debrided. However, once the child's position is established, additional photos exploring the child's dimensions in relation to environmental hazards and reconstructing the child's position are helpful. For example, if it is reported that the child reached up to pull a pot off the stove, a photo of the child standing and reaching, accompanied by a ruler, is helpful when compared with police-obtained environmental

Burn Estimate: Age Versus Area

	Birth–1 y	1–4 y	5–9 y	10–14 y	15 y	2°	3°	Total
Head	19	17	13	11	9			
Neck	2	2	2	2	2			
Anterior trunk	13	13	13	13	13			
Posterior trunk	13	13	13	13	13			
Right buttock	2½	2½	2½	2½	2½			
Left buttock	2½	2½	2½	2½	2½			
Genitalia	1	1	1	1	1			
Right upper arm	4	4	4	4	4			
Left upper arm	4	4	4	4	4			
Right lower arm	3	3	3	3	3			
Left lower arm	3	3	3	3	3			
Right hand	2½	2½	2½	2½	2½			
Left hand	2½	2½	2½	2½	2½			
Right thigh	5½	6½	8	8½	9			
Left thigh	5½	6½	8	8½	9			
Right leg	5	5	5½	6	6½			
Left leg	5	5	5½	6	6½			
Right foot	3½	3½	3½	3½	3½			
Left foot	3½	3½	3½	3½	3½			
					Total			

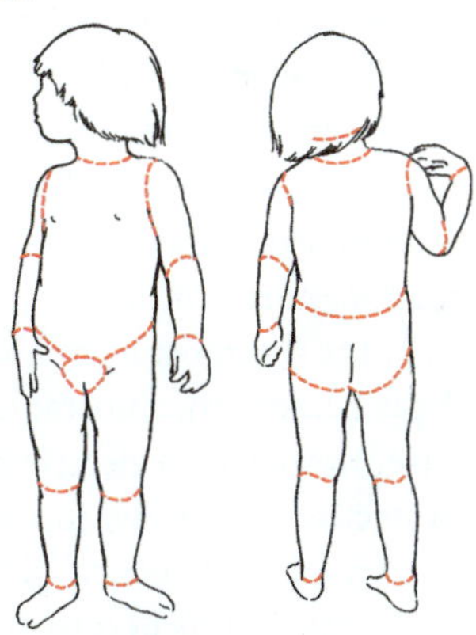

FIGURE 3.33

Regional percentages of body surface area in children, by age. Note how proportions change with age.

From Sheridan RL. Thermal injuries. In: McInerny TK, Adam HM, Campbell DE, DeWitt TG, Foy JM, Kamat DM, eds. *American Academy of Pediatrics Textbook of Pediatric Care*. 2nd ed. Elk Grove Village, IL: American Academy of Pediatrics; 2017:2987–2994.

photos. Children 12 to 23 months old may be expected to be able to reach above a 36" countertop while standing on tiptoes; some may be able to reach as much as 8" above it.[114] Photos from the time of presentation can instruct a jury about the initial severity of the injury and how delay in care may have led to complications such as infection. This can convince jurors that the parents were not acting as reasonable caregivers by delaying care. Additionally, photos that follow the child's injuries through healing are better measures of the severity of the burn injury depth than the presenting photos alone and may be helpful in further elucidating the mechanism of the burn.

When burn injuries are being investigated for possible abuse, it is important to use CPS and/or the police to conduct a scene investigation and photograph the scene. Although the scene and event may be inferred from the history, nothing is as reliable as direct observation (Figure 3.34). Sizes and heights of tubs, sinks, faucets, and other fixtures should be documented for comparison with the child's height and reach.[114] The type of faucet (single vs dual handle) should be determined, along with an estimate of whether a child's strength could turn it on. If the faucet has temperature- or flow-limiting devices, they should be noted. The temperature of the cold water alone and tap water temperature and flow volumes over time after only the hot water is turned on are needed. The maximum temperature should be documented. Water temperatures attained at various sites within the tub should be measured in this process. The water-heating system should be examined and the heater's type, settings, and distance from the tub documented and photographed. The heater's distance from the tub and the temperature of the environment through which piping travels will modify the time until the maximum water temperature is reached. In some water systems, flushing a toilet will reduce the faucet's cold-water flow, causing sudden undiluted hot water. Modern gas and electric water heaters should have been preset by the manufacturer and/or installer at about 48.9°C (120°F) to minimize scald risk. The thermostats of both types of heaters are descriptively calibrated. A gas heater's thermostat is easily read because it is located outside its base. However, an electric heater has 2 (top and bottom) thermostats under protective panels and insulation. When checking them, it is important to turn off the electrical power, because bare 220-V wiring enters the thermostats. It is best to provide investigators with a documentation form for the site visit (see Figure 3.34).

When children have patterned contact injuries, it is important to anticipate what object might have caused the injury and to inform investigators what implement(s) they should be seeking (see Figure 3.19).

Photography of a reconstructed scene and an injury reenactment are helpful. If legal hearings about complex injuries, such as tap water immersions, are likely, it is helpful to collaborate with a medical illustrator to delineate areas of different burn depth on body diagrams and to provide a reconstruction of the child's position at the time of injury (Figure 3.35).

Evidence Worksheet for Hot Water Burns

! — **Items needed for scene investigation**

☐ **Thermometer** (Use of a scientific thermometer designed to measure liquid temperatures and which as been calibrated for accuracy is recommended.)

Brand: ____________________

☐ **Tape Measure**
☐ **Timer/Stopwatch**
☐ **Camera (film/digital)**

A

Case No.
Present Date:
Suspect Name:
Victim's Name:
Incident Location (within dwelling):
Address:
City/State/Zip:

A1 Type of Burn: ☐ Immersion ☐ Splash ☐ Running water ☐ Other (spill, splatter, etc.)

B Water Heater Temperature Measurement: (Electric – Disconnect power before removing plates!)

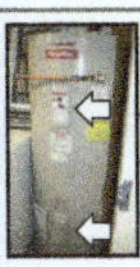

Electric Water Heater
Brand:
Capacity:
Upper plate temp:
Lower plate temp:

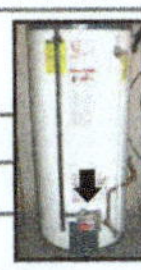

Gas Water Heater
Brand:
Capacity:
Temperature Setting:

Pre-injury hot water usage (prior hour): None __ <6 small amounts __ >6 small amounts __
1 shower/bath/laundry __ >1 shower/bath/laundry __

C Incident Location Measurements (in inches): ☐ Bathtub ☐ Basin/Sink ☐ Other

Inside Width:	Inside Depth to drain:	Sketch scene on separate page and photograph using tape measure. If site of injury unclear, complete B & C for both sink and tub. Check whether such a child's strength could turn handles.
Inside Length:	Height of Rim from Floor:	
Inside Depth to faucet handles:	Construction: (porcelain, fiberglass, single/double faucet handles)	

D

Running Water Temperatures (Hot) (in Fahrenheit or Celsius)

Seconds	Degrees	Seconds	Degrees
0	____	45	____
5	____	60	____
10	____	120	____
20	____	180	____
30	____	____	____

Maximum Temp

(Full hot running water)		(Full H/C running water)**	
Peak temp.	Seconds	Peak temp.	Seconds
____	____	____	____

**(For a single handle faucet-use middle position)

Standing Hot Water in Incident Location (temp. measured in middle of location, mid-depth)

Water Depth Inches	Min/Second	Minutes	Water Temp Degrees
		0	____
1	____	1	____
2	____	2	____
3	____	3	____
4	____	4	____
5	____	5	____
____	____	10	____
____	____	30	____
		____	____

E ____________ ran water in ____________ identified as source of burn injury.
Results: ________ inches of water. One minute after water turned off the mid-depth temperature is ________ degrees F/C.

Investigator #1: ____________________ ID #: ________ Department: ____________________
Investigator #2: ____________________ ID #: ________ Department: ____________________

FIGURE 3.34
Tap water burn investigation form.

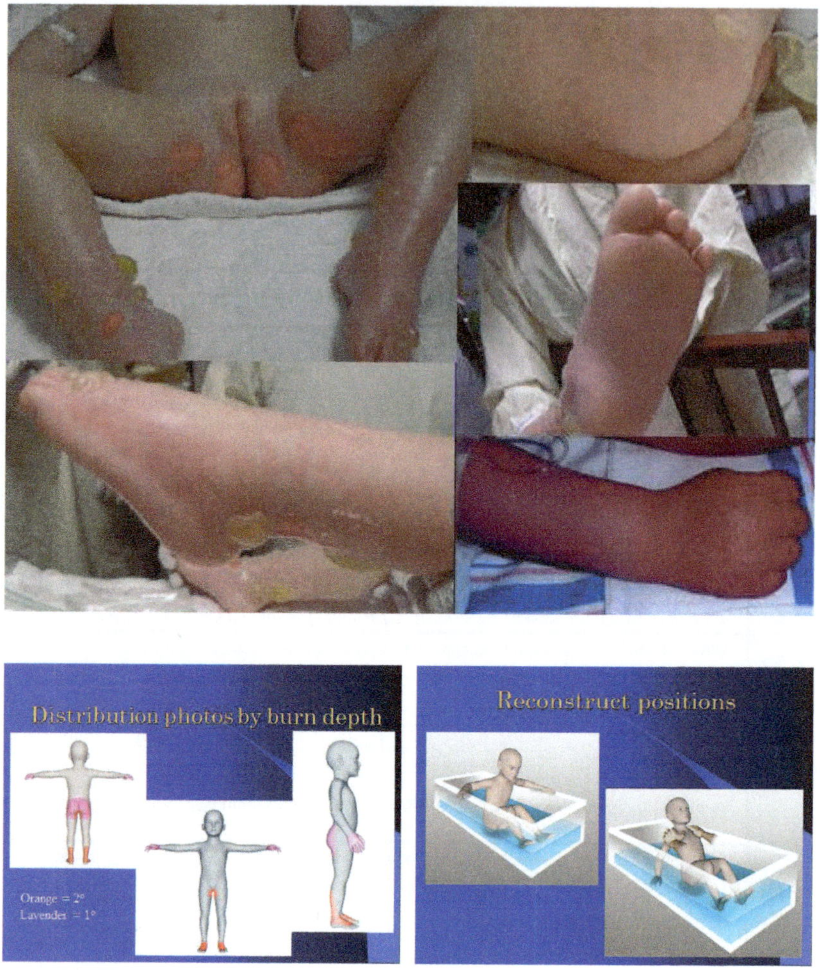

FIGURE 3.35

This 3-year-old girl's father reported that she had wet her pants. He ran a tub of only hot water. He responded to a phone call before he could dilute it with cold. After he heard her scream, he found her standing in the water. The burn pattern has a mix of epidermal burns of her hands and upper buttocks and partial-thickness dermal burns of the convexity of her buttocks and feet. Her foot burn margins are not horizontal. The burn diagrams document her burn distribution. They suggest a biphasic injury. By holding the edge of the tub, she could keep most of her buttocks out of the water, but her feet are immersed at an angle. The shallower burns suggest she sustained briefer exposures of hands and upper buttocks after being forced down into the tub and trying to tripod out with her hands in the water. Her left clavicle was acutely broken, but at trial, it was attributed to a playground fall a few days before. The father was acquitted.
Medical illustration by Kate Sweeney.

Burn Morbidity and Mortality

Purdue et al reported that the delayed burn care associated with abusive burn injuries resulted in increased burn mortality.[115] Among 607 children with non-abusive burn injuries there were no deaths, while 6% (4/71) of children with abusive burn injuries died. In a more recent paper from Parkland Hospital in Dallas, TX, 5% of children hospitalized with burns had been abused. Mortality with abuse was greater (5.4% vs 2.3%).[116] As seen in other studies, children who had experienced abuse were younger, and 90% of children who had experienced abuse had scalds, versus 42% of those who had been injured unintentionally.[116] Children who had experienced abuse more commonly had hand, bilateral feet, buttock, and perineal injuries. From the 1970s to the 1990s and early 2000s, burn death rates in dedicated burn centers dramatically decreased, so that almost no toddlers who were not abused died of injuries affecting less than 60% BSA.[117,118] However, deaths continue in about one-fourth of children with inhalation injuries. Deaths in the field are usually related to inhalation injuries or immolation. Early in-hospital burn deaths usually result from hypovolemic burn shock, while later deaths are more often the result of sepsis, acute respiratory distress syndrome, or multiorgan failure. The failure of abusive parents to seek expeditious care increases early and late burn deaths.

Abusive Burn Mimics and Other Burn-Like Injuries

Cultural and religious practices or substances may result in unintentional or non-abusive burn or burn-like injuries. In Chinese moxibustion, the moxa herb is lit to smoldering and either applied directly to skin or held adjacent to skin as a curative folk medical practice[119] (Figure 3.36). It may be self-administered or administered by a practitioner. Some consider a blistering burn necessary for efficacy.[120] Cases may be seen from a variety of Asian and Horn of Africa countries. These burn patterns often appear to have a purposeful distribution or to be logically related to the patient's complaints. In Nigeria, foot burning has been used to "treat" seizure disorders.[121] In some cultures, garlic poultices used for treatment can cause delayed blistering, looking like partial-thickness burns (Figure 3.37).[122,123]

Buttock burns, sparing the gluteal cleft but involving the convexities of the perineum and buttocks, are known to happen in diapered children who have been given or who have self-ingested senna-containing laxatives, causing irritating diarrhea. These injuries lack the circumferential immersion water lines of immersion scalds. This type of burn was first reported by Leventhal et al in 2001 shortly after the US Food and Drug Administration removed the ingredient phenolphthalein from over-the-counter laxatives; senna was used as a replacement[124,125] (Figure 3.38). Spiller et al reported that 33% of children who received senna laxatives

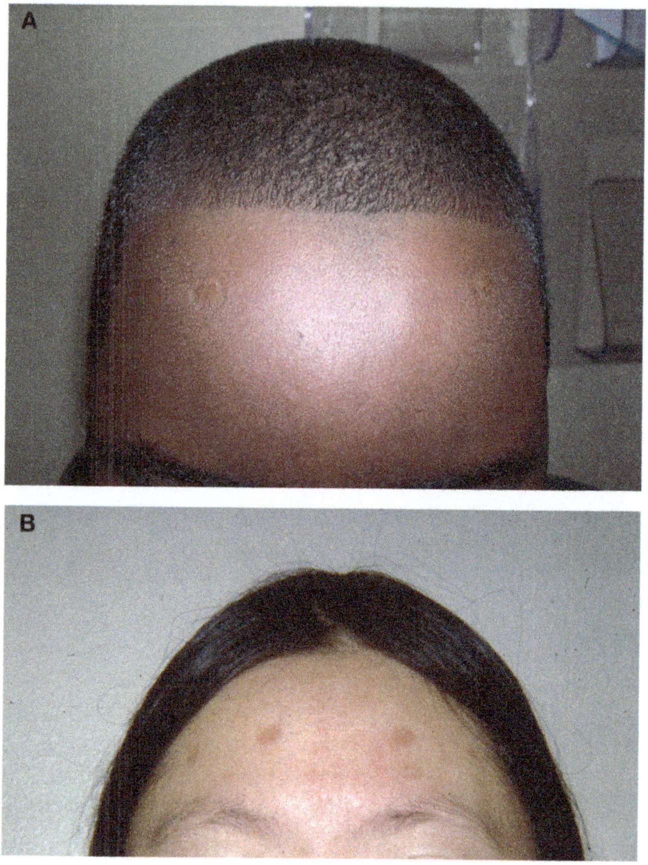

FIGURE 3.36

A, While still in East African refugee camps, this Somali child was treated for a "big head" by bitemporal burning. B, This Vietnamese woman reported treatment with bitemporal moxibustion for her migraine headaches.

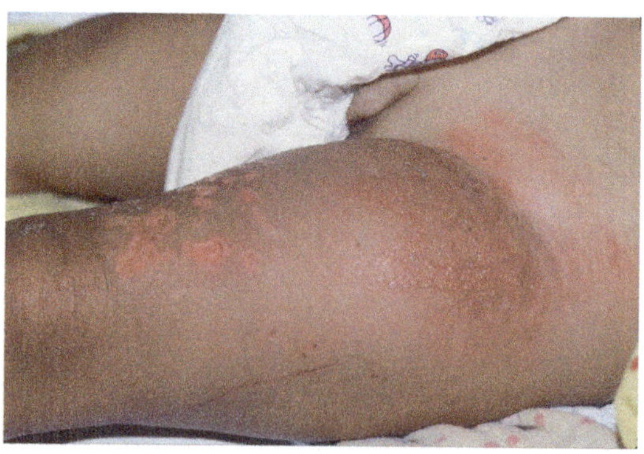

FIGURE 3.37

This 1½-year-old Hispanic child's parents had treated a presumed leg ailment with a poultice of mashed garlic. It caused a chemical dermatitis.

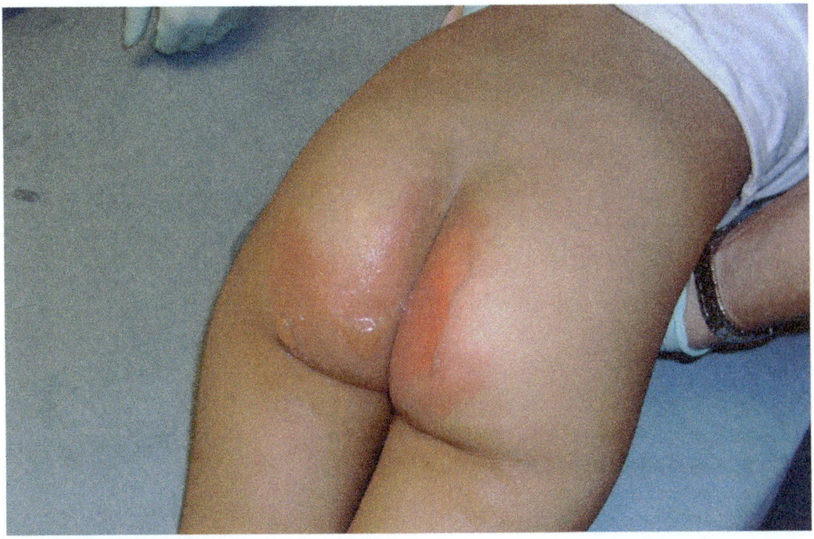

FIGURE 3.38
This child developed diarrhea after receiving senna-containing laxatives. The diarrhea had been contained within the diaper, causing the chemical burn. The margins of the gluteal cleft and buttock convexities are typically more injured than the depth of the gluteal cleft.

developed severe diaper rash and 11% had blistering and sloughing of skin.[126] These reactions were significantly more likely if the child was in diapers (72%) and developed diarrhea. The reactions were not dose related. Ingestions were either therapeutic or self-inflicted; some preparations come in a chocolate formulation that may be appealing to children. Diarrhea alone, without a history of senna ingestion, has also been seen to cause similar burns in a few children.

Silver nitrate cautery of umbilical granulomas has been recognized to cause chemical burns of the surrounding abdominal skin.[127] In diapered children, ulcerative "ammoniacal" burn-like lesions can occur and the dermatologic conditions of Jacquet diaper dermatitis or pseudo-verrucous papules and pustules, a more severe erosive and/or proliferative diaper dermatitis, can result (Figure 3.39). Bullous impetigo with staphylococcal infection can cause shallow burn-like bullae at the site of infection, which could be confused with scalds[128] (Figure 3.40). Toxigenic staphylococcal infection also causes toxin-mediated generalized erythroderma, intradermal cleavage, positive Nikolsky sign, and denuding epidermis in children with more distant and sometimes inconsequential-appearing staphylococcal infections. Toxic epidermolysis has a similar appearance but is usually a drug-induced, bullous dermatitis.[129] Perianal streptococcal infections are also a source of superficially denuded and weepy perineal skin, which looks like a superficial scald (Figure 3.41).

Inflicted ligatures or binding can cause pressure injuries reflecting the shape of the injuring object (Figure 3.42). However, unintentional sock top or elastic injuries also can initially look like mummified pressure burns and tend to heal with significant hyperpigmentation[130] (Figure 3.43). The "salt and ice challenge" popularized by teens on the internet involves their demonstrating bravery by placing salt and an ice cube on the skin for as long as they can stand the pain. Partial-thickness skin injuries similar to frostbite can result.[131]

A variety of plant chemicals, mostly psoralens, such as those found in citrus and celery, are sun sensitizers, capable of causing blistering or hyperpigmented skin lesions called *phytophotodermatitis,* which can suggest acute burn injury or residual postburn pigmentation (Figure 3.44). The epidermolysis bullosa diseases are congenital disorders resulting in various depths of epidermal to dermal cleavage. Bullae result from minor

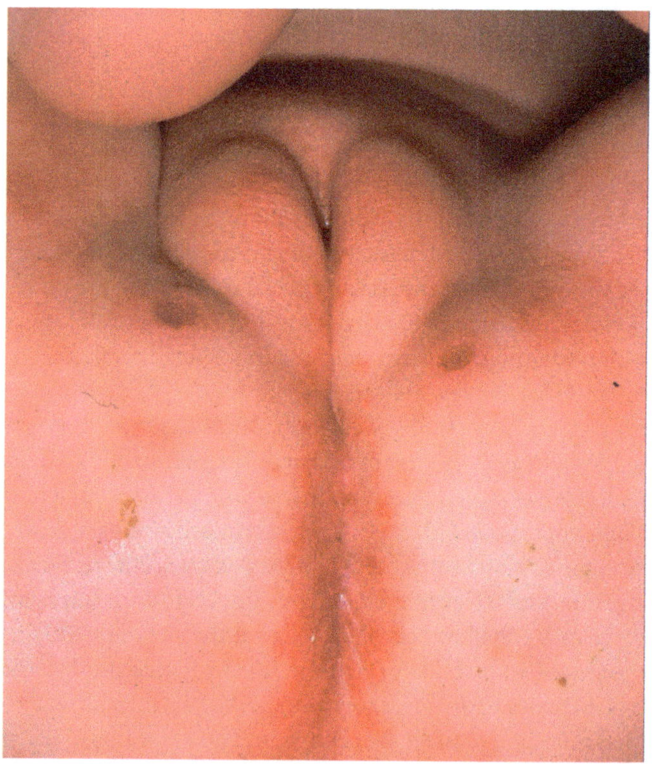

FIGURE 3.39

This infant had a severe diaper rash, Jacquet diaper dermatitis. Two areas of deeper ulceration could be confused with cigarette burns. Such rashes were more common with the use of home-laundered cloth diapers. They are more common with stool-incontinent children.

trauma that, if seen in isolation, could be confused with burn injuries. Autoimmune congenital bullous dermatoses also might cause confusion, but two-thirds are present in neonates, most have additional skin findings, and one-third have mucosal involvement. Most mothers of affected neonates also are recognizably affected.[132] Bullous erythema multiforme leads to widespread blistering. The associated characteristic erythematous target lesions will usually allow recognition. Contact dermatitis causes erythematous plaques that are often associated with fine vesiculation. The plaques usually appear distinctly different from superficial burns. Henna preparations and their ingredients can cause contact or photodermatitis. These and other mimics are noted in Table 3.4.

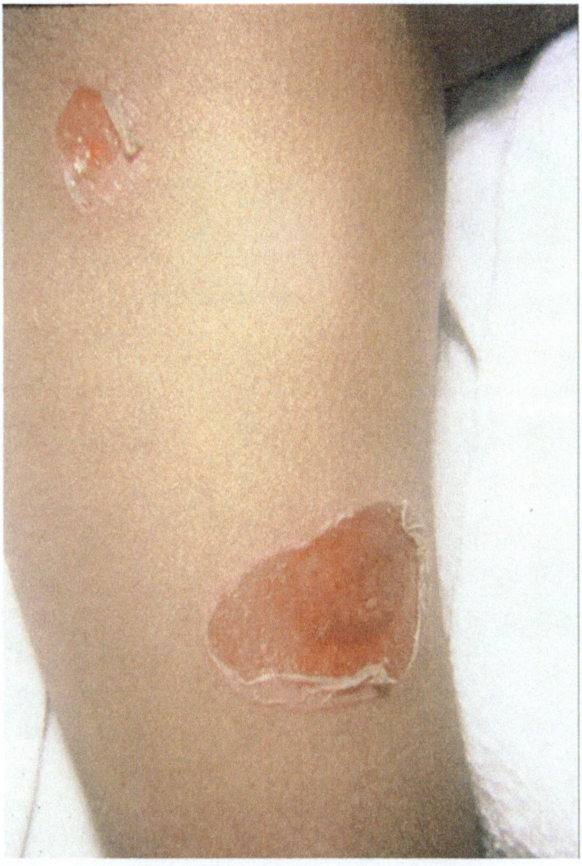

FIGURE 3.40
This child developed the superficial blisters typical of staphylococcal bullous impetigo. *Staphylococcus* was cultured from the wound base.

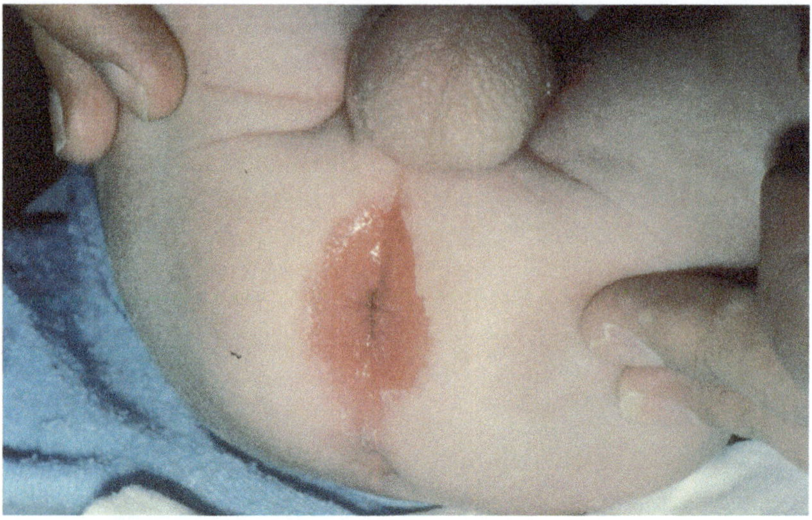

FIGURE 3.41
Perianal streptococcal infection presents as slickly denuded perineal skin, which could be confused with a scald burn.

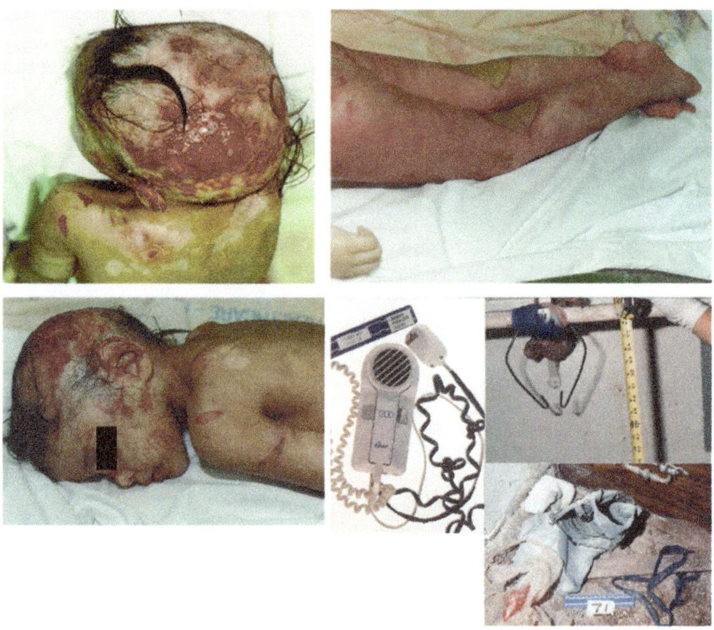

FIGURE 3.42
This 4½-year-old girl had previously sustained a scalp scald. Thereafter, she was hung by her caregiver aunt and uncle in a closet at night and her legs were bound to keep her from scratching. She had multiple contact burns from hair dryer grids and curling irons. Terminally, she sustained a forced lower body bath immersion burn (note popliteal sparing) and had abusive head trauma with subdural hemorrhage. The deep pressure injuries over her heel cords caused by her binding are apparent. Note tools of her torture: electric hair dryer for contact burns, closet apparatus by which she was hung at night, and straps used to bind her ankles.

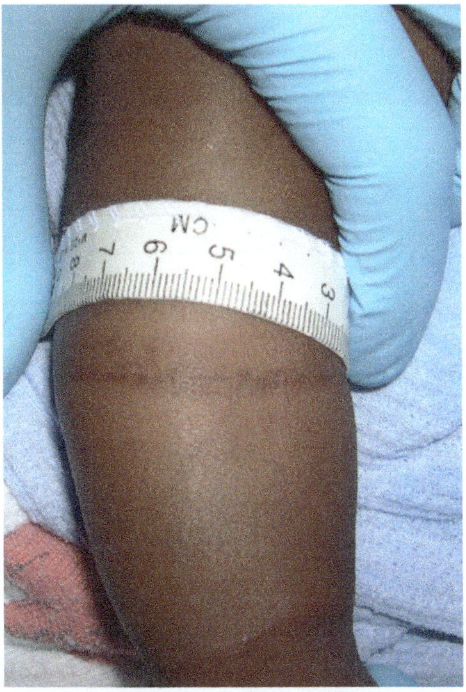

FIGURE 3.43

This infant sustained 2 clothing elastic constriction injuries on the back of her calf. This is a well-recognized, innocent injury that results in linear skin erosion and/or secondary pigmentary change from pressure injury. It could be confused with a linear contact burn.

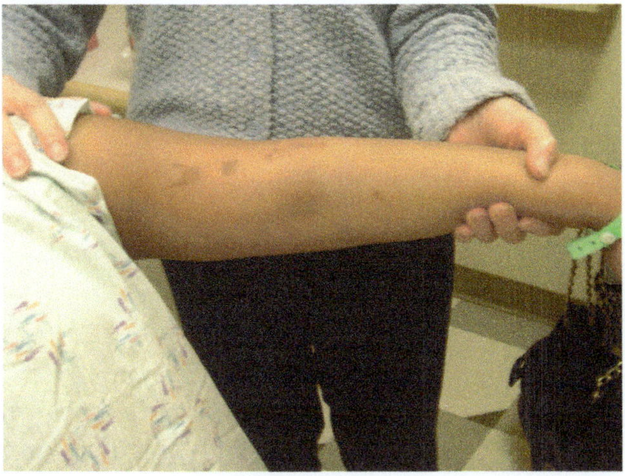

FIGURE 3.44

Phytophotodermatitis. Children exposed to photosensitizing compounds, such as the psoralens in limes and celery, can sustain hyperpigmented to blistering skin lesions after sun exposure.

Photo courtesy of Dr Rebecca Wiester.

TABLE 3.4
Skin Lesions Sometimes Confused With Inflicted Burns

Burn Pattern	Mimicking Lesions	References
Circular or patterned burns	Moxibustion	118,119
	Garlic burns	121,122
	Impetigo/bullous impetigo	127
	Erythema multiforme	133
	Therapeutic burns for seizures/convulsions by African healers	120
	Innocent (elastic/sock line) pressure injuries	129
	Phytophotodermatitis	134
	Enuresis alarm burn	135
	Maqua	136
	Dermatitis herpetiformis	134
	Fixed drug eruption	137
	Urticaria pigmentosa	138
	Accidental contact burns, car seat and/or buckle	134,139
Unpatterned burns	Senna burn	123–125
	Diaper dermatitis: Jacquet or pseudo-verrucous papules and pustules	137
	Staphylococcal scalded skin syndrome	127,140
	Toxic epidermolysis	128
	Perianal streptococcus	141
	Epidermolysis bullosa	134,142
	Autoimmune bullous dermatoses	131
	"Salt and ice challenge"	130
	Allergic contact burns	
	Dishwasher effluent burns	143
	Accidental scald burns	39,104,144
	Silver nitrate burns	126
	Congenital indifference to pain	145
	Superglue/methacrylate burns	146
	Chilblain	88,137
	Sunburn	147
	Home remedy chemical burns	134

References

1. World Health Organization. Burns. https://www.who.int/en/news-room/fact-sheets/detail/burns. Published March 6, 2018. Accessed April 22, 2019
2. Hummel RP III, Greenhalgh DG, Barthel PP, et al. Outcome and socioeconomic aspects of suspected child abuse scald burns. *J Burn Care Rehabil*. 1993;14(1):121–126 PMID: 8454659 https://doi.org/10.1097/00004630-199301000-00026
3. Peck MD, Priolo-Kapel D. Child abuse by burning: a review of the literature and an algorithm for medical investigations. *J Trauma*. 2002;53(5):1013–1022 PMID: 12435962 https://doi.org/10.1097/00005373-200211000-00036
4. Centers for Disease Control and Prevention. Injury prevention and control. Welcome to WISQARS. https://www.cdc.gov/injury/wisqars/index.html. Reviewed March 21, 2019. Accessed April 22, 2019
5. D'Souza AL, Nelson NG, McKenzie LB. Pediatric burn injuries treated in US emergency departments between 1990 and 2006. *Pediatrics*. 2009;124(5):1424–1430 PMID: 19805456 https://doi.org/10.1542/peds.2008-2802
6. National Safety Council. Injury facts. https://injuryfacts.nsc.org. Accessed April 22, 2019
7. Kemp AM, Jones S, Lawson Z, Maguire SA. Patterns of burns and scalds in children. *Arch Dis Child*. 2014;99(4):316–321 PMID: 24492796 https://doi.org/10.1136/archdischild-2013-304991
8. Thombs BD. Patient and injury characteristics, mortality risk, and length of stay related to child abuse by burning: evidence from a national sample of 15,802 pediatric admissions. *Ann Surg*. 2008;247(3):519–523 PMID: 18376198 https://doi.org/10.1097/SLA.0b013e31815b4480
9. Laitakari E, Koljonen V, Pyörälä S, Rintala R. Outpatient treated burns in infants younger than 1 year in Helsinki during 2005-2009. *Burns*. 2014;40(3):489–494 PMID: 24001919 https://doi.org/10.1016/j.burns.2013.08.007
10. Burlinson CE, Wood FM, Rea SM. Patterns of burn injury in the preambulatory infant. *Burns*. 2009;35(1):118–122 PMID: 18947932 https://doi.org/10.1016/j.burns.2008.02.005
11. Nguyen DQ, Tobin S, Dickson WA, Potokar TS. Infants under 1 year of age have a significant risk of burn injury. *Burns*. 2008;34(6):863–867 PMID: 18378092 https://doi.org/10.1016/j.burns.2007.11.011
12. Sahu SA, Agrawal K, Patel PK. Scald burn, a preventable injury: analysis of 4306 patients from a major tertiary care center. *Burns*. 2016;42(8):1844–1849 PMID: 27436508 https://doi.org/10.1016/j.burns.2016.06.022
13. Collier ZJ, Ramaiah V, Glick JC, Gottlieb LJA. A 6-year case-control study of the presentation and clinical sequelae for noninflicted, negligent, and inflicted pediatric burns. *J Burn Care Res*. 2017;38(1):e101–e124 PMID: 28009699 https://doi.org/10.1097/BCR.0000000000000408
14. Lorch M, Goldberg J, Wright J, Burd RS, Ryan LM. Epidemiology and disposition of burn injuries among infants presenting to a tertiary-care pediatric emergency department. *Pediatr Emerg Care*. 2011;27(11):1022–1026 PMID: 22068061 https://doi.org/10.1097/PEC.0b013e318235e0e4
15. Sheridan RL, Ryan CM, Petras LM, Lydon MK, Weber JM, Tompkins RG. Burns in children younger than two years of age: an experience with 200 consecutive admissions. *Pediatrics*. 1997;100(4):721–723 PMID: 9310533 https://doi.org/10.1542/peds.100.4.721
16. Yasti AC, Tumer AR, Atli M, Tutuncu T, Derinoz A, Kama NA. A clinical forensic scientist in the burns unit: necessity or not? A prospective clinical study. *Burns*. 2006;32(1):77–82 PMID: 16380212 https://doi.org/10.1016/j.burns.2005.07.006

17. Saeman MR, Hodgman EI, Burris A, et al. Epidemiology and outcomes of pediatric burns over 35 years at Parkland Hospital. *Burns*. 2016;42(1):202–208 PMID: 26613626 https://doi.org/10.1016/j.burns.2015.10.011
18. Daria S, Sugar NF, Feldman KW, Boos SC, Benton SA, Ornstein A. Into hot water head first: distribution of intentional and unintentional immersion burns. *Pediatr Emerg Care*. 2004;20(5):302–310 PMID: 15123901 https://doi.org/10.1097/01.pec.0000125658.05196.b1
19. Rawlins JM, Khan AA, Shenton AF, Sharpe DT. Epidemiology and outcome analysis of 208 children with burns attending an emergency department. *Pediatr Emerg Care*. 2007;23(5):289–293 PMID: 17505269 https://doi.org/10.1097/01.pec.0000248698.42175.2b
20. Shah M, Orton E, Tata LJ, Gomes C, Kendrick D. Risk factors for scald injury in children under 5 years of age: a case-control study using routinely collected data. *Burns*. 2013;39(7):1474–1478 PMID: 23639223 https://doi.org/10.1016/j.burns.2013.03.022
21. Jugmohan B, Loveland J, Doedens L, Moore RL, Welthagen A, Westgarth-Taylor CJ. Mortality in paediatric burns victims: a retrospective review from 2009 to 2012 in a single centre. *S Afr Med J*. 2016;106(2):189–192 PMID: 26821901 https://doi.org/10.7196/SAMJ.2016.v106i2.8942
22. McLoughlin E, Clarke N, Stahl K, Crawford JD. One pediatric burn unit's experience with sleepwear-related injuries. *Pediatrics*. 1977;60(4):405–409 PMID: 905002
23. Kumar S, Ali W, Verma AK, Pandey A, Rathore S. Epidemiology and mortality of burns in the Lucknow Region, India—a 5 year study. *Burns*. 2013;39(8):1599–1605 PMID: 23663899 https://doi.org/10.1016/j.burns.2013.04.008
24. Kumar S, Singh US, Verma AK, Ali W, Krishna A. Intentional and non-intentional burn related deaths: a comparative study of socio-demographic profile. *Burns*. 2015;41(2):265–270 PMID: 25000816 https://doi.org/10.1016/j.burns.2014.06.006
25. Mashreky SR, Rahman A, Svanström L, Khan TF, Rahman F. Burn mortality in Bangladesh: findings of national health and injury survey. *Injury*. 2011;42(5):507–510 PMID: 20031124 https://doi.org/10.1016/j.injury.2009.11.020
26. Tarim A, Nursal TZ, Basaran O, et al. Scalding in Turkish children: comparison of burns caused by hot water and hot milk. *Burns*. 2006;32(4):473–476 PMID: 16621318 https://doi.org/10.1016/j.burns.2005.11.004
27. Chen XJ, Sun WJ, Wang J, et al. Epidemiology of bedside stove burns in a retrospective cohort of 5089 pediatric patients. *Burns*. 2014;40(8):1761–1769 PMID: 24863713 https://doi.org/10.1016/j.burns.2014.03.018
28. Haynes WM, ed. *CRC Handbook of Chemistry and Physics*. 97th ed. CRC Press; 2016
29. Chiu TW, Ng DC, Burd A. Properties of matter in assessment of scald injuries. *Burns*. 2007;33(2):185–188 PMID: 17118563 https://doi.org/10.1016/j.burns.2006.06.013
30. McChesney PM. Preventing burns from insulating pipes. *Chem Eng*. 1981;88:59–64
31. Hettiaratchy S, Papini R. Initial management of a major burn: II—assessment and resuscitation. *BMJ*. 2004;329(7457):101–103 PMID: 15242917 https://doi.org/10.1136/bmj.329.7457.101
32. Moritz AR, Henriques FC. Studies of thermal injury: II. The relative importance of time and surface temperature in the causation of cutaneous burns. *Am J Pathol*. 1947;23(5):695–720 PMID: 19970955
33. Abraham JP, Plourde B, Vallez L, Stark J, Diller KR. Estimating the time and temperature relationship for causation of deep-partial thickness skin burns. *Burns*. 2015;41(8):1741–1747 PMID: 26188899 https://doi.org/10.1016/j.burns.2015.06.002
34. Henriques FC Jr. Studies of thermal injury; the predictability and the significance of thermally induced rate processes leading to irreversible epidermal injury. *Arch Pathol (Chic)*. 1947;43(5):489–502 PMID: 20243514

35. Pollitzer MJ, Whitehead MD, Reynolds EO, Delpy D. Effect of electrode temperature and in vivo calibration on accuracy of transcutaneous estimation of arterial oxygen tension in infants. *Pediatrics*. 1980;65(3):515–522 PMID: 7360538
36. Feldman KW. Help needed on hot water burns. *Pediatrics*. 1983;71(1):145–146 PMID: 6848972
37. Henriques FC, Moritz AR. Studies of thermal injury: I. The conduction of heat to and through skin and the temperatures attained therein. A theoretical and an experimental investigation. *Am J Pathol*. 1947;23(4):530–549 PMID: 19970945
38. Seidenari S, Giusti G, Bertoni L, Magnoni C, Pellacani G. Thickness and echogenicity of the skin in children as assessed by 20-MHz ultrasound. *Dermatology*. 2000;201(3): 218–222 PMID: 11096192 https://doi.org/10.1159/000018491
39. Stoll AM, Greene LC. Relationship between pain and tissue damage due to thermal radiation. *J Appl Physiol*. 1959;14(3):373–382 PMID: 13654166 https://doi.org/10.1152/jappl.1959.14.3.373
40. Feldman KW, Clarren SK, McLaughlin JF. Tap water burns in handicapped children. *Pediatrics*. 1981;67(4):560–562 PMID: 6454880
41. Lagunju IA, Oyinlade AO, Babatunde OD. Seizure-related injuries in children and adolescents with epilepsy. *Epilepsy Behav*. 2016;54:131–134 PMID: 26708062 https://doi.org/10.1016/j.yebeh.2015.11.019
42. Hammond J, Perez-Stable A, Ward CG. Predictive value of historical and physical characteristics for the diagnosis of child abuse. *South Med J*. 1991;84(2):166–168 PMID: 1990446 https://doi.org/10.1097/00007611-199102000-00004
43. Allasio D, Fischer H. Immersion scald burns and the ability of young children to climb into a bathtub. *Pediatrics*. 2005;115(5):1419–1421 PMID: 15867058 https://doi.org/10.1542/peds.2004-1550
44. Pawlik MC, Kemp A, Maguire S, Nuttall D, Feldman KW, Lindberg DM; ExSTRA investigators. Children with burns referred for child abuse evaluation: burn characteristics and co-existent injuries. *Child Abuse Negl*. 2016;55:52–61 PMID: 27088728 https://doi.org/10.1016/j.chiabu.2016.03.006
45. Klaassen Z, Go PH, Mansour EH, et al. Pediatric genital burns: a 15-year retrospective analysis of outcomes at a level 1 burn center. *J Pediatr Surg*. 2011;46(8):1532–1538 PMID: 21843720 https://doi.org/10.1016/j.jpedsurg.2011.02.050
46. Baggott K, Rabbitts A, Leahy NE, Bourke P, Yurt RW. Pediatric sink-bathing: a risk for scald burns. *J Burn Care Res*. 2013;34(6):639–643 PMID: 23412329 https://doi.org/10.1097/BCR.0b013e31827e5049
47. Loller C, Buxton GA, Kerzmann TL. Hot soup! Correlating the severity of liquid scald burns to fluid and biomedical properties. *Burns*. 2016;42(3):589–597 PMID: 26796241 https://doi.org/10.1016/j.burns.2015.10.016
48. Cassell OC, Hubble M, Milling MA, Dickson WA. Baby walkers—still a major cause of infant burns. *Burns*. 1997;23(5):451–453 PMID: 9426918 https://doi.org/10.1016/S0305-4179(97)89768-9
49. Sheridan RL. Recognition and management of hot liquid aspiration in children. *Ann Emerg Med*. 1996;27(1):89–91 PMID: 8572457 https://doi.org/10.1016/S0196-0644(96)70302-5
50. Faller-Marquardt M, Pollak S, Schmidt U. Cigarette burns in forensic medicine. *Forensic Sci Int*. 2008;176(2-3):200–208 PMID: 17976935 https://doi.org/10.1016/j.forsciint.2007.09.006
51. Hammig BJ, Henry J. Pediatric injuries associated with fireplaces, United States, 2002-2007. *Pediatr Emerg Care*. 2011;27(2):106–109 PMID: 21252811 https://doi.org/10.1097/PEC.0b013e31820943d0

52. Dunst CM, Scott EC, Kraatz JJ, Anderson PM, Twomey JA, Peltier GL. Contact palm burns in toddlers from glass enclosed fireplaces. *J Burn Care Rehabil*. 2004;25(1):67–70 PMID: 14726741 https://doi.org/10.1097/01.BCR.0000105093.55037.63
53. Wibbenmeyer L, Gittelman MA, Kluesner K, et al. A multicenter study of preventable contact burns from glass fronted fireplaces. J Burn Care Res. 2015;36(1):240–245 PMID: 25559733 https://doi.org/10.1097/BCR.0000000000000215
54. Simons M, Brady D, McGrady M, Plaza A, Kimble R. Hot iron burns in children. *Burns*. 2002;28(6):587–590 PMID: 12220918 https://doi.org/10.1016/S0305-4179(02)00077-3
55. Qazi K, Gerson LW, Christopher NC, Kessler E, Ida N. Curling iron-related injuries presenting to U.S. emergency departments. *Acad Emerg Med*. 2001;8(4):395–397 PMID: 11282678 https://doi.org/10.1111/j.1553-2712.2001.tb02121.x
56. Berger LR, Kalishman S. Floor furnace burns to children. *Pediatrics*. 1983;71(1):97–99 PMID: 6848984
57. Harel S, Burkey B, Nanassy AD, et al. Flame time of a cigarette lighter to achieve temperature capable of inflicting a burn. *Burns*. 2017;43(6):1227–1232 PMID: 28279515 https://doi.org/10.1016/j.burns.2017.02.002
58. Knox BL, Starling SP, Feldman KW, Kellogg ND, Frasier LD, Tiapula SL. Child torture as a form of child abuse. *J Child Adolesc Trauma*. 2014;7(1):37–49 https://doi.org/10.1007/s40653-014-0009-9
59. Ngu F, Patel B, McBride C. Epidemiology of isolated foot burns in children presenting to a Queensland paediatric burns centre—a two-year study in warmer climate. *Burns Trauma*. 2017;5(1):6 PMID: 28261623 https://doi.org/10.1186/s41038-017-0070-3
60. Sinha M, Salness R, Foster KN, Fenn R, Hannasch C. Accidental foot burns in children from contact with naturally heated surfaces during summer months: experience from a regional burn center. *J Trauma*. 2006;61(4):975–978 PMID: 17033571 https://doi.org/10.1097/01.ta.0000229810.36074.36
61. Hemington-Gorse S, Pellard S, Wilson-Jones N, Potokar T. Foot burns: epidemiology and management. *Burns*. 2007;33(8):1041–1045 PMID: 17433550 https://doi.org/10.1016/j.burns.2006.11.014
62. Goltsman D, Li Z, Connolly S, Meyerowitz-Katz D, Allan J, Maitz PKM. Pediatric treadmill burns: assessing the effectiveness of prevention strategies. *Burns*. 2016;42(7):1581–1587 PMID: 27522637 https://doi.org/10.1016/j.burns.2016.02.007
63. Kemp AM, Maguire SA, Lumb RC, Harris SM, Mann MK. Contact, cigarette and flame burns in physical abuse: a systematic review. *Child Abuse Rev*. 2014;23(1):35–47 https://doi.org/10.1002/car.2278
64. Hicks RA, Stolfi A. Skeletal surveys in children with burns caused by child abuse. *Pediatr Emerg Care*. 2007;23(5):308–313 PMID: 17505273 https://doi.org/10.1097/01.pec.0000270174.39228.30
65. Brywczynski J, Arnold DH. Shower steamer burns in a toddler: case report and brief review of steam burns in children. *Pediatr Emerg Care*. 2008;24(11):782–784 PMID: 19018224 https://doi.org/10.1097/PEC.0b013e31818d3b61
66. Wallis BA, Turner J, Pearn J, Kimble RM. Scalds as a result of vapour inhalation therapy in children. *Burns*. 2008;34(4):560–564 PMID: 17954012 https://doi.org/10.1016/j.burns.2007.07.016
67. Al Himdani S, Javed MU, Hughes J, et al. Home remedy or hazard?: management and costs of paediatric steam inhalation therapy burn injuries. *Br J Gen Pract*. 2016;66(644):e193–e199 PMID: 26917659 https://doi.org/10.3399/bjgp16X684289
68. Prescott PR. Hair dryer burns in children. *Pediatrics*. 1990;86(5):692–697 PMID: 2235221

69. Wilson Jones N, Wong P, Potokar T. Electric hair straightener burns an epidemiological and thermodynamic study. *Burns*. 2008;34(4):521–524 PMID: 17949917 https://doi.org/10.1016/j.burns.2007.07.013
70. Ortega HW, Vander Velden H, Smith GA. Grill-related injuries in children treated in US emergency departments, 1990-2009. *Pediatr Emerg Care*. 2016;32(12):835–839 PMID: 27753713 https://doi.org/10.1097/PEC.0000000000000939
71. Lowell G, Quinlan K. Not child's play: national estimates of microwave-related burn injuries among young children. *J Trauma Acute Care Surg*. 2016;81(4 suppl 1):S20–S24 PMID: 26998780 https://doi.org/10.1097/TA.0000000000001050
72. Puczynski M, Rademaker D, Gatson RL. Burn injury related to the improper use of a microwave oven. *Pediatrics*. 1983;72(5):714–715 PMID: 6634275
73. Bagirathan S, Rao K, Al-Benna S, O'Boyle CP. Facial burns from exploding microwaved foods: case series and review. *Burns*. 2016;42(2):e9–e12 PMID: 26120085 https://doi.org/10.1016/j.burns.2015.02.014
74. Wu C, Tan AL, Maze DA, Holland AJ. Instant hot noodles: do they need to burn? *Burns*. 2013;39(2):363–368 PMID: 22975407 https://doi.org/10.1016/j.burns.2012.06.005
75. Alexander RC, Surrell JA, Cohle SD. Microwave oven burns to children: an unusual manifestation of child abuse. *Pediatrics*. 1987;79(2):255–260 PMID: 3808798
76. Hibbard RA, Blevins R. Palatal burn due to bottle warming in a microwave oven. *Pediatrics*. 1988;82(3):382–384 PMID: 3405668
77. Nemethy M, Clore ER. Microwave heating of infant formula and breast milk. *J Pediatr Health Care*. 1990;4(3):131–135 PMID: 2189981 https://doi.org/10.1016/0891-5245(90)90050-G
78. Guerrero L. Burns due to acid assaults in Bogotá, Colombia. *Burns*. 2013;39(5):1018–1023 PMID: 23260999 https://doi.org/10.1016/j.burns.2012.10.022
79. Dinis-Oliveira RJ, Carvalho F, Moreira R, et al. Clinical and forensic signs related to chemical burns: a mechanistic approach. *Burns*. 2015;41(4):658–679 PMID: 25280586 https://doi.org/10.1016/j.burns.2014.09.002
80. Cowan D, Ho B, Sykes KJ, Wei JL. Pediatric oral burns: a ten-year review of patient characteristics, etiologies and treatment outcomes. *Int J Pediatr Otorhinolaryngol*. 2013;77(8):1325–1328 PMID: 23786788 https://doi.org/10.1016/j.ijporl.2013.05.026
81. Lang C, Cox M. Pediatric cutaneous bleach burns. *Child Abuse Negl*. 2013;37(7):485–488 PMID: 23545350 https://doi.org/10.1016/j.chiabu.2013.02.009
82. Pandey S, Sivakumar DK, Chittoria RK, Mohapatra DP, Friji MT. Camphor burns over the forehead: socially relevant non-homicidal injury in a child. *Indian J Plast Surg*. 2016;49(2):289–291 PMID: 27833304 https://doi.org/10.4103/0970-0358.191292
83. D'Cruz R, Pang TC, Harvey JG, Holland AJ. Chemical burns in children: aetiology and prevention. *Burns*. 2015;41(4):764–769 PMID: 25468474 https://doi.org/10.1016/j.burns.2014.10.020
84. Etemesi BA. Impact of hair relaxers in women in Nakuru, Kenya. *Int J Dermatol*. 2007;46(suppl 1):23–25 PMID: 17919201 https://doi.org/10.1111/j.1365-4632.2007.03458.x
85. Meizoso JP, Ramaley SR, Ray JJ, et al. Scald burns from hair braiding. *J Burn Care Res*. 2016;37(1):e7–e9 PMID: 26594857 https://doi.org/10.1097/BCR.0000000000000316
86. Rabban JT, Blair JA, Rosen CL, Adler JN, Sheridan RL. Mechanisms of pediatric electrical injury. New implications for product safety and injury prevention. *Arch Pediatr Adolesc Med*. 1997;151(7):696–700 PMID: 9232044 https://doi.org/10.1001/archpedi.1997.02170440058010
87. Tomkins KL, Holland AJA. Electrical burn injuries in children. *J Paediatr Child Health*. 2008;44(12):727–730 https://doi.org/10.1111/j.1440-1754.2008.01414.x

88. Güzey S, Dal AD, Şahin İ, Nişancı M, Yavan İ. A new experimental burn model with an infrared heater. *Ulus Travma Acil Cerrahi Derg*. 2016;22(5):412–416 PMID: 27849315
89. Nizamoglu M, Tan A, Vickers T, Segaren N, Barnes D, Dziewulski P. Cold burn injuries in the UK: the 11-year experience of a tertiary burns centre. *Burns Trauma*. 2016;4(1):36 PMID: 27843971 https://doi.org/10.1186/s41038-016-0060-x
90. Feldman KW, Monastersky C, Feldman GK. When is childhood drowning neglect? *Child Abuse Negl*. 1993;17(3):329–336 PMID: 8330219 https://doi.org/10.1016/0145-2134(93)90055-A
91. Hayek SN, Wibbenmeyer LA, Kealey LD, et al. The efficacy of hair and urine toxicology screening on the detection of child abuse by burning. *J Burn Care Res*. 2009;30(4):587–592 PMID: 19506505 https://doi.org/10.1097/BCR.0b013e3181abfd30
92. Burke BA, Lewis RW II, Latenser BA, et al. Methamphetamine-related burns in the cornbelt. *J Burn Care Res*. 2008;29(4):574–579 PMID: 18535481 https://doi.org/10.1097/BCR.0b013e31817db832
93. Campos JK, Wong YM, Hasty BN, McElligott KA, Mosier MJ. The effect of socioeconomic status and parental demographics on activation of Department of Child and Family Services in pediatric burn injury. *J Burn Care Res*. 2017;38(4):e722–e733 PMID: 27893581
94. Morrongiello BAMB, McArthur BA, Goodman S, Bell M. Don't touch the gadget because it's hot! Mothers' and children's behavior in the presence of a contrived hazard at home: implications for supervising children. *J Pediatr Psychol*. 2015;40(1):85–95 PMID: 25060600 https://doi.org/10.1093/jpepsy/jsu056
95. Runyan CW, Bangdiwala SI, Linzer MA, Sacks JJ, Butts J. Risk factors for fatal residential fires. *N Engl J Med*. 1992;327(12):859–863 PMID: 1508246 https://doi.org/10.1056/NEJM199209173271207
96. Squires T, Busuttil A. Child fatalities in Scottish house fires 1980-1990: a case of child neglect? *Child Abuse Negl*. 1995;19(7):865–873 PMID: 7583744 https://doi.org/10.1016/0145-2134(95)00050-I
97. Mierley MCBS, Baker SP. Fatal house fires in an urban population. *JAMA*. 1983;249(11):1466–1468 PMID: 6827724 https://doi.org/10.1001/jama.1983.03330350042024
98. Chester DL, Jose RM, Aldlyami E, King H, Moiemen NS. Non-accidental burns in children—are we neglecting neglect? *Burns*. 2006;32(2):222–228 PMID: 16448766 https://doi.org/10.1016/j.burns.2005.08.018
99. Anderst J, Dowd MD, Schnitzer P, Tryon T. Preliminary development of a rapid assessment of supervision scale for young children. *Pediatrics*. 2012;129(6):e1517–e1524 PMID: 22566419 https://doi.org/10.1542/peds.2011-2880
100. James-Ellison M, Barnes P, Maddocks A, et al. Social health outcomes following thermal injuries: a retrospective matched cohort study. *Arch Dis Child*. 2009;94(9):663–667 PMID: 19531525 https://doi.org/10.1136/adc.2008.143727
101. Duke JM, Rea S, Boyd JH, Randall SM, Wood FM. Mortality after burn injury in children: a 33-year population-based study. *Pediatrics*. 2015;135(4):e903–e910 PMID: 25802351 https://doi.org/10.1542/peds.2014-3140
102. Zaloga WF, Collins KA. Pediatric homicides related to burn injury: a retrospective review at the medical university of South Carolina. *J Forensic Sci*. 2006;51(2):396–399 PMID: 16566778 https://doi.org/10.1111/j.1556-4029.2006.00066.x
103. Abel EL. Childhood homicide in Erie County, New York. *Pediatrics*. 1986;77(5):709–713 PMID: 3703638
104. Maguire S, Moynihan S, Mann M, Potokar T, Kemp AM. A systematic review of the features that indicate intentional scalds in children. *Burns*. 2008;34(8):1072–1081 PMID: 18538478 https://doi.org/10.1016/j.burns.2008.02.011

105. Feldman KW, Schaller RT, Feldman JA, McMillon M. Tap water scald burns in children. *Pediatrics*. 1978;62(1):1–7 PMID: 683765
106. Clark KD, Tepper D, Jenny C. Effect of a screening profile on the diagnosis of nonaccidental burns in children. *Pediatr Emerg Care*. 1997;13(4):259–261 PMID: 9291513 https://doi.org/10.1097/00006565-199708000-00005
107. Bousema S, Stas HG, van de Merwe MH, et al; Dutch Burn Repository Group, Maasstad Hospital Rotterdam. Epidemiology and screening of intentional burns in children in a Dutch burn centre. *Burns*. 2016;42(6):1287–1294 PMID: 27211360 https://doi.org/10.1016/j.burns.2016.01.009
108. Kemp AM, Hollen L, Emond AM, Nuttall D, Rea D, Maguire S. Raising suspicion of mistreatment from burns: derivation and validation of the BuRN-Tool. *Burns*. 2018;44(2):335–343 PMID: 28918905
109. DeGraw M, Hicks RA, Lindberg D; Using Liver Transaminases to Recognize Abuse (ULTRA) Study Investigators. Incidence of fractures among children with burns with concern regarding abuse. *Pediatrics*. 2010;125(2):e295–e299 PMID: 20083520 https://doi.org/10.1542/peds.2009-1478
110. Fagen KE, Shalaby-Rana E, Jackson AM. Frequency of skeletal injuries in children with inflicted burns. *Pediatr Radiol*. 2015;45(3):396–401 PMID: 25238809 https://doi.org/10.1007/s00247-014-3163-1
111. Belfer RA, Klein BL, Orr L. Use of the skeletal survey in the evaluation of child maltreatment. *Am J Emerg Med*. 2001;19(2):122–124 PMID: 11239255 https://doi.org/10.1053/ajem.2001.21345
112. Seifert D, Krohn J, Larson M, Lambe A, Püschel K, Kurth H. Violence against children: further evidence suggesting a relationship between burns, scalds, and the additional injuries. *Int J Legal Med*. 2010;124(1):49–54 PMID: 19399513 https://doi.org/10.1007/s00414-009-0347-6
113. Sheridan RL. Burn care for children. *Pediatr Rev*. 2018;39(6):273–286 PMID: 29858290 https://doi.org/10.1542/pir.2016-0179
114. Allasio D, Fischer H. How far can toddlers reach onto a standard kitchen countertop? *Clin Pediatr (Phila)*. 2011;50(3):262–263 PMID: 20926841 https://doi.org/10.1177/0009922810382573
115. Purdue GF, Hunt JL, Prescott PR. Child abuse by burning—an index of suspicion. *J Trauma*. 1988;28(2):221–224 PMID: 3346922 https://doi.org/10.1097/00005373-198802000-00018
116. Hodgman EI, Pastorek RA, Saeman MR, et al. The Parkland Burn Center experience with 297 cases of child abuse from 1974 to 2010. *Burns*. 2016;42(5):1121–1127 PMID: 27268012 https://doi.org/10.1016/j.burns.2016.02.013
117. Sheridan RL, Remensnyder JP, Schnitzer JJ, Schulz JT, Ryan CM, Tompkins RG. Current expectations for survival in pediatric burns. *Arch Pediatr Adolesc Med*. 2000;154(3):245–249 PMID: 10710021 https://doi.org/10.1001/archpedi.154.3.245
118. Kraft R, Herndon DN, Al-Mousawi AM, Williams FN, Finnerty CC, Jeschke MG. Burn size and survival probability in paediatric patients in modern burn care: a prospective observational cohort study. *Lancet*. 2012;379(9820):1013–1021 PMID: 22296810 https://doi.org/10.1016/S0140-6736(11)61345-7
119. Feldman KW. Pseudoabusive burns in Asian refugees. *Child Abuse Negl*. 1995;19(5):657–658 PMID: 7664144
120. Yoon C, Cho YS, Park S, Chung SP, Choi YH. Epidemiology of burns caused by moxibustion in Korea. *Burns*. 2016;42(7):1588–1592 PMID: 27156790 https://doi.org/10.1016/j.burns.2016.04.015

121. Alabi GH, Omolase CO. Feet burning: a traditional medical practice associated with significant burns in patients with seizures: 4 case reports. *Burns*. 2012;38(1):e5–e8 PMID: 22035887 https://doi.org/10.1016/j.burns.2011.09.019
122. Keles MK, Bayram Y, Durmus M. How fast can a naturopathic medicine cause skin burn? A case report of garlic burn. *Ann Burns Fire Disasters*. 2015;28(3):228–229 PMID: 27279812
123. Zazzera E. A 7-month-old infant with plantar garlic burns. *J Emerg Nurs*. 2017;43(5): 467–468 PMID: 27181193
124. MacDuff S, Sun J, Bell DE, Lentz CW, Kahn SA. Accidental burn by intentional laxative use. *Pediatr Emerg Care*. 2016;32(8):541–543 PMID: 27490728 https://doi.org/10.1097/PEC.0000000000000855
125. Leventhal JM, Griffin D, Duncan KO, Starling S, Christian CW, Kutz T. Laxative-induced dermatitis of the buttocks incorrectly suspected to be abusive burns. *Pediatrics*. 2001;107(1):178–179 PMID: 11134455 https://doi.org/10.1542/peds.107.1.178
126. Spiller HA, Winter ML, Weber JA, Krenzelok EP, Anderson DL, Ryan ML. Skin breakdown and blisters from senna-containing laxatives in young children. *Ann Pharmacother*. 2003;37(5):636–639 PMID: 12708936 https://doi.org/10.1345/aph.1C439
127. Majjiga VS, Kumaresan P, Glass EJ. Silver nitrate burns following umbilical granuloma treatment. *Arch Dis Child*. 2005;90(7):674 PMID: 15970607 https://doi.org/10.1136/adc.2004.067918
128. Knox BL, Petska HW, DeMuri GP, Feldman KW. Staphylococcal infection mimicking child abuse: what is the differential diagnosis and appropriate evaluation? *Pediatr Emerg Care*. 2011;27(6):547–549 PMID: 21642794 https://doi.org/10.1097/PEC.0b013e31821dc717
129. Schwartz RA. Toxic epidermal necrolysis. *Cutis*. 1997;59(3):123–128 PMID: 9071550
130. Feldman KW. Confusion of innocent pressure injuries with inflicted dry contact burns. *Clin Pediatr (Phila)*. 1995;34(2):114–115 PMID: 7729107 https://doi.org/10.1177/000992289503400210
131. Roussel LO, Bell DE. Tweens feel the burn: "salt and ice challenge" burns. *Int J Adolesc Med Health*. 2016;28(2):217–219 PMID: 25901711
132. Zhao CY, Chiang YZ, Murrell DF. Neonatal autoimmune blistering diseases: a systemic review. *Pediatr Dermatol*. 2016;33(4):367–374 PMID: 27086740 https://doi.org/10.1111/pde.12859
133. Adler R, Kane-Nussen B. Erythema multiforme: confusion with child battering syndrome. *Pediatrics*. 1983;72(5):718–720 PMID: 6634277
134. Bays J. Conditions mistaken for physical abuse. In: *Child Abuse: Medical Diagnosis and Management*. 2nd ed. Philadelphia, PA: Lippincott, Williams and Wilkins; 2001:287–306
135. Diez F Jr, Berger TG. Scarring due to an enuresis blanket. *Pediatr Dermatol*. 1988;5(1): 58–60 PMID: 3380764 https://doi.org/10.1111/j.1525-1470.1988.tb00886.x
136. Stewart GM, Rosenberg NM. Conditions mistaken for child abuse: part II. *Pediatr Emerg Care*. 1996;12(3):217–221 PMID: 8806151 https://doi.org/10.1097/00006565-199606000-00019
137. Wheeler DM, Hobbs CJ. Mistakes in diagnosing non-accidental injury: 10 years' experience. *Br Med J (Clin Res Ed)*. 1988;296(6631):1233–1236 PMID: 3133026 https://doi.org/10.1136/bmj.296.6631.1233
138. Gordon EM, Bernat JR Jr, Ramos-Caro FA. Urticaria pigmentosa mistaken for child abuse. *Pediatr Dermatol*. 1998;15(6):484–485 PMID: 9875978 https://doi.org/10.1046/j.1525-1470.1998.1998015484.x
139. Schmitt BD, Gray JD, Britton HL. Car seat burns in infants: avoiding confusion with inflicted burns. *Pediatrics*. 1978;62(4):607–609 PMID: 714595
140. Ginsburg CM. Staphylococcal toxin syndromes. *Pediatr Infect Dis J*. 1991;10(4):319–321 PMID: 2062629 https://doi.org/10.1097/00006454-199104000-00011

141. Winterton PM. Perianal infection with beta haemolytic streptococcus. *Arch Dis Child*. 1995;72(6):544 PMID: 7618949 https://doi.org/10.1136/adc.72.6.544-a
142. Winship IM, Winship WS. Epidermolysis bullosa misdiagnosed as child abuse. A report of 3 cases. *S Afr Med J*. 1988;73(6):369–370 PMID: 3353812
143. Sheridan RL, Sheridan MG, Tompkins RG. Dishwasher effluent burns in infants. *Pediatrics*. 1993;91(1):142–144 PMID: 8416479
144. Titus MO, Baxter AL, Starling SP. Accidental scald burns in sinks. *Pediatrics*. 2003;111(2):E191–E194 PMID: 12563095 https://doi.org/10.1542/peds.111.2.e191
145. Spencer JA, Grieve DK. Congenital indifference to pain mistaken for non-accidental injury. *Br J Radiol*. 1990;63(748):308–310 PMID: 1693303 https://doi.org/10.1259/0007-1285-63-748-308
146. Eyth CP, Echlin K, Jones I. Cyanoacrylate burn injuries: two unusual cases and a review of the literature. *Wounds*. 2016;28(12):E53–E59 PMID: 28054930
147. Wardinsky TD, Vizcarrondo FE, Cruz BK. The mistaken diagnosis of child abuse: a three-year USAF Medical Center analysis and literature review. *Mil Med*. 1995;160(1):15–20 PMID: 7746427 https://doi.org/10.1093/milmed/160.1.15

CHAPTER 4

Skeletal Manifestations of Child Abuse

Suzanne B. Haney, MD, FAAP
Assistant Professor of Pediatrics
University of Nebraska Medical Center
Children's Hospital and Medical Center
Omaha, NE

Susan A. Scherl, MD, FAAP
Professor
Department of Orthopaedics
University of Nebraska Medical Center
Attending Physician
Section of Pediatric Orthopaedics
Children's Hospital and Medical Center
Omaha, NE

Historical Perspective

Skeletal injuries as a result of child abuse were first reported by Ambrose Tardieu in Paris in an 1860 report on children who experienced neglect and abuse.[1] In 1946, John Caffey noted the correlation between long bone fractures and subdural hematomas in infants.[2] This was even better described in his later article on shaken infants.[3] Subsequently, C. Henry Kempe coined the term "battered child syndrome" and included a number of children who had fractures and other bony injuries as a result of abuse in his seminal article.[4]

Presentation/Diagnosis

The most common presentation of a child with a fracture is when a child is brought in with a chief concern of a fall or other injury and has subsequent pain on manipulation or a gross deformity.[5] Infants are more difficult to evaluate because they are unable to properly localize and/or express pain. Although infants may also present with pain on movement or a gross deformity, they may present with only inconsolable crying and no obvious source. Fractures are a very common accidental injury and can occur in all ages. However, fractures in younger, nonambulatory infants and children are more concerning for abuse. Almost 25% of infants who present with fractures are found to be abused, while only 3% of children aged 2 to 3 years who present with fractures are found to have experienced abuse.[6]

History of Present Illness

Whether or not a history is consistent with an injury is a strong indicator of whether the injury was the result of abuse. It is prudent for the medical professional to obtain a detailed history of the injury from the caregiver. This would include the circumstances surrounding the injury, how the child was injured, how the child landed, the flooring, other involved children and adults, and how the child reacted to the injury.[7] The child's developmental abilities will also assist in determining if the child's injury was accidental or not. Children who are nonambulatory (ie, not yet cruising) and especially those who are nonmobile are less likely to sustain a fracture accidentally. A lack of a detailed history of injury, a mechanism that is not consistent with the injury, a history that changes over time, and a delay in care are all historical indicators that are concerning for inflicted injury.[8] In instances where there is limited or no history of injury, obtaining the history of when the child was last well (uninjured) can help narrow the timing of the injury.

A past medical history should include medical conditions that would predispose a child to fragile bones and to injuries that are commonly seen in cases of abuse. This would include other injuries or fractures, hearing deficits, bruising history, and any other medical concerns. It is also necessary to obtain a complete birth history for prematurity, birth injuries, and prenatal conditions.

A thorough family history includes assessing if there are any other family members with a number of fractures or with fractures as a result of minor trauma. In addition, it is important to obtain the medical history of the parents and siblings as well as assess for dental and auditory issues.

The social history in suspected abuse cases includes any and all caregivers, including child care and babysitters and any other adults living in the home, and any prior contact with authorities. Social stressors such as money, job pressures, mental health conditions, and other children in the household should be evaluated. Families should be asked about prior social services contact, prescription and illegal drug use, and domestic violence because these can all contribute to abusive situations.

Physical Examination

The physical examination of children with fractures includes a thorough skin examination assessing the child for bruises, burns, or other marks concerning for inflicted injury, with special attention paid to oral and auricular injuries. A lack of bruising directly associated with the fractures does not rule out abuse; in fact, fewer than 20% of inflicted fractures have associated bruises.[9] A detailed examination to determine if there are other areas of tenderness, crepitus, or swelling can assist in looking for other fractures. Features such as blue sclera, dentinogenesis imperfecta, gum disease, and bowed extremities can assist in identifying other conditions such as osteogenesis imperfecta (OI), which might predispose a child to fractures.

Radiographic Assessment

There are 2 main reasons to perform additional testing in children with suspected abuse. The first is to evaluate for other abusive injuries; the second is to rule out other causes for the child's condition. While some of the evaluation can be done in conjunction with other testing (eg, laboratory assessment), remember that the child's medical care takes priority; for example, a skeletal survey can be postponed until a child is clinically stable.

Imaging

In children with a fracture that is concerning for abuse, ensuring appropriate imaging of the fracture itself is paramount. This includes 2 or more views of the injured area and should also include views of adjacent joints or bones. Imaging the contralateral side may aid in diagnosing an injury. In a child for which plain radiograph results are negative, but for whom there is continued concern for bony injury, repeating radiographs in 10 to 14 days is prudent. An occult fracture will frequently become visible in that time frame through callus formation and/or remodeling.

Skeletal Survey

The skeletal survey is the most common study done to evaluate children for occult bony injuries or abnormalities. The skeletal survey is a series of images performed of each area of the body: at least 19 separate images as recommended by the American College of Radiology (ACR) (Box 4.1).[10] Some institutions add more studies, including oblique ribs, and may also reimage individual areas as needed. Unfortunately, there are still institutions (typically adult, more rural hospitals) that perform suboptimal studies. If a child is being transferred to a larger center, the skeletal survey can wait until after the transfer. The skeletal survey is recommended by the American Academy of Pediatrics and the ACR in children younger than 24 months, although newer research suggests that there may be yield in children up to 36 months or older.[8,10,11] There is little to support the utility of a skeletal survey in a child older than 5 years.

BOX 4.1
Complete Skeletal Survey Table

Appendicular Skeleton

Humeri (AP)

Forearms (AP)

Hands (PA)

Femurs (AP)

Lower legs (AP)

Feet (PA or AP)

Axial Skeleton

Thorax (AP and lateral), to include ribs, thoracic, and upper lumbar spine

Pelvis (AP), to include the mid lumbar spine

Lumbosacral spine (lateral)

Cervical spine (AP and lateral)

Skull (frontal and lateral)

Abbreviations: AP, anteroposterior; PA, posteroanterior.

From American College of Radiology. ACR practice guideline for skeletal surveys in children (res. 47, 17, 35). In: *ACR Standards.* Reston, VA: American College of Radiology; 2006:203-207.

Follow-up Skeletal Survey

In cases where child abuse is strongly suspected, a follow-up skeletal survey (FUSS) 2 weeks later is recommended by the American Academy of Pediatrics.[8] Acute fractures, especially in the ribs and metaphyses, are easily missed and will become apparent later as the callus and/or periosteal elevation appear. A study by Harper and colleagues found that FUSSs yielded new information in 21.5% of children who had been referred to a hospital child protection team.[12] Radiation exposure is a common concern when repeating the skeletal survey, and more recent studies have shown that excluding the head, spine, and pelvis on the FUSS decreases radiation and has no significant effect on the yield.[13]

Postmortem skeletal surveys can be performed after death in cases of suspected abuse. Routine autopsy protocols do not include the appendicular skeleton, and injuries can be missed if they are not found prior to autopsy. As with routine skeletal surveys, these studies should be done under the observation of a trained radiologist according to the ACR recommendations.[10] Because each jurisdiction has different policies for consent and authority in such cases, a hospital should have preexisting protocols on how to handle postmortem skeletal surveys. In addition, there must be consideration of trauma to the staff in performing these studies.

Ultrasonography

Ultrasonography is particularly useful in diagnosing injury at the costochondral junction and in demonstrating subperiosteal abscess prior to the appearance of fracture or periosteal reaction on plain radiograph.[14–16] It can also be used to visualize the non-ossified epiphysis in cases of trans-physeal distal humerus fracture.[17] Advantages of ultrasonography are that it is quick and noninvasive and does not involve radiation. However, it is operator dependent, and the quality and interpretation of the studies vary with practitioner experience.

Magnetic Resonance Imaging

Magnetic resonance imaging (MRI) can be used as an adjunctive study in cases in which clinical suspicion of diaphyseal fracture is high but plain radiographs are negative. However, whole-body MRI should not be used as a stand-alone screening test or in lieu of the skeletal survey, because it is not sensitive in picking up rib fractures or classic metaphyseal lesions (CMLs), both of which are injuries highly specific for abuse.[18] Magnetic resonance imaging has the advantage of not involving radiation, but it has the drawback of typically needing to be done under sedation or anesthesia in young children.

Positron Emission Tomography

Positron emission tomography scanning using sodium fluorine-18 can be a useful adjunct for the diagnosis of abusive fractures, although it does not replace the need for an initial skeletal survey.[19] One study has shown that it is more sensitive than initial skeletal survey in the diagnosis of thoracic and rib fractures, although less sensitive for visualizing CMLs.[20] Done in conjunction with the skeletal survey, it can, therefore, sometimes provide additional information prior to the 2-week waiting time for a FUSS. This can be helpful in cases in which follow-up cannot be assured or in which it is necessary to make immediate decisions about disposition. However, the test does involve radiation, generally requires sedation or anesthesia, and may not be available at all centers. Traditional bone scan is no longer commonly used in the diagnosis of non-accidental trauma, because it involves radiation, takes a significant amount of time to perform, and is not sensitive for skull fractures, CMLs, fractures in the vicinity of growth plates, and symmetrical bilateral fractures. It also gives no information on the age or stage of healing of fractures.

Evaluation of Siblings

Siblings and other children in the same environment (eg, child care) where the patient was injured are also at risk for inflicted injury and should be appropriately evaluated. This evaluation includes a thorough physical examination and a radiologic evaluation depending on age. Skeletal surveys should be strongly considered for young (<2 years or so) siblings and other children in the same environment with a child who has experienced abuse, and head imaging should be considered in infants younger than 6 months.[8] A study by Lindberg and colleagues found that 16% of contacts of children who had experienced abuse had an occult fracture. Twin siblings were at highest risk.[21]

Laboratory Assessment

Laboratory evaluation should be done to rule out any medical conditions that might predispose a child to fracture more easily than expected. Calcium, phosphorus, and alkaline phosphatase levels can determine basic bone metabolism, although an elevated alkaline phosphatase level can be present with multiple healing fractures.[22] Occult abdominal injuries should be screened for with liver and pancreatic testing as well as a urinalysis. Other useful laboratory studies include 25-hydroxy vitamin D levels, parathyroid hormone levels, and urine calcium/creatinine excretion ratios in children with clear osteopenia or concerns for rickets. Serum copper, vitamin C, and genetic testing for medical conditions can be guided by the history and physical examination.

Dating of Injuries

Fractures of long bones and ribs commonly heal in an expected pattern. On radiograph, it is easy to distinguish acute fractures from those with clear callus formation. In most children, callus formation occurs about 7 to 10 days after the initial fracture. Periosteal reaction, a more accurate finding for dating fractures, is not present acutely and appears around 11 days' post-injury. More subtle findings, such as the presence of a fracture line and hard versus soft callus formation, are not useful for dating fractures[23] (Table 4.1).

TABLE 4.1
Estimating Fracture Age

Radiographic finding	Time From Injury
Periosteal new bone	10–14 d
Resorption of fracture line	14–21 d
Early callus	14–21 d
Bridging callus	21–42 d
Remodeling	≥6–12 mo

Adapted from Halliday KE, Broderick NJ, Somers JM, Hawkes R. Dating fractures in infants. *Clin Radiol.* 2011;66(11):1049–1054, with permission from Elsevier.

Biomechanics

Biomechanics is the scientific discipline that qualifies and quantifies the complex interplay between the structure and function of the musculoskeletal system. The human body is subject to a wide variety of internal and external forces.[24] *Internal forces* are those exerted by one part of the body on another (eg, muscle on bone). *External forces* are exerted on the body by the environment. In vivo, these interactions are extremely complex. In experimental or hypothetical settings, the goal is to control for enough variables to obtain meaningful, reproducible data without oversimplifying to the point where relevance to a clinical setting is compromised.

Material properties of a substance, such as bone, are independent of shape and include elasticity, brittleness, and toughness. They characterize the mechanical function and structural limitations of a substance.[24] Structural properties are dependent on the substance and its shape. Stiffness, which is the ability to resist failure in torsion, axial load, or bending, is a structural property. Bone is also anisotropic, meaning that its mechanical properties differ depending on the type of load applied to it. Bone is weakest in withstanding shear, followed by tension, and is strongest in compression. Cortical and cancellous bone have differing abilities to withstand force, and an individual's bone mineral density also plays a role. Another biomechanical feature of bone is that it is viscoelastic; its deformation characteristics depend on the rate of loading. An example is the trabecular bone, which is stiffer in compression the faster it is loaded.[25]

All these interacting variables complicate the ability to design in vitro experiments and laboratory models of fracture that accurately reproduce in vivo conditions.[24] It is challenging to reproduce the conditions of living bone that are present in a live human being, including a soft tissue envelope and blood flow, by using cadaver or artificial bone in a laboratory setting. Animal and computer models are useful but also have limitations. This is why it can be challenging to definitively answer questions in the clinical setting about how a fracture occurred or how much force it took to cause a fracture.

However, fracture morphology does give very basic information about the type of force that causes a fracture. Tension causes transverse fractures, axial load or compression causes torus or oblique fractures, bending causes transverse fractures with or without a butterfly fragment, and torsion causes spiral fractures.[25] Orthopedists typically use this simplified scheme to aid in planning surgical constructs (eg, a fracture that occurs in tension is fixed with a plate applied with compression).

Classic metaphyseal lesions are typically described as the result of shear, but a porcine model has reproduced CMLs via lateral bend, which is a tensile force.[26] Any of the types of forces described herein can be generated via accidental and intentional mechanisms.

The amount of force necessary to load a bone to failure in vivo is subject to many variables, including the size and shape of the bone, its cortical thickness and trabecular architecture, and the direction and speed of the force.

Fracture Specificity

Kleinman has delineated a pattern of specificity of abuse in childhood fractures (Box 4.2). In this scheme, he describes high-, mid-, and low-specificity fractures.[27]

High-Specificity Fractures

Long Bone Fractures in Nonambulatory Children

Any long bone fracture (diaphyseal, metaphyseal, or physeal) in a child who is too young to walk should raise concern for child abuse. A single, isolated, transverse long bone fracture is the most common fracture pattern in abusive trauma; it occurs in 13% of cases.[28] Various series show the humerus, tibia, and femur to be most commonly affected.[28–31] While earlier literature postulated that spiral fractures were particularly suspicious for abuse, numerous, more recent studies have found transverse fractures more common in cases of abuse, particularly in the femur.[7,28,32,33] One large meta-analysis showed no significant differences in distribution between spiral, transverse, and oblique patterns in abusive femur fractures.[30]

Other, more recent studies have focused on child age and developmental stage as a diagnostic aid. For femur fractures, nonambulatory status is the single most important predictive factor for likelihood of inflicted injury.[30,34,35] Abuse accounts for up to 80% of femur fractures in infants younger than 1 year.[29,36,37] In a study of 139 children aged 4 years or younger, Schwend et al found that 42% of diaphyseal femur fractures in nonambulatory children were attributable to abuse, compared with only 2.6% in the ambulatory cohort.[34] Another study, looking at a total of 138 femur fractures in children up to 4 years old, found that 74.1% of fractures in infants 12 months or younger were secondary to abuse, compared with 14.3%, 8.9%, and 5.3% in the 13- to 24-month-old, 25- to 36-month-old, and 37- to 48-month-old cohorts, respectively. There was also a statistically significant difference in the rate of abuse in infants 12 months or younger compared with all the other cohorts.[35] The American Academy of Orthopaedic Surgeons clinical practice guidelines on pediatric diaphyseal femur fractures recommends evaluation

BOX 4.2
Fracture Specificity

High-Specificity Fractures

Long bone fractures in nonambulatory children

- Trans-physeal distal humerus fractures
- Classic metaphyseal lesions
- Rib fractures
- Sternum, scapula, or pelvic fractures without history of major trauma

Multiple fractures

- In various stages of healing
- Bilateral symmetrical fractures (acute or healing)
- Fractures associated with other injuries

Mid-Specificity Fractures

Spine fractures

Fractures of the hands and feet

Skull fractures

Clavicle fractures

Isolated long bone fractures in ambulatory children without a plausible history

Low-Specificity Fractures

Toddler fracture

Distal radial and ulnar torus fractures

Supracondylar humerus fractures

Isolated long bone fractures in ambulatory children with a plausible history

From Kleinman PK, ed. *Diagnostic Imaging of Child Abuse.* 3rd ed. Cambridge, United Kingdom: Cambridge University Press; 2015.

for child abuse for all children younger than 36 months with a femur fracture (Figure 4.1).[38] Although several studies make similar recommendations, most acknowledge that infants younger than 1 year, and children who have not yet achieved ambulation, are most at risk.[32,34,39] Subsequently, this guideline was made by consensus, because of a lack of sufficient evidence-based medicine to support a specific evaluation age cutoff.

Two studies have looked at complete transverse metaphyseal fractures of the distal femur. Arkader et al found that these fractures were a "harbinger" of abuse in children younger than walking age, with 75% of patients younger than 1 year presenting with this injury found to have experienced abuse.[40] However, Haney et al determined a much lower rate of abuse (28%) in a series of comparable size and similar fractures. They proposed a "plausible accidental mechanism" for such fractures (eg, the parent falls while carrying the child straddled across one hip,

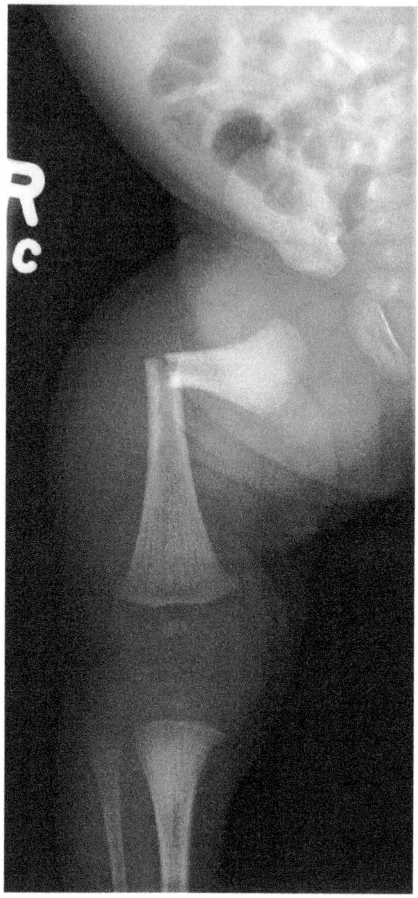

FIGURE 4.1
Diaphyseal femur fracture.

compressing the child's distal femur, which lands beneath the parent's body), particularly if there are no other concerning corroborative findings on the physical examination or skeletal survey.[41] Of note, all 5 of the infants in their series who had experienced abuse were younger than 1 year, once again highlighting the need to maintain a low threshold to investigate long bone fractures in nonambulatory children. Coffey et al found that 96% of tibia and fibular fractures in a cohort of children younger than 18 months were secondary to abuse.[42] Similarly, 54% of humerus fractures in children younger than 3 years are likely the result of abuse, with the prevalence statistically significantly higher in children 15 months or younger.[30,43,44]

Displaced physeal fractures are sometimes referred to as "epiphyseal separations," although most orthopedists prefer to describe these injuries more specifically by using the Salter-Harris classification.[45] The Salter-Harris classification has strong intra- and interobserver reliability and is generally prognostic (ie, a Salter-Harris type 1 fracture usually has a better prognosis than a Salter-Harris type 2 fracture, and so on).[45,46] An example of a physeal fracture frequently associated with abuse is the trans-physeal distal humerus fracture (figures 4.2 and 4.3). The fracture pattern is usually a displaced Salter-Harris type 1 fracture of the distal humeral physis. However, these fractures typically occur in infants younger than 1 year, in whom the distal humeral epiphysis is completely non-ossified; therefore, the entire distal fracture fragment is not visible on plain radiograph, making diagnosis challenging. Subsequently, these fractures are often diagnosed late, once periosteal reaction is visible on plain radiograph. Acutely, ultrasonography, MRI, or arthrogram can aid in diagnosis. A recent study found the diagnosis missed on 56% of plain radiographs but confirmed by ultrasonography in 100% of cases, with 38% of cases (all in infants younger than 1 month) secondary to birth trauma and 40% the result of abuse.[17]

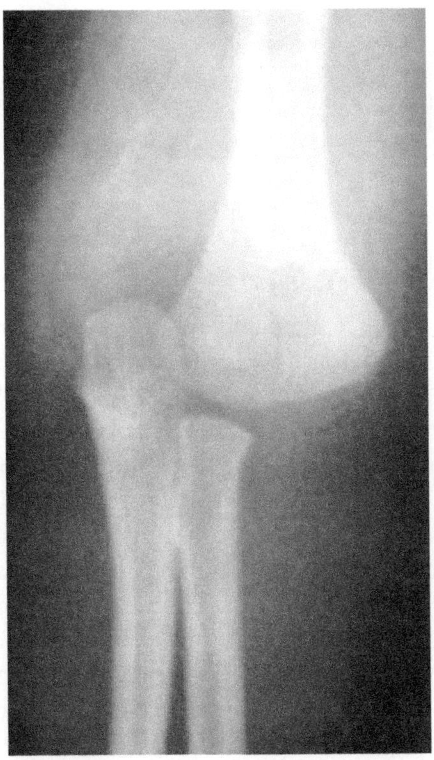

FIGURE 4.2
Trans-physeal distal humerus fracture.

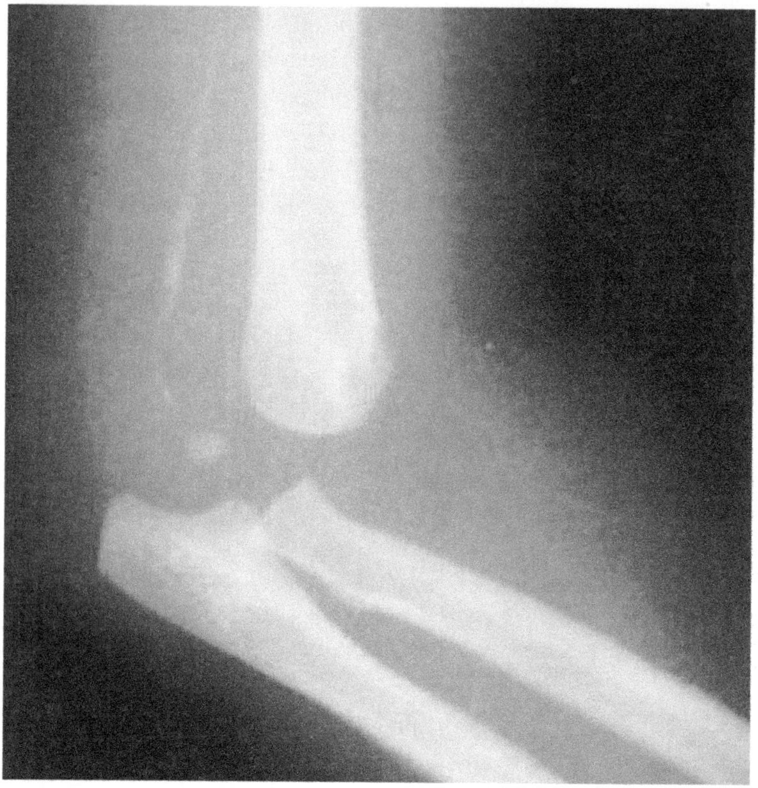

FIGURE 4.3
Trans-physeal distal humerus fracture.

Classic Metaphyseal Lesions

Classic metaphyseal lesions, although relatively uncommon, are highly specific for abuse, particularly if they are found to be present in more than 1 long bone.[47–49] They account for up to 28% of abusive long bone fractures.[28,50,51] They are speculated to occur via a mechanism of combined traction and torsion, causing shearing forces through the periphery of the metaphysis.[52] However, an experimental porcine model has produced CMLs by applying a tensile stress through varus and valgus loading.[26] The resultant fracture consists of a peripheral fragment of metaphysis, which includes the subperiosteal bone collar, and abuts but does not affect the physis (figures 4.4 and 4.5). The fragment is typically discoid and wider peripherally than centrally. Fragment appearance on radiography depends on the view and is the source of the historical descriptions of the CML: on a tangential anteroposterior or lateral view, the fracture appears as wedge-shaped fragments at the edge of the metaphysis ("corner" fracture); on an oblique or angulated view, curvilinear fragments adjacent to the metaphysis are visible (bucket-handle fracture) (figures 4.6 and 4.7). Classic metaphyseal lesions also have a characteristic histological appearance of sub-physeal microfractures through the primary spongiosa and calcified cartilage of the metaphysis.[53]

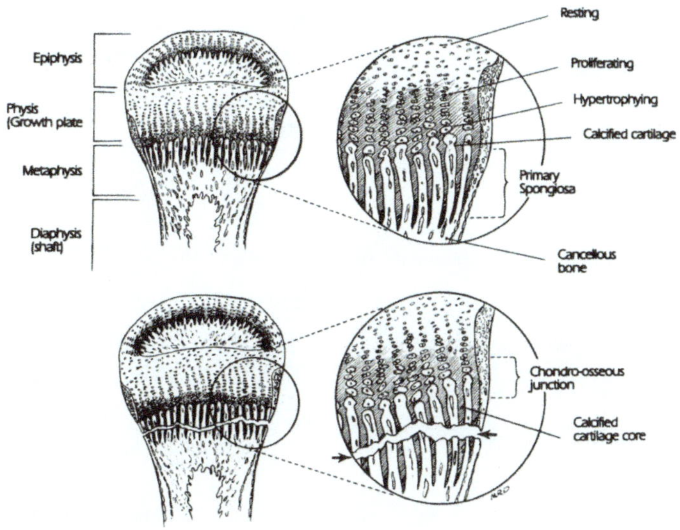

FIGURE 4.4
Common metaphyseal lesion.

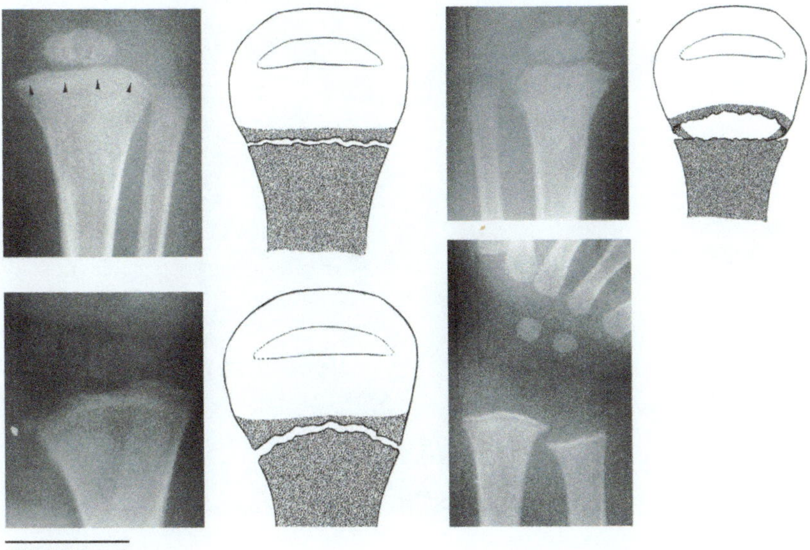

FIGURE 4.5
Common metaphyseal lesions.

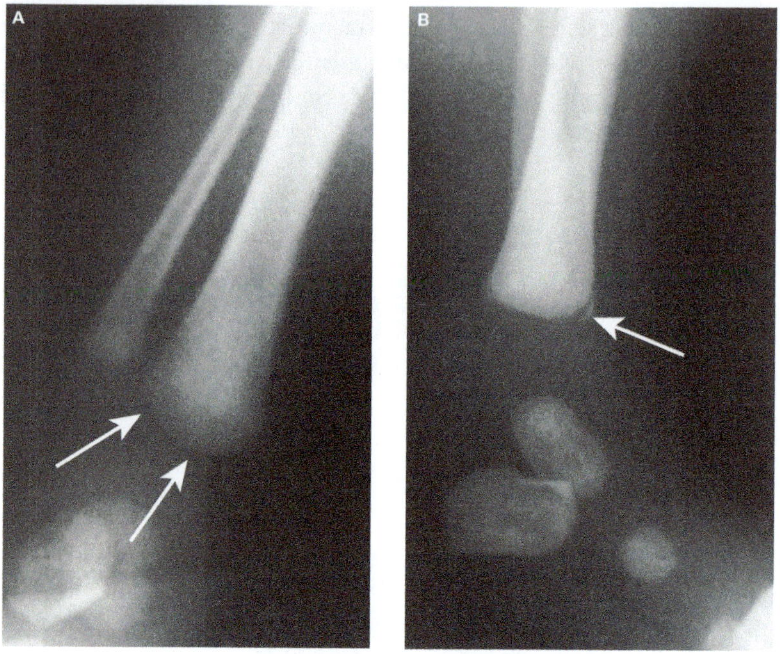

FIGURE 4.6
A 1-month-old had a swollen left leg. A, Radiography shows a bucket-handle fracture (arrows) of the distal tibial metaphysis. B, Viewed in a lateral projection, it appears as a "corner" fracture (arrow).

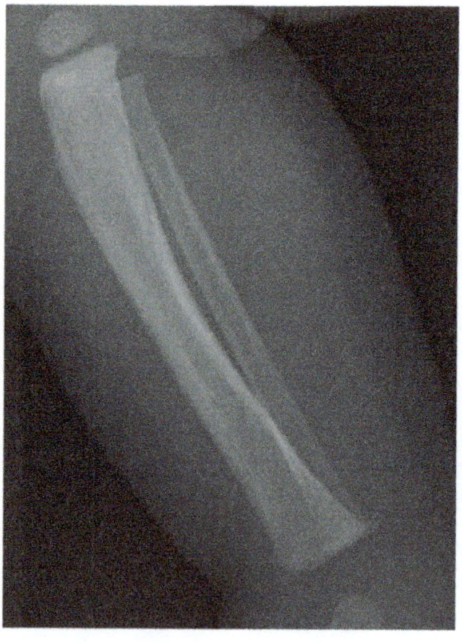

FIGURE 4.7
Distal tibia classic metaphyseal lesion with a "chip" appearance.

Because the periosteum is firmly adherent to the bone in the region where CMLs typically occur, they sometimes produce little subperiosteal hemorrhage. Subsequently, it is possible for them to heal without generating a large amount of periosteal reaction. However, in such cases, it is often possible to visualize healing of the fracture on plain radiograph by using highly detailed radiographic techniques.[54,55] Because CMLs are highly specific for abusive trauma in infants, it has been suggested that high-detail radiography and histologic evaluation of metaphyseal bone samples be a part of the postmortem evaluation of infants in cases of suspected abuse or unexplained death.[54] Although the traction-torsion mechanism thought to be responsible for most CMLs is rare in the setting of accidental trauma, particularly in infants younger than 1 year,[40] there have been reports of CMLs occurring accidentally during cesarean delivery and during therapeutic manipulation and casting of clubfeet being treated by the Ponseti method.[56,57]

Rib Fractures

Rib fractures are highly specific for abusive trauma (Figure 4.8). A meta-analysis calculated the probability of abuse in a child with a rib fracture at 71% (95% CI, 42%–91%).[30] Similarly to the case of long bone fractures, prevalence of abuse associated with rib fractures increases as the age of the child decreases, with 80% of rib fractures in infants younger than 1 year found to be inflicted.[58] Historically, a classic pattern of 3 or 4 posterior fractures of consecutive ribs, corresponding with the placement of the perpetrator's fingers while squeezing or shaking the child, has been described[47,59] (Figure 4.9). However, in Kemp's meta-analysis, 2 included studies[60,61] showed anterior rib fractures to be most common in abuse, and the predictive value of posterior rib fractures was not consistent.[60–62] Overall, the specific location of the rib fractures was not directly correlated to the likelihood of abuse.[30]

Children's ribs are relatively strong and flexible; therefore, rib fractures are a marker for high-energy trauma, with an increased risk of mortality.[47] It is imperative to carefully examine children with rib fractures for other fractures, head trauma, and visceral injuries. Chest compressions administered while performing cardiopulmonary resuscitation have not been found to result in rib fractures.[59,63,64] A study in 2014 reviewed 546 chest radiographs in 80 infants who received cardiopulmonary resuscitation via the "2-thumb" technique and identified no rib fractures.[65] In the absence of a documented high-energy injury, such as a motor vehicle crash or a fall from a significant height, rib fractures in young children should raise concern for child abuse.[47,48,66]

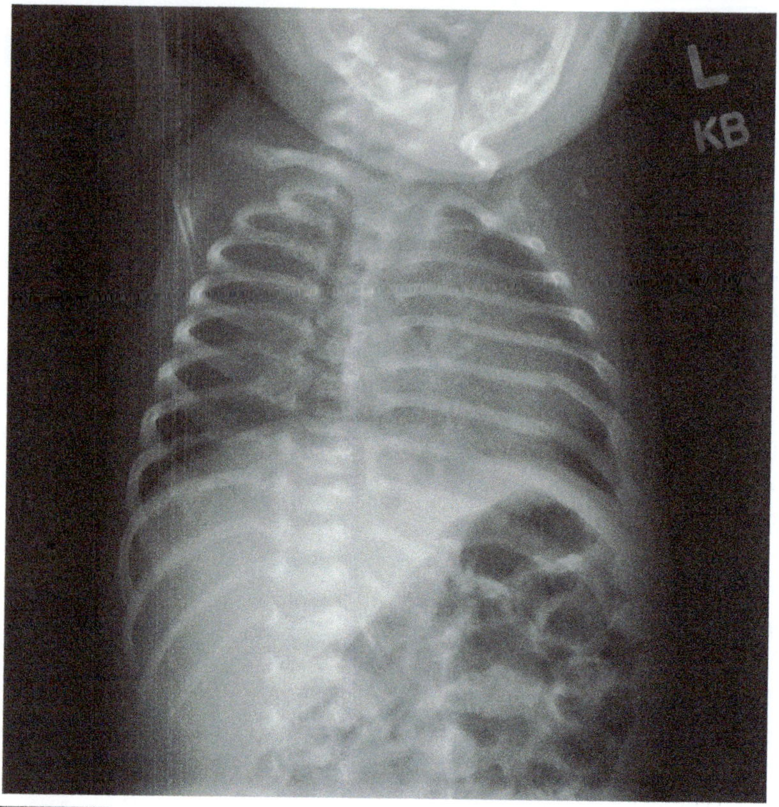

FIGURE 4.8
Rib fractures.

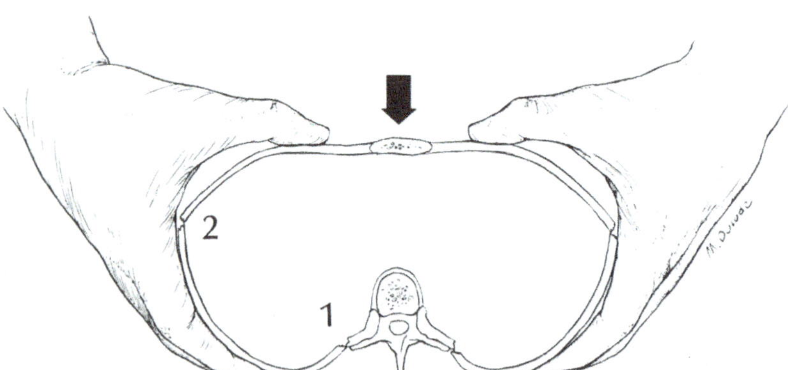

FIGURE 4.9
With anteroposterior compression of the chest, rib fractures occur initially in the proximal rib over the transverse process of the adjacent vertebrae (1) and more laterally along the posterior arc of the rib to the midaxillary line (2).

Sternum, Scapula, and Pelvic Fractures

Fractures of the sternum, scapula, and pelvis are rare in children and are almost always the result of high-energy trauma. They should trigger concern for abuse in the absence of a verifiable, plausible mechanism, such as a motor vehicle crash or a fall from a significant height.[47,67–71]

Multiple Fractures

Multiple fractures, either acute or in various stages of healing, are highly specific for abuse.[6,30,72] (Figure 4.10). Fifty percent overall of children who have experienced abuse, and 80% of those younger than 1 year, will be diagnosed with more than 1 fracture.[47,49,73] There is an odds ratio for likelihood of abuse of 4 to 6 for children with 3 or more fractures, compared with those with only 1 fracture.[6] A specific common pattern is bilateral acute femoral, tibial, or humeral fractures, consistent with the child being held and shaken by the extremities.[3,74–76]

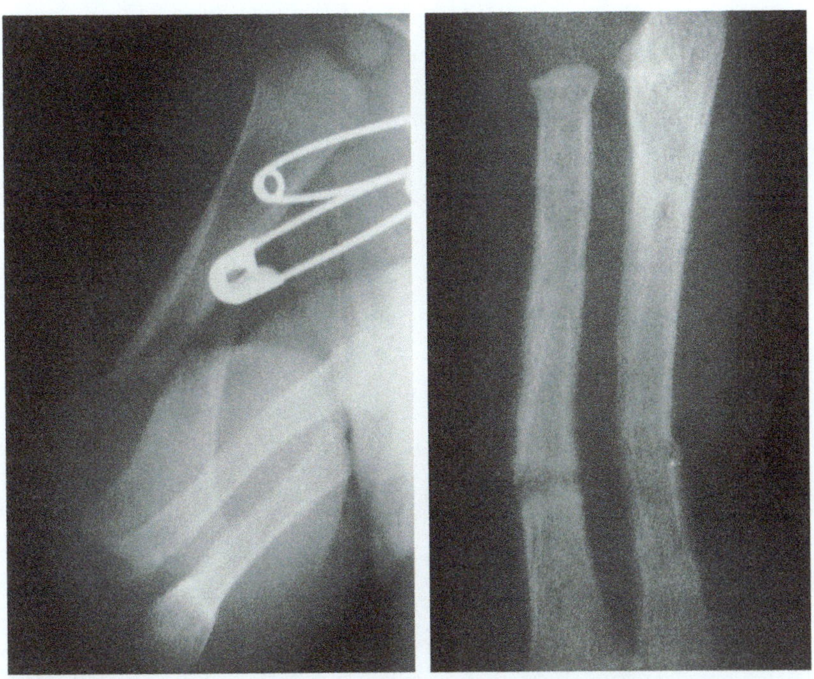

FIGURE 4.10
Multiple fractures in various stages of healing in the same individual. The humerus is acute in appearance with no signs of healing, while the radius and ulna have periosteal elevation and callus formation.

Fractures Associated With Other Injuries

Acute or healing fractures diagnosed in conjunction with other corroborative injuries are indicative of abuse. Examples of other suspicious or sentinel injuries include burns, bruises, frenulum tears, intracranial hemorrhage, subconjunctival hemorrhage, and abdominal or genital injury.[77]

Mid-Specificity Fractures

Spine Fractures

Like fractures of the sternum and scapula, traumatic spine fractures are unusual in children and typically are the result of a high-energy injury. They can result from a direct impact or indirectly from flexion and extension forces.[78] In the absence of a verifiable accident, they are concerning for abuse but not as specifically as the high-specificity fractures discussed previously. Spinal fractures account for about 1% to 3% of accidental and abusive pediatric fractures.[78] Anterior compression fractures secondary to axial load are most common and are frequently asymptomatic. They are often an incidental finding on skeletal survey[79] (Figure 4.11). However, compression can be forceful enough to cause

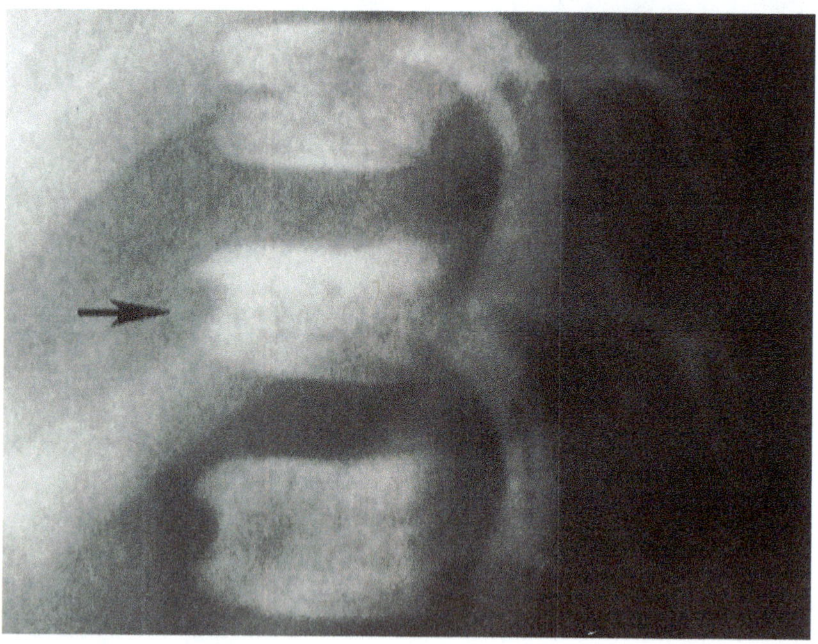

FIGURE 4.11
Compression fracture of a lumbar vertebral body.

retropulsion of bone fragments into the spinal canal (burst fracture), which can result in spinal cord compression and neurologic disability. Flexion or extension mechanisms cause a variety of fracture patterns of the posterior elements of the vertebrae, typically in the cervical spine or at the cervicothoracic or thoracolumbar junctions. They are more likely to be symptomatic and cause neurologic compromise.[80–82]

Fractures of the Hands and Feet

Accidental fractures of the hands and feet are uncommon in nonambulatory children and should raise concern if diagnosed in children younger than walking age. They are found on up to 10% of skeletal surveys performed with dedicated coned-down views of the hands and feet[79] (Figure 4.12).

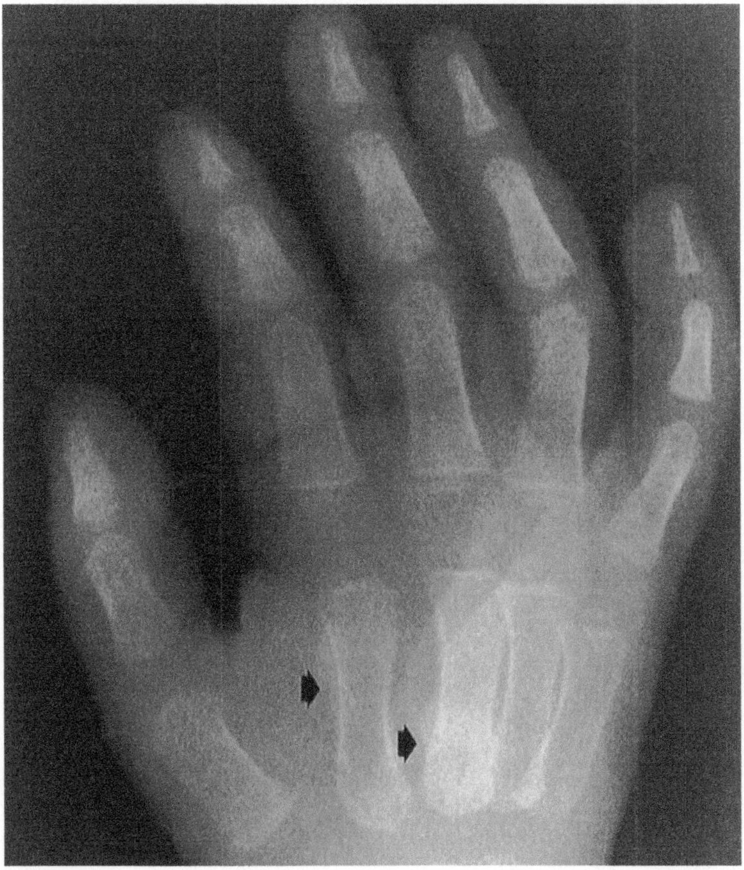

FIGURE 4.12
Healing fractures of the second and third carpel bones.

Skull Fractures

Corroborative history is important in the evaluation of skull fractures, because the most common fracture pattern is the same in accidental and abusive trauma: a simple, linear parietal fracture.[83–85] Abuse should be suspected in cases of inconsistent or implausible history. The literature varies on whether or not more complex skull fractures (stellate, depressed, diastatic, multiple, bilateral, or crossing suture lines) are more likely than simple fractures to be associated with abuse[83,85–87] (Figure 4.13). Short falls (<3 feet) are unlikely to cause a complex skull fracture.[88,89]

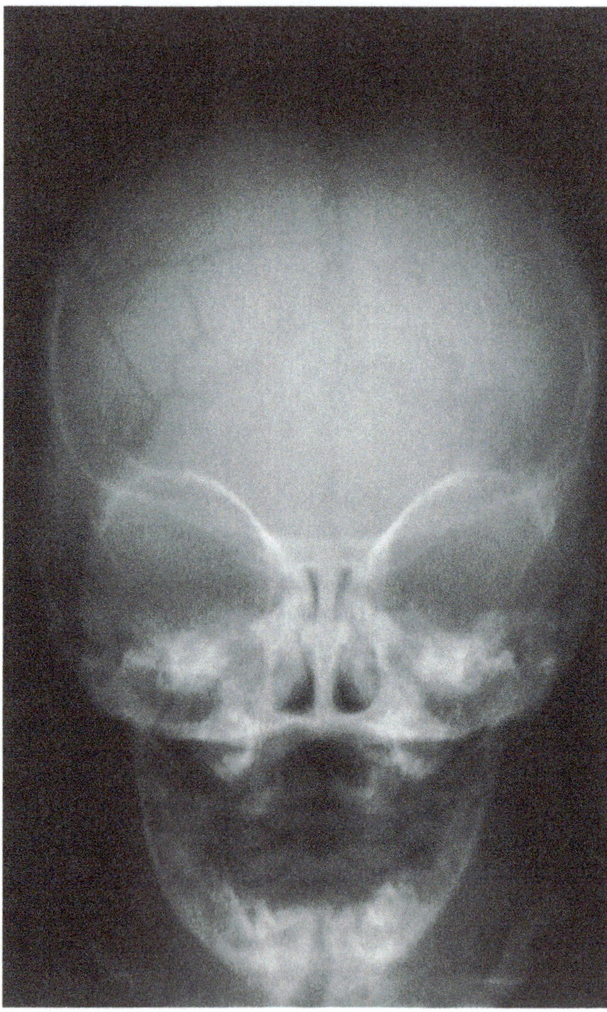

FIGURE 4.13
Complex or stellate skull fracture.

Clavicle Fractures

Fractures of the clavicle are a common result of birth trauma. In such cases, callus formation will be visible on radiography when the baby is 7 to 10 days old. An acute clavicle fracture (Figure 4.14), without evidence of healing callus, in a neonate older than 10 days should raise concern for abuse. Most clavicle fractures, both accidental and inflicted, occur in the mid-shaft region. Distal and proximal clavicle fractures are uncommon in children younger than 3 years; in this cohort, they can be the result of shaking.[68] In various studies, clavicle fractures have been reported in 3% to 10% of cases of abuse.[28,67,90,91]

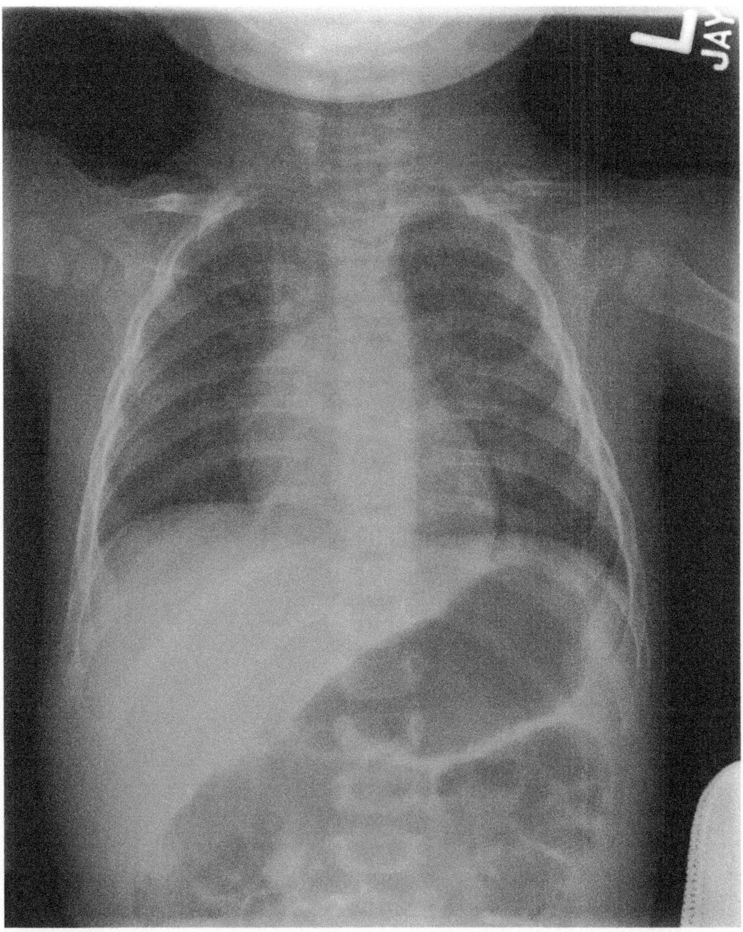

FIGURE 4.14

A 6-month-old presents after 2 episodes of altered breathing and cyanosis. Evaluation revealed a biparietal skull fracture, bilateral subdural hematomas, left clavicular fracture with minimal callus formation, and bruising of the leg, forehead, and foot. No history of trauma was offered.

Isolated Long Bone Fracture in an Ambulatory Child Without a Plausible History

A long bone fracture in an ambulatory child that results from an unwitnessed injury or for which no plausible explanation is given presents a diagnostic challenge. It should raise concern for abuse and, therefore, should be evaluated with a workup for abuse. However, this situation is not as suspicious as that of a nonambulatory child with a fracture. In all these cases, a thorough history and physical examination, including a detailed social history, can assist in determining the likelihood of an accidental or abusive injury.

Low-Specificity Fractures

Toddler Fracture

A toddler fracture typically presents as an isolated, non-displaced spiral fracture of the distal tibial metaphysis, although it can be diaphyseal as well. Often, it is necessary to obtain an oblique radiograph of the tibia to adequately visualize the fracture. These fractures are sustained by ambulatory children and can result from seemingly trivial injury; parents often report a misstep off a stair or curb or a simple standing-height fall. A well-documented etiology for this fracture pattern is a child getting his or her foot caught along the edge of a playground slide while going down the slide seated on an adult's lap.[92] This particular mechanism can occur in nonambulatory children. However, keep in mind that a radiology report of "toddler fracture" is by no means a guarantee of accidental etiology, and, with the exception of the slide mechanism noted previously, a child must be ambulatory to sustain a true toddler fracture. Another low-specificity variation of tibia fracture is a transverse or torus fracture of the proximal tibial metaphysis, caused by the recoil of the mat of a trampoline.[93]

Distal Radial and Ulnar Torus Fractures

Buckle fractures of the distal radius and ulna are the result of compressive forces that typically occur from a fall on an outstretched arm or from running into a barrier with the arm outstretched. They are extremely common and are almost always accidental.

Supracondylar Humerus Fractures

Supracondylar humerus fractures are typically accidental and occur from a fall, often from playground equipment or a trampoline.[43,44,94] In one study of 388 supracondylar humerus fractures, the mechanism was a fall in 79% and child abuse in 0.5%.[94] However, as is the case with other types of fractures, it is still necessary to maintain a higher index of suspicion the younger the child is. Another study found 30% (3 of 10) supracondylar fractures in children younger than 3 years to be abusive.[44]

Differential Diagnosis

Fracture mechanisms other than abuse should always be considered as part of the evaluation. A thorough past medical and family history can help to narrow down possible medical conditions that may contribute to fractures. The workup and management of medical conditions can be improved with the assistance of other subspecialties including orthopedic surgery, endocrinology, and genetics.

The most common cause of a fracture in a child is an accidental injury. Medical conditions such as OI, rickets, and disuse osteopenia can predispose children to fracture with minimal force. These conditions are commonly brought up by families and defense attorneys in cases of suspected child abuse. It is important that medical professionals evaluate each suspected abuse case individually to ensure that alternate causes have been properly ruled in or out. However, a child who is found to have a medical condition can still experience abuse.

Accidental Fractures

Accidental fractures represent a significant number of injuries every year. In children younger than 3 years, more than 70% of fractures are the result of an accidental injury.[6] It is not uncommon in cases of inflicted injury for the caregiver to provide a false history of injury, most commonly involving a household fall. However, children can be unpredictable and have been reported to have some rather unexpected injuries from normal play. The presenting history must be carefully considered in light of the child's developmental abilities and the pattern of fracture presented.

Obstetric Trauma

Birth trauma, especially clavicular fractures, can be occult and missed in the newborn period. Clavicular fractures are very common in typical newborn deliveries and should be considered in an infant who presents within a month or two of delivery. Long bone and skull fractures are rarer and are usually only seen in traumatic deliveries. Rib fractures have been reported as a result of birth trauma but are rare and associated with large neonates and traumatic deliveries.[62]

Nutritional and Metabolic Causes

Rickets

Vitamin D deficiency rickets is rare in developed countries. While children may be found to have laboratory evidence of vitamin D deficiency or insufficiency, rickets and the resultant increase in bony fragility is only seen when there are clear findings on radiography.[95] These findings include demineralization, loss of zone of provisional calcification, widening of the physes, and metaphyseal cupping (Figure 4.15).

Abnormal bone metabolism can also be the result of renal disease (renal osteodystrophy). Chronic kidney disease results in abnormalities in phosphorus, calcium, vitamin D, and parathyroid levels in the bones.[96] Patients can develop significant bony fragility, especially if their condition is inadequately managed. These conditions are rarely confused with abuse because of the clear medical history of renal disease.

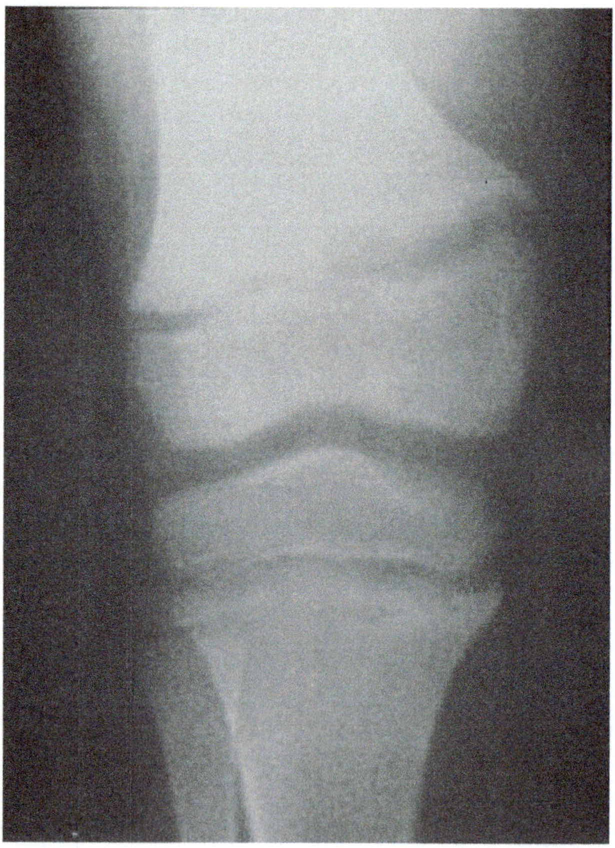

FIGURE 4.15
Rickets with widening of the physes and metaphyseal cupping.

Preterm Birth

Preterm birth, especially when the child is severely preterm or very ill, can result in bony fragility as a result of inadequate bone mineralization.[97] The third trimester is the period during which a fetus's bony skeleton is mineralized; the loss of that trimester can contribute to poor bone development. In addition, use of diuretics or prolonged parenteral nutrition can also contribute to poor bone mineralization. Some of these neonates even sustain iatrogenic fractures while hospitalized.

Osteogenesis Imperfecta

Skeletal dysplasias such as OI are rare genetic conditions that may result in fragile bones that are more prone to fracture. Osteogenesis imperfecta is caused by defects in the formation of type I collagen. The most common mutations are seen in the *COL1A1* and *COL1A2* genes. Depending on the variant, these can present at or near birth with in utero fractures and severe bowing of the extremities, conditions that are unlikely to be mistaken for abuse (Figure 4.16). Less severe types of OI typically manifest with fractures that could be mistaken for abuse, including extremity

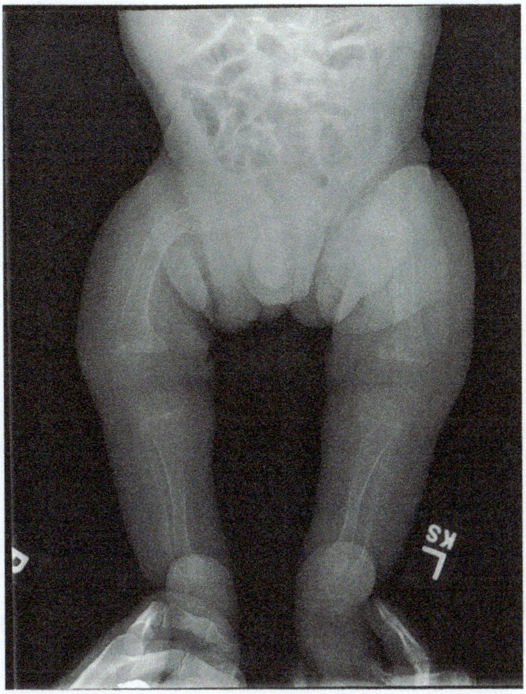

FIGURE 4.16
Osteogenesis imperfecta as shown with severe osteopenia and bowing of the long bones.

fractures; however, these typically present in ambulatory children. Common findings include wormian bones in the skull (Figure 4.17), blue sclera, and dentinogenesis imperfecta.[98] A family history of easily fractured bones or dental anomalies may assist in determining if the child is at risk for a skeletal dysplasia; however, many of these are de novo genetic abnormalities, and the lack of a family history does not rule out a skeletal dysplasia. In cases where there is significant concern for bony fragility, consultation with a geneticist and/or more detailed genetic testing for the common genetic findings in OI can assist in diagnosis.

Other Conditions

Scurvy, or vitamin C deficiency, is rare with appropriate nutrition but is still seen in cases of food fads and other limited diets.[99] Children with scurvy have metaphyseal changes that may mimic CMLs, but other findings, including the diet history, osteopenia, and mucous membrane hemorrhages, can assist in assigning the proper diagnosis.[100] Menkes disease is a rare x-linked recessive genetic condition that results from a defect in copper metabolism. Metaphyseal changes and subperiosteal new bone formation may be seen on radiographs. However, children with Menkes disease commonly have identifiable sparse, kinky hair as well as

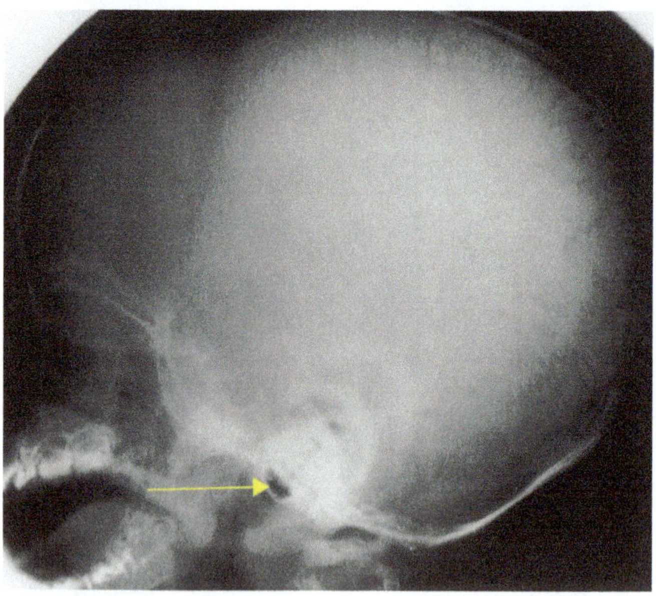

FIGURE 4.17
Osteogenesis imperfecta with wormian bones.

failure to thrive, developmental delay, wormian bones, and anterior rib flaring.[101] There are other rare genetic diseases that can predispose infants and children to fractures. These are usually readily apparent with physical examination and radiographs.[102]

Infection/Neoplasm

Bony infections (osteomyelitis) and neoplasms can lead to bony fragility and pathologic fractures. These are usually easy to distinguish from abuse with history, physical examination, laboratory evaluation, and radiography. Osteomyelitis can be present with septic arthritis and may have irregularities at the metaphyses that may resemble CMLs. Examination and laboratory assessment will reveal systemic concerns such as fever, elevated white blood cell count, erythrocyte sedimentation rate, C-reactive protein, and other markers for infection.[8] Lytic bony lesions can be malignant or benign but are usually clearly visible on radiograph, especially to a trained radiologist. Bony metastases can also cause bony fragility and leave children more prone to fracture, but again, these conditions should be readily identified with routine laboratory assessment.

Disuse Osteopenia

Children with musculoskeletal conditions that prohibit them from typical ambulation and movement are at risk for demineralization as a result of the lack of weight-bearing and movement.[103] These children can develop fractures as a result of routine caregiving, such as physical therapy and transfers. Difficulty also arises because these children are at increased risk of abuse due to their vulnerable status.[22]

Normal Variants

Some normal variation in bony structure on radiography can be misinterpreted as a fracture or a sign of abuse. The most common finding misinterpreted as abuse is subperiosteal new bone formation (Figure 4.18). While this is a frequent finding in healing fractures, it may also be present in normal, uninjured infants, especially when the finding is bilateral and does not extend to the metaphysis.[104] There are many variations in the appearance of the metaphysis in infants. Some of these, like a beaked appearance, can mimic a CML. Vessel tracts in the bones can have the appearance of non-displaced fractures. Obtaining repeat radiographs in 2 to 3 weeks can assist in determining if the irregularities are indeed fractures (with interval healing or bony changes) or bony variants (no interval changes).[105]

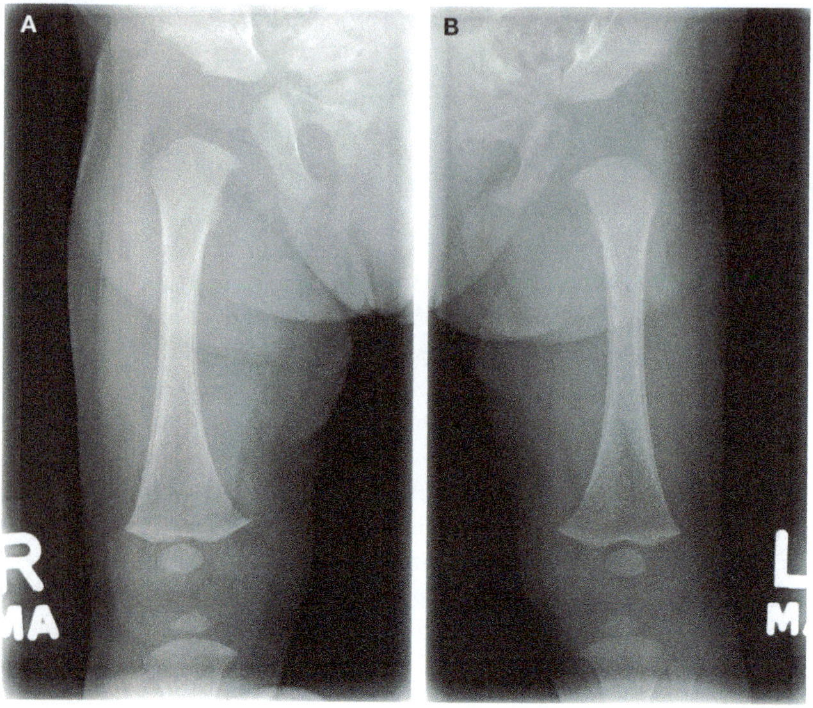

FIGURE 4.18
Femur periosteal reaction. A, Right. B, Left.

Management and Follow-up of Fractures

Because closed fractures in very young children have great healing and remodeling potential, most fractures secondary to inflicted injury can be treated nonoperatively. Asymptomatic, healing fractures (ie, those exhibiting periosteal reaction or callus formation), as are often found on skeletal survey, may not require any acute treatment or immobilization. For acute, symptomatic fractures, casts or splints may be used. Femur fractures in infants younger than 6 months can be treated in a Pavlik harness.[38] Proximal humerus or clavicle fractures in infants can be immobilized with a simple, non-constricting swathe or by connecting the long sleeve of the child's shirt to the front of the shirt with a safety pin. Fractures that may require operative treatment include open fractures, intraarticular fractures, or displaced physeal fractures. An example would be a displaced trans-physeal distal humerus fracture, which, if diagnosed acutely, usually requires operative reduction and pinning.

Short-term complications and long-term sequelae from childhood fractures are uncommon, although delay in diagnosis holds up initiation of appropriate pain management. Most uncomplicated fractures are fully healed within 3 months and completely remodeled within 1 year. Fractures involving the physis are typically followed with serial radiographs for 1 to 2 years, depending on the age of the child, to monitor growth plate function. If premature physeal arrest does occur, treatment is typically surgical but depends on the age of the child, location of the injury, and extent of limb length difference or angular deformity.

Conclusion

Fractures are a frequent physical finding in cases of child abuse, second in incidence only to cutaneous soft tissue injuries.[106] Up to 55% of children who have experienced physical abuse are reported to have sustained an inflicted fracture.[28,47] These children are generally quite young; 85% of non-accidental fractures are diagnosed in children younger than 3 years, with 69% diagnosed in infants younger than 12 months.[28,67,83] Developmental stage consistent with the ability to independently ambulate is an important factor; until children can walk on their own, they are far less likely to engage in activities in which an accidental injury can occur.

Despite fractures being a common manifestation of inflicted trauma, they can pose a diagnostic dilemma. There is no fracture pattern, location, or morphology that is pathognomonic for child abuse. However, certain fractures and fracture patterns are more or less suggestive of inflicted trauma. Knowing the differences between the high-, mid-, and low-specificity fractures can aid in workup and diagnosis.

References

1. Tardieu A. Ėtude mėdio lėgale sur les sėrvices et mauvais traitments exercės sur des enfants. *Annales d'hygiene publique et de mėdicine lėgale*. 1860;13:355–366
2. Caffey J. Multiple fractures in the long bones of infants suffering from chronic subdural hematoma. *Am J Roentgenol Radium Ther*. 1946;56(2):163–173 PMID: 20995763
3. Caffey J. On the theory and practice of shaking infants. Its potential residual effects of permanent brain damage and mental retardation. *Am J Dis Child*. 1972;124(2):161–169 PMID: 4559532 https://doi.org/10.1001/archpedi.1972.02110140011001
4. Kempe CH, Silverman FN, Steele BF, Droegemueller W, Silver HK. The battered-child syndrome. *JAMA*. 1962;181:17–24 PMID: 14455086
5. Rivara FP, Parish RA, Mueller BA. Extremity injuries in children: predictive value of clinical findings. *Pediatrics*. 1986;78(5):803–807 PMID: 3763294
6. Leventhal JM, Martin KD, Asnes AG. Incidence of fractures attributable to abuse in young hospitalized children: results from analysis of a United States database. *Pediatrics*. 2008;122(3):599–604 PMID: 18762531 https://doi.org/10.1542/peds.2007-1959
7. Pierce MC, Bertocci GE, Janosky JE, et al. Femur fractures resulting from stair falls among children: an injury plausibility model. *Pediatrics*. 2005;115(6):1712–1722 PMID: 15930236 https://doi.org/10.1542/peds.2004-0614

8. Flaherty EG, Perez-Rossello JM, Levine MA, Hennrikus WL; American Academy of Pediatrics Committee on Child Abuse and Neglect, Section on Radiology, Section on Endocrinology, and Section on Orthopaedics; Society for Pediatric Radiology. Evaluating children with fractures for child physical abuse. *Pediatrics*. 2014;133(2): e477–e489 PMID: 24470642 https://doi.org/10.1542/peds.2013-3793
9. Peters ML, Starling SP, Barnes-Eley ML, Heisler KW. The presence of bruising associated with fractures. *Arch Pediatr Adolesc Med*. 2008;162(9):877–881 PMID: 18762607 https://doi.org/10.1001/archpedi.162.9.877
10. American College of Radiology. ACR practice guideline for skeletal surveys in children (res. 47, 17, 35). In: ACR Standards. Reston, VA: American College of Radiology; 2006:203–207 https://www.acr.org/-/media/ACR/Files/Practice-Parameters/Skeletal-Survey.pdf
11. Lindberg DM, Berger RP, Reynolds MS, Alwan RM, Harper NS; Examining Siblings to Recognize Abuse Investigators. Yield of skeletal survey by age in children referred to abuse specialists. *J Pediatr*. 2014;164(6):1268–1273.e1 PMID: 24630357 https://doi.org/10.1016/j.jpeds.2014.01.068
12. Harper NS, Eddleman S, Lindberg DM; ExSTRA Investigators. The utility of follow-up skeletal surveys in child abuse. *Pediatrics*. 2013;131(3):e672–e678 PMID: 23400607 https://doi.org/10.1542/peds.2012-2608
13. Harlan SR, Nixon GW, Campbell KA, Hansen K, Prince JS. Follow-up skeletal surveys for nonaccidental trauma: can a more limited survey be performed? *Pediatr Radiol*. 2009;39(9):962–968 PMID: 19565233 https://doi.org/10.1007/s00247-009-1313-7
14. Chapman S. Radiological aspects of non-accidental injury. *J R Soc Med*. 1990;83(2):67–71 PMID: 2181137 https://doi.org/10.1177/014107689008300204
15. Rao P, Carty H. Non-accidental injury: review of the radiology. *Clin Radiol*. 1999;54(1): 11–24 PMID: 9915505 https://doi.org/10.1016/S0009-9260(99)91234-5
16. Smeets AJ, Robben SG, Meradji M. Sonographically detected costo-chondral dislocation in an abused child. A new sonographic sign to the radiological spectrum of child abuse. *Pediatr Radiol*. 1990;20(7):566–567 PMID: 2216598 https://doi.org/10.1007/BF02011396
17. Supakul N, Hicks RA, Caltoum CB, Karmazyn B. Distal humeral epiphyseal separation in young children: an often-missed fracture-radiographic signs and ultrasound confirmatory diagnosis. *AJR Am J Roentgenol*. 2015;204(2):W192–W198 PMID: 25615780 https://doi.org/10.2214/AJR.14.12788
18. Perez-Rossello JM, Connolly SA, Newton AW, Zou KH, Kleinman PK. Whole-body MRI in suspected infant abuse. *AJR Am J Roentgenol*. 2010;195(3):744–750 PMID: 20729455 https://doi.org/10.2214/AJR.09.3364
19. Drubach LA, Sapp MV, Laffin S, Kleinman PK. Fluorine-18 NaF PET imaging of child abuse. *Pediatr Radiol*. 2008;38(7):776–779 PMID: 18504566 https://doi.org/10.1007/s00247-008-0885-y
20. Drubach LA, Johnston PR, Newton AW, Perez-Rossello JM, Grant FD, Kleinman PK. Skeletal trauma in child abuse: detection with 18F-NaF PET. *Radiology*. 2010;255(1): 173–181 PMID: 20308455 https://doi.org/10.1148/radiol.09091368
21. Lindberg DM, Shapiro RA, Laskey AL, Pallin DJ, Blood EA, Berger RP; ExSTRA Investigators. Prevalence of abusive injuries in siblings and household contacts of physically abused children. *Pediatrics*. 2012;130(2):193–201 PMID: 22778300 https://doi.org/10.1542/peds.2012-0085
22. Jenny C; American Academy of Pediatrics Committee on Child Abuse and Neglect. Evaluating infants and young children with multiple fractures. *Pediatrics*. 2006;118(3):1299–1303 PMID: 16951031 https://doi.org/10.1542/peds.2006-1795

23. Halliday KE, Broderick NJ, Somers JM, Hawkes R. Dating fractures in infants. *Clin Radiol*. 2011;66(11):1049–1054 PMID: 21763645 https://doi.org/10.1016/j.crad.2011.06.001
24. Bottlang M, Fitzpatrick DC, Augat P. Musculoskeletal biomechanics. In: Flynn J, ed. Orthopaedic Knowledge Update 10. Vol 10. Rosemont, IL: American Academy of Orthopaedic Surgeons; 2011:59–72
25. Le T, Benedetti GE, eds. Biomechanics of Fracture and Fixation. Orthopaedic Core Curriculum. Rosemont, IL: Orthopaedic Trauma Association; 2009
26. Thompson A, Bertocci G, Kaczor K, Smalley C, Pierce MC. Biomechanical investigation of the classic metaphyseal lesion using an immature porcine model. *AJR Am J Roentgenol*. 2015;204(5):W503–W509 PMID: 25905956 https://doi.org/10.2214/AJR.14.13267
27. Kleinman PK, ed. *Diagnostic Imaging of Child Abuse*. 3rd ed. Cambridge, United Kingdom: Cambridge University Press; 2015
28. King J, Diefendorf D, Apthorp J, Negrete VF, Carlson M. Analysis of 429 fractures in 189 battered children. *J Pediatr Orthop*. 1988;8(5):585–589 PMID: 3170740
29. Beals RK, Tufts E. Fractured femur in infancy: the role of child abuse. *J Pediatr Orthop*. 1983;3(5):583–586 PMID: 6655054 https://doi.org/10.1097/01241398-198311000-00004
30. Kemp AM, Dunstan F, Harrison S, et al. Patterns of skeletal fractures in child abuse: systematic review. *BMJ*. 2008;337(oct02 1):a1518 PMID: 18832412 https://doi.org/10.1136/bmj.a1518
31. Pandya NK, Baldwin K, Wolfgruber H, Christian CW, Drummond DS, Hosalkar HS. Child abuse and orthopaedic injury patterns: analysis at a level I pediatric trauma center. *J Pediatr Orthop*. 2009;29(6):618–625 PMID: 19700994 https://doi.org/10.1097/BPO.0b013e3181b2b3ee
32. Hui C, Joughin E, Goldstein S, et al. Femoral fractures in children younger than three years: the role of nonaccidental injury. *J Pediatr Orthop*. 2008;28(3):297–302 PMID: 18362793 https://doi.org/10.1097/BPO.0b013e3181653bf9
33. Scherl SA, Miller L, Lively N, Russinoff S, Sullivan CM, Tornetta P 3rd. Accidental and nonaccidental femur fractures in children. *Clin Orthop Relat Res*. 2000;(376):96–105 PMID: 10906863
34. Schwend RM, Werth C, Johnston A. Femur shaft fractures in toddlers and young children: rarely from child abuse. *J Pediatr Orthop*. 2000;20(4):475–481 PMID: 10912603 https://doi.org/10.1097/01241398-200007000-00010
35. Son-Hing JP, Deniz Olgun Z. The frequency of nonaccidental trauma in children under the age of 3 years with femur fractures: is there a better cutoff point for universal workups? *J Pediatr Orthop B*. 2018;27(4):366–368 PMID: 28926487 https://doi.org/10.1097/BPB.0000000000000495
36. Gross RH, Stranger M. Causative factors responsible for femoral fractures in infants and young children. *J Pediatr Orthop*. 1983;3(3):341–343 PMID: 6874931 https://doi.org/10.1097/01241398-198307000-00012
37. McClelland CQ, Heiple KG. Fractures in the first year of life. A diagnostic dilemma. *Am J Dis Child*. 1982;136(1):26–29 PMID: 7055105 https://doi.org/10.1001/archpedi.1982.03970370028006
38. Kocher MS, Sink EL, Blasier RD, et al; American Academy of Orthopaedic Surgeons. American Academy of Orthopaedic Surgeons clinical practice guideline on treatment of pediatric diaphyseal femur fracture. *J Bone Joint Surg Am*. 2010;92(8):1790–1792 PMID: 20660244 https://doi.org/10.2106/JBJS.J.00137
39. Taitz J, Moran K, O'Meara M. Long bone fractures in children under 3 years of age: is abuse being missed in emergency department presentations? *J Paediatr Child Health*. 2004;40(4):170–174 PMID: 15009543 https://doi.org/10.1111/j.1440-1754.2004.00332.x

40. Arkader A, Friedman JE, Warner WC Jr, Wells L. Complete distal femoral metaphyseal fractures: a harbinger of child abuse before walking age. *J Pediatr Orthop*. 2007;27(7): 751–753 PMID: 17878779 https://doi.org/10.1097/BPO.0b013e3181558b13
41. Haney SB, Boos SC, Kutz TJ, Starling SP. Transverse fracture of the distal femoral metadiaphysis: a plausible accidental mechanism. *Pediatr Emerg Care*. 2009;25(12):841–844 PMID: 19952971 https://doi.org/10.1097/PEC.0b013e3181c330f0
42. Coffey C, Haley K, Hayes J, Groner JI. The risk of child abuse in infants and toddlers with lower extremity injuries. *J Pediatr Surg*. 2005;40(1):120–123 PMID: 15868570 https://doi.org/10.1016/j.jpedsurg.2004.09.003
43. Shaw BA, Murphy KM, Shaw A, Oppenheim WL, Myracle MR. Humerus shaft fractures in young children: accident or abuse? *J Pediatr Orthop*. 1997;17(3):293–297 PMID: 9150014 https://doi.org/10.1097/01241398-199705000-00005
44. Strait RT, Siegel RM, Shapiro RA. Humeral fractures without obvious etiologies in children less than 3 years of age: when is it abuse? *Pediatrics*. 1995;96(4 Pt 1):667–671 PMID: 7567328
45. Salter RB, Harris WR. Injuries involving the epiphyseal plate. *J Bone Joint Surg*. 1963;45(3):587–622 https://doi.org/10.2106/00004623-196345030-00019
46. Slongo T, Audigé L, Schlickewei W, Clavert JM, Hunter J; International Association for Pediatric Traumatology. Development and validation of the AO pediatric comprehensive classification of long bone fractures by the Pediatric Expert Group of the AO Foundation in collaboration with AO Clinical Investigation and Documentation and the International Association for Pediatric Traumatology. *J Pediatr Orthop*. 2006;26(1):43–49 PMID: 16439900 https://doi.org/10.1097/01.bpo.0000187989.64021.ml
47. Kocher MS, Kasser JR. Orthopaedic aspects of child abuse. *J Am Acad Orthop Surg*. 2000;8(1):10–20 PMID: 10666649 https://doi.org/10.5435/00124635-200001000-00002
48. Offiah A, van Rijn RR, Perez-Rossello JM, Kleinman PK. Skeletal imaging of child abuse (non-accidental injury). *Pediatr Radiol*. 2009;39(5):461–470 PMID: 19238374 https://doi.org/10.1007/s00247-009-1157-1
49. Stewart GM, Rosenberg NM. Conditions mistaken for child abuse: part I. *Pediatr Emerg Care*. 1996;12(2):116–121 PMID: 8859923 https://doi.org/10.1097/00006565-199604000-00014
50. Worlock P, Stower M, Barbor P. Patterns of fractures in accidental and non-accidental injury in children: a comparative study. *Br Med J (Clin Res Ed)*. 1986;293(6539):100–102 PMID: 3089406 https://doi.org/10.1136/bmj.293.6539.100
51. Loder RT, Bookout C. Fracture patterns in battered children. *J Orthop Trauma*. 1991;5(4):428–433 PMID: 1762003 https://doi.org/10.1097/00005131-199112000-00007
52. Pierce MC, Bertocci GE, Vogeley E, Moreland MS. Evaluating long bone fractures in children: a biomechanical approach with illustrative cases. *Child Abuse Negl*. 2004;28(5):505–524 PMID: 15206413 https://doi.org/10.1016/j.chiabu.2003.01.001
53. Kleinman PK, Marks SC, Blackbourne B. The metaphyseal lesion in abused infants: a radiologic-histopathologic study. *AJR Am J Roentgenol*. 1986;146(5):895–905 PMID: 3485907 https://doi.org/10.2214/ajr.146.5.895
54. Kleinman PK, Blackbourne BD, Marks SC, Karellas A, Belanger PL. Radiologic contributions to the investigation and prosecution of cases of fatal infant abuse. *N Engl J Med*. 1989;320(8):507–511 PMID: 2915652 https://doi.org/10.1056/NEJM198902233200807
55. Paddock M, Sprigg A, Offiah AC. Imaging and reporting considerations for suspected physical abuse (non-accidental injury) in infants and young children. Part 1: initial considerations and appendicular skeleton. *Clin Radiol*. 2017;72(3):179–188 PMID: 28063602 https://doi.org/10.1016/j.crad.2016.11.016
56. Grayev AM, Boal DK, Wallach DM, Segal LS. Metaphyseal fractures mimicking abuse during treatment for clubfoot. *Pediatr Radiol*. 2001;31(8):559–563 PMID: 11550767 https://doi.org/10.1007/s002470100497

57. Lysack JT, Soboleski D. Classic metaphyseal lesion following external cephalic version and cesarean section. *Pediatr Radiol*. 2003;33(6):422–424 PMID: 12709748 https://doi.org/10.1007/s00247-003-0914-9
58. Paine CW, Fakeye O, Christian CW, Wood JN. Prevalence of abuse among young children with rib fractures: a systematic review. *Pediatr Emerg Care*. 2019;35(2):96–103 PMID: 27749806 https://doi.org/10.1097/PEC.0000000000000911
59. Betz P, Liebhardt E. Rib fractures in children—resuscitation or child abuse? *Int J Legal Med*. 1994;106(4):215–218 PMID: 8038115 https://doi.org/10.1007/BF01371340
60. Barsness KA, Cha ES, Bensard DD, et al. The positive predictive value of rib fractures as an indicator of nonaccidental trauma in children. *J Trauma*. 2003;54(6):1107–1110 PMID: 12813330 https://doi.org/10.1097/01.TA.0000068992.01030.A8
61. Cadzow SP, Armstrong KL. Rib fractures in infants: red alert! The clinical features, investigations and child protection outcomes. *J Paediatr Child Health*. 2000;36(4): 322–326 PMID: 10940163 https://doi.org/10.1046/j.1440-1754.2000.00515.x
62. Bulloch B, Schubert CJ, Brophy PD, Johnson N, Reed MH, Shapiro RA. Cause and clinical characteristics of rib fractures in infants. *Pediatrics*. 2000;105(4):E48 PMID: 10742369 https://doi.org/10.1542/peds.105.4.e48
63. Feldman KW, Brewer DK. Child abuse, cardiopulmonary resuscitation, and rib fractures. *Pediatrics*. 1984;73(3):339–342 PMID: 6701057
64. Spevak MR, Kleinman PK, Belanger PL, Primack C, Richmond JM. Cardiopulmonary resuscitation and rib fractures in infants. A postmortem radiologic-pathologic study. *JAMA*. 1994;272(8):617–618 PMID: 8057518 https://doi.org/10.1001/jama.1994.03520080059044
65. Franke I, Pingen A, Schiffmann H, et al; for Arbeitsgemeinschaft Kinderschutz in der Medizin. Cardiopulmonary resuscitation (CPR)-related posterior rib fractures in neonates and infants following recommended changes in CPR techniques. *Child Abuse Negl*. 2014;38(7):1267–1274 PMID: 24636360 https://doi.org/10.1016/j.chiabu.2014.01.021
66. Garcia VF, Gotschall CS, Eichelberger MR, Bowman LM. Rib fractures in children: a marker of severe trauma. *J Trauma*. 1990;30(6):695–700 PMID: 2352299 https://doi.org/10.1097/00005373-199006000-00007
67. Akbarnia B, Torg JS, Kirkpatrick J, Sussman S. Manifestations of the battered-child syndrome. *J Bone Joint Surg Am*. 1974;56(6):1159–1166 PMID: 4436352 https://doi.org/10.2106/00004623-197456060-00005
68. Kogutt MS, Swischuk LE, Fagan CJ. Patterns of injury and significance of uncommon fractures in the battered child syndrome. *Am J Roentgenol Radium Ther Nucl Med*. 1974;121(1):143–149 PMID: 4833902 https://doi.org/10.2214/ajr.121.1.143
69. Merten DF, Radkowski MA, Leonidas JC. The abused child: a radiological reappraisal. *Radiology*. 1983;146(2):377–381 PMID: 6849085 https://doi.org/10.1148/radiology.146.2.6849085
70. Ablin DS, Greenspan A, Reinhart MA. Pelvic injuries in child abuse. *Pediatr Radiol*. 1992;22(6):454–457 PMID: 1437374 https://doi.org/10.1007/BF02013511
71. Starling SP, Heller RM, Jenny C. Pelvic fractures in infants as a sign of physical abuse. *Child Abuse Negl*. 2002;26(5):475–480 PMID: 12079085 https://doi.org/10.1016/S0145-2134(02)00323-X
72. McGraw EP, Pless JE, Pennington DJ, White SJ. Postmortem radiography after unexpected death in neonates, infants, and children: should imaging be routine? *AJR Am J Roentgenol*. 2002;178(6):1517–1521 PMID: 12034631 https://doi.org/10.2214/ajr.178.6.1781517
73. Krishnan J, Barbour PJ, Foster BK. Patterns of osseous injuries and psychosocial factors affecting victims of child abuse. *Aust N Z J Surg*. 1990;60(6):447–450 PMID: 2346440 https://doi.org/10.1111/j.1445-2197.1990.tb07400.x

74. Caffey J. The parent-infant traumatic stress syndrome; (Caffey-Kempe syndrome), (battered babe syndrome). *Am J Roentgenol Radium Ther Nucl Med*. 1972;114(2):218–229 PMID: 5058509
75. Caffey J. The whiplash shaken infant syndrome: manual shaking by the extremities with whiplash-induced intracranial and intraocular bleedings, linked with residual permanent brain damage and mental retardation. *Pediatrics*. 1974;54(4):396–403 PMID: 4416579
76. Kleinman PK. Diagnostic imaging in infant abuse. *AJR Am J Roentgenol*. 1990;155(4): 703–712 PMID: 2119097 https://doi.org/10.2214/ajr.155.4.2119097
77. Lindberg DM, Beaty B, Juarez-Colunga E, Wood JN, Runyan DK. Testing for abuse in children with sentinel injuries. *Pediatrics*. 2015;136(5):831–838 PMID: 26438705 https://doi.org/10.1542/peds.2015-1487
78. Akbarnia BA. Pediatric spine fractures. *Orthop Clin North Am*. 1999;30(3):521–536, x PMID: 10393772 https://doi.org/10.1016/S0030-5898(05)70103-6
79. Lindberg DM, Harper NS, Laskey AL, Berger RP; ExSTRA Investigators. Prevalence of abusive fractures of the hands, feet, spine, or pelvis on skeletal survey: perhaps "uncommon" is more common than suggested. *Pediatr Emerg Care*. 2013;29(1):26–29 PMID: 23283258 https://doi.org/10.1097/PEC.0b013e31827b475e
80. Diamond P, Hansen CM, Christofersen MR. Child abuse presenting as a thoracolumbar spinal fracture dislocation: a case report. *Pediatr Emerg Care*. 1994;10(2):83–86 PMID: 8029116 https://doi.org/10.1097/00006565-199404000-00005
81. Gabos PG, Tuten HR, Leet A, Stanton RP. Fracture-dislocation of the lumbar spine in an abused child. *Pediatrics*. 1998;101(3 Pt 1):473–477 PMID: 9481017 https://doi.org/10.1542/peds.101.3.473
82. Rooks VJ, Sisler C, Burton B. Cervical spine injury in child abuse: report of two cases. *Pediatr Radiol*. 1998;28(3):193–195 PMID: 9561545 https://doi.org/10.1007/s002470050330
83. Leventhal JM, Thomas SA, Rosenfield NS, Markowitz RI. Fractures in young children. Distinguishing child abuse from unintentional injuries. *Am J Dis Child*. 1993;147(1):87–92 PMID: 8418609 https://doi.org/10.1001/archpedi.1993.02160250089028
84. Harwood-Nash DC, Hendrick EB, Hudson AR. The significance of skull fractures in children. A study of 1,187 patients. *Radiology*. 1971;101(1):151–156 PMID: 5111967 https://doi.org/10.1148/101.1.151
85. Meservy CJ, Towbin R, McLaurin RL, Myers PA, Ball W. Radiographic characteristics of skull fractures resulting from child abuse. *AJR Am J Roentgenol*. 1987;149(1):173–175 PMID: 3495978 https://doi.org/10.2214/ajr.149.1.173
86. Arnholz D, Hymel KP, Hay TC, Jenny C. Bilateral pediatric skull fractures: accident or abuse? *J Trauma*. 1998;45(1):172–174 PMID: 9680036 https://doi.org/10.1097/00005373-199807000-00039
87. Hobbs CJ. Skull fracture and the diagnosis of abuse. *Arch Dis Child*. 1984;59(3):246–252 PMID: 6712273 https://doi.org/10.1136/adc.59.3.246
88. Helfer RE, Slovis TL, Black M. Injuries resulting when small children fall out of bed. *Pediatrics*. 1977;60(4):533–535 PMID: 905018
89. Tarantino CA, Dowd MD, Murdock TC. Short vertical falls in infants. *Pediatr Emerg Care*. 1999;15(1):5–8 PMID: 10069302 https://doi.org/10.1097/00006565-199902000-00002
90. Galleno H, Oppenheim WL. The battered child syndrome revisited. *Clin Orthop Relat Res*. 1982;(162):11–19
91. Herndon WA. Child abuse in a military population. *J Pediatr Orthop*. 1983;3(1):73–76 PMID: 6841606 https://doi.org/10.1097/01241398-198302000-00012

92. Gaffney JT. Tibia fractures in children sustained on a playground slide. *J Pediatr Orthop*. 2009;29(6):606–608 PMID: 19700991 https://doi.org/10.1097/BPO.0b013e3181b2ba2f
93. Kakel R. Trampoline fracture of the proximal tibial metaphysis in children may not progress into valgus: a report of seven cases and a brief review. *Orthop Traumatol Surg Res*. 2012;98(4):446–449 PMID: 22579506 https://doi.org/10.1016/j.otsr.2012.02.007
94. Farnsworth CL, Silva PD, Mubarak SJ. Etiology of supracondylar humerus fractures. *J Pediatr Orthop*. 1998;18(1):38–42 PMID: 9449099 https://doi.org/10.1097/01241398-199801000-00008
95. Perez-Rossello JM, Feldman HA, Kleinman PK, et al. Rachitic changes, demineralization, and fracture risk in healthy infants and toddlers with vitamin D deficiency. *Radiology*. 2012;262(1):234–241 PMID: 22106354 https://doi.org/10.1148/radiol.11110358
96. Kemper MJ, van Husen M. Renal osteodystrophy in children: pathogenesis, diagnosis and treatment. *Curr Opin Pediatr*. 2014;26(2):180–186 PMID: 24553631 https://doi.org/10.1097/MOP.0000000000000061
97. Christian CW, States LJ. Medical mimics of child abuse. *AJR Am J Roentgenol*. 2017;208(5):982–990 PMID: 28225649 https://doi.org/10.2214/AJR.16.17450
98. Ablin DS, Greenspan A, Reinhart M, Grix A. Differentiation of child abuse from osteogenesis imperfecta. *AJR Am J Roentgenol*. 1990;154(5):1035–1046 PMID: 2108539 https://doi.org/10.2214/ajr.154.5.2108539
99. Shetty AK, Steele RW, Silas V, Dehne R. A boy with a limp. *Lancet*. 1998;351(9097):182 PMID: 9449874 https://doi.org/10.1016/S0140-6736(97)10235-5
100. Strelling MK. Infantile scurvy. *BMJ*. 1960;1(5174):701–703 PMID: 13835207 https://doi.org/10.1136/bmj.1.5174.701
101. Arita JH, Faria EC, Peruchi MM, Lin J, Rodrigues Masruha M, Vilanova LC. Menkes disease as a differential diagnosis of child abuse. *Arq Neuropsiquiatr*. 2009;67(2B): 507–509 PMID: 19623454 https://doi.org/10.1590/S0004-282X2009000300026
102. Bronicki LM, Stevenson RE, Spranger JW. Beyond osteogenesis imperfecta: causes of fractures during infancy and childhood. *Am J Med Genet C Semin Med Genet*. 2015;169(4):314–327 PMID: 26531771 https://doi.org/10.1002/ajmg.c.31466
103. Henderson RC, Lark RK, Gurka MJ, et al. Bone density and metabolism in children and adolescents with moderate to severe cerebral palsy. *Pediatrics*. 2002;110(1 Pt 1):e5 PMID: 12093986 https://doi.org/10.1542/peds.110.1.e5
104. Carty HM. Fractures caused by child abuse. *J Bone Joint Surg Br*. 1993;75(6):849–857 PMID: 8245070 https://doi.org/10.1302/0301-620X.75B6.8245070
105. Harper NS, Lewis T, Eddleman S, Lindberg DM; ExSTRA Investigators. Follow-up skeletal survey use by child abuse pediatricians. *Child Abuse Negl*. 2016;51:336–342 PMID: 26342432 https://doi.org/10.1016/j.chiabu.2015.08.015
106. McMahon P, Grossman W, Gaffney M, Stanitski C. Soft-tissue injury as an indication of child abuse. *J Bone Joint Surg Am*. 1995;77(8):1179–1183 PMID: 7642662 https://doi.org/10.2106/00004623-199508000-00006

CHAPTER 5

Visceral Manifestations of Child Abuse

M. Katherine Henry, MD, MSCE, FAAP
Fellow
Department of Pediatrics
Perelman School of Medicine at the University of Pennsylvania
Safe Place: The Center for Child Protection and Health
Division of General Pediatrics
Children's Hospital of Philadelphia
Philadelphia, PA

Daniel M. Lindberg, MD
Associate Professor
Department of Emergency Medicine
Department of Pediatrics
University of Colorado School of Medicine
Attending Physician
Kempe Center for the Prevention and Treatment of Child Abuse and Neglect
Children's Hospital Colorado
Aurora, CO

Introduction

Traumatic thoracic and abdominal injuries are rare compared with other forms of inflicted injuries but can be deadly. While none are reported exclusively in abuse, identification of these injuries can dramatically affect abuse recognition and subsequent protection of a child. Because these injuries can be easily missed, routine or protocolized screening should be used to improve injury detection and prevent bias.

The clinician caring for these children faces 2 primary decisions: when to evaluate for occult thoracic or abdominal injuries in a child for whom there is concern for abuse, and when to consider abuse in a child presenting with abdominal or thoracic injuries.

Epidemiology of Abdominal and Thoracic Trauma

Abdominal Trauma

Abuse accounts for roughly a quarter of serious abdominal injuries in infants, and approximately 2% to 3% of children evaluated for abuse will have an abdominal injury.[1–3] While abdominal trauma is relatively uncommon among children who have experienced abuse, it is second only to abusive head trauma (AHT) as a cause of death in fatal child abuse.[4] Research from the 1980s found that 45% to 50% of children with major blunt abdominal trauma attributed to abuse died.[5,6] More recent data have shown lower mortality rates, but children who have experienced abuse are still at increased risk. In a study of children 0 to 9 years of age hospitalized with abdominal trauma, 9.0% of children with abusive and 3.4% of children with accidental abdominal trauma died.[7] Another study found a mortality rate of 11% in children with inflicted abdominal trauma.[2] Along with improvements in care, increased testing for occult abdominal trauma has probably identified more minor, clinically subtle injuries, increasing prevalence and decreasing the case to fatality ratio. Like all abusive injuries, mild abusive visceral trauma is more likely to be missed than accidental injuries because caregivers may be more likely to avoid medical care and may not provide an accurate history.

Abusive abdominal injuries are most common in older infants and toddlers. This is younger than the distribution of accidental abdominal injuries but slightly older than other, more common abusive injuries, such as fractures and AHT, which predominate in young infants. On the whole, children with abusive abdominal injuries are generally younger than those with accidental abdominal injuries; indeed, among children younger than 5 years, abuse is second only to motor vehicle crashes as a cause of blunt abdominal injury.[8]

Although no single type of abdominal trauma is pathognomonic for abuse, certain types of intra-abdominal injuries are overrepresented in children who have experienced abuse. Both hollow viscus and pancreatic injuries are observed more commonly in children who have experienced abuse and warrant high concern for inflicted trauma in the absence of a plausible mechanism.[8–12] In one study of children with abusive abdominal trauma, 50% had hollow visceral injuries, most frequently to the duodenum, jejunum, and ileum (Figure 5.1).[13] Among children younger than 5 years with intra-abdominal injury, pancreatic trauma was identified in 25.4% of children with abusive injuries compared with 5.71% of accidental falls.[8] Pancreatic injuries due to abuse include pancreatitis, pseudocyst, and pancreatic fractures (Figure 5.2).[14]

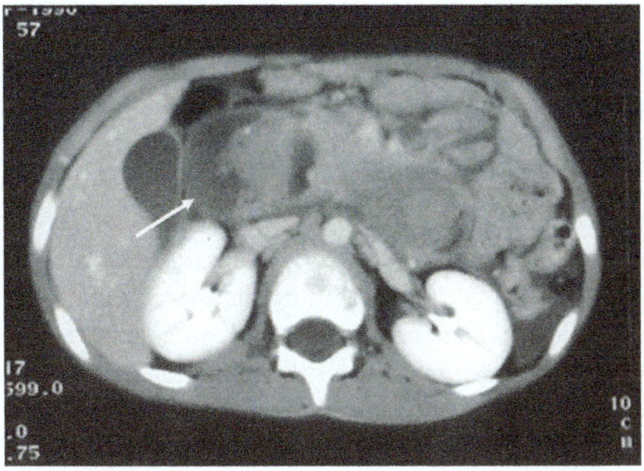

FIGURE 5.1
Computed tomography scan demonstrating a duodenal hematoma (white arrow) from a fist to the epigastrium.

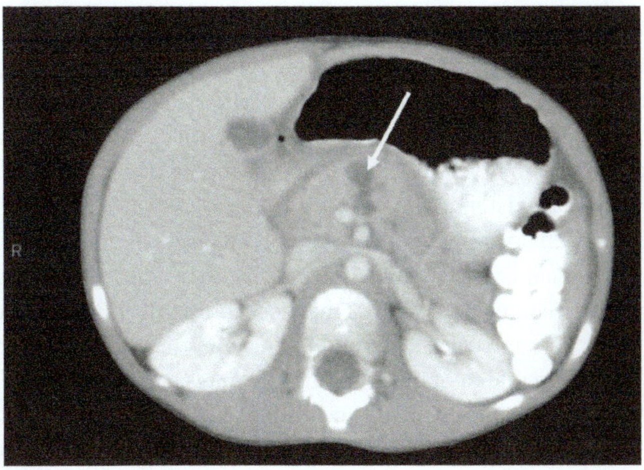

FIGURE 5.2
Typical findings in a transection of the pancreas caused by blunt force. Note fracture line (white arrow) through the mid-body of the pancreas as it overlies the spine.

Because hollow viscus and pancreatic injuries are the least likely to heal spontaneously, their overrepresentation in children who have experienced abuse may be an artifact resulting from missed solid organ injuries, could reflect increased vulnerability of the pancreas and bowel to abusive injury mechanisms like a direct blow, or could be a combination of these factors.

Thoracic Trauma

Abusive thoracic injuries include rib fractures (which are more common) and internal thoracic organs (which are relatively rare). Among 2,890 subspecialty evaluations for physical abuse in the Examining Siblings to Recognize Abuse (ExSTRA) cohort, only 23 (0.8%) were found to have internal thoracic injuries, while 82 (2.8%) were found to have abdominal injuries and 250 (8.7%) had rib fractures.

Thoracic injuries are found more commonly in young children with non-accidental trauma compared with those with accidental trauma. An institutional trauma registry of children younger than 18 years found that 17% of children with non-accidental trauma had thoracic injuries (including both fractures and pulmonary contusions) compared with 6.0% of children presenting with accidental mechanisms.[15] Among children with rib fractures, accidental mechanisms occur more often in older children (mean age 20 months) compared with inflicted injuries (mean age 4 months).[16]

Types of Injuries

Abdominal Trauma

Unlike some types of abuse, the abdominal injuries seen in abuse are not qualitatively different than what is seen in severe accidental injury. While some abdominal injuries are overrepresented in abuse, no abdominal injury has the specificity for abuse of a classic metaphyseal lesion or characteristic retinal hemorrhages.

Abuse has been documented to cause injury to every abdominal organ and structure, including solid organ and hollow viscus injury.[17] Without stratifying by mechanism of trauma, the most commonly injured abdominal organs are the liver and spleen, although injuries to the kidneys, adrenal glands, and pancreas are not uncommon. Estimates of frequencies of hollow viscus injuries vary but are generally overrepresented in abuse (Table 5.1).

Thoracic Trauma

Bony thoracic injuries include fractures of the sternum, ribs, clavicles, and vertebrae. When contiguous ribs are fractured in more than one

TABLE 5.1
Frequency of Injury Types Among Children With Abdominal Injuries[1,2,9,13,18]

Organ	All Patients (%)	Abused Only (%)
Spleen	47	9–10
Liver	33	49–64
Kidney/adrenal	17	19–20
Pancreas	3	7–20
Hollow viscus/mesentery	18	12–50

location, this can result in *flail chest,* an isolated segment of fractured ribs moving paradoxically to the remaining chest wall, and is associated with high mortality. Internal injuries include cardiac and pulmonary trauma, as well as injuries to the mediastinum, thoracic duct, pleura, and pericardium. Cardiac injuries encompass cardiac contusions, traumatic pericardial effusion, aneurysms, and rupture, as well as commotio cordis, which occurs when blunt chest trauma causes ventricular fibrillation.[19–22] Pulmonary trauma includes contusions, pleural effusions, pulmonary edema, lacerations, and pneumomediastinum.[19] In addition, significant blunt impact to the chest may result in small lacerations to the lung parenchyma and subsequent development of post-traumatic pulmonary pseudocysts.[23] Injury to the thoracic duct can result in traumatic chylothorax, where lymphatic leakage leads to accumulation of milky, white fluid in the (usually left) pleural space.[24]

Clinical Presentation

Abdominal Trauma

Presentation of children with abusive abdominal injuries can range from completely asymptomatic to obvious critical illness. Diagnosis may be hindered by the lack of an accurate history and the limits of the abdominal examination in the young or severely injured child. Abdominal injuries can manifest with a wide range of nonspecific signs and symptoms, including fussiness, fever, vomiting, constipation, hematochezia, hematuria, and hematemesis, among others; in children with a history of abdominal trauma or concern for inflicted trauma, these should prompt consideration of intra-abdominal injury. The absence of these signs and symptoms should not prevent screening when there is a reasonable concern for abuse and a significant injury.[22]

Abdominal tenderness, bruising, and/or distention are the most specific signs of abdominal injury; children with these symptoms should be evaluated for abdominal injury. Nevertheless, none of these findings alone or in combination are sufficiently sensitive to rule out abusive abdominal injuries (Figure 5.3). In one large study, abdominal pain or tenderness was only 79% sensitive for abdominal injury in children, and sensitivity declined rapidly with small changes in Glasgow Coma Scale. Abdominal bruising is concerning when present (pretest probability 40% in one sample) but not sensitive enough to rule out injury.[25,26]

Because the signs of abdominal injury can be subtle, delay in seeking care occurs in children with accidental and abusive abdominal injury. Initial examination findings may be falsely reassuring, particularly in

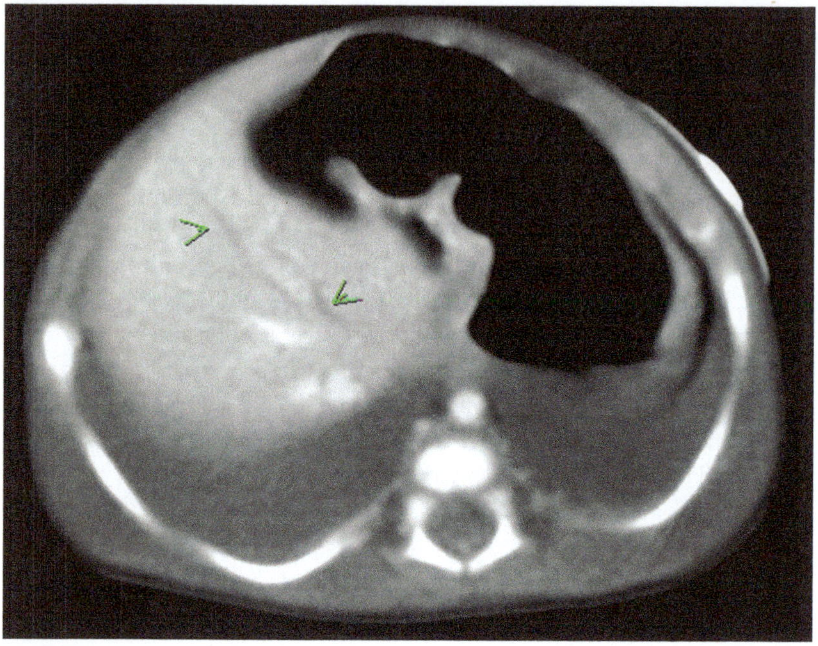

FIGURE 5.3

Grade 2 liver laceration in a 6-week-old who presented for bronchiolitis and respiratory distress and who was found to have more than 20 rib and clavicle fractures, pleural effusions, and pulmonary contusions on post-intubation chest radiography. Head computed tomography (CT) showed intracranial bleed. Abdominal examination findings were normal, but aspartate aminotransferase/alanine aminotransferase was 139/102 IU/L. Abdominal CT showed grade 2 liver laceration.

Image courtesy of Daniel M. Lindberg, MD, Children's Hospital Colorado.

injuries caused by a direct blow from bicycle handlebars.[27] Accordingly, delay in seeking care alone should not be used to determine whether a subtle or mild abdominal injury was the result of abuse because delays of longer than 12 hours have shown only modest specificity and relatively low positive predictive values for abuse.[9]

Thoracic Trauma

Thoracic injury is often difficult to diagnose by clinical examination alone. Rib or clavicle fractures may present with crepitus or palpable callus or may be completely asymptomatic. Infants with rib fractures may also present with paradoxical fussiness, characterized by worsening irritability when held. Rib fractures commonly manifest with nonspecific symptoms that are easily confused with common diseases like reflux, respiratory symptoms, colic, or constipation, making them easy to miss.[28] While many thoracic injuries are occult and require a high level of suspicion, children may present with respiratory distress if they have pneumothorax or flail chest[29] or present in malignant arrhythmia or cardiac arrest from commotio cordis.[19,20]

Evaluation

Abdominal Trauma

The approach to screening for occult abdominal injuries differs substantially in cases of accidental and abusive trauma. In accidental injuries, in which there is no forensic significance to injury identification, the algorithm proposed by the Pediatric Emergency Care Applied Research Network has been shown to be highly sensitive for clinically significant injuries.[30] This approach is expected to miss some minor injuries but is reasonable because identifying abdominal injuries without clinical significance is unlikely to prevent further accidental injuries. However, in cases with concern for abuse, it is the forensic significance of these injuries that necessitates routine screening because the identification of an occult injury can profoundly affect abuse recognition and future child protection.[30]

In cases with concern for abuse, the American Academy of Pediatrics (AAP) recommendation to perform laboratory testing for abdominal injury in children evaluated for physical abuse with serious injury should be followed.[22] Based on experience, *serious injury* is defined in this chapter to include AHT; fractures more significant than simple, isolated skull fractures; and children who require critical care or who have other injuries specific for abuse. For children with a history of significant abdominal injury or concerning physical examination findings such as significant abdominal bruising or tenderness, clinical evaluations should begin with imaging rather than laboratory testing.

Laboratory Evaluation

Currently, there is some controversy about whether laboratory testing should be conducted routinely, in most cases with concern for abuse, or only when there are specific signs of abdominal injury or severe cases of abuse. Authors who recommend routine laboratory testing do so because abdominal injuries are easy to miss and because screening hepatic transaminases (aspartate aminotransferase [AST] and alanine aminotransferase [ALT]) have been shown to improve detection (Figure 5.4).[2,3,31,32]

Coant and colleagues found that 3 of 49 children (6%) with suspected abuse had occult abdominal trauma, with liver lacerations identified in 3 of 4 children with elevated liver enzymes.[31] Lindberg and colleagues found

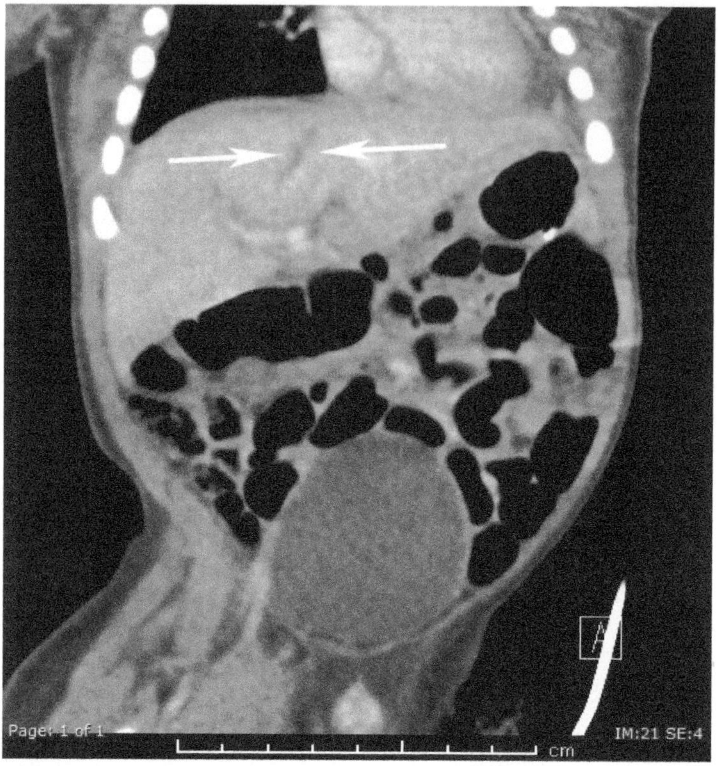

FIGURE 5.4

A 44-day-old who presented with seizure activity and altered mental status after a report that he suddenly stopped breathing during a diaper change. He was found to have small subdural hematoma and aspartate aminotransferase/alanine aminotransferase of 146/70 IU/L. Abdominal computed tomography showed multiple, acute rib fractures and this grade 2 liver laceration (white arrows). Retinal examination showed characteristic retinal hemorrhages. The boy's father confessed to handling him "too roughly."

Image courtesy of Daniel M. Lindberg, Children's Hospital Colorado

that, among all children younger than 5 years evaluated for physical abuse (pretest probability of abdominal injury of 3%), the threshold of an AST or ALT greater than 80 IU/L has a sensitivity and specificity of 77% and 82%, respectively, and a positive predictive value of 16%.[3] In a secondary analysis of a similar but separate population, this threshold of 80 IU/L similarly demonstrated a sensitivity of 83.9%, specificity of 83.1%, and positive predictive value of 20% (Figure 5.5).[2] A routine approach can therefore increase detection and also may decrease risks of practice variation and bias that have been shown in other abuse screening.[33,34]

Conversely, clinicians who oppose routine testing or favor a higher threshold do so because of concerns of over-testing and radiation risk. In the 2 large series cited previously, the first (Using Liver Transaminases to

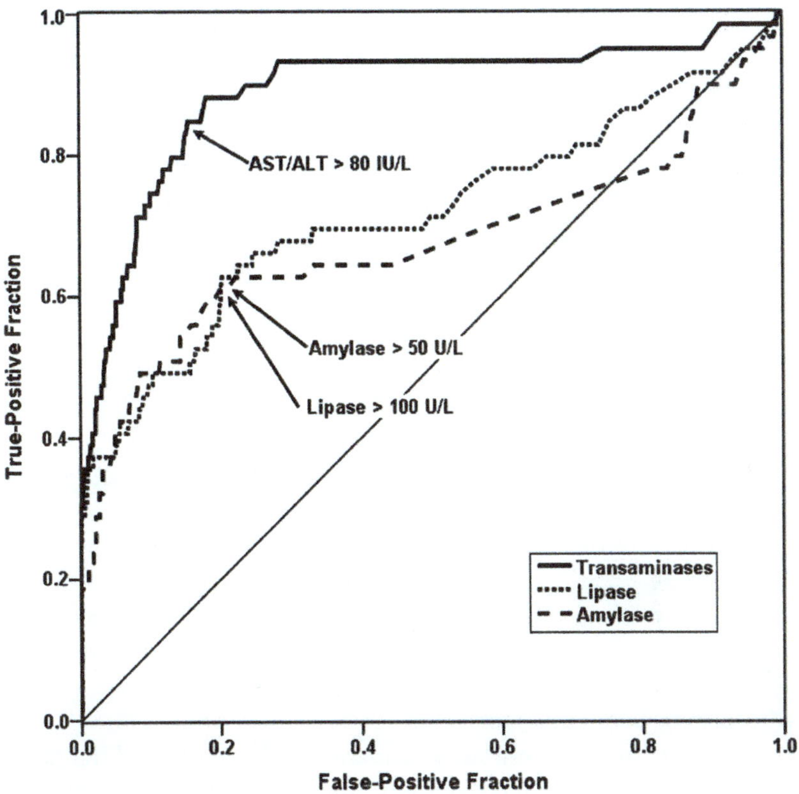

FIGURE 5.5

Receiver operating characteristic curve of aspartate aminotransferase (AST)/alanine aminotransferase (ALT), amylase, and lipase from Examining Siblings to Recognize Abuse[2] study.

From Lindberg DM, Shapiro RA, Blood EA, Steiner RD, Berger RP; Examining Siblings to Recognize Abuse Investigators. Utility of hepatic transaminases in children with concern for abuse. *Pediatrics.* 2013;131(2):268–275.

Recognize Abuse, or ULTRA[3]) recommended universal testing for study subjects, while the second (ExSTRA[2]) was a secondary analysis of a study of children who underwent testing at medical professionals' discretion. In the first series, AST/ALT was obtained in 76% of subjects and definitive testing (computed tomography [CT], magnetic resonance imaging [MRI], laparotomy, or autopsy) was performed in 16%. In the second series, AST/ALT was obtained in only 53% of subjects and definitive testing in only 11%. Nevertheless, the rate of abdominal injury identification was similar between the 2 studies (3.2% with routine screening and 2.8% using medical professional discretion). The authors suggested that a routine approach would require an additional 47 AST/ALT tests and an additional 10 to 11 CT scans to identify each additional abdominal injury.

To put these numbers in perspective, studies have suggested additional risk of cancer from a single abdominal CT scan to be between 1:300 and 1:760.[35] In comparison with this low cancer risk, the transaminase results led to changes in social or legal management, such as the decision to report to child protective services, safety planning, or the conclusion of whether a child was abused, in 15% of children with abdominal injuries.[3] Evidence therefore supports that the risk of malignancy is low compared with the benefit of identifying an injury that may ensure child protection.

Advocates of targeted testing also note that a protocolized approach does not account for other factors that can increase transaminases, such as shock, viral infection, or muscle injury. Finally, a single AST/ALT threshold may not be appropriate for patients with different pretest probabilities of abuse. For example, some clinicians may suggest imaging all children with AST/ALT greater than 120 IU/L, and children with AST/ALT greater than 80 IU/L when there are other symptoms that raise concern for abdominal injury.

Ultimately, routine testing at a single AST/ALT threshold will minimize missed abuse, prevent disproportionate testing as a result of implicit bias, and be relatively easy to implement. Clinicians who choose a more discretionary approach might use periodic audits to ensure that screening does not wane over time or is not dependent on demographic factors such as race or socioeconomic status.

Pancreatic enzymes (amylase and lipase) are also markers of trauma but carry a lower sensitivity and specificity compared with transaminases in cases of suspected abuse. There is insufficient evidence to support routine screening with pancreatic enzymes as part of the evaluation for occult inflicted trauma. Prior work has found limited sensitivity and specificity for these tests even at the optimal thresholds. Amylase has a sensitivity of only 62.5% and specificity of 77.9% at a threshold of 50 U/L, while lipase has a sensitivity of only 61.5% and specificity of 79.2% at a threshold of 100 U/L (see Figure 5.5).[2] Notably, these "optimal" thresholds were within the reference ranges for both tests, implying that to obtain even these relatively low test characteristics would require imaging for many children with laboratory values within reference range.

Because gross or microscopic hematuria may be seen in renal trauma, urinalysis has been suggested in the evaluation for occult abdominal trauma. Hematuria is not universally reported in children with blunt renal injuries.[36,37] Among children undergoing an evaluation for abuse in one study, urine testing was performed uncommonly. While any degree of hematuria had low sensitivity for abdominal injury (28%), it had a relatively high positive predictive value (24%), although it is not clear how many abdominal injuries are identified by urine testing that would have been missed by clinical examination and transaminases.[3]

Imaging Modalities

Computed tomography with intravenous (IV) contrast is the criterion standard imaging study for abusive abdominal injury.[22,38,39] Intravenous contrast increases the sensitivity of CT in detecting injuries and improves visualization of vasculature and solid organs. If there is concern for renal trauma, delayed excretory phase CT images may be considered as well.[39] Although abdominal CT does not capture the entire rib cage, the lower ribs are often imaged and may be evaluated for fracture.

While ultrasonography is an appealing modality because of lack of radiation, it can be falsely reassuring if results are negative. Conventional ultrasonography is not sensitive for solid organ injuries compared with CT and is operator dependent, with sensitivities ranging from approximately 39% to 82%.[40–43]

Focused assessment with sonography in trauma (FAST) examination is a general ultrasonographic screen for hemoperitoneum that is commonly used in adult trauma patients. In children, FAST ultrasonography for intraperitoneal fluid carries a sensitivity of 52% to 80% for hemoperitoneum and 66% for intra-abdominal injuries.[43,44] A recent randomized controlled trial demonstrated that FAST examinations (compared to standard care) did not improve clinical care or decrease the percentage of children who ultimately underwent CT.[45] It is difficult to extrapolate this literature to children who have experienced abuse for whom non-clinically significant injuries may carry forensic implications.

Contrast-enhanced ultrasound (CEUS) is emerging as a promising tool in abdominal imaging (Figure 5.6), yet more research is needed before CEUS can be used routinely in lieu of CT in young children. In CEUS, the contrast agent differs from that used in CT and consists of microbubbles of gas encased in a phospholipid or albumin shell.[46] The gas is exhaled by the lungs without nephrotoxicity. Limitations of CEUS include poor performance in identification of active bleeding, hollow visceral trauma, and some renal injuries.[47] While CEUS has been studied in large numbers of adolescents and adults, few data exist on the use of CEUS in detection of abdominal trauma in young children.[40,48–55]

Magnetic resonance imaging is proposed as another radiation-free imaging alternative to CT. However, it is often not readily available in the acute setting and commonly requires sedation. A growing body of literature suggests that the risks of sedation to cognitive ability are at least as great as the risks of neoplasia from radiation.[56] While data about the sensitivity and specificity of MRI for pediatric abdominal trauma have not been published, MRI is a reasonable alternative modality when there is a high level of concern about radiation, when there are other contraindications to CT, or for children who require sedation or MRI for other reasons.

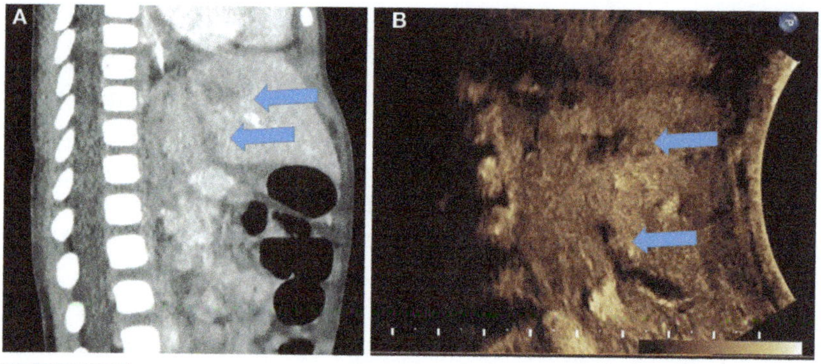

FIGURE 5.6
Toddler who presented after a reported fall from a bed but was found to have intracranial trauma, retinal hemorrhages, and multiple rib fractures of different stages of healing. Sagittal contrast-enhanced computed tomography image of the abdomen (A) raised concern for a liver laceration (blue arrows) with multiple geometric hypoattenuating (dark) regions in the parenchyma. Sagittal contrast-enhanced ultrasound image of the liver (B) (rotated 90 degrees clockwise for anatomic comparison) obtained approximately 20 hours later confirmed the presence of a grade 3 liver laceration with linear hypoechoic (dark) geometric regions as a result of disruption of parenchymal perfusion (blue arrows).
Image courtesy of Susan J. Back, MD, and M. Katherine Henry, MD.

Computed tomography with IV contrast is recommended by the AAP as the initial imaging study for most children with moderate to high suspicion for intra-abdominal injury by history, examination findings, or laboratory testing.[38] While the risk of radiation is real and important, the risk can be considered acceptable in this population when balanced against the risks of missing an abusive injury and the risks associated with other testing modalities.

Thoracic Trauma

Laboratory Evaluation

There are no laboratory studies that are widely used to detect thoracic injury, which is overwhelmingly diagnosed with imaging. Troponin I, cardiac form (cTnI), has been proposed as a marker of myocardial injury in children with suspected inflicted trauma.[57,58] Injured children undergoing an evaluation for physical abuse have higher levels of cTnI compared with uninjured children.[58] Whether cTnI levels differ between injured children with inflicted versus accidental trauma is not known.

Imaging Modalities

Chest radiography with dedicated oblique views of the ribs are the highest yield views in the skeletal survey, which should be obtained in all children younger than 2 years with concern for physical abuse.[22]

However, rib fractures are also the most likely fracture to be missed on the initial skeletal survey.[59] The AAP recommends a follow-up skeletal survey for children whose initial skeletal survey is equivocal or when there is moderate or high suspicion of abuse after the initial skeletal survey.[38] When waiting 2 weeks for a follow-up skeletal survey is impossible or impractical, low-dose CT, 18F bone scan, or MRI can be considered, although each has additional risks from radiation and/or sedation.[60–62] With regard to cardiac contusions, electrocardiography and echocardiography can be considered, with further guidance from pediatric cardiologists or trauma specialists for advanced imaging modalities and interpretation.

Differential Diagnosis

The differential diagnosis for children undergoing an evaluation for abdominal or thoracic trauma includes both medical and traumatic causes. Before coming to a final diagnosis of abusive thoracic or abdominal injury, clinicians should exclude nontraumatic medical entities and accidental injury. Thoracic or abdominal injuries generally require a forceful, direct blow and are therefore vanishingly rare as a result of common household trauma.

Nontraumatic Conditions That Mimic Trauma

Laboratory Findings

The differential diagnosis for elevated transaminases is broad and includes infection, shock, medication effects, and genetic and metabolic causes, as well as extrahepatic etiologies such as myopathies, hemolysis, and endocrinopathies.[63] Elevated pancreatic enzymes and pancreatitis can be the result of shock, medication effects, biliary pathology, infections, or scorpion stings; they may be hereditary in origin and can also be idiopathic, although each of these is rare in children.[64,65] In children, pancreatitis without other medical explanation is highly concerning for trauma and should trigger a thorough search for history of recent focal, forceful abdominal injury, as well as testing for occult abusive injuries.

Abdominal Free Fluid

Isolated abdominal free fluid is a nonspecific finding and can be difficult to interpret in the pediatric trauma patient. Isolated free fluid could represent abdominal injury not detected on imaging or be physiologic in origin.[66] Isolated free fluid is found in 8% to 14% of children with blunt abdominal trauma.[67,68] Children with intra-abdominal fluid who later require operative management or who are later found to have intra-abdominal injuries commonly have decreased level of consciousness or abdominal pain on initial examination.[67,68] In isolation, therefore, small amounts of abdominal free fluid should not raise concern for abuse unless the child is clearly symptomatic or progresses to peritonitis.

Sternal Ossification Centers

A rotated projection or oblique rib views can cause sternal ossification centers to overlap with ribs and appear like healing fractures (Figure 5.7).[69] Confusion can be avoided by routinely assessing rotation of chest radiographs or by comparing alternate projections.

Idiopathic Gastric Rupture

Rarely, spontaneous gastric rupture not associated with trauma has been reported in the early neonatal period.[70] Infants typically present with abdominal distention that may progress to respiratory distress. Idiopathic gastric rupture has also been reported in preschool-aged children and is thought to result from gastric distention compromising

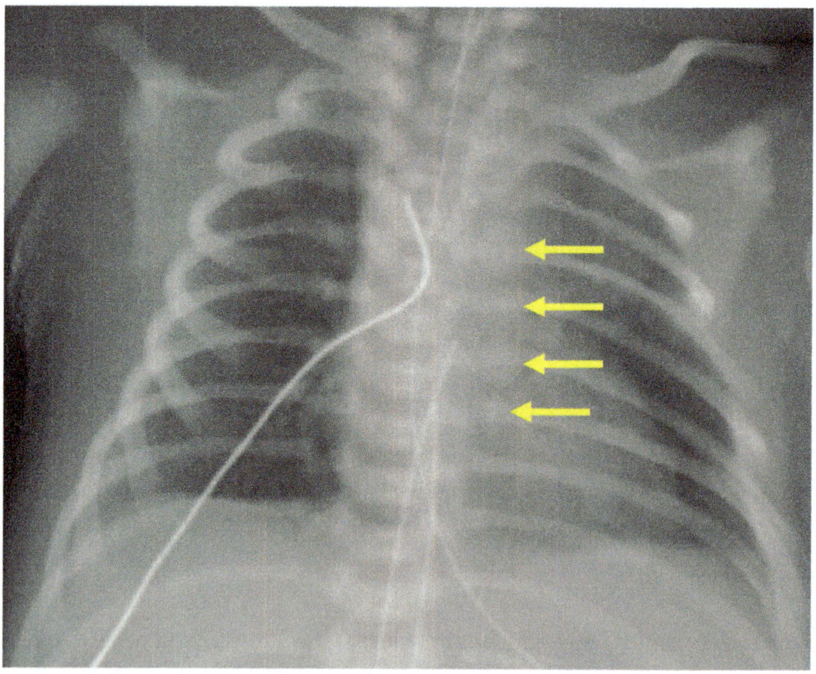

FIGURE 5.7
Sternal ossification centers (yellow arrows) mimic rib fractures.
Image courtesy of Laura Fenton, MD, Children's Hospital of Colorado.

vascular patency.[71] Given the rare incidence relative to abuse, this would be considered a diagnosis of exclusion in an infant who has been discharged from the hospital after birth. It should only be considered after a thorough evaluation for other traumatic injuries and a careful assessment of the safety of the infant's environment.

Imaging Artifacts

Imaging artifacts, including poor contrast timing, can create false positives. Variations in solid organ perfusion can result in false positives in CT if findings do not clinically correlate. In ultrasonography, edge artifact can mimic free fluid or parenchymal injury when ultrasound waves impact the edge of a fluid-filled structure and create shadowing.

Diagnoses Commonly Associated With Medical Conditions

Pneumatosis Intestinalis

Pneumatosis intestinalis and portal venous gas are classically associated with necrotizing enterocolitis in neonates. However, pneumatosis intestinalis has been associated with accidental[72] and non-accidental trauma.[73] The source of pneumatosis should be identified for any child. Unless a nontraumatic etiology is identified (eg, necrotizing enterocolitis), the patient should receive a thorough evaluation for abusive injuries or a dangerous home environment.

Pleural Effusion

Pleural effusion is commonly caused by medical conditions as well as inflicted and accidental trauma.[74] The identification of a new, significant pleural effusion should trigger a search for its etiology, and a thoracentesis may be appropriate. Non-abusive causes of pleural effusion include parapneumonic effusion, viral pleurisy, renal disease, subdiaphragmatic irritation, and neoplastic effusions. While a pleural effusion in isolation is not pathognomonic for trauma, it should prompt an evaluation for additional injuries when there is no clear medical etiology.

Chylothorax

While chylothorax has been described as the result of abusive injury to the thoracic duct,[17,24] the list of non-abusive etiologies is long. Medical etiologies include lymphatic disorders, congenital anomalies, and postoperative complications in children with congenital heart disease. Chylothorax may also be idiopathic. A thorough evaluation for inflicted injury should be conducted in young children with unexplained chylothorax (including dedicated history, physical examination, and skeletal survey), but without other signs of maltreatment, a diagnosis of abuse should not be assigned based on an isolated chylothorax.[17,24]

Injury Mechanism and Expected Injuries

Abdominal Injury

As in all cases, clinicians faced with estimating the likelihood of abuse in a child with a known abdominal injury must consider the likelihood of the injury occurring as the result of the reported history and whether the injury could have occurred as the result of unwitnessed trauma that occurred despite reasonable supervision. No one type of abdominal injury is pathognomonic for abuse. In assessing the likelihood of abdominal injury from a given mechanism, clinicians should consider the amount of force and the application (focal or diffuse) of the force. For example, some highly focal mechanisms (eg, handlebar injuries) have high risk of injury even with a relatively low amount of force, while high-energy mechanisms (eg, a car striking a pedestrian) can cause injury even without a focal force. The most concerning mechanisms for injury are those that combine high energy with focal force, such as a direct blow to the abdomen or a fall onto a focal object such as a railing, handlebar, or sawhorse (Figure 5.8).

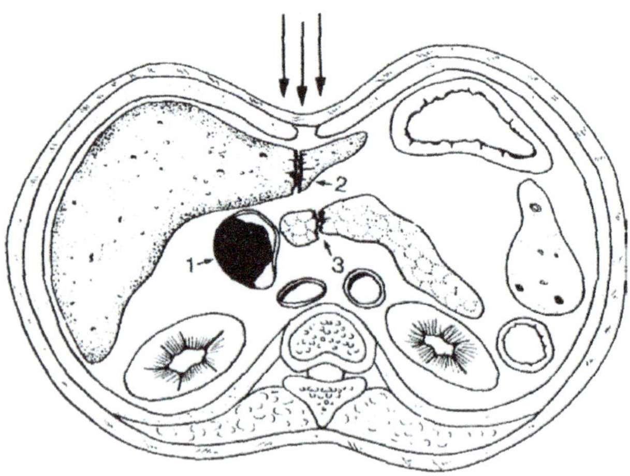

FIGURE 5.8

Common injury mechanism in child abuse. Blunt force (eg, from a fist) crushes organs against the rigid spine. Organs at risk include the duodenum (1), liver (2), and pancreas (3).

From Nimkin K, Kleinman PK. Visceral trauma. In: Kleinman PK, ed. *Diagnostic Imaging of Child Abuse*. 3rd ed. Cambridge, United Kingdom: Cambridge University Press; 2015:563–607.

The presence of significant intra-abdominal injury warrants high concern for abuse in the absence of a plausible, accidental, focal or high-energy mechanism.

Uncommon Causes of Abdominal Injuries

Falls are often a reported mechanism of injury, but short household falls are an unlikely cause of significant abdominal trauma (Figure 5.9). While studies have described truncal injuries in 2% to 4% of children

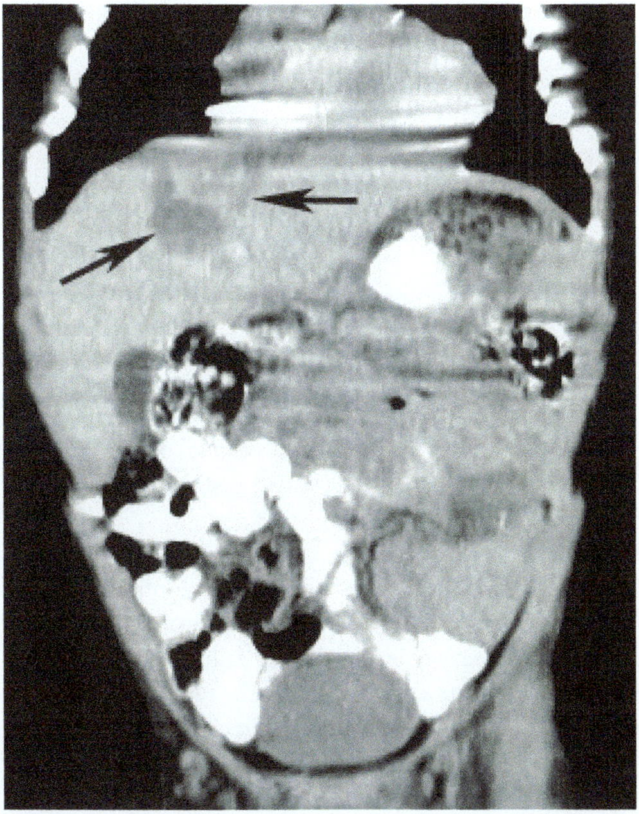

FIGURE 5.9

Twenty-eight–month-old boy who was noted by the primary care pediatrician to have facial bruising. Reported history was for a short fall onto tile. Examination showed a handful of other, nonspecific bruising but normal abdominal examination. Aspartate aminotransferase/alanine aminotransferase was 46/134 IU/L. Abdominal ultrasonography showed an equivocal finding, and computed tomography showed grade 3 liver laceration (black arrows). The mother was later found to have struck the child with a pack of frozen hot dogs and was recorded threatening a witness to the assault on a phone line from prison.

Image courtesy of Daniel M. Lindberg, MD, Children's Hospital Colorado.

presenting with accidental stairway falls, the type and severity of truncal injuries were not described.[75–77] Even if all injuries were significant, intra-abdominal injury rates are low. Hollow viscus injuries are especially unlikely to result from short falls or stairway falls. One study reviewed 677 published cases of stairway falls and 312 published cases of hollow viscus injuries and demonstrated that no cases overlapped.[77] While one study reported 16 hollow viscus injuries from "low-velocity accidents," this category included falls up to 10 feet and bicycle crashes.[9]

Significant intra-abdominal trauma is also uncommon after high-level falls. In one study of more than 300 children falling 15 feet or greater, only 0.9% of these falls resulted in bowel injuries. Hepatic, splenic, and renal injuries were reported in 1.2%, 2.4%, and 0.9% of these high-level falls, respectively.[78]

Cardiopulmonary resuscitation (CPR) is, at times, proposed as a cause of abdominal injury, but this should be interpreted with skepticism. Among 211 deceased children who underwent CPR, 2 retroperitoneal hematomas, 1 splenic contusion, 1 stomach perforation, and 1 finding of trace hemoperitoneum were identified.[79] Notably, these were children with a mean duration of CPR of 45 minutes who did not survive their resuscitation.

High Risk

High-energy, focal trauma is most likely to cause intra-abdominal injury. Among children with witnessed mechanisms, common sources of significant abdominal injury include motor vehicle collisions, direct blows, significant falls (>20 feet), automobile versus pediatrician or bike, and motorcycle injuries.[45,80,81]

Focal trauma, high-energy trauma, and a combination of the 2 can result in hollow viscus injury. Hollow viscus injury commonly results from a focal or localized blow, such as a handlebar injury or direct blow,[82] or crush injury such as a heavy object or dresser falling on a child.[77] Go-kart and motor vehicle accidents are examples of the type of high-energy trauma that may result in bowel perforation in children.[77,81,83]

Thoracic Trauma

Given that the intrathoracic structures are protected by the ribs, focal trauma is less of a concern, and injuries to the heart, lungs, and thoracic duct require significant force, beyond the force of typical household accidents. Children presenting with thoracic and intrathoracic trauma in the absence of a significant history of trauma should, therefore, be assessed carefully for evidence of abuse.

Falls uncommonly cause internal thoracic trauma. In one study of more than 700 children who were treated for falls by a pediatric trauma surgery service, children with high-level falls (≥15 feet) were rarely found to have cardiac contusion (0.9%), pulmonary contusion (3.3%), and pneumothorax (2.4%).[78]

Blunt cardiac trauma, such as cardiac contusions or traumatic ventricular septal defects, requires significant force and has been reported in cases of assault, motor vehicle collisions, and significant blunt force, such as being kicked by a cow or a blow from a falling 10" to 12" diameter tree limb.[21,84] Falls are a reported cause of traumatic ventricular septal defects and include a fall from a horse with the child's anterior chest striking a stone and chest trauma from a fall in a bathtub.

Commotio cordis, in contrast, occurs after blunt trauma to the precordium but is a function of the timing of the impact in the cardiac cycle rather than the degree of force. In older children, impacts commonly occur in sports from projectiles such as baseballs and hockey pucks and do not appear to bystanders to be outside the normal for the sport.[85]

Pulmonary trauma in the setting of rib fractures is highly concerning for abuse in the absence of a plausible accidental mechanism. In a series of 65 children younger than 3 years with rib fractures, mechanisms associated with accidental rib fractures included motor vehicle collisions, multistory window falls, and crush injuries. Internal pulmonary thoracic trauma was observed in 12.8% of children with abuse compared with 55.6% of children with accidental trauma in this series.[16]

Birth trauma is an uncommon but reported cause of rib fractures. In one review of the literature, only 13 cases of perinatal mid-posterior rib fractures were identified, most commonly in large neonates with difficult deliveries.[86] While rib fractures are very likely to be asymptomatic and could be missed in neonates who do not undergo radiography, incidental identification of healing rib fractures in neonates who have radiography for other reasons is rare.[87] A thorough birth history should be obtained in young infants with rib fractures whose radiographic healing patterns are consistent with fractures that occurred at birth.

Management and Prognosis

Abdominal Injury

To date, there is no abuse-specific management of intra-abdominal injury other than reporting suspected abuse to ensure protection of the child. In general, children with solid organ injuries tend to improve without specific treatment, while those with injuries to the small bowel frequently deteriorate without operative management. In cases with identified traumatic intra-abdominal injury, a surgeon should be consulted.

The standard of care for most pediatric liver and spleen injuries is nonoperative management. In 2000, the American Pediatric Surgical Association published guidelines for resource utilization in hemodynamically stable children with isolated grade 1 through 4 liver or spleen injury (Table 5.2).[88] These guidelines recommended intensive care unit monitoring only among children with a grade 4 injury because those with lower grade injuries required operative management in fewer than 3% of cases. Similarly, most children with renal trauma are now managed nonoperatively.[89] Nonoperative management for solid organ injuries is successful in approximately 95% of cases.[18,90] Failure of nonoperative management has been reported for reasons including persistent hemorrhage, vascular injury, shock, pancreatic injury (eg, transection, avulsion, pseudocyst), peritonitis, free air, and concurrent injuries (eg, hollow visceral injuries, ruptured diaphragm).[18,90] Among children with any type of intra-abdominal injury, nearly two-thirds of children requiring operative management have hollow viscus injuries.[91]

The prognosis for solid organ injury is generally excellent, with a mortality rate of 0.8% for cases with solid organ injuries and without severe brain injury.[90] Higher mortality is reported in children with hollow viscus injury. Mortality among 214 children who required operative management for hollow viscus injury or who died prior to operative management was 6.1%.[92] Children with abusive abdominal injuries have worse outcomes relative to accidental injuries,[7,10] with mortality rates ranging from 9% to 50%.[2,5–7] This increased mortality may be the result of increased injury severity, delay in seeking care or in diagnosis, increased prevalence of the most dangerous abdominal injuries (pancreatic and hollow viscus injuries), repeated injury, and/or the presence of extra-abdominal injuries.

Thoracic Injury

As with abdominal trauma, there is no abuse-specific management of thoracic injury beyond reporting to child protective services. Unless contiguous rib fractures are present causing flail chest, rib fractures heal without intervention beyond pain control. Tension pneumothorax is managed emergently by tube or needle thoracostomy to normalize pleural pressure. Small, hemodynamically stable pneumothoraxes may be managed with observation alone. Pneumomediastinum is generally self-limited.

TABLE 5.2
Spleen and Liver Injury Scales From the American Pediatric Surgical Association

Grade[a]	Injury Type	Spleen Description	Liver Description
1	Hematoma	Subcapsular, <10% surface area	Subcapsular, <10% surface area
	Laceration	Capsular tear, <1 cm parenchymal depth	Capsular tear, <1 cm parenchymal depth
2	Hematoma	Subcapsular, 10%–50% surface area; intraparenchymal, <5 cm in diameter	Subcapsular, 10%–50% surface area; intraparenchymal, <10 cm in diameter
	Laceration	1–3 cm parenchymal depth which does not involve a trabecular vessel	1–3 cm parenchymal depth, <10 cm in length
3	Hematoma	Subcapsular, >50% surface area or expanding; ruptured subcapsular or parenchymal hematoma Intraparenchymal hematoma >5 cm or expanding	Subcapsular, >50% surface area or expanding; ruptured subcapsular or parenchymal hematoma Intraparenchymal hematoma >10 cm or expanding
	Laceration	>3 cm parenchymal depth or involving trabecular vessels	>3 cm parenchymal depth
4	Laceration	Laceration involving segmental or hilar vessels producing major devascularization (>25% of spleen)	Parenchymal disruption involving 25%–75% of hepatic lobe or 1–3 Couinaud segments within a single lobe
5	Laceration	Completely shattered spleen	Parenchymal disruption involving >75% of hepatic lobe or >3 Couinaud segments within a single lobe
	Vascular	Hilar vascular injury which causes devascularized spleen	Juxtahepatic venous injuries (ie, retrohepatic vena cava/central major hepatic veins)
6	Vascular	NA	Hepatic avulsion

Abbreviation: NA, not applicable.

[a] Advance one grade for multiple injuries, up to grade 3.

Derived from Moore EE, Cogbill TH, Jurkovich GJ, Shackford SR, Malangoni MA, Champion HR. Organ injury scaling: spleen and liver (1994 revision). *J Trauma.* 1995;38(3):323–324 PMID: 7897707 https://doi.org/10.1097/00005373-199503000-00001.

Conclusion

Abusive intrathoracic and abdominal injuries are neither as common as abusive fractures or cutaneous injuries nor as deadly as AHT. Nevertheless, a typical child protection team will encounter a handful of abusive abdominal or intrathoracic injuries each year, with important medical and forensic implications. Most thoracic injuries will be identified with a history and physical examination supplemented by plain radiography, as in the skeletal survey. Conversely, abdominal injuries may be clinically subtle, and children with significant injuries should be screened with laboratory testing of AST/ALT followed by CT scanning for children with elevated transaminases or other high-risk signs of injury. Significant abdominal or thoracic injuries rarely result from ordinary household trauma. Plausible accidental mechanisms require high energy and/or focal force. Hemodynamically stable children with solid organ injury are typically treated expectantly, while those with hollow viscus injury, pancreatic injury, or hemodynamic instability require emergent surgery.

References

1. Lane WG, Dubowitz H, Langenberg P, Dischinger P. Epidemiology of abusive abdominal trauma hospitalizations in United States children. *Child Abuse Negl*. 2012;36(2):142–148 PMID: 22398302 https://doi.org/10.1016/j.chiabu.2011.09.010
2. Lindberg DM, Shapiro RA, Blood EA, Steiner RD, Berger RP; ExSTRA Investigators. Utility of hepatic transaminases in children with concern for abuse. *Pediatrics*. 2013;131(2):268–275 PMID: 23319537 https://doi.org/10.1542/peds.2012-1952
3. Lindberg D, Makoroff K, Harper N, et al; ULTRA Investigators. Utility of hepatic transaminases to recognize abuse in children. *Pediatrics*. 2009;124(2):509–516 PMID: 19620197 https://doi.org/10.1542/peds.2008-2348
4. Schnitzer PG, Ewigman BG. Child deaths resulting from inflicted injuries: household risk factors and perpetrator characteristics. *Pediatrics*. 2005;116(5):e687–e693 PMID: 16263983 https://doi.org/10.1542/peds.2005-0296
5. Cooper A, Floyd T, Barlow B, et al. Major blunt abdominal trauma due to child abuse. *J Trauma*. 1988;28(10):1483–1487 PMID: 3172310 https://doi.org/10.1097/00005373-198810000-00015
6. Sivit CJ, Taylor GA, Eichelberger MR. Visceral injury in battered children: a changing perspective. *Radiology*. 1989;173(3):659–661 PMID: 2813769 https://doi.org/10.1148/radiology.173.3.2813769
7. Lane WG, Lotwin I, Dubowitz H, Langenberg P, Dischinger P. Outcomes for children hospitalized with abusive versus noninflicted abdominal trauma. *Pediatrics*. 2011;127(6):e1400–e1405 PMID: 21555490 https://doi.org/10.1542/peds.2010-2096
8. Carter KW, Moulton SL. Pediatric abdominal injury patterns caused by "falls": a comparison between nonaccidental and accidental trauma. *J Pediatr Surg*. 2016;51(2):326–328 PMID: 26850907 https://doi.org/10.1016/j.jpedsurg.2015.10.056
9. Wood J, Rubin DM, Nance ML, Christian CW. Distinguishing inflicted versus accidental abdominal injuries in young children. *J Trauma*. 2005;59(5):1203–1208 PMID: 16385300 https://doi.org/10.1097/01.ta.0000196437.07011.b1
10. Trokel M, DiScala C, Terrin NC, Sege RD. Blunt abdominal injury in the young pediatric patient: child abuse and patient outcomes. *Child Maltreat*. 2004;9(1):111–117 PMID: 14871002 https://doi.org/10.1177/1077559503260310
11. Gaines BA, Shultz BS, Morrison K, Ford HR. Duodenal injuries in children: beware of child abuse. *J Pediatr Surg*. 2004;39(4):600–602 PMID: 15065036 https://doi.org/10.1016/j.jpedsurg.2003.12.010
12. Trokel M, Discala C, Terrin NC, Sege RD. Patient and injury characteristics in abusive abdominal injuries. *Pediatr Emerg Care*. 2006;22(10):700–704 PMID: 17047468 https://doi.org/10.1097/01.pec.0000238734.76413.do

13. Roaten JB, Partrick DA, Bensard DD, et al. Visceral injuries in nonaccidental trauma: spectrum of injury and outcomes. *Am J Surg*. 2005;190(6):827–829 PMID: 16307928 https://doi.org/10.1016/j.amjsurg.2005.05.049
14. Servaes S, Haller JO. Characteristic pancreatic injuries secondary to child abuse. *Emerg Radiol*. 2003;10(2):90–93 PMID: 15290514 https://doi.org/10.1007/s10140-002-0258-z
15. Roaten JB, Partrick DA, Nydam TL, et al. Nonaccidental trauma is a major cause of morbidity and mortality among patients at a regional level 1 pediatric trauma center. *J Pediatr Surg*. 2006;41(12):2013–2015 PMID: 17161194 https://doi.org/10.1016/j.jpedsurg.2006.08.028
16. Darling SE, Done SL, Friedman SD, Feldman KW. Frequency of intrathoracic injuries in children younger than 3 years with rib fractures. *Pediatr Radiol*. 2014;44(10):1230–1236 PMID: 24771095 https://doi.org/10.1007/s00247-014-2988-y
17. Maguire SA, Upadhyaya M, Evans A, et al. A systematic review of abusive visceral injuries in childhood—their range and recognition. *Child Abuse Negl*. 2013;37(7):430–445 PMID: 23306146 https://doi.org/10.1016/j.chiabu.2012.10.009
18. Tataria M, Nance ML, Holmes JH 4th, et al. Pediatric blunt abdominal injury: age is irrelevant and delayed operation is not detrimental. *J Trauma*. 2007;63(3):608–614 PMID: 18073608 https://doi.org/10.1097/TA.0b013e318142d2c2
19. Denton JS, Kalelkar MB. Homicidal commotio cordis in two children. *J Forensic Sci*. 2000;45(3):734–735 PMID: 10855990
20. Baker AM, Craig BR, Lonergan GJ. Homicidal commotio cordis: the final blow in a battered infant. *Child Abuse Negl*. 2003;27(1):125–130 PMID: 12510035 https://doi.org/10.1016/S0145-2134(02)00511-2
21. Karpas A, Yen K, Sell LL, Frommelt PC. Severe blunt cardiac injury in an infant: a case of child abuse. *J Trauma*. 2002;52(4):759–764 PMID: 11956397 https://doi.org/10.1097/00005373-200204000-00026
22. Christian CW; American Academy of Pediatrics Committee on Child Abuse and Neglect. The evaluation of suspected child physical abuse. *Pediatrics*. 2015;135(5):e1337–e1354 PMID: 25917988 https://doi.org/10.1542/peds.2015-0356
23. Wyvill V, Starling SP, Clayton M. Posttraumatic pulmonary pseudocysts as a manifestation of child abuse. *Pediatr Emerg Care*. 2012;28(2):178–179 PMID: 22307189 https://doi.org/10.1097/PEC.0b013e3182447de3
24. Anderst JD. Chylothorax and child abuse. *Pediatr Crit Care Med*. 2007;8(4):394–396 PMID: 17545935
25. Barnes PM, Norton CM, Dunstan FD, Kemp AM, Yates DW, Sibert JR. Abdominal injury due to child abuse. *Lancet*. 2005;366(9481):234–235 PMID: 16023514 https://doi.org/10.1016/S0140-6736(05)66913-9
26. Hilmes MA, Hernanz-Schulman M, Greeley CS, Piercey LM, Yu C, Kan JH. CT identification of abdominal injuries in abused pre-school-age children. *Pediatr Radiol*. 2011;41(5):643–651 PMID: 21107556 https://doi.org/10.1007/s00247-010-1899-9
27. Lam JP, Eunson GJ, Munro FD, Orr JD. Delayed presentation of handlebar injuries in children. *BMJ*. 2001;322(7297):1288–1289 PMID: 11375234 https://doi.org/10.1136/bmj.322.7297.1288
28. Kondis JS, Muenzer J, Luhmann JD. Missed fractures in infants presenting to the emergency department with fussiness. *Pediatr Emerg Care*. 2017;33(8):538–543 PMID: 28350717 https://doi.org/10.1097/PEC.0000000000001106
29. Gipson CL, Tobias JD. Flail chest in a neonate resulting from nonaccidental trauma. *South Med J*. 2006;99(5):536–538 PMID: 16711322 https://doi.org/10.1097/01.smj.0000216471.54786.e5

30. Lindberg DM, Berger RP, Lane WG. PECARN abdominal injury rule should exclude potentially abused children. *Ann Emerg Med.* 2013;62(3):276–277 PMID: 23969129 https://doi.org/10.1016/j.annemergmed.2013.02.031
31. Coant PN, Kornberg AE, Brody AS, Edwards-Holmes K. Markers for occult liver injury in cases of physical abuse in children. *Pediatrics.* 1992;89(2):274–278 PMID: 1734396
32. Lane WG, Dubowitz H, Langenberg P. Screening for occult abdominal trauma in children with suspected physical abuse. *Pediatrics.* 2009;124(6):1595–1602 PMID: 19933726 https://doi.org/10.1542/peds.2009-0904
33. Wood JN, French B, Song L, Feudtner C. Evaluation for occult fractures in injured children. *Pediatrics.* 2015;136(2):232–240 PMID: 26169425 https://doi.org/10.1542/peds.2014-3977
34. Trokel M, Waddimba A, Griffith J, Sege R. Variation in the diagnosis of child abuse in severely injured infants. *Pediatrics.* 2006;117(3):722–728 PMID: 16510652 https://doi.org/10.1542/peds.2004-2731
35. Brenner DJ, Hall EJ. Computed tomography—an increasing source of radiation exposure. *N Engl J Med.* 2007;357(22):2277–2284 PMID: 18046031 https://doi.org/10.1056/NEJMra072149
36. Fitzgerald CL, Tran P, Burnell J, Broghammer JA, Santucci R. Instituting a conservative management protocol for pediatric blunt renal trauma: evaluation of a prospectively maintained patient registry. *J Urol.* 2011;185(3):1058–1064 PMID: 21256524 https://doi.org/10.1016/j.juro.2010.10.045
37. Broghammer JA, Langenburg SE, Smith SJ, Santucci RA. Pediatric blunt renal trauma: its conservative management and patterns of associated injuries. *Urology.* 2006;67(4):823–827 PMID: 16566992 https://doi.org/10.1016/j.urology.2005.11.062
38. American Academy of Pediatrics Section on Radiology. Diagnostic imaging of child abuse. *Pediatrics.* 2009;123(5):1430–1435 PMID: 19403511 https://doi.org/10.1542/peds.2009-0558
39. Wootton-Gorges SL, Soares BP, Alazraki AL, et al; Expert Panel on Pediatric Imaging. ACR Appropriateness Criteria® suspected physical abuse—child. *J Am Coll Radiol.* 2017;14(5S):S338–S349 PMID: 28473090 https://doi.org/10.1016/j.jacr.2017.01.036
40. Menichini G, Sessa B, Trinci M, Galluzzo M, Miele V. Accuracy of contrast-enhanced ultrasound (CEUS) in the identification and characterization of traumatic solid organ lesions in children: a retrospective comparison with baseline US and CE-MDCT. *Radiol Med (Torino).* 2015;120(11):989–1001 PMID: 25822953 https://doi.org/10.1007/s11547-015-0535-z
41. Valentino M, Ansaloni L, Catena F, Pavlica P, Pinna AD, Barozzi L. Contrast-enhanced ultrasonography in blunt abdominal trauma: considerations after 5 years of experience. *Radiol Med (Torino).* 2009;114(7):1080–1093 PMID: 19774445 https://doi.org/10.1007/s11547-009-0444-0
42. Karam O, La Scala G, Le Coultre C, Chardot C. Liver function tests in children with blunt abdominal traumas. *Eur J Pediatr Surg.* 2007;17(5):313–316 PMID: 17968786 https://doi.org/10.1055/s-2007-965533
43. Holmes JF, Gladman A, Chang CH. Performance of abdominal ultrasonography in pediatric blunt trauma patients: a meta-analysis. *J Pediatr Surg.* 2007;42(9):1588–1594 PMID: 17848254 https://doi.org/10.1016/j.jpedsurg.2007.04.023
44. Fox JC, Boysen M, Gharahbaghian L, et al. Test characteristics of focused assessment of sonography for trauma for clinically significant abdominal free fluid in pediatric blunt abdominal trauma. *Acad Emerg Med.* 2011;18(5):477–482 PMID: 21569167 https://doi.org/10.1111/j.1553-2712.2011.01071.x

45. Holmes JF, Kelley KM, Wootton-Gorges SL, et al. Effect of abdominal ultrasound on clinical care, outcomes, and resource use among children with blunt torso trauma: a randomized clinical trial. *JAMA*. 2017;317(22):2290–2296 PMID: 28609532 https://doi.org/10.1001/jama.2017.6322
46. Laugesen NG, Nolsoe CP, Rosenberg J. Clinical applications of contrast-enhanced ultrasound in the pediatric work-up of focal liver lesions and blunt abdominal trauma: a systematic review. *Ultrasound Int Open*. 2017;3(1):E2–E7 PMID: 28255580 https://doi.org/10.1055/s-0042-124502
47. Miele V, Piccolo CL, Trinci M, Galluzzo M, Ianniello S, Brunese L. Diagnostic imaging of blunt abdominal trauma in pediatric patients. *Radiol Med (Torino)*. 2016;121(5):409–430 PMID: 27075018 https://doi.org/10.1007/s11547-016-0637-2
48. Catalano O, Aiani L, Barozzi L, et al. CEUS in abdominal trauma: multi-center study. *Abdom Imaging*. 2009;34(2):225–234 PMID: 18682877 https://doi.org/10.1007/s00261-008-9452-0
49. Clevert DA, Weckbach S, Minaifar N, Clevert DA, Stickel M, Reiser M. Contrast-enhanced ultrasound versus MS-CT in blunt abdominal trauma. *Clin Hemorheol Microcirc*. 2008;39(1–4):155–169 PMID: 18503121
50. Manetta R, Pistoia ML, Bultrini C, Stavroulis E, Di Cesare E, Masciocchi C. Ultrasound enhanced with sulphur-hexafluoride-filled microbubbles agent (SonoVue) in the follow-up of mild liver and spleen trauma. *Radiol Med (Torino)*. 2009;114(5):771–779 PMID: 19484583 https://doi.org/10.1007/s11547-009-0406-6
51. Thorelius L. Emergency real-time contrast-enhanced ultrasonography for detection of solid organ injuries. *Eur Radiol*. 2007;17(suppl 6):F107–F111 PMID: 18376464 https://doi.org/10.1007/s10406-007-0235-4
52. Valentino M, Serra C, Pavlica P, et al. Blunt abdominal trauma: diagnostic performance of contrast-enhanced US in children–initial experience. *Radiology*. 2008;246(3):903–909 PMID: 18195385 https://doi.org/10.1148/radiol.2463070652
53. Oldenburg A, Hohmann J, Skrok J, Albrecht T. Imaging of paediatric splenic injury with contrast-enhanced ultrasonography. *Pediatr Radiol*. 2004;34(4):351–354 PMID: 14652701 https://doi.org/10.1007/s00247-003-1092-5
54. Valentino M, Serra C, Zironi G, De Luca C, Pavlica P, Barozzi L. Blunt abdominal trauma: emergency contrast-enhanced sonography for detection of solid organ injuries. *AJR Am J Roentgenol*. 2006;186(5):1361–1367 PMID: 16632732 https://doi.org/10.2214/AJR.05.0027
55. Armstrong LB, Mooney DP, Paltiel H, et al. Contrast enhanced ultrasound for the evaluation of blunt pediatric abdominal trauma. *J Pediatr Surg*. 2018;53(3):548–552 PMID: 28351519
56. Jevtovic-Todorovic V. Anesthetics and cognitive impairments in developing children: what is our responsibility? *JAMA Pediatr*. 2017;171(12):1135–1136 PMID: 28973500 https://doi.org/10.1001/jamapediatrics.2017.3033
57. Bennett BL, Mahabee-Gittens M, Chua MS, Hirsch R. Elevated cardiac troponin I level in cases of thoracic nonaccidental trauma. *Pediatr Emerg Care*. 2011;27(10):941–944 PMID: 21960096 https://doi.org/10.1097/PEC.0b013e3182307afe
58. Bennett BL, Steele P, Dixon CA, et al. Serum cardiac troponin I in the evaluation of nonaccidental trauma. *J Pediatr*. 2015;167(3):669–673.e1 PMID: 26141552
59. Harper NS, Eddleman S, Lindberg DM; ExSTRA Investigators. The utility of follow-up skeletal surveys in child abuse. *Pediatrics*. 2013;131(3):e672–e678 PMID: 23400607 https://doi.org/10.1542/peds.2012-2608
60. Sanchez TR, Grasparil AD, Chaudhari R, Coulter KP, Wootton-Gorges SL. Characteristics of rib fractures in child abuse—the role of low-dose chest computed

tomography. *Pediatr Emerg Care*. 2018;34(2):81–83 PMID: 26760828 https://doi.org/10.1097/PEC.0000000000000608
61. Drubach LA, Johnston PR, Newton AW, Perez-Rossello JM, Grant FD, Kleinman PK. Skeletal trauma in child abuse: detection with 18F-NaF PET. *Radiology*. 2010;255(1):173–181 PMID: 20308455 https://doi.org/10.1148/radiol.09091368
62. Bainbridge JK, Huey BM, Harrison SK. Should bone scintigraphy be used as a routine adjunct to skeletal survey in the imaging of non-accidental injury? A 10 year review of reports in a single centre. *Clin Radiol*. 2015;70(8):e83–e89 PMID: 26055408 https://doi.org/10.1016/j.crad.2015.04.012
63. Lamireau T, McLin V, Nobili V, Vajro P. A practical approach to the child with abnormal liver tests. *Clin Res Hepatol Gastroenterol*. 2014;38(3):259–262 PMID: 24736033 https://doi.org/10.1016/j.clinre.2014.02.010
64. Kandula L, Lowe ME. Etiology and outcome of acute pancreatitis in infants and toddlers. *J Pediatr*. 2008;152(1):106–110, 110.e1
65. Oracz G, Kolodziejczyk E, Sobczynska-Tomaszewska A, et al. The clinical course of hereditary pancreatitis in children—a comprehensive analysis of 41 cases. *Pancreatology*. 2016;16(4):535–541 PMID: 27179762 https://doi.org/10.1016/j.pan.2016.04.009
66. Berona K, Kang T, Rose E. Pelvic free fluid in asymptomatic pediatric blunt abdominal trauma patients: a case series and review of the literature. *J Emerg Med*. 2016;50(5):753–758 PMID: 26884127 https://doi.org/10.1016/j.jemermed.2016.01.003
67. Holmes JF, London KL, Brant WE, Kuppermann N. Isolated intraperitoneal fluid on abdominal computed tomography in children with blunt trauma. *Acad Emerg Med*. 2000;7(4):335–341 PMID: 10805620 https://doi.org/10.1111/j.1553-2712.2000.tb02232.x
68. Christiano JG, Tummers M, Kennedy A. Clinical significance of isolated intraperitoneal fluid on computed tomography in pediatric blunt abdominal trauma. *J Pediatr Surg*. 2009;44(6):1242–1248 PMID: 19524748 https://doi.org/10.1016/j.jpedsurg.2009.02.045
69. McAloon J, O'Neill C. Ossification centres, not rib fractures. *Arch Dis Child*. 2011;96(3):284 PMID: 21252063 https://doi.org/10.1136/adc.2010.207951
70. Shashikumar VL, Bassuk A, Pilling GP IV, Cresson SL. Spontaneous gastric rupture in the newborn: a clinical review of nineteen cases. *Ann Surg*. 1975;182(1):22–25 PMID: 1147704 https://doi.org/10.1097/00000658-197507000-00004
71. Libeer F, Vanhamel N, Huyghe M, Verlinden E. Spontaneous gastric rupture in non-neonatal children: a case report. *Acta Chir Belg*. 2007;107(5):560–563 PMID: 18074921 https://doi.org/10.1080/00015458.2007.11680124
72. Jona JZ. Benign pneumatosis intestinalis coli after blunt trauma to the abdomen in a child. *J Pediatr Surg*. 2000;35(7):1109–1111 PMID: 10917307 https://doi.org/10.1053/jpsu.2000.7837
73. Deutsch SA, Christian CW. Pneumatosis intestinalis due to child abuse. *Pediatr Emerg Care*. 2016 PMID: 27902668 https://doi.org/10.1097/PEC.0000000000000976
74. Sagar M, Shukla S, Bradley-Dodds K. Nonaccidental trauma presenting with respiratory distress and pleural effusion. *Pediatr Emerg Care*. 2012;28(1):61–63 PMID: 22217891 https://doi.org/10.1097/PEC.0b013e3182417a77
75. Joffe M, Ludwig S. Stairway injuries in children. *Pediatrics*. 1988;82(3 Pt 2):457–461 PMID: 3405681
76. Chiaviello CT, Christoph RA, Bond GR. Stairway-related injuries in children. *Pediatrics*. 1994;94(5):679–681 PMID: 7936895
77. Huntimer CM, Muret-Wagstaff S, Leland NL. Can falls on stairs result in small intestine perforations? *Pediatrics*. 2000;106(2 Pt 1):301–305 PMID: 10920155 https://doi.org/10.1542/peds.106.2.301

78. Wang MY, Kim KA, Griffith PM, et al. Injuries from falls in the pediatric population: an analysis of 729 cases. *J Pediatr Surg*. 2001;36(10):1528–1534 PMID: 11584402 https://doi.org/10.1053/jpsu.2001.27037
79. Bush CM, Jones JS, Cohle SD, Johnson H. Pediatric injuries from cardiopulmonary resuscitation. *Ann Emerg Med*. 1996;28(1):40–44 PMID: 8669737 https://doi.org/10.1016/S0196-0644(96)70137-3
80. Alkan M, Iskit SH, Soyupak S, et al. Severe abdominal trauma involving bicycle handlebars in children. *Pediatr Emerg Care*. 2012;28(4):357–360 PMID: 19680164 https://doi.org/10.1097/PEC.0b013e3181acd30f
81. Arbogast KB, Moll EK, Morris SD, Anderko RL, Durbin DR, Winston FK. Factors influencing pediatric injury in side impact collisions. *J Trauma*. 2001;51(3):469–477 PMID: 11535893 https://doi.org/10.1097/00005373-200109000-00008
82. Canty TG Sr, Canty TG Jr, Brown C. Injuries of the gastrointestinal tract from blunt trauma in children: a 12-year experience at a designated pediatric trauma center. *J Trauma*. 1999;46(2):234–240 PMID: 10029026 https://doi.org/10.1097/00005373-199902000-00005
83. Abbas SM, Upadhyay V. Hollow viscus injury in children: Starship Hospital experience. *World J Emerg Surg*. 2007;2(1):14 PMID: 17547770 https://doi.org/10.1186/1749-7922-2-14
84. Knapp JF, Sharma V, Wasserman G, Hoover CJ, Walsh I. Ventricular septal defect following blunt chest trauma in childhood: a case report. *Pediatr Emerg Care*. 1986;2(4):242–243 PMID: 3797270 https://doi.org/10.1097/00006565-198612000-00009
85. Maron BJ. Sudden death in young athletes. *N Engl J Med*. 2003;349(11):1064–1075 PMID: 12968091 https://doi.org/10.1056/NEJMra022783
86. van Rijn RR, Bilo RA, Robben SG. Birth-related mid-posterior rib fractures in neonates: a report of three cases (and a possible fourth case) and a review of the literature. *Pediatr Radiol*. 2009;39(1):30–34 PMID: 18941740 https://doi.org/10.1007/s00247-008-1035-2
87. Goldberg A, Ruest S, Kannan G, Moore J. Rib fracture prevalence in infants and children. Paper presented at: Annual Meeting of the Helfer Society; 2018; Nashville, TN
88. Stylianos S; The APSA Trauma Committee. Evidence-based guidelines for resource utilization in children with isolated spleen or liver injury. *J Pediatr Surg*. 2000;35(2):164–169 PMID: 10693659 https://doi.org/10.1016/S0022-3468(00)90003-4
89. Dangle PP, Fuller TW, Gaines B, et al. Evolving mechanisms of injury and management of pediatric blunt renal trauma—20 years of experience. *Urology*. 2016;90:159–163 PMID: 26825488 https://doi.org/10.1016/j.urology.2016.01.017
90. Holmes JH 4th, Wiebe DJ, Tataria M, et al. The failure of nonoperative management in pediatric solid organ injury: a multi-institutional experience. *J Trauma*. 2005;59(6):1309–1313 PMID: 16394902 https://doi.org/10.1097/01.ta.0000197366.38404.79
91. Arbra CA, Vogel AM, Zhang J, et al. Acute procedural interventions after pediatric blunt abdominal trauma: a prospective multicenter evaluation. *J Trauma Acute Care Surg*. 2017;83(4):597–602 PMID: 28930954 https://doi.org/10.1097/TA.0000000000001533
92. Letton RW, Worrell V; APSA Committee on Trauma Blunt Intestinal Injury Study Group. Delay in diagnosis and treatment of blunt intestinal injury does not adversely affect prognosis in the pediatric trauma patient. *J Pediatr Surg*. 2010;45(1):161–166 PMID: 20105598 https://doi.org/10.1016/j.jpedsurg.2009.10.027

CHAPTER 6

Maxillofacial, Neck, and Dental Manifestations of Child Abuse

Ryan Brown, MD, FAAP
Clinical Associate Professor
Department of Pediatrics
The University of Oklahoma College of Medicine
Medical Director, Child Protection Team
The Children's Hospital at OU Medical Center
Oklahoma City, OK

Larissa Hines, MD, FAAP
Child Protection and Family Health, Department of Pediatrics
University of Utah School of Medicine
Salt Lake City, UT

Introduction

Physical injuries to the structures of the face, mouth, and neck are among the most common seen in children who have experienced abuse. Studies have shown that 65% to 75% of all physical abuse involves injuries to the head, neck, and face, with approximately half involving some form of orofacial injury.[1–3] For example, Willging et al[4] reviewed the medical records of 4,340 children who experienced abuse who were seen at a large urban hospital over 5 years. Injuries to the head and neck were seen in 49% of these children, and of those, the head or neck was the primary injury site in 82% of cases. In another retrospective analysis of hospitalized children who experienced abuse, Leavitt et al[5] found the incidence of otolaryngological findings to be 56%, more than half of which were directly related to physical abuse or neglect. Craniofacial injuries also are the most common injuries sustained by children who intervene in domestic violence.[6]

Abusive injuries to the face and mouth typically are caused by blunt trauma by a hand or object, although penetrating trauma to facial cavities is well described. Most documented injuries are mild, with ecchymoses, abrasions, and lacerations most common.[4] Overall, boys and girls suffer from maltreatment at the same rate.[7] However, among emergency department visits for physical abuse, boys are more likely to be seen than girls (56% vs 46%).[8] Many of the injuries are mild, requiring outpatient treatment only. In the early part of child abuse literature, extensive facial injuries were described.[9] Orofacial injuries are not commonly isolated and often are associated with more severe internal injuries.

Certain injuries, such as those to the ear, nose, or throat, should arouse suspicion of abuse, especially in infants and young children. The TEN-4 rule specifies that bruising to the *t*orso, *e*ars, or *n*eck, or bruising in infants younger than 4 months, are significant indicators of abuse.[10] When recurrent, these injuries are almost always inflicted.[11] Cutaneous injuries are easily recognized, but injuries to the oral cavity may be overlooked by physicians who do not routinely examine the structures within the mouth.[2,12]

Injuries to the Face

Bruising and Burns

Contusions are the most common injury seen in children who have experienced abuse and are the most common injury sustained to the head and face.[1,2] The specificity for abuse of facial bruising is highest in young children. Facial bruising is notably uncommon during infancy and is even more atypical in nonambulatory infants.[13–15] In contrast with accidental injuries, bruises to the head and face are common in infants who have experienced abuse.[16,17] Pacifiers and bottles have been used by frustrated caregivers to inflict such injuries (Figure 6.1). These injuries should always elicit concern.

One key component to the child abuse evaluation is the inquiry of past injuries to a child. *Sentinel events* are injuries that are discovered in hindsight after a child has experienced abuse (see Chapter 1, Sentinel Injuries). In a large institutional study, 27.5% of children who had experienced abusive head injuries had a sentinel injury, with nearly two-thirds of all bruises noted on the face, forehead, or ear. Also, tears to the upper labial frenulum should raise concerns for abuse, especially in children who are not mobile.[18]

McMahon et al[19] reviewed soft tissue injuries in 341 hospitalized children reported for abuse and compared patterns of injury by age. Although infants averaged only one soft tissue injury, approximately 50% of those injuries were to the head and face. In contrast, children older than 2 years averaged 3 soft tissue injuries, of which 25% were to the head and face. Labbé and Caouette[20] performed 2,040 physical examinations in a 1-year period on children 0 to 17 years old to identify patterns of recent skin injuries in children who had not experienced abuse. While injuries in ambulatory

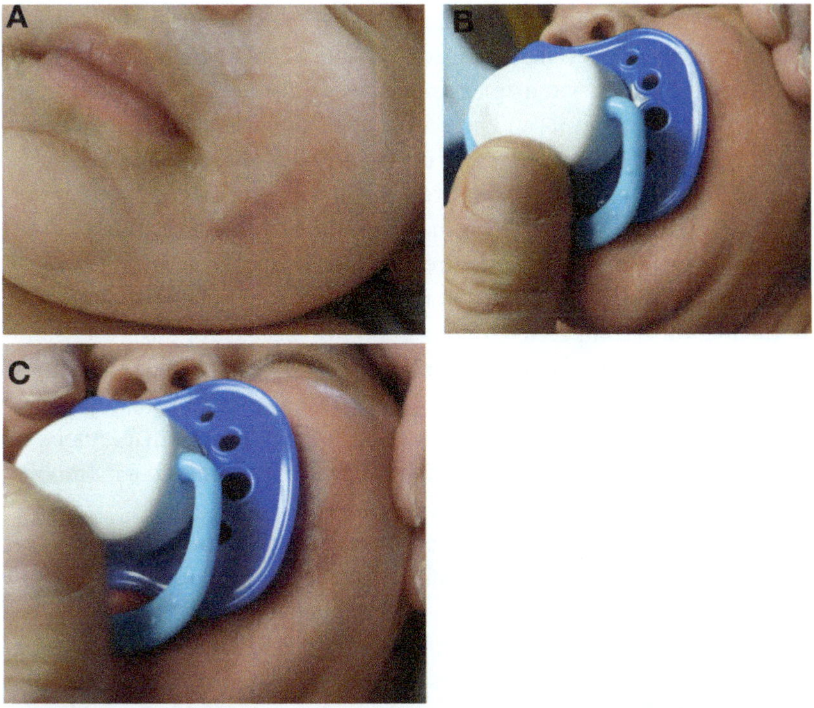

FIGURE 6.1
A 4-month-old with cheek bruising (A), which matched the shape of his favorite pacifier (B, C).

children were common, fewer than 1% of all children examined had injuries to the chin, ears, or neck. Injuries in those locations, while not diagnostic of child abuse, should be scrutinized. Nonambulatory infants were least likely to have any injury on the body, although in the 11% who did have an injury, most were self-inflicted fingernail scratches. Bruises were very uncommon in this age; only 1% of nonambulatory infants had any bruise to the body at all. Facial bruising in infants may be the only external indication of trauma and is often associated with skeletal or other internal injuries.[14]

Inflicted facial burns may result from scalding or contact with hot objects and represent approximately 20% of inflicted burns identified. Immersion facial injuries are occasionally reported.[21] In a reported series of inflicted facial immersion burns, children's faces were submerged into sinks, bathtubs, or containers of hot liquids. Mortality from immersion in sinks or tubs was extremely high.

Fractures

Facial fractures are uncommon pediatric injuries. Approximately 5% of all facial fractures occur before the age of 12 years, and only 1% occur in the first 5 years after birth.[22] The frequency of facial fractures is higher among the adolescent population, and in this age group the pattern of fractures begins to resemble that seen in adults. Fractures to the mid-third of the facial skeleton are uncommon in preadolescent children and extremely rare in infants and preschool-aged children.[15,23] Fractures of the zygoma or maxillary fractures of the Le Fort type are rare pediatric injuries[24] and have not been reported in children who have experienced abuse. Mandibular fractures are more common. The pediatric mandible, however, is protected from fracture by the elasticity of the developing mandible; the relatively thick, soft tissue of the face; and the small size of the mandible compared with the cranium.[25] Because of the protection the frontal bone affords the smaller mandible, major head trauma is more likely to be transmitted to the frontal bone than the mandible.[15] When mandibular fractures occur, they are likely to be located in the premolar or subcondylar region, and more than one fracture site within the mandible is common throughout childhood (Figure 6.2).[17]

Mandibular fractures are uncommon but well described in children who have experienced abuse. Neonatal mandibular fracture inflicted by a mother who has postpartum psychosis has been reported.[26] In a review by Siegel et al[25] of 73 mandibular fractures seen at an urban children's hospital over 10 years, mandibular fractures were most common in adolescents and least common in infants and preschoolers. Altercation, with direct blow to the jaw, was the most frequent cause of fracture. Child abuse accounted for 14% of the injuries, with an equal distribution throughout childhood. The authors concluded that child abuse should be strongly considered when infants present with isolated mandibular fractures.

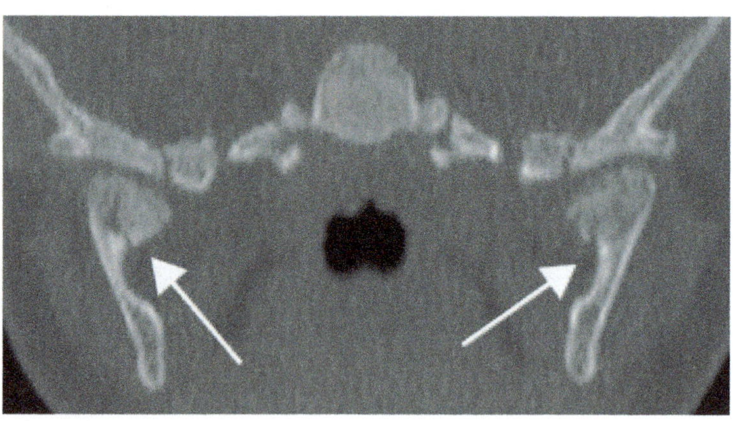

FIGURE 6.2
A 4-month-old with bilateral, non-displaced subcondylar fractures of the mandible (arrows). The baby had bruising to the chin after falling from a changing table onto a hard tile surface.

Clinically, mandibular fractures in the premolar area are not severely painful. Those involving the subcondylar region are associated with trismus and pain and tenderness in the region of the temporomandibular joint. A contusion in the floor of the mouth may denote a fracture of the mandible. An irregularity in the mandibular arch may be noted, including alteration of the dental occlusion. Treatment varies by age and severity of the fracture.[19]

Injuries to the Ear

Injuries to the external and internal structures of the ear are well described in children who have experienced abuse and may result from direct or penetrating trauma. Figure 6.3 shows the anatomical structures of the ear. Blows to the ear may cause bruising or hematomas of the pinna (figures 6.4 and 6.5), abrasions, scarring, or, less commonly, meatal wall lacerations, hemotympanum, or perforation of the tympanic membrane.[5] Bruises caused by pinching or pulling the ear may reveal a matching bruise on the posterior surface.[27] Auricular perichondritis (cauliflower ear) can be caused by repetitive trauma such as pulling of the pinna or direct blows.[27] Other

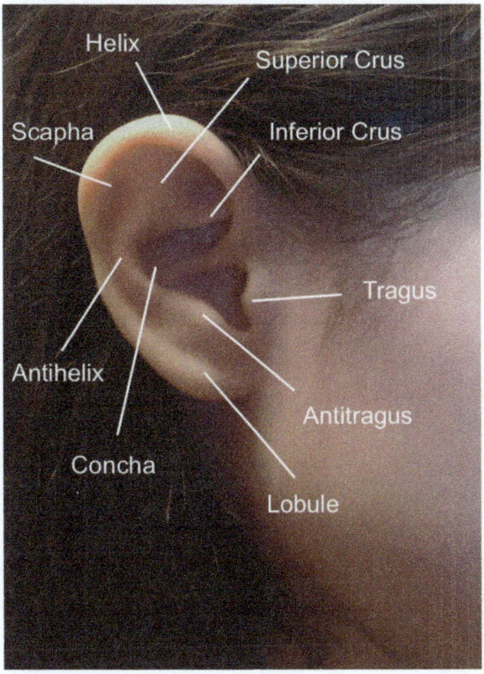

FIGURE 6.3
Anatomical landmarks of the ear.

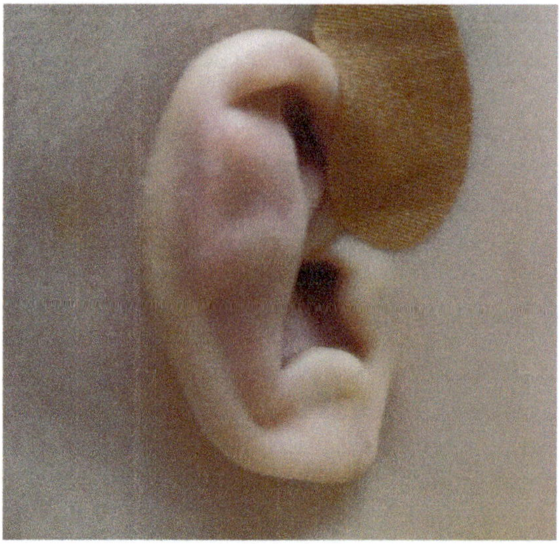

FIGURE 6.4
Auricular hematoma in a 3-year-old resulting from repeated pulling of and direct blows to the pinna.

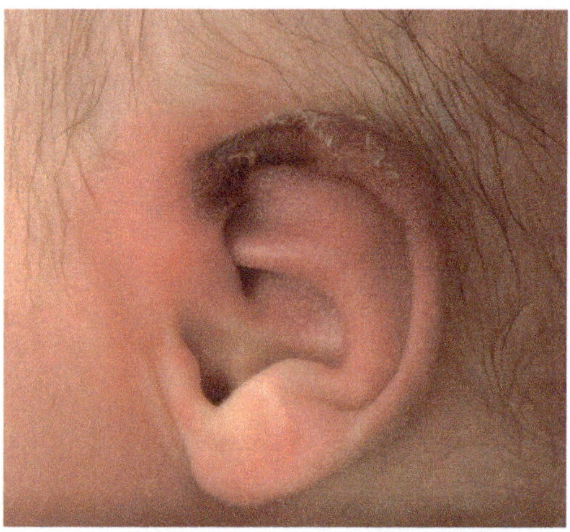

FIGURE 6.5
A 2-week-old with ear bruising caused by biting of the ear by caregiver. The baby had multiple other injuries.

unusual injuries include a report of ossicular discontinuity (fractured stapes) from a blow to the ear and simulation of recurrent ear bleeding using beet juice.[11] Instillation of caustic substances into the external ear canal can manifest with ataxia, nystagmus, and facial nerve dysfunction and can lead to otorrhea, burns, and inflammation of the external auditory canal and perforation of the tympanic membrane.[28,29] Penetrating trauma with a pointed instrument may result in direct injury to the external meatus, tympanic membrane, or middle or inner ear. Repeated penetrating injuries are rarely accidental and are described in cases of medical child abuse.[30] Other aural manifestations of medical child abuse include trauma to the auditory canal resulting in bloody otorrhea or otitis externa and repeated placement of foreign bodies or substances, such as saliva, in the ear canal.[31–34] Like other orofacial injuries, aural injuries are unlikely to be isolated.

The tin ear syndrome is a pathognomonic triad of abuse consisting of unilateral ear bruising, radiographic evidence of ipsilateral cerebral edema with loss of the basilar cistern, and retinal hemorrhage.[35] The ear injuries described in the original report consisted of purpuric hemorrhages in the antitragus, helix, triangular fossa, and the interior folds of the ear. Internal ear injury was not present. All 3 children described died, and autopsy revealed the presence of an ipsilateral thin layer subdural hemorrhage. The mechanism postulated was blunt injury to the ear, resulting in rotational acceleration of the head and subsequent brain injury.

Injuries to the Nose

Abusive trauma to the nose, like other inflicted facial trauma, is often associated with extracranial injury. Blunt trauma to the nose can result in superficial abrasions, bruises, or nasal fractures.[4] Figure 6.6 shows the anatomical structures of the nose. The development of a hematoma and abscess of the nasal septum after direct trauma is a rare complication of abuse. Canty and Berkowitz[36] noted 2 children who had experienced abuse in their case series of septal hematoma and abscess. Unlike the older children who developed hematoma and abscess of the nasal septum after minor, isolated nasal trauma, the children who experienced abuse were young (< 2 years); had severe facial, neck, and nasal injuries; and had a history of previous abuse. Nasal bone fractures are less common in children than soft tissue injuries because of the compliant nature of the pediatric bone.[37] Failure to treat nasal injury appropriately potentially leads to disturbances in growth and development of the nose and surrounding structures.[36–39]

Columella destruction and septal perforation, while uncommon, are documented in the abuse literature.[38,39] Fischer and Allasio[40] reported 6-month-old twins with traumatic destruction of the nose. One infant had loss of the nasal tip, columella, and distal nasal septum, with collapse of the nares; the other had loss of the alar rim and collapse of the nostril. Further investigation revealed nasal deformities in a 2-year-old sister. The nasal injuries to all 3 children were isolated and thought to be caused by forceful, repeated nasal rubbing or picking (Figure 6.7).

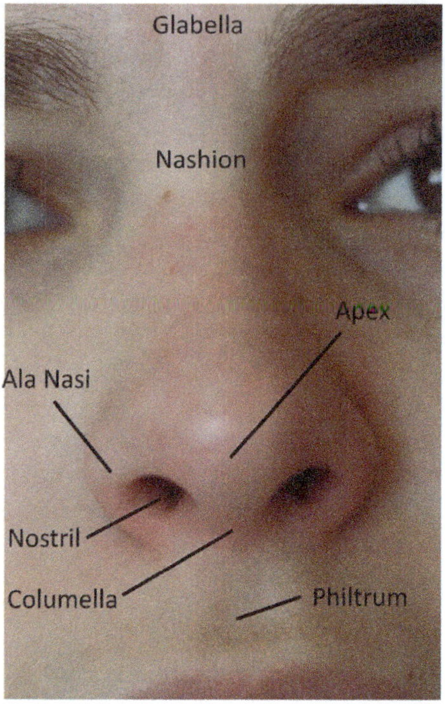

FIGURE 6.6
Anatomical landmarks of the nose.

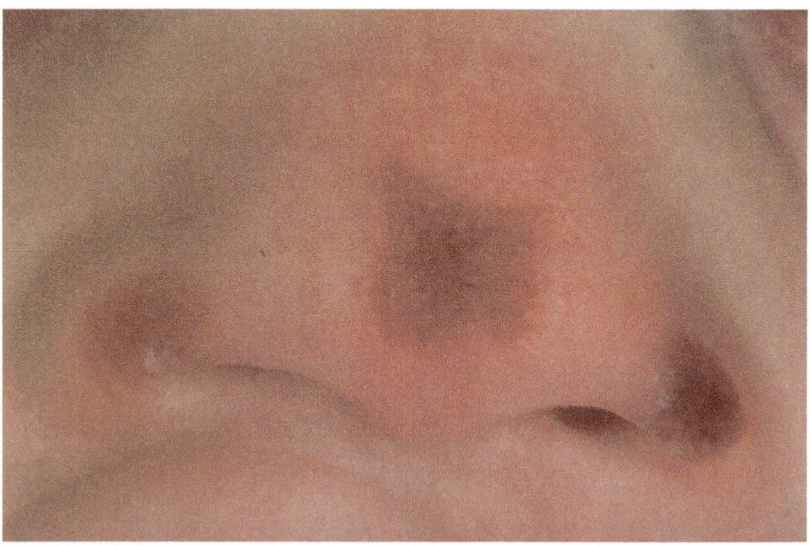

FIGURE 6.7
A 2-week-old with deep abrasions of bilateral nasal alae and nasal apex. The baby had multiple other injuries.

Nosebleeds, although common in the pediatric population, can be a sign of abuse, especially in the very young. Rees et al compiled a literature search to determine the proportion of children younger than 2 years who had been asphyxiated and presented with epistaxis. In 3 studies, the proportion of children presenting with epistaxis who had been asphyxiated was between 7% and 24%. Other features associated with asphyxia in live children were altered skin color, abnormalities on chest radiograph, respiratory difficulty, and malaise. It was recommended that a thorough investigation as to the etiology of epistaxis in an infant with unexplained epistaxis should be performed.[41]

Injuries to the Pharynx, Larynx, and Esophagus

Iatrogenic pharyngeal and cervical esophageal perforation in infants is uncommon and usually related to instrumentation of the oropharynx. A diagram of the anatomical structures of the oropharynx is shown in Figure 6.8. The incidence of oral, jaw, or neck injury during intubation is less than 1%; injuries found in these areas are significantly associated with abuse.[42] The anatomical weakness of the hypopharyngeal-esophageal junction predisposes this area to perforation.[43] Similar perforations due to child abuse are occasionally reported in the literature and are typically caused by penetrating trauma to the child's mouth.[44–46] In a systematic review, Reece et al described pharyngeal perforations to be the abusive injury most frequently seen by otolaryngologists.[46] These injuries were more common in younger infants and manifested with subcutaneous emphysema, drooling, dysphagia, and hemoptysis. Additional injuries were found in more than half of these patients, with external ear injuries being the most common. Pharyngeal or esophageal lacerations introduce air, oral secretions, and bacteria into the soft tissues of the neck and mediastinum, with potentially life-threatening sequelae.[43,47] Such consequences of injury are well described. In 1971, Morris and Reay[48] described a battered baby with respiratory and feeding difficulties. Investigation revealed pharyngeal atresia, in which the soft palate was fused with the posterior pharyngeal wall. The authors suggest that the atresia was congenital, although they considered the more probable traumatic etiology. Inflicted tears to the palate, pharynx, tonsillar fossa, and high posterior cervical esophagus have resulted in the development of esophageal abscesses, pneumomediastinum, and a mediastinal pseudocyst.[49,50] Bansal and Abramo[51] reported a 2-month-old who had experienced abuse with severe subcutaneous emphysema of the scalp, neck, and anterior and posterior

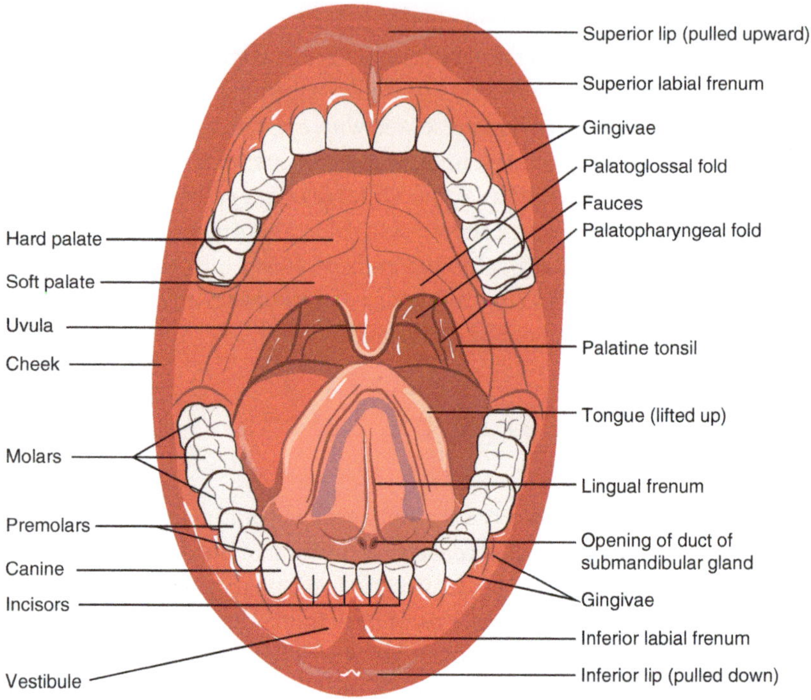

FIGURE 6.8
Anatomical landmarks of the oropharynx.

chest, with pneumomediastinum and subsequent *Moraxella catarrhalis* sepsis caused by traumatic pharyngeal laceration.

Children with perforating injuries may present with fever, drooling, respiratory distress, erythematous cervical swelling, dysphagia, dysphonia, subcutaneous emphysema, or pneumomediastinum.[47] Infants with perforating pharyngeal injuries may have concomitant acute rib fractures, which may be missed on initial skeletal survey (Figure 6.9). These fractures are most likely due to forceful chest squeezing during the oral trauma. Although most traumatic perforations associated with abuse occur in infants, exceptions exist.[52] Ablin and Reinhart[53] describe a 6-year-old who had experienced abuse whose avulsed tooth was impacted through the esophageal wall, leading to a retropharyngeal and mediastinal abscess. The authors suggest the possibility of sexual assault as the cause of the initial injury.

Oral and esophageal foreign bodies in children who have experienced abuse are well described.[11] In a series of abusive ingestions and foreign bodies, Friedman[54] reported a 6-month-old who was found to have a metallic foreign body in the esophagus and lower gastrointestinal tract and an 8-year-old boy who drank a glass of lye, causing extensive caustic burns and

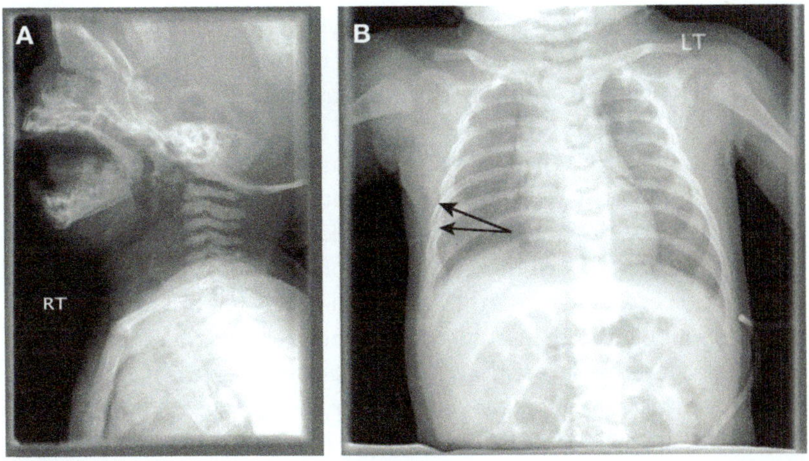

FIGURE 6.9
A, A 3-month-old who presented with hemoptysis, stridor, and respiratory distress. Lateral neck radiograph shows retropharyngeal swelling and air in the retropharyngeal space. In the operating room, the baby was found to have injury with eschar formation to the posterior pharynx. B, Chest radiograph of the same 3-month-old shows pneumomediastinum and acute fractures of the right lateral fourth through sixth ribs (arrows).

subsequent esophageal strictures. Intentional poisonings by caregivers can be inflicted with poisons or normal household substances (eg, water, salt) and can be associated with medical child abuse.[55] Krugman et al describes 4 infants with aspiration of baby wipes due to forced suffocation.[56] Foreign bodies being forced into the esophagus as a form of fatal child abuse is rare. Nolte[57] described repeated introduction of coins into the esophagus of a 5-month-old who ultimately died with multiple coins found in the esophagus.

Vocal cord paralysis can be a complication of strangulation or abusive head trauma.[58] The paralysis is due to central or peripheral neuropathology. Children with unilateral paralysis may have few acute symptoms other than a weak voice or cry but are at risk for aspiration. Children with bilateral vocal cord paralysis usually have stridor or signs of upper airway obstruction. Bilateral cord paralysis can be an overlooked cause of extubation failure in patients with severe head injuries.

Injuries to the Neck

Neck injuries in children who have experienced abuse are less well studied than those of the head, although case reports of inflicted neck injuries are well documented. Cutaneous injuries, usually contusions or abrasions, are reported in a series of children who were abused.[59] More unusual injuries have also been documented. Ng et al[60] reported a 1-year-old who was found to have multiple needles embedded in her neck. This was discovered after an autopsy of the child's 1-month-old sister revealed multiple needles in the brain and body. The authors speculate that the ethnic and cultural origins of the patients reported (Indian and African) may be relevant in this form of injury.[61] Although bruises are familiar injuries, Williams and colleagues[62] reported a child whose apparent cervical bruising was found to represent a cystic lymphangioma of the neck.

Strangulation is a well-described cause of child homicide.[63] The physical examination of a child who has been strangled may reveal linear or circumferential ligature marks. Isolated venous obstruction from more mild neck compression may lead to petechiae over the skin of the face and posterior-auricular region, the conjunctivae, or oral mucosa.[64] There also may be intense facial congestion, especially in fatal cases. The petechiae are due to increased vascular pressure, which ruptures small venules. Petechiae will not be seen if the strangulation causes simultaneous venous and arterial obstruction. Direct radiologic evidence of strangulation is rare. Carty[65] described the radiologic finding of calcification in the supraclavicular soft tissues of a 3-month-old who had experienced abuse. The calcification was thought to be caused by fat necrosis from previous strangulation of the baby. Although strangulation or suffocation of a child may cause petechial hemorrhages of the face or neck, this is not a reliable finding. In a series of 14 patients who were intentionally suffocated during covert video surveillance, no child had facial markings that lasted more than 30 to 60 seconds after the attempted suffocation.[66] Meadow[67] reviewed the records of 81 children who were fatally smothered. Blood in the mouth or nose or on the face was reported in 39% of the children, and only 10 children had either bruises or petechiae on the face or neck. More than half of the victims had neither bruises, petechiae, nor a history or finding of bleeding. Accidental strangulation from a mother's long hair during co-sleeping also has been described in the literature.[68]

Injuries to the Cervical Spine

Cervical spine and spinal cord injuries were once thought to be uncommon findings in children who had experienced abuse, but they have been found to occur in 15% of young children with inflicted injuries.[69–72] Injuries to the cervical spine and cord may escape detection if not properly evaluated. With the improved and increased use of magnetic resonance imaging (MRI) in the evaluation of children involved in trauma, both accidental and non-accidental, the once perceived low rates of injury have increased.

Cervical spinal cord injury without radiographic abnormality is a well-known phenomenon in young children and is related to the mechanical tolerances of the young spine. Plain radiographs and computed tomography will fail to detect such cord injuries, although MRI may detect abnormalities such as those of the ligaments or spinal cord.[73] Concomitant brain injury in some children who experienced abuse may obscure signs of cervical cord injury.[71] Some injuries to the spine are asymptomatic and are identified only with MRI or even autopsy.

Spinal cord injuries in children, either accidental or inflicted, occur most commonly in the upper region. One study showed that about 74% of injuries in a study of 504 children involved the C1 and/or C2 vertebrae. In recent years, an association of cervical cord injury and inflicted head injury has been noted. Most of the findings point to ligamentous injuries.[74] In a comparative study of 183 infants younger than 48 months, cervical injuries were found in a majority. Cervical spine ligamentous injuries were found to be present in 78% of infants with abusive head trauma, 46% of infants who had a traumatic injury not associated with abuse, and only 1% of infants in a non-accidental control group. The majority of the cervical injuries involved the nuchal, atlanto-occipital, and atlantoaxial ligaments.[75]

Fractures

Despite the frequency of abusive head trauma attributed to shaking, fractures to the cervical spine are rare. One study of cervical injuries in patients with abusive head trauma revealed that 71% of the children had a cervical cord injury, but none of the 52 children studied had a cervical fracture.[76] Cervical spine fractures associated with abuse are reported in infants and are postulated to be caused by forced hyperflexion or hyperextension of the neck during shaking or a direct blow. The actual mechanism of these injuries remains speculative, and concomitant intracranial injury is typically absent.[77] Cervical spine fractures may manifest with symptoms related to cord compression but are often asymptomatic, identified during skeletal survey.[78,79] In almost all case reports, additional skeletal injuries are present. Compression fractures, fracture dislocations, and anterior subluxations all may result from abuse. A hangman's fracture, which results from traumatic spondylolysis of the C2 vertebrae, is a rare manifestation of abuse.[80–82] Like other cervical fractures, it is thought to be caused by severe hyperflexion or hyperextension of the neck. Congenital spondylolysis can be confused with a hangman's fracture, and serial radiographic studies may be needed to distinguish the two.[83,84] A large cohort study found that intracranial injuries were present in up to 70% of children who had spinal fractures due to abuse.[85] This highlights the importance of a maltreatment workup in children with spinal fractures.

Injuries Resulting From Sexual Abuse

The oral cavity is frequently involved in child sexual abuse cases.[86] Forced oral sex, or fellatio, can cause palatal erythema, petechiae, and bruising; repeated fellatio can cause deep palatal ulcerations.[87] Similar injuries can also be seen on the floor of the mouth.[88] Sexually transmitted infections can have variable appearances in the oral cavity, making identification difficult for practitioners.[89] For example, oral gonorrhea may present with pharyngitis, exudative tonsillitis, or gingivitis but is most often asymptomatic in children.[90] However, confirmed oral gonorrhea in preadolescent children is pathognomonic for sexual abuse.[90,91] Condyloma acuminatum may be found in the mucosa of the lip, cheek, palate, gingiva, or tongue but is infrequently considered in the differential diagnosis of oral lesions in children.[87,92] The primary chancre of syphilis can be located on the lip, although this is rare in children.

A careful examination of the oral cavity in children who have been sexually abused is warranted and, on occasion, may reveal evidence to substantiate the diagnosis. If the child is verbal, a forensic interview can be helpful to augment the physical examination.

Injuries to the Oral Cavity

Many injuries to facial structures are within the scope of dentistry or easily observed by the dental professional in the course of routine dental treatment. Some types of injuries are pathognomonic for abuse and easily identified by the dentist. Injuries of this type include those that appear simultaneously on multiple body planes.[93] The anatomical tooth structure is shown in Figure 6.10. Injuries that exhibit patterned marks, implements, or an adult's hand, or bilateral injuries to the face, carry a high index of suspicion of abuse and can occur on easily observable areas of the child's body.[94] Various explanations for the mouth as a target of abuse are possible. Injuries to the mouth represent an assault on the communicative "self" of the child and can be a compelling reason behind abuse directed at the mouth. Another factor is the adult's easy access to the head of a child, which is often well within reach. Also, any physical injury or emotional trauma may elicit a cry from the child. Efforts to silence the crying often can result in injuries to the mouth. The oral cavity is not only significant in communication but also in the nutrition of the child, which is felt to be a reason for physical abuse in this region.[95]

While treatment of oral injuries is usually referred to a general dentist, pediatric dentist, or oral surgeon, proper evaluation of the child who has experienced abuse cannot be completed without a thorough examination by the primary care clinician. Various types of oral injuries

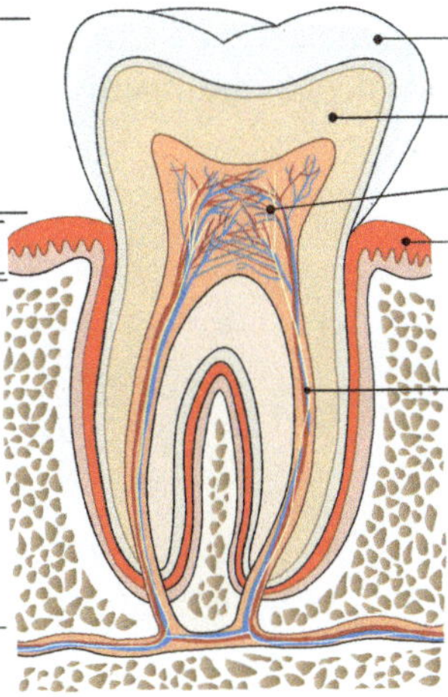

FIGURE 6.10
Anatomical structures of the tooth.

may be encountered in any clinical setting. Orofacial injuries that may be encountered in child abuse include trauma to the teeth, supporting structures, and surrounding tissues. The principal intraoral injuries of child abuse include missing and fractured teeth, oral contusions, oral lacerations, jaw fractures, and oral burns. Naidoo reported the most common location for inflicted mouth injuries was the lips (54%), with less frequent injuries of the oral mucosa, teeth, gingiva, and tongue.[12]

Oral Injuries to Infants

Inflicted injuries to oral structures of the infant should be considered separately from those of older children. Infants generally do not have teeth before 4 to 6 months of age. The pattern of eruption of primary teeth varies widely and is usually not important in deciding whether child abuse has occurred. Delayed eruption of primary teeth may, however, be seen in cases of child neglect resulting from poor nutrition or may be a result of poor prenatal nutrition during fetal development.

The difficulties and frustrations surrounding an infant's feeding may lead to abuse. Intraoral lacerations have long been recognized as possible indicators of forced feeding and abuse.[96] Injury can occur when excessive pressure is used while feeding with a bottle or when a utensil is misdirected during feeding. If the adult feels that the infant is uncooperative during bottle-feeding, the adult may use excessive force to introduce the nipple into the infant's mouth or press too firmly against oral structures. This can cause mild to severe contusions of the lips, gingivae, and floor of the mouth, as well as lacerations of the labial frenula (Figure 6.11). Forced feeding with a utensil can lacerate the tongue, the floor of the mouth, or the lips (Figure 6.12).

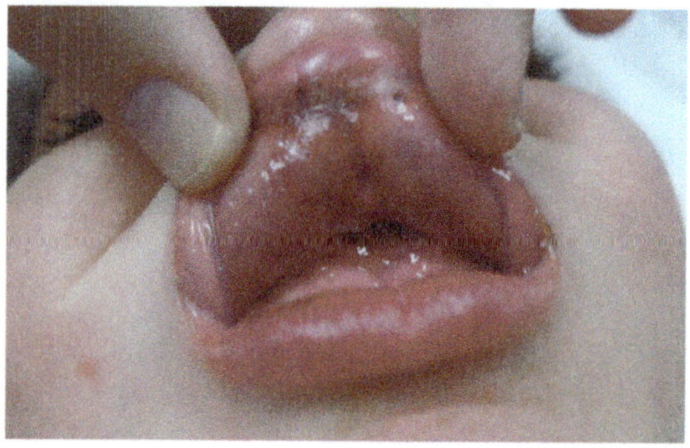

FIGURE 6.11
A 6-month-old with a laceration of the upper labial frenula extending beyond the upper alveolar ridge from forced feeding.

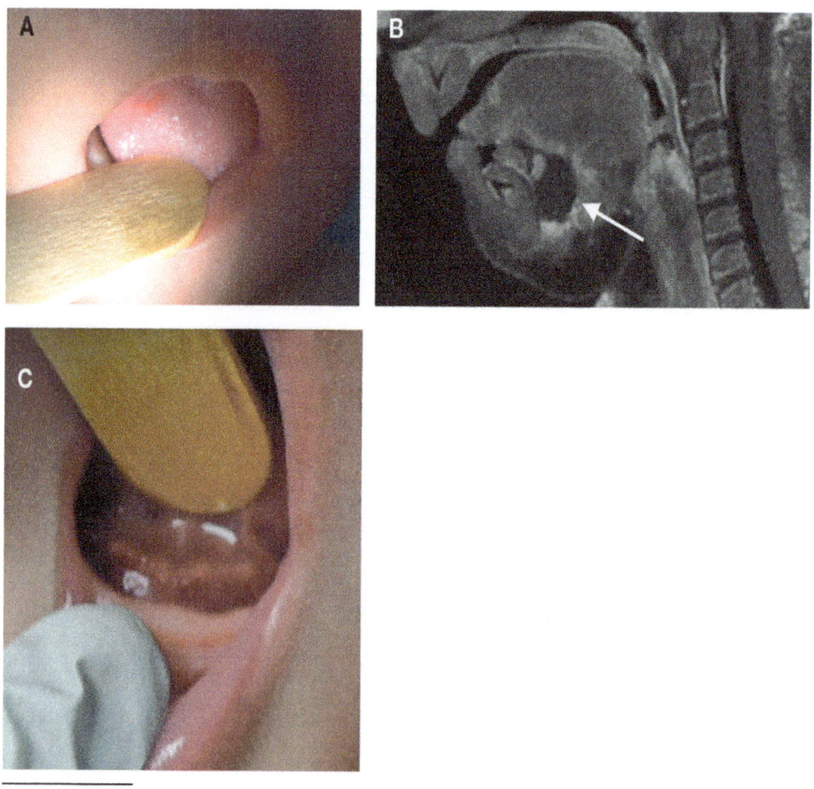

FIGURE 6.12
A 2-month-old with a curvilinear abrasion on the tongue (A), a large sublingual hematoma causing feeding difficulties (B), and sublingual bruising caused by forced feeding (C).

Injuries to Teeth

All injuries to teeth and supporting structures should be referred to a dentist as soon as possible. Abuse-related injuries to teeth can include movement of the teeth within the socket, fracture, or loss. Any trauma to a tooth that does not result in loss of the tooth may, however, move the tooth sufficiently to result in loss of the tooth's vitality. Even relatively minor trauma may disrupt the neurovascular supply of the pulp, resulting in pulp necrosis.[97] Evidence of tooth injury may not be evident immediately after the trauma. However, after several weeks or months, non-vital teeth are often characterized by slight to severe color changes of the tooth resulting from the necrotic pulp tissue within. The non-vital tooth appears discolored or markedly darker compared with the adjacent teeth. Differential diagnosis of discolored teeth should also include a history of exposure to tetracycline or heavy metals during formation of the tooth enamel. Teeth affected in this manner, and not by trauma, will show similar discoloration for all teeth forming during the exposure.

Tooth Fractures

Fractures of teeth can involve the crown, the root, or both. While tooth fractures are sometimes seen in abusive injuries, they can also be accidental. Fractures occur either when the tooth is struck with a hard object or when the face comes into contact with a hard surface (Figure 6.13).

Fractures can involve only the enamel, extend into the dentin layer, or involve the tooth's pulp. Also, teeth may fracture, even bodily through the entire tooth, and still remain held in place by the surrounding bone, periodontal ligament, and gingival tissues. Timely referral to a dentist is mandatory for treatment of tooth fractures. Modern restorative materials and bonding procedures can save teeth with enamel or dentin fractures that only a decade ago would have required full crowns or extraction (Table 6.1).[98,99]

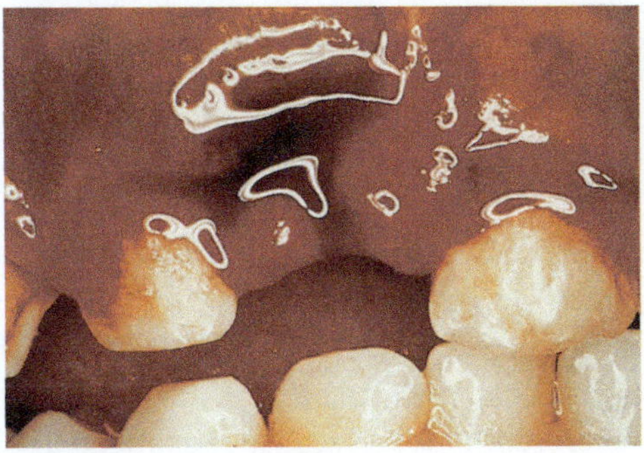

FIGURE 6.13
An 11-year-old with a traumatic avulsion of a permanent central incisor from a beating.

TABLE 6.1
Dental Fractures

Fracture Type	Definition[a]	Clinical Findings
Enamel infraction	Incomplete fracture (crack) of the enamel without loss of tooth substance	Nontender
Enamel fracture	Fracture with loss of tooth substance confined to the enamel	Loss of enamel, no visible sign of exposed dentin Nontender, normal mobility
Enamel dentin fracture	Fracture with loss of tooth substance confined to the enamel and dentin but not involving the pulp	Loss of enamel and dentin, no visible sign of exposed dentin Nontender, normal mobility
Complicated crown fracture	Fracture involving enamel and dentin and exposing the pulp	Crown fracture, does not extend to gingival margin
Uncomplicated crown-root fracture	Fracture involving the enamel, dentin, and cementum but not exposing the pulp	Crown fracture extending below the gingival margin Coronal fragment is mobile.
Complicated crown-root fracture	Fracture involving enamel, dentin, and cementum and exposing the pulp	Crown fracture extending below the gingival margin with exposed pulp Coronal fragment is mobile.
Root fracture	Fracture involving dentin, cementum, and the pulp. Can further be classified according to the displacement of the coronal fragment as horizontal, oblique, and vertical.	Bleeding from the gingival sulcus may be noted. Tooth may be tender.
Alveolar fracture	Fracture involving the alveolar bone; may extend to adjacent bone	Segment mobility and dislocation with several teeth moving together are common findings. Occlusal change due to misalignment of the fractured alveolar segment is often noted.

[a] International Association of Dental Traumatology. International Association of Dental Traumatology guidelines for the management of traumatic dental injuries. *Dent Traumatol.* 2012;28(1):2–12, 88–96, 174–182

Displaced or Avulsed Teeth

A tooth that has been moved within its socket often causes tears of the periodontal ligament and may bleed into the tooth's sulcus. Teeth traumatized in this way may also exhibit more mobility than normal. Normal, healthy teeth should move no more than 1 mm within the socket. Palpation to test tooth mobility must be conducted using 2 metal instruments or wooden tongue blades, and the examiner should not rely on moving the tooth with fingers to judge the tooth's mobility. This is because the miniscule movement of teeth is virtually impossible to detect with the soft tissue of the fingers.

A traumatized tooth can be displaced in any direction. Teeth can be bodily moved anteriorly or posteriorly, intruded into or avulsed from the socket, or moved medially or distally if adjacent teeth are not in tight contact. This can happen with accidental injuries as well as with abuse. Contact directly on the tooth or from a blow to the face that transfers energy to the teeth can cause the displacement. Either the abuser's hand or an object can deliver sufficient force to displace one or several teeth (Table 6.2).[98,99]

In severe cases, the entire tooth can be forcefully expelled from the alveolar bone (Figure 6.14). The tendency for a tooth to be avulsed is related to the force and direction of the trauma as well as the anatomy of the tooth. Single-rooted teeth and teeth with conically shaped roots are more easily avulsed without being fractured. Therefore, anterior teeth, especially

TABLE 6.2
Displacement Injuries

Injury Type	Definition[a]	Clinical Findings
Concussion	Injury to the tooth-supporting structures without abnormal loosening or displacement of the tooth but with marked redaction to percussion	Tender to touch Normal mobility and no bleeding
Subluxation (loosening)	Injury to the tooth-supporting structures with abnormal loosening but without displacement of the tooth	Increased mobility, not displaced Bleeding from gingival crevice may be present.
Extrusive luxation (peripheral dislocation, peripheral avulsion)	Partial displacement of the tooth out of its socket	Tooth appears elongated. May be excessively mobile
Lateral luxation	Displacement of the tooth in a direction other than axially Accompanied by comminution or fracture of the alveolar socket	Tooth is displaced, usually in palatal/lingual or labial direction. Immobile
Intrusive luxation (central dislocation)	Displacement of the tooth into the alveolar bone Accompanied by comminution or fracture of the alveolar socket	Tooth is displaced through the labial bone plate or can impinge on the succedaneous tooth bud.
Avulsion (exarticulation)	Complete displacement of the tooth out of its socket	Tooth is completely out of socket.

[a] International Association of Dental Traumatology. International Association of Dental Traumatology guidelines for the management of traumatic dental injuries. *Dent Traumatol.* 2012;28(1):2–12, 88–96, 174–182

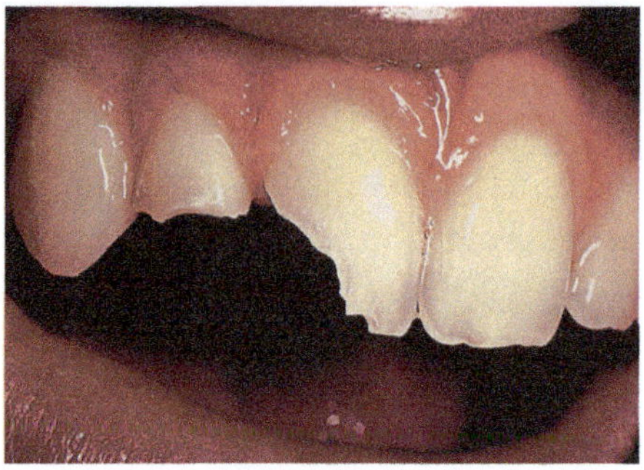

FIGURE 6.14
Fractured teeth sustained when a 16-year-old hit his mouth against a piece of furniture during a beating.

incisors, are most likely to be avulsed, but some premolars (bicuspids) also may have cone-shaped roots. Multi-rooted, posterior teeth are less likely to be avulsed, because of their location in the mouth and the physics involved in forcing a multi-rooted tooth bodily out of the alveolar bone. Because root anatomy of a primary tooth is likely to be less conical in form than its permanent counterpart, expulsion of teeth during physical violence is less common in children with primary dentition. Severe trauma can, of course, remove or shatter any tooth.

At least 2 cases have been reported of children who were abused by having permanent teeth extracted by the parents. In these cases, one adult held the child while another removed the intact teeth using pliers without anesthesia.[97]

Traumatic tooth avulsion of adult or secondary teeth requires immediate dental consultation. The tooth must be kept moist in isotonic saline solution or milk. The chances for successful reimplantation are best if the procedure is accomplished within 30 minutes of the avulsion. No attempt should be made to clean or remove tissue tags from the tooth before the dentist reimplants it. Removing anything from the tooth may result in loss of tissue important for periodontal ligament regeneration. Reimplanted teeth must be stabilized for an absolute minimum of 7 to 10 days with intraoral fixation.

Injuries to Oral Soft Tissues

Gingiva

Trauma that affects teeth is also likely to affect the surrounding gingivae. In addition, trauma from an object striking the child can produce contusions or lacerations of the gingivae without apparent trauma to adjacent teeth. Radiographic examination is necessary in all cases of gingival trauma to properly diagnose any damage to adjacent teeth or alveolar bone.

Lingual and Labial Frenula

Inflicted trauma can cause mild to extensive damage of the attachment tissues of the tongue and lips. Along with lacerations caused by forced feeding discussed previously, many forms of abusive trauma can tear these tissues. Blows to the face can displace the lip far enough to stretch the lip's attachment tissue beyond its elastic limit, causing laceration of the frenulum itself. Invasive trauma that introduces a hard or sharp object, including fingers and hands, into the mouth can also lacerate these areas. Forceful pulling at the lips is thought to cause labial frenula lacerations as well.

While accidental frenulum tears are common in the 8- to 18-month-old who is learning to walk, similar injuries in young infants (< 6 months) and in older, more stable children should raise a suspicion of abuse. Lingular frenulum injuries in young infants may result in a hematoma under the tongue that can be misdiagnosed as a hemangioma or other nontraumatic finding.[100] Sublingual hematomas may present as a rapidly growing mass, inability to feed, or respiratory compromise due to the size of the mass[101] (see Figure 6.12B). Sublingual hematomas or bruising can occur with or without obvious frenula injury.[102] Proposed mechanisms for lingular frenulum tear and sublingual hematoma include forced feeding and forcefully shoving objects or hands into the mouth. Healing frenula tears may form a sharply defined white eschar. Frenula injuries in very young infants are often associated with skeletal or other inflicted injuries and, when identified, require a thorough injury evaluation and involvement of child protective services to ensure the future safety of the infant.[100] Frenula tears will almost always heal on their own, although they may require sutures if the wound is large, the alveolar bone is exposed, or the wound separates when the lip is pulled upward.[103]

Lips

Any trauma to the mouth can cause contusions and lacerations of the upper or lower lip. Inflicted injuries to the lips are evidenced by marks from either the offending object or the child's own teeth. A study from Brazil noted that the maxilla area was affected more than half the time (55.6%) in physical abuse cases. Nearly all the injuries involved soft tissue lacerations (94.8%), and half of those were located on the upper lip (46.4%).[104]

When a blow is directed at the face or lips, the oral tissues can come into forceful contact with the child's teeth. The lips may show resulting "bite marks" from the child's own teeth. Bruising or laceration at the corners of the lips can also result from the use of a rope or other material to gag and silence the child. This can also result in lichenification or scarring at the corners of the lips.[105] Burns or scarring at the commissures of the lips may result from electrical burns from biting an electrical cord and are more likely to be caused accidentally.

In addition, fixed and removable orthodontic appliances can damage lips during trauma. The clinician must exercise caution when examining the child's mouth if orthodontic appliances are in place because lips can become trapped in the wires or brackets.

Tongue

Laceration of the tongue can occur from abuse involving forcing an object in the mouth. Starr presented a case report of a 10-month-old found to have a 3-cm metallic rod embedded in the tongue requiring surgical removal.[104]

Most abusive injuries to the tongue are a result of the child biting the tongue inadvertently. Any blow to the jaw can trap the tongue between upper and lower teeth. These injuries usually involve the lateral or anterior surfaces of the tongue and resemble jagged indentations seen with any bite mark in soft tissue. If the bite involves posterior areas of the tongue, the marks may appear more like crushed tissue and not show definite bite marks. Bite marks to the tongue inflicted by the child's own teeth are likely to show a curvature consistent with the child's own arch. A bite mark on the tongue from an abuser may show a curve in the direction opposite to the curve of the child's dental arch.

Burns

Burns can affect any oral soft tissue. Abusive burns result from the introduction of a hot object into the mouth, forced feeding of a food or liquid that is too hot, or the use of caustic or acidic materials such as drain cleaner.

Dental Implications of Child Neglect

Typically, dental neglect is but one manifestation of the general neglect of a child. The American Academy of Pediatric Dentistry (AAPD) has defined *dental neglect* as a "willful failure of parent or guardian, despite adequate access to care, to seek and follow through with treatment necessary to ensure a level of oral health essential for adequate function and freedom from pain and infection."[105] Untreated dental problems are as serious as an untreated wound to any other part of the body, in part because neglected oral health can lead to complications that affect the entire body. Also, children may withdraw from peers due to emotional aspects of poor oral health, such as embarrassment.

Also included in the AAPD definition is the failure to follow through on treatment needs once the caregiver has been informed that treatment is needed. Many parents are unaware of conditions in their children's mouths. It is only after caregivers follow the dentist's diagnosis that they are aware that a problem is present or even serious. However, if parents are informed of serious dental conditions and refuse to address these problems according to their personal resources, they have neglected their child. Therefore, parents' failure to follow through with necessary treatment is probably more important in determining reportable dental neglect than parents' lack of knowledge. Also, most practitioners would agree that no neglect may exist if parents are providing for their children's oral health needs in a manner consistent with their own financial situation or available economic existence. The argument has also been made that if parents have even taken the child to the dentist who diagnosed a dental problem, the parents are not neglecting the child. However, episodic pain relief is not appropriate dental care when adequate resources exist for more comprehensive care and definitive treatment.

The AAPD definitions of dental neglect serve neither as law nor as a standard of practice for reporting suspected cases of child neglect. They are merely a guideline for practitioners evaluating a patient's oral health in light of societal norms and fiscal realities. It is up to the medical professional to weigh the guidelines and legal definitions against such issues as finances, transportation, and access to dental care.

Rampant caries involves gross carious lesions, including the mandibular anterior teeth. These teeth are the least likely to decay and are easily seen by even untrained observers. The most common form of dental neglect is failure to provide treatment of carious teeth. Multiple carious lesions can debilitate an otherwise healthy child, while untreated caries can lead to more serious problems of severe pain, fever, malaise, and lethargy. Pulpal infections can penetrate alveolar bone and exit through the gingiva, usually at or near the tooth's apex, resulting in a parulis or gum boil. Severe untreated lesions can lead to infection of fascial planes leading to serious, even fatal, consequences.

Baby bottle tooth decay, a form of early childhood caries, is a severe form of rampant caries resulting from the habit of putting a child to bed with a nursing bottle or letting the child fall asleep at the breast. The remnants of milk in the child's mouth allow for bacterial growth, leading to carious lesions that can amputate teeth at the gingival crest. The clinical pattern of baby bottle tooth decay is typically different from other forms of rampant caries because the most seriously affected teeth are the maxillary anterior teeth. While genetics does play a role in a person's susceptibility to caries, deleterious feeding habits can overcome even optimum genetic disposition. Medical professionals should keep in mind that baby bottle tooth decay is preventable; recurrence could be considered a form of child neglect and reported as such.

Other conditions may constitute dental neglect if left untreated. These include severe malocclusions, abnormal tongue position, cleft lip or palate, missing teeth, or other manifestations that may lead to speech or eating difficulties.

Role of Dentistry in Preventing Abuse and Neglect

Dentists and other medical professionals in all 50 states and the District of Columbia are required by statute to report suspected cases of child abuse and neglect.[106] Studies have shown that despite this mandate, dentists are unlikely to report suspected abuse or neglect.[1,107–109] Survey data from Becker et al[1] showed that only 18% of cases that were recognized as child abuse by the dental professional were reported. More recent survey data have shown improvements in reporting; however, one-third of cases recognized by dentists still go unreported.[109] Dentists have reported uncertainty and fear of litigation as the leading reasons for not reporting suspected cases.[107]

A concern of the dentist or oral health care professional is that there are no clear guidelines that exactly define what brings dental neglect to the level of reporting. Also, state agencies often place dental problems and concerns as low priorities if compared in isolation to other forms of abuse.[110] However, the importance of the recognition of severe dental caries was pointed out by Sillevis Smitt et al. In their study from the Netherlands, there was a strong correlation between severe dental caries and child abuse and neglect. Forty-seven out of 205 children (23%) who had to have tooth extractions under general anesthesia due to severe caries were found to have been neglected or abused.[111]

In an effort to change dentists' involvement with child protective services, the American Dental Association (ADA) added the required recognition and reporting of suspected child abuse to its *Principles of Ethics and Code of*

Professional Conduct in 1993.[112] Official ADA policy states that dentists should become familiar with all physical signs of child abuse that are observable in the course of the normal dental visit. In 1999, the ADA further refined its policy to encourage dentists to become better educated about all forms of abuse and neglect and to learn about state-specific legal considerations for reporting suspected victims of abuse and neglect of all ages.[113]

The Prevent Abuse and Neglect Through Dental Awareness (PANDA) Coalition was established to better educate dental professionals about child abuse prevention. The PANDA Coalition is a public/private partnership between the dental community, public health and social services agencies, and a dental insurance company. Increased reporting by dentists of suspected cases of child abuse and neglect since the coalition's educational program premiered in 1992 has proven the success of the initiative. In the first 4 years since the inception of PANDA education and awareness programs, the reporting by dentists of suspected child abuse and neglect rose by 160%.[114]

References

1. Becker DB, Needleman HL, Kotelchuck M. Child abuse and dentistry: orofacial trauma and its recognition by dentists. *J Am Dent Assoc*. 1978;97(1):24–28 PMID: 28343 https://doi.org/10.14219/jada.archive.1978.0447
2. da Fonseca MA, Feigal RJ, ten Bensel RW. Dental aspects of 1248 cases of child maltreatment on file at a major county hospital. *Pediatr Dent*. 1992;14(3):152–157 PMID: 1528783
3. Cameron JM, Johnson HR, Camps FE. The battered child syndrome. *Med Sci Law*. 1966;6(1):2–21 PMID: 5907350 https://doi.org/10.1177/002580246600600102
4. Willging JP, Bower CM, Cotton RT. Physical abuse of children. A retrospective review and an otolaryngology perspective. *Arch Otolaryngol Head Neck Surg*. 1992;118(6):584–590 PMID: 1637535 https://doi.org/10.1001/archotol.1992.01880060032010
5. Leavitt EB, Pincus RL, Bukachevsky R. Otolaryngologic manifestations of child abuse. *Arch Otolaryngol Head Neck Surg*. 1992;118(6):629–631 PMID: 1637540 https://doi.org/10.1001/archotol.1992.01880060079017
6. Christian CW, Scribano P, Seidl T, Pinto-Martin JA. Pediatric injury resulting from family violence. *Pediatrics*. 1997;99(2):E8 PMID: 9099765 https://doi.org/10.1542/peds.99.2.e8
7. US Administration for Children and Families. Child Maltreatment 2015. Washington, DC: US Department of Health and Human Services;2017. http://www.acf.hhs.gov/programs/cb/research-data-technology/statistics-research/child-maltreatment
8. King AJ, Farst KJ, Jaeger MW, Onukwube JI, Robbins JM. Maltreatment-related emergency department visits among children 0 to 3 years old in the United States. *Child Maltreat*. 2015;20(3):151–161 PMID: 25631298 https://doi.org/10.1177/1077559514567176
9. Tate RJ. Facial injuries associated with the battered child syndrome. *Br J Oral Surg*. 1971;9(1):41–45 PMID: 5315395 https://doi.org/10.1016/S0007-117X(71)80007-0

10. Pierce MC, Kaczor K, Aldridge S, O'Flynn J, Lorenz DJ. Bruising characteristics discriminating physical child abuse from accidental trauma. *Pediatrics*. 2010;125(1): 67–74 PMID: 19969620 https://doi.org/10.1542/peds.2008-3632
11. Grace A, Grace S. Child abuse within the ear, nose and throat. *J Otolaryngol*. 1987;16(2):108–111 PMID: 3599153
12. Naidoo S. A profile of the oro-facial injuries in child physical abuse at a children's hospital. *Child Abuse Negl*. 2000;24(4):521–534 PMID: 10798841 https://doi.org/10.1016/S0145-2134(00)00114-9
13. Sugar NF, Taylor JA, Feldman KW; Puget Sound Pediatric Research Network. Bruises in infants and toddlers: those who don't cruise rarely bruise. *Arch Pediatr Adolesc Med*. 1999;153(4):399–403 PMID: 10201724 https://doi.org/10.1001/archpedi.153.4.399
14. Carpenter RF. The prevalence and distribution of bruising in babies. *Arch Dis Child*. 1999;80(4):363–366 PMID: 10086945 https://doi.org/10.1136/adc.80.4.363
15. Mortimer PE, Freeman M. Are facial bruises in babies ever accidental? *Arch Dis Child*. 1983;58(1):75–76 PMID: 6830281 https://doi.org/10.1136/adc.58.1.75-b
16. Dunstan FD, Guildea ZE, Kontos K, Kemp AM, Sibert JR. A scoring system for bruise patterns: a tool for identifying abuse. *Arch Dis Child*. 2002;86(5):330–333 PMID: 11970921 https://doi.org/10.1136/adc.86.5.330
17. Maguire S, Mann MK, Sibert J, Kemp A. Are there patterns of bruising in childhood which are diagnostic or suggestive of abuse? A systematic review. *Arch Dis Child*. 2005;90(2):182–186 PMID: 15665178 https://doi.org/10.1136/adc.2003.044065
18. Sheets LK, Leach ME, Koszewski IJ, Lessmeier AM, Nugent M, Simpson P. Sentinel injuries in infants evaluated for child physical abuse. *Pediatrics*. 2013;131(4):701–707 PMID: 23478861 https://doi.org/10.1542/peds.2012-2780
19. McMahon P, Grossman W, Gaffney M, Stanitski C. Soft-tissue injury as an indication of child abuse. *J Bone Joint Surg Am*. 1995;77(8):1179–1183 PMID: 7642662 https://doi.org/10.2106/00004623-199508000-00006
20. Labbé J, Caouette G. Recent skin injuries in normal children. *Pediatrics*. 2001;108(2): 271–276 PMID: 11483787 https://doi.org/10.1542/peds.108.2.271
21. Daria S, Sugar NF, Feldman KW, Boos SC, Benton SA, Ornstein A. Into hot water head first: distribution of intentional and unintentional immersion burns. *Pediatr Emerg Care*. 2004;20(5):302–310 PMID: 15123901 https://doi.org/10.1097/01.pec.0000125658.05196.b1
22. Rowe NL. Fractures of the facial skeleton in children. *J Oral Surg*. 1968;26(8):505–515 PMID: 5243132
23. Kaban LB, Mulliken JB, Murray JE. Facial fractures in children: an analysis of 122 fractures in 109 patients. *Plast Reconstr Surg*. 1977;59(1):15–20 PMID: 831236 https://doi.org/10.1097/00006534-197701000-00002
24. Waite DE. Pediatric fractures of jaw and facial bones. *Pediatrics*. 1973;51(3):551–559 PMID: 4707870
25. Siegel MB, Wetmore RF, Potsic WP, Handler SD, Tom LW. Mandibular fractures in the pediatric patient. *Arch Otolaryngol Head Neck Surg*. 1991;117(5):533–536 PMID: 2021472 https://doi.org/10.1001/archotol.1991.01870170079017
26. Chidzonga MM. Mandibular fracture in a neonate: report of a case. *Int J Oral Maxillofac Surg*. 2006;35(2):186–187 PMID: 16153807 https://doi.org/10.1016/j.ijom.2005.07.011
27. Welbury RR, Murphy JM. The dental practitioner's role in protecting children from abuse. 2. The orofacial signs of abuse. *Br Dent J*. 1998;184(2):61–65 PMID: 9489211 https://doi.org/10.1038/sj.bdj.4809545

28. Cuesta L, Betlloch I, Bañuls J, Toledo F. "Cauliflower ear" in a teenager: a possible sign of child abuse. *Pediatr Dermatol*. 2012;29(2):226–227 PMID: 22150252 https://doi.org/10.1111/j.1525-1470.2011.01416.x
29. Kini N, Lazoritz S, Ott C, Conley SF. Caustic instillation into the ear as a form of child abuse. *Am J Emerg Med*. 1997;15(4):442–443 PMID: 9217549 https://doi.org/10.1016/S0735-6757(97)90149-2
30. Grace A, Kalinkiewicz M, Drake-Lee AB. Covert manifestations of child abuse. *Br Med J (Clin Res Ed)*. 1984;289(6451):1041–1042 PMID: 6435763 https://doi.org/10.1136/bmj.289.6451.1041-a
31. DiBiase P, Timmis H, Bonilla JA, Szeremeta W, Post JC. Munchausen syndrome by proxy complicating ear surgery. *Arch Otolaryngol Head Neck Surg*. 1996;122(12):1377–1380 PMID: 8956754 https://doi.org/10.1001/archotol.1996.01890240083018
32. Zohar Y, Avidan G, Shvili Y, Laurian N. Otolaryngologic cases of Munchausen's syndrome. *Laryngoscope*. 1987;97(2):201–203 PMID: 3807622 https://doi.org/10.1288/00005537-198702000-00011
33. Griffiths H, Cuddihy PJ, Marnane C. Bleeding ears: a case of Munchausen syndrome by proxy. *Int J Pediatr Otorhinolaryngol*. 2001;57(3):245–247 PMID: 11223457 https://doi.org/10.1016/S0165-5876(00)00415-8
34. Bennett AM, Bennett SM, Prinsley PR, Wickstead M. Spitting in the ear: a falsified disease using video evidence. *J Laryngol Otol*. 2005;119(11):926–927 PMID: 16354350 https://doi.org/10.1258/002221505774783502
35. Hanigan WC, Peterson RA, Njus G. Tin ear syndrome: rotational acceleration in pediatric head injuries. *Pediatrics*. 1987;80(5):618–622 PMID: 3670962
36. Canty PA, Berkowitz RG. Hematoma and abscess of the nasal septum in children. *Arch Otolaryngol Head Neck Surg*. 1996;122(12):1373–1376 PMID: 8956753 https://doi.org/10.1001/archotol.1996.01890240079017
37. Haug RH, Foss J. Maxillofacial injuries in the pediatric patient. *Oral Surg Oral Med Oral Pathol Oral Radiol Endod*. 2000;90(2):126–134 PMID: 10936829 https://doi.org/10.1067/moe.2000.107974
38. Orton CI. Loss of columella and septum from an unusual form of child abuse. Case report. *Plast Reconstr Surg*. 1975;56(3):345–346 PMID: 1153551 https://doi.org/10.1097/00006534-197509000-00021
39. Pincus RL, Bukachevsky RP. Medially based horizontal nasolabial flaps for reconstruction of columellar defects. *Arch Otolaryngol Head Neck Surg*. 1990;116(8):973–974 PMID: 2378728 https://doi.org/10.1001/archotol.1990.01870080095025
40. Fischer H, Allasio D. Nasal destruction due to child abuse. *Clin Pediatr (Phila)*. 1996;35(3):165–166 PMID: 8904493 https://doi.org/10.1177/000992289603500311
41. Rees P, Kemp A, Carter B, Maguire S. A systematic review of the probability of asphyxia in children aged <2 years with unexplained epistaxis. *J Pediatr*. 2016;168:178–84.e10 PMID: 26507155 https://doi.org/10.1016/j.jpeds.2015.09.043
42. Lopez MR, Abd-Allah S, Deming DD, et al. Oral, jaw, and neck injury in infants and children: from abusive trauma or intubation? *Pediatr Emerg Care*. 2014;30(5):305–310
43. Tostevin PM, Hollis LJ, Bailey CM. Pharyngeal trauma in children—accidental and otherwise. *J Laryngol Otol*. 1995;109(12):1168–1175 PMID: 8551149 https://doi.org/10.1017/S0022215100132359
44. McDowell HP, Fielding DW. Traumatic perforation of the hypopharynx—an unusual form of abuse. *Arch Dis Child*. 1984;59(9):888–889 PMID: 6486867 https://doi.org/10.1136/adc.59.9.888

45. Golova N. An infant with fever and drooling: infection or trauma? *Pediatr Emerg Care*. 1997;13(5):331–333 PMID: 9368246 https://doi.org/10.1097/00006565-199710000-00008
46. Reece RM, Arnold J, Splain J. Pharyngeal perforation as a manifestation of child abuse. *Child Maltreat*. 1996;1(4):364–367 https://doi.org/10.1177/1077559596001004009
47. Ramnarayan P, Qayyum A, Tolley N, Nadel S. Subcutaneous emphysema of the neck in infancy: under-recognized presentation of child abuse. *J Laryngol Otol*. 2004;118(6): 468–470 PMID: 15285869 https://doi.org/10.1258/00222150432319635
48. Morris TM, Reay HA. A battered baby with pharyngeal atresia. *J Laryngol Otol*. 1971;85(7):729–731 PMID: 5090116 https://doi.org/10.1017/S0022215100074016
49. Ablin DS, Reinhart MA. Esophageal perforation with mediastinal abscess in child abuse. *Pediatr Radiol*. 1990;20(7):524–525 PMID: 2216586 https://doi.org/10.1007/BF02011381
50. Kleinman PK, Spevak MR, Hansen M. Mediastinal pseudocyst caused by pharyngeal perforation during child abuse. *AJR Am J Roentgenol*. 1992;158(5):1111–1113 PMID: 1566677 https://doi.org/10.2214/ajr.158.5.1566677
51. Bansal BC, Abramo TJ. Subcutaneous emphysema as an uncommon presentation of child abuse. *Am J Emerg Med*. 1997;15(6):573–575 PMID: 9337364 https://doi.org/10.1016/S0735-6757(97)90160-1
52. Morzaria S, Walton JM, MacMillan A. Inflicted esophageal perforation. *J Pediatr Surg*. 1998;33(6):871–873 PMID: 9660218 https://doi.org/10.1016/S0022-3468(98)90663-7
53. Ablin DS, Reinhart MA. Esophageal perforation by a tooth in child abuse. *Pediatr Radiol*. 1992;22(5):339–341 PMID: 1408439 https://doi.org/10.1007/BF02016250
54. Friedman EM. Caustic ingestions and foreign body aspirations: an overlooked form of child abuse. *Ann Otol Rhinol Laryngol*. 1987;96(6):709–712 PMID: 3688764 https://doi.org/10.1177/000348948709600621
55. Dine MS, McGovern ME. Intentional poisoning of children—an overlooked category of child abuse: report of seven cases and review of the literature. *Pediatrics*. 1982;70(1): 32–35 PMID: 7088630
56. Krugman SD, Lantz PE, Sinal S, De Jong AR, Coffman K. Forced suffocation of infants with baby wipes: a previously undescribed form of child abuse. *Child Abuse Negl*. 2007;31(6):615–621 PMID: 17617455 https://doi.org/10.1016/j.chiabu.2006.12.012
57. Nolte KB. Esophageal foreign bodies as child abuse. Potential fatal mechanisms. *Am J Forensic Med Pathol*. 1993;14(4):323–326 PMID: 8116592 https://doi.org/10.1097/00000433-199312000-00010
58. Myer CM III, Fitton CM. Vocal cord paralysis following child abuse. *Int J Pediatr Otorhinolaryngol*. 1988;15(2):217–220 PMID: 3397242 https://doi.org/10.1016/0165-5876(88)90074-2
59. Jessee SA. Physical manifestations of child abuse to the head, face and mouth: a hospital survey. *ASDC J Dent Child*. 1995;62(4):245–249 PMID: 7593881
60. Ng CS, Hall CM, Shaw DG. The range of visceral manifestations of non-accidental injury. *Arch Dis Child*. 1997;77(2):167–174 PMID: 9301362 https://doi.org/10.1136/adc.77.2.167
61. Hadley GP, Bösenberg AT, Wiersma R, Grant H. Needle implantation ascribed to "tikoloshe" [letter]. *Lancet*. 1993;342(8882):1304 PMID: 7901614 https://doi.org/10.1016/0140-6736(93)92397-C
62. Williams CM, Spector R, Braun M. Cervical bruises—a battered child? Cystic lymphangioma. *Arch Dermatol*. 1986;122(9):1066–1067, 1069–1070 PMID: 3740889 https://doi.org/10.1001/archderm.122.9.1066

63. Fornes P, Druilhe L, Lecomte D. Childhood homicide in Paris, 1990-1993: a report of 81 cases. *J Forensic Sci*. 1995;40(2):201–204 PMID: 7602277 https://doi.org/10.1520/JFS15341J
64. Greenbaum J, Christian CW. Asphyxiation in children. In: David TJ, ed. Recent Advances in Paediatrics. London, United Kingdom: Royal Society of Medicine Press Ltd; 2006:93–112
65. Carty H. Case report: child abuse—necklace calcification—a sign of strangulation. *Br J Radiol*. 1993;66(792):1186–1188 PMID: 8293265 https://doi.org/10.1259/0007-1285-66-792-1186
66. Samuels MP, McClaughlin W, Jacobson RR, Poets CF, Southall DP. Fourteen cases of imposed upper airway obstruction. *Arch Dis Child*. 1992;67(2):162–170 PMID: 1543373 https://doi.org/10.1136/adc.67.2.162
67. Meadow R. Unnatural sudden infant death. *Arch Dis Child*. 1999;80(1):7–14 PMID: 10325752 https://doi.org/10.1136/adc.80.1.7
68. Milkovich SM, Owens J, Stool D, Chen X, Beran M. Accidental childhood strangulation by human hair. *Int J Pediatr Otorhinolaryngol*. 2005;69(12):1621–1628 PMID: 15985296 https://doi.org/10.1016/j.ijporl.2005.04.029
69. Piatt JH Jr, Steinberg M. Isolated spinal cord injury as a presentation of child abuse. *Pediatrics*. 1995;96(4 Pt 1):780–782 PMID: 7567347
70. Towbin A. Sudden infant death (cot death) related to spinal injury [letter]. *Lancet*. 1967;290(7522):940 https://doi.org/10.1016/S0140-6736(67)90254-1
71. Sneed RC, Stover SL. Undiagnosed spinal cord injuries in brain-injured children. *Am J Dis Child*. 1988;142(9):965–967 PMID: 3414628 https://doi.org/10.1001/archpedi.1988.02150090063023
72. Baerg J, Thirumoorthi A, Hazboun R, Vannix R, Krafft P, Zouros A. Cervical spine injuries in young children: pattern and outcomes in accidental versus inflicted trauma. *J Surg Res*. 2017;219:366–373 PMID: 29078907 https://doi.org/10.1016/j.jss.2017.06.053
73. Cirak B, Ziegfeld S, Knight VM, Chang D, Avellino AM, Paidas CN. Spinal injuries in children. *J Pediatr Surg*. 2004;39(4):607–612 PMID: 15065038 https://doi.org/10.1016/j.jpedsurg.2003.12.011
74. Kadom N, Khademian Z, Vezina G, Shalaby-Rana E, Rice A, Hinds T. Usefulness of MRI detection of cervical spine and brain injuries in the evaluation of abusive head trauma. *Pediatr Radiol*. 2014;44(7):839–848 PMID: 24557483 https://doi.org/10.1007/s00247-014-2874-7
75. Choudhary AK, Ishak R, Zacharia TT, Dias MS. Imaging of spinal injury in abusive head trauma: a retrospective study. *Pediatr Radiol*. 2014;44(9):1130–1140 PMID: 24687620 https://doi.org/10.1007/s00247-014-2959-3
76. Brennan LK, Rubin D, Christian CW, Duhaime AC, Mirchandani HG, Rorke-Adams LB. Neck injuries in young pediatric homicide victims. *J Neurosurg Pediatr*. 2009;3(3):232–239 PMID: 19338471 https://doi.org/10.3171/2008.11.PEDS0835
77. Shannon P, Smith CR, Deck J, Ang LC, Ho M, Becker L. Axonal injury and the neuropathology of shaken baby syndrome. *Acta Neuropathol*. 1998;95(6):625–631 PMID: 9650755 https://doi.org/10.1007/s004010050849
78. Rooks VJ, Sisler C, Burton B. Cervical spine injury in child abuse: report of two cases. *Pediatr Radiol*. 1998;28(3):193–195 PMID: 9561545 https://doi.org/10.1007/s002470050330
79. Thomas NH, Robinson L, Evans A, Bullock P. The floppy infant: a new manifestation of nonaccidental injury. *Pediatr Neurosurg*. 1995;23(4):188–191 PMID: 8835208 https://doi.org/10.1159/000120957
80. Kleinman PK, Shelton YA. Hangman's fracture in an abused infant: imaging features. *Pediatr Radiol*. 1997;27(9):776–777 PMID: 9285748 https://doi.org/10.1007/s002470050227

81. McGrory BE, Fenichel GM. Hangman's fracture subsequent to shaking in an infant. *Ann Neurol*. 1977;2(1):82 PMID: 900911 https://doi.org/10.1002/ana.410020116
82. Ranjith RK, Mullett JH, Burke TE. Hangman's fracture caused by suspected child abuse. A case report. *J Pediatr Orthop B*. 2002;11(4):329–332 PMID: 12370585
83. Parisi M, Lieberson R, Shatsky S. Hangman's fracture or primary spondylolysis: a patient and a brief review. *Pediatr Radiol*. 1991;21(5):367–368 PMID: 1891266 https://doi.org/10.1007/BF02011491
84. van Rijn RR, Kool DR, de Witt Hamer PC, Majoie CB. An abused five-month-old girl: hangman's fracture or congenital arch defect? *J Emerg Med*. 2005;29(1):61–65 PMID: 15961011 https://doi.org/10.1016/j.jemermed.2005.01.008
85. Barber I, Perez-Rossello JM, Wilson CR, Silvera MV, Kleinman PK. Prevalence and relevance of pediatric spinal fractures in suspected child abuse. *Pediatr Radiol*. 2013;43(11):1507–1515 PMID: 23812002 https://doi.org/10.1007/s00247-013-2726-x
86. Fisher-Owens SA, Lukefahr JL, Tate AR; American Academy of Pediatrics Section on Oral Health and Committee on Child Abuse and Neglect; American Academy of Pediatric Dentistry Council on Clinical Affairs and Council on Scientific Affairs; Ad Hoc Work Group on Child Abuse and Neglect. Oral and dental aspects of child abuse and neglect. *Pediatrics*. 2017;140(2):e20171487 PMID: 28771417 https://doi.org/10.1542/peds.2017-1487
87. Heitzler GD, Cranin AN, Gallo L. Sexual abuse of the oral cavity in children. *J Mich Dent Assoc*. 1994;76(6):28–30 PMID: 9508927
88. Jessee SA. Orofacial manifestations of child abuse and neglect. *Am Fam Physician*. 1995;52(6):1829–1834 PMID: 7484693
89. Casamassimo PS. Child sexual abuse and the pediatric dentist. *Pediatr Dent*. 1986; 8(1 Spec No):102–106 PMID: 2941722
90. De Jong AR. Sexually transmitted diseases in sexually abused children. *Sex Transm Dis*. 1986;13(3):123–126 PMID: 3764623 https://doi.org/10.1097/00007435-198607000-00002
91. Everett VD, Ingram DL, Flick LAR, Russell TA, Tropez-Sims ST, McFadden AY. A comparison of sexually transmitted diseases (STDs) found in a total of 696 boys and 2973 girls evaluated for sexual abuse [abstract]. *Pediatr Res*. 1998;43(4 pt 2):91A https://doi.org/10.1203/00006450-199804001-00542
92. Kui LL, Xiu HZ, Ning LY. Condyloma acuminatum and human papilloma virus infection in the oral mucosa of children. *Pediatr Dent*. 2003;25(2):149–153 PMID: 12723841
93. Schmitt BD, Kempe CH. The pediatrician's role in child abuse and neglect. *Curr Probl Pediatr*. 1975;5(5):3–47 PMID: 1149491 https://doi.org/10.1016/S0045-9380(75)80020-X
94. Mouden LD. The role for dental professionals in preventing child abuse and neglect. *J Calif Dent Assoc*. 1998;26(10):737–739, 741–743 PMID: 9879241
95. Thompson LA, Tavares M, Ferguson-Young D, Ogle O, Halpern LR. Violence and abuse: core competencies for identification and access to care. *Dent Clin North Am*. 2013;57(2):281–299 PMID: 23570806 https://doi.org/10.1016/j.cden.2013.01.003
96. Kempe CH. Uncommon manifestations of the battered child syndrome. *Am J Dis Child*. 1975;129(11):1265 PMID: 1190156 https://doi.org/10.1001/archpedi.1975.02120480003001
97. Zaleckiene V, Peciuliene V, Brukiene V, Drukteinis S. Traumatic dental injuries: etiology, prevalence and possible outcomes. *Stomatologija*. 2014;16(1):7–14 PMID: 24824054
98. World Health Organization. *Application of the International Classification of Diseases to Dentistry and Stomatology (ICD-SA)*. Geneva, Switzerland: World Health Organization; 1995

99. International Association of Dental Traumatology. International Association of Dental Traumatology guidelines for the management of traumatic dental injuries. *Dent Traumatol*. 2012;28(1):2–12, 88–96, 174–182
100. Carrotte PV. An unusual case of child abuse. *Br Dent J*. 1990;168(11):444–445 PMID: 2361086 https://doi.org/10.1038/sj.bdj.4807234
101. Kudek MR, Knox BL. Sublingual hematoma: when to suspect child abuse. *Clin Pediatr (Phila)*. 2014;53(8):809–812 PMID: 24707018 https://doi.org/10.1177/0009922814529184
102. Mehra M, Chiesa AE, Sirotnak AP. Two cases of sublingual hematoma as a manifestation of child abuse. *Ear Nose Throat J*. 2015;94(12):494–496 PMID: 26670756
103. Lin HW, Wieland AM, Ostrower ST. Child abuse presenting as oral cavity bruising. *Otolaryngol Head Neck Surg*. 2009;141(2):290–291 PMID: 19643269 https://doi.org/10.1016/j.otohns.2009.03.018
104. Starr M, Klein EJ, Sugar N. A perplexing case of child abuse: oral injuries in abuse and physician reporting responsibilities. Pediatr Emerg Care. 2015;31:581–583
105. American Academy of Pediatric Dentistry. Definition of dental neglect. https://www.aapd.org/research/oral-health-policies--recommendations/dental-neglect. Accessed February 22, 2019</eref>
106. Mouden LD, Bross DC. Legal issues affecting dentistry's role in preventing child abuse and neglect. *J Am Dent Assoc*. 1995;126(8):1173–1180 PMID: 7560576 https://doi.org/10.14219/jada.archive.1995.0339
107. Kenney JP, Spencer DE. Child abuse and neglect. In: Bowers CM, Bell G, eds. Manual of Forensic Odontology. 3rd ed. Colorado Springs, CO: American Society of Forensic Odontology; 1996
108. Cotton EE. Steps in child protection: reporting, social services and the judicial system (part of a panel presentation). Presented at: Proceedings: Dentists C.A.R.E. (Child Abuse Recognition and Education) Conference; July 31 to August 1, 1998; Chicago, IL
109. Saxe MD, McCourt JW. Child abuse: a survey of ASDC members and a diagnostic-data-assessment for dentists. *ASDC J Dent Child*. 1991;58(5):361–366 PMID:1834710
110. Bhatia SK, Maguire SA, Chadwick BL, et al. Characteristics of child dental neglect: a systematic review. *J Dent*. 2014;42(3):229–239 PMID: 24140926 https://doi.org/10.1016/j.jdent.2013.10.010
111. Sillevis Smitt H, de Leeuw J, de Vries T. Association between severe dental caries and child abuse and neglect. *J Oral Maxillofac Surg*. 2017;75(11):2304–2306
112. American Dental Association. Resolution 44–1999. Adopted by the 1999 ADA House of Delegates. October 1999; Honolulu, Hawaii
113. Mouden LD. Dentistry preventing family violence. *Mo Dent J*. 1996;76(6):21–22, 24, 27 PMID:9564320
114. Moden LD. Dentistry addressing family violence. *Mo Dent J*. 1996;76(6):21–27

CHAPTER 7

Abusive Head Trauma

Stephen C. Boos, MD, FAAP
Associate Professor of Pediatrics
University of Massachusetts Medical School–Baystate
Springfield, MA
Adjunct Associate Professor of Pediatrics
Tufts University School of Medicine
Boston, MA

Mark S. Dias, MD, FAAP, FAANS
Professor of Neurosurgery and Pediatrics
Penn State College of Medicine
Penn State Health Children's Hospital
Hershey, PA

The term *abusive head trauma* (AHT) can potentially refer to a wide range of inflicted injuries involving the head. The concept of AHT, and the related concept of *shaken baby syndrome,* have received a great deal of attention in the medical and lay press. Not surprisingly, as definitions have varied, so too have findings. This chapter focuses on neurotrauma inflicted on children during impact to, or violent motion of, the head resulting in intracranial injuries to the meninges, intracranial blood vessels, brain and upper cervical spinal cord, and retinae. Literature on AHT is replete with terms to differentiate these injuries from those that arise from accidental or unintentional means. Whereas some authors have referred to "accidental head trauma" and "non-accidental head trauma," most presently refer to AHT and non-AHT. Details of bruises, skull and cervical fractures, direct orbital trauma, oral injuries, and other organ trauma that commonly co-occur with AHT will be discussed elsewhere in this textbook.

Epidemiology

Incidence of Abusive Head Trauma

Reports on the incidence of AHT vary by the age groups, definitions of AHT, locations, and periods of the studies. The incidence is highest in the first year after birth (13.0–40.5 per 100,000 per year) with a much lower incidence (as low as 2.4 per 100,000 per year) during the second year.[1–14]

Incidence of Shaking Events

Since the early writings of Caffey and Guthkelch, authors have associated AHT with violent infant shaking,[15,16] and this has been corroborated by studies of perpetrator statements.[17–19] In a survey of mothers from the United States, 2.6% admitted to shaking a child younger than 2 years.[20] Combining this figure with data from Niederkrotenthaler et al on US incidence of AHT in children younger than 2 years[8] suggests that potentially many more children are shaken than are brought to medical attention from their injuries, with a maximal occurrence of 8.1 significant injury events per 1,000 children younger than 2 years who were shaken.

Identified Risk Factors (Crying, Family Composition/Perpetrator)

Perpetrator, family, and child characteristics have been linked to AHT. When identified, perpetrators are mostly male, with fathers or another male romantic partner of the child's mother being the most frequently identified perpetrator.[11,17,21–24] Babysitters, most of whom are female, and mothers follow in frequency. Families involved in AHT are disproportionately from historically disenfranchised racial or ethnic groups, such as African Americans in the United States and Maori in New Zealand.[4–6,10,11,25] Abusive head trauma is also more common in populations affected by poverty, reliance on public insurance, and recent economic challenges.[6,8,10–12,23–30] Social issues associated with AHT often covary, creating differences between studies, but include mental illness, substance use disorder, domestic violence, criminal histories, compromised prenatal care, attachment disorders, and developmentally inappropriate beliefs and expectations about the child.[26,31,32] Factors associated with the child who has experienced AHT may also affect risk. For example, virtually all studies find male infants at modest to significant increased risk. Indirect and perpetrator report evidence suggests that infant crying often provokes abusive events.[18,33–35] Twin gestation, preterm birth, newborns who are small for gestational age, and obstetric complications may also place a baby at risk.[26,35,36]

Clinical Presentation

Most commonly, the infant with AHT presents with acute and severe neurological deterioration, including varying degrees of stupor or coma with or without focal neurological deficits, apnea or disordered breathing often requiring resuscitation and ventilatory support, and multiple and prolonged seizure activity.[37–41] Others may present with nonspecific findings such as irritability or inconsolable crying, vomiting, brief resolved unexplained event (previously called an acute life-threatening event), or anemia or thrombocytosis that may be more difficult to associate with abuse.[42–44] Yet others are identified by later sequelae of their injuries,[45,46] with some presenting with multiple subdural collections of varying ages.[45] In all these cases, the history obtained most commonly lacks any mention of trauma or reports a minor event such as a short fall that is inadequate to explain the severity of the findings.[25,45,47,48] A changing history in an attempt to account for additional findings as they arise is also common.

The most frequent history given in AHT is an abrupt onset of symptoms with no reported trauma. A short fall from an elevated surface is the next most frequent, and a fall from or in an adult's arms follows.[25,42,47,49] In cases of non-AHT, absence of trauma history is much less common and a fall is the most common explanation, sometimes with the fall distance not stated.[25,47,49] A study by Amagasa et al[48] divided presenting trauma history for intracranial hemorrhage into absent, low risk, and middle to high risk. Children with absent or low-risk trauma history had *more* severe injuries, including seizures, retinal hemorrhages (RHs), subdural hemorrhage (SDH), and poor neurological outcome than children with middle- to high-risk histories. Third-party witnesses, skull fractures, and subarachnoid hemorrhage were *less* common in these groups. Children with unknown histories were the most likely to have a child abuse evaluation and referral for protective services, followed by those with low-risk histories. The authors of this study suggest that some children who had possibly experienced abuse were not reported.[48]

Classical Acute Presentation

Comparative studies clearly demonstrate that those who experience AHT have a greater degree of neurological impairment and are more critically injured than those who are unintentionally injured, are more likely to require resuscitation and ventilatory support, and are more likely to experience seizures that may be multiple and difficult to treat in the acute phase. Acute or mixed density SDH, most often of small volume, is the most common (averaging approximately 80% of cases) and the most statistically specific intracranial imaging finding in AHT (Figure 7.1). In contrast, epidural, subarachnoid, parenchymal, and intraventricular hemorrhages are not statistically more common in AHT than non-AHT.[19] Impaired consciousness, ranging from irritability to stupor or coma, reflects underlying parenchymal brain injury that is usually evident on computed tomography (CT), as brain swelling with obliteration of sulci and basal cisterns as well as loss of gray-white differentiation, and on

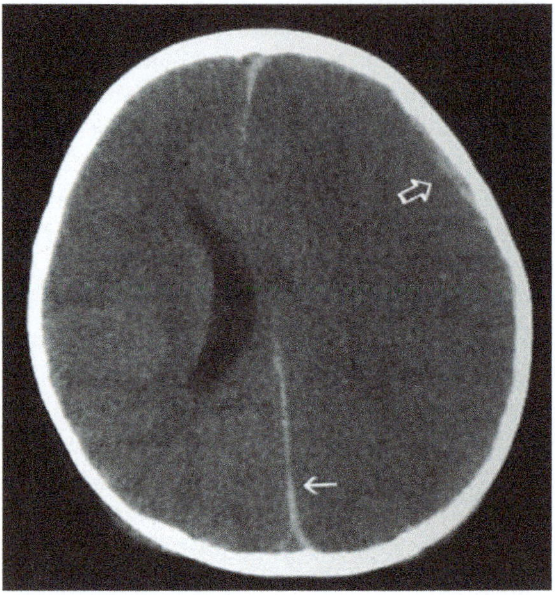

FIGURE 7.1
Small convexity (open arrow) and parafalcine subdural hemorrhage (solid arrow) with swelling and hypodensity of the left cerebral hemisphere, effacement of the left lateral ventricle and midline shift.

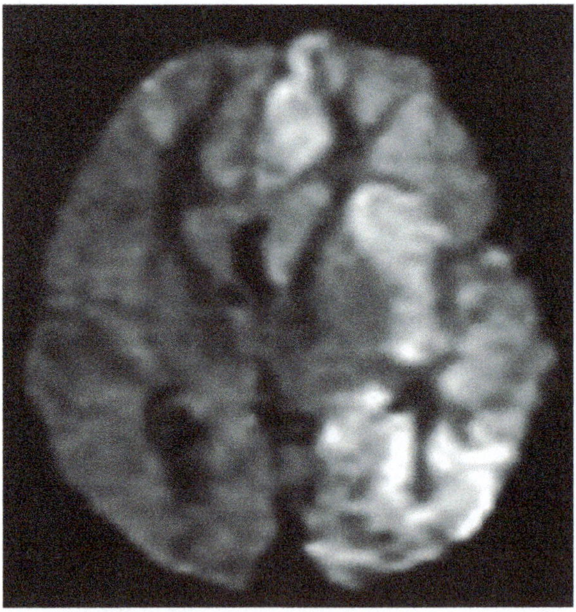

FIGURE 7.2
Restricted diffusion on magnetic resonance imaging, apparent diffusion coefficient map, seen as bright signal throughout the left cerebral hemisphere and less so on the right. This is the same patient as in Figure 7.1.

magnetic resonance (MR) imaging, as T2 prolongation (leading to increased brightness) and restricted diffusion (Figure 7.2).[50–52] Interestingly, children with AHT are significantly less likely than those who are unintentionally injured to have isolated skull fractures. Studies of impact injury have demonstrated that infants are more susceptible to skull fracture than are older children, so their younger age should make the population who have experienced AHT more susceptible to skull fracture from impact. This finding, therefore, becomes important when discussing the degree to which shaking is an important contributory mechanism in AHT.[53,54]

Retinal hemorrhages are apparent in 38% to 100% of children with AHT and average approximately 80% across multiple studies[55–60]; they are more common and more severe than those in children who experience unintentional trauma. Retinal hemorrhages in children who have experienced AHT are commonly too numerous to count, are widely spread throughout the retina, involve multiple retinal layers,[57–61] and may be associated with retinoschisis (a traumatic tear within the retinal layers leading to a blood [schisis] cavity or retinal fold[62]); the severity of RH often correlates with the severity of the brain injury (Figure 7.3).[56,61] Other associated injuries, such as bruising of body regions that are uncommonly bruised in day-to-day activities, rib fractures, and fractures of long bones such as those involving the metaphyseal end plates, may also distinguish children who have experienced AHT from those who have experienced unintentional injuries.

Distinguishing findings from 5 meta-analytic studies and their frequency from 3 large series among the AHT population are summarized in Table 7.1.

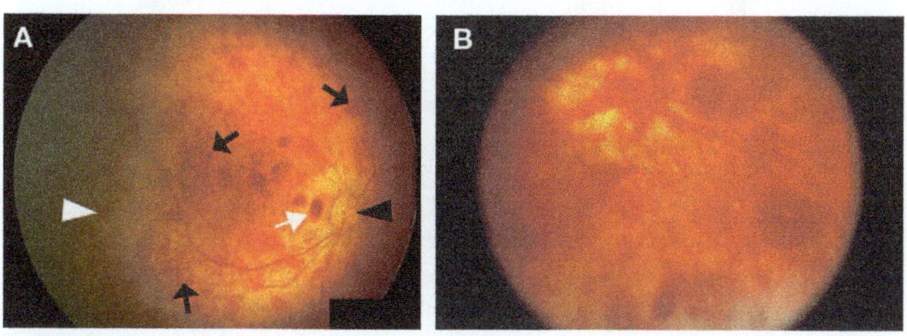

FIGURE 7.3

A, Moderate retinal hemorrhage in a child with abusive head trauma. Too-numerous-to-count intraretinal hemorrhages (black arrows), extending into the periphery (white arrowhead) with limited preretinal hemorrhage (white arrow). Optic disc (black arrowhead). B, Extensive and confluent intraretinal and preretinal hemorrhages throughout the posterior pole and extending into the periphery.

A, From Binenbaum G, Rogers DL, Forbes BJ, et al. Patterns of retinal hemorrhage associated with increased intracranial pressure in children. *Pediatrics.* 2013;132(2):e430–e434. B, From Zenel JA. An infant who has head trauma. *Pediatr Rev.* 2000;21(6):210–214.

TABLE 7.1
Findings That May Help Distinguish Children With Abusive Head Trauma (AHT) From Those With Non-AHT Injuries

Finding	Bhardwaj et al[37]	Kemp et al[41]	Maguire et al[38]	Piteau et al[40]	Maguire et al[39]	Feldman et al[63]	Keenan et al[49]	Kelly et al[25]
	Specificity	OR	OR	OR	OR	Incidence	Incidence	Incidence
Seizure			**5.08**	**7.25**			48.8%	
Apnea			**6.95**	**5.31**			38.8%	
SDH		**8.230**		**8.92**		IC	93.8%	88.90%
SAH		0.979		1.42			11.3%	19.40%
EDH		**0.112**		**0.15**			1.3%	1.67%
Cerebral ischemia				**4.79**			18.8%	26.70%
Cerebral edema		**2.160**		**2.17**				6.67%
Skull fx + ICH				**7.76**			17.5% combined	
Skull fx only				**0.01**				
Any bruise				**4.77**		54.0%		
Head and neck bruise			**4.54**	**0.42**				
Rib fx			**42.75**	**27.10**			27.5%	15.00%
Any acute fx						27.9%		
Any healing fx						27.0%		
Long bone fx			**13.95**	**4.23**			18.8%	18.30%
CML				**11.80**			17.5%	
RH	**94%**		**31.50**		**14.7**	65.1%	76.3%	65.00%

Bold numbers indicate a statistically significant difference.

Abbreviations: CML, classic fracture of the metaphyseal end plate; EDH, epidural hemorrhage; fx, fracture; IC, inclusion criterion for study (rate, thus, is 100%); ICH, intracranial hemorrhage; OR, odds ratio; RH, retinal hemorrhage; SAH, subarachnoid hemorrhage; SDH, subdural hemorrhage.

Individual studies have identified other findings that distinguish the neurologically injured population diagnosed with AHT. These studies have been collected and subjected to systematic review and, where possible, meta-analysis, in an online resource.[64]

Two research groups have derived and validated clinical prediction rules as a means to identify hospitalized children with head injuries with a substantial likelihood of having experienced abuse.[65,66] Hymel and colleagues studied multiple clinical features, all identifiable at initial presentation, to identify those that were associated with AHT and would, therefore, inform a decision to undertake a child abuse workup.

They identified 4 features: 1) SDH that was bilateral or involved the interhemispheric fissure; 2) respiratory compromise on the scene; 3) bruising of the torso, ear, or neck; and 4) skull fracture other than single, simple, unilateral, parietal fractures. The presence of any one of these features had a sensitivity of 96% and specificity of 43% for AHT.[65] Cowley and colleagues studied features that were initially apparent or revealed on subsequent child abuse workup to identify those that, singly or in combination, were associated with AHT. They found that the presence of 3 of 6 findings—bruising of the head or neck, any documented seizure, any identified apnea, rib fracture, long bone fracture, and RH—had a sensitivity of 72.3% and a specificity of 85.6% for AHT.[66]

Symptom Onset

In addition to the nature and diagnostic specificity of presenting symptoms, their timing can be critical in evaluating AHT to determine when primary injury occurred. The infant's environment may include multiple caregivers who might be potential perpetrators of the abuse. Pinpointing when the injury occurred may be the key to identifying who inflicted it, freeing other caregivers from suspicion. In many situations, symptom onset may be the best way to identify the period during which the injury occurred, thereby narrowing the range of possible perpetrators.

Multiple studies have documented that children with the most severe presentation, and those with the worst clinical outcomes (including death), become rapidly and persistently symptomatic in most cases. Children with moderate injury may deteriorate with posttraumatic seizure or expanding intracranial mass, principally epidural hemorrhage (EDH). These outcomes, however, are very uncommon (Table 7.2).

The rarity of severe neurological outcomes for children who present to the emergency department with initially good neurological scores (Glasgow Coma Scale [GCS] 13–15) has been well documented in derivation data for the Pediatric Emergency Care Applied Research Network, Canadian Assessment of Tomography for Childhood Head Injury, and Children's Head Injury Algorithm for the Prediction of Important Clinical Events head imaging clinical prediction rules. Children who present as lucid and neurologically normal rarely have significant intracranial findings, rarely require medical intervention, and rarely have poor outcomes.[74,75]

The possibility of delayed deterioration after infliction of serious neurological injury cannot be absolutely refuted. It can, however, be contextualized. Although rare, there are reports of children with significant or even fatal head injuries who have experienced a "lucid"

TABLE 7.2
Findings of Significant Studies of Abusive Head Trauma

Author	Population	Finding
Arbogast et al[67]	Fatal head injury in those <4 y	93.2% had initial GCS <7. 98.1% of all and 96.8% of those who experienced abuse <24 mo of age had initial GCS <13.
Gilliland[68]	Infants and young children with fatal AHT	71% had severe symptoms within 24 h. 13% additional with lethargy.
Biron and Shelton[69]	Severe AHT with "reliable observer"	68.8% had immediate deterioration. Additional 18.8% comatose after being with perpetrator.
Willman et al[70]	Non-abusive child head injury fatalities	1.2% had initial GCS of 15 (a case of epidural hematoma).
Jaquet et al[71]	Children <16 y of age with non-abusive intracranial injury (GCS 9–15)	3.4% deteriorated and none died. Deterioration occurred with seizure, status epilepticus, expanding epidural hematoma.
De Leeuw et al[72]	Confessed AHT	100% with confessed shaking immediately unconscious. 50% of confessed impact conscious but symptomatic for a period.
Starling et al[17]	AHT with perpetrator statements	91% immediately symptomatic. 9% unobserved after trauma, then found symptomatic.
Adamsbaum et al[73]	AHT with perpetrator statements	100% immediate symptoms. 35% seizure, vomiting, neurological deficits within 30 min.

Abbreviations: AHT, abusive head trauma; GCS, Glasgow Coma Scale.

interval during which there were either neurologically normal or were nearly normal and subsequently deteriorated. Snoek et al[76] identified 42 (4.3%) of 967 children with head injuries who deteriorated neurologically after an initial lucid period. Posttraumatic seizures (with full recovery) accounted for 13 cases, transient neurological signs with full recovery accounted for an additional 25 cases, and one child deteriorated from an expanding epidural hematoma and recovered following surgery. The 3 remaining children died, unfortunately, without a description of their intracranial findings. Humphreys et al[77] described 4 children who died following a period in which the child "verbalized to some degree," although all were symptomatic and only one achieved a maximum GCS of 13 prior to deterioration. In addition to non–mass-occupying intracranial bleeding, each child had brain swelling and 2 had extensive cerebral contusions. Choudhry et al[78] reported 31 (4.1%) of 757 children with head injuries and adults with initial GCS at or above 13. Expanding intracranial hemorrhage accounted for 21 cases and systemic medical causes explained the other 10. Hamilton et al[79] identified 2 children among 17,962 children with minor head trauma who suffered delayed deterioration from expanding intracranial hemorrhage (one epidural and one intraparenchymal). As discussed previously, the one child with delayed deterioration and death in the study by Willman et al also had a large EDH.[70]

Immediate posttraumatic seizures (defined as those that occur within the first 24 hours following injury) may complicate accidental brain injuries, but they are almost universally benign, do not contribute to the ultimate neurological outcome, and do not portend future epilepsy. Early posttraumatic seizure (occurring within 7 days of injury) occurs with all severities of head trauma but is more likely in children with severe head injury, low GCS, loss of consciousness, and prolonged loss of consciousness.[80–86]

Other rare causes of delayed neurological deterioration include traumatic hyponatremia due to syndrome of inappropriate antidiuretic hormone (SIADH) secretion or cerebral salt wasting, and vascular dissection or occlusion with cerebrovascular accident. Absent a complicating condition, there is a greater than 95% likelihood that a child with classically presenting acute AHT developed symptoms within a few minutes of the inciting trauma.

Dating RHs is generally unreliable, although one study suggested that the presence of too-numerous-to-count intraretinal splinter and flame hemorrhages may indicate injury that occurred within a few days, whereas their absence may indicate injury that occurred at least 1 week prior.[87] Identifying the time of injury based on CT or MR imaging appearances of intracranial injury or hemorrhage is also problematic and is discussed further as follows.

Mild, Subacute, and Chronic Presentation

Other children who have experienced AHT may present with a milder encephalopathy and nonspecific symptoms or signs such as a brief alteration in consciousness, brief resolved unexplained event, irritability or somnolence, anorexia or vomiting, or seizure with rapid recovery.[45,88–90] The diagnosis of AHT is most commonly entertained when the evaluation leads to the identification of an SDH. Unfortunately, a significant proportion of these children are missed at initial presentation[91] and may present later with more serious or life-threatening injuries. Others present with progressive macrocephaly or bulging fontanelles and are found on neuroimaging to have hypodense or mixed density subdural collections[45,46] (Figure 7.4). Although mixed density SDH was previously thought to represent evidence of multiple injury episodes and recent studies have confirmed that mixed density SDH are more common in AHT than in unintentional injuries,[52,92] a study of 18 infants with SDH who died in traffic crashes confirmed that mixed density SDH can arise as the result of a single injury (Figure 7.5).[93] Mixed density subdural collections may represent acute SDH with serum extrusion, acute subdural blood mixed with cerebrospinal fluid (CSF), chronic SDH or subdural hygroma (defined as a subdural collection, the principal component of which appears to be CSF and which is clear, xanthochromic, or faintly pink tinged and generally lacking any surrounding membranes) with a small amount of rebleeding, or acute traumatic SDH in a child with preexisting subdural hygroma or chronic SDH.[94]

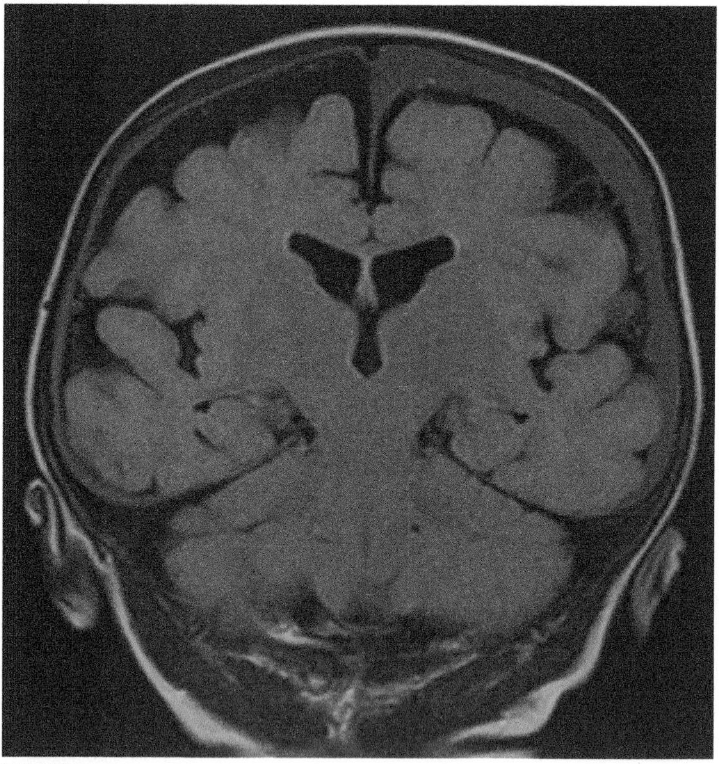

FIGURE 7.4
Fluid attenuated inversion recovery sequence coronal T1 magnetic resonance imaging scan demonstrating bilateral subdural collections with different signal characteristics.

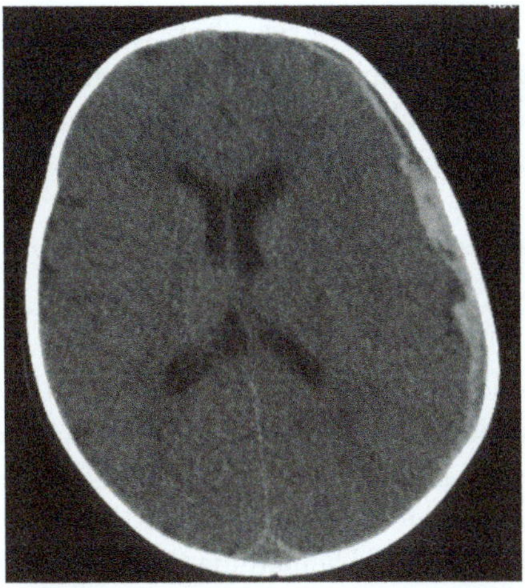

FIGURE 7.5
Axial computed tomography scan. Mixed density is seen within a left convexity acute subdural hematoma. Also seen is a subdural hemorrhage within the interhemispheric fissure.

Despite their milder symptoms, the evidence for AHT in children presenting in this manner is substantial. When children with small extra-axial hemorrhage under a skull fracture are excluded, more than half, and as many as 80%, of these cases are found to involve abuse.[45,46,90]

Intracranial injuries may be identified even in children who have no clinical symptoms of AHT. Intracranial imaging of young children for evaluation of extracranial abusive injuries may show additional intracranial injuries in 1% to 29%.[42-44] Whether these children were asymptomatic from their cranial injuries or were initially symptomatic and allowed to recover before additional abusive injuries brought them to medical care is unknown. Current American College of Radiology (ACR) Appropriateness Criteria state that intracranial neuroimaging "may be appropriate" for children younger than 24 months without neurological signs and symptoms who potentially have experienced physical abuse.[95]

Biomechanics and Pathophysiology

Biomechanics and Primary Traumatic Brain Injury

An understanding of the circumstances, pathophysiology, and biomechanics of traumatic brain injury (TBI) must incorporate an explanation for the intracranial bleeding that is almost universally seen and the brain injuries that result in mortality and long-term morbidity for the child. Before discussing injury biomechanics, it is helpful to first interpret basic terminology and to understand the various mechanisms and classifications of AHT injuries. These include concepts of injury severity, injury type, injury mechanism, and tissue tolerance. Once these are understood, generalizations about the mechanisms that produce specific injuries can be made.

Injury Severity

It is important to distinguish between the *severity* and the *type* of cranial injuries, especially when communicating with social service and law enforcement officials who may have less familiarity with these concepts. For example, while a skull fracture may constitute a severe injury to a nonmedical professional, it is, in and of itself, not the cause of acute neurological deterioration or long-term disability. Similarly, a large or rapidly expanding epidural hematoma (Figure 7.6) can cause coma from increased intracranial pressure (ICP) without the need for any direct parenchymal brain injury. That these types of injuries can occur as a consequence of low-height falls can confuse those who are not medical

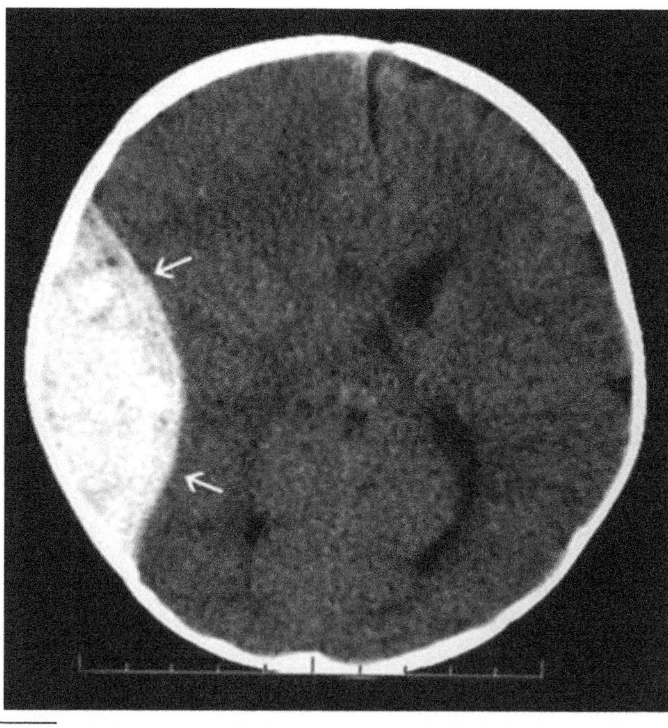

FIGURE 7.6
Axial computed tomography scan demonstrating right-sided acute epidural hematoma with mass effect and midline shift.

professionals and lead to an erroneous conclusion that such injuries "must have occurred" from more forceful or inflicted injury.

In general, the grading of TBI uses the GCS, which is assessed during the acute post-injury period, after trauma resuscitation. The GCS ranges from 3 to 15 depending on the patient's eye-opening, motor, and verbal responses (Table 7.3). Patients with a GCS of 13 to 15 are considered to have mild injuries; scores of 9 to 12 are considered moderate; and scores of 3 to 8 are considered severe. Although the GCS is validated in older children and adults, it has substantial limitations in the evaluation of infants. Other infant coma scores have, therefore, been developed, such as the Infant Coma Scale[96–99] (see Table 7.3). In addition, many children have been pharmacologically sedated, paralyzed, or intubated before arriving at the hospital, which also changes their GCS; the GCS in intubated patients is, therefore, usually calculated using only the best motor and eye-opening scores followed by the letter T (for intubated). Finally, seizures, some of which can be difficult to identify clearly in infants, can also confound the assessment.

TABLE 7.3
Adult and Infant Glasgow Coma Scores

	Glasgow Coma Scale	Infant Coma Scale
Eyes	**4:** Opens eyes spontaneously	**4:** Opens eyes spontaneously
	3: Opens eyes in response to voice	**3:** Opens eyes in response to speech
	2: Opens eyes in response to painful stimuli	**2:** Opens eyes in response to painful stimuli
	1: Does not open eyes	**1:** Does not open eyes
Verbal	**5:** Oriented, converses normally	**5:** Smiles, orients to sounds, follows objects, interacts
	4: Confused, disoriented	**4:** Cries but consolable, inappropriate interactions
	3: Utters incoherent words	**3:** Inconsistently inconsolable, moaning
	2: Incomprehensible sounds	**2:** Inconsolable, agitated
	1: Makes no sounds	**1:** No verbal response
Motor	**6:** Obeys commands	**6:** Moves spontaneously or purposefully
	5: Localizes to painful stimuli	**5:** Withdraws from touch
	4: Flexion/withdrawal to painful stimuli	**4:** Withdraws from pain
	3: Abnormal flexion to painful stimuli (decorticate response)	**3:** Abnormal flexion to pain for an infant (decorticate response)
	2: Extension to painful stimuli (decerebrate response)	**2:** Extension to pain (decerebrate response)
	1: Makes no movements	**1:** No motor response

Injury Type

It is critical to properly and completely identify the type and location of all cranial injuries on neuroimaging studies or at autopsy. Skull fractures can be identified by their location (which bones are involved) and their type (linear vs complex). Complex fracture may be comminuted (having multiple branches), diastatic (having fracture edges that are separated), depressed (having an edge or fragment that is pressed in toward the brain or lifted outward), or basilar; cross suture lines into adjacent skull bones; or have other unusual features. Extra-axial blood collections should, whenever possible, be specified by type and location. Types include epidural (between the skull and dura mater), subdural (between the dura mater and arachnoid), subarachnoid (deep to the arachnoid and lying within the CSF compartment), and/or subpial (below the pia mater and abutting the cortical surface). The location may be overlying the convexity of each or both cerebral hemispheres, within the interhemispheric fissure and adjacent to the falx cerebri separating the 2 hemispheres, overlying or beneath the tentorium cerebri separating the cerebral hemispheres from the posterior fossa structures, within the posterior fossa, or within the basal cisterns.

Parenchymal brain injuries should similarly be described by type and location. Injuries may include superficial cortical contusions, deep white matter injuries, intracerebral or intraventricular hemorrhage, cerebral edema (seen as loss of the distinction between gray and white matter on CT scans), and/or ischemic-anoxic injuries (represented as hypodensities on CT scans and hyperintensities on diffusion-weighted MR images). Locations include the specific cerebral hemispheric lobes (frontal, parietal, temporal, occipital), deep hemispheric white matter tracts (centrum semiovale, corpus callosum), basal ganglia (caudate, putamen, and/or globus pallidus), thalamus, and/or hypothalamus.

It is important to be aware that most patients with AHT have more than 1 injury type, that many injury types are graded in severity, and that most injury types can arise by more than a single mechanism. Failing to understand these distinctions can lead to erroneous assumptions about the possible causes of a given injury.

Injury Mechanisms

The study of what mechanisms result in which injuries has a long and evolving history; a full discussion of this subject is beyond the constraints of this chapter and has been the subject of a number of reviews.[54,60,100–103] However, some generalizations can be made that may be of use to the medical professional called on to assess and care for children presenting with AHT. Discussions of these generalizations with lay investigators and in court must be nuanced and guarded to avoid overstating the certainty of what is known.

The anatomical components of the head, including the brain, can be injured by direct contact to the head, as well as by motion of the structures within the intracranial compartment. *Contact* (also called *impact*) forces occur when the head is struck by or impacts an object or surface. Contact events cause damage when structures deform adjacent to the site at which the contact occurs. Examples include scalp abrasions, bruises, hematomas, or lacerations; skull fractures; epidural hematomas; localized subdural or subarachnoid bleeding; and localized brain surface contusions.

In contrast, *inertial* forces occur when structures inside the skull are set in motion, either when a stationary head *accelerates* or when a moving head *decelerates*. Differential motion between structures during acceleration and deceleration results in deformation of those intracranial tissues. The occurrence of deformation, called *strain*, can result in tissue injury when it exceeds the tolerance of that particular tissue stretch over a given time, the *strain rate*. Altered consciousness (eg, concussion), rupture of parasagittal bridging veins leading to SDH, and traumatic axonal injury are examples of injuries caused by inertial forces. Inertial injuries may be further subdivided into those that are linear, called *translational* deceleration, in which the brain moves in a straight line, and *rotational* or *angular* deceleration, in which the brain moves around a center of rotation.

Inertial events can occur with or without actual impact. Examples of noncontact inertial events include instances of whiplash in automobile crashes in which the head moves but does not strike any surface, or shaking an infant with no head impact. Likewise, *contact* events can occur with or without inertial injuries, such as when a TV falls on a child who is then pinned to the floor. It should be stressed that in most clinical trauma, contact and inertial forces occur, although their relative importance varies by event. Whether these various types of forces result in a specific injury type depends on the magnitude and direction of the force and the tissue tolerance.

The absence of visible contact injuries often causes confusion in interpreting injury events. Whereas visible contact injuries confirm that contact has occurred, the absence of surface contact injuries does not rule out contact. In children who die from AHT, contact injuries may be found at autopsy that were not apparent on the clinical examination of the living child.[104] This is particularly important in AHT, in which the absence of impact injuries does not mean that shaking was the sole causal mechanism.

Tissue Tolerance

Whether a particular mechanism results in a particular injury, and that injury's severity, depends on whether the tolerance of each involved tissue is exceeded. Tissue tolerances are defined by the magnitude of forces, measured as stress (the forces per unit volume) or strain (deformity in percent); the direction and nature of the force (contact vs initial, transverse vs rotational acceleration, and axial vs coronal vs sagittal rotation); and the time over which those forces develop. When tolerances are exceeded, tissues may fail mechanically, such as a tearing bridging vessel leading to SDH. They may also fail physiologically, such as the neuron that loses the ability to regulate transmembrane ion and water flux, resulting in axonal injury. Tissue tolerances are influenced by several variables, including age, anatomical variation, prior injury, and surgical intervention. Thus, patients with temporal arachnoid cysts may sustain SDH from relatively minor impacts, presumably due to bridging veins that are stretched over a long distance and more prone to tearing. Some children with shunted hydrocephalus and/or enlarged subarachnoid spaces seem to have a lower threshold for sustaining SDH, as do some elderly individuals with brain atrophy.

Infants and small children have specific biomechanical features that influence injury susceptibility. One important example is infant skull deformability due to the thinness of the skull and open sutures. Infants sustaining head impacts can have significant deformation of the underlying brain and vessels, leading to different types of injuries. Tearing of surface or deep vessels can occur from skull deformation, such as in SDHs related to delivery.[105] There is evidence to support increased susceptibility to inertial events and decreased susceptibility to focal brain surface deformation in infant gyrencephalate animals compared with more mature animals.[106,107] Mechanically, immature tissue also has a higher water content, which causes it to be more resistant to deformation.[108]

Most experimental data on tissue tolerance has been studied with single strains developed at a limited range of strain rates. There are some data to indicate that once strained, tissue is altered and may experience a repeat strain differently. Alterations may be physical/mechanical and/or physiologic/functional and may be immediate and/or sustained. These factors create additional complexity in the evaluation of the biomechanics of a single shaking event involving repeated, rhythmic, rotational acceleration events, which might recur multiple times over days, weeks, and months.[18]

Mechanisms of Specific Injuries

Data from clinical series, accident reconstructions, and experimental models have furthered the understanding of what mechanisms generally cause what injury types.[55,102,109–126] Table 7.4 outlines the typical mechanisms and magnitude of the various injury types seen in infants and children.

Scalp and skull injuries and brain surface contusions are caused by contact forces, although some brain surface contusions can be caused by inertial events (eg, contrecoup contusions caused by the brain moving within the skull). Similarly, EDH is almost always associated with an impact and may be accompanied by scalp bruising or skull fractures, particularly fractures that cross the middle meningeal artery in the temporal fossa or the dural venous sinuses. However, infants with thin, pliable skulls may have an epidural hematoma without a corresponding skull fracture.[127] This is a good example of the same strain exceeding the tissue tolerance of one tissue (the meningeal artery) while not exceeding the tissue tolerance of an adjacent tissue (the infant skull). Small focal convexity SDH, focal subarachnoid hemorrhage, and superficial cortical contusions are also more likely caused by impact injuries, especially when associated with scalp swelling and/or skull fracture. Subdural hemorrhage may also arise from the application of slow, static forces, such as during child birth[128–132] or from crush injuries[133] that tear venous sinuses or cortical bridging veins.

TABLE 7.4
Injury Types and Mechanisms

Injury Type	Mechanism	Magnitude of Force
Scalp laceration	Contact	Variable (low to high)
Scalp hematoma	Contact	Variable (low to high)
Skull fracture	Contact or crush (static loading)	Variable (low to high)
Epidural hematoma	Contact	Variable (low to high)
Cortical contusion	Contact or inertial (contrecoup)	Usually moderate to high
Cortical laceration	Contact	High
Focal subarachnoid hemorrhage	Contact (cortical vessel or venous tear), static loading (eg, birth injuries)	Moderate to high
Subdural hematoma, focal convexity	Inertial (usually, especially in older children/adults), contact (cortical vessel or venous tear), static loading (eg, birth injuries)	Moderate to high
Subdural hematoma, diffuse, bilateral or interhemispheric	Inertial (usually, especially in older children/adults)	Moderate to high
Diffuse axonal injury	Inertial	High

Diffuse, interhemispheric, and perifalcine SDH and traumatic axonal injury are the result of inertial events that include large angular accelerations. Infant head injury models have shown that the inertial forces generated by impacts, even from short falls, are many times greater than those that can be achieved by shaking alone.[104,109] This has led some to conclude that shaking alone cannot generate forces sufficient to achieve injury thresholds. However, it must be emphasized that these thresholds were derived from adult primate studies,[134] and their applicability to human infants has been questioned.[54,108,135] Moreover, the results of these studies do not comport with the benign nature of falls in children, most of which result in little or no visible injury. The models themselves vary in their construction, particularly with regard to neck flexibility, which varies widely between models. The effects of repetitive oscillatory loading, as would occur during bouts of shaking, have not been fully examined. The contribution of upper cervical spinal cord injuries[136–138] producing disordered breathing or apnea as possible contributors to the pathophysiology of AHT also remains to be studied. An ovine model of pure nonimpact shaking has produced intracranial injuries similar to AHT and even death.[139–142] Many perpetrator statements in AHT consistently describe violent shaking as a causal mechanism; virtually all of these cases lack any evidence of impact injury such as scalp bruising/swelling or skull fracture, yet they demonstrate SDH and brain injuries in the same frequency as those with impact mechanisms.[17,18] Finally, a case of witnessed adult SDH and brain injury similar to AHT caused by violent nonimpact shaking has been reported.[143]

Experimental Biomechanics of Falls and Shaking

As noted, the prior discussion incorporates generalizations. These concepts result from experience with adults and children and from various experimental methods. Animal and human cadaver tissue, whole animal and whole cadaver, anthropomorphic test mannequin, mathematical modeling, and computer-based finite element analysis have been applied to this problem. All such methods are, in some way, removed from the actual trauma and injury event of a real child, and all involve approximations and assumptions. As such, best practice is to validate models against known events before attempting to predict the outcome of posited events. At the current level of understanding, it is likely premature to make bold assertions of certitude in settings that lack scientific understanding and nuance, such as legal proceedings. Unfortunately, the cautious clinician may still need to face the strong assertions of others, which will require a better understanding of research methods and results.

The biomechanics of both violent shaking and impacts have been evaluated using a variety of test dummies and computer simulations. For example, Prange and colleagues[109] studied the maximum rotational velocity and deceleration sustained by a biofidelic doll undergoing free falls, inflicted impacts, and shaking. In this study, angular velocities and decelerations increased with fall height and surface hardness (concrete > carpeted pad over concrete > foam padding), as would be expected.[109] The values obtained from a 1-foot fall onto carpeted floor or foam are low enough that cranial injuries of any type would be highly unlikely, whereas a 1-foot fall onto concrete or a 3-foot fall onto carpet might be expected to produce a skull fracture. Whether the biomechanical forces from these types of falls are sufficient to produce significant intracranial injuries, such as axonal injury and SDH, is debatable, with various studies providing conflicting evidence.[109,144–146]

Mannequins with varying degrees of biofidelity have been used to evaluate whether isolated infant shaking is sufficient to cause the injuries found in AHT. While one such published study has predicted concussion, none have predicted the severe brain injury and SDH typical of classic AHT.[104,109,110,147,148] In contrast, finite element models have predicted SDH following shaking events.[149,150] A significant limitation with all these biomechanical studies is that the injury thresholds for axonal injury and SDH were derived from studies of adult primates undergoing single, nonimpact accelerations[134,144,151] and extrapolated to infant humans based solely on mass scaling. Until we gain a better understanding of how these material properties contribute to the thresholds for injury in human infants, it is unlikely that biomechanical simulations will provide accurate information on which to base any firm conclusions.

A number of animal models have been developed and tested, each involving limitations and assumptions. A lamb model, developed by Finnie and colleagues,[140–142] is particularly germane because it involves direct human shaking, without impact, of an immature, gyrencephalate animal. While the pattern of injury in the lambs was different from the findings in infants with AHT, the model has demonstrated retinal injury, SDH, brain injury, and death as a result of this violent shaking.

Reports of violent shaking without impact from many perpetrators[17,18] support shaking as a pathophysiological mechanism for these injuries and is at odds with the results of biomechanical studies. Although some reporting perpetrators may be lying, it seems inconceivable that all are consistently lying about the same thing. These facts have led many authors to maintain that shaking alone, without impact, also can lead to brain injury.[54]

Pathophysiology, Secondary Brain Injuries, and the Biochemical Response to Traumatic Brain Injury

In addition to the primary biomechanical injuries discussed previously, TBI produces a cascade of pathophysiological and metabolic changes, which are collectively referred to as *secondary* brain injuries. Primary damage to the brain stem and extracranial injuries may produce apnea, hypotension, bradycardia, or cardiac arrest, resulting in hypoxia and ischemia to other brain tissues. Changes in vascular flow regulation following primary strain of brain tissues may produce decreased brain perfusion; ischemia, or increased brain perfusion; and interstitial edema. Accumulation of blood within an epidural or SDH may increase ICP or compress blood vessels, compromising brain circulation. Primary injury to draining veins and sinuses may initiate venous thrombosis,[152,153] leading to venous infarction. Primary damage to neurons may disrupt membrane regulation of ion and water flux, producing cytotoxic edema and increased ICP. Injured neurons may also release excitotoxic neurotransmitters such as glutamate; inflammatory mediators such as tumor necrosis factor, interleukins, and quinolinic acid; oxidative stress and free radical damage; and regulators of apoptosis (programmed cell death) such as bcl-2 and cytochrome c.[154–170] Studies have demonstrated greater changes in the concentration of these agents within CSF after AHT compared with unintentional trauma,[162,169–172] and others have demonstrated an increased susceptibility of the infant brain to these abnormalities.[173] Hypoxic-ischemic parenchymal brain injury, as manifest on diffusion weighted MR imaging sequences, is common in AHT and likely responsible for the relatively poor outcome of patients with AHT.[50]

Hypoxia and hypotension are common in severe TBI and contribute significantly to underlying primary mechanical brain injuries. In particular, cytotoxic edema from ischemia, as manifest on diffusion weighted MR imaging sequences, is common in AHT; although the cause of this ischemia is multifactorial, it likely involves systemic hypoxemia due to apnea or disordered breathing, hypoperfusion due to altered cerebrovascular autoregulation, and increased metabolic demands as injured tissues attempt to repair or expend energy during seizure.

Chronic Subdural Hemorrhage and Subdural Hygroma

The mechanism and pathophysiology for the formation of chronic SDH is a matter of debate. Chronic SDH are composed partially or entirely of fluid rather than clot and are hypodense to brain parenchyma on CT scans.

The fluid may evolve over days to weeks from red, to purple-brown (also called crankcase oil), to straw or tea colored, and finally to faint yellow. Classic teaching holds that chronic subdural collections evolve over time from acute subdural blood that is undergoing gradual dissolution and resorption. Studies of serial neuroimaging in AHT, in which some acute subdural hematomas evolve to chronic collections over time, support this conclusion.[51,52] Subdural fluid contains antifibrinolytic agents that promote micro-hemorrhages. In addition, membranes form on outer and inner sides of the SDH during the first 3 weeks after injury; the outer membrane in particular becomes neovascularized, and small micro-hemorrhages into the subdural fluid develop over this time.[174]

In adults, chronic subdural collections may also evolve from subdural hygromas.[175–177] The proposal is that acute trauma produces a rent in the arachnoid, perhaps with minimal associated bleeding, that allows CSF, with minimal or no acute blood components, to escape from the subarachnoid space and collect within the subdural space; this subdural collection, which is hypodense to brain parenchyma on CT scans, is referred to as a subdural hygroma. Magnetic resonance imaging may distinguish chronic SDH and subdural hygroma because the former, containing various blood products, differs in intensity from CSF on 1 or more sequences, whereas the latter, containing exclusively or largely CSF, is most commonly isointense to CSF on all sequences. Over time, vascularized pseudomembranes surround the SDH just as they do with chronic SDH, and repeated micro-hemorrhages contribute to expansion of the hygroma and a change in its radiological appearance.[175–177] Whether this mechanism applies to infants and children is unknown. Mixed density subdural collections have been described on initial CT scans performed after motor vehicle crashes in infants[93] and were proposed to represent an admixture of blood, serum, and CSF. To further test the relationship between the subdural and CSF spaces, Zouros et al injected radio-labeled indium In 111 into the lumbar thecal space after placing a subdural catheter to drain mixed density or fluid density subdural collections; the tracer appeared within the subdural fluid within 3 to 24 hours.[178] This developing science justifies caution in attempts to date mixed or low-density subdural collections on CT.

Mechanisms of Retinal Hemorrhage

While the previous discussion of TBI is applicable to abusive and severe unintentional injury, the biomechanics and pathophysiology of RH must account for significant differences in the incidence and nature of RH between severe unintentional injury and abuse. Theories that have been advanced include tracking of blood from the cranial cavity into the globe, increased ICP, vascular transmission of ICP from high intrathoracic pressure, and vitreoretinal traction during rotational acceleration of the eye. There are several reasons to accept the theory that RH in abuse occurs by primary mechanical injury and vitreoretinal traction. Severe vehicular crashes may produce RHs resembling those of AHT.[179] A single, rapid rotational event in 3- to 5-day-old piglets produced ocular hemorrhages involving the vitreous, vitreous base, peripheral retina, ciliary body, and optic nerve sheath; most hemorrhages involved areas of strong vitreoretinal attachment.[180] Manual shaking of infant lambs also produced limited RH in a few animals, although not in the classic pattern associated with AHT.[142] A more thorough discussion of biomechanics and RH can be found in Chapter 8, Ocular Manifestations of Child Abuse. Mathematical modeling via finite element analysis has begun to describe the vitreoretinal traction model as well.[181–183]

Evaluation

History

It is best to get a broad and complete history as early as possible, preferably even before AHT has become the focus of concern. Uncovering an explanatory medical condition or trauma event history will prevent unnecessary suspicion, evaluation, and reporting, all of which would be unnecessary to properly care for the underlying medical condition and painful for the family. A history of other medical conditions and concerns, the birth narrative, previous injury events, and custodial arrangements will be more credible when provided by the family before suspicion has been raised or occult injuries are identified. In more concerning situations, it may be preferable to interview each potential informant separately whenever possible.

Once a finding that may be the consequence of trauma is identified, the history will immediately turn to questions about recent and remote traumatic events. This history should be broad in the range of trauma and the time frame covered, probing explanatory possibilities for the known injury and potential findings that might be found on subsequent workup. Any traumatic event needs to be described in detail—what exactly occurred, what the infant's position and activity were when he or she became symptomatic or was injured, how the infant reacted, how the symptoms became known and by whom, how high a fall was, what symptoms were present after the injury, and how they progressed. What did the caregiver do in response to the infant's symptoms? What was the time sequence from onset of symptoms to medical care?

Similarly, the onset of symptoms should be documented in detail. Current symptoms should be tracked back until 2 independent witnesses can verify that the child was fully awake, acting normally, and eating normally. The development and pace of symptoms, and any period when symptoms may not have been observed, such as sleep, should be documented and correlated with the presence of each caregiver and the time frame of events. A similar analysis should also be performed for any past symptoms that might represent similar, prior trauma.

A detailed history of the pregnancy and birth process should be sought. Did the mother experience any unusual trauma while pregnant? Were there any prenatal concerns or prepartum imaging findings? What was the gestational age and weight of the newborn? What was the route of delivery, and was assistance necessary to extract the newborn, such as forceps or vacuum extractor? What was the baby's head and neurological condition after delivery?

The child's past medical history can reveal clues to differential diagnostic concerns, symptoms of previously unrecognized injury, and sentinel injuries that may have been dismissed as minor and unimportant, such as bruises in infancy. Signs of coagulation deserve particular focus; delayed separation and bleeding of the umbilical stump, abnormal bleeding after circumcision or other procedures, nosebleeds, gingival bleeding with minor trauma, and a history of bruising or petechiae should be specifically sought. Metabolic disorders may manifest as a large head circumference at birth, prolonged or severe neonatal jaundice, unusually significant response to minor illnesses, inability to tolerate normal fasting, or neurodevelopmental delays. Failure to thrive may signal an underlying illness or chronic neglect. Fever is not typical for AHT and should raise concern for infection. A history of prior meningitis may explain a subdural hygroma. To be sufficiently broad, a complete review of systems should be performed.

The previous developmental abilities of the child should be documented and considered when evaluating a trauma history. A history of a fall for an infant who cannot yet crawl or sit will be more difficult to accept than the same history obtained for a child who can stand or jump. Although infants who do not yet roll can manage to make their way over and off of surfaces, this will be less likely than a baby who can roll or crawl. Preexisting developmental delays may also indicate underlying disease, previous neurotrauma, or chronic neglect. Prior developmental capacity will form the baseline for judging subsequent outcome. Finally, parents who express unrealistic developmental expectations may have a higher likelihood for abuse.

Family medical history presents another chance to search for underlying medical conditions. It is not enough to ask if there is a family history of a named condition, such as hemophilia. The conditions should be described and specific symptoms elicited. Asking about people who bleed or bruise easily or excessively, nosebleeds, gingival bleeding, bleeding following surgical or dental procedures, menstrual blood flow, anemia, and transfusion will further probe a coagulopathy history. Parental heights, fracture histories, quick inspection of the sclerae and dental enamel, and inquiry about hearing loss will advance the consideration of osteogenesis imperfecta or related diseases. A family history of macrocephaly may suggest metabolic conditions or benign expansion of the subarachnoid space. The health and neurodevelopmental condition of other related children may uncover metabolic diseases. A history of intracranial hemorrhage in related children may raise the possibility of either an underlying medical condition or serial child abuse.

The social history is very important in evaluating and caring for families. At a minimum, knowing who cares for the child in what settings identifies possible historians as well as possible perpetrators. Social risk factors include domestic violence, prior involvement with child protective services, parental mental illness including substance abuse, and parental stressors such as acute financial and relationship issues. Some of these questions are sensitive, making them awkward to ask and alarming to the family. Additionally, these issues create opportunity for social biases to enter into the evaluation and diagnosis of the child. Social biases have been shown to influence both the vigor with which child abuse is evaluated and the ultimate diagnosis and management of abuse, although this finding is inconsistent.[184–186] Regardless, these issues are important in the overall assessment of risk and safety.

Physical Examination

Like the history, the physical examination should be comprehensive rather than problem focused. Additional injuries are commonly identified in children with AHT.[45,63,187,188] Bruising occurs in approximately 50% but may occur in easily overlooked locations such as the ears, scalp, folds of the neck, and diaper area (Figure 7.7). Bruising of the trunk, ear, or neck, or in young infants, creates substantial concern for abuse.[189] Intraoral injuries such as frenula tears, contusion of the buccal or labial mucosa, tooth avulsion, and palatal or pharyngeal injury should be sought; resuscitative efforts and intubation must be considered when evaluating intraoral, nuchal, and anterior thoracic injuries. While minor oral, facial, or anterior thoracic injuries may be seen, serious or fatal internal injuries, rib fractures, and RHs seldom, if ever, occur in pediatric cardiopulmonary resuscitation.[190–195] Inspection and palpation of the skeleton will establish whether skeletal injuries are outwardly evident, and observation of the child's behavior and activity will establish whether they are symptomatic; abdominal palpation will do the same for visceral injury.

The eye examination is crucial to the proper evaluation of AHT and has been recommended by the American Academy of Pediatrics (AAP) in the evaluation of young children who are suspected to have experienced child physical abuse, and particularly those with intracranial findings.[196] Evaluating children who are suspected to have experienced abuse but who do not have intracranial findings is seldom fruitful, although isolated retinal findings have been reported.[197–199] Non-ophthalmologists can and do identify RHs when they look.[200] The extent and nature of RH are better evaluated by a trained ophthalmologist. Because RH can begin evolving early after trauma,[87] an ophthalmological examination by dilated indirect ophthalmoscopy should be performed as soon as is feasible.[196] A detailed retinal drawing or digital retinal imaging will memorialize the findings; retinal imaging or fluorescein angiography may allow for secondary review or remote consultation.[201,202] Scoring and descriptive systems for RH have been developed, and good inter-rater reliability established, for

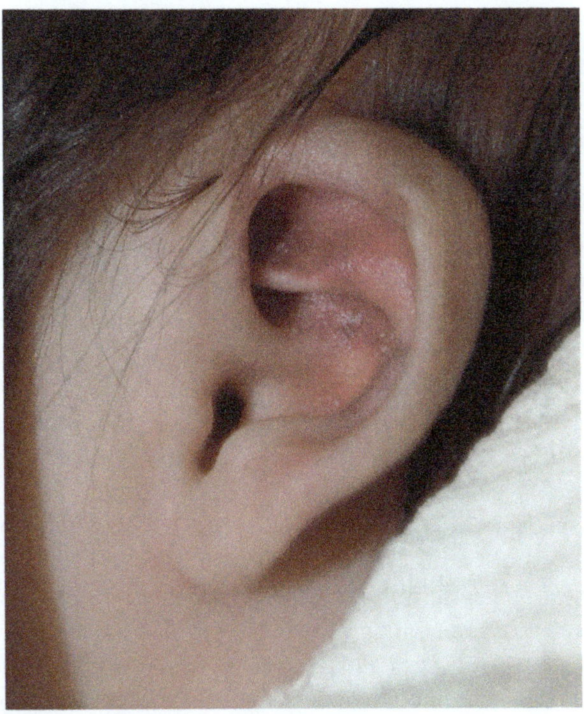

FIGURE 7.7
Ear bruising in an infant with ipsilateral subdural hemorrhage and parenchymal brain injury.

ophthalmologists grading RH.[203–205] Retinal hemorrhage can also be detected on MR imaging,[206,207] but the details are best documented by ophthalmoscopy to establish the specificity of abuse and consider other diagnostic possibilities.

Ocular pathology in the deceased child is also an important facet of documenting abuse. At least 3 methods for examining the eye have been used: an anterior approach, a superior approach from the intracranial cavity, and a superior approach with en bloc removal of the orbital contents. In addition to demonstrating RHs and vitreous hemorrhages that are visible to the ophthalmologist, blood and/or hemosiderin may also be demonstrated in the optic nerve and sheath, ocular muscles and their insertion sites, and periorbital fat.[208–211]

Neuroimaging

Neuroimaging is a critical component in evaluating AHT, with 4 potential aims: 1) identifying the extent and nature of the injuries; 2) creating a differential diagnosis and excluding other conditions; 3) establishing the time of the injury; and 4) contributing to the overall prognosis or outcome. Standard neuroimaging modalities include plain radiography, ultrasonography, CT, and MR imaging.

Types of Neuroimaging

The utility of plain radiography has been largely supplanted by cross-sectional CT and/or MR imaging, but plain radiography can provide useful information for the evaluation of AHT. Radiography may identify scalp swelling, calvarial and/or facial fractures, sutural diastasis, and spine fractures or instability, as well as congenital skull and spinal abnormalities (Figure 7.8) and wormian bones suggestive of osteogenesis imperfecta. Cervical spine radiographs can identify subluxation or bone fractures; they are inexpensive and easy to obtain urgently, but their sensitivity is lower than CT or MR imaging, and they cannot directly identify ligamentous injuries.

Ultrasonographic imaging can only be used in the infant with an open fontanelle, and its utility in the evaluation of AHT is limited because much more detailed information can be obtained using CT or MR imaging. The primary utility of ultrasonography is in the screening evaluation of the asymptomatic infant with macrocephaly, in whom the differential diagnosis includes hydrocephalus, benign expansion of the subarachnoid spaces (BESS), and chronic subdural collections (hematoma or hygroma). Ultrasonography can reliably differentiate hematoma and hygroma by identifying the cortical bridging vessels crossing the subarachnoid space (BESS) or closely applied to the cortical surface (SDH or hygroma).

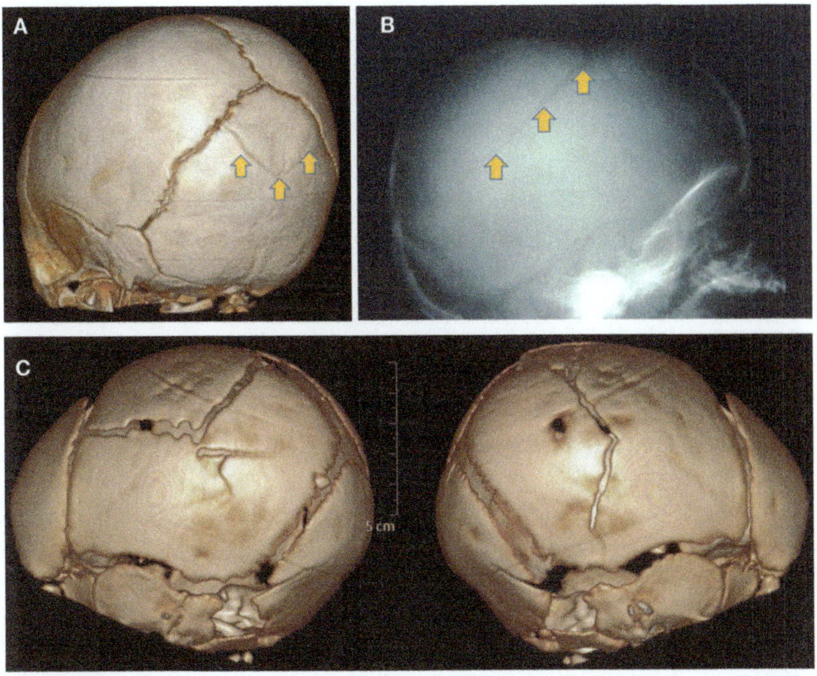

FIGURE 7.8
A, 3-dimensional surface reconstruction from computed tomography scan demonstrates typical skull with accessory occipital suture (arrows). B, Lateral skull radiograph; simple linear parietal skull fracture. C, 3-dimensional surface reconstructions from computed tomography scan; complex, biparietal branching skull fracture.

Ultrasonography may also be helpful in identifying cortical lacerations, although MR imaging is preferred.[212]

Computed tomography is the most commonly used acute imaging modality, particularly in the child who has been severely injured; it can delineate bone and soft tissue abnormalities and is particularly useful in identifying bone injuries and acute intracranial blood.

The ability to display various abnormalities depends on the slice thickness, the computer algorithm used to acquire the information, and the window used to view the resultant images (the last of which can be readily modified by the viewer by selecting a preestablished window setting such as "brain" or "bone" or manipulating a roller ball or cursor). Subtle bone fractures, particularly those involving the skull base or spine, are best imaged using thin (0.5- to 1-mm thick) slices and specific bone algorithms that highlight the interface between bone and soft tissues. Unfortunately, this algorithm is poor for imaging soft tissues such as the brain, so additional soft tissue algorithms are added. Thin extra-axial hematomas are best imaged using soft tissue algorithms that are windowed for blood, whereas the differentiation of gray and white matter and the identification of subtle hypodensities within the brain parenchyma are best imaged using soft tissue algorithms that are windowed for brain. Thin sections also allow 3-dimensional reconstructions that may be extremely helpful in identifying and characterizing skull fractures, accessory ossification centers,[213] and congenital malformations of the skull and/or spine. Although most institutions use reduced radiation doses to image children, these supplemental sequences may be warranted in specific circumstances. Contrast may be helpful to identify subdural membranes in cases of hypodense subdural collections. Computed tomographic angiography may be useful to evaluate the brain vasculature for vascular injury or occlusion, aneurysms, or arteriovenous malformations (AVMs) in select cases (Figure 7.9).

Magnetic resonance imaging has historically been undertaken after the child has been stabilized to supplement and expand on CT findings. Fast-sequence MR imaging techniques that allow for MR imaging without sedation have been used in some institutions for the initial evaluation of the injured child, but the sensitivity is generally not as great as CT or the complete complement of MR imaging sequences.[214] A full MR imaging examination yields much more detailed information than CT or fast-sequence MR imaging about intracranial contents and has become especially important in identifying ligamentous, spinal cord, and nerve root injuries as well as spinal subdural blood.[137,215–217]

Various MR imaging sequences are available, and each has strengths and weaknesses (Table 7.5). The traditional T1, T2, and fluid attenuated inversion recovery (FLAIR) imaging sequences have more recently been supplemented by an increasing number of sequences, including diffusion weighted images (DWIs) and apparent diffusion coefficient (ADC) imaging sequences that identify cytotoxic edema due to hypoxic-ischemic encephalopathy (HIE); gradient echo (GRE) and susceptibility weighted imaging (SWI) sequences that better identify small areas of hemorrhage and slow-moving venous blood; short tau inversion recovery fat-saturation sequences that eliminate fat signal and reveal subtle spinal ligamentous or soft tissue injuries; MR vascular imaging such as MR arteriography and MR venography that can identify vascular dissection or occlusion, aneurysms and vascular malformations, bridging vein disruption and thrombosis,[152,153] or venous sinus thrombosis; and MR spectroscopy that can identify elevated tissue levels of lactate, glutamate, and N-acetyl aspartate that have been correlated with outcome.[218,219] Because MR imaging in infants involves anesthesia, and these additional sequences

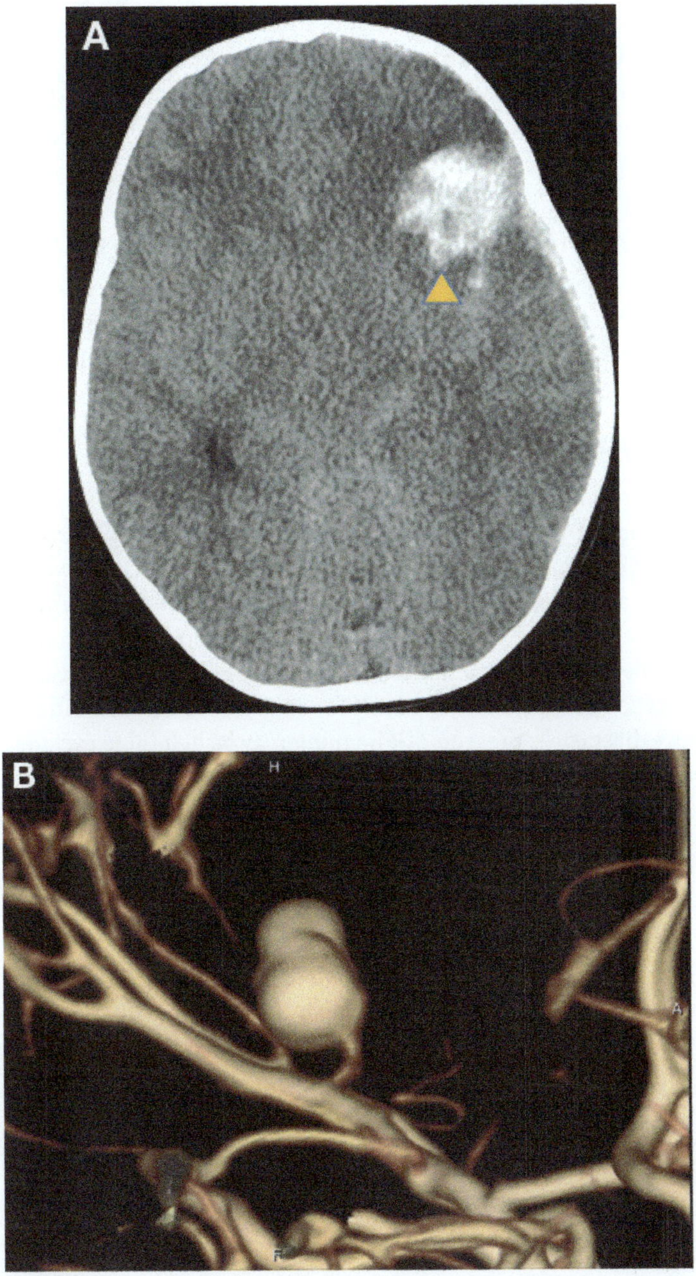

FIGURE 7.9

A, Axial computed tomography scan demonstrating focal intracerebral hematoma near the sylvian fissure, an adjacent small convexity extra-axial hemorrhage, and subarachnoid hemorrhage within the ambient cistern adjacent to the midbrain (arrowhead). B, Accompanying computed tomography angiogram demonstrates a multilobulated middle cerebral artery aneurysm.

usually add only a small amount of additional imaging time, many hospitals have implemented protocols that incorporate cranial and spinal imaging (at least cervical and, in some institutions, the entire spine), as well as many of these additional sequences, to obtain the most detailed and comprehensive information possible.

Neuroimaging Findings in Abusive Head Trauma

A number of excellent recent reviews have analyzed the neuroimaging of AHT in detail.[94,220–222] The basic findings are reviewed in the following sections; the interested reader is referred to these reviews for further information.

Scalp Injuries

Scalp injuries are important to identify because their presence confirms direct contact injury to the head. Skin contusions are not generally identified on neuroimaging, but sub-scalpal injuries such as swelling (manifest as localized increase in scalp thickness), subgaleal hematomas (located between the galea and pericranium), or cephalohematoma (located between the pericranium and skull) should prompt close examination of the underlying bone for skull fractures. If significant fracture diastasis is present, MR imaging may be helpful to exclude an associated dural tear with herniation of brain through the bone defect, which may result in an arachnoid cyst (also known as a leptomeningeal cyst or growing skull fracture).[223]

TABLE 7.5
Appearance of Subdural Hemorrhage on Computed Tomography and Magnetic Resonance Imaging Scans at Various Times

Stage	Time	CT	T1	T2
Hyperacute	<12–24 h	hyper	hypo/iso	hyper
Acute	1–3 d	hyper	hypo/iso	very hypo
Early subacute	2 d–2 wk	iso at 2–3 wk	hyper	very hypo
Late subacute	1 wk–2 mo		very hyper	hyper
Chronic SDH membrane	≥3 wk	hyper	iso	very hyper
Chronic fluid	≥3 wk	hypo	hypo (>CSF)	hyper

Abbreviations: CSF, cerebrospinal fluid; CT, computed tomography; hyper, hyperdense (CT) or hyperintense (magnetic resonance imaging); hypo, hypodense (CT) or hypointense (magnetic resonance imaging); iso, isodense; SDH, subdural hemorrhage.

Adapted by permission from Springer Nature: Vezina G. Assessment of the nature and age of subdural collections in nonaccidental head injury with CT and MRI. *Pediatr Radiol.* 2009;39(6):586–590, copyright 2009.

Skull Fractures

Skull fractures are of several types depending on their morphology: linear, comminuted or stellate (having multiple branches), diastatic (having bone edges that are separated), depressed, basilar, or sutural (involving a suture line). Both skull radiography and CT identify skull fractures. One disadvantage of CT scans has been their relative insensitivity in identifying fractures that run parallel to the axial sections. However, spiral CT scanning, thinner slice thickness, post-image reformatting of coronal and sagittal sequences, and 3-dimensional reformatting have all improved the sensitivity of CT significantly. In one study of 177 children with suspected abuse undergoing skull radiography and CT scans with 3-dimensional reconstructions, CT was 97% sensitive and 94% specific for identifying skull fractures, and interobserver agreement was significantly greater for CT than plain radiography. The authors questioned the need for plain radiography in cases in which CT scans were obtained.[224]

Skull fractures are identified in 25% to 40% of cases of AHT.[52,63,225–228] They are also common following non-AHT from short or intermediate falls, where they are most commonly linear and parietal in location; generally are not associated with significant intracranial injuries except for small underlying focal epidural, subarachnoid, or subpial hemorrhages; and have a good outcome. A number of studies have examined the specificity of skull fracture type in identifying AHT. Linear skull fractures are the most frequently observed, occur in unintentional and abusive injuries, are most commonly parietal, and are, therefore, in themselves relatively nonspecific in differentiating non-AHT from AHT. Some authors have suggested that multiple fractures and those that cross suture lines may have higher specificity for AHT,[229,230] although studies have not consistently identified any specific pattern that predicts AHT.[231]

Care must be taken to differentiate skull fractures from other bony abnormalities and even normal bone variations. Vascular channels or grooves in the skull may simulate fractures, although these are usually not conspicuous in infants. Variations in the sutures, especially those involving the occipital bone, can also generate confusion; knowing the embryology and common developmental variants of the occipital bone is helpful.[213] Localized scalp swelling above the bony abnormality suggests a fracture rather than a developmental variant.

Epidural Hemorrhage

The specificity of intracranial hemorrhage has been reported in a number of studies, and Kemp and colleagues more recently have performed a meta-analysis of the existing literature.[41] Epidural hemorrhage occurs in 0% to 9% (averaging 4%) of cases of AHT and significantly less often following AHT than following non-AHT injuries (odds ratio [OR], 0.1; 95% CI, 0.07–0.18; $P < 0.0001$) (see Figure 7.6).[41] The bleeding source may be arterial, from the meningeal vessels (typically the middle meningeal artery or its branches), or venous, from fracture fragments associated with an overlying skull fracture. The former typically produces a larger, lentiform (football-shaped) hyperdense clot, whereas the latter may be atypical and difficult to distinguish from subdural blood in some cases. Mixed density in an EDH may represent active, hyperacute bleeding with a mixture of clotted and unclotted blood, or a subacute clot with partial liquefaction; the former usually occurs in the setting of acute and rapid neurological deterioration, whereas the latter usually is minimally symptomatic or asymptomatic.

Subdural Hemorrhage

Subdural hemorrhage is simultaneously the most common intracranial finding and the most strongly associated with AHT (see Figure 7.1).[41,57] An average of 80% of children with AHT have identified SDH, according to multiple studies.[52,57,232–235] In the analysis by Kemp and colleagues of 10 comparative studies, SDH occurred in 41% to 94% (average 68%) and was significantly more common in AHT that accidental trauma (OR, 8.2; 95% CI, 6.1–11; $P < 0.0001$).[41] Subdural hemorrhages are most commonly located in or adjacent to the interhemispheric fissure and/or adjacent to the tentorium,[51] are typically small (2–5 mm in greatest thickness), follow the contour of the skull, do not cause significant mass effect, and are rarely a primary cause of neurological deterioration. On CT, interhemispheric SDH may be difficult to distinguish from an infant's normally hyperdense falx cerebri; the presence of unilateral or irregular hyperdensities on CT, or blood products adjacent to the falx on GRE MR imaging sequences, confirms SDH. Similarly, SDH resting on the tentorium, when cut tangentially on axial CT images, often looks "feathered" and diffuse and may be missed by the unwary; coronal or sagittal reconstructions are helpful to identify blood above or below the tentorium.

Subdural hemorrhages can have 4 different imaging characteristics on CT (see Table 7.4); they may be hyperdense, isodense, or hypodense to brain, or they may be of mixed density. Acute blood (within hours) is hyperdense in the absence of significant anemia (hemoglobin level < 8 g/dL). Most reabsorb and disappear over a short time.[51,52] The remainder generally lose their hyperdensity over 3 to 12 days' post-injury, becoming isodense and then hypodense to brain.[51,52,92,236] Like EDH, mixed density SDH may also occur under different circumstances, even when present on the initial scan. On the one hand, mixed density SDH may reflect ongoing active (hyperacute) subdural bleeding with a mixture of clotted and unclotted blood; the SDH in this circumstance is usually large and the child is deteriorating rapidly.[237,238] On the other hand, mixed density SDH may be present on the initial or subsequent CT scans and may represent an admixture of acutely clotted blood, serum, and CSF from acute bleeding; subacute or chronic collections from prior trauma, where clotted blood has begun to liquefy; the result of multiple injuries, including at least 1 prior cranial trauma; or rebleeding into an established SDH with an admixture of acute and chronic blood. It is, therefore, difficult at best to firmly establish whether a mixed density SDH on initial scans is acute, subacute, or chronic based solely on neuroimaging, and some have discouraged the use of these terms in describing SDH, instead advising the use of descriptive terms only.

On MR imaging, blood has characteristic imaging intensities at various times (see Table 7.4) that depend largely on the oxygen state of the hemoglobin molecule (oxygenated vs deoxygenated) and its location (intracellular or extracellular), as well as the presence of hemoglobin degradation products such as methemoglobin and hemosiderin. The appearance of blood on MR imaging changes over time, and this evolution was originally studied[239] and most reliably chronicled in adults with intracerebral hematomas. Some have suggested that the evolution of blood on MR imaging occurs more slowly in subdural compared with intracerebral hematomas, because of a higher oxygen tension in the subdural space and dilution of blood products by CSF.[94] Moreover, the evolution is imperfect and inadequately studied in young children (where subarachnoid CSF is more abundant). The presence of serum and CSF admixed with the blood may also change its MR imaging signal characteristics. Finally, SDH often redistributes over time in infants due to gravity, migrating posteriorly along the falx or even the convexity on subsequent scans, and separates into supernatant and precipitate fractions that have different characteristics seen on MR imaging.[52,94] The difficulties inherent in this analysis are discussed in greater detail in the Timing Injuries Based on Neuroimaging section.

Acute SDH are thought to arise from ruptures or tears of bridging veins that traverse the subarachnoid space from the medial convexity to the superior sagittal sinus and parasagittal dura. Recent studies have identified bridging vein ruptures on MR imaging, appearing as hypointense linear or curvilinear structures having a rounded head near the midline convexity on GRE or SWI sequences; a small perivascular clot at the end of the torn bridging vein has been referred to as the "tadpole"[153] or "lollipop"[152] sign. A more recent study using highly detailed coronal susceptibility weighted MR imaging sequences reported a poor correlation between these signs and bridging vein thrombosis and suggested that these findings may reflect deformation of torn bridging veins rather than intraluminal thrombosis per se.[240]

Chronic SDHs are hypodense to brain on CT and T1-hypointense and T2-FLAIR-hyperintense on MR imaging; they may appear to have CSF density and intensity, although often the CSF within the subjacent subarachnoid space has a different density and intensity, particularly on MR imaging FLAIR sequences (Figure 7.10). Each of the compartments may have a different intensity on MR imaging. Again, chronic subdural membranes may develop within the collection and may be visible, particularly on contrast-enhanced MR imaging scans. Rarely, subdural hygromas—subdural collections of CSF having little or no blood products and mildly increased protein—may be present and are completely or nearly isodense or isointense to CSF on all imaging sequences.[241] Unlike chronic SDH, subdural hygromas do not generally have membranes.[241] The origin of chronic SDH and subdural hygromas is debated. The consensus is that hygromas are the result of arachnoid tears that allow CSF to dissect from the subarachnoid to the subdural space. The traditional understanding, supported by imaging evidence, is that chronic SDH, at least in AHT, can certainly evolve over time from acute SDH[51,52]; however, at least in adults, an alternative mechanism is that chronic SDHs arise from micro-hemorrhages within subdural hygromas.[174–177] Whether this occurs in AHT is more a matter of speculation.[241]

Subarachnoid and Intracerebral Hemorrhages

Subarachnoid hemorrhage occurs in both AHT and unintentional injuries; in the meta-analysis of 8 comparative studies by Kemp and colleagues, subarachnoid hemorrhage was present in 2.8% to 35.5% of AHT cases (average 15.2%) and was not significantly more common in AHT than in non-AHT injuries (OR, 0.98; 95% CI, 0.47–2.0; $P = 0.95$). Similarly, intracerebral hemorrhage or contusion was not present more frequently in AHT than non-AHT injuries (OR, 0.96; 95% CI, 0.6–1.6; $P = 0.86$).[41]

Parenchymal Injuries

One of the hallmarks in many cases of AHT is parenchymal injuries. Impact and inertial injuries may produce different patterns of injury.[220] Isolated impact injuries generally result in focal parenchymal abnormalities such as subpial hemorrhages along the cortical surface; focal micro-hemorrhages within the superficial cortical layers, gray-white junction, subcortical U fibers, or deeper white matter; or localized

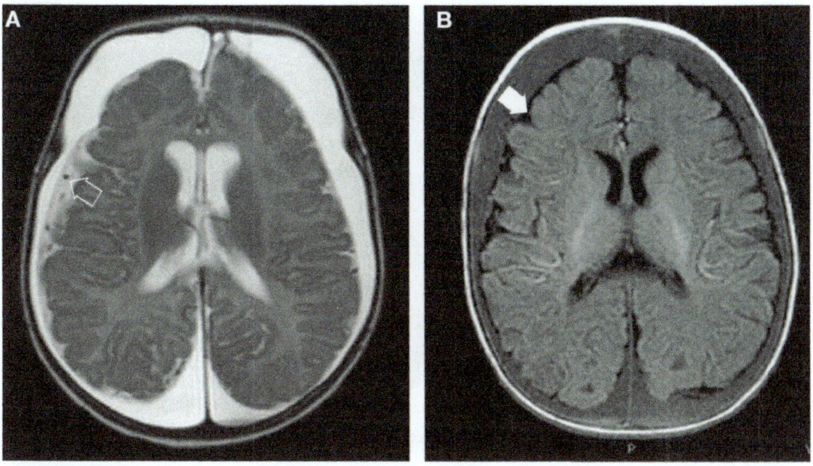

FIGURE 7.10
T2 (A) and fluid attenuated inversion recovery (B) axial magnetic resonance images demonstrate chronic subdural collections in children following abusive head trauma. The subarachnoid space is present beneath the subdural fluid (arrows).

vasogenic edema from contusion injuries (Figure 7.11). Focal lesions often underlie skull fractures and/or scalp injuries, confirming their nature as impact injuries; contrecoup injuries may be present. Gliding cortical contusions along the inferior frontal and anterior temporal lobes may be present from movement of the cortex along the adjacent skull base, although these are less common in infants because the adjacent bone is smoother and less irregular than in adults (Figure 7.12). Cortical tears or lacerations may be visible as slits or clefts within the gyri.[212]

Impulsive brain injuries follow a somewhat different pattern, with more diffuse and widespread injuries that are not limited to impact sites. Deeper parenchymal injuries are often present in areas of axonal abundance, such as the corpus callosum (particularly the splenium), deep cortical white matter (centrum semiovale), and cerebral peduncles; these lesions are often hemorrhagic (Figure 7.13), particularly on GRE or SWI sequences, and their number correlates with poor outcome.[242] There is often a loss of the interface between the gray and white matter from edema[52]; this is significantly associated with AHT (OR, 2.16; 95% CI, 1.04–4.46; $P = 0.04$).[41] The most conspicuous parenchymal injury, however, is evident as CT hypodensity with a corresponding T2/FLAIR hyperintensity, DWI hypo-intensity, and ADC hyperintensity on MR imaging.[50–52,243] (Figure 7.14). In the review by Kemp et al of 3 comparative studies, this finding was present in 19% to 37% (average 24%) and was significantly more common in cases of AHT than in non-AHT cases (OR, 3.7; 95% CI, 1.4–10; $P = 0.01$).[41] The DWI and ADC

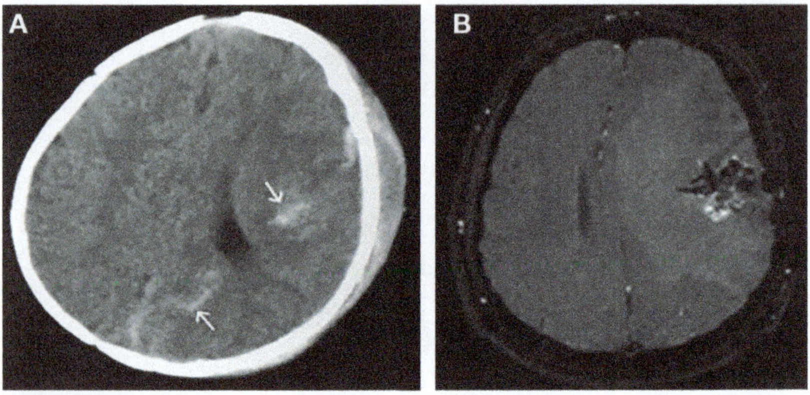

FIGURE 7.11
Axial computed tomography (A) and susceptibility weighted imaging axial magnetic resonance imaging (B) scans demonstrating left parietal cerebral contusions. Computed tomography shows hyperdense intraparenchymal and subarachnoid blood (arrows). Susceptibility weighted imaging shows paramagnetic effects as black signal, representing blood products.

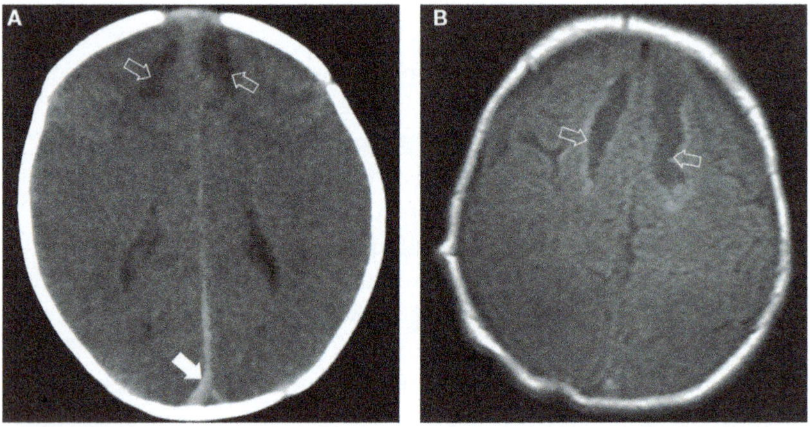

FIGURE 7.12
Axial computed tomography (A) and T1-weighted magnetic resonance imaging (B) studies demonstrating bifrontal cortical lacerations (open arrows). Interhemispheric subdural hemorrhage is also apparent (solid arrow).

abnormalities reflect cytotoxic edema from HIE and correlate closely with outcome.[41,242,244] The changes may follow a watershed distribution where the distal vascular territories (arterial border zones) from the anterior, middle, and posterior cerebral arteries merge and where the tissues are, therefore, particularly vulnerable to global hypoperfusion or hypoxia.[50,245] At the extreme, global hemispheric hypodensities with relative sparing of either the basal ganglia and thalamus and/or cerebellum is known as the "reversal sign"[246] or "big black brain."[247]

Spine Injuries

Spine injuries were previously thought to be rare in AHT. However, more recent neuroradiological and autopsy studies using newer imaging and/or autopsy techniques have much more frequently demonstrated ligamentous, spinal cord, and cervical nerve root and ganglion injuries in AHT.[136,137,215,217,248–251] Cervical spine and spinal cord injuries, in particular, have been observed in 71% of fatal AHT cases at autopsy[136] and 78% of nonfatal cases on MR imaging.[137] Autopsy findings include cervical spinal cord contusions, lacerations, or transections; meningeal hemorrhages; and nerve root avulsions and/or dorsal root ganglion hemorrhages. Neuroimaging studies in nonfatal cases reveal predominantly ligamentous injuries and spinal SDHs; evidence of direct cervical cord or dorsal root injuries is less common. Ligamentous injuries are best demonstrated as hyperintensities on short-tau inversion recovery fat suppression MR imaging sequences (Figure 7.15); the fat suppression allows edema and/or

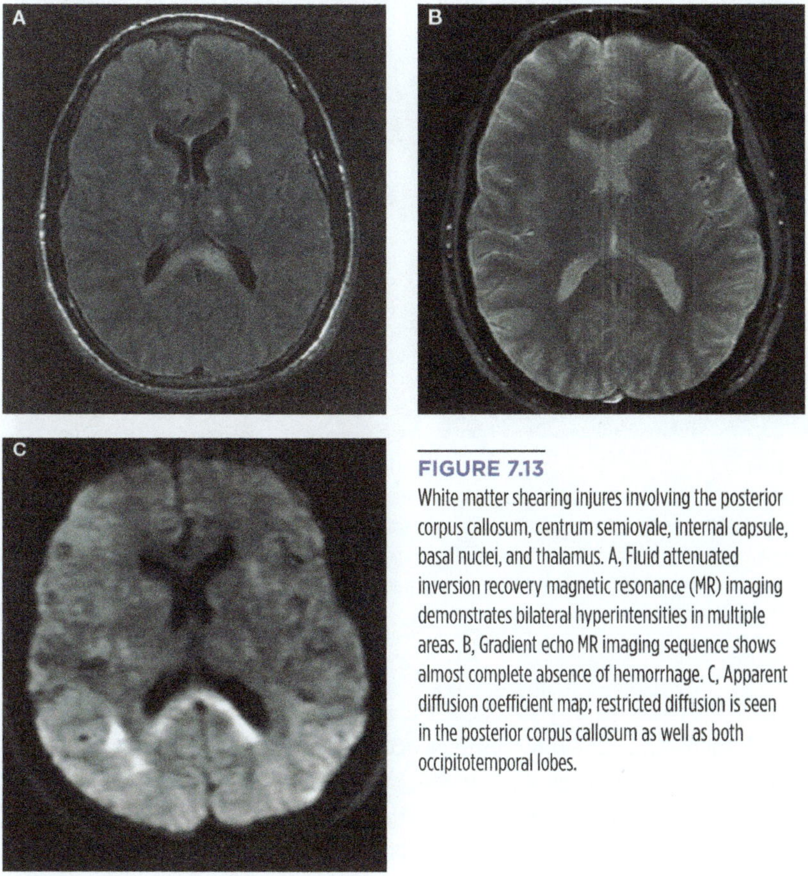

FIGURE 7.13
White matter shearing injures involving the posterior corpus callosum, centrum semiovale, internal capsule, basal nuclei, and thalamus. A, Fluid attenuated inversion recovery magnetic resonance (MR) imaging demonstrates bilateral hyperintensities in multiple areas. B, Gradient echo MR imaging sequence shows almost complete absence of hemorrhage. C, Apparent diffusion coefficient map; restricted diffusion is seen in the posterior corpus callosum as well as both occipitotemporal lobes.

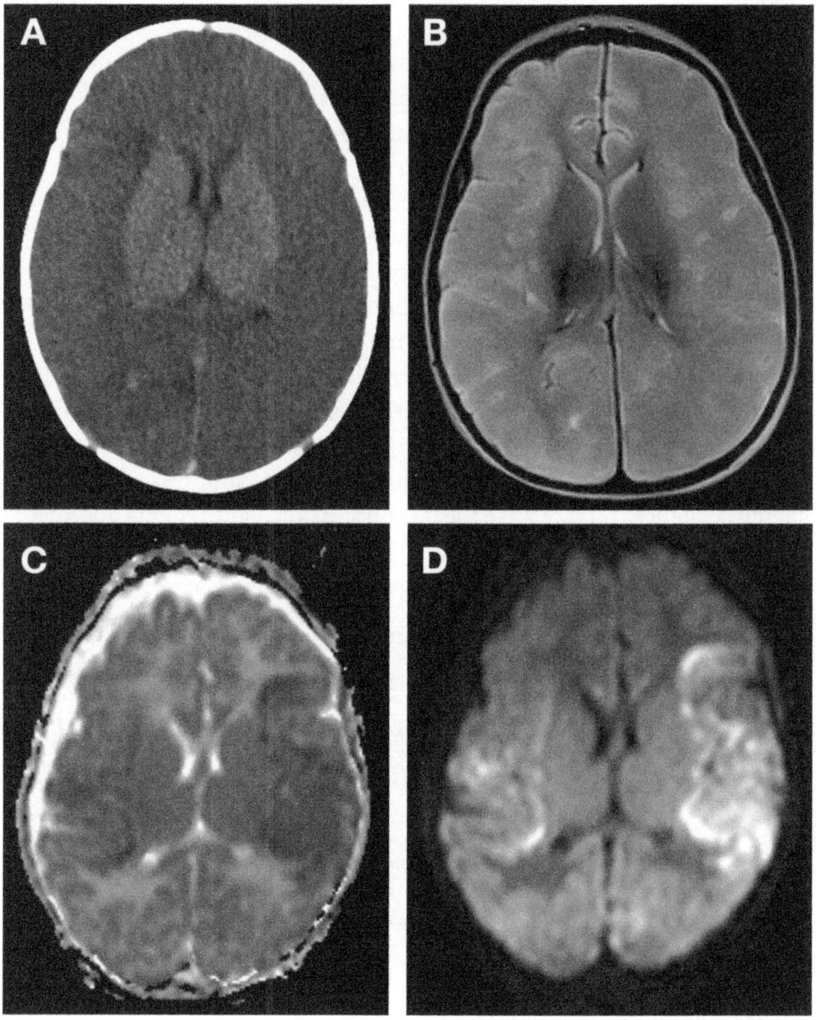

FIGURE 7.14
Parenchymal brain injuries. A, Axial computed tomography scan demonstrates cerebral hypodensity with relative preservation of the basal ganglia, constituting the "reversal sign." B, Corresponding T2-weighted magnetic resonance (MR) imaging sequence demonstrates global cerebral hyperintensity with preservation of deep structures. C–D, Diffusion and apparent diffusion coefficient MR images, from another patient, demonstrate restricted diffusion indicative of cytotoxic edema.

hemorrhage to be better visualized. The nuchal ligament is most commonly injured, followed by the interspinous, occipitoatlantal, and atlantoaxial ligaments. Bone fractures occur in 6% of cases of AHT.[137] Retroclival collections are rare but significant additional findings in children with AHT and reflect injury to the anterior occipital-cervical ligaments, including the tectorial membrane.[252] The preponderance of ligamentous injuries at the occipitocervical junction (occiput to C2) and the rarity of injuries to the subaxial spine (C3–C7) reflect the vulnerability of the upper infant spine and spinal cord to injury.[253] A significant correlation between occipitocervical ligamentous injuries and hypoxic-ischemic brain injuries on MR imaging is consistent with the conclusion that upper cervical spinal cord injury may lead to disordered breathing and HIE.[137]

Spinal SDH is demonstrated by MR imaging in about half of AHT cases.[137,215] Spinal SDHs may be located anywhere along the spinal cord but are more common in the thoracolumbar spine, and as many as half may be missed if the entire spine is not imaged. They are rarely symptomatic, although priapism has been reported.[215] The origin of spinal SDH is unclear; some authors have interpreted spinal SDH to be the consequence of gravity-dependent inferior migration of posterior fossa SDH into the spinal compartment because, as the spinal dura has no corresponding intradural venous plexus, there is usually no evidence of local trauma at the site of the SDH (particularly in thoracolumbar collections), and the attenuation of the cranial and spinal SDH are congruent.[137,215] Interestingly, spinal SDH is significantly less common among cases of unintentional trauma with clinical suspicion of spinal injury[137]; whether, and how, this speaks to the mechanism of injury in AHT remains unclear and is the focus of further study.

Timing Injuries Based on Neuroimaging

It has long been hoped that neuroimaging in general, and MR imaging in particular, could provide a reliable time frame for trauma. Unfortunately, this may be more problematic than previously thought.[51,52,92,236] In particular, the aging of SDH based on neuroimaging is problematic given a lack of information on the evolution of SDH over time, even in infants with unintentional injuries and known injury times; the uncertainty as to the exact injury time in AHT; the extent to which an admixture of clotted and unclotted blood, serum, and CSF may change the imaging characteristics of SDH; variability in the evolution of SDH and significant temporal overlap among various imaging findings and between different individuals; methodological limitations of the available studies—specifically, variability in the timing of follow-up imaging based on clinical reasons; and the influence of subdural rebleeding over time, which may further change the imaging characteristics of SDH. This difficulty has led some to suggest that medical professionals simply describe the attenuation subdural of collections on CT scans or MR imaging and avoid using terms such as *acute* and *chronic*.

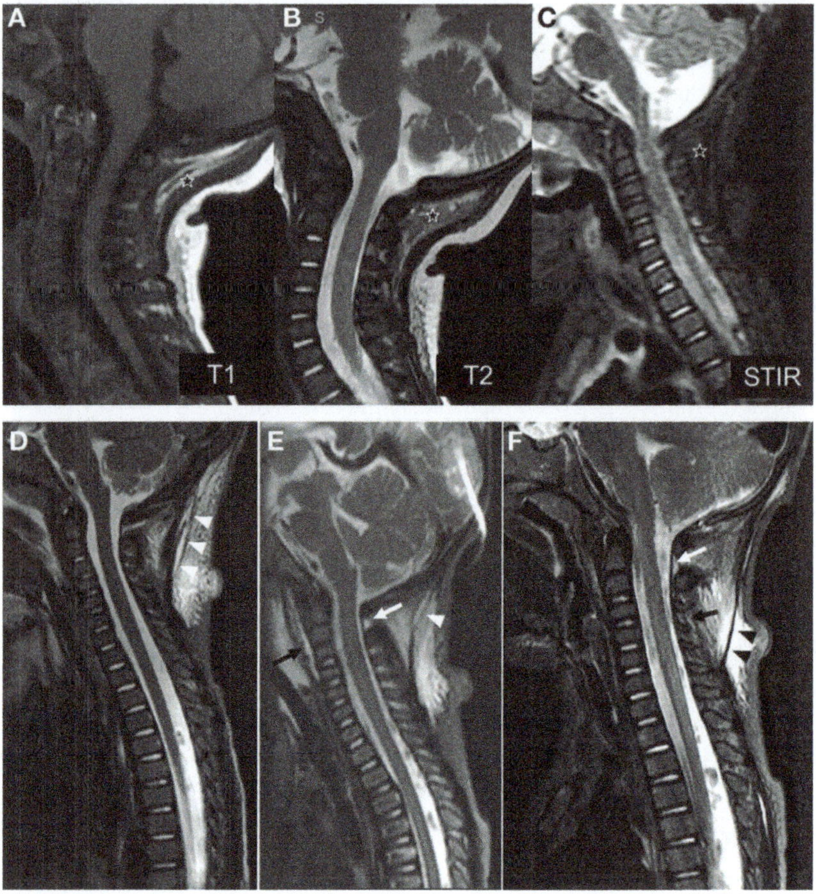

FIGURE 7.15

Appearance of normal upper nuchal ligament and ligamentous injuries on magnetic resonance (MR) images. Upper row demonstrates normal appearance of the nuchal (stars) and other cervical ligaments. A, Sagittal T1 MR image. B, Sagittal T2 MR image. C, Sagittal short-tau inversion recovery sequence.

Lower row (D–F) demonstrates nuchal ligamentous injuries on sagittal short-tau inversion recovery MR imaging sequences in 3 different children with head trauma. D, Child with abusive head trauma and injury to the nuchal ligament. E, Child with abusive head trauma and nuchal ligament injury, including a tear in the outer (lamellar) portion; prevertebral soft tissue swelling and atlantoaxial ligamentous injury are also present. F, Child with accidental head trauma with nuchal ligament injury, including partial disruption of the lamellar portion; atlantoaxial ligament and interspinous ligament injuries are also present.

Images E and F are reproduced from Choudhary AK, Ishak R, Zacharia TT, Dias MS. Imaging of spinal injury in abusive head trauma: a retrospective study. *Pediatr Radiol.* 2014;44(9):1130–1140.

However, certain broad generalizations can be made based on these recent studies. First, acute blood is initially hyperdense to brain on CT scans and becomes progressively less dense over time; uniformly hyperdense SDH generally takes between 3 and 14 days to become hypodense to brain.[51,52,92,94,236] Second, in general, T1 hyperintense and T2 hypointense SDH on MR imaging (the "early subacute phase") appears earlier (1–5 days) than T1 and T2 hyperintensity (the "late subacute phase," 1–30 days), although there is significant overlap.[52] Collections that are uniformly or substantially hypodense on CT scan and T1 hypointense and T2 hyperintense on MR imaging (similar to CSF) reflect chronicity; the consensus is that these appear at least 2 to 4 weeks after injury,[51,52,92,236] especially in an infant who is asymptomatic with progressive head enlargement; has slow, progressive deterioration; and/or shows evidence of prior (healing) extracranial trauma. Subdural membranes may appear on post-contrast MR imaging within an acute SDH in adults[254]; whether this is true in infants has not been rigorously studied.

Mixed density SDHs have long been interpreted as evidence of repeated cranial trauma. Mixed density SDH on initial neuroimaging occurs in up to 53% of children who experience AHT[19,51,52] and is more common after AHT than after non-AHT,[19] and some children with mixed density SDH have evidence of older extra-cerebral trauma such as healing fractures, all of which support this interpretation. However, Vinchon et al have reported infants with mixed density SDH on initial CT scans after known unintentional trauma from motor vehicle crashes, suggesting that mixed density SDH may occur acutely and reflects an admixture of clot, serum, and CSF.[93] In one study, infants undergoing simultaneous burr hole drainage of subacute or chronic SDH and an injection of a radiotracer into the lumbar CSF demonstrated rapid appearance of the tracer in the subdural drain, suggesting free communication between the subdural and subarachnoid CSF spaces.[178] Finally, some SDHs on serial MR imaging are of different intensities in different regions of the collection on the same scan[52,92] and have both supernatant and precipitant layers,[236] suggesting that migration of blood products within the subdural space is common[92,236] and may account for some mixed collections. These studies have cast doubt on the significance of mixed density SDH as a marker of prior injury.

Abusive parenchymal injuries, particularly hypodensities, may be more accurately timed (at least as a minimum time between the injury and imaging). Recent studies have demonstrated the appearance of parenchymal hypodensities (and corresponding DWI and ADC abnormalities on MR imaging) as early as 1 hour (and commonly within several hours) of the reporting of injury.[51,52] Edema (loss of gray-white differentiation on CT scans) may be apparent within 1 hour and is usually apparent (67% of cases) within the first 24 hours following report of injury. Parenchymal hemorrhages also appear most commonly on the first or second scans performed within hours of the injury.[51,52]

It has become increasingly apparent that interpreting the imaging studies in isolation—that is, without clinical correlation—to establish the timing of the injury is problematic. However, when interpreted in light of a detailed clinical timeline, neuroimaging can provide important clues to the time of the injury.

Skeletal Surveys

Children with AHT commonly have extracranial skeletal injuries. A skeletal survey has been recommended by the AAP and ACR for all children younger than 2 years with suspected physical abuse.[95,255] In addition, children aged 2 to 5 years may be candidates for imaging if they cannot report a history, show evidence of disability, or report pain and tenderness. Specific consensus recommendations for skeletal surveys have been developed by the AAP and ACR for children with AHT[256] and include all infants younger than 6 months with intracranial hemorrhage; all infants 6 to 11 months old with intracranial hemorrhage except well-appearing infants with epidural or small extra-axial hemorrhage underlying a skull fracture with a report of a high fall; and children 12 to 24 months old with SDH, other than a small hemorrhage underlying a skull fracture, and external signs of head trauma or clinical signs of brain injury. The AAP and ACR recommend repeating the skeletal survey in 2 weeks for further clinical information and clarification of findings on initial skeletal survey.[95,255]

Laboratory Assessment

A number of laboratory tests should be considered, depending on the circumstances and physical findings, to evaluate the likelihood of abuse and/or exclude other disorders. A complete blood cell count with differential may identify leukemia, signs of systemic infection, and thrombocytopenia or thrombocytosis. Anemia and thrombocytosis have been statistically associated with AHT; one study comparing 429 children with AHT with 700 children with accidental TBI revealed that a hematocrit of less than 30% and platelet count greater than 400,000/µL were significantly more common in AHT (although nearly 20% of children with unintentional brain injuries had anemia and 27% had thrombocytosis).[257] American Academy of Pediatrics–recommended testing for coagulopathy in children with intracranial hemorrhage includes prothrombin time, activated partial thromboplastin time, factor VIII level, factor IX level, and a disseminated intravascular coagulation panel (dimerized plasmin fragment D and fibrinogen).[258] To this panel, many clinicians have added various tests such as factor XI, factor XIII, thrombin time, von Willebrand disease studies, and others depending on the circumstances. In addition to their diagnostic utility, coagulation studies predict poor outcomes in TBI.[259,260]

A metabolic panel may be necessary. Serum sodium levels should be followed serially after TBI and may either decline due to SIADH or cerebral salt wasting or rise due to diabetes insipidus. In particular, the development of secondary hyponatremia may precipitate delayed clinical deterioration. Aspartate aminotransferase, alanine aminotransferase, and possibly lipase or amylase may be elevated with occult intra-abdominal injury.[261–263] While there are no firm recommendations regarding screens for metabolic diseases, birth screening for glutaric aciduria type 1 should be sought and serum amino acids, urine organic acids, and acyl-carnitine panel should be considered for those having no prior newborn screening and clinical concerns. Testing for collagen diseases, osteogenesis imperfecta, or Ehlers-Danlos syndrome vascular type should also be considered under the appropriate clinical circumstances, as described in the following Differential Diagnosis of Abusive Head Trauma section. Whenever an initial laboratory test or clinical probe results in concern, consultation with a specialist in the specific area of interest is highly desirable.

Differential Diagnosis of Abusive Head Trauma

Although clinicians rightly seek to solidify a single explanation for a child's findings, it should be remembered that a concurrent illness or unintentional injury may coexist with, and does not completely exclude, abuse. The differential diagnosis of AHT can be conveniently divided into 3 categories depending on the history provided. In the first instance, in which there is no history of trauma but clear indicia of cranial impact trauma, AHT remains foremost in the differential diagnosis. In the second instance, in which there is no history of trauma with intracranial injuries or RH or clear evidence of cranial impact injury, one should consider other medical conditions that might produce such injuries without trauma. In the third instance, in which a history of trauma is provided to account for the identified injuries, the extent and type of injuries must be considered in the context of the history provided and the infant's developmental milestones. If the history and injuries match, it is plausible to consider an unintentional injury. On the other hand, injuries associated with a higher energy mechanism than described in the history; injuries of multiple natures or ages, such as unexplained bruising or fractures, geographically separate injuries, and both old and new injuries; or a history that is inconsistent with the developmental age of the child all support the diagnosis of abuse. The history provided usually involves some sort of household or unintentional fall; the discussion, therefore, begins with the outcomes of unintentional falls.

Differential diagnoses of AHT are summarized in Box 7.1.

Injuries From Unintentional Short Falls

Multiple studies have documented the outcomes from falls from various heights—short falls from less than 4 to 6 feet, falls from intermediate height (typically between 6 and 15 feet), and falls from significant height (>15 feet). Specific types of falls, such as falls from windows, beds, bunk beds, stairs (with and without walkers), and, most importantly, hospital beds and cribs, have also been studied. A review of multiple studies of unintentional falls from various heights involving 1,902 children found 23 fatal injuries, 18 of which were due to falls from 3 stories or more. The aggregate odds of dying from falls of less than 3 stories is, therefore, 5 out of 1,902, or 0.26%.[264] Common injuries in these studies included skull fractures, EDH, contusions, subarachnoid hemorrhage, and focal (or contact) SDHs.[264] The following discussion highlights a few of the larger studies involving infants and toddlers:

BOX 7.1
Differential Diagnosis of Abusive Head Trauma

Unintentional Trauma

- Short falls
- Stairway falls
- Falls in walkers
- Motor vehicle crash
- Birth trauma

Medical Causes

- Coagulopathy
- Vascular disorders
- Collagen disorders
- Glutaric aciduria type 1
- Menkes disease (kinky hair syndrome)
- Alagille syndrome
- Other rare metabolic causes
- Benign expansion of the subarachnoid fluid space
- Shunted hydrocephalus
- Arachnoid cyst

Among 916 falls in infants younger than 1 year, of whom 25% rolled from a couch or bed, 33% fell from baby equipment or a table, 16% dropped from caregivers' arms, 11% fell from a standing height, and 13% fell from other devices or down stairs, only 12% were admitted to the hospital and there was only 1 death (0.11%). Skull fractures were present in 75.5%, either in isolation (46.2%) or combined with an intracranial injury (29.2%) and most commonly involving one (82.5%) or both (2.5%) parietal bones. Epidural hemorrhage occurred in 2% and SDH in 1.2%.[53]

Among 278 children younger than 2 years, 85% of whom fell from 1 to 30 feet, 6% had a skull fracture and 2% had intracranial injuries, including SDH, EDH, or subarachnoid hemorrhage; cerebral contusions; or cerebral edema. The overall mortality in this series was 0.4%. Young age correlated significantly with the likelihood of skull fracture and intracranial injury.[265]

A prospective study of 154 children younger than 2 years (mean age 10.1 months) who sustained falls from 0.3 to 9.0 m (0.98–29.53 ft) (median 0.9 m [2.95 ft]), 88% of whom fell 1.6 m or less (≤5.25 ft), identified skull fractures in 79% (86% of which were linear). Intracranial injuries were present in 16 children (10.4%) and included 14 with epidural hematomas, 1 with subarachnoid hemorrhage and cerebral contusion, and 1 with cerebral contusion only. All children were evaluated by an ophthalmologist; 3 children had RH, all associated with significant midline shift and large EDH.[266]

Ibrahim and colleagues studied 285 children, including 157 infants younger than 1 year and 128 toddlers 1 to 4 years of age, who fell from varying heights (low: ≤ 0.9 m [3 ft] [n = 98]; intermediate: 1.2–2.7 m [4–9 ft] [n = 96]; high: ≥ 3.0 m [10 ft] [n = 24]; and down stairs [n = 67]) and had neuroimaging. Among low height falls, skull fractures were present in 73% of infants and 23% of toddlers ($P < 0.05$); intracranial injuries (not otherwise specified or stratified by height) were present in 55% of infants and 42% of toddlers (not statistically significant). Despite the higher proportion of intracranial injuries compared with other series, the mean GCS in the low height group was 14.2 among infants and 14.5 among toddlers. Among intermediate fall heights, skull fractures were present in 69% of infants and 49% of toddlers ($P < 0.05$) and primary intracranial injury (not otherwise specified or stratified by height) was present in 49% of infants and 36% of toddlers (not statistically significant). Retinal hemorrhages were present in only 1 child from a short fall (unilateral RH associated with a large EDH) and 2 from intermediate falls (posterior pole RH following a fall of 8–10 ft, unspecified bilateral RH following a lethal fall from 15 ft onto concrete). This study also revealed that 11% of children with falls and skull fracture had no clinically or radiographically visible soft tissue swelling.[125]

Chadwick et al studied mortality from falls in child care centers that employ multiple providers, encourage line-of-sight visibility, and discourage isolation of children with individual caregivers to minimize the risk of unattended injury. In a review of 25 published studies involving more than 6 million children in child care, there were 2 fall-related deaths, a frequency of less than 0.00003%. Moreover, among 2.5 million children younger than 5 years suffering falls of less than 1.4 m (4.7 ft) in the California EpiCenter online injury database, only 6 deaths were identified, a mortality of 0.48 per 1 million children per year.[267]

Finally, a study by Plunkett of more than 75,000 reports to the US Consumer Product Safety Commission of children injured from playground falls identified 18 deaths (5 younger than 2 years). Although most children in this study were older, 6 were younger than 36 months and fell between 0.6 and 1.8 m (2 and 6 ft); one case also had a possible additional crush injury from an adult falling on the child. Although this study has been cited in court to support the possibility of death following "short" falls, the overall mortality (< 0.024%) supports that fatal short falls are extraordinarily rare (the true mortality is likely much lower, as falls without injury would not have been reported). Moreover, one-third of the deaths had large associated extra-axial hematomas requiring surgical evacuation (Figure 7.16) and 3 had other conditions (thrombocytopenia, cerebral AVM, carotid dissection) that contributed to, or accounted for, the deaths.[118]

Witnessed Short Falls

Several studies have specifically analyzed children with witnessed or highly monitored falls from various heights, thereby reducing the possibility of a false fall history and being less likely to reflect a selection bias for unusually injurious falls. Six studies have collectively examined 1,113 children falling while in the hospital. These 6 studies identified a total of 10 children (7 of whom were newborns) with skull fractures, 1 newborn with a cerebral contusion, and 1 newborn with SDH (as discussed in the Birth Trauma section, SDH is identified relatively commonly after typical delivery, so its presence could be incidental to the fall). There were no clinically recognized brain injuries or deaths.[112,268–271] Unfortunately, in none of these studies was intracranial imaging (CT or MR imaging) universally performed, so asymptomatic intracranial pathology may have been missed. Nonetheless, these studies overwhelmingly confirm the clinical benignity of short falls in children.

In another study of 106 children younger than 3 years who sustained witnessed falls, none lost consciousness, 3 (2.8%) suffered skull fractures,

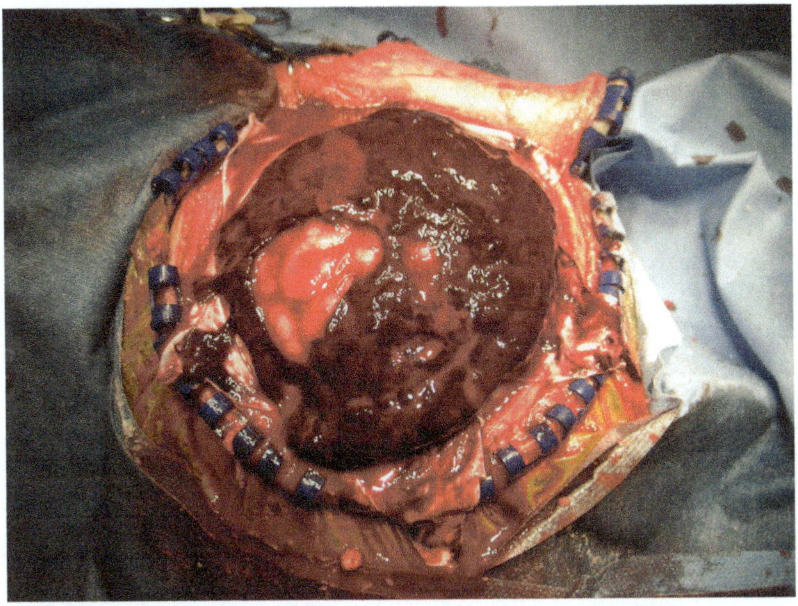

FIGURE 7.16
Intraoperative image of a large space-occupying subdural hemorrhage. Subarachnoid hemorrhage is also visible overlying the exposed cortical gyri.

and none died. In contrast, 34% of children with unwitnessed falls of less than 1.5 m (5 ft) suffered severe (but not otherwise specified) intracranial injuries with a mortality of 3.8%. The authors of this study concluded that some of the short-fall stories in the unwitnessed group were likely missed AHT.[272]

Finally, a review of 829 children (77% < 5 years) reported to the National Pediatric Trauma Registry who fell from windows (96% from ≥ 2 stories) demonstrated a mortality of 1.7%.[273] This stands in stark contrast to the reported 13% to 33% mortality from AHT.[51,233,234]

Special Circumstances: Stairway Falls and Walker-Related Injuries

Stairway falls and walker injuries deserve special mention because they are biomechanically complex and have the potential for significant rotational acceleration. The head is particularly vulnerable to injury in stairway falls. In a review of more than 90,000 stairway injuries among children younger than 5 years, 94% of which occur in the home, head injuries were identified in 32% of infants younger than 12 months, 24% of 1-year-olds, and 17% of 2-year-olds. However, overall, only 5% required hospitalization. Infants were more likely to be injured in a walker or while being carried.[274] Three additional studies, involving a total of 671 children who sustained stairway injuries, identified 6 skull fractures, 2 cerebral contusions, and 1 SDH.[116,275,276] More frequent and severe injuries occurred after falling down stairs in the arms of an adult.[276]

In contrast to these results, another study of 67 infant- and toddler-related stairway falls identified skull fractures in 73% and 23% of infants and toddlers, respectively ($P < 0.05$), and primary brain injury in 60% and 30% of infants and toddlers, respectively ($P < 0.05$).[125] Finally, a single case report described a 7-month-old who fell down a flight of stairs and sustained a large convexity and tentorial SDH, with numerous multilayered RHs and optic nerve sheath hemorrhages. An elevated prothrombin time (17.6 s) and partial thromboplastin time (>200 s) may have accentuated the hemorrhages.[277]

Walkers are likely to cause more frequent and severe injuries compared with simple stairway falls; one study demonstrated a 4-fold increase in overall injuries and a 2-fold increase in fractures among walker-related stairway falls compared with stairway falls without walkers.[278] In another study of 65 infants and children aged 3 to 17 months sustaining walker-related injuries, of whom 46 (71%) sustained walker-associated falls down stairs, skull fractures occurred in 10 (15%), concussions in 8 (12%), and intracranial hemorrhage in 5 (8%); 1 infant died with SDH, skull fracture, and spinal cord injury.[279]

Rare Serious Outcomes Following Short Falls

There are rare instances wherein children died or sustained severe head injuries from short falls.[113,280,281] The largest series of fatal fall injuries included 44 children (mean age 2.4 y, 64% < 3 y), 18 of whom fell less than 0.9 m (3 ft); 14 of the 18 (76%) had large mass lesions that contributed to, or caused, their deaths. The intracranial findings and fall heights for the remaining 4 children were not further described.[113] A second series of "incontrovertible" unintentional fatal injuries included a short fall from a barstool in a child who also had a 1-cm-thick SDH that required surgical evacuation, with diffuse bilateral cerebral hypodensities and no RH.[280] Backward falls with occipital impacts may also engender more severe injuries, possibly because of the inability of the child to cushion the fall with outstretched arms. Among 8 children younger than 24 months with occipital impacts from witnessed falls, none had skull fractures, but all had SDH, 2 with significant mass effect. Two children had additional brain infarction, and 7 had RH. Six children returned to baseline within 24 hours, but 2 children were comatose, 1 required surgical evacuation of a large SDH, and 1 died. The authors were aware of 14 similar cases.[282]

From the available data, one can reach a number of reasonable conclusions. First, accidental falls are almost always benign occurrences, although skull fractures can be expected in perhaps as many as 73% and are more common among infants than in toddlers.[125] Most skull fractures are linear and parietal. Second, serious intracranial injury and prolonged neurological dysfunction are uncommon. Intracranial hemorrhage is more common after intermediate level (1.8–4.6 m [6–15 ft]) than short (<1.2–1.8 m [4–6 ft]) falls in most studies. Epidural hemorrhage is more common following unintentional injuries and is usually small, underlying a fracture and, therefore, likely venous in origin. When present, SDH is usually focal rather than diffuse or interhemispheric. Less commonly, large mass effect EDH or SDH, subarachnoid hemorrhage, or intraparenchymal contusions can occur. How commonly asymptomatic intracranial pathology can appear after short falls is unknown because neuroimaging in many studies is not universally performed. Third, mortality from short falls is low, estimated at 1 fatality per 2 million children younger than 5 years per year.

Fourth, and perhaps most importantly, the pathology and mode of injury or death following short falls is usually fundamentally different from that following higher energy head injuries or AHT. Many deaths from short falls are caused by large mass effect extra-axial hematomas,[113] vascular dissection and stroke, severe hyponatremia, or other readily explainable reasons, and lack other indicia of abuse, such as extensive multilayered RHs or retinoschisis, long bone or multiple rib fractures, and/or unexplained bruising. On the other hand, small EDH, thin diffuse SDH, subarachnoid hemorrhage, or limited and focal cerebral contusions do not, in and of themselves, cause severe neurological deterioration or death. Diffuse cerebral edema and widespread ischemic/anoxic injuries, so common in children with AHT, are incredibly rare after short falls.

Birth Trauma

A careful review of the pregnancy and birth history should be obtained when evaluating children with AHT. Cranial trauma is sometimes evident at birth. Visible injuries may include scalp lacerations, caput succedaneum, cephalohematoma or subgaleal hematomata, and depressed skull fractures; intracranial injuries may include all manner of intracranial hemorrhages and parenchymal brain injury.[131,132] In one large study by Towner and colleagues, cranial injuries were more frequent among infants who underwent assisted (vacuum or forceps) deliveries compared with spontaneous vaginal deliveries; the incidence among those undergoing cesarean deliveries before the onset of labor was lower than those delivered by cesarean delivery after the onset of labor.[131]

Peri-tentorial SDHs are the most common intracranial injury and likely reflect traction forces that deform the head with bleeding from the deep venous system.[283] Subdural hemorrhages accounts for 4% to 73% of symptomatic neonatal intracranial hemorrhage.[132,284,285] Cephalopelvic disproportion, preterm birth, maternal primiparity and grand multiparity, and both precipitous and prolonged, difficult labors have all been implicated.[286] Occipital osteodiastasis is a particularly severe birth injury characterized by separation of the occipital squama from the lateral or condylar parts of the occipital bone, leading to upward displacement of the occipital bone into the posterior fossa with dural, tentorial, or venous sinus tears and resultant posterior fossa hemorrhage and injury. Osteodiastasis is most often associated with a breech presentation and significant neck hyperextension.[286–289]

Of greater concern for the evaluation of AHT are birth-related cranial injuries that are asymptomatic and, therefore, occult. Several studies have confirmed that SDH may be present in 8% to 50% of asymptomatic newborns.[128–130,290,291] Subdural hemorrhages are more frequently in the posterior interhemispheric fissure, tentorium, or occipital convexity, with or without associated posterior fossa hemorrhage; isolated posterior fossa SDH is uncommon.[128,130] Complete resolution occurs in 94% to 100% of those imaged within 4 weeks,[128,130] and there is no published peer-reviewed case of acute deterioration or death in a child following an initially occult birth-related SDH. Similarly, birth-related RHs are present in 13% to 40% of asymptomatic newborns but resolve within 4 to 6 postnatal weeks.[60,292–295] It can therefore be concluded from these studies that birth trauma is not responsible for acute neurological deterioration or death that occurs later in childhood.

Coagulopathy

Coagulopathy is an important differential diagnostic concern, the evaluation of which is complicated by the fact that disseminated intravascular coagulopathy may occur following parenchymal brain injury.[296–298] A number of conditions may be considered. Hemorrhagic disease of the newborn from vitamin K deficiency, particularly its late form occurring several weeks postnatal,[299–301] may occur when parents refuse vitamin K at the time of birth.[302,303] Inherited coagulopathies may also manifest with intracranial hemorrhage, although this is rarely confused with abuse; among 189 children with inherited coagulopathies in one study, 15.3% presented in a manner concerning for child abuse, although only 2 of these (1.1% of the entire cohort) had intracranial bleeding, both having von Willebrand disease and one with concerns for coexistent abuse.[304] Intracranial hemorrhages have been described in various factor deficiencies (II, V, VII,

X, XI, and XIII[305,306]), von Willebrand disease,[307] hypoprothrobinemia[307] and afibrinogenemia,[308] and congenital platelet dysfunction.[307]

Acquired coagulopathy and thrombocytopenia may also result in intracranial hemorrhage. Intracranial bleeding from immune thrombocytopenic purpura (ITP) is well known, occurring in 0.4% of children. Intracranial bleeding is more frequent with chronic ITP[309]; severe bleeding is more frequent with platelet counts ofless than 30,000/µL (30 x 10^9/L). Intracranial hemorrhage may also be provoked when children with ITP experience head trauma, although the threshold platelet counts to produce intracranial hemorrhage appear to be similar for spontaneous and posttraumatic hemorrhages.[310] Recognized trauma does not appear to affect the anticipated number of platelets associated with severe hemorrhage. Intracerebral and subarachnoid hemorrhage are more common with ITP, although both acute and chronic SDHs have, on rare occasions, been reported.

Children who are severely ill with sepsis, leukemia, or an acquired coagulopathy may have RHs. These are typically less severe than those in AHT, but severe RHs, and even retinal folds and retinoschisis, have been reported.[311,312] While not strictly a coagulopathy, leukemia is commonly discussed in this light; both coagulopathy and thrombophilia have been reported with leukemia, and subdural collections, other intracranial bleeding, cerebrovascular lesions, and venous sinus thrombosis have all been reported.[313,314]

Vascular Disorders

Vascular and meningeal abnormalities may lead to subarachnoid and/or intracerebral hemorrhage and parenchymal brain injury; however, SDH is rarely seen. In one study of 85 children with nontraumatic intracranial hemorrhage, AVMs and aneurysms (see Figure 7.9) accounted for 28% and led to subarachnoid and intracerebral hemorrhage but not SDH.[315]

Collagen Disorders

The collagen disorders Ehlers-Danlos syndrome and osteogenesis imperfecta may rarely lead to intracranial hemorrhage and be confused with AHT. Vascular type Ehlers-Danlos syndrome (formerly type IV) is caused by a heterozygous mutation in the *COL3A1* gene (Figure 7.17). Subdural hemorrhage, stroke, and intracranial aneurysmal rupture have been reported in adolescence and early adulthood.[316,317] Osteogenesis imperfecta has numerous subtypes but is most commonly caused by autosomal dominant mutations in the *COL1A1* or *COL1A2* gene. Retinal hemorrhages following minor trauma, acute and chronic SDH, and epidural hematomas have all been reported with osteogenesis imperfecta.[318–320]

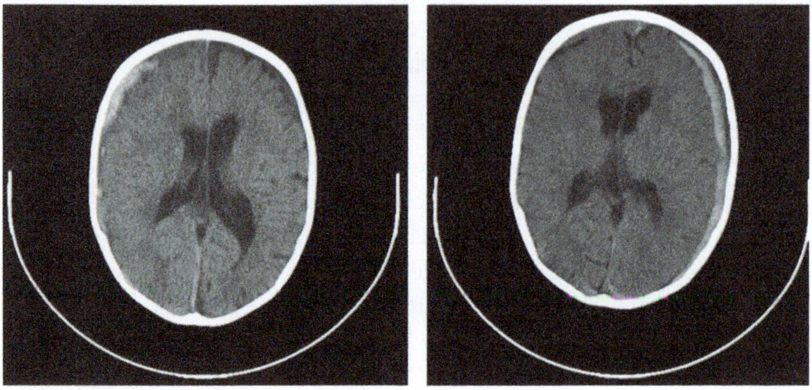

FIGURE 7.17
Axial computed tomography scan demonstrating mixed density convexity and posterior interhemispheric bilateral subdural hemorrhage and mild ventricular enlargement in a child with vascular type Ehlers-Danlos syndrome.

Metabolic Disorders

Glutaricaciduria

Glutaricaciduria is the result of mutations in the glutaryl-CoA dehydrogenase gene, which is involved in the metabolism of the amino acids lysine, hydroxylysine, and tryptophan. In newborns, the most common feature is isolated macrocephaly, present in 70%.[321] Over 2 to 18 months, children develop acute neurological crises, often precipitated by an infection, with profound hypotonia, rigidity or dystonia, behavioral arrest, diminished consciousness, and/or seizures. The neuroimaging hallmark includes acute necrosis involving the basal ganglia (initially in the putamen and advancing later to the caudate head and globus pallidus). Other radiological features include edema, enlarged extra-axial CSF spaces, widened sylvian fissures, and bilateral middle fossa arachnoid cysts (Figure 7.18). These crises are repeated if the diagnosis is not made and treatment begun. Progressive dystonia with periventricular gliosis, atrophy, and ex vacuo ventricular enlargement may ensue in chronic cases. In one study, 13% of patients developed acute SDH after minor head trauma, with RH and papilledema in 2.[321] The condition is readily detected on routine postnatal metabolic screening examinations. If this screen has not been performed or there is ongoing clinical suspicion, urinary organic acids can be obtained and will demonstrate increased levels of glutaric acid, 3-hydroxyglutaric acid, and glutaconic acid. Plasma carnitine and glutarylcarnitine are also elevated in glutaricaciduria.

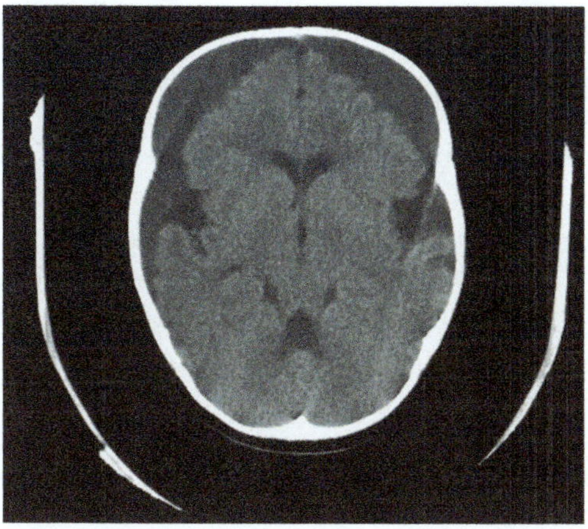

FIGURE 7.18

Axial computed tomography scan in a child with glutaricaciduria type I. Note the pointed frontal lobes and widened sylvian fissures, characteristic of front-temporal atrophy in this condition.

Menkes Disease (Kinky Hair Syndrome)

Menkes disease (kinky hair syndrome) is an X-linked disorder involving mutations of the *ATP7* gene, which is involved in maintenance of serum copper levels. Menkes disease occurs in 1 in 100,000 to 1 in 250,000 infants.[322] One-third of the occurrences are caused by new mutations. The disease results in maldistribution of copper in various organs; the kidney and small intestine have greater amounts, while brain and other tissues become depleted. The reduction in copper interferes with copper-mediated enzymes necessary for proper growth and functioning of bone, skin, hair, blood vessels, and the central nervous system. A less severe form, called occipital horn syndrome, appears later in life.

Symptoms of Menkes disease appear during infancy with mild developmental delays for the initial 2 to 3 months, followed by subsequent progressive and severe regression of milestones with severe and universal hypotonia, hypothermia or temperature dysregulation, growth failure, and seizures. The hair is characteristically kinky, colorless or steel-colored, brittle, and easily broken; it is often less abundant and even shorter on the sides and the back of the head than on the top. Microscopic examination reveals characteristic flattened shaft with narrowing and twists at irregular intervals (called *pili torti*). There is a characteristic facies with "sagging jowls," chubby cheeks, and large ears; delayed dental eruption is common. Bone involvement may result in osteopenia, bone fractures, and metaphyseal widening. Involvement of the intracranial arteries can result in intracranial bleeding, including SDH; the combination of SDH and multiple bone fractures raises concern for abuse. Other neuroimaging findings include white matter dysmyelination, atrophy, widened extra-axial CSF spaces, and ex vacuo ventricular enlargement. Patients rarely live beyond 3 years of age. Pathological examination of the brain reveals extensive degeneration and atrophy. Clinical and pathological features such as fractures, spurring of long bone metaphyses, brain atrophy, and SDH may raise concerns for abuse. The diagnosis is confirmed by documenting diminished serum copper and ceruloplasmin levels.[323–326]

Alagille Syndrome

Alagille syndrome typically presents with jaundice and liver damage in the neonatal period. Children develop cardiopulmonary vascular issues and have a characteristic facial appearance with a broad prominent forehead, deep-set eyes, and a small pointed chin. Liver abnormalities may uncommonly be absent. The combination of a bleeding tendency and the development of intracranial vascular abnormalities may result in intracranial bleeding, typically subarachnoid.[327,328]

Other Rare Conditions

Cases of SDH, RH, or both may occur in association with other rare congenital disorders, including congenital disorders of glycosylation, combined methylmalonic acidosis with homocystinuria, and malignant atrophic papulosis (Degos disease).[329–331] The acquired condition hemophagocytic lymphohistiocytosis has also been reported to present in a manner similar to AHT.[332] The rarity of these cases makes it difficult to rule out coexistent AHT when evaluating these reports.

Disorders of Cerebrospinal Fluid Circulation

Children with disordered CSF flow such as hydrocephalus, benign extra-axial collections of infancy, or arachnoid cysts may, as a consequence, be at increased risk for SDH with minimal or even absent identifiable trauma.

Benign Expansion of the Subarachnoid Spaces

Benign expansion of the subarachnoid spaces (also called benign expansion of the extra-axial spaces, benign extra-axial collections of infancy, and benign external hydrocephalus) involves the accumulation of CSF within the cortical subarachnoid space such that the subarachnoid space measures greater than 4 mm.[333] Head growth typically accelerates smoothly during the first 15 to 18 postnatal months, on average crossing the 95th percentile at about 3 to 4 months of age and continuing to rise slowly, tapering off, and paralleling or decelerating toward the normal curve thereafter.[334] The anterior fontanelle is commonly flat or sunken (although it may be large), the cranial sutures are apposed, and the infant is asymptomatic with no symptoms or signs of elevated ICP and normal developmental milestones (gross motor skills may be slightly delayed during the first postnatal year due to the macrocephaly that is thought to hinder the infant's head control and ability to roll and crawl).

It is important to differentiate BESS, in which the fluid is subarachnoid, from chronic subdural hematomas or hygromas, which are subdural; this distinction is best made on neuroimaging studies. On CT scans and MR imaging, the subarachnoid spaces have attenuation values identical to CSF, are usually symmetrical, overlie the frontal lobes, and do not cause gyral flattening or displacement of the brain. The sulci are widened as would be expected with increased extra-axial CSF; in fact, a mistaken diagnosis of "cerebral atrophy" is sometimes made. If the infant were to be imaged prone, the collections would shift toward the occipital lobes. Most importantly, blood vessels can be visualized crossing the subarachnoid space between the cortical surface and the dura, best appreciated on contrasted CT scans and T2 weighted MR images. Magnetic resonance imaging, in particular, demonstrates the vessels quite readily as flow voids (Figure 7.19). The brain parenchyma is otherwise normal.

In contrast, children with chronic subdural collections usually have symptoms and/or signs of elevated ICP. In contrast to the smooth acceleration seen in BESS, children with chronic subdural collections often have an inflection point that may reflect the time of the abuse. Chronic subdural collections often have slightly different attenuations compared with CSF on CT scans and, particularly, on 1 or more MR imaging sequences. Finally, because both the arachnoid and cortical vessels in the subarachnoid space are displaced toward the cortical surface by an overlying chronic subdural collection, there are no visible blood vessels crossing the collection until the collection reaches the parasagittal dura where the vessels, as they approach the superior sagittal sinus and parasagittal dura, abruptly lift off the cortical surface to enter the sinus and parasagittal dura. Magnetic resonance imaging and post-contrast CT scans may also identify chronic subdural membranes along the inner surface of the collection. Additional signs of prior traumatic cranial injury on MR imaging, such as encephalomalacia or global cerebral atrophy, thinning of the corpus callosum, blood products on GRE or SWI sequences, and T2/FLAIR changes in the cerebral hemispheric white matter, may also be present.

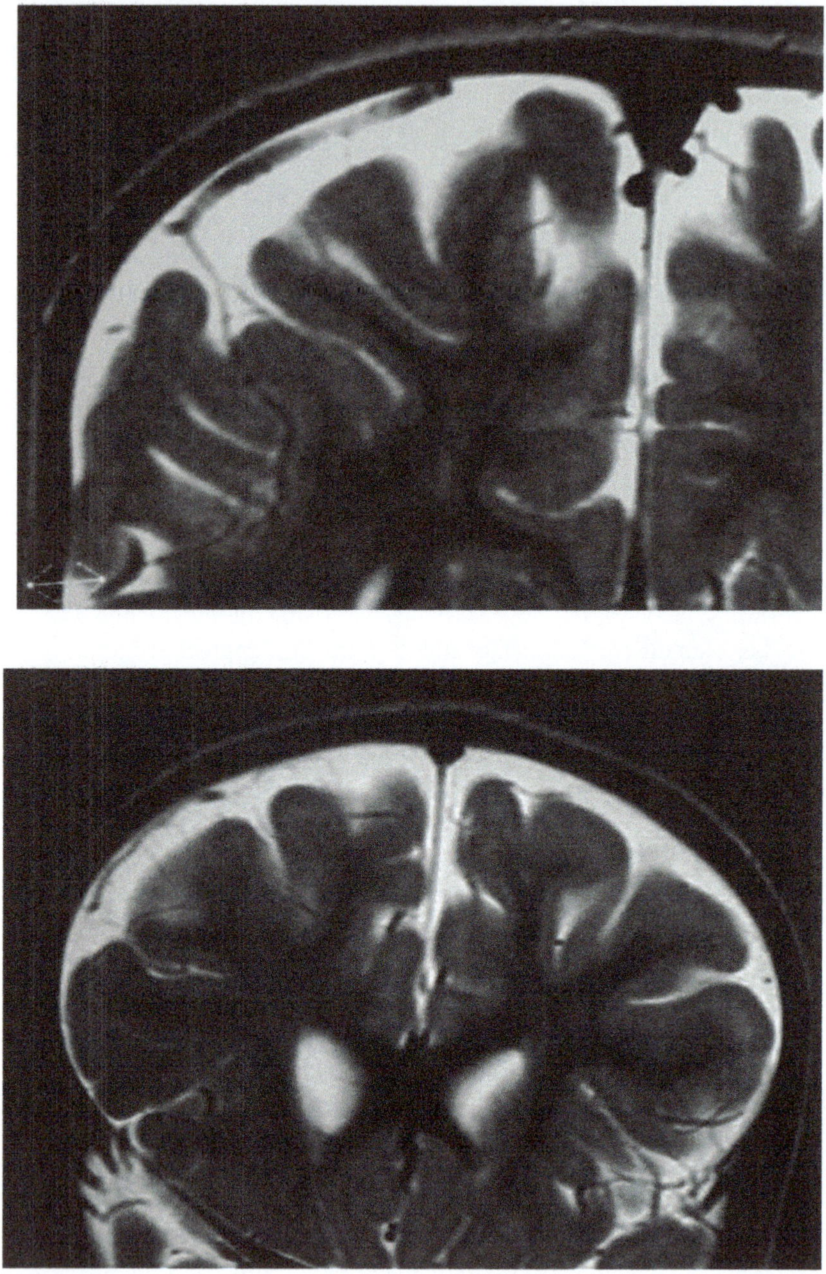

FIGURE 7.19

Coronal T2-weighted magnetic resonance (MR) imaging scans in 2 children with benign extra-axial collections of infancy. Blood vessels cross the subarachnoid cerebrospinal fluid space, which is isointense to cerebrospinal fluid on all MR imaging sequences (not shown). There is no distortion or flattening of the gyri. Rather, the gyri are widened.

Another particularly vexing scenario is the coexistence of a subdural collection in an infant with BESS (Figure 7.20). Formerly described only in isolated case reports and small series of infants,[335–337] subdural collections have been demonstrated in more recent studies in approximately 2% of infants with BESS and no prior history of trauma,[338,339] suggesting that infants with BESS are at greater risk for isolated SDH. Neuroimaging shows a mixed attenuation extra-axial fluid collection having an outer convexity subdural collection that overlies a deeper, subarachnoid CSF collection. Mixed density subdural collections, and even bilateral collections having different densities, may be present. These infants virtually always present with asymptomatic macrocephaly. The increased susceptibility to SDH among children with BESS has been attributed to

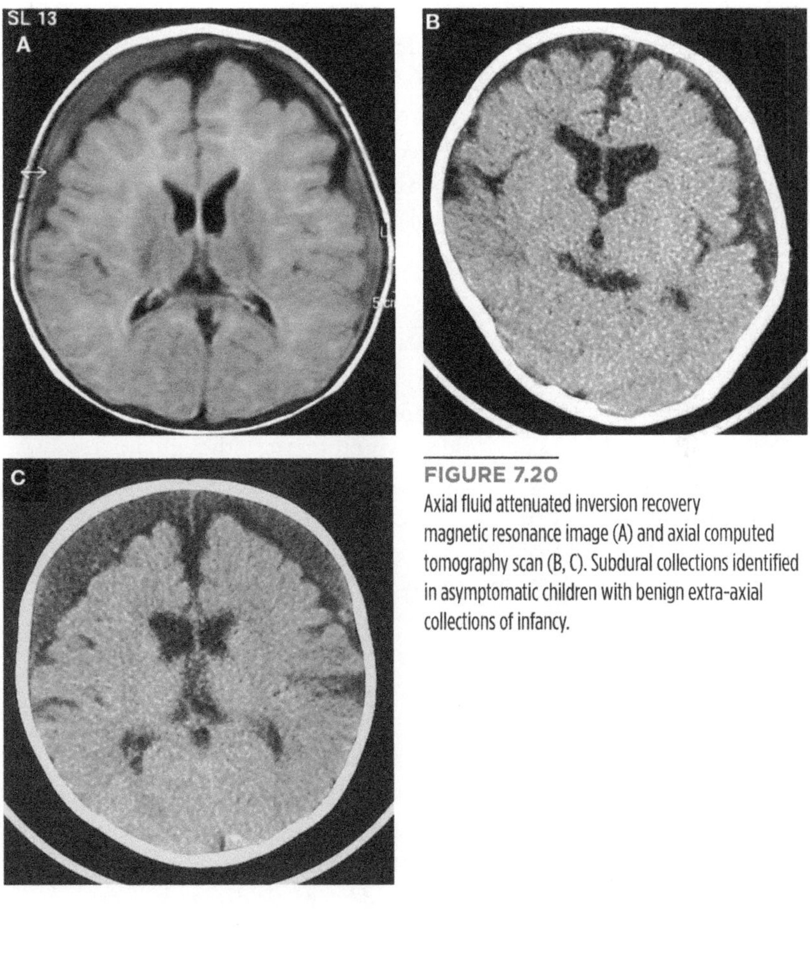

FIGURE 7.20
Axial fluid attenuated inversion recovery magnetic resonance image (A) and axial computed tomography scan (B, C). Subdural collections identified in asymptomatic children with benign extra-axial collections of infancy.

longitudinal tension on bridging veins during relatively greater movement between the brain and dura,[340] particularly in association with rotational movements. This is an attractive hypothesis because other conditions that increase extra-axial CSF spaces, such as arachnoid cysts, hydrocephalus, and brain atrophy; metabolic disorders such as glutaric aciduria; and old age are also associated with an increased risk for SDH.

Shunted Hydrocephalus

Patients with shunted hydrocephalus may, on occasion, experience subdural bleeding, spontaneously or as a consequence of over-shunting or relatively minor trauma.[341,342] Most commonly, over-shunting results in ventricular and cortical mantle collapse, generating extra-axial subdural collections that are hypodense to brain and consist mostly of displaced CSF and small amounts of hemorrhage; these chronic subdural collections may calcify over time.[341] In most cases, these collections are asymptomatic and are noted on routine follow-up images. Of a study of 336 children with shunted hydrocephalus followed for a mean of 4 years, 17 (5%) developed subdural fluid collections, of whom only 5 (1.5% of the entire cohort) were "severely symptomatic" from acute subdural bleeding. Intracerebral bleeding remote from the shunt catheter tract may also occur, particularly among neonates with severe hydrocephalus and a rapid decrease in ventricular size.[343]

Arachnoid Cysts

Arachnoid cysts arise because of a focal embryonic splitting of the meninges into 2 layers with an intervening CSF collection. They most frequently arise in the middle fossa anterior to the temporal lobe. Most children with middle fossa cysts are asymptomatic, although progressive or chronic headaches or seizures may occur.

Displaced and stretched temporal veins along the outer wall of the arachnoid cyst are a source of spontaneous or posttraumatic bleeding. Acute and chronic SDH,[344,345] as well as intracystic hemorrhage with or without accompanying subdural collections,[346–348] have been reported as complications. Subdural fluid collections overlie the arachnoid cyst; virtually all are ipsilateral to the cyst, although bilateral collections have been reported.[348,349] In a study of 41 children younger than 16 years (mean age 10 years, youngest 2 years) with arachnoid cysts and associated bleeding, 37 (90%) had middle fossa cysts; a history of minor head trauma was described in 24 (59%) and ranged from 2 days to 16 weeks (mean 40 days) before presentation. All had SDH, and 28 had additional intracystic hemorrhage. Surgery included burr hole drainage of the subdural collections (suggesting a chronicity to them), and the outcome was almost universally good. There were no cases of coma or death.[344]

Management of Abusive Head Trauma

In most ways, the management of AHT mirrors the management of TBI in general. After initial resuscitation in the emergency department, the child who is acutely ill and has a GCS less than 8 and/or significant intracranial pathology is generally admitted to the pediatric intensive care unit; intubation is commonly performed to protect the airway and manage disordered breathing. A cervical collar is applied until the cervical spine is cleared; plain radiography or CT scan of the cervical spine is done. Given the recent discovery of ligamentous cervical spine injuries in a high proportion of these infants,[137,249] a cervical spine MR imaging examination should be considered (although it appears that most of the injuries are stable and do not require surgical treatment). Early correction of coagulopathy is important to prevent progression of intracranial hemorrhage; fresh frozen plasma and platelet transfusions have been the mainstay of resuscitation, although their effect on outcomes have been inconsistent.[350] More recently, multifactor solutions such as factor IX complex (also known as prothrombin complex concentrate) have been increasingly used in high-risk patients and may hold some promise in restricting ongoing bleeding and reducing time to operative intervention.[351,352] Prophylactic anticonvulsants should be strongly considered for at least the first week following TBI.[240] A number of studies have demonstrated a significantly increased incidence of seizures during the first 72 hours among children with AHT compared with other types of TBI[353,354]; continuous electroencephalographic monitoring should be considered because of the high incidence of subclinical seizures and even status epilepticus.[354]

Management of increased ICP is a mainstay of treatment and is based on the Monro-Kellie doctrine, wherein the cranial compartment is considered to be of fixed volume containing brain, blood, and CSF, an increase in any of which, without a compensatory reduction in another component, will result in elevated ICP. Intracranial pressure monitoring should be considered for those patients with a GCS less than 8 and can be accomplished by inserting an intraparenchymal fiberoptic monitor or an external ventricular drain.

Guidelines for the management of pediatric TBI have been published[355]; the interested reader is referred to this resource for more detailed information. General measures to control ICP include sedation (with or without pharmacological paralysis), maintaining euvolemia and avoiding hypotension to maintain cerebral perfusion pressure, elevating the head of the bed to encourage venous drainage from the brain, avoiding prolonged hyperventilation and hypocapnia in the absence of clinical evidence of transtentorial herniation (fixed dilated pupil and/or contralateral hemiplegia), and avoiding jugular vein neck compression by an overly tight cervical collar.

Specific treatments to control ICP are generally introduced when the ICP is sustained above 15 to 20 mm Hg for longer than 5 minutes (even lower thresholds may be considered for infants). Primary treatments include CSF drainage from an external ventricular drain and/or administering either hypertonic (3%) saline or an osmotic diuretic such as mannitol. Prolonged hyperventilation should be avoided.[355] Second-tier therapies should be considered for persistently elevated ICP despite primary treatments and may include decompressive hemicraniectomy, pentobarbital coma, or continuous lumbar drainage.

Additional surgical considerations include elevation of depressed skull fractures that are open, cosmetically apparent, or depressed greater than the thickness of the skull, and evacuation of extra-axial or intracerebral hematomas. Surgical evacuation of SDH is not commonly required in AHT, as these SDHs are usually thin (< 5–6 mm) and not contributing to the infant's clinical condition. Brain shift greater than the thickness of the SDH suggests underlying brain injury and/or swelling. Larger SDHs are evacuated to remove a potential source of ICP elevations and eliminate focal brain compression. Chronic SDH with significant mass effect can be drained by serial fontanelle taps or placement of subdural drain(s). The fluid may be cherry red or deep violet, crankcase oil, tea colored, or xanthochromic; no studies have systematically evaluated the appearance of the fluid as a function of time from the injury. Serial taps or external drains are associated with a 50% to 82% ultimate failure rate,[356] and a subdural shunt is often needed for longer term management.[356]

Prognosis and Outcome

Many studies have reported that children with AHT have worse outcomes than matched children with non-AHT injuries (Figure 7.21). Overall mortality from AHT ranges from 7.7% to 37.5% with a mean of 19%.[8,357–361] Significant neurological impairments are evident in at least 50% of survivors. In one study, 5% were vegetative, 34% were severely disabled, 25% were moderately disabled, and only 13% had a good outcome. Specific disabilities included hemiparesis (19%), quadriparesis (35%), cranial nerve impairment (20%), early posttraumatic seizure (32%–79%), epilepsy (30%), blindness (15%) and visual impairment (30%), microcephaly (50%),

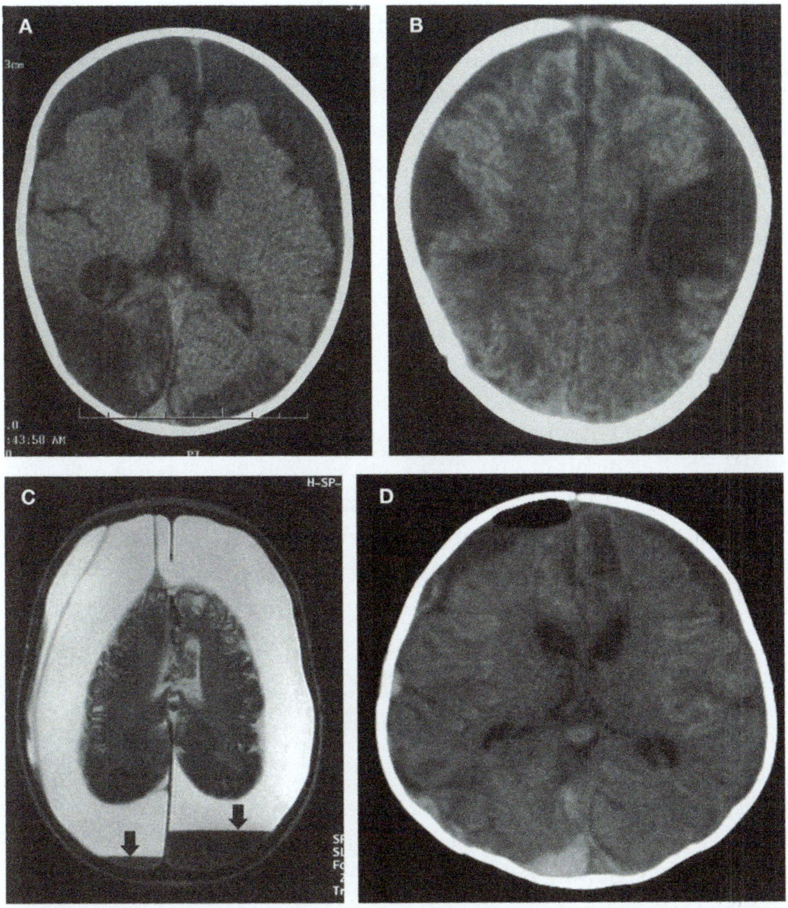

FIGURE 7.21

Late sequelae of parenchymal brain injuries following abusive head trauma. A, Axial computed tomography (CT) scan demonstrates overall brain atrophy with bilateral expanded subarachnoid spaces and overlying chronic subdural collections; focal encephalomalacia involving both occipital and right frontal lobes is also present. B, Axial CT scan demonstrates bilateral frontoparietal encephalomalacia and white matter gliosis. C, Axial T2-weighted magnetic resonance image demonstrates severe global atrophy with huge bilateral multicompartmental extra-axial mixed intensity collections; note fluid-fluid level (arrows). D, Axial CT scan shows cortical laminar necrosis as serpiginous high density paralleling the cortical surface.

intellectual or cognitive deficits (54%), and severe behavioral disorders (38%).[361] Early predictors of poor outcome include previous medical or developmental disabilities, repeated abuse, low parental socioeconomic status, lower GCS at presentation, occurrence and duration of coma, need for resuscitation, extent of parenchymal brain injury and hypoxic-ischemic brain injury, brain perfusion, and presence of coagulopathy.[259,260,361–363]

The economic consequences of AHT are significant.[10,364,365] Initial medical costs are estimated at $27,939 to $34,513, with lifetime projected medical costs of $224,500 to $506,193.[10,364–366] A case with lifetime medical costs exceeding $1 million was reported in 1996.[367] Legal and child protective costs, estimated at $195,471 to $281,280, and educational costs, estimated at $455,988 to $1,790,068,[364,366] add to this burden. The most recent US data identified $5.7 million for each AHT death and $2.6 million for each AHT survivor.[364]

Prevention

Given the heartbreaking clinical outcomes and extraordinary cost of AHT, the best way to deal with it would be to prevent it in the first place. There are 3 types of prevention programs: primary prevention, with the aim of addressing all elements of a population (eg, teaching parents of all newborns about crying and the danger of violent shaking); secondary prevention, with the aim of targeting those at higher risk (eg, home visitation by nurses for families at high risk for abuse); and tertiary prevention, which seeks to protect children from identified perpetrators and prevent recidivism. Efforts to prevent AHT and other forms of abuse are discussed in greater detail in Chapter 33, Evidence-based Child Abuse and Neglect Prevention Programs.

Conclusion

An enormous amount of research has been performed in the decades since Guthkelch[16] and Caffey[15,368] first described the entity now referred to as AHT. The overwhelming bulk of this research has upheld the diagnostic accuracy of the various clinical features of AHT and the specificity of those features in differentiating AHT from other conditions such as unintentional trauma. Research and experience have provided strong evidence that shaking alone can injure infants and that injurious impact can occur without evidence of impact. Changes in autopsy and imaging techniques have revealed cervical ligamentous and spinal cord injuries that may well underlie the commonly reported disordered breathing and provide the substrate for intracranial hypoxic-ischemic injuries in these cases. Advanced neuroimaging has opened a window into the molecular underpinnings of primary and secondary cellular injury, and analysis of CSF and other bodily fluids holds the promise of identifying cellular brain injury much as troponins now identify cellular cardiac injury. Although a suitable animal model of AHT has not, and probably never will be, discovered, it is now incontrovertible that manual shaking (at least of infant lambs) can result in neuronal injury, subdural bleeding, and even death. Although biomechanical and computational models of AHT have been hindered by a lack of infant-specific tissue physical properties, progress is being made in this area as well.

References

1. Ellingson KD, Leventhal JM, Weiss HB. Using hospital discharge data to track the incidence of inflicted traumatic brain injury in infants: a comparison of population-based studies. Paper presented at: Measuring the Incidence of Inflicted Childhood Neurotrauma; October 5–6, 2006; Seattle, WA
2. Forjuoh SN. Child maltreatment related injuries: incidence, hospital charges, and correlates of hospitalization. *Child Abuse Negl*. 2000;24(8):1019–1025 PMID: 10983812 https://doi.org/10.1016/S0145-2134(00)00163-0
3. Parks SE, Annest JL, Hill HA, Karch DL. *Pediatric Abusive Head Trauma: Recommended Definitions for Public Health Surveillance and Research*. Atlanta, GA: Centers for Disease Control and Prevention; 2012
4. Parks SE, Kegler SR, Annest JL, Mercy JA. Characteristics of fatal abusive head trauma among children in the USA: 2003-2007: an application of the CDC operational case definition to national vital statistics data. *Inj Prev*. 2012;18(3):193–199 PMID: 22015935 https://doi.org/10.1136/injuryprev-2011-040128
5. Parks S, Sugerman D, Xu L, Coronado V. Characteristics of non-fatal abusive head trauma among children in the USA, 2003-2008: application of the CDC operational case definition to national hospital inpatient data. *Inj Prev*. 2012;18(6):392–398 PMID: 22328632 https://doi.org/10.1136/injuryprev-2011-040234
6. Selassie AW, Borg K, Busch C, Russell WS. Abusive head trauma in young children: a population-based study. *J Trauma Nurs*. 2014;21(2):72–82 PMID: 24614297 https://doi.org/10.1097/JTN.0000000000000038
7. Shanahan ME, Zolotor AJ, Parrish JW, Barr RG, Runyan DK. National, regional, and state abusive head trauma: application of the CDC algorithm. *Pediatrics*. 2013;132(6):e1546–e1553 PMID: 24276842 https://doi.org/10.1542/peds.2013-2049
8. Niederkrotenthaler T, Xu L, Parks SE, Sugerman DE. Descriptive factors of abusive head trauma in young children—United States, 2000-2009. *Child Abuse Negl*. 2013;37(7):446–455 PMID: 23535075 https://doi.org/10.1016/j.chiabu.2013.02.002
9. Xiang J, Shi J, Wheeler KK, Yeates KO, Taylor HG, Smith GA. Paediatric patients with abusive head trauma treated in US emergency departments, 2006-2009. *Brain Inj*. 2013;27(13-14):1555–1561 PMID: 24102484 https://doi.org/10.3109/02699052.2013.831126
10. Boop S, Axente M, Weatherford B, Klimo P Jr. Abusive head trauma: an epidemiological and cost analysis. *J Neurosurg Pediatr*. 2016;18(5):542–549 PMID: 27402215 https://doi.org/10.3171/2016.1.PEDS15583
11. Kesler H, Dias MS, Shaffer M, Rottmund C, Cappos K, Thomas NJ. Demographics of abusive head trauma in the Commonwealth of Pennsylvania. *J Neurosurg Pediatr*. 2008;1(5):351–356 PMID: 18447667 https://doi.org/10.3171/PED/2008/1/5/351
12. Minns RA, Brown JK. Neurological perspectives of non-accidental head injury and whiplash/shaken baby syndrome: an overview. In: Minns RA, Brown JK, eds. *Shaking and Other Non-Accidental Head Injuries in Children*. London, United Kingdom: Cambridge University Press; 2005:1–105
13. Fujiwara T, Barr RG, Brant RF, Rajabali F, Pike I. Using International Classification of Diseases, 10th Edition, codes to estimate abusive head trauma in children. *Am J Prev Med*. 2012;43(2):215–220 PMID: 22813688

14. Talvik I, Männamaa M, Jüri P, et al. Outcome of infants with inflicted traumatic brain injury (shaken baby syndrome) in Estonia. *Acta Paediatr*. 2007;96(8):1164–1168 PMID: 17578492 https://doi.org/10.1111/j.1651-2227.2007.00362.x
15. Caffey J. On the theory and practice of shaking infants. Its potential residual effects of permanent brain damage and mental retardation. *Am J Dis Child*. 1972;124(2):161–169 PMID: 4559532 https://doi.org/10.1001/archpedi.1972.02110140011001
16. Guthkelch AN. Infantile subdural haematoma and its relationship to whiplash injuries. *BMJ*. 1971;2(5759):430–431 PMID: 5576003 https://doi.org/10.1136/bmj.2.5759.430
17. Starling SP, Patel S, Burke BL, Sirotnak AP, Stronks S, Rosquist P. Analysis of perpetrator admissions to inflicted traumatic brain injury in children. *Arch Pediatr Adolesc Med*. 2004;158(5):454–458 PMID: 15123478 https://doi.org/10.1001/archpedi.158.5.454
18. Adamsbaum C, Grabar S, Mejean N, Rey-Salmon C. Abusive head trauma: judicial admissions highlight violent and repetitive shaking. *Pediatrics*. 2010;126(3):546–555 PMID: 20696720 https://doi.org/10.1542/peds.2009-3647
19. Vinchon M, de Foort-Dhellemmes S, Desurmont M, Delestret I. Confessed abuse versus witnessed accidents in infants: comparison of clinical, radiological, and ophthalmological data in corroborated cases. *Childs Nerv Syst*. 2010;26(5):637–645 PMID: 19946688 https://doi.org/10.1007/s00381-009-1048-7
20. Runyan DK, Shankar V, Hassan F, et al. International variations in harsh child discipline. *Pediatrics*. 2010;126(3):e701–e711 PMID: 20679301 https://doi.org/10.1542/peds.2008-2374
21. Starling SP, Holden JR, Jenny C. Abusive head trauma: the relationship of perpetrators to their victims. *Pediatrics*. 1995;95(2):259–262 PMID: 7838645
22. Flaherty EG. Analysis of caretaker histories in abuse: comparing initial histories with subsequent confessions. *Child Abuse Negl*. 2006;30(7):789–798 PMID: 16844217 https://doi.org/10.1016/j.chiabu.2005.12.008
23. Dias MS, Smith K, DeGuehery K, Mazur P, Li V, Shaffer ML. Preventing abusive head trauma among infants and young children: a hospital-based, parent education program. *Pediatrics*. 2005;115(4):e470–e477 PMID: 15805350 https://doi.org/10.1542/peds.2004-1896
24. Scribano PV, Makoroff KL, Feldman KW, Berger RP. Association of perpetrator relationship to abusive head trauma clinical outcomes. *Child Abuse Negl*. 2013;37(10):771–777 PMID: 23735871 https://doi.org/10.1016/j.chiabu.2013.04.011
25. Kelly P, John S, Vincent AL, Reed P. Abusive head trauma and accidental head injury: a 20-year comparative study of referrals to a hospital child protection team. *Arch Dis Child*. 2015;100(12):1123–1130 PMID: 26130384 https://doi.org/10.1136/archdischild-2014-306960
26. Kelly P, Thompson JMD, Koh J, et al. Perinatal risk and protective factors for pediatric abusive head trauma: a multicenter case-control study. *J Pediatr*. 2017;187:240–246.e4 PMID: 28550953 https://doi.org/10.1016/j.jpeds.2017.04.058
27. Ettaro L, Berger RP, Songer T. Abusive head trauma in young children: characteristics and medical charges in a hospitalized population. *Child Abuse Negl*. 2004;28(10):1099–1111 PMID: 15519438 https://doi.org/10.1016/j.chiabu.2004.06.006
28. Wood JN, French B, Fromkin J, et al. Association of pediatric abusive head trauma rates with macroeconomic indicators. *Acad Pediatr*. 2016;16(3):224–232 PMID: 26183000 https://doi.org/10.1016/j.acap.2015.05.008
29. Berger RP, Fromkin JB, Stutz H, et al. Abusive head trauma during a time of increased unemployment: a multicenter analysis. *Pediatrics*. 2011;128(4):637–643 PMID: 21930535 https://doi.org/10.1542/peds.2010-2185

30. Huang MI, O'Riordan MA, Fitzenrider E, McDavid L, Cohen AR, Robinson S. Increased incidence of nonaccidental head trauma in infants associated with the economic recession. *J Neurosurg Pediatr*. 2011;8(2):171–176 PMID: 21806359 https://doi.org/10.3171/2011.5.PEDS1139
31. Ricci L, Giantris A, Merriam P, Hodge S, Doyle T. Abusive head trauma in Maine infants: medical, child protective, and law enforcement analysis. *Child Abuse Negl*. 2003;27(3):271–283 PMID: 12654325 https://doi.org/10.1016/S0145-2134(03)00006-1
32. Barr RG. Preventing abusive head trauma resulting from a failure of normal interaction between infants and their caregivers. *Proc Natl Acad Sci USA*. 2012;109(suppl 2): 17294–17301 PMID: 23045677 https://doi.org/10.1073/pnas.1121267109
33. Barr RG, Trent RB, Cross J. Age-related incidence curve of hospitalized shaken baby syndrome cases: convergent evidence for crying as a trigger to shaking. *Child Abuse Negl*. 2006;30(1):7–16 PMID: 16406023 https://doi.org/10.1016/j.chiabu.2005.06.009
34. Lee C, Barr RG, Catherine N, Wicks A. Age-related incidence of publicly reported shaken baby syndrome cases: is crying a trigger for shaking? *J Dev Behav Pediatr*. 2007;28(4):288–293 PMID: 17700080 https://doi.org/10.1097/DBP.0b013e3180327b55
35. Talvik I, Alexander RC, Talvik T. Shaken baby syndrome and a baby's cry. *Acta Paediatr*. 2008;97(6):782–785 PMID: 18397351 https://doi.org/10.1111/j.1651-2227.2008.00778.x
36. Sieswerda-Hoogendoorn T, Bilo RA, van Duurling LL, et al. Abusive head trauma in young children in the Netherlands: evidence for multiple incidents of abuse. *Acta Paediatr*. 2013;102(11):e497–e501 PMID: 23909838 https://doi.org/10.1111/apa.12377
37. Bhardwaj G, Chowdhury V, Jacobs MB, Moran KT, Martin FJ, Coroneo MT. A systematic review of the diagnostic accuracy of ocular signs in pediatric abusive head trauma. *Ophthalmology*. 2010;117(5):983–992.e17 PMID: 20347153 https://doi.org/10.1016/j.ophtha.2009.09.040
38. Maguire SA, Kemp AM, Lumb RC, Farewell DM. Estimating the probability of abusive head trauma: a pooled analysis. *Pediatrics*. 2011;128(3):e550–e564 PMID: 21844052 https://doi.org/10.1542/peds.2010-2949
39. Maguire SA, Watts PO, Shaw AD, et al. Retinal haemorrhages and related findings in abusive and non-abusive head trauma: a systematic review. *Eye (Lond)*. 2013;27(1):28–36 PMID: 23079748 https://doi.org/10.1038/eye.2012.213
40. Piteau SJ, Ward MG, Barrowman NJ, Plint AC. Clinical and radiographic characteristics associated with abusive and nonabusive head trauma: a systematic review. *Pediatrics*. 2012;130(2):315–323 PMID: 22778309 https://doi.org/10.1542/peds.2011-1545
41. Kemp AM, Jaspan T, Griffiths J, et al. Neuroimaging: what neuroradiological features distinguish abusive from non-abusive head trauma? A systematic review. *Arch Dis Child*. 2011;96(12):1103–1112 PMID: 21965812 https://doi.org/10.1136/archdischild-2011-300630
42. Rubin DM, Christian CW, Bilaniuk LT, Zazyczny KA, Durbin DR. Occult head injury in high-risk abused children. *Pediatrics*. 2003;111(6 Pt 1):1382–1386 PMID: 12777556 https://doi.org/10.1542/peds.111.6.1382
43. Laskey AL, Holsti M, Runyan DK, Socolar RR. Occult head trauma in young suspected victims of physical abuse. *J Pediatr*. 2004;144(6):719–722 PMID: 15192615
44. Shaikh H, Wrotniak BH, Mazur PM; Women and Children's Hospital of Buffalo. Occult head injury in children less than 2 years with suspected child abuse in the emergency department. *Pediatr Emerg Care*. 2017;1 PMID: 28562465 https://doi.org/10.1097/PEC.0000000000001187
45. Feldman KW, Sugar NF, Browd SR. Initial clinical presentation of children with acute and chronic versus acute subdural hemorrhage resulting from abusive head trauma. *J Neurosurg Pediatr*. 2015;16(2):177–185 PMID: 25932780 https://doi.org/10.3171/2014.12.PEDS14607

46. Morris MW, Smith S, Cressman J, Ancheta J. Evaluation of infants with subdural hematoma who lack external evidence of abuse. *Pediatrics*. 2000;105(3 Pt 1):549–553 PMID: 10699108 https://doi.org/10.1542/peds.105.3.549
47. Hettler J, Greenes DS. Can the initial history predict whether a child with a head injury has been abused? *Pediatrics*. 2003;111(3):602–607 PMID: 12612243 https://doi.org/10.1542/peds.111.3.602
48. Amagasa S, Matsui H, Tsuji S, Moriya T, Kinoshita K. Accuracy of the history of injury obtained from the caregiver in infantile head trauma. *Am J Emerg Med*. 2016;34(9): 1863–1867 PMID: 27422215 https://doi.org/10.1016/j.ajem.2016.06.085
49. Keenan HT, Runyan DK, Marshall SW, Nocera MA, Merten DF. A population-based comparison of clinical and outcome characteristics of young children with serious inflicted and noninflicted traumatic brain injury. *Pediatrics*. 2004;114(3):633–639 PMID: 15342832 https://doi.org/10.1542/peds.2003-1020-L
50. Ichord RN, Naim M, Pollock AN, Nance ML, Margulies SS, Christian CW. Hypoxic-ischemic injury complicates inflicted and accidental traumatic brain injury in young children: the role of diffusion-weighted imaging. *J Neurotrauma*. 2007;24(1):106–118 PMID: 17263674 https://doi.org/10.1089/neu.2006.0087
51. Dias MS, Backstrom J, Falk M, Li V. Serial radiography in the infant shaken impact syndrome. *Pediatr Neurosurg*. 1998;29(2):77–85 PMID: 9792961 https://doi.org/10.1159/000028694
52. Bradford R, Choudhary AK, Dias MS. Serial neuroimaging in infants with abusive head trauma: timing abusive injuries. *J Neurosurg Pediatr*. 2013;12(2):110–119 PMID: 23799250 https://doi.org/10.3171/2013.4.PEDS12596
53. Mulligan CS, Adams S, Tzioumi D, Brown J. Injury from falls in infants under one year. *J Paediatr Child Health*. 2017;53(8):754–760 PMID: 28653434 https://doi.org/10.1111/jpc.13568
54. Dias MS. The case for shaking. In: Jenny C, ed. *Child Abuse and Neglect: Diagnosis, Treatment, and Evidence*. St. Louis, MO: Elsevier; 2011:364–372 https://doi.org/10.1016/B978-1-4160-6393-3.00041-5
55. Duhaime AC, Alario AJ, Lewander WJ, et al. Head injury in very young children: mechanisms, injury types, and ophthalmologic findings in 100 hospitalized patients younger than 2 years of age. *Pediatrics*. 1992;90(2 Pt 1):179–185 PMID: 1641278
56. Morad Y, Kim YM, Armstrong DC, Huyer D, Mian M, Levin AV. Correlation between retinal abnormalities and intracranial abnormalities in the shaken baby syndrome. *Am J Ophthalmol*. 2002;134(3):354–359 PMID: 12208246 https://doi.org/10.1016/S0002-9394(02)01628-8
57. Bechtel K, Stoessel K, Leventhal JM, et al. Characteristics that distinguish accidental from abusive injury in hospitalized young children with head trauma. *Pediatrics*. 2004;114(1):165–168 PMID: 15231923 https://doi.org/10.1542/peds.114.1.165
58. Binenbaum G, Mirza-George N, Christian CW, Forbes BJ. Odds of abuse associated with retinal hemorrhages in children suspected of child abuse. *J AAPOS*. 2009;13(3): 268–272 PMID: 19541267 https://doi.org/10.1016/j.jaapos.2009.03.005
59. Minns RA, Jones PA, Tandon A, Fleck BW, Mulvihill AO, Elton RA. Prediction of inflicted brain injury in infants and children using retinal imaging. *Pediatrics*. 2012;130(5): e1227–e1234 PMID: 23045566 https://doi.org/10.1542/peds.2011-3274
60. Levin AV. Retinal haemorrhages and child abuse. In: David TJ, ed. *Recent Advances in Paediatrics. 18*. Edinburgh: Churchill Livingstone; 2000:151–219
61. Binenbaum G, Christian CW, Ichord RN, et al. Retinal hemorrhage and brain injury patterns on diffusion-weighted magnetic resonance imaging in children with head

trauma. *J AAPOS*. 2013;17(6):603–608 PMID: 24215807 https://doi.org/10.1016/j.jaapos.2013.09.002

62. Greenwald MJ, Weiss A, Oesterle CS, Friendly DS. Traumatic retinoschisis in battered babies. *Ophthalmology*. 1986;93(5):618–625 PMID: 3725321 https://doi.org/10.1016/S0161-6420(86)33688-1
63. Feldman KW, Bethel R, Shugerman RP, Grossman DC, Grady MS, Ellenbogen RG. The cause of infant and toddler subdural hemorrhage: a prospective study. *Pediatrics*. 2001;108(3):636–646 PMID: 11533330 https://doi.org/10.1542/peds.108.3.636
64. Royal College of Paediatrics and Child Health. *Child Protection Evidence: Systematic Review on Neurological Injuries*. Royal College of Paediatrics and Child Health; 2015. https://www.rcpch.ac.uk/sites/default/files/2018-07/child_protection_evidence_-_neurological_injuries.pdf. Accessed June 10, 2019
65. Hymel KP, Armijo-Garcia V, Foster R, et al; Pediatric Brain Injury Research Network (PediBIRN) Investigators. Validation of a clinical prediction rule for pediatric abusive head trauma. *Pediatrics*. 2014;134(6):e1537–e1544 PMID: 25404722 https://doi.org/10.1542/peds.2014-1329
66. Cowley LE, Morris CB, Maguire SA, Farewell DM, Kemp AM. Validation of a prediction tool for abusive head trauma. *Pediatrics*. 2015;136(2):290–298 PMID: 26216332 https://doi.org/10.1542/peds.2014-3993
67. Arbogast KB, Margulies SS, Christian CW. Initial neurologic presentation in young children sustaining inflicted and unintentional fatal head injuries. *Pediatrics*. 2005;116(1):180–184 PMID: 15995050 https://doi.org/10.1542/peds.2004-2671
68. Gilliland MGF. Interval duration between injury and severe symptoms in nonaccidental head trauma in infants and young children. *J Forensic Sci*. 1998;43(3):723–725 PMID: 9608715 https://doi.org/10.1520/JFS16211J
69. Biron DL, Shelton D. Functional time limit and onset of symptoms in infant abusive head trauma. *J Paediatr Child Health*. 2007;43(1-2):60–65 PMID: 17207058 https://doi.org/10.1111/j.1440-1754.2007.01004.x
70. Willman KY, Bank DE, Senac M, Chadwick DL. Restricting the time of injury in fatal inflicted head injuries. *Child Abuse Negl*. 1997;21(10):929–940 PMID: 9330794 https://doi.org/10.1016/S0145-2134(97)00054-9
71. Jacquet C, Boetto S, Sevely A, Sol JC, Chaix Y, Cheuret E. Monitoring criteria of intracranial lesions in children post mild or moderate head trauma. *Neuropediatrics*. 2018;49(6):385–391 PMID: 30223286 https://doi.org/10.1055/s-0038-1668138
72. De Leeuw M, Beuls E, Parizel P, Jorens P, Jacobs W. Confessed abusive blunt head trauma. *Am J Forensic Med Pathol*. 2013;34(2):130–132 PMID: 23629386 https://doi.org/10.1097/PAF.0b013e31828629ca
73. Adamsbaum C, Morel B, Ducot B, Antoni G, Rey-Salmon C. Dating the abusive head trauma episode and perpetrator statements: key points for imaging. *Pediatr Radiol*. 2014;44(S4)(suppl 4):S578–S588 PMID: 25501730 https://doi.org/10.1007/s00247-014-3171-1
74. Babl FE, Borland ML, Phillips N, et al; Paediatric Research in Emergency Departments International Collaborative. Accuracy of PECARN, CATCH, and CHALICE head injury decision rules in children: a prospective cohort study. 2017;389(10087):2393–2402 PMID: 28410792
75. Lee LK, Monroe D, Bachman MC, et al; Traumatic Brain Injury (TBI) Working Group of Pediatric Emergency Care Applied Research Network (PECARN). Isolated loss of consciousness in children with minor blunt head trauma. *JAMA Pediatr*. 2014;168(9):837–843 PMID: 25003654 https://doi.org/10.1001/jamapediatrics.2014.361

76. Snoek JW, Minderhoud JM, Wilmink JT. Delayed deterioration following mild head injury in children. *Brain*. 1984;107(Pt 1):15–36 PMID: 6697152 https://doi.org/10.1093/brain/107.1.15
77. Humphreys RP, Hendrick EB, Hoffman HJ. The head-injured child who "talks and dies". A report of 4 cases. *Childs Nerv Syst*. 1990;6(3):139–142 PMID: 2357710 https://doi.org/10.1007/BF00308490 PMID: 2357710
78. Choudhry OJ, Prestigiacomo CJ, Gala N, Slasky S, Sifri ZC. Delayed neurological deterioration after mild head injury: cause, temporal course, and outcomes. *Neurosurgery*. 2013;73(5):753–760 PMID: 23867298 https://doi.org/10.1227/NEU.0000000000000105
79. Hamilton M, Mrazik M, Johnson DW. Incidence of delayed intracranial hemorrhage in children after uncomplicated minor head injuries. *Pediatrics*. 2010;126(1):e33–e39 PMID: 20566618 https://doi.org/10.1542/peds.2009-0692
80. Chiaretti A, De Benedictis R, Polidori G, Piastra M, Iannelli A, Di Rocco C. Early post-traumatic seizures in children with head injury. *Childs Nerv Syst*. 2000;16(12):862–866 PMID: 11156302 https://doi.org/10.1007/s003810000368
81. Ateş O, Ondül S, Onal C, et al. Post-traumatic early epilepsy in pediatric age group with emphasis on influential factors. *Childs Nerv Syst*. 2006;22(3):279–284 PMID: 15889309
82. Liesemer K, Bratton SL, Zebrack CM, Brockmeyer D, Statler KD. Early post-traumatic seizures in moderate to severe pediatric traumatic brain injury: rates, risk factors, and clinical features. *J Neurotrauma*. 2011;28(5):755–762 PMID: 21381863 https://doi.org/10.1089/neu.2010.1518
83. Arndt DH, Goodkin HP, Giza CC. Early posttraumatic seizures in the pediatric population. *J Child Neurol*. 2016;31(1):46–56 PMID: 25564481 https://doi.org/10.1177/0883073814562249
84. Dias MS, Carnevale F, Li V. Immediate posttraumatic seizures: is routine hospitalization necessary? *Pediatr Neurosurg*. 1999;30(5):232–238 PMID: 10461069 https://doi.org/10.1159/000028803
85. Keret A, Bennett-Back O, Rosenthal G, et al. Posttraumatic epilepsy: long-term follow-up of children with mild traumatic brain injury. *J Neurosurg Pediatr*. 2017;20(1):64–70 PMID: 28474982 https://doi.org/10.3171/2017.2.PEDS16585
86. Huguenard AL, Miller BA, Sarda S, Capasse M, Reisner A, Chern JJ. Mild traumatic brain injury in children is associated with a low risk for posttraumatic seizures. *J Neurosurg Pediatr*. 2016;17(4):476–482 PMID: 26613272 https://doi.org/10.3171/2015.7.PEDS14723
87. Binenbaum G, Chen W, Huang J, Ying GS, Forbes BJ. The natural history of retinal hemorrhage in pediatric head trauma. *J AAPOS*. 2016;20(2):131–135 PMID: 27079593 https://doi.org/10.1016/j.jaapos.2015.12.008
88. Parker K, Pitetti R. Mortality and child abuse in children presenting with apparent life-threatening events. *Pediatr Emerg Care*. 2011;27(7):591–595 PMID: 21712749 https://doi.org/10.1097/PEC.0b013e3182225563
89. Stark W, Rominger A, Warkentine F, Caperell K. The utility of head computed tomography in the evaluation of apparent life-threatening event. *Pediatr Emerg Care*. 2018;34(9):623–627 PMID: 27741078
90. Hansen JB, Frazier T, Moffatt M, Zinkus T, Anderst JD. Evaluations for abuse in young children with subdural hemorrhages: findings based on symptom severity and benign enlargement of the subarachnoid spaces. *J Neurosurg Pediatr*. 2018;21(1):31–37 PMID: 29099352 https://doi.org/10.3171/2017.7.PEDS17317

91. Jenny C, Hymel KP, Ritzen A, Reinert SE, Hay TC. Analysis of missed cases of abusive head trauma. *JAMA*. 1999;281(7):621–626 PMID: 10029123 https://doi.org/10.1001/jama.281.7.621
92. Vinchon M, Desurmont M, Soto-Ares G, De Foort-Dhellemmes S. Natural history of traumatic meningeal bleeding in infants: semiquantitative analysis of serial CT scans in corroborated cases. *Childs Nerv Syst*. 2010;26(6):755–762 PMID: 19946689 https://doi.org/10.1007/s00381-009-1047-8
93. Vinchon M, Noizet O, Defoort-Dhellemmes S, Soto-Ares G, Dhellemmes P. Infantile subdural hematomas due to traffic accidents. *Pediatr Neurosurg*. 2002;37(5):245–253 PMID: 12411716 https://doi.org/10.1159/000066216
94. Vezina G. Assessment of the nature and age of subdural collections in nonaccidental head injury with CT and MRI. *Pediatr Radiol*. 2009;39(6):586–590 PMID: 19305988 https://doi.org/10.1007/s00247-009-1212-y
95. Wootton-Gorges SL, Soares BP, Alazraki AL, et al; Expert Panel on Pediatric Imaging. ACR appropriateness criteria suspected physical abuse—child. *J Am Coll Radiol*. 2017;14(5S):S338–S349 PMID: 28473090 https://doi.org/10.1016/j.jacr.2017.01.036
96. Durham SR, Clancy RR, Leuthardt E, et al. CHOP Infant Coma Scale ("Infant Face Scale"): a novel coma scale for children less than two years of age. *J Neurotrauma*. 2000;17(9):729–737 PMID: 11011813 https://doi.org/10.1089/neu.2000.17.729
97. Raimondi AJ, Hirschauer J. Head injury in the infant and toddler. Coma scoring and outcome scale. *Childs Brain*. 1984;11(1):12–35 PMID: 6705608
98. Yager JY, Johnston B, Seshia SS. Coma scales in pediatric practice. *Am J Dis Child*. 1990;144(10):1088–1091 PMID: 2403089
99. Simpson DA, Cockington RA, Hanieh A, Raftos J, Reilly PL. Head injuries in infants and young children: the value of the Paediatric Coma Scale. Review of literature and report on a study. *Childs Nerv Syst*. 1991;7(4):183–190 PMID: 1933914 https://doi.org/10.1007/BF00249393
100. Reece RM. Differential diagnosis of inflicted childhood neurotrauma. In: Reece RM, Nicholson CE, eds. *Inflicted Childhood Neurotrauma*. Elk Grove Village, IL: American Academy of Pediatrics; 2003
101. American Academy of Pediatrics Committee on Child Abuse and Neglect. Shaken baby syndrome: rotational cranial injuries-technical report. *Pediatrics*. 2001;108(1):206–210 PMID: 11433079 https://doi.org/10.1542/peds.108.1.206
102. Hymel KP, Bandak FA, Partington MD, Winston KR. Abusive head trauma? A biomechanics-based approach. *Child Maltreat*. 1998;3(2):116–128 https://doi.org/10.1177/1077559598003002006
103. Pierce MC, Bertocci GE, Berger R, Vogeley E. Injury biomechanics for aiding in the diagnosis of abusive head trauma. *Neurosurg Clin N Am*. 2002;13(2):155–168 PMID: 12391701 https://doi.org/10.1016/S1042-3680(01)00006-7
104. Duhaime AC, Gennarelli TA, Thibault LE, Bruce DA, Margulies SS, Wiser R. The shaken baby syndrome. A clinical, pathological, and biomechanical study. *J Neurosurg*. 1987;66(3):409–415 PMID: 3819836 https://doi.org/10.3171/jns.1987.66.3.0409
105. Menezes AH, Smith DE, Bell WE. Posterior fossa hemorrhage in the term neonate. *Neurosurgery*. 1983;13(4):452–456 PMID: 6633841 https://doi.org/10.1227/00006123-198310000-00021
106. Raghupathi R, Mehr MF, Helfaer MA, Margulies SS. Traumatic axonal injury is exacerbated following repetitive closed head injury in the neonatal pig. *J Neurotrauma*. 2004;21(3):307–316 PMID: 15115605 https://doi.org/10.1089/089771504322972095

107. Duhaime A-C, Margulies SS, Durham SR, et al. Maturation-dependent response of the piglet brain to scaled cortical impact. *J Neurosurg*. 2000;93(3):455–462 PMID: 10969944 https://doi.org/10.3171/jns.2000.93.3.0455
108. Prange MT, Margulies SS. Regional, directional, and age-dependent properties of the brain undergoing large deformation. *J Biomech Eng*. 2002;124(2):244–252 PMID: 12002135
109. Prange MT, Coats B, Duhaime A-C, Margulies SS. Anthropomorphic simulations of falls, shakes, and inflicted impacts in infants. *J Neurosurg*. 2003;99(1):143–150 PMID: 12854757 https://doi.org/10.3171/jns.2003.99.1.0143
110. Massi M, Jenny C. Biomechanics of the shaken baby. a comparison of the APRICA 2.5 and APRICA 3.4 anthropomorphic test devices. Paper presented at: Pediatric Abusive Head Trauma: Medical, Forensic, and Scientific Advances and Prevention; July 12–13, 2007; Hershey, PA
111. Helfer RE, Slovis TL, Black M. Injuries resulting when small children fall out of bed. *Pediatrics*. 1977;60(4):533–535 PMID: 905018
112. Nimityongskul P, Anderson LD. The likelihood of injuries when children fall out of bed. *J Pediatr Orthop*. 1987;7(2):184–186 PMID: 3558802 https://doi.org/10.1097/01241398-198703000-00014
113. Hall JR, Reyes HM, Horvat M, Meller JL, Stein R. The mortality of childhood falls. *J Trauma*. 1989;29(9):1273–1275 PMID: 2769810 https://doi.org/10.1097/00005373-198909000-00015
114. Musemeche CA, Barthel M, Cosentino C, Reynolds M. Pediatric falls from heights. *J Trauma*. 1991;31(10):1347–1349 PMID: 1942140 https://doi.org/10.1097/00005373-199110000-00004
115. Reiber GD. Fatal falls in childhood. How far must children fall to sustain fatal head injury? Report of cases and review of the literature. *Am J Forensic Med Pathol*. 1993;14(3):201–207 PMID: 8311050 https://doi.org/10.1097/00000433-199309000-00005
116. Chiaviello CT, Christoph RA, Bond GR. Stairway-related injuries in children. *Pediatrics*. 1994;94(5):679–681 PMID: 7936895
117. Tarantino CA, Dowd MD, Murdock TC. Short vertical falls in infants. *Pediatr Emerg Care*. 1999;15(1):5–8 PMID: 10069302 https://doi.org/10.1097/00006565-199902000-00002
118. Plunkett J. Fatal pediatric head injuries caused by short-distance falls. *Am J Forensic Med Pathol*. 2001;22(1):1–12 PMID: 11444653 https://doi.org/10.1097/00000433-200103000-00001
119. Johnson K, Fischer T, Chapman S, Wilson B. Accidental head injuries in children under 5 years of age. *Clin Radiol*. 2005;60(4):464–468. PMID: 15767104 PMID: 15767104 https://doi.org/10.1016/j.crad.2004.09.013
120. Thompson A, Bertocci G, Pierce MC. Assessment of injury potential in pediatric bed fall experiments using an anthropomorphic test device. *Accid Anal Prev*. 2013;50:16–24 PMID: 23131474 https://doi.org/10.1016/j.aap.2012.09.011
121. Batterbee DC, Sims ND, Becker W, Worden K, Rowson J. Computational model of an infant brain subjected to periodic motion simplified modelling and Bayesian sensitivity analysis. *Proc Inst Mech Eng H*. 2011;225(11):1036–1049 PMID: 22292202 https://doi.org/10.1177/0954411911420002
122. Bertocci GE, Pierce MC, Deemer E, Aguel F, Janosky JE, Vogeley E. Using test dummy experiments to investigate pediatric injury risk in simulated short-distance falls. *Arch Pediatr Adolesc Med*. 2003;157(5):480–486 PMID: 12742885 https://doi.org/10.1001/archpedi.157.5.480

123. Cheng J, Howard IC, Rennison M. Study of an infant brain subjected to periodic motion via a custom experimental apparatus design and finite element modelling. *J Biomech*. 2010;43(15):2887–2896 PMID: 20708735 https://doi.org/10.1016/j.jbiomech.2010.07.023
124. Coats B, Margulies SS. Potential for head injuries in infants from low-height falls. *J Neurosurg Pediatr*. 2008;2(5):321–330 PMID: 18976102 https://doi.org/10.3171/PED.2008.2.11.321
125. Ibrahim NG, Wood J, Margulies SS, Christian CW. Influence of age and fall type on head injuries in infants and toddlers. *Int J Dev Neurosci*. 2012;30(3):201–206 PMID: 22079853 https://doi.org/10.1016/j.ijdevneu.2011.10.007
126. Margulies SS, Thibault KL. Infant skull and suture properties: measurements and implications for mechanisms of pediatric brain injury. *J Biomech Eng*. 2000;122(4): 364–371 PMID: 11036559 https://doi.org/10.1115/1.1287160
127. Irie F, Le Brocque R, Kenardy J, Bellamy N, Tetsworth K, Pollard C. Epidemiology of traumatic epidural hematoma in young age. *J Trauma*. 2011;71(4):847–853 PMID: 21336188 https://doi.org/10.1097/TA.0b013e3182032c9a
128. Rooks VJ, Eaton JP, Ruess L, Petermann GW, Keck-Wherley J, Pedersen RC. Prevalence and evolution of intracranial hemorrhage in asymptomatic term infants. *AJNR Am J Neuroradiol*. 2008;29(6):1082–1089 PMID: 18388219 https://doi.org/10.3174/ajnr.A1004
129. Looney CB, Smith JK, Merck LH, et al. Intracranial hemorrhage in asymptomatic neonates: prevalence on MR images and relationship to obstetric and neonatal risk factors. *Radiology*. 2007;242(2):535–541 PMID: 17179400 https://doi.org/10.1148/radiol.2422060133
130. Whitby EH, Griffiths PD, Rutter S, et al. Frequency and natural history of subdural haemorrhages in babies and relation to obstetric factors. *Lancet*. 2004;363(9412):846–851 PMID: 15031028 https://doi.org/10.1016/S0140-6736(04)15730-9
131. Towner D, Castro MA, Eby-Wilkens E, Gilbert WM. Effect of mode of delivery in nulliparous women on neonatal intracranial injury. *N Engl J Med*. 1999;341(23):1709–1714 PMID: 10580069 https://doi.org/10.1056/NEJM199912023412301
132. Pollina J, Dias MS, Li V, Kachurek D, Arbesman M. Cranial birth injuries in term newborn infants. *Pediatr Neurosurg*. 2001;35(3):113–119 PMID: 11641618 https://doi.org/10.1159/000050403
133. Gnanaraj L, Gilliland MGF, Yahya RR, et al. Ocular manifestations of crush head injury in children. *Eye (Lond)*. 2007;21(1):5–10 PMID: 16311527 https://doi.org/10.1038/sj.eye.6702174
134. Gennarelli TA, Thibault LE, Adams JH, Graham DI, Thompson CJ, Marcincin RP. Diffuse axonal injury and traumatic coma in the primate. *Ann Neurol*. 1982;12(6):564–574 PMID: 7159060 https://doi.org/10.1002/ana.410120611
135. Margulies S, Coats B. Biomechanics of pediatric TBI. In: Anderson V, Yeates K, eds. *Pediatric Traumatic Brain Injury: New Frontiers in Clinical and Translational Research*. Cambridge, United Kingdom: Cambridge University Press; 2010 https://doi.org/10.1017/CBO9780511676383.002
136. Brennan LK, Rubin D, Christian CW, Duhaime A-C, Mirchandani HG, Rorke-Adams LB. Neck injuries in young pediatric homicide victims. *J Neurosurg Pediatr*. 2009;3(3): 232–239 PMID: 19338471 https://doi.org/10.3171/2008.11.PEDS0835
137. Choudhary AK, Ishak R, Zacharia TT, Dias MS. Imaging of spinal injury in abusive head trauma: a retrospective study. *Pediatr Radiol*. 2014;44(9):1130–1140 PMID: 24687620 https://doi.org/10.1007/s00247-014-2959-3

138. Hadley MN, Sonntag VKH, Rekate HL, Murphy A. The infant whiplash-shake injury syndrome: a clinical and pathological study. *Neurosurgery*. 1989;24(4):536–540 PMID: 2710298 https://doi.org/10.1227/00006123-198904000-00008
139. Anderson RW, Sandoz B, Dutschke JK, et al. Biomechanical studies in an ovine model of non-accidental head injury. *J Biomech*. 2014;47(11):2578–2583 PMID: 24974335 https://doi.org/10.1016/j.jbiomech.2014.06.002
140. Finnie JW, Blumbergs PC, Manavis J, et al. Neuropathological changes in a lamb model of non-accidental head injury (the shaken baby syndrome). *J Clin Neurosci*. 2012;19(8):1159–1164 PMID: 22705132 https://doi.org/10.1016/j.jocn.2011.12.019
141. Finnie JW, Blumbergs PC, Manavis J, Vink R. Pattern of cerebrospinal immediate early gene c-fos expression in an ovine model of non-accidental head injury. *J Clin Neurosci*. 2013;20(12):1759–1761 PMID: 24035422 https://doi.org/10.1016/j.jocn.2013.03.010
142. Finnie JW, Manavis J, Blumbergs PC. Diffuse neuronal perikaryal amyloid precursor protein immunoreactivity in an ovine model of non-accidental head injury (the shaken baby syndrome). *J Clin Neurosci*. 2010;17(2):237–240 PMID: 20036546 https://doi.org/10.1016/j.jocn.2009.07.001
143. Pounder DJ. Shaken adult syndrome. *Am J Forensic Med Pathol*. 1997;18(4):321–324 PMID: 9430280 https://doi.org/10.1097/00000433-199712000-00001
144. Abel JM, Gennarelli TA, Segawa H, eds. Incidence and severity of cerebral concussion in the rhesus monkey following sagittal plane angular acceleration. In: Proceeding of 22nd Stapp Car Crash Conference; 1978; Warrendale, PA https://doi.org/10.4271/780886
145. Margulies SS, Thibault LE, Gennarelli TA. Physical model simulations of brain injury in the primate. *J Biomech*. 1990;23(8):823–836 PMID: 2384494 https://doi.org/10.1016/0021-9290(90)90029-3
146. Nahum AM, Smith RW, eds. An experimental model for closed head impact injury. In: Proceedings of 20th Stapp Car Crash Conference; 1976; Dearborn, MI https://doi.org/10.4271/760825
147. Wolfson DR, McNally DS, Clifford MJ, Vloeberghs M. Rigid-body modelling of shaken baby syndrome. *Proc Inst Mech Eng H*. 2005;219(1):63–70 PMID: 15777058 https://doi.org/10.1243/095441105X9237
148. Cory CZ, Jones BM. Can shaking alone cause fatal brain injury? A biomechanical assessment of the Duhaime shaken baby syndrome model. *Med Sci Law*. 2003;43(4):317–333 PMID: 14655963 https://doi.org/10.1258/rsmmsl.43.4.317
149. Couper Z, Albermani F. Mechanical response of infant brain to manually inflicted shaking. *Proc Inst Mech Eng H*. 2010;224(1):1–15 PMID: 20225453 https://doi.org/10.1243/09544119JEIM587
150. Roth S, Raul JS, Ludes B, Willinger R. Finite element analysis of impact and shaking inflicted to a child. *Int J Legal Med*. 2007;121(3):223–228 PMID: 17091312 https://doi.org/10.1007/s00414-006-0129-3
151. Gennarelli TA, Thibault LE. Biomechanics of acute subdural hematoma. *J Trauma*. 1982;22(8):680–686 PMID: 7108984 https://doi.org/10.1097/00005373-198208000-00005
152. Choudhary AK, Bradford R, Dias MS, Thamburaj K, Boal DKB. Venous injury in abusive head trauma. *Pediatr Radiol*. 2015;45(12):1803–1813 PMID: 26150078 https://doi.org/10.1007/s00247-015-3399-4
153. Hahnemann ML, Kinner S, Schweiger B, et al. Imaging of bridging vein thrombosis in infants with abusive head trauma: the "tadpole sign." *Eur Radiol*. 2015;25(2):299–305 PMID: 25274619 https://doi.org/10.1007/s00330-014-3443-z
154. Bayir H, Kagan VE, Tyurina YY, et al. Assessment of antioxidant reserves and oxidative stress in cerebrospinal fluid after severe traumatic brain injury in infants and children.

Pediatr Res. 2002;51(5):571–578 PMID: 11978879 https://doi.org/10.1203/00006450-200205000-00005

155. Bell MJ, Kochanek PM, Doughty LA, et al. Interleukin-6 and interleukin-10 in cerebrospinal fluid after severe traumatic brain injury in children. *J Neurotrauma*. 1997;14(7):451–457 PMID: 9257663 https://doi.org/10.1089/neu.1997.14.451
156. Bell MJ, Kochanek PM, Heyes MP, et al. Quinolinic acid in the cerebrospinal fluid of children after traumatic brain injury. *Crit Care Med*. 1999;27(3):493–497 PMID: 10199527 https://doi.org/10.1097/00003246-199903000-00023
157. Berger RP, Adelson PD, Pierce MC, Dulani T, Cassidy LD, Kochanek PM. Serum neuron-specific enolase, S100B, and myelin basic protein concentrations after inflicted and noninflicted traumatic brain injury in children. *J Neurosurg*. 2005;103(1)(suppl):61–68 PMID: 16122007 https://doi.org/10.3171/ped.2005.103.1.0061
158. Berger RP, Pierce MC, Wisniewski SR, et al. Neuron-specific enolase and S100B in cerebrospinal fluid after severe traumatic brain injury in infants and children. *Pediatrics*. 2002;109(2):E31 PMID: 11826241 https://doi.org/10.1542/peds.109.2.e31
159. Clark RS, Kochanek PM, Adelson PD, et al. Increases in bcl-2 protein in cerebrospinal fluid and evidence for programmed cell death in infants and children after severe traumatic brain injury. *J Pediatr*. 2000;137(2):197–204 PMID: 10931412 https://doi.org/10.1067/mpd.2000.106903
160. Han YY, Carcillo JA, Ruppel RA, et al. Cerebrospinal fluid procalcitonin and severe traumatic brain injury in children. *Pediatr Crit Care Med*. 2002;3(1):39–44 PMID: 12793921 https://doi.org/10.1097/00130478-200201000-00010
161. Satchell MA, Lai Y, Kochanek PM, et al. Cytochrome c, a biomarker of apoptosis, is increased in cerebrospinal fluid from infants with inflicted brain injury from child abuse. *J Cereb Blood Flow Metab*. 2005;25(7):919–927 PMID: 15744250 https://doi.org/10.1038/sj.jcbfm.9600088
162. Lai Y, Kochanek PM, Adelson PD, Janesko K, Ruppel RA, Clark RSB. Induction of the stress response after inflicted and non-inflicted traumatic brain injury in infants and children. *J Neurotrauma*. 2004;21(3):229–237 PMID: 15115598 https://doi.org/10.1089/089771504322972022
163. Robertson CL, Bell MJ, Kochanek PM, et al. Increased adenosine in cerebrospinal fluid after severe traumatic brain injury in infants and children: association with severity of injury and excitotoxicity. *Crit Care Med*. 2001;29(12):2287–2293 PMID: 11801827 https://doi.org/10.1097/00003246-200112000-00009
164. Robertson CL, Minamino N, Ruppel RA, et al. Increased adrenomedullin in cerebrospinal fluid after traumatic brain injury in infants and children. *J Neurotrauma*. 2001;18(9):861–868 PMID: 11565598 https://doi.org/10.1089/089771501750451785
165. Ruppel RA, Kochanek PM, Adelson PD, et al. Endothelin-1 is increased in cerebrospinal fluid following traumatic brain injury in children. *Crit Care Med*. 1999;27(suppl):A76 https://doi.org/10.1097/00003246-199912001-00188
166. Ruppel RA, Kochanek PM, Adelson PD, et al. Excitatory amino acid concentrations in ventricular cerebrospinal fluid after severe traumatic brain injury in infants and children: the role of child abuse. *J Pediatr*. 2001;138(1):18–25 PMID: 11148507 https://doi.org/10.1067/mpd.2001.110979
167. Shore PM, Jackson EK, Wisniewski SR, Clark RSB, Adelson PD, Kochanek PM. Vascular endothelial growth factor is increased in cerebrospinal fluid after traumatic brain injury in infants and children. *Neurosurgery*. 2004;54(3):605–611 PMID: 15028134 https://doi.org/10.1227/01.NEU.0000108642.88724.DB

168. Whalen MJ, Carlos TM, Kochanek PM, et al. Interleukin-8 is increased in cerebrospinal fluid of children with severe head injury. *Crit Care Med*. 2000;28(4):929–934 PMID: 10809261 https://doi.org/10.1097/00003246-200004000-00003
169. Kochanek PM, Clark RSB, Ruppel RA, et al. Biochemical, cellular, and molecular mechanisms in the evolution of secondary damage after severe traumatic brain injury in infants and children: lessons learned from the bedside. *Pediatr Crit Care Med*. 2000;1(1):4–19 PMID: 12813280 https://doi.org/10.1097/00130478-200007000-00003
170. Berger RP, Kochanek PM, Pierce MC. Biochemical markers of brain injury: could they be used as diagnostic adjuncts in cases of inflicted traumatic brain injury? *Child Abuse Negl*. 2004;28(7):739–754 PMID: 15261469 https://doi.org/10.1016/j.chiabu.2004.01.007
171. Ruppel RA, Clark RSB, Bayir H, Satchell MA, Kochanek PM. Critical mechanisms of secondary damage after inflicted head injury in infants and children. *Neurosurg Clin N Am*. 2002;13(2):169–182, v PMID: 12391702 https://doi.org/10.1016/S1042-3680(01)00005-5
172. Wagner AK, Bayir H, Ren D, Puccio A, Zafonte RD, Kochanek PM. Relationships between cerebrospinal fluid markers of excitotoxicity, ischemia, and oxidative damage after severe TBI: the impact of gender, age, and hypothermia. *J Neurotrauma*. 2004;21(2):125–136 PMID: 15000754 https://doi.org/10.1089/089771504322778596
173. Bittigau P, Sifringer M, Pohl D, et al. Apoptotic neurodegeneration following trauma is markedly enhanced in the immature brain. *Ann Neurol*. 1999;45(6):724–735 PMID: 10360764 https://doi.org/10.1002/1531-8249(199906)45:6<724::AID-ANA6>3.0.CO;2-P
174. Lee KS, Bae WK, Bae HG, Doh JW, Yun IG. The computed tomographic attenuation and the age of subdural hematomas. *J Korean Med Sci*. 1997;12(4):353–359 PMID: 9288636 https://doi.org/10.3346/jkms.1997.12.4.353
175. Lee K-S. The pathogenesis and clinical significance of traumatic subdural hygroma. *Brain Inj*. 1998;12(7):595–603 PMID: 9653522 https://doi.org/10.1080/026990598122359
176. Lee KS, Bae WK, Doh JW, Bae HG, Yun IG. Origin of chronic subdural haematoma and relation to traumatic subdural lesions. *Brain Inj*. 1998;12(11):901–910 PMID: 9839025 https://doi.org/10.1080/026990598121972
177. Lee K-S, Bae W-K, Bae H-G, Yun IG. The fate of traumatic subdural hygroma in serial computed tomographic scans. *J Korean Med Sci*. 2000;15(5):560–568 PMID: 11068995 https://doi.org/10.3346/jkms.2000.15.5.560
178. Zouros A, Bhargava R, Hoskinson M, Aronyk KE. Further characterization of traumatic subdural collections of infancy. Report of five cases. *J Neurosurg*. 2004;100(5 suppl):512–518 PMID: 15287465
179. Kivlin JD, Currie ML, Greenbaum VJ, Simons KB, Jentzen J. Retinal hemorrhages in children following fatal motor vehicle crashes: a case series. *Arch Ophthalmol*. 2008;126(6):800–804 PMID: 18541842 https://doi.org/10.1001/archopht.126.6.800
180. Coats B, Binenbaum G, Peiffer RL, Forbes BJ, Margulies SS. Ocular hemorrhages in neonatal porcine eyes from single, rapid rotational events. *Invest Ophthalmol Vis Sci*. 2010;51(9):4792–4797 PMID: 20435592 https://doi.org/10.1167/iovs.10-5211
181. Yoshida M, Yamazaki J, Mizunuma H. A finite element analysis of the retinal hemorrhages accompanied by shaken baby syndrome/abusive head trauma. *J Biomech*. 2014;47(14):3454–3458 PMID: 25282076 https://doi.org/10.1016/j.jbiomech.2014.09.014
182. Nadarasa J, Deck C, Meyer F, Raul JS, Willinger R. Infant eye finite element model to investigate retinal hemorrhages after fall and shaking events. *Comput Methods Biomech Biomed Engin*. 2015;18(sup1)(suppl 1):2016–2017 PMID: 26230636 https://doi.org/10.1080/10255842.2015.1069602
183. Rangarajan N, Kamalakkannan SB, Hasija V, et al. Finite element model of ocular injury in abusive head trauma. *J AAPOS*. 2009;13(4):364–369 PMID: 19419890 https://doi.org/10.1016/j.jaapos.2008.11.006

184. Rojas M, Walker-Descartes I, Laraque-Arena D. An experimental study of implicit racial bias in recognition of child abuse. *Am J Health Behav.* 2017;41(3):358–367 PMID: 28376980 https://doi.org/10.5993/AJHB.41.3.15
185. Wood JN, Hall M, Schilling S, Keren R, Mitra N, Rubin DM. Disparities in the evaluation and diagnosis of abuse among infants with traumatic brain injury. *Pediatrics.* 2010;126(3):408–414 PMID: 20713477 https://doi.org/10.1542/peds.2010-0031
186. Keenan HT, Campbell KA, Page K, Cook LJ, Bardsley T, Olson LM. Perceived social risk in medical decision-making for physical child abuse: a mixed-methods study. *BMC Pediatr.* 2017;17(1):214 PMID: 29273019 https://doi.org/10.1186/s12887-017-0969-7
187. Atwal GS, Rutty GN, Carter N, Green MA. Bruising in non-accidental head injured children; a retrospective study of the prevalence, distribution and pathological associations in 24 cases. *Forensic Sci Int.* 1998;96(2-3):215–230 PMID: 9854835 https://doi.org/10.1016/S0379-0738(98)00126-1
188. Hymel KP, Willson DF, Boos SC, et al; Pediatric Brain Injury Research Network (PediBIRN) Investigators. Derivation of a clinical prediction rule for pediatric abusive head trauma. *Pediatr Crit Care Med.* 2013;14(2):210–220 PMID: 23314183 https://doi.org/10.1097/PCC.0b013e3182712b09
189. Pierce MC, Kaczor K, Aldridge S, O'Flynn J, Lorenz DJ. Bruising characteristics discriminating physical child abuse from accidental trauma. *Pediatrics.* 2010;125(1): 67–74 PMID: 19969620 https://doi.org/10.1542/peds.2008-3632
190. Odom A, Christ E, Kerr N, et al. Prevalence of retinal hemorrhages in pediatric patients after in-hospital cardiopulmonary resuscitation: a prospective study. *Pediatrics.* 1997;99(6):E3 PMID: 9164799 https://doi.org/10.1542/peds.99.6.e3
191. Maguire S, Mann M, John N, Ellaway B, Sibert JR, Kemp AM; Welsh Child Protection Systematic Review Group. Does cardiopulmonary resuscitation cause rib fractures in children? A systematic review. *Child Abuse Negl.* 2006;30(7):739–751 PMID: 16857258 https://doi.org/10.1016/j.chiabu.2005.12.007
192. Matshes EW, Lew EO. Do resuscitation-related injuries kill infants and children? *Am J Forensic Med Pathol.* 2010;31(2):178–185 PMID: 20436339 https://doi.org/10.1097/PAF.0b013e3181df62ee
193. Martin PS, Jones MD, Maguire SA, Theobald PS, Kemp AM. Increased incidence of CPR-related rib fractures in infants—is it related to changes in CPR technique? *Resuscitation.* 2012;83(4):e109 PMID: 22269097 https://doi.org/10.1016/j.resuscitation.2011.08.034
194. Franke I, Pingen A, Schiffmann H, et al; for Arbeitsgemeinschaft Kinderschutz in der Medizin. Cardiopulmonary resuscitation (CPR)-related posterior rib fractures in neonates and infants following recommended changes in CPR techniques. *Child Abuse Negl.* 2014;38(7):1267–1274 PMID: 24636360 https://doi.org/10.1016/j.chiabu.2014.01.021
195. Ondruschka B, Baier C, Siekmeyer M, Buschmann C, Dreßler J, Bernhard M. Cardiopulmonary resuscitation-associated injuries in still-/newborns, infants and toddlers in a German forensic collective. *Forensic Sci Int.* 2017;279:235–240 PMID: 28926779 https://doi.org/10.1016/j.forsciint.2017.09.007
196. Levin AV, Christian CW; American Academy of Pediatrics Committee on Child Abuse and Neglect, Section on Ophthalmology. The eye examination in the evaluation of child abuse. *Pediatrics.* 2010;126(2):376–380 PMID: 20660545 https://doi.org/10.1542/peds.2010-1397
197. Thackeray JD, Scribano PV, Lindberg DM. Yield of retinal examination in suspected physical abuse with normal neuroimaging. *Pediatrics.* 2010;125(5):e1066–e1071 PMID: 20385633 https://doi.org/10.1542/peds.2009-2184
198. Li S, Mitchell E, Fromkin J, Berger RP. Retinal hemorrhages in low-risk children evaluated for physical abuse. *Arch Pediatr Adolesc Med.* 2011;165(10):913–917 PMID: 21969393 https://doi.org/10.1001/archpediatrics.2011.150

199. Greiner MV, Berger RP, Thackeray JD, Lindberg DM; Examining Siblings to Recognize Abuse (ExSTRA) Investigators. Dedicated retinal examination in children evaluated for physical abuse without radiographically identified traumatic brain injury. *J Pediatr.* 2013;163(2):527–531 PMID: 23498157 https://doi.org/10.1016/j.jpeds.2013.01.063
200. Morad Y, Kim YM, Mian M, Huyer D, Capra L, Levin AV. Nonophthalmologist accuracy in diagnosing retinal hemorrhages in the shaken baby syndrome. *J Pediatr.* 2003;142(4):431–434 PMID: 12712063 https://doi.org/10.1067/mpd.2003.161
201. Saleh M, Schoenlaub S, Desprez P, et al. Use of digital camera imaging of eye fundus for telemedicine in children suspected of abusive head injury. *Br J Ophthalmol.* 2009;93(4):424–428 PMID: 19019943 https://doi.org/10.1136/bjo.2008.147561
202. Yusuf IH, Barnes JK, Fung THM, Elston JS, Patel CK; Medscape. Non-contact ultra-widefield retinal imaging of infants with suspected abusive head trauma. *Eye (Lond).* 2017;31(3):353–363 PMID: 28234351 https://doi.org/10.1038/eye.2017.2
203. Tandon A, McIntyre S, Yu A, et al. Retinal haemorrhage description tool. *Br J Ophthalmol.* 2011;95(12):1719–1722 PMID: 21984780 https://doi.org/10.1136/bjophthalmol-2011-300248
204. Ng WS, Watts P, Lawson Z, Kemp A, Maguire S. Development and validation of a standardized tool for reporting retinal findings in abusive head trauma. *Am J Ophthalmol.* 2012;154(2):333–339.e5 PMID: 22542369 https://doi.org/10.1016/j.ajo.2012.02.007
205. Chhabra MS, Bonsall DJ, Cassedy AE, Wallace GH, Schoenberger SD, West CE. Reliability of grading retinal hemorrhages in abusive head trauma. *J AAPOS.* 2013;17(4):343–346 PMID: 23911129 https://doi.org/10.1016/j.jaapos.2013.03.022
206. Beavers AJ, Stagner AM, Allbery SM, Lyden ER, Hejkal TW, Haney SB. MR detection of retinal hemorrhages: correlation with graded ophthalmologic exam. *Pediatr Radiol.* 2015;45(9):1363–1371 PMID: 25737098 https://doi.org/10.1007/s00247-015-3312-1
207. Hwang M, Shin SS, Thimm MA, et al. Apparent diffusion coefficient (ADC) of the vitreous humor and susceptibility weighted imaging (SWI) of the retina in abused children with retinal hemorrhages. *Clin Imaging.* 2017;44:38–41 PMID: 28399448 https://doi.org/10.1016/j.clinimag.2017.03.017
208. Wygnanski-Jaffe T, Levin AV, Shafiq A, et al. Postmortem orbital findings in shaken baby syndrome. *Am J Ophthalmol.* 2006;142(2):233–240 PMID: 16876502 https://doi.org/10.1016/j.ajo.2006.03.038
209. Matschke J, Püschel K, Glatzel M. Ocular pathology in shaken baby syndrome and other forms of infantile non-accidental head injury. *Int J Legal Med.* 2009;123(3):189–197 PMID: 18936952 https://doi.org/10.1007/s00414-008-0293-8
210. Del Bigio MR, Phillips SM. Retroocular and subdural hemorrhage or hemosiderin deposits in pediatric autopsies. *J Neuropathol Exp Neurol.* 2017;76(4):313–322 PMID: 28340081 https://doi.org/10.1093/jnen/nlx010
211. Puanglumyai S, Lekawanvijit S. The importance of optic nerve sheath hemorrhage as a postmortem finding in cases of fatal abusive head trauma: a 13-year study in a tertiary hospital. *Forensic Sci Int.* 2017;276:5–11 PMID: 28458085 https://doi.org/10.1016/j.forsciint.2017.04.008
212. Palifka LA, Frasier LD, Metzger RR, Hedlund GL. Parenchymal brain laceration as a predictor of abusive head trauma. *AJNR Am J Neuroradiol.* 2016;37(1):163–168 PMID: 26471745 https://doi.org/10.3174/ajnr.A4519
213. Choudhary AK, Jha B, Boal DK, Dias M. Occipital sutures and its variations: the value of 3D-CT and how to differentiate it from fractures using 3D-CT? *Surg Radiol Anat.* 2010;32(9):807–816 PMID: 20174986 https://doi.org/10.1007/s00276-010-0633-5

214. Kralik SF, Yasrebi M, Supakul N, et al. Diagnostic performance of ultrafast brain MRI for evaluation of abusive head trauma. *AJNR Am J Neuroradiol*. 2017;38(4):807–813 PMID: 28183837 https://doi.org/10.3174/ajnr.A5093
215. Choudhary AK, Bradford RK, Dias MS, Moore GJ, Boal DKB. Spinal subdural hemorrhage in abusive head trauma: a retrospective study. *Radiology*. 2012;262(1): 216–223 PMID: 22069156 https://doi.org/10.1148/radiol.11102390
216. Feldman KW, Weinberger E, Milstein JM, Fligner CL. Cervical spine MRI in abused infants. *Child Abuse Negl*. 1997;21(2):199–205 PMID: 9056099 https://doi.org/10.1016/S0145-2134(96)00145-7
217. Kadom N, Khademian Z, Vezina G, Shalaby-Rana E, Rice A, Hinds T. Usefulness of MRI detection of cervical spine and brain injuries in the evaluation of abusive head trauma. *Pediatr Radiol*. 2014;44(7):839–848 PMID: 24557483 https://doi.org/10.1007/s00247-014-2874-7
218. Ashwal S, Tong KA, Ghosh N, Bartnik-Olson B, Holshouser BA. Application of advanced neuroimaging modalities in pediatric traumatic brain injury. *J Child Neurol*. 2014;29(12):1704–1717 PMID: 24958007 https://doi.org/10.1177/0883073814538504
219. Ashwal S, Wycliffe ND, Holshouser BA. Advanced neuroimaging in children with nonaccidental trauma. *Dev Neurosci*. 2010;32(5-6):343–360 PMID: 20938158 https://doi.org/10.1159/000316801
220. Wright JN. CNS injuries in abusive head trauma. *AJR Am J Roentgenol*. 2017;208(5): 991–1001 PMID: 28245144 https://doi.org/10.2214/AJR.16.17602
221. Hedlund GL, Frasier LD. Neuroimaging of abusive head trauma. Forensic Sci Med Pathol. 2009;5(4):280–290 PMID: 20012715
222. Fernando S, Obaldo RE, Walsh IR, Lowe LH. Neuroimaging of nonaccidental head trauma: pitfalls and controversies. *Pediatr Radiol*. 2008;38(8):827–838 PMID: 18176805 https://doi.org/10.1007/s00247-007-0729-1
223. Guler I, Buyukterzi M, Oner O, Tolu I. Post-traumatic leptomeningeal cyst in a child: computed tomography and magnetic resonance imaging findings. *J Emerg Med*. 2015;48(5):e121–e122 PMID: 25662419 https://doi.org/10.1016/j.jemermed.2014.12.042
224. Culotta PA, Crowe JE, Tran QA, et al. Performance of computed tomography of the head to evaluate for skull fractures in infants with suspected non-accidental trauma. *Pediatr Radiol*. 2017;47(1):74–81 PMID: 27744559 https://doi.org/10.1007/s00247-016-3707-7
225. Case ME, Graham MA, Handy TC, Jentzen JM, Monteleone JA; National Association of Medical Examiners Ad Hoc Committee on Shaken Baby Syndrome. Position paper on fatal abusive head injuries in infants and young children. *Am J Forensic Med Pathol*. 2001;22(2):112–122 PMID: 11394743 https://doi.org/10.1097/00000433-200106000-00002
226. Rorke LB. Neuropathology. In: Kornberg AE, ed. *Child Abuse A Medical Reference*. New York, NY: Churchill Livingstone; 1992:403–422
227. King WJ, MacKay M, Sirnick A; Canadian Shaken Baby Study Group. Shaken baby syndrome in Canada: clinical characteristics and outcomes of hospital cases. *CMAJ*. 2003;168(2):155–159 PMID: 12538542
228. Alexander R, Sato Y, Smith W, Bennett T. Incidence of impact trauma with cranial injuries ascribed to shaking. *Am J Dis Child*. 1990;144(6):724–726 PMID: 2346156 https://doi.org/10.1001/archpedi.1990.02150300124032
229. Hobbs CJ. Skull fracture and the diagnosis of abuse. *Arch Dis Child*. 1984;59(3):246–252 PMID: 6712273 https://doi.org/10.1136/adc.59.3.246
230. Meservy CJ, Towbin R, McLaurin RL, Myers PA, Ball W. Radiographic characteristics of skull fractures resulting from child abuse. *AJR Am J Roentgenol*. 1987;149(1):173–175 PMID: 3495978 https://doi.org/10.2214/ajr.149.1.173

231. Barber I, Kleinman PK. Imaging of skeletal injuries associated with abusive head trauma. *Pediatr Radiol*. 2014;44(S4)(suppl 4):S613–S620 PMID: 25501733 https://doi.org/10.1007/s00247-014-3099-5
232. Hymel KP, Rumack CM, Hay TC, Strain JD, Jenny C. Comparison of intracranial computed tomographic (CT) findings in pediatric abusive and accidental head trauma. *Pediatr Radiol*. 1997;27(9):743–747 PMID: 9285736 https://doi.org/10.1007/s002470050215
233. Sinal SH, Ball MR. Head trauma due to child abuse: serial computerized tomography in diagnosis and management. *South Med J*. 1987;80(12):1505–1512 PMID: 3423894 https://doi.org/10.1097/00007611-198712000-00006
234. Zimmerman RA, Bilaniuk LT, Bruce D, Schut L, Uzzell B, Goldberg HI. Computed tomography of craniocerebral injury in the abused child. *Radiology*. 1979;130(3):687–690 PMID: 424539 https://doi.org/10.1148/130.3.687
235. Zimmerman RA, Bilaniuk LT, Bruce D, Schut L, Uzzell B, Goldberg HI. Interhemispheric acute subdural hematoma: a computed tomographic manifestation of child abuse by shaking. *Neuroradiology*. 1978;16(1):39–40 PMID: 740207 https://doi.org/10.1007/BF00395197
236. Vinchon M, Noulé N, Tchofo PJ, Soto-Ares G, Fourier C, Dhellemmes P. Imaging of head injuries in infants: temporal correlates and forensic implications for the diagnosis of child abuse. *J Neurosurg*. 2004;101(1)(suppl):44–52 PMID: 16206971 https://doi.org/10.3171/ped.2004.101.2.0044
237. Sargent S, Kennedy JG, Kaplan JA. "Hyperacute" subdural hematoma: CT mimic of recurrent episodes of bleeding in the setting of child abuse. *J Forensic Sci*. 1996;41(2):314–316 PMID: 8871392 https://doi.org/10.1520/JFS15434J
238. Barnes PD, Robson CD. CT findings in hyperacute nonaccidental brain injury. *Pediatr Radiol*. 2000;30(2):74–81 PMID: 10663515 https://doi.org/10.1007/s002470050018
239. Gomori JM, Grossman RI, Goldberg HI, Zimmerman RA, Bilaniuk LT. Intracranial hematomas: imaging by high-field MR. *Radiology*. 1985;157(1):87–93 PMID: 4034983 https://doi.org/10.1148/radiology.157.1.4034983
240. Temkin NR, Dikmen SS, Wilensky AJ, Keihm J, Chabal S, Winn HR. A randomized, double-blind study of phenytoin for the prevention of post-traumatic seizures. *N Engl J Med*. 1990;323(8):497–502 PMID: 2115976 https://doi.org/10.1056/NEJM199008233230801
241. Wittschieber D, Karger B, Niederstadt T, Pfeiffer H, Hahnemann ML. Subdural hygromas in abusive head trauma: pathogenesis, diagnosis, and forensic implications. *AJNR Am J Neuroradiol*. 2015;36(3):432–439 PMID: 24948499 https://doi.org/10.3174/ajnr.A3989
242. Colbert CA, Holshouser BA, Aaen GS, et al. Value of cerebral microhemorrhages detected with susceptibility-weighted MR Imaging for prediction of long-term outcome in children with nonaccidental trauma. *Radiology*. 2010;256(3):898–905 PMID: 20720073 https://doi.org/10.1148/radiol.10091842
243. Biousse V, Suh DY, Newman NJ, Davis PC, Mapstone T, Lambert SR. Diffusion-weighted magnetic resonance imaging in shaken baby syndrome. *Am J Ophthalmol*. 2002;133(2):249–255 PMID: 11812430 https://doi.org/10.1016/S0002-9394(01)01366-6
244. Foster KA, Recker MJ, Lee PS, Bell MJ, Tyler-Kabara EC. Factors associated with hemispheric hypodensity after subdural hematoma following abusive head trauma in children. *J Neurotrauma*. 2014;31(19):1625–1631 PMID: 24693985 https://doi.org/10.1089/neu.2014.3372
245. Zimmerman RA, Bilaniuk LT, Farina L. Non-accidental brain trauma in infants: diffusion imaging, contributions to understanding the injury process. *J Neuroradiol*. 2007;34(2):109–114 PMID: 17445894 https://doi.org/10.1016/j.neurad.2007.01.124

246. Han BK, Towbin RB, De Courten-Myers G, McLaurin RL, Ball WS Jr. Reversal sign on CT: effect of anoxic/ischemic cerebral injury in children. *AJNR Am J Neuroradiol.* 1989;10(6):1191–1198 PMID: 2512781
247. Duhaime AC, Durham S. Traumatic brain injury in infants: the phenomenon of subdural hemorrhage with hemispheric hypodensity ("Big Black Brain"). *Prog Brain Res.* 2007;161:293–302 PMID: 17618985 https://doi.org/10.1016/S0079-6123(06)61020-0
248. Peterson JE, Love JC, Pinto DC, Wolf DA, Sandberg G. A novel method for removing a spinal cord with attached cervical ganglia from a pediatric decedent. *J Forensic Sci.* 2016;61(1):241–244 PMID: 26296423 https://doi.org/10.1111/1556-4029.12925
249. Governale LS, Brink FW, Pluto CP, et al. A retrospective study of cervical spine MRI findings in children with abusive head trauma. *Pediatr Neurosurg.* 2018;53(1):36–42 PMID: 29084406 https://doi.org/10.1159/000481511
250. Henry MK, Zonfrillo MR, French B, Song L, Feudtner C, Wood JN. Hospital variation in cervical spine imaging of young children with traumatic brain injury. *Acad Pediatr.* 2016;16(7):684–691 PMID: 26854208 https://doi.org/10.1016/j.acap.2016.01.017
251. Baerg J, Thirumoorthi A, Vannix R, Taha A, Young A, Zouros A. Cervical spine imaging for young children with inflicted trauma: Expanding the injury pattern. *J Pediatr Surg.* 2017;52(5):816–821 PMID: 28190553 https://doi.org/10.1016/j.jpedsurg.2017.01.049
252. Silvera VM, Danehy AR, Newton AW, et al. Retroclival collections associated with abusive head trauma in children. *Pediatr Radiol.* 2014;44(S4)(suppl 4):S621–S631 PMID: 25501734 https://doi.org/10.1007/s00247-014-3170-2
253. Hadley MN, Zabramski JM, Browner CM, Rekate H, Sonntag VK. Pediatric spinal trauma. Review of 122 cases of spinal cord and vertebral column injuries. *J Neurosurg.* 1988;68(1):18–24 PMID: 3335907 https://doi.org/10.3171/jns.1988.68.1.0018
254. Williams VL, Hogg JP. Magnetic resonance imaging of chronic subdural hematoma. *Neurosurg Clin N Am.* 2000;11(3):491–498 PMID: 10918019 https://doi.org/10.1016/S1042-3680(18)30112-8
255. American Academy of Pediatrics Section on Radiology. Diagnostic imaging of child abuse. *Pediatrics.* 2009;123(5):1430–1435 PMID: 19403511 https://doi.org/10.1542/peds.2009-0558
256. Paine CW, Scribano PV, Localio R, Wood JN. Development of guidelines for skeletal survey in young children with intracranial hemorrhage. *Pediatrics.* 2016;137(4):137 PMID: 26956102 https://doi.org/10.1542/peds.2015-3024
257. Acker SN, Partrick DA, Ross JT, Nadlonek NA, Bronsert M, Bensard DD. Head injury and unclear mechanism of injury: initial hematocrit less than 30 is predictive of abusive head trauma in young children. *J Pediatr Surg.* 2014;49(2):338–340 PMID: 24528981 https://doi.org/10.1016/j.jpedsurg.2013.10.008
258. Anderst JD, Carpenter SL, Abshire TC; American Academy of Pediatrics Section on Hematology/Oncology and Committee on Child Abuse and Neglect. Evaluation for bleeding disorders in suspected child abuse. *Pediatrics.* 2013;131(4):e1314–e1322 PMID: 23530182 https://doi.org/10.1542/peds.2013-0195
259. Scavarda D, Gabaudan C, Ughetto F, et al. Initial predictive factors of outcome in severe non-accidental head trauma in children. *Childs Nerv Syst.* 2010;26(11):1555–1561 PMID: 20461522 https://doi.org/10.1007/s00381-010-1150-x
260. Leeper CM, Nasr I, McKenna C, Berger RP, Gaines BA. Elevated admission international normalized ratio strongly predicts mortality in victims of abusive head trauma. *J Trauma Acute Care Surg.* 2016;80(5):711–716 PMID: 27100929 https://doi.org/10.1097/TA.0000000000000954

261. Coant PN, Kornberg AE, Brody AS, Edwards-Holmes K. Markers for occult liver injury in cases of physical abuse in children. *Pediatrics*. 1992;89(2):274–278 PMID: 1734396
262. Lindberg D, Makoroff K, Harper N, et al; ULTRA Investigators. Utility of hepatic transaminases to recognize abuse in children. *Pediatrics*. 2009;124(2):509–516 PMID: 19620197 https://doi.org/10.1542/peds.2008-2348
263. Lindberg DM, Lindsell CJ, Shapiro RA. Variability in expert assessments of child physical abuse likelihood. *Pediatrics*. 2008;121(4):e945–e953 PMID: 18381522 https://doi.org/10.1542/peds.2007-2485
264. Dias MS. Inflicted head injury: future directions and prevention. *Neurosurg Clin N Am*. 2002;13(2):247–257 PMID: 12391709 https://doi.org/10.1016/S1042-3680(01)00009-2
265. Gruskin KD, Schutzman SA. Head trauma in children younger than 2 years: are there predictors for complications? *Arch Pediatr Adolesc Med*. 1999;153(1):15–20 PMID: 9894994 https://doi.org/10.1001/archpedi.153.1.15
266. Trenchs V, Curcoy AI, Morales M, Serra A, Navarro R, Pou J. Retinal haemorrhages in-head trauma resulting from falls: differential diagnosis with non-accidental trauma in patients younger than 2 years of age. *Childs Nerv Syst*. 2008;24(7):815–820 PMID: 18270718 https://doi.org/10.1007/s00381-008-0583-y
267. Chadwick DL, Bertocci G, Castillo E, et al. Annual risk of death resulting from short falls among young children: less than 1 in 1 million. *Pediatrics*. 2008;121(6):1213–1224 PMID: 18519492 https://doi.org/10.1542/peds.2007-2281
268. Lyons TJ, Oates RK. Falling out of bed: a relatively benign occurrence. *Pediatrics*. 1993;92(1):125–127 PMID: 8516057
269. Levene S, Bonfield G. Accidents on hospital wards. *Arch Dis Child*. 1991;66(9):1047–1049 PMID: 1929510 https://doi.org/10.1136/adc.66.9.1047
270. Monson SA, Henry E, Lambert DK, Schmutz N, Christensen RD. In-hospital falls of newborn infants: data from a multihospital health care system. *Pediatrics*. 2008;122(2):e277–e280 PMID: 18676512 https://doi.org/10.1542/peds.2007-3811
271. Ruddick C, Platt MW, Lazaro C. Head trauma outcomes of verifiable falls in newborn babies. *Arch Dis Child Fetal Neonatal Ed*. 2010;95(2):F144–F145. PMID: 20231220 PMID: 20231220
272. Williams RA. Injuries in infants and small children resulting from witnessed and corroborated free falls. *J Trauma*. 1991;31(10):1350–1352 PMID: 1942141 https://doi.org/10.1097/00005373-199110000-00005
273. Benoit R, Watts DD, Dwyer K, Kaufmann C, Fakhry S. Windows 99: a source of suburban pediatric trauma. *J Trauma*. 2000;49(3):477–482 PMID: 11003326 https://doi.org/10.1097/00005373-200009000-00015
274. Zielinski AE, Rochette LM, Smith GA. Stair-related injuries to young children treated in US emergency departments, 1999-2008. *Pediatrics*. 2012;129(4):721–727 PMID: 22412031 https://doi.org/10.1542/peds.2011-2314
275. Joffe M, Ludwig S. Stairway injuries in children. *Pediatrics*. 1988;82(3 Pt 2):457–461 PMID: 3405681
276. Docherty E, Hassan A, Burke D. Things that go bump...bump...bump: an analysis of injuries from falling down stairs in children based at Sheffield Children's Hospital. *Emerg Med J*. 2010;27(3):207–208 PMID: 20304888 https://doi.org/10.1136/emj.2008.069179
277. Greeley C. Commentary on: Lantz PE, Couture DE. Fatal acute intracranial injury, subdural hematoma, and retinal hemorrhages caused by stairway fall. J Forensic Sci 2011;56(6):1648-53. *J Forensic Sci*. 2012;57(2):560–561 PMID: 22356693 https://doi.org/10.1111/j.1556-4029.2012.02060.x

278. Partington MD, Swanson JA, Meyer FB. Head injury and the use of baby walkers: a continuing problem. *Ann Emerg Med*. 1991;20(6):652–654 PMID: 2039104 https://doi.org/10.1016/S0196-0644(05)82386-8
279. Chiaviello CT, Christoph RA, Bond GR. Infant walker-related injuries: a prospective study of severity and incidence. *Pediatrics*. 1994;93(6 Pt 1):974–976 PMID: 8190586
280. Steinbok P, Singhal A, Poskitt K, Cochrane DD. Early hypodensity on computed tomographic scan of the brain in an accidental pediatric head injury. *Neurosurgery*. 2007;60(4):689–695 PMID: 17415206 https://doi.org/10.1227/01.NEU.0000255398.00410.6B
281. Denton S, Mileusnic D. Delayed sudden death in an infant following an accidental fall: a case report with review of the literature. *Am J Forensic Med Pathol*. 2003;24(4):371–376 PMID: 14634479 https://doi.org/10.1097/01.paf.0000097851.18478.16
282. Atkinson N, van Rijn RR, Starling SP. Childhood falls with occipital impacts. *Pediatr Emerg Care*. 2018;34(12):837–847 PMID: 28590993 https://doi.org/10.1097/PEC.0000000000001186
283. Wigglesworth JS, Pape KE. Pathophysiology of intracranial haemorrhage in the newborn. *J Perinat Med*. 1980;8(3):119–133 PMID: 6999146
284. Leblanc R, O'Gorman AM. Neonatal intracranial hemorrhage. A clinical and serial computerized tomographic study. *J Neurosurg*. 1980;53(5):642–651 PMID: 7431073 https://doi.org/10.3171/jns.1980.53.5.0642
285. Bergman I, Bauer RE, Barmada MA, et al. Intracerebral hemorrhage in the full-term neonatal infant. *Pediatrics*. 1985;75(3):488–496 PMID: 3975118
286. Hovind KH. Traumatic birth injuries. In: Raimondi AJ, Choux M, DiRocco C, eds. *Head Injuries in the Newborn and Infant*. New York: Springer Verlag; 1986:87–109 https://doi.org/10.1007/978-1-4615-7183-4_7
287. Takagi T, Fukuoka H, Wakabayashi S, Nagai H, Shibata T. Posterior fossa subdural hemorrhage in the newborn as a result of birth trauma. *Childs Brain*. 1982;9(2):102–113 PMID: 7094671 https://doi.org/10.1159/000120042
288. Wigglesworth JS, Husemeyer RP. Intracranial birth trauma in vaginal breech delivery: the continued importance of injury to the occipital bone. *Br J Obstet Gynaecol*. 1977;84(9):684–691 PMID: 911720 https://doi.org/10.1111/j.1471-0528.1977.tb12681.x
289. Currarino G. Occipital osteodiastasis: presentation of four cases and review of the literature. *Pediatr Radiol*. 2000;30(12):823–829 PMID: 11149088 https://doi.org/10.1007/s002470000337
290. Holden KR, Titus MO, Van Tassel P. Cranial magnetic resonance imaging examination of normal term neonates: a pilot study. *J Child Neurol*. 1999;14(11):708–710 PMID: 10593546 https://doi.org/10.1177/088307389901401104
291. Heibel M, Heber R, Bechinger D, Kornhuber HH. Early diagnosis of perinatal cerebral lesions in apparently normal full-term newborns by ultrasound of the brain. *Neuroradiology*. 1993;35(2):85–91 PMID: 8433799 https://doi.org/10.1007/BF00593960
292. Hughes LA, May K, Talbot JF, Parsons MA. Incidence, distribution, and duration of birth-related retinal hemorrhages: a prospective study. *J AAPOS*. 2006;10(2):102–106 PMID: 16678742 https://doi.org/10.1016/j.jaapos.2005.12.005
293. Watts P, Maguire S, Kwok T, et al. Newborn retinal hemorrhages: a systematic review. *J AAPOS*. 2013;17(1):70–78 PMID: 23363882 https://doi.org/10.1016/j.jaapos.2012.07.012
294. Goyal P, Padhi TR, Das T, et al. Outcome of universal newborn eye screening with wide-field digital retinal image acquisition system: a pilot study. *Eye (Lond)*. 2018;32(1):67–73 PMID: 28737759 https://doi.org/10.1038/eye.2017.129

295. Yanli Z, Qi Z, Yu L, Haike G. Risk factors affecting the severity of full-term neonatal retinal hemorrhage. *J Ophthalmol*. 2017;2017:4231489 PMID: 28804645 https://doi.org/10.1155/2017/4231489
296. Peiniger S, Nienaber U, Lefering R, et al; Trauma Registry of the Deutsche Gesellschaft für Unfallchirurgie. Glasgow Coma Scale as a predictor for hemocoagulative disorders after blunt pediatric traumatic brain injury. *Pediatr Crit Care Med*. 2012;13(4):455–460 PMID: 22422166 https://doi.org/10.1097/PCC.0b013e31823893c5
297. Hymel KP, Abshire TC, Luckey DW, Jenny C. Coagulopathy in pediatric abusive head trauma. *Pediatrics*. 1997;99(3):371–375 PMID: 9041291 https://doi.org/10.1542/peds.99.3.371
298. Liras IN, Caplan HW, Stensballe J, Wade CE, Cox CS, Cotton BA. Prevalence and impact of admission acute traumatic coagulopathy on treatment intensity, resource use, and mortality: an evaluation of 956 severely injured children and adolescents. *J Am Coll Surg*. 2017;224(4):625–632 PMID: 28131925 https://doi.org/10.1016/j.jamcollsurg.2016.12.046
299. Rutty GN, Smith CM, Malia RG. Late-form hemorrhagic disease of the newborn: a fatal case report with illustration of investigations that may assist in avoiding the mistaken diagnosis of child abuse. *Am J Forensic Med Pathol*. 1999;20(1):48–51 PMID: 10208337 https://doi.org/10.1097/00000433-199903000-00012
300. Ozdemir MA, Karakukcu M, Per H, Unal E, Gumus H, Patiroglu T. Late-type vitamin K deficiency bleeding: experience from 120 patients. *Childs Nerv Syst*. 2012;28(2):247–251 PMID: 21928065 https://doi.org/10.1007/s00381-011-1575-x
301. Brousseau TJ, Kissoon N, McIntosh B. Vitamin K deficiency mimicking child abuse. *J Emerg Med*. 2005;29(3):283–288 PMID: 16183447 https://doi.org/10.1016/j.jemermed.2005.02.009
302. Siauw C, Wirbelauer J, Schweitzer T, Speer CP. Late vitamin K deficient bleeding in 2 young infants—renaissance of a preventable disease. *Z Geburtshilfe Neonatol*. 2015;219(5):238–242 PMID: 26556811 https://doi.org/10.1055/s-0035-1555873
303. Kassis KL, Wada KJ, Milton A. Another disease re-emerges due to parental shot refusal: case report of a fussy infant with blood in stool. *J Emerg Med*. 2015;49(1):e15–e17 PMID: 25841290 https://doi.org/10.1016/j.jemermed.2015.02.022
304. Jackson J, Carpenter S, Anderst J. Challenges in the evaluation for possible abuse: presentations of congenital bleeding disorders in childhood. *Child Abuse Negl*. 2012;36(2):127–134 PMID: 22398301 https://doi.org/10.1016/j.chiabu.2011.09.009
305. Acharya SS. Rare bleeding disorders in children: identification and primary care management. *Pediatrics*. 2013;132(5):882–892 PMID: 24127475 https://doi.org/10.1542/peds.2012-3662
306. Paroskie A, Carpenter SL, Lowen DE, Anderst J, DeBaun MR, Sidonio RF Jr. A two-center retrospective review of the hematologic evaluation and laboratory abnormalities in suspected victims of non-accidental injury. *Child Abuse Negl*. 2014;38(11):1794–1800 PMID: 24928052 https://doi.org/10.1016/j.chiabu.2014.05.012
307. Shih SL, Lin JC, Liang DC, Huang JK. Computed tomography of spontaneous intracranial haemorrhage due to haemostatic disorders in children. *Neuroradiology*. 1993;35(8):619–621 PMID: 8278046 https://doi.org/10.1007/BF00588410
308. Vorstman EB, Anslow P, Keeling DM, Haythornthwaite G, Bilolikar H, McShane MT. Brain haemorrhage in five infants with coagulopathy. *Arch Dis Child*. 2003;88(12):1119–1121 PMID: 14670783 https://doi.org/10.1136/adc.88.12.1119
309. Neunert C, Noroozi N, Norman G, et al. Severe bleeding events in adults and children with primary immune thrombocytopenia: a systematic review. *J Thromb Haemost*. 2015;13(3):457–464 PMID: 25495497 https://doi.org/10.1111/jth.12813

310. Alterkait A, Jamjoom R, Ratnapalan S. Head trauma and intracranial hemorrhage in children with idiopathic thrombocytopenic purpura. *Pediatr Emerg Care*. 2015;31(6): 454–458 PMID: 26035504 https://doi.org/10.1097/PEC.0000000000000499
311. Adams GGW, Agrawal S, Sekhri R, Peters MJ, Pierce CM. Appearance and location of retinal haemorrhages in critically ill children. *Br J Ophthalmol*. 2013;97(9):1138–1142 PMID: 23645820 https://doi.org/10.1136/bjophthalmol-2012-302429
312. Agrawal S, Peters MJ, Adams GGW, Pierce CM. Prevalence of retinal hemorrhages in critically ill children. *Pediatrics*. 2012;129(6):e1388–e1396 PMID: 22614777 https://doi.org/10.1542/peds.2011-2772
313. Ulu EMK, Töre HG, Bayrak A, Güngör D, Coşkun M. MRI of central nervous system abnormalities in childhood leukemia. *Diagn Interv Radiol*. 2009;15(2):86–92 PMID: 19517377
314. Ranta S, Tuckuviene R, Mäkipernaa A, et al. Cerebral sinus venous thromboses in children with acute lymphoblastic leukaemia—a multicentre study from the Nordic Society of Paediatric Haematology and Oncology. *Br J Haematol*. 2015;168(4):547–552 PMID: 25288392 https://doi.org/10.1111/bjh.13162
315. Lo WD, Lee J, Rusin J, Perkins E, Roach ES. Intracranial hemorrhage in children: an evolving spectrum. *Arch Neurol*. 2008;65(12):1629–1633 PMID: 19064750 https://doi.org/10.1001/archneurol.2008.502
316. Kato T, Hattori H, Yorifuji T, Tashiro Y, Nakahata T. Intracranial aneurysms in Ehlers-Danlos syndrome type IV in early childhood. *Pediatr Neurol*. 2001;25(4):336–339 PMID: 11704406 https://doi.org/10.1016/S0887-8994(01)00315-0
317. Malfait F, De Paepe A. Bleeding in the heritable connective tissue disorders: mechanisms, diagnosis and treatment. *Blood Rev*. 2009;23(5):191–197 PMID: 19592142 https://doi.org/10.1016/j.blre.2009.06.001
318. Ganesh A, Jenny C, Geyer J, Shouldice M, Levin AV. Retinal hemorrhages in type I osteogenesis imperfecta after minor trauma. *Ophthalmology*. 2004;111(7):1428–1431 PMID: 15234150 https://doi.org/10.1016/j.ophtha.2003.10.028
319. Groninger A, Schaper J, Messing-Juenger M, Mayatepek E, Rosenbaum T. Subdural hematoma as clinical presentation of osteogenesis imperfecta. *Pediatr Neurol*. 2005;32(2):140–142 PMID: 15664779 https://doi.org/10.1016/j.pediatrneurol.2004.07.011
320. Sasaki-Adams D, Kulkarni A, Rutka J, Dirks P, Taylor M, Drake JM. Neurosurgical implications of osteogenesis imperfecta in children. Report of 4 cases. *J Neurosurg Pediatr*. 2008;1(3):229–236 PMID: 18352768 https://doi.org/10.3171/PED/2008/1/3/229
321. Strauss KA, Puffenberger EG, Robinson DL, Morton DH. Type I glutaric aciduria, part 1: natural history of 77 patients. *Am J Med Genet C Semin Med Genet*. 2003;121C(1):38–52 PMID: 12888985 https://doi.org/10.1002/ajmg.c.20007
322. Amador E, Domene R, Fuentes C, Carreño JC, Enríquez G. Long-term skeletal findings in Menkes disease. *Pediatr Radiol*. 2010;40(8):1426–1429 PMID: 20180106 https://doi.org/10.1007/s00247-010-1551-8
323. Jayawant S, Halpin S, Wallace S. Menkes kinky hair disease: an unusual case. *Eur J Paediatr Neurol*. 2000;4(3):131–134 PMID: 10872109 https://doi.org/10.1053/ejpn.2000.0281
324. Bacopoulou F, Henderson L, Philip SG. Menkes disease mimicking non-accidental injury. *Arch Dis Child*. 2006;91(11):919 PMID: 17056864 https://doi.org/10.1136/adc.2005.081836
325. Koprivsek K, Lucic M, Kozic D, Djordjevic M, Kravljanac R. Basal ganglia lesions in the early stage of Menkes disease. *J Inherit Metab Dis*. 2010;33(3):301–302 PMID: 20352341 https://doi.org/10.1007/s10545-010-9063-0

326. Droms RJ, Rork JF, McLean R, Martin M, Belazarian L, Wiss K. Menkes disease mimicking child abuse. *Pediatr Dermatol*. 2017;34(3):e132–e134 PMID: 28318055 https://doi.org/10.1111/pde.13106
327. Lykavieris P, Crosnier C, Trichet C, Meunier-Rotival M, Hadchouel M. Bleeding tendency in children with Alagille syndrome. *Pediatrics*. 2003;111(1):167–170 PMID: 12509572 https://doi.org/10.1542/peds.111.1.167
328. Emerick KM, Krantz ID, Kamath BM, et al. Intracranial vascular abnormalities in patients with Alagille syndrome. *J Pediatr Gastroenterol Nutr*. 2005;41(1):99–107 PMID: 15990638 https://doi.org/10.1097/01.MPG.0000162776.67758.2F
329. Cohn RD, Eklund E, Bergner AL, et al. Intracranial hemorrhage as the initial manifestation of a congenital disorder of glycosylation. *Pediatrics*. 2006;118(2):e514–e521 PMID: 16816004 https://doi.org/10.1542/peds.2005-1307
330. Francis PJ, Calver DM, Barnfield P, Turner C, Dalton RN, Champion MP. An infant with methylmalonic aciduria and homocystinuria (cblC) presenting with retinal haemorrhages and subdural haematoma mimicking non-accidental injury. *Eur J Pediatr*. 2004;163(7):420–421 PMID: 15221473 https://doi.org/10.1007/s00431-004-1440-y
331. Moss C, Wassmer E, Debelle G, et al. Degos disease: a new simulator of non-accidental injury. *Dev Med Child Neurol*. 2009;51(8):647–650 PMID: 19549203 https://doi.org/10.1111/j.1469-8749.2009.03349.x
332. Rooms L, Fitzgerald N, McClain KL. Hemophagocytic lymphohistiocytosis masquerading as child abuse: presentation of three cases and review of central nervous system findings in hemophagocytic lymphohistiocytosis. *Pediatrics*. 2003;111(5 Pt 1):e636–e640 PMID: 12728123 https://doi.org/10.1542/peds.111.5.e636
333. Blaser S. Enlarged subarachnoid spaces. In: Osborn A, ed. *Diagnostic Imaging: Brain*. Salt Lake City, UT: Amirsys; 2004
334. Dias MS, Li V. Pediatric neurosurgical disease. *Pediatr Clin North Am*. 1998;45(6): 1539–1578, x PMID: 9889766 https://doi.org/10.1016/S0031-3955(05)70103-6
335. Kapila A, Trice J, Spies WG, Siegel BA, Gado MH. Enlarged cerebrospinal fluid spaces in infants with subdural hematomas. *Radiology*. 1982;142(3):669–672 PMID: 6977789 https://doi.org/10.1148/radiology.142.3.6977789
336. Laubscher B, Deonna T, Uske A, van Melle G. Primitive megalencephaly in children: natural history, medium term prognosis with special reference to external hydrocephalus. *Eur J Pediatr*. 1990;149(7):502–507 PMID: 2347345 https://doi.org/10.1007/BF01959405
337. Ravid S, Maytal J. External hydrocephalus: a probable cause for subdural hematoma in infancy. *Pediatr Neurol*. 2003;28(2):139–141 PMID: 12699866 https://doi.org/10.1016/S0887-8994(02)00500-3
338. Greiner MV, Richards TJ, Care MM, Leach JL. Prevalence of subdural collections in children with macrocrania. *AJNR Am J Neuroradiol*. 2013;34(12):2373–2378 PMID: 23868166 https://doi.org/10.3174/ajnr.A3588
339. McKeag H, Christian CW, Rubin D, Daymont C, Pollock AN, Wood J. Subdural hemorrhage in pediatric patients with enlargement of the subarachnoid spaces. *J Neurosurg Pediatr*. 2013;11(4):438–444 PMID: 23394356 https://doi.org/10.3171/2012.12.PEDS12289
340. Papasian NC, Frim DM. A theoretical model of benign external hydrocephalus that predicts a predisposition towards extra-axial hemorrhage after minor head trauma. *Pediatr Neurosurg*. 2000;33(4):188–193 PMID: 11124635 https://doi.org/10.1159/000055951
341. Sharma RR, Mahapatra A, Pawar SJ, Sousa J, Athale SD. Symptomatic calcified subdural hematomas. *Pediatr Neurosurg*. 1999;31(3):150–154 PMID: 10708357 https://doi.org/10.1159/000028851

342. Faulhauer K, Schmitz P. Overdrainage phenomena in shunt treated hydrocephalus. *Acta Neurochir (Wien)*. 1978;45(1-2):89–101 PMID: 742440 https://doi.org/10.1007/BF01774384
343. Oushy S, Parker JJ, Campbell K, et al. Frontal and occipital horn ratio is associated with multifocal intraparenchymal hemorrhages in neonatal shunted hydrocephalus. *J Neurosurg Pediatr*. 2017;20(5):432–438 PMID: 28885094 https://doi.org/10.3171/2017.6.PEDS16481
344. Liu Z, Xu P, Li Q, Liu H, Chen N, Xu J. Arachnoid cysts with subdural hematoma or intracystic hemorrhage in children. *Pediatr Emerg Care*. 2014;30(5):345–351 PMID: 24786991 https://doi.org/10.1097/PEC.0000000000000128
345. Auer LM, Gallhofer B, Ladurner G, Sager WD, Heppner F, Lechner H. Diagnosis and treatment of middle fossa arachnoid cysts and subdural hematomas. *J Neurosurg*. 1981;54(3):366–369 PMID: 7463138 https://doi.org/10.3171/jns.1981.54.3.0366
346. Albuquerque FC, Giannotta SL. Arachnoid cyst rupture producing subdural hygroma and intracranial hypertension: case reports. *Neurosurgery*. 1997;41(4):951–956 PMID: 9316060 https://doi.org/10.1097/00006123-199710000-00036
347. Gelabert-González M, Fernández-Villa J, Cutrín-Prieto J, Garcìa Allut A, Martínez-Rumbo R. Arachnoid cyst rupture with subdural hygroma: report of three cases and literature review. *Childs Nerv Syst*. 2002;18(11):609–613 PMID: 12420120 https://doi.org/10.1007/s00381-002-0651-7
348. Donaldson JW, Edwards-Brown M, Luerssen TG. Arachnoid cyst rupture with concurrent subdural hygroma. *Pediatr Neurosurg*. 2000;32(3):137–139 PMID: 10867560 https://doi.org/10.1159/000028918
349. Choong CT, Lee SH. Subdural hygroma in association with middle fossa arachnoid cyst: acetazolamide therapy. *Brain Dev*. 1998;20(5):319–322 PMID: 9761002 https://doi.org/10.1016/S0387-7604(98)00039-4
350. Maegele M. Coagulopathy after traumatic brain injury: incidence, pathogenesis, and treatment options. *Transfusion*. 2013;53(suppl 1):28S–37S PMID: 23301970 https://doi.org/10.1111/trf.12033
351. Joseph B, Hadjizacharia P, Aziz H, et al. Prothrombin complex concentrate: an effective therapy in reversing the coagulopathy of traumatic brain injury. *J Trauma Acute Care Surg*. 2013;74(1):248–253 PMID: 23271101
352. Joseph B, Pandit V, Khalil M, et al. Use of prothrombin complex concentrate as an adjunct to fresh frozen plasma shortens time to craniotomy in traumatic brain injury patients. *Neurosurgery*. 2015;76(5):601–607 PMID: 25886249 https://doi.org/10.1227/NEU.0000000000000685
353. Chung MG, O'Brien NF. Prevalence of early posttraumatic seizures in children with moderate to severe traumatic brain injury despite levetiracetam prophylaxis. *Pediatr Crit Care Med*. 2016;17(2):150–156 PMID: 26669640 https://doi.org/10.1097/PCC.0000000000000588
354. O'Neill BR, Handler MH, Tong S, Chapman KE. Incidence of seizures on continuous EEG monitoring following traumatic brain injury in children. *J Neurosurg Pediatr*. 2015;16(2):167–176 PMID: 25955809 https://doi.org/10.3171/2014.12.PEDS14263
355. Kochanek PM, Carney N, Adelson PD, et al; et al. Guidelines for the acute medical management of severe traumatic brain injury in infants, children, and adolescents—second edition. *Pediatr Crit Care Med*. 2012;13(suppl 1):S1–S82 PMID: 22217782 https://doi.org/10.1097/PCC.0b013e318259ee85
356. Melo JR, Di Rocco F, Bourgeois M, et al. Surgical options for treatment of traumatic subdural hematomas in children younger than 2 years of age. *J Neurosurg Pediatr*. 2014;13(4):456–461 PMID: 24559279 https://doi.org/10.3171/2014.1.PEDS13393

357. Alexander R, Crabbe L, Sato Y, Smith W, Bennett T. Serial abuse in children who are shaken. *Am J Dis Child.* 1990;144(1):58–60 PMID: 2294721 https://doi.org/10.1001/archpedi.1990.02150250068033
358. Bonnier C, Nassogne MC, Evrard P. Outcome and prognosis of whiplash shaken infant syndrome; late consequences after a symptom-free interval. *Dev Med Child Neurol.* 1995;37(11):943–956 PMID: 8566455 https://doi.org/10.1111/j.1469-8749.1995.tb11949.x
359. Lowen DE. Neurodevelopmental outcomes of abusive head trauma. In: Frasier L, Rauth-Farley K, Alexander R, Parrish R, eds. *Abusive Head Trauma in Infants and Children.* St Louis, MO: G.W. Medical Publishing Co; 2006:455–469
360. Nuño M, Pelissier L, Varshneya K, Adamo MA, Drazin D. Outcomes and factors associated with infant abusive head trauma in the US. *J Neurosurg Pediatr.* 2015;16(5):515–522 PMID: 26230462 https://doi.org/10.3171/2015.3.PEDS14544
361. Chevignard MP, Lind K. Long-term outcome of abusive head trauma. *Pediatr Radiol.* 2014;44(S4)(suppl 4):S548–S558 PMID: 25501726 https://doi.org/10.1007/s00247-014-3169-8
362. Wong AM, Yeh CH, Liu HL, et al. Arterial spin-labeling perfusion imaging of children with subdural hemorrhage: Perfusion abnormalities in abusive head trauma. *J Neuroradiol.* 2017;44(4):281–287 PMID: 28341000 https://doi.org/10.1016/j.neurad.2017.02.003
363. Khan NR, Fraser BD, Nguyen V, et al. Pediatric abusive head trauma and stroke. *J Neurosurg Pediatr.* 2017;20(2):183–190 PMID: 28574318 https://doi.org/10.3171/2017.4.PEDS16650
364. Miller TR, Steinbeigle R, Lawrence BA, et al. Lifetime cost of abusive head trauma at ages 0–4, USA. *Prev Sci.* 2018;19(6):695–704 PMID: 28685210
365. Peterson C, Xu L, Florence C, Parks SE. Annual cost of U.S. hospital visits for pediatric abusive head trauma. *Child Maltreat.* 2015;20(3):162–169 PMID: 25911437 https://doi.org/10.1177/1077559515583549
366. Friedman J, Reed P, Sharplin P, Kelly P. Primary prevention of pediatric abusive head trauma: a cost audit and cost-utility analysis. *Child Abuse Negl.* 2012;36(11-12):760–770 PMID: 23141137 https://doi.org/10.1016/j.chiabu.2012.07.008
367. Showers J, ed. Executive summary. Paper presented at: The National Conference on Shaken Baby Syndrome: A Medical, Legal, and Prevention Challenge; 1996; Salt Lake City, UT
368. Caffey J. The whiplash shaken infant syndrome: manual shaking by the extremities with whiplash-induced intracranial and intraocular bleedings, linked with residual permanent brain damage and mental retardation. *Pediatrics.* 1974;54(4):396–403 PMID: 4416579

CHAPTER 8

Ocular Manifestations of Child Abuse

Brooke D. Saffren, OMS-IV
Philadelphia College of Osteopathic Medicine
Philadelphia, PA

Yair Morad, MD
Department of Ophthalmology
Assaf Harofeh Medical Center
Tel Aviv University
Tel Aviv, Israel

Alex V. Levin, MD, MHSc, FRCSC, FAAP, FAAO
Chief, Pediatric Ophthalmology and Ocular Genetics
Wills Eye Hospital
Philadelphia, PA

Introduction

Ocular abnormalities may be found in all forms of child abuse. In one study, the eye was the presenting sign for child physical abuse in 4% to 6% of cases.[1] Ophthalmology consultations are an important tool in identifying child abuse or differentiating the child who has not experienced abuse. This is particularly important in physical abuse, although ocular abnormalities may be found as manifestations in nonorganic failure to thrive, child neglect, sexual abuse, medical child abuse, and perhaps emotional abuse.

Too often in the medical literature and other settings, comments are made about the specificity or implications of "retinal hemorrhages." The use of this rather generic term is no more helpful in determining a diagnosis of non-inflicted versus inflicted injury than the use of the term "fracture" without describing the involved bone and type of fracture. The non-ophthalmologist is at a distinct disadvantage in achieving an adequate description of intraocular hemorrhage because of infrequency of performing retinal examination, unfamiliarity with retinal anatomy, failure to dilate the pupil pharmacologically, and the optical limitations of the direct ophthalmoscope, particularly in the awake and uncooperative infant. Non-ophthalmologists are very good at recognizing the presence or absence of retinal hemorrhages; however, they are less facile at careful description.[2,3] False-positive and false-negative reports do occur.

Abusive Head Trauma

Ocular involvement joins skeletal and brain injury as a cardinal manifestation of abusive head trauma (AHT), especially when the traumatic event is characterized by repeated acceleration-deceleration with or without blunt impact to the head. Retinal hemorrhages are seen in approximately 85% of infants who have experienced abusive head trauma. Vitreoretinal traction and perhaps acceleration-deceleration injury to the orbital contents appear to be key factors in the pathogenesis of the hemorrhagic retinopathy and other eye findings. Elevation of intracranial pressure (ICP), hypoxia, anemia, and increased intrathoracic pressure may also contribute to appearance of the intraocular abnormalities, although the unique mechanics of repetitive acceleration-deceleration forces seems to be the critical factor; the other factors rarely result in significant hemorrhagic retinopathy themselves. Recent studies clearly indicate that isolated elevated ICP does not cause extensive retinal hemorrhage.[4,5] Please see Chapter 7, Abusive Head Trauma, for a lengthier discussion of the pathogenesis of retinal hemorrhage in AHT.[6–8]

Anatomy

Describing hemorrhagic retinopathy in detail affords the examiner information that is critical to recognizing potential etiologies. The retina lines the inside of the eye. It is a vascularized, multilayered structure. It is separated from the sclera (white of the eye) by an interposed vascular layer called the *choroid*. The area of the retina straight back from the pupil and in the center of the visual axis is known as the *fovea* (Figure 8.1). This area has specialized anatomy and functions as the source of central vision. The line of sight (visual axis) is along this pupil-fovea line. The area of retina that surrounds the fovea posteriorly is known as the *macula* (see Figure 8.1). The optic disc is located just nasal to the macula. The optic nerve represents the collection of nerve fibers emanating from the retina to carry the vision messages to the brain. The arterial supply to and venous drainage from the retina enter and exit the eye through the center of the optic nerve. These vessels branch out over the superficial retinal layers, starting as 4 major branches (arcades), 2 temporal (superior and inferior) and 2 nasal (superior and inferior) (see Figure 8.1). The superior and inferior temporal arcades surround the macula. The retina extends along the inner surface

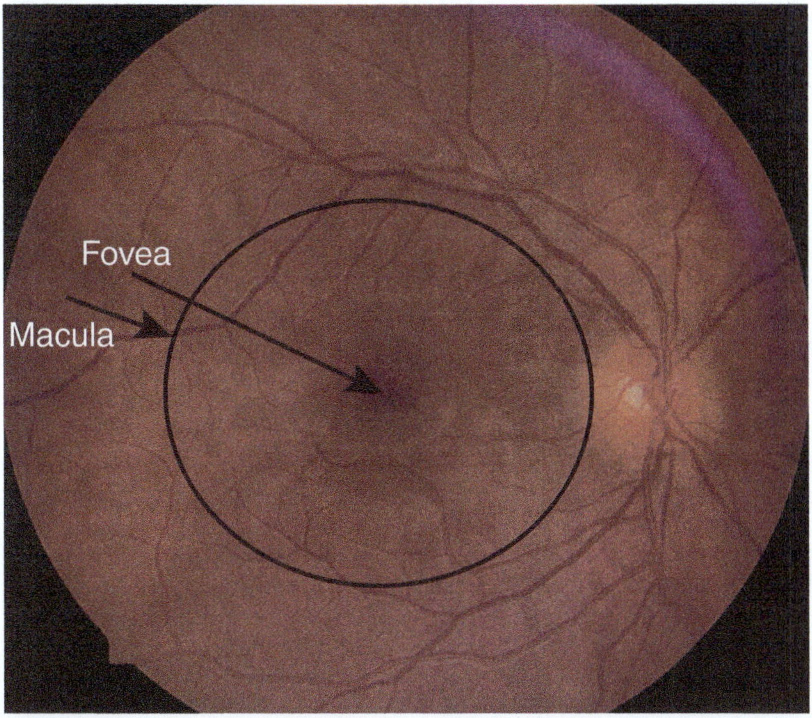

FIGURE 8.1
The posterior pole. This area of the retina encompasses the optic nerve and macula as well as the immediately surrounding retina.

of the globe almost up to the back of the iris. The retinal edge is known as the *ora serrata*. The area of retina leading up to the ora is known as the *peripheral retina* and is not easily visible with the direct ophthalmoscope.

Injury Description

Hemorrhage may be found lying on, within, or underneath the retina. These hemorrhages are identified as *preretinal*, *intraretinal*, and *subretinal* hemorrhages, respectively (Figure 8.2). Hemorrhages have different shapes and morphology according to the level of the retina affected. Intraretinal hemorrhages within the superficial layer of the retina (nerve fiber layer) assume a somewhat linear "splinter" or "flame" shape. *Dot* and *blot* hemorrhages refer to deeper intraretinal hemorrhages that tend to have a round or amorphous geographic appearance (see Figure 8.2). Dot hemorrhages are generally smaller than blot hemorrhages, but there is no specific size cutoff point for the use of either term. Some have white centers. Although well recognized as a manifestation of endocarditis (Roth spots), this nonspecific sign may be observed in virtually any

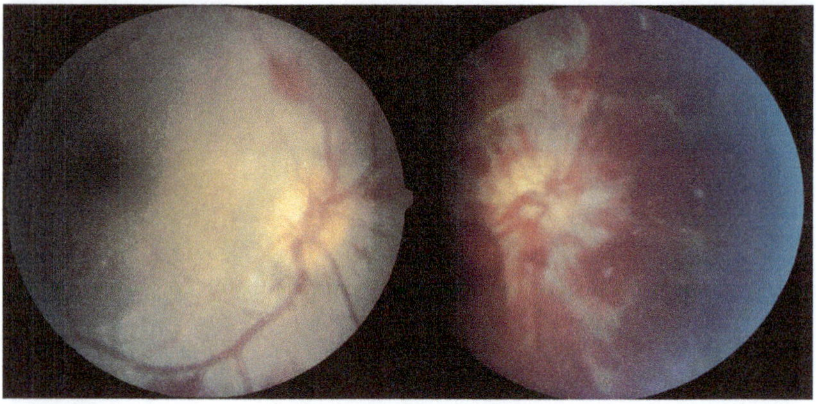

FIGURE 8.2
Retinal hemorrhages of various types in abusive head trauma. Note the asymmetry between the eyes, as may sometimes occur, as well as the variety of hemorrhages. The image on the right (left eye) demonstrates a severe hemorrhagic retinopathy that is very concerning for abuse head trauma with too-numerous-to-count preretinal, subretinal, and intraretinal hemorrhages. The image on the left (right eye) is a more nonspecific retinopathy with approximately 10 intraretinal hemorrhages largely confined to the peripapillary area with flame, dot, and blot hemorrhages.

cause or condition associated with retinal hemorrhage, including AHT.[3] Hemorrhages can also occur in the gel (vitreous) that fills the back part of the eye (*vitreous hemorrhage*).

There is no current universally accepted classification system for retinal hemorrhages. The number of hemorrhages can be counted or described using general terms such as "too numerous to count." Subjective terms, such as "mild," "moderate," and "severe," may be open to different interpretations. Hemorrhages may involve the entire retina or one or more specific regions. Hemorrhages can be described as being immediately around the optic nerve (peripapillary) or confined to the posterior pole, which includes the peripapillary region and the macula. The midperipheral retina describes the region between the posterior pole and peripheral retina. Perivascular hemorrhages lie along major branches of the vascular tree. The retinal hemorrhages of AHT may be unilateral or asymmetrical between the eyes.[7,8]

Traumatic retinoschisis (Figure 8.3) is a retinal abnormality that is highly specific for AHT (shaken baby syndrome), because it is otherwise rarely reported in infants and young children. In the AHT age group, the vitreous has especially strong attachment to the macula, peripheral retina, and blood vessels.[9] In one computer-based finite element analysis of the eye in AHT, the importance of forces generated at the macula and the peripheral retina was observed.[10] In the setting of repetitive acceleration-deceleration forces associated with AHT, the vitreous exerts increased traction on the retina in these locations, and in the macula can cause the retina layers to split, resulting

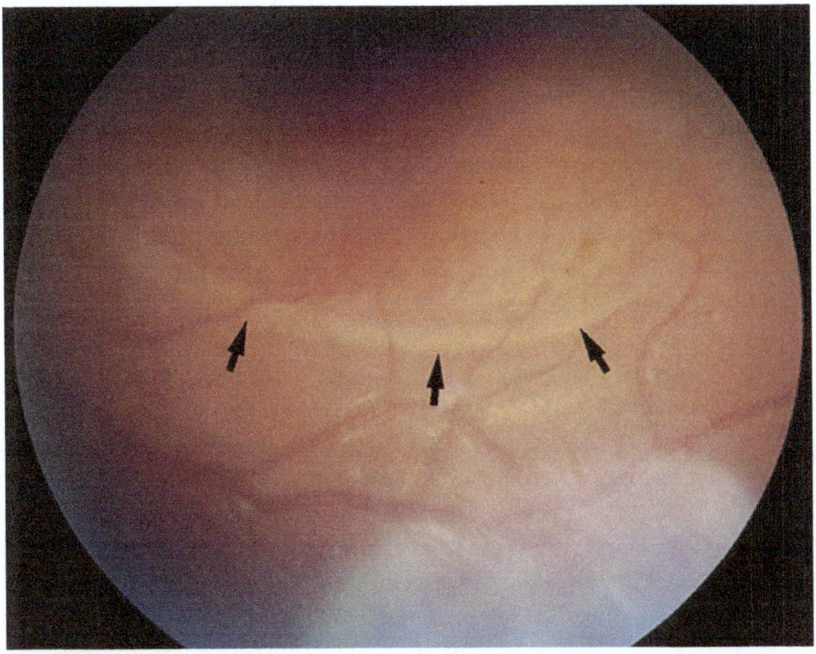

FIGURE 8.3
Paramacular fold. Note the white line (arrows) over which blood vessels are elevated, caused by traction on the retina by the vitreous (vitreous not visible in photograph). This produces mechanical disruption of the pigment layer underlying the retina, resulting in the hypopigmentation. The paramacular fold is often found at the edges of a traumatic retinoschisis cystic cavity or may be isolated, as seen here.

in a cystic cavity that may be partially or completely filled with blood. Usually, the split is at the internal limiting membrane. Retinoschisis can easily be mistaken for preretinal hemorrhages, and it is important to make clinical distinctions between them. Recognition of traumatic retinoschisis is aided by the identification of circumlinear ridges (paramacular folds) or lines at the edges of the lesion (see Figure 8.3). The folds may or may not be present and can also be observed in the absence of a retinoschisis cavity or remain after a schisis cavity has settled. Lines may be hemorrhagic or hypopigmented. Imaging modalities such as optical coherence tomography and intravenous fluorescein angiography can be useful in the evaluation of patients with AHT.[11] Intravenous fluorescein angiography may be useful in the diagnosis of retinal non-perfusion, which is a potential complication of vitreous traction.[12,13] Postmortem gross and histologic examination can also demonstrate physical evidence of vitreoretinal traction.[14]

Other than AHT, traumatic retinoschisis has been observed in only 2 instances of head crush injury[15,16] but was not observed when larger samples of patients with head crush injury were studied.[17] Paramacular folds have also been reported in fatal motor vehicle crashes[18,19] and in an 11-m fall.[19] However, these observations had several morphological distinctions from injury typically seen in AHT, and the clinical scenarios are easily distinguishable on the basis of known history of the precipitating events.[20] Schisis-like cavities can also form directly over blood vessels (Figure 8.4), although this is a less-specific finding that may be mimicked by virtually any disorder in which a major vessel can have a local bleed (eg, vasculitis, leukemia). The blood within a retinoschisis cavity may leak into the vitreous and compromise vision, making careful monitoring and follow-up essential.

Further evidence linking acceleration-deceleration forces (shaking) to retinal hemorrhage comes from studies[21,22] that reveal orbital injury and/or optic nerve–scleral junction hemorrhage. Those who have experienced AHT show more hemorrhages in the orbital fat and optic nerve dura than those who have experienced accidental trauma,[14,21] which may play a role in generating intraocular bleeding. The injuries observed in the orbit may help to explain the long-term visual effects of AHT. Direct injury to the nerve causes optic atrophy, which is second only to cortical injury as the cause of permanent visual loss or blindness in survivors. Postmortem examination of the entire orbital contents,

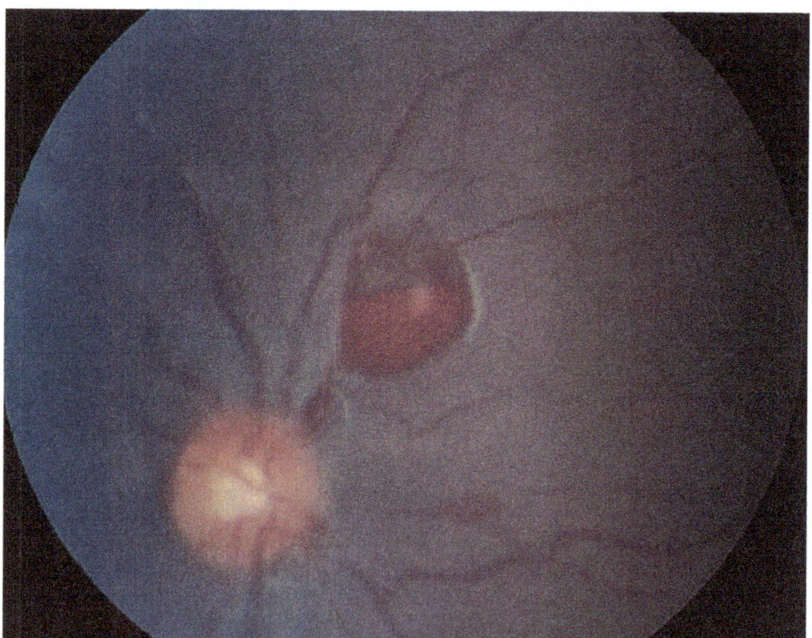

FIGURE 8.4

A schisis-like blood collection in front of a blood vessel may be a sign of vessel shearing due to abusive head trauma but can also be due to other causes.

preferably with sections taken after removal en bloc by a combined transconjunctival and intracranial route, may have specific utility in understanding the cause of a child's death.[23]

Etiology and Differential Diagnosis

There are many causes of retinal hemorrhages in children (Box 8.1).[4] Birth can result in retinal hemorrhages in up to 45% of healthy babies at term examined in the first 24 hours after birth[24] and 20% of healthy babies within the first 48 hours.[25] Retinal hemorrhage can occur after any type of delivery but is more common after spontaneous vaginal and vacuum-assisted parturition[26] and least common after cesarean.[27,28] Studies in virtually every demographic setting have shown collectively that flame hemorrhages resolve within 7 days after birth (usually within 72 hours).[24,29] Intraretinal dot/blot hemorrhages usually resolve by 6 weeks (usually within 2–3 weeks) but have been reported to last as long as 8 to 10 weeks, especially when located in the fovea.[25,26,29] Preretinal and vitreous hemorrhage may also last longer. Although hemorrhagic retinopathy of normal birth, which may even be extensive and extending to the ora, may be difficult to distinguish from the retina of AHT before 4 weeks of age, normal babies do not demonstrate traumatic retinoschisis or paramacular folds, and other evidence of AHT is absent. Subretinal hemorrhage is rare as a result of birth. After the time limitations for resolution of birth hemorrhage have expired, AHT is the most common cause of retinal hemorrhage in children younger than 5 years.

Increased ICP creates disruption in axoplasmic flow and capillary nonperfusion, which leads to papilledema. However, fewer than 8% of patients who have experienced AHT have papilledema even when increased ICP is present.[7,30] Papilledema may result in peripapillary flame or other intraretinal hemorrhages which are few in number, or pre-papillary hemorrhage.[4] Increased ICP alone does not cause the extensive, multilayered retinal hemorrhages typically associated with AHT.[5] Likewise, intracranial hemorrhage alone, although not uncommonly associated with intraocular hemorrhage in adults (Terson syndrome), occurs in fewer than 8% of children with intracranial bleeding.[31]

Purtscher retinopathy is associated with increased intrathoracic pressure and is seen, for example, in chest crush injuries in adults. It is categorized by polygonal white retinal patches. It is rarely reported in AHT, even with the presence of rib fractures.[7,32] Multiple studies show that retinal hemorrhage is rare after cardiopulmonary resuscitation with chest compression, and when it does occur, it is confined to very few hemorrhages in the posterior pole.[6,33,34] The increased intrathoracic pressure produced by the Valsalva maneuver during cough or excessive vomiting can cause distinctive isolated preretinal hemorrhage in the posterior pole of adults[35,36]; however, studies show that it is rare in children.[37,38] Retinal hemorrhage is also not seen associated with the increased intrathoracic pressure during seizures in childhood.[39–41]

Accidental injury that involves severe rotational and acceleration-deceleration forces, such as a rollover multiple-impact motor vehicle crash,[18] can induce unique shearing forces within the eye that may cause severe intraocular hemorrhage, and even retinoschisis, to develop. Retinal hemorrhages in the setting of accidental trauma are otherwise rare, and the hemorrhages are almost always limited to the posterior pole, predominantly intraretinal and preretinal, and relatively few in number.[6,42] The presence of hemorrhage in the peripheral retina is also important in recognizing AHT versus accidental head trauma.[43–46] Retinal hemorrhages may be more common after accidental head injury with epidural hemorrhage[47] and perhaps with occipital impact, but they still present as predominantly intraretinal, limited in number and confined to the posterior pole. Severe and life-threatening trauma may rarely result in more extensive retinal hemorrhages, but the accidental injury mechanism is usually obvious. One paper suggested that significant hemorrhagic retinopathy might develop following short falls,[33] but it had many flaws, including a lack of formal ophthalmology consultation within the study population.[6] Other sources have observed mild to moderate retinal hemorrhages following falls,[48–51] but these cases are reported as extremely rare[49] and not all sources completely ruled out child abuse.[48,50,51] Even after motor vehicle crash, the incidence of retinal hemorrhage is only 14% in young children.[52]

BOX 8.1
Select[a] Causes of Retinal Hemorrhage[b] in Children

Abusive head injury
Accidental trauma
Anemia
Birth
Carbon monoxide
Cerebral aneurysm
Coagulopathy
Extracorporeal membrane oxygenation
Glutaricaciduria
Hypertension
Hypo/hypernatremia
Hypoxia/hypotension

(continued)

BOX 8.1 *(continued)*

Increased intracranial pressure
Leukemia
Malaria
Meningitis/sepsis/endocarditis
Osteogenesis imperfecta with trauma
Retinal diseases
Retinal infection
Retinopathy of prematurity (active)
Vasculitis

[a] This box is not an exhaustive list of causes.
[b] The term *retinal hemorrhage* is used here generically. Describing the number, location, patterns, and distribution of the hemorrhages helps with differential diagnosis along with systemic evaluation and history.

Examination Protocol

Ophthalmology consultation is necessary in all cases of suspected AHT and unexplained sudden infant death, preferably within the first 24 hours of the infant's presentation and no later than 72 hours whenever possible.[53] Evaluation should consist of full, indirect ophthalmoscopy examination through a dilated pupil. The indirect ophthalmoscope provides a wide field of view that can extend to the ora serrata, which is not visible with direct ophthalmoscopy. If there are concerns with pharmacologic dilation regarding preservation of pupillary reactivity for neurologic monitoring, options include the use of short-acting agents (phenylephrine, 2.5%; tropicamide, 1%), which will wear off within 4 to 6 hours; dilating one pupil at a time; or, if no other options exist, using small pupil indirect ophthalmoscopy. Number, type, patterns, location, and extent of retinal hemorrhages should be documented by the ophthalmologist, as well as the presence of retinoschisis or paramacular folds. Retinal abnormalities can be photographed or illustrated with detailed drawings.[6] In fatal cases involving children younger than 5 years, eye removal along with orbital contents for histopathology examination is recommended when AHT is suspected or the cause is unknown.[52,53]

Forensic Implications: Timing and Resolution of Retinal Hemorrhages

Criminal investigators may request a defined window of time within which the abuse may have occurred. Although timing of retinal hemorrhages with exact precision cannot be determined, intraretinal hemorrhages are likely to resolve more rapidly than preretinal hemorrhage. Intraretinal hemorrhages resolve typically within days up to 2 weeks, and preretinal hemorrhages take several weeks.[54,55] Therefore, the presence of extensive intraretinal hemorrhage suggests that the trauma happened a few days prior, and the presence of preretinal hemorrhage in the absence of intraretinal hemorrhage suggests trauma days to weeks prior. Although retinal hemorrhage progression has been reported,[55,56] it is rare and likely results from preretinal hemorrhage or blood within a retinoschisis cavity, extending into the vitreous. Some data from adults[57,58] and clinical experience in children who have experienced abuse[6] suggest perhaps a 2- to 3-day delay in the development of vitreous hemorrhage, particularly after traumatic retinoschisis, but these data are "soft" and should not be used to rule out the possibility of vitreous hemorrhages occurring at the moment of shaking.

The timing of papilledema after increases in ICP also is not well understood and may take hours to days to develop. Old injuries may have particular morphology, such as retinal pigmentary clumping, the fixed fold in a retinal detachment, or the whitened residual vitreous collection representing prior hemorrhage. A hypopigmented circumlinear line in the posterior pole may be a sign of prior retinoschisis due to AHT.

Prognosis and Visual Outcomes

Other ocular injuries are less common after shaking, including cataract, hyphema, ptosis, retinal edema, retinal detachment, and total disruption of the ocular contents.[6] Some of these injuries may reflect coincidental blunt trauma to the eye, either during or in addition to the shaking. Although some authors have suggested that blunt impact is necessary to generate enough acceleration-deceleration to cause severe, particularly fatal, AHT injury,[59] numerous others have concluded to the contrary that severe injury and death can result from shaking alone.[6,42,60] Furthermore, the fact that shaking alone is enough to cause severe neurotrauma is supported by perpetrator accounts.[61–63] Retinal hemorrhages due to shaking in the presence of normal neuroimaging have been reported,[64] and computed tomography scans showing edema without hemorrhage have also been observed.[65] Mild hemorrhagic retinopathy in the absence of neurotrauma is likely not enough to bring a child to medical attention, and early signs of abuse have a high risk of missed diagnosis.[66] Those who have experienced AHT may make their first presentation to the medical system with relatively few or nonspecific symptoms and signs,[67] and AHT symptoms can often be mistaken for other common diseases in children.[68] Although retinal examination is not used as screening for AHT, it is a specific sign and can be used for situations with a high clinical suspicion of abuse.

Even the severe retinal hemorrhages and traumatic retinoschisis often resolve without long-term visual sequelae.[69] Less commonly, visual impairment can result from retinal fibrosis, retinal scarring, amblyopia, and consequences of vitreous hemorrhage.[70] More often, long-term visual impairment results from optic atrophy[6] or cortical damage,[71–75] both as a direct result of the acceleration-deceleration forces characteristic of AHT. Posterior fossa subdural hemorrhage, cerebral edema, and hypoxic-ischemic injury are highly characteristic of AHT[76] and may further contribute to the long-term sequela such as neurologic injury and visual impairment.[77] Caregivers may not be able to observe visual impairment in alert and interactive children, despite the presence of retinal hemorrhage. This is particularly true if only one eye has sustained the brunt of the ocular injury.[3] In most instances, young children will seem to function normally unless both eyes have severe visual damage that is enough to interfere with the relatively few visual demands in their lives. Therefore, a history of normal visual function, as observed by caregivers in the home, does not rule out the possibility that hemorrhagic retinopathy has taken place and long-term visual impairment from retina and/or optic nerve injury, which can affect global development, may still occur.[78] Ophthalmology follow-up is necessary to identify developmental visual delay and potentially rule out other sources of neurocognitive disabilities.[79] Those who have experienced AHT are at risk for long-term visual effects even in the absence of retinal hemorrhage. Initial visual responsiveness after injury has been found to be positively correlated with survival.[74] Multiple studies[7,55,80] have noted a positive correlation between the severity of retinopathy and the severity of intracranial injury.

Other Forms of Physical Abuse

Virtually any ocular injury could possibly result from an act of child abuse. The face is involved in up to 45% of child abuse cases, with the eyes affected in up to 61%. It has been estimated that 4% to 6% of those who have experienced physical abuse first present to the ophthalmologist.[81] Determining the cause of pediatric eye injury requires a history and complete physical examination, with appropriate diagnostic testing. Certain eye injuries are virtually always indicators of trauma, even in the absence of a history of trauma, whereas others must at least invoke the consideration of trauma.

TABLE 8.1
Specificity of Ocular Findings to Indicate Trauma

Always Trauma	Usually Trauma	Consider Trauma
• Conjunctival/lid abrasion/laceration • Corneal/scleral laceration • Commotio retinae (Berlin edema, "retinal bruise") • Vitreous base avulsion	• Periorbital ecchymosis • Hyphema	• Unilateral ectopia lentis/cataract/corneal scar/iritis • Unilateral infantile cataract • Unilateral optic atrophy • Retinal detachment

Table 8.1 offers some diagnostic guidelines for considering a possible traumatic nature of an observed ocular finding. Items that are listed as having a cause that is always traumatic do not necessarily imply abuse, but abuse should be considered if no history of significant trauma is given. Sequelae of unknown etiology, such as corneal scar or old retinal detachment or vitreous hemorrhage, can be observed in a child who has sustained visual loss at some time substantially before the examination. Further investigations, such as neuroimaging, may be useful.

Particular attention should be paid to the common error of attempting to date periocular hemorrhage in trying to establish a time of injury. The skin of the periorbita has looser attachments to the underlying tissue compared with other areas on the body. As a result, larger quantities of blood can accumulate with injury, thus giving periorbital ecchymosis darker color and less predictable resolution time. Therefore, dating systems, which are already subject to inaccuracy and were designed with other body parts in mind, are largely inaccurate. In addition, the loose skin around the eye allows tracking of blood in the subcutaneous planes from areas on the forehead or scalp to lower areas on the face. A single blow to the forehead or anterior scalp can result in tracking of blood to the tissues around both eyes, thus giving the false impression of bilateral injury (Figure 8.5).

A particularly troublesome situation arises when the eye is injured "accidentally" during physical discipline. Anecdotally, one of this chapter's authors has seen 9 cases of hyphema (blood in the anterior chamber of the eye between the cornea and pupil) during a belt beating in which the child had squirmed or the caregiver had lost positional control of the child and the belt or its buckle struck the eye. One child was rendered permanently blind in that eye, another lost the eye, and one did not experience sequelae until 30 years later when she presented with late-onset traumatic glaucoma (angle-recession glaucoma).

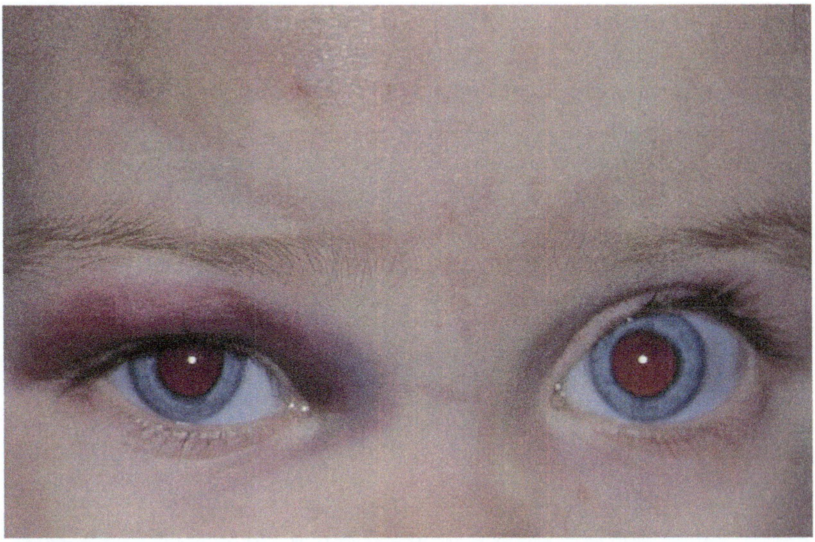

FIGURE 8.5
Bilateral periorbital ecchymosis from accidental blunt trauma to the right central forehead.

Medical Child Abuse

Ocular injury may be a primary or secondary manifestation of medical child abuse (previously known as Munchausen syndrome by proxy or factitious disorder by proxy). Direct ocular injury from medical child abuse has taken the form of covert instillation of a noxious substance onto the ocular surface, resulting in conjunctivitis or corneal scarring,[82–84] atropine sprayed onto the ocular surface resulting in factitious unilateral pupillary dilation,[85] and periorbital/orbital cellulitis due to the injection of noxious substances into the periorbita.[86] An examining physician might suspect covert chemical instillation when there is predominant involvement of the inferior half of the cornea and conjunctiva or when a child presents with chronic recurrent red eye of unknown cause. The predilection for inferior corneal involvement results from the upgaze induced by forced opening of a resisting eye (Bell phenomenon), thus exposing only the inferior corneal and conjunctival surfaces to the bulk of the noxious agent. Pharmacologic testing is available to help sort out the causes of anisocoria.[8] Careful inspection of the involved skin in an area of periorbital cellulitis may reveal needle-puncture marks.

Subconjunctival hemorrhage or periocular petechiae may result from covert suffocation.[87] Although there are other possible causes, such as normal birth and pertussis (which often yields a more severe

360° hemorrhage), and there has been one reported case of subconjunctival hemorrhage as a result of adenovirus serotype 3 infection,[88] subconjunctival hemorrhage beyond the neonatal period is actually quite uncommon in the absence of direct blunt trauma to the eye. In any baby or child with sudden unexplained seizure, altered mental status, or unexplained signs of anoxia, a full eye examination should be requested to rule out not only the retinal hemorrhages of AHT but also the possibility of covert suffocation, as indicated by subconjunctival hemorrhage. Ophthalmic findings may otherwise go unobserved. The ophthalmologist must be alerted to inspect the conjunctiva before proceeding with retinal examination, which itself may induce subconjunctival hemorrhage if instrumentation is used.

Other indirect effects of medical child abuse include those that result from covert poisoning that affects the central nervous system. The pupils may become bilaterally constricted or enlarged.[89,90] Asymmetry of the pupils (anisocoria) may result from elevated ICP. Eye-movement disorders, including strabismus[91] and nystagmus,[92] can be seen. In addition, the patient who has been covertly poisoned may be visually inattentive and seem to not be focusing.

Neglect

Nonorganic failure to thrive has no specific ocular manifestations, although anecdotal reports exist of blindness due to bilateral corneal scarring in a child left to die in a latrine in a third-world country and of bilateral corneal erosions due to exposure in a severely wasted and neglected child who was left listless and unattended for a prolonged period before coming to medical attention. The lids were incompletely closed during this period and the blink rate reduced, thus leaving characteristic exposure desiccation injury involving the lower third of each cornea. In one reported case of severe social isolation and neglect, a young girl had been limited to the confines of her bedroom for her first 13 years. This reportedly resulted in a limited ability to focus her vision past 10 feet, corresponding to the size of the room in which she was kept.[93]

It is more common that the ophthalmologist is confronted with the chronic but perhaps less dramatic issue of medical neglect and noncompliance. For example, if the caregiver does not adhere to the prescribed regimen of patching to treat amblyopia, the child may be left with a permanently legally blind eye. Although noncompliance with patching regimens can be seen in otherwise normative families, complete failure to comply with patching is particularly troublesome, especially considering that amblyopia is a treatable disorder. Failure to seek prompt medical attention for injury or other obvious ocular disorders also may result in blindness. Consultations and collaboration between ophthalmologists and pediatricians and family physicians are essential in managing such situations.

Sexual Abuse

Although rare, there is one reported case of retinal hemorrhage presumably due to an extreme Valsalva effect in resisting a sexual assault, and there have been reports of children with severe retinal hemorrhages from fatal AHT in which sexual assault also occurred.[94]

Ocular involvement from sexually transmitted infection is also rare in children. Syphilis, "the great imitator," can result in a wide variety of ocular manifestations, including keratitis, uveitis, retinal abnormalities, and optic nerve changes. It is always transmitted sexually, with the exception of transmission to the fetus or through the birth canal. Congenital syphilis has a different profile of ocular manifestations than does acquired infection and should be distinguishable by the ophthalmologist as well as other generalists and specialists.

Although non-neonatal transmission of gonorrhea to the urethra, vagina, oropharynx, and rectum occurs exclusively through sexual contact, there is some evidence that the conjunctiva might represent a unique "externalized" mucosal membrane that may make nonsexual transmission by fomites possible.[95,96] One child was reported to develop mild gonorrheal conjunctivitis after her mother, who had an active vaginal discharge later proven to be from gonorrhea, used a washcloth to clean her own genitals and then directly applied that same washcloth to her child's face during a joint shower. Full sexual abuse evaluation, including examination and culture of other orifices and interview by a trained sexual abuse social worker and physician, as well as a child protective services investigation of the family and home, failed to uncover any evidence to support sexual abuse. However, the child was preverbal. Lewis et al have reported 2 other similar cases.[96]

Although there have been no reported cases, it is theoretically possible that non-neonatal chlamydia conjunctivitis can result from nonsexual transmission, similarly to gonorrhea.[97] Human papillomavirus can result in conjunctival lesions, and pubic lice can infest the eyelashes. Cases due to sexual abuse are known, but there are no studies evaluating the possibility of alternate routes of transmission. HIV can have a wide range of primary and secondary ocular manifestations, but these are less common in infected children compared with infected adults. Of course, children may acquire HIV through routes other than sexual transmission.

Nonsexual routes more frequently transmit herpes simplex and molluscum contagiosum than direct sexual contact. In these instances, the consideration of sexual abuse is usually a low priority in the absence of other risk factors.

In the absence of neonatal transmission or voluntary sexual contact in an older adolescent, a full workup for sexual abuse should be undertaken for ocular manifestations of syphilis, gonorrhea, chlamydia, human papillomavirus, pubic lice, and, in the absence of other clear risk factors, HIV. At the very least, this intervention may have public health advantages in identifying infected adults in the child's home.

Emotional Abuse

Although perhaps not truly an ophthalmic manifestation of abuse, one must consider the psychosocial damage induced by harmful visual experiences in childhood. Caregivers or other adults may subject children to viewing sexual activity or drug-abuse behaviors. In a national survey of 1,000 children aged 2 to 17 years, one-third had witnessed some form of violence. Of these children, 20% had witnessed violence with a weapon; 9.6% had witnessed shooting, bombs, or riots; and 0.6% had witnessed murder.[98] The rates of exposure to violence are reportedly worse in more urban areas.[99] There is certain to be an adverse emotional effect of such visual experiences. Children also may present with functional visual loss and an otherwise normal eye examination as a result of unrevealed physical, emotional, or sexual abuse in the home.[100,101] Clearly, such causes are far less common than the other adverse childhood experiences, but it is important to include child abuse in the differential diagnosis.

References

1. Jensen A, Smith R, Olson M. Ocular clues to child abuse. *J Pediatr Ophthalmol.* 1971;8(4):270–272
2. Morad Y, Kim YM, Mian M, Huyer D, Capra L, Levin AV. Nonophthalmologist accuracy in diagnosing retinal hemorrhages in the shaken baby syndrome. *J Pediatr.* 2003;142(4):431–434 PMID: 12712063 https://doi.org/10.1067/mpd.2003.161
3. Kivlin JD, Simons KB, Lazoritz S, Ruttum MS. Shaken baby syndrome. *Ophthalmology.* 2000;107(7):1246–1254 PMID: 10889093 https://doi.org/10.1016/S0161-6420(00)00161-5
4. Binenbaum G, Rogers DL, Forbes BJ, et al. Patterns of retinal hemorrhage associated with increased intracranial pressure in children. *Pediatrics.* 2013;132(2):e430–e434 PMID: 23878052 https://doi.org/10.1542/peds.2013-0262
5. Shiau T, Levin AV. Retinal hemorrhages in children: the role of intracranial pressure. *Arch Pediatr Adolesc Med.* 2012;166(7):623–628 PMID: 22393175 https://doi.org/10.1001/archpediatrics.2012.46

6. Levin A. Retinal haemorrhage and child abuse. In: David T, ed. *Recent Advances in Paediatrics*. Vol 18. London, United Kingdom: Churchill Livingstone; 2000:151–219
7. Morad Y, Kim YM, Armstrong DC, Huyer D, Mian M, Levin AV. Correlation between retinal abnormalities and intracranial abnormalities in the shaken baby syndrome. *Am J Ophthalmol*. 2002;134(3):354–359 PMID: 12208246 https://doi.org/10.1016/S0002-9394(02)01628-8
8. Levin AV. Retinal hemorrhage in abusive head trauma. *Pediatrics*. 2010;126(5):961–970 PMID: 20921069 https://doi.org/10.1542/peds.2010-1220
9. Sebag J. Age-related differences in the human vitreoretinal interface. *Arch Ophthalmol*. 1991;109(7):966–971 PMID: 2064577 https://doi.org/10.1001/archopht.1991.01080070078039
10. Rangarajan N, Kamalakkannan SB, Hasija V, et al. Finite element model of ocular injury in abusive head trauma. *J AAPOS*. 2009;13(4):364–369 PMID: 19419890 https://doi.org/10.1016/j.jaapos.2008.11.006
11. Muni RH, Kohly RP, Sohn EH, Lee TC. Hand-held spectral domain optical coherence tomography finding in shaken-baby syndrome. *Retina*. 2010;30(4 suppl):S45–S50 PMID: 20386092 https://doi.org/10.1097/IAE.0b013e3181dc048c
12. Hayden A, Tawansy K, Gonzales J, Patel P, Chung M. Peripheral retinal non-perfusion in the shaken baby syndrome. *Invest Ophthalmol Vis Sci*. 2004;45:E-abstract 271
13. Goldenberg DT, Wu D, Capone A Jr, Drenser KA, Trese MT. Nonaccidental trauma and peripheral retinal nonperfusion. *Ophthalmology*. 2010;117(3):561–566 PMID: 20036009 https://doi.org/10.1016/j.ophtha.2009.08.013
14. Abed Alnabi W, Tang GJ, Eagle RC Jr, Gulino S, Thau A, Levin AV. Pathology of perimacular folds due to vitreoretinal traction in abusive head trauma. *Retina*. 2018 PMID: 30048385 https://doi.org/10.1097/IAE.0000000000002273
15. Lantz PE, Sinal SH, Stanton CA, Weaver RG Jr. Perimacular retinal folds from childhood head trauma. *BMJ*. 2004;328(7442):754–756 PMID: 15044292 https://doi.org/10.1136/bmj.328.7442.754
16. Lueder GT, Turner JW, Paschall R. Perimacular retinal folds simulating nonaccidental injury in an infant. *Arch Ophthalmol*. 2006;124(12):1782–1783 PMID: 17159043 https://doi.org/10.1001/archopht.124.12.1782
17. Gnanaraj L, Gilliland MG, Yahya RR, et al. Ocular manifestations of crush head injury in children. *Eye (Lond)*. 2007;21(1):5–10 PMID: 16311527 https://doi.org/10.1038/sj.eye.6702174
18. Kivlin JD, Currie ML, Greenbaum VJ, Simons KB, Jentzen J. Retinal hemorrhages in children following fatal motor vehicle crashes: a case series. *Arch Ophthalmol*. 2008;126(6):800–804 PMID: 18541842 https://doi.org/10.1001/archopht.126.6.800
19. Moran K, Reddie I, Jacobs M. Severe haemorrhagic retinopathy and traumatic retinoschisis in a 2 year old infant, after an 11 metre fall onto concrete. *Acta Paediatr*. 2008;97(suppl 459):149
20. Levin AV. Retinal hemorrhages of crush head injury: learning from outliers. *Arch Ophthalmol*. 2006;124(12):1773–1774 PMID: 17159039 https://doi.org/10.1001/archopht.124.12.1773
21. Wygnanski-Jaffe T, Levin AV, Shafiq A, et al. Postmortem orbital findings in shaken baby syndrome. *Am J Ophthalmol*. 2006;142(2):233–240 PMID: 16876502 https://doi.org/10.1016/j.ajo.2006.03.038
22. Elner SG, Elner VM, Albert DM, Arnall M. The medicolegal implications of detecting hemosiderin in the eyes of children who are suspected of being abused—reply. *Arch Ophthalmol*. 1991;109(3):322 https://doi.org/10.1001/archopht.1991.01080030023020

23. Gilliland MG, Levin AV, Enzenauer RW, et al. Guidelines for postmortem protocol for ocular investigation of sudden unexplained infant death and suspected physical child abuse. *Am J Forensic Med Pathol*. 2007;28(4):323–329 PMID: 18043020 https://doi.org/10.1097/PAF.0b013e31815b4c00
24. Giles CL. Retinal hemorrhages in the newborn. *Am J Ophthalmol*. 1960;49(5):1005–1011 PMID: 13850047 https://doi.org/10.1016/0002-9394(60)91824-9
25. Callaway NF, Ludwig CA, Blumenkranz MS, Jones JM, Fredrick DR, Moshfeghi DM. Retinal and optic nerve hemorrhages in the newborn infant: one-year results of the Newborn Eye Screen Test study. *Ophthalmology*. 2016;123(5):1043–1052 PMID: 26875004 https://doi.org/10.1016/j.ophtha.2016.01.004
26. Hughes LA, May K, Talbot JF, Parsons MA. Incidence, distribution, and duration of birth-related retinal hemorrhages: a prospective study. *J AAPOS*. 2006;10(2):102–106 PMID: 16678742 https://doi.org/10.1016/j.jaapos.2005.12.005
27. Zhao Q, Zhang Y, Yang Y, et al. Birth-related retinal hemorrhages in healthy full-term newborns and their relationship to maternal, obstetric, and neonatal risk factors. *Graefes Arch Clin Exp Ophthalmol*. 2015;253(7):1021–1025 PMID: 25981120 https://doi.org/10.1007/s00417-015-3052-9
28. Watts P, Maguire S, Kwok T, et al. Newborn retinal hemorrhages: a systematic review. *J AAPOS*. 2013;17(1):70–78 PMID: 23363882 https://doi.org/10.1016/j.jaapos.2012.07.012
29. Sezen F. Retinal haemorrhages in newborn infants. *Br J Ophthalmol*. 1971;55(4):248–253 PMID: 5103091 https://doi.org/10.1136/bjo.55.4.248
30. Kivlin J. Ophthalmic manifestations of shaken baby syndrome. In: Lazoritz S, Palusci V, eds. *The Shaken Baby Syndrome: A Multidisciplinary Approach*. New York, NY: The Hayworth Press, Inc; 2001:137–153
31. Schloff S, Mullaney PB, Armstrong DC, et al. Retinal findings in children with intracranial hemorrhage. *Ophthalmology*. 2002;109(8):1472–1476 PMID: 12153798 https://doi.org/10.1016/S0161-6420(02)01086-2
32. Tomasi LG, Rosman NP. Purtscher retinopathy in the battered child syndrome. *Am J Dis Child*. 1975;129(11):1335–1337 PMID: 1190166 https://doi.org/10.1001/archpedi.1975.02120480051012
33. Plunkett J. Fatal pediatric head injuries caused by short-distance falls. *Am J Forensic Med Pathol*. 2001;22(1):1–12 PMID: 11444653 https://doi.org/10.1097/00000433-200103000-00001
34. Pham H, Enzenauer RW, Elder JE, Levin AV. Retinal hemorrhage after cardiopulmonary resuscitation with chest compressions. *Am J Forensic Med Pathol*. 2013;34(2):122–124 PMID: 23629401 https://doi.org/10.1097/PAF.0b013e31828c38f9
35. Ladjimi A, Zaouali S, Messaoud R, et al. Valsalva retinopathy induced by labour. *Eur J Ophthalmol*. 2002;12(4):336–338 PMID: 12220009 https://doi.org/10.1177/112067210201200417
36. Chapman-Davies A, Lazarevic A. Valsalva maculopathy. *Clin Exp Optom*. 2002;85(1):42–45 PMID: 11952395 https://doi.org/10.1111/j.1444-0938.2002.tb03071.x
37. Herr S, Pierce MC, Berger RP, Ford H, Pitetti RD. Does Valsalva retinopathy occur in infants? An initial investigation in infants with vomiting caused by pyloric stenosis. *Pediatrics*. 2004;113(6):1658–1661 PMID: 15173487 https://doi.org/10.1542/peds.113.6.1658
38. Goldman M, Dagan Z, Yair M, Elbaz U, Lahat E, Yair M. Severe cough and retinal hemorrhage in infants and young children. *J Pediatr*. 2006;148(6):835–836 PMID: 16769399 https://doi.org/10.1016/j.jpeds.2005.12.052
39. Sandramouli S, Robinson R, Tsaloumas M, Willshaw HE. Retinal haemorrhages and convulsions. *Arch Dis Child*. 1997;76(5):449–451 PMID: 9196364 https://doi.org/10.1136/adc.76.5.449

40. Curcoy AI, Trenchs V, Morales M, Serra A, Pineda M, Pou J. Do retinal haemorrhages occur in infants with convulsions? *Arch Dis Child*. 2009;94(11):873–875 PMID: 19666457 https://doi.org/10.1136/adc.2007.132522
41. Tyagi AK, Scotcher S, Kozeis N, Willshaw HE. Can convulsions alone cause retinal haemorrhages in infants? *Br J Ophthalmol*. 1998;82(6):659–660 PMID: 9797668 https://doi.org/10.1136/bjo.82.6.659
42. Alexander R, Sato Y, Smith W, Bennett T. Incidence of impact trauma with cranial injuries ascribed to shaking. *Am J Dis Child*. 1990;144(6):724–726 PMID: 2346156 https://doi.org/10.1001/archpedi.1990.02150300124032
43. Bechtel K, Stoessel K, Leventhal JM, et al. Characteristics that distinguish accidental from abusive injury in hospitalized young children with head trauma. *Pediatrics*. 2004;114(1):165–168 PMID: 15231923 https://doi.org/10.1542/peds.114.1.165
44. Togioka BM, Arnold MA, Bathurst MA, et al. Retinal hemorrhages and shaken baby syndrome: an evidence-based review. *J Emerg Med*. 2009;37(1):98–106 PMID: 19081701 https://doi.org/10.1016/j.jemermed.2008.06.022
45. Maguire SA, Watts PO, Shaw AD, et al. Retinal haemorrhages and related findings in abusive and non-abusive head trauma: a systematic review. Eye (Lond). 2013;27(1):28–36 PMID: 23079748
46. Binenbaum G, Mirza-George N, Christian CW, Forbes BJ. Odds of abuse associated with retinal hemorrhages in children suspected of child abuse. *J AAPOS*. 2009;13(3): 268–272 PMID: 19541267 https://doi.org/10.1016/j.jaapos.2009.03.005
47. Forbes BJ, Cox M, Christian CW. Retinal hemorrhages in patients with epidural hematomas. *J AAPOS*. 2008;12(2):177–180 PMID: 18258466 https://doi.org/10.1016/j.jaapos.2007.07.009
48. Scheller J, Huisman TA. Moderate bilateral retinal hemorrhages in an infant following a short fall. Clin Pediatr (Phila). 2015;54(10):999–1002 PMID: 25316220
49. Trenchs V, Curcoy AI, Morales M, Serra A, Navarro R, Pou J. Retinal haemorrhages in-head trauma resulting from falls: differential diagnosis with non-accidental trauma in patients younger than 2 years of age. *Childs Nerv Syst*. 2008;24(7):815–820 PMID: 18270718 https://doi.org/10.1007/s00381-008-0583-y
50. Gardner HB. A witnessed short fall mimicking presumed shaken baby syndrome (inflicted childhood neurotrauma). *Pediatr Neurosurg*. 2007;43(5):433–435 PMID: 17786015 https://doi.org/10.1159/000106399
51. Aoki N, Masuzawa H. Infantile acute subdural hematoma. Clinical analysis of 26 cases. *J Neurosurg*. 1984;61(2):273–280 PMID: 6737052 https://doi.org/10.3171/jns.1984.61.2.0273
52. Vinchon M, Noizet O, Defoort-Dhellemmes S, Soto-Ares G, Dhellemmes P. Infantile subdural hematomas due to traffic accidents. *Pediatr Neurosurg*. 2002;37(5):245–253 PMID: 12411716 https://doi.org/10.1159/000066216
53. Levin AV, Christian CW; American Academy of Pediatrics Committee on Child Abuse and Neglect and Section on Ophthalmology. The eye examination in the evaluation of child abuse. *Pediatrics*. 2010;126(2):376–380 PMID: 20660545 https://doi.org/10.1542/peds.2010-1397
54. Binenbaum G, Chen W, Huang J, Ying GS, Forbes BJ. The natural history of retinal hemorrhage in pediatric head trauma. *J AAPOS*. 2016;20(2):131–135 PMID: 27079593 https://doi.org/10.1016/j.jaapos.2015.12.008
55. Matthews GP, Das A. Dense vitreous hemorrhages predict poor visual and neurological prognosis in infants with shaken baby syndrome. *J Pediatr Ophthalmol Strabismus*. 1996;33(4):260–265 PMID: 8827564 https://doi.org/10.3928/0191-3913-19960701-13

56. Gilles EE, McGregor ML, Levy-Clarke G. Retinal hemorrhage asymmetry in inflicted head injury: a clue to pathogenesis? *J Pediatr*. 2003;143(4):494–499 PMID: 14571228 https://doi.org/10.1067/S0022-3476(03)00416-5
57. Muller PJ, Deck JH. Intraocular and optic nerve sheath hemorrhage in cases of sudden intracranial hypertension. *J Neurosurg*. 1974;41(2):160–166 PMID: 4366848 https://doi.org/10.3171/jns.1974.41.2.0160
58. Vanderlinden RG, Chisholm LD. Vitreous hemorrhages and sudden increased intracranial pressure. *J Neurosurg*. 1974;41(2):167–176 PMID: 4842785 https://doi.org/10.3171/jns.1974.41.2.0167
59. Duhaime AC, Gennarelli TA, Thibault LE, Bruce DA, Margulies SS, Wiser R. The shaken baby syndrome. A clinical, pathological, and biomechanical study. *J Neurosurg*. 1987;66(3):409–415 PMID: 3819836 https://doi.org/10.3171/jns.1987.66.3.0409
60. Cory CZ, Jones BM. Can shaking alone cause fatal brain injury? A biomechanical assessment of the Duhaime shaken baby syndrome model. *Med Sci Law*. 2003;43(4):317–333 PMID: 14655963 https://doi.org/10.1258/rsmmsl.43.4.317
61. Biron D, Shelton D. Perpetrator accounts in infant abusive head trauma brought about by a shaking event. *Child Abuse Negl*. 2005;29(12):1347–1358 PMID: 16289688 https://doi.org/10.1016/j.chiabu.2005.05.003
62. Starling SP, Holden JR, Jenny C. Abusive head trauma: the relationship of perpetrators to their victims. *Pediatrics*. 1995;95(2):259–262 PMID: 7838645
63. Adamsbaum C, Grabar S, Mejean N, Rey-Salmon C. Abusive head trauma: judicial admissions highlight violent and repetitive shaking. *Pediatrics*. 2010;126(3):546–555 PMID: 20696720 https://doi.org/10.1542/peds.2009-3647
64. Morad Y, Avni I, Benton SA, et al. Normal computerized tomography of brain in children with shaken baby syndrome. *J AAPOS*. 2004;8(5):445–450 PMID: 15492737 https://doi.org/10.1016/j.jaapos.2004.06.007
65. Morad Y, Avni I, Capra L, et al. Shaken baby syndrome without intracranial hemorrhage on initial computed tomography. *J AAPOS*. 2004;8(6):521–527 PMID: 15616498 https://doi.org/10.1016/j.jaapos.2004.07.009
66. Oral R, Yagmur F, Nashelsky M, Turkmen M, Kirby P. Fatal abusive head trauma cases: consequence of medical staff missing milder forms of physical abuse. *Pediatr Emerg Care*. 2008;24(12):816–821 PMID: 19050665 https://doi.org/10.1097/PEC.0b013e31818e9f5d
67. Ludwig S, Warman M. Shaken baby syndrome: a review of 20 cases. *Ann Emerg Med*. 1984;13(2):104–107 PMID: 6691610 https://doi.org/10.1016/S0196-0644(84)80571-5
68. Lopes NR, Eisenstein E, Williams LC. Abusive head trauma in children: a literature review. *J Pediatr (Rio J)*. 2013;89(5):426–433 PMID: 23850113 https://doi.org/10.1016/j.jped.2013.01.011
69. Greenwald MJ, Weiss A, Oesterle CS, Friendly DS. Traumatic retinoschisis in battered babies. *Ophthalmology*. 1986;93(5):618–625 PMID: 3725321 https://doi.org/10.1016/S0161-6420(86)33688-1
70. Chevignard MP, Lind K. Long-term outcome of abusive head trauma. *Pediatr Radiol*. 2014;44(S4)(suppl 4):S548–S558 PMID: 25501726 https://doi.org/10.1007/s00247-014-3169-8
71. Han DP, Wilkinson WS. Late ophthalmic manifestations of the shaken baby syndrome. *J Pediatr Ophthalmol Strabismus*. 1990;27(6):299–303 PMID: 2086746
72. Haviland J, Russell RI. Outcome after severe non-accidental head injury. *Arch Dis Child*. 1997;77(6):504–507 PMID: 9496184 https://doi.org/10.1136/adc.77.6.504

73. Makaroff KL, Putnam FW. Outcomes of infants and children with inflicted traumatic brain injury. *Dev Med Child Neurol*. 2003;45(7):497–502 PMID: 12828406 https://doi.org/10.1111/j.1469-8749.2003.tb00947.x
74. McCabe CF, Donahue SP. Prognostic indicators for vision and mortality in shaken baby syndrome. *Arch Ophthalmol*. 2000;118(3):373–377 PMID: 10721960 https://doi.org/10.1001/archopht.118.3.373
75. Case ME. Inflicted traumatic brain injury in infants and young children. *Brain Pathol*. 2008;18(4):571–582 PMID: 18782169 https://doi.org/10.1111/j.1750-3639.2008.00204.x
76. Kemp AM, Jaspan T, Griffiths J, et al. Neuroimaging: what neuroradiological features distinguish abusive from non-abusive head trauma? A systematic review. *Arch Dis Child*. 2011;96(12):1103–1112 PMID: 21965812 https://doi.org/10.1136/archdischild-2011-300630
77. King WJ, MacKay M, Sirnick A; Canadian Shaken Baby Study Group. Shaken baby syndrome in Canada: clinical characteristics and outcomes of hospital cases. *CMAJ*. 2003;168(2):155–159 PMID: 12538542
78. Hansen RM, Fulton AB. *Taylor and Hoyt's Pediatric Ophthalmology and Strabismus*. 5th ed. Edinburgh, Scotland: Elsevier Inc; 2017
79. Illingworth RS. Delayed visual maturation. *Arch Dis Child*. 1961;36(188):407–409 PMID: 13717539 https://doi.org/10.1136/adc.36.188.407
80. Wilkinson WS, Han DP, Rappley MD, Owings CL. Retinal hemorrhage predicts neurologic injury in the shaken baby syndrome. *Arch Ophthalmol*. 1989;107(10):1472–1474 PMID: 2803095 https://doi.org/10.1001/archopht.1989.01070020546037
81. Friendly DS. Ocular manifestations of physical child abuse. *Trans Am Acad Ophthalmol Otolaryngol*. 1971;75(2):318–332 PMID: 5557171
82. Taylor D, Bentovim A. Recurrent nonaccidentally inflicted chemical eye injuries to siblings. *J Pediatr Ophthalmol*. 1976;13(4):238–242 PMID: 1018209
83. Baskin DE, Stein F, Coats DK, Paysse EA. Recurrent conjunctivitis as a presentation of Munchausen syndrome by proxy. *Ophthalmology*. 2003;110(8):1582–1584 PMID: 12917177 https://doi.org/10.1016/S0161-6420(03)00489-5
84. Taylor D. Unnatural injuries. *Eye (Lond)*. 2000;14(Pt 2):123–150 PMID: 10845007 https://doi.org/10.1038/eye.2000.44
85. Wood PR, Fowlkes J, Holden P, Casto D. Fever of unknown origin for six years: Munchausen syndrome by proxy. *J Fam Pract*. 1989;28(4):391–395 PMID: 2703809
86. Feenstra J, Merth IT, Treffers PD. [A case of Munchausen syndrome by proxy]. *Tijdschr Kindergeneeskd*. 1988;56(4):148–153 PMID: 3176014
87. Meadow R. ABC of child abuse. Suffocation. *BMJ*. 1989;298(6687):1572–1573 PMID: 2503121 https://doi.org/10.1136/bmj.298.6687.1572
88. Chiu CH, Chuang YY, Su LH. Subconjunctival haemorrhage and respiratory distress. *Lancet*. 2001;358(9283):724 PMID: 11551580 https://doi.org/10.1016/S0140-6736(01)05841-X
89. Deonna T, Marcoz JP, Meyer HU, de Techtermann F, Bianchi F. [Factitious epilepsy: Munchausen syndrome by proxy. Another aspect of child abuse: recurrent coma in a 4-year-old child caused by nonaccidental poisoning]. *Rev Med Suisse Romande*. 1985;105(11):995–1002 PMID: 4089391
90. Rogers D, Tripp J, Bentovim A, Robinson A, Berry D, Goulding R. Papers and originals. *Br Med J*. 1976;1(6013):793–796 PMID: 1260335 https://doi.org/10.1136/bmj.1.6013.793

91. Kahn G, Goldman E. Munchausen syndrome by proxy: mother fabricates infant's hearing impairment. *J Speech Hear Res.* 1991;34(4):957–959 PMID: 1956202 https://doi.org/10.1044/jshr.3404.957
92. Rosenberg DA. Web of deceit: a literature review of Munchausen syndrome by proxy. *Child Abuse Negl.* 1987;11(4):547–563 PMID: 3322516 https://doi.org/10.1016/0145-2134(87)90081-0
93. Curtiss S. *Genie: A Psycholinguistic Study of a Modern-Day "Wild Child."* New York, NY: Academic Press; 1977
94. San Martin R, Steinkuller PG, Nisbet RM. Retinopathy in the sexually abused battered child. *Ann Ophthalmol.* 1981;13(1):89–91 PMID: 7247165
95. Levin A. Ocular manifestations of child abuse. *Ophthalmol Clin North Am.* 1990;3(2):249–264
96. Lewis LS, Glauser TA, Joffe MD. Gonococcal conjunctivitis in prepubertal children. *Am J Dis Child.* 1990;144(5):546–548 PMID: 2109929
97. Goodyear-Smith F. What is the evidence for non-sexual transmission of gonorrhoea in children after the neonatal period? A systematic review. *J Forensic Leg Med.* 2007;14(8):489–502 PMID: 17961874 https://doi.org/10.1016/j.jflm.2007.04.001
98. Finkelhor D, Ormrod R, Turner H, Hamby SL. The victimization of children and youth: a comprehensive, national survey. *Child Maltreat.* 2005;10(1):5–25 PMID: 15611323 https://doi.org/10.1177/1077559504271287
99. Stein BD, Jaycox LH, Kataoka S, Rhodes HJ, Vestal KD. Prevalence of child and adolescent exposure to community violence. *Clin Child Fam Psychol Rev.* 2003;6(4):247–264 PMID: 14719637 https://doi.org/10.1023/B:CCFP.0000006292.61072.d2
100. Catalono RA, Simon JW, Krohel GB, Rosenberg PN. Functional visual loss in children. *Ophthalmology.* 1986;93(3):385–390 PMID: 3703508 https://doi.org/10.1016/S0161-6420(86)33730-8
101. Lim SA, Siatkowski RM, Farris BK. Functional visual loss in adults and children patient characteristics, management, and outcomes. *Ophthalmology.* 2005;112(10):1821–1828 PMID: 16140382 https://doi.org/10.1016/j.ophtha.2005.05.009

PART 2

Sexual Abuse

CHAPTER 9

Taking Forensically Sound Histories in Cases of Alleged Sexual Abuse

Jenna Spagnuolo, DCFI
Forensic Interviewer Supervisor
Child Abuse Program
Children's Hospital of The King's Daughters
Norfolk, VA

Suzanne P. Starling, MD, FAAP
Medical Director, Chadwick Center for Children & Families
Rady Children's Hospital of San Diego
Clinical Professor of Pediatrics, University of California San Diego
San Diego, CA

Introduction

In 2015, the US Department of Health and Human Services estimated that child protective services (CPS) received 4 million referrals involving 7.2 million children. Of those children, 311,000 were served in a child advocacy center (CAC), with two-thirds of them disclosing sexual abuse.[1] Although parents and caregivers often warn children of "stranger danger," a survey of 63,000 sexual abuse cases that were substantiated by CPS in 2013 indicated approximately 80% of perpetrators were a parent and 6% were other relatives.[2,3] Children who have experienced sexual abuse regularly present to medical practices for care. Such children may come to the attention of a medical professional secondary to physical sequelae of sexual abuse or to behavioral or emotional manifestations of having experienced sexual abuse, or for reasons seemingly unrelated to concerns about sexual abuse.[4]

This chapter will help medical professionals develop the skills they need to effectively respond when an incident of alleged sexual abuse has occurred. It will discuss the dynamics behind taking forensically sound histories in cases of alleged child sexual abuse and identify when it is appropriate for a medical professional to question the child. In addition, forensic interview best practices and accurate record keeping will be discussed.

Location of the Interview

Although interviews of children who have experienced sexual abuse can occur in many locations, forensic interviews conducted at a CAC are considered best practice throughout the United States.[5,6] A *forensic interview* is a developmentally sensitive and legally sound method of gathering factual information about allegations of abuse or exposure to violence. This interview is conducted by a trained and neutral medical professional using research and practice-informed techniques as part of a larger investigative process.[2]

A CAC is a safe, child-friendly facility where children can come with a non-offending caregiver for evaluation and treatment of suspected child abuse. The child and family are provided services that may include child advocacy, forensic interviews, medical examinations, therapy, and courtroom preparation. The individuals who provide these services, along with law enforcement, child protective agencies, attorneys, and others, make up the multidisciplinary team. In many communities, multidisciplinary and multiagency teams develop policies about how mandated reporters should respond to possible sexual abuse, including which members of the team should question children. There are 1,036 CACs across the United States to assist in decision-making regarding children who have experienced child abuse. The National Children's Advocacy Center website (www.nationalcac.org/find-a-cac) lists all the CACs in the United States.

For localities without access to a CAC, medical professionals may be called on to take a history from a child. Many factors influence the decision for a medical professional to question a child suspected of experiencing sexual abuse. Medical professionals need to consider their local policy and practice. While it may be a challenge to develop skills for interviewing children who are reporting sexual abuse, it is important to understand the fundamental principles of questioning children with a technique that is sensitive and appropriate so children can disclose in a way that does not interfere with the criminal investigation. Consideration should also be taken to identify the child's developmental stage in the disclosure process.

Understanding the Disclosure Process

Abuse disclosure is a process, not an event. Many factors determine how and when children disclose and if they disclose at all. These factors include family relationships, having a protective caregiver, gender, feelings of culpability, social and cultural norms, and perpetrator-child relationship.[7–10]

There are 2 types of disclosure: purposeful and accidental. A *purposeful disclosure* is one in which the child makes a conscious decision to make someone else aware of the event(s). An *accidental disclosure* is one in which others are made aware of the abuse unintentionally.[11] Accidental disclosures could occur if another individual witnesses the abuse or sees videos or pictures of the abusive event, if the child has a positive test result for sexually transmitted infections, or if text messages or other communications between the child and the alleged offender are intercepted. It is important for the professional who is interviewing to know the type of disclosure because it may affect the child's ability to fully participate in an interview. For example, if a child has not told anyone about the abuse and is unaware that other individuals know about the event, a full disclosure to a professional is unlikely.

Whether purposeful or accidental, a child may be in 1 of 4 stages of disclosure as identified by Sorensen and Snow.[11] The first stage is *denial*, in which the child's initial statement indicates that no abuse occurred. The second stage is *disclosure*; this can be either a tentative disclosure, showing reluctance or providing a partial disclosure, or an active disclosure, with the child providing his or her own account of the alleged sexual abuse event(s). *Retraction* is the third stage and is identified as the withdrawal of any disclosure or parts of a disclosure that have been made. Finally, a child may *reaffirm or reassert* their abuse disclosure. While it is important to understand the concept of these stages, not all children will experience every stage. Additionally, children may vacillate between these stages when in the disclosure process.

Even in confirmed cases of sexual abuse, children may not disclose immediately or may never disclose at all. Various studies have looked at the rates of disclosure of children who have experienced sexual abuse (Table 9.1).

TABLE 9.1
Abuse Disclosure Rates

Type of Study	Disclosed Immediately	Delayed Disclosure	Disclosed as an Adult or Older Child
Adult Retrospective Studies			
Hébert et al, 2009[12]	21.3% (up to 1 mo)	21.2% (up to 5 y)	57.5% (>5 y)
Smith et al, 2000[13]	27% (up to 1 y)	19% (>1 y)	28% (not until survey administered)
Studies of Adolescents and Children			
Schönbucher et al, 2012[14]	33% (first week)	33% (up to 5 y)	33% (>5 y)
Kogan, 2004[15]	43% (up to 1 mo)	31% (>1 mo but during childhood)	26% (not until survey administered)

From Townsend C. Child sexual abuse disclosure: what practitioners need to know. Darkness to Light website. https://www.d2l.org/wp-content/uploads/2016/10/ChildSexualAbuseDisclosurePaper_20160217_v.1.pdf. Published February 2016. Accessed July 11, 2019.

While the body of research indicates it is difficult for children to disclose sexual abuse, the advice for medical professionals is to employ forensically sound questioning techniques. Such techniques will help avoid eliciting false allegations from children about possible sexual abuse or otherwise contaminating a child's disclosure.

Responding to a Disclosure of Child Sexual Abuse

Obtaining forensically sound histories in cases of alleged sexual abuse is very different from the typical history-taking strategies medical professionals use. In a general medical examination, the medical professional typically employs direct questions such as, "How long have you had a fever?" and "What did you eat this morning?" The techniques for eliciting a history in cases of suspected abuse involves use of open-ended questions. There are at least 2 reasons for this. First, children's free recall memory is the most accurate when open-ended questions are asked. Second, if only closed-ended inquiries are employed, such as direct, leading, and coercive questions, the child's disclosures may be inaccurate, guided more by the questioner than by the child. Such

BOX 9.1
Response to an Abuse Disclosure

Do

- Allow the child to talk without interruption, allowing the child to tell what happened in his/her own words.
- Reassure the child he/she has done the right thing by telling you and that what happened is not his/her fault.
- Believe the child.
- Contact the local or state child protective services hotline and local law enforcement.

Do not

- Pressure the child to talk or overwhelm him/her with questions.
- Overreact or become emotional; children may interpret that your anger or disgust is directed at them, and children who feel they are in trouble often stop talking.
- Blame the child or minimize the child's feelings.
- Make promises you cannot keep or that are out of your control, such as telling the child you will keep this information a secret or predicting the outcome of an investigation.
- Confront the offender.

disclosures are less valid in a CPS and legal setting. If the content of the interview and the child's statements are challenged, the child may not be adequately protected.

When a child makes a disclosure of abuse, there are critical actions (Box 9.1) to ensure the child's safety and the integrity of an investigation.

Children's Language Development and Linguistics

The basic concepts of child development and linguistics are important when speaking with children.[16] There are 2 divisions of language, expressive and receptive. *Expressive language* involves the individual's ability to write, speak, or otherwise communicate thoughts, feelings, wants, and needs. *Receptive language* is the ability to understand words and language, such as reading signs and other written information and understanding the meaning of sounds and time. From infancy to adolescence, there are developmental milestones for language development and acquisition.

Chronological age alone does not predict a child's ability to understand, interpret, and respond with accuracy to questions. Other factors should be taken into consideration when speaking with a child, such as the age and ability of the child's parents, the number and age of the child's siblings, participation in a child care or school setting, the family's culture, mental and physical health conditions, and developmental disabilities. Allison Foster developed the adapted guidelines for age-appropriate questioning (Figure 9.1).[17–20]

Just as there are limitations to children's responses to abstract concepts, there are limitations to their understanding of language and the concept of time. Children at different developmental levels have different interpretations and understanding of language.

Children who are 3 to 6 years old may use words without full comprehension of their meaning. Therefore, clarification of the terms used by this age group is necessary. If a child states, "I had to watch the show that was inappropriate," follow-up questions such as, "What does inappropriate mean?" or "What made the show inappropriate?" will help provide clarification without relying on the medical professional to apply his or her own understanding of the word. Also, children within this age range are typically concrete and have difficulty seeing situations from someone else's perspective. Asking "why" questions to these children ("Why did you go in the bedroom?" or "Why did he tell you to take off your pants?") may elicit a guess from the child instead of a recall of the actual

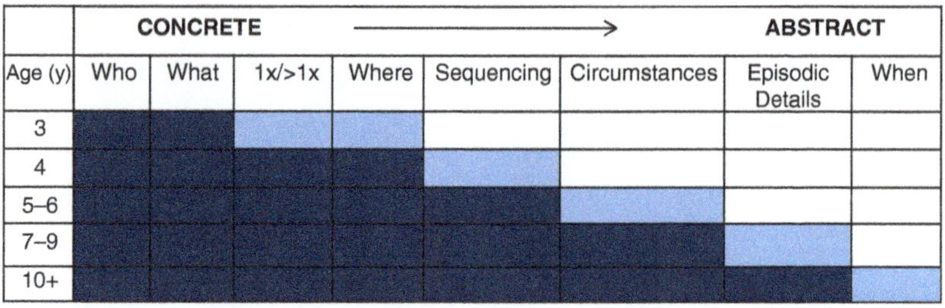

FIGURE 9.1

Guidelines for age-appropriate interview questions. The darker shading represents what children may be able to answer if they are developing normally. Lighter shading represents question types that some children at the indicated age may have the capacity to answer.

From Questioning children. Gundersen Health System website. https://www.gundersenhealth.org/app/files/public/2527/NCPTC-Questioning-Children-binder.pdf. Published 2016. Accessed January 23, 2019.

events. Instead, keep questions as simple and concrete as possible while minimizing the number of words used in each question. These children will generally be able to express who was there, what happened, and where it happened but may have confusion about the temporal order of the events that took place.

Additionally, children who are between 3 and 6 years of age do not generally understand the meaning of words used to describe time. "Yesterday" could mean the event happened several days ago or that simply it happened before the conversation that the child is currently having. Asking a child of this age, especially in situations of chronic abuse, to tell how many times an event occurred will likely force a guess. A better approach is to have the child tell you if something happened one time or more than one time. The duration of an event is also difficult for children in this age range: "How long were you in the bathroom?" or "How many minutes did you have to do that?" are question types that should be avoided. It is also important to use proper names and places when speaking with children in this age range. It is difficult for them to understand pronouns such as *he, she, them,* or *themselves.* Children within this age range can typically recognize commonly used prepositions such as *before, on,* or *in.* However, they should be used with caution, and less common prepositions such as *beyond* and *toward* should be avoided.[17]

From ages 7 to 11 years, children continue to emulate speech of those around them; while they have a better understanding of word meanings, it is still necessary to seek clarification of the terms they use. For example, a child provided the statement, "My stepdad raped me." On further clarification, it was determined the child's stepfather touched her breast on top of her clothing while play-fighting. The child told a friend about the incident and the friend provided her with the word "rape." Children in this age range also begin to apply their knowledge and are beginning to apply more abstract thinking. They have more language and cognitive abilities to describe an abusive event and should typically be able to answer who was present, what happened, where the event occurred, the sequence of a particular event, circumstances that led up to the event, and what happened after. These children also begin to recognize cause and effect and have a basic understanding of the legal system. Therefore, their disclosure or lack thereof factors in the dynamics of their family/perpetrator relationships, whether or not they have a protective caregiver, and any feelings of culpability.[7–10,17]

Adolescents begin to view events from multiple perspectives and continue to develop a more abstract view of situations. Although they may physically resemble adults, their brains are still developing and their emotional development may not match their physical development. Adolescents aged 13 years and older may begin to focus more on themselves and are influenced by their peer groups and other groups or persons who make them feel special. Because of this, they may be more susceptible to grooming by older perpetrators, including those they meet online. *Grooming* may include extra attention, gift buying, and flattery and is individualized to the specific child. Teens may begin to develop feelings for the perpetrator and engage as a compliant victim in sexual acts or by granting requests by the perpetrator for sexually explicit photos or videos. Speaking with teens who were compliant (ie, adolescents who do not identify as a victim) is different than other conversations with children who have experienced sexual abuse and may include questions like, "Tell me how you met your boyfriend," or "What do you and your girlfriend like to do together?"

Some basic principles to remember when speaking with a child or teen include

- Use words in their most basic form (house vs residence).
- Translate difficult words and avoid jargon (gender, genitals, perpetrator).
- Use proper names and places.
- Use one idea per question and stay on task.
- Avoid questions that limit a child to 2 choices; offer an alternative to the binary ("Were your clothes on, or off, or something else?").

Minimal Facts Interview

When there is access to a CAC or when the local protocol recommends a formal forensic interview, the medical professional may still gather minimal facts about the alleged abuse to provide as a mandated reporter. A *minimal facts interview* includes

- Type of abusive activity that occurred
- Identity of the alleged perpetrator(s), including relationship to the child, date of birth, address, and race
- Presence of witnesses and/or other children
- Child's physical and emotional safety, such as suicidal ideation
- Need for immediate medical attention, either for the child's health or to gather physical evidence

Minimal facts may be gathered from an adult; questioning the child may not be necessary.

When a minimal facts interview is necessary, medical professionals should begin by developing a rapport with the child and assessing the child's capacity to communicate. A good practice is to use open-ended questions during the rapport-building stage, such as, "Tell me all about school." The child's responses in the rapport-building phase can inform the medical professional about the child's ability to respond to open-ended questions. When developing rapport, questions should remain neutral with the intent of soliciting a narrative from the child. The narrative topic should be one that the child is familiar with and not fantasy or oriented in make-believe concepts. Children's ability to report events that happened to them in the past and their knowledge of their environment, such as who lives at their house, are other capacities to assess during the beginning phase of the interview. Other examples of open-ended questions include

- "Tell me about your family."
- "Tell me more about you."
- "Tell me some things you like about your family; tell me some things you do not like about your family."

If the child cannot provide responses to open-ended questions, the professional should employ more closed-ended questions during rapport building, such as, "Who lives with you?" to learn what kinds of questions the child can understand.

Following the rapport-building phase in a minimal facts interview, a transition is made to identify the abusive activity that allegedly occurred. Questions may include

- "Tell me what we are here to talk about today."
- "I understand something may have happened to you. Tell me what happened."
- "I see a bruise on your face. Tell me about how that happened."

Once a child makes a disclosure of abuse, further exploration is needed to make a mandated report. Obtaining this information is critical in assessing the safety of the child and includes identifying the alleged offender and their relationship with the child, presence of witnesses and/or other children, and the need for immediate medical attention. Open-ended questions that elicit free narrative and event recall should continue to be used and then funneled into more closed-ended questions as needed to obtain information. After asking a closed-ended question, the medical professional should then follow up by asking one that is open-ended. For example

Professional: You said Uncle Tommy touched you one time. Where were you when Uncle Tommy touched you?

Child: In my bedroom.

Professional: Tell me everything that happened in the bedroom when Uncle Tommy touched you.

Children may provide broad accounts of their experiences when disclosing repeated or chronic abuse. Generic prompts elicit information about what usually happened during repeated similar events. If a child provides information about what typically occurred, generic prompts can be used. Episodic prompts elicit details about specific individual events.[21] (See Box 9.2.) If the child is capable of differentiating between events, or if it is identified as a one-time occurrence, the professional may use episodic prompts.

While question types are important, the manner in which the professional speaking with the child conducts herself or himself is also vital. A key practice is providing children the time they need to answer the question. Once a child is providing an account of an event, let the narrative end before asking clarifying questions and avoid interrupting the child. Also, guessing or assuming what a child may have said or was alluding to can inhibit an investigation. If a response is unclear, it is acceptable to ask the child to provide clarifying information or to repeat his or her response.

Word usage and usage of developmentally appropriate language by interviewers also affect the quality of the interview. Proper pronunciation of words should be used when speaking with a child instead of mimicking the child's pronunciation or baby talk.[21]

BOX 9.2
Generic Versus Episodic Interview Prompts

Generic prompts

- Tell me what happened.
- Then what happens?
- What happens next?
- What happens when [child's words for the repeated action to other information that identifies the topic, eg, "...the other children leave"]?
- You said [child's words; eg, "He tells you to come sit on his lap"]. Then what happens?
- You said sometimes [child's words; eg, "She uses a belt"]. Tell me what happens when [child's words; eg, "She uses a belt"].
- Tell me what happened that time.
- Then what happened?

Episodic prompts

- What happened the last time?
- What else happened when [child's words for the event or other information that identifies the topic, eg, "...the other children left"]?
- You said [child's words; eg, "He told me to sit on his lap"]. Then what happened?
- You said once [child's words; eg, "She used a belt"]. Tell me about that time.

However, the child's word for body parts or the term the child uses for identifying people should not be changed by the interviewer. For example, if the child identifies her grandmother as "Memaw," the interviewer should use the child's word when referring to the grandmother. In the same vein, the interviewer should avoid introducing new words until the child uses them first. If, for example, the child identifies her vagina as a "cookie," the interviewer should also use the same terminology when referring to the genitalia.

More questions may be asked to provide the child with an opportunity to ask his or her own questions and for the medical professional to assess safety. Questions may include

- "Do you have any questions for me?"
- "Is there anything that we have not talked about yet that you want to talk about?"
- "Does anyone else know about what happened?"
- "Who are safe people that you can talk to?"

This conversation is intended to gather only the minimal facts needed to provide to law enforcement and CPS. If a child is reluctant to disclose, do not pressure the child to interact or overwhelm the child with questions. Instead, make a formal report of what information is obtained during the interaction.

To assist medical professionals and other mandated reporters when speaking with children who have allegedly experienced abuse, Anne Graffam Walker developed the Checklist for Interviewing/Questioning Children[17] (Box 9.3).

BOX 9.3
Checklist for Interviewing/Questioning Children

I. Framing the Event

- ☐ Did I tell the child my name and what my job is—in nontechnical words?
- ☐ Did I help the child become familiar with the surroundings of the interview?
- ☐ Did I tell the child the purpose of our talk, and why it is important, and what will happen afterward?
- ☐ Did I give the child a chance to ask me questions about this talk?
- ☐ Did I ask the child to narrate fully on a neutral topic? Did I try to establish a common vocabulary for the things we talk about? Was I listening to the kinds of words and sentences the child used?

II. Using Clear Language

- ☐ Did I use easy words instead of hard ones?
- ☐ Did I avoid legal words and phrases?
- ☐ Did I avoid using words that mean one thing in everyday life but another in law (like "court"?)
- ☐ Did I question the assumption that because a child uses a word, he or she understands the concept it represents?
- ☐ Was I as redundant as possible? That is, did I use specific names and places instead of pronouns (like "he" and "we") and vague referents (like "it," that," and "there")?

III. Asking Questions

- ☐ Did I keep all my questions and sentences simple? Did I try for one main (new) thought per utterance?
- ☐ Did I avoid asking "Do you remember" questions?
- ☐ When I shifted topics, and when I moved from the present to the past or vice versa, did I alert the child I was going to do so?
- ☐ Did I give the child the necessary help to organize his or her story?

(continued)

BOX 9.3 (*continued*)

- ☐ Did I avoid asking the child about abstract concepts like, "What is the difference between truth and lies?" Did I choose instead to give the child everyday, concrete examples and let him or her demonstrate rather than articulate knowledge of abstract concepts, right and wrong?
- ☐ Did I use as few negatives as possible in questions I asked?

IV. Listening to the Answers

- ☐ Were the child's RESPONSES to my questions ANSWERS to my questions? Am I sure?
- ☐ If the child's answers were inconsistent, did I ask myself if
  - I or someone else had asked the same question repeatedly?
  - I had changed the wording of a question I had asked before?
  - I was forgetting that children can be very literal in their interpretation of language?
  - The child's processing of language might not be as mature as mine?

V. Global Checks

- ☐ Did I stay in the child's world by framing my questions in terms of the child's experience?
- ☐ Did I make sure not to take the child's understanding of language for granted?
- ☐ Was I listening to my OWN language, my OWN questions?

Adapted from Walker AG. *Handbook on Questioning Children: A Linguistic Perspective*. 3rd ed. Washington, DC: American Bar Association Center on Children and the Law; 2013.

Forensic Interview Structure

The formal *forensic interview* is similar to a minimal facts interview in that it uses open-ended, non-leading questions to explore allegations of abuse. However, the purpose and structure of a forensic interview is very different from a minimal facts interview. It is a developmentally sensitive and legally sound method of gathering factual information conducted by a specially trained and neutral professional child forensic interviewer; the interviewer uses research and practice-informed techniques as part of a larger investigative process.[2]

Individuals from all the nation's major forensic interview training programs[22] convened in 2010 in an effort to reach consensus on best practices for forensic interviewing of children. The result was a paper published in 2015 by the Office of Juvenile Justice and Delinquency Prevention, a branch of the US Department of Justice. This publication indicated that all models of interviews, whether highly structured or semi-structured, included 3 phases: the initial rapport-building phase, the substantive phase, and the closure phase.

The *initial rapport-building phase* typically comprises introductions with an age- and context-appropriate explanation of documentation methods, a review of interview instructions, a discussion of the importance of telling the truth, and practice providing narratives and episodic memory training. The *substantive phase* most often includes a narrative description of events, detail-seeking strategies, clarification, and testing of alternative hypotheses, when appropriate. The *closure phase* gives more attention to the socioemotional needs of a child, transitioning to non-substantive topics, allowing for questions, and discussing safety or educational messages.[22]

Use of Demonstrative Communication and Media

The goal of a forensic interview is to have the child verbally describe his or her experience. A question remains, however, as to whether limiting children to verbal responses allows all children to fully recount their experiences or whether media (eg, paper, markers, anatomically detailed drawings or dolls) may be used during the interview to aid in description. The use of media varies greatly by model and professional training.[23]

Forensic interviewers employ many different tools to assist them in an interview. Some children lack verbal communication skills or are reluctant or distressed when asked to respond verbally to questions about alleged sexual abuse. In these situations, and for clarification purposes, demonstrative communication such as human figure drawings and anatomical dolls may be used to assist the child. In addition, media such as photos of the child or alleged offender and copies of text messages or other communications between the alleged offender and the child may be employed. In some cases, other modes of communication, such as having the child write down her disclosure or drawing a picture of the room where the abuse occurred, may be useful. These techniques are for clarification purposes only and are not used to elicit a disclosure of abuse. It is important the medical professional is not interpreting the child's written words or drawings but, rather, following up with questions that provide clarification. For example, if a child writes, "Tommy hurt me," the medical professional may respond with, "Did Tommy hurt you one time or more than one time?" or "Tell me more about Tommy hurting you."

The use of demonstrative communication devices, media, and other modes of communication when speaking with a child about alleged sexual abuse is not considered best practice for a minimal facts interview that would be performed by a medical professional. Such techniques are best employed by well-trained child forensic interviewers.

Record Keeping for Medical Professionals

Accurate and complete records are important when medical professionals document what a child or caregiver has told them about allegations of sexual abuse. The record should specify as much of the conversation as possible, including the presenting reason for the child's visit to the medical professional and who made the initial statement of the alleged abuse. The medical professional would document whether or not the statement was made spontaneously by the child and document any information the caregiver provided about the allegation. It is essential that notes include the child's *verbatim* statements about the sexual abuse and the specific questions the medical professional employed to gather information.[16,24]

Mandated Reporting

The federal Child Abuse Prevention and Treatment Act (CAPTA)[25] defines *child abuse and neglect* as

- Any recent act or failure to act on the part of a parent or caregiver which results in death, serious physical or emotional harm, sexual abuse, or exploitation
- An act or failure to act which presents an imminent risk of serious harm

Many medical professionals have genuine concerns about reporting abuse. In 2015,[26] a survey including 556 medical professionals, teachers, and therapists identified factors that may hinder a professional from reporting suspected or alleged child abuse. These factors include concern that reporting will not help the family (51%), concern that reporting would damage the relationship with the family (49%), previous poor experience with CPS (47%), and not knowing what happens after a report is made (42%). Although these barriers may be in place, reporting remains the first step in the healing process for a child who has experienced abuse. If a report is delayed or not made, additional harm could come to the child. Additionally, individual states may enforce penalties against mandated reporters who fail to report child abuse or neglect.[27]

Mandated reporting of child abuse and neglect in a timely manner is vital to the child's safety and to the subsequent investigation by law enforcement and child protection agencies. Medical professionals should develop a written policy on how to appropriately respond to and report suspected child sexual abuse. Such a policy could include the reporting process, the time frame in which a report must be made, and the identification of the appropriate law enforcement and child protection agencies to which the report will be made.

Conclusion

Medical professionals are in a unique position to help children who have experienced sexual abuse. Because of their role in the lives and well-being of their patients, medical professionals are likely to be sought out by caregivers and trusted by children. Medical professionals can improve the lives and futures of their patients by taking a forensically sound history of the incident being reported. While it may be a challenge to develop skills for interviewing children who are reporting sexual abuse, it is important to understand the fundamental principles of questioning children in a sensitive and appropriate way so that children can disclose the sexual abuse they experienced and receive the assistance they need to recover and heal.

References

1. US Administration for Children and Families. *Child Maltreatment 2015*. Washington, DC: US Department of Health and Human Services;2017. http://www.acf.hhs.gov/programs/cb/research-data-technology/statistics-research/child-maltreatment
2. Finkelhor D, Shattuck A. Characteristics of crimes against juveniles. University of New Hampshire Crimes against Children Research Center website. http://www.unh.edu/ccrc/pdf/CV26_Revised%20Characteristics%20of%20Crimes%20against%20Juveniles_5-2-12.pdf. Published May 2012. Accessed January 23, 2019
3. US Department of Health and Human Services Administration for Children and Families, Administration on Children, Youth and Families, Children's Bureau. *Child Maltreatment 2013*. https://www.acf.hhs.gov/sites/default/files/cb/cm2013.pdf. Accessed January 23, 2019
4. Bays J, Chadwick D. Medical diagnosis of the sexually abused child. *Child Abuse Negl.* 1993;17(1):91–110 PMID: 8435791 https://doi.org/10.1016/0145-2134(93)90011-S
5. Cross TP, Jones LM, Walsh WA, Simone M, Kolko D. Child forensic interviewing in children's advocacy centers: empirical data on a practice model. *Child Abuse Negl.* 2007;31(10):1031–1052 PMID: 17996298 https://doi.org/10.1016/j.chiabu.2007.04.007
6. Cross TP, Jones LM, Walsh WA, et al. *Evaluating Children's Advocacy Centers' Response to Child Sexual Abuse. Juvenile Justice Bulletin No. 218530*. Washington, DC: US Dept of Justice, Office of Juvenile Justice and Delinquency Prevention; 2008

7. Alaggia R. Many ways of telling: expanding conceptualizations of child sexual abuse disclosure. *Child Abuse Negl.* 2004;28(11):1213–1227 PMID: 15567025 https://doi.org/10.1016/j.chiabu.2004.03.016
8. Bottoms B, Quas J, Davis S. The influence of interviewer-provided social support on children's suggestibility, memory, and disclosures. In: Pipe M-E, Lamb ME, Orbach Y, Cederborg A, eds. *Child Sexual Abuse: Disclosure, Delay, and Denial.* Mahwah, NJ: Lawrence Erlbaum Associates; 2007
9. Hershkowitz I, Orbach Y, Lamb ME, Sternberg KJ, Horowitz D. Dynamics of forensic interviews with suspected abuse victims who do not disclose abuse. *Child Abuse Negl.* 2006;30(7):753–769 PMID: 16846642 https://doi.org/10.1016/j.chiabu.2005.10.016
10. Lyon TD, Ahern EC. Disclosure of child sexual abuse. In: Myers JEB, ed. *The APSAC Handbook on Child Maltreatment.* 3rd ed. Newbury Park, CA: Sage; 2010:233–252
11. Sorensen T, Snow B. How children tell: the process of disclosure in child sexual abuse. *Child Welfare.* 1991;70(1):3–15 PMID: 1997290
12. Hébert M, Tourigny M, Cyr M, McDuff P, Joly J. Prevalence of childhood sexual abuse and timing of disclosure in a representative sample of adults from Quebec. *Can J Psychiatry.* 2009;54(9):631–636 PMID: 19751552 https://doi.org/10.1177/070674370905400908
13. Smith DW, Letourneau EJ, Saunders BE, Kilpatrick DG, Resnick HS, Best CL. Delay in disclosure of childhood rape: results from a national survey. *Child Abuse Negl.* 2000;24(2):273–287 PMID: 10695522 https://doi.org/10.1016/S0145-2134(99)00130-1
14. Schönbucher V, Maier T, Mohler-Kuo M, Schnyder U, Landolt MA. Disclosure of child sexual abuse by adolescents: a qualitative in-depth study. *J Interpers Violence.* 2012;27(17):3486–3513 PMID: 22821848 https://doi.org/10.1177/0886260512445380
15. Kogan SM. Disclosing unwanted sexual experiences: results from a national sample of adolescent women. *Child Abuse Negl.* 2004;28(2):147–165 PMID: 15003399 https://doi.org/10.1016/j.chiabu.2003.09.014
16. American Professional Society on the Abuse of Children. Practice guidelines: forensic interviewing in cases of suspected child abuse. https://www.apsac.org. Published 2012. Accessed January 23, 2019
17. Walker AG. *Handbook on Questioning Children: A Linguistic Perspective.* 3rd ed. Washington, DC: American Bar Association Center on Children and the Law; 2013
18. Massengale J. Child development: a primer for child abuse professionals. *NCPCA Update Newsletter.* 2001;14(8):1–4
19. Bourg W, Broderick R, Flagor R, Kelly DM, Ervin DL, Butler J. Posing appropriate questions. In: *A Child Interviewer's Guidebook.* Thousand Oaks, CA: Sage Publications; 1999:78–98
20. Saywitz KJ, Lyon TD, Goodman GS. Interviewing children. In: Myers JEB, ed. *The APSAC Handbook on Child Maltreatment.* 3rd ed. Newbury Park, CA: Sage; 2010:337–360
21. Poole DA. *Interviewing Children: The Science of Conversation in Forensic Contexts.* Washington, DC: American Psychological Association; 2016 https://doi.org/10.1037/14941-000
22. Newlin C, Steele LC, Chamberlin A, et al. Child forensic interviewing: best practices. *Juvenile Justice Bull.* 2015;2–17
23. Gundersen National Child Protection Training Center. Anatomical dolls and diagrams: a position paper from Gundersen National Child Protection Training Center and the ChildFirst/Finding Words Forensic Interview Training Programs. https://www.gundersenhealth.org/app/files/public/3580/NCPTC-Anatomical-Dolls-and-Diagrams-position-paper.pdf. Published 2016. Accessed January 23, 2019

24. American Professional Society on the Abuse of Children. Practice guidelines: psychosocial evaluation of suspected sexual abuse in children. 2nd ed. https://apsac.memberclicks.net/assets/documents/PracticeGuidelines/psychosocial%20evaluation%20of%20suspected%20sexual%20abuse%20in%20children%20second%20edition.pdf. Published 1997. Accessed January 23, 2019
25. Child Abuse Prevention and Treatment Act, 42 USC §5101–5119 (1974), as amended by the CAPTA Reauthorization Act of 2010, Pub L No. 111–320
26. Walsh WA, Jones LM. Factors that influence child abuse reporting: a survey of child-serving professionals. University of New Hampshire Crimes against Children Research Center website. http://www.unh.edu/ccrc/pdf/Final%20Reporting%20Bulletin%20Professional%20Perceptions.pdf. Published September 2015. Accessed January 23, 2019
27. Child Welfare Information Gateway. *Penalties for Failure to Report and False Reporting of Child Abuse and Neglect.* Washington DC; US Dept of Health and Human Services, Children's Bureau; 2016. https://www.childwelfare.gov/topics/systemwide/laws-policies/statutes/report. Accessed January 23, 2019

CHAPTER 10

Medical Evaluation of Suspected Sexual Abuse in Prepubertal Children

Molly Curtin Berkoff, MD, FAAP
Associate Professor of Pediatrics
Division of General Pediatrics and Adolescent Medicine
Department of Pediatrics
University of North Carolina at Chapel Hill
Chapel Hill, NC

Martin A. Finkel, DO, FACOP, FAAP
Professor of Pediatrics
Institute Codirector
Child Abuse Research Education & Service (CARES) Institute
School of Osteopathic Medicine
Rowan University
Stratford, NJ

Diagnostic Considerations

The medical diagnosis and treatment of children exposed to inappropriate sexual contact is only one of the many aspects of the evaluation of child sexual abuse. The collective insights of many disciplines interacting with mutual respect and understanding is essential to ensure an understanding of what a child may have experienced if abuse has occurred as well as the child's ongoing treatment needs.

The medical diagnosis and treatment of suspected child sexual abuse has evolved over the past 40 years.[1–14] During this period, medical professionals have enhanced their knowledge and skills in evaluating children alleged to be abused.[15] Most of the literature has been focused on responding to the challenges of diagnosing sexual abuse in girls, with significantly less attention to boys. Much of the approach to the medical assessment is the same whether the child who has experienced abuse is a boy or a girl.[16]

Medical professionals (eg, physicians, nurse practitioners, physician assistants) define their role in treating children who have experienced sexual abuse in terms of prevention, identification, assessment and management, treatment, and interaction with the professional systems responsible for the safety and protection of children who have been sexually abused. Some medical professionals see their role limited only to referring suspected sexual abuse cases to a local or regional diagnostic clinic or center that has been developed to serve the needs of these children. Others see an opportunity to participate actively in evaluating children and have learned much from the child protective services (CPS), law enforcement, and mental health communities about the best practice methods of assessment and treatment of children who have experienced abuse.

A successful medical evaluation requires an understanding of the varied clinical presentations of child sexual abuse and how to ensure the appropriate assessment, including the need for a complete medical history, technical skills to conduct an examination, and documentation of the evaluation. The medical professional who understands age-appropriate development and behaviors, the dynamics of how children are engaged in sexually inappropriate contact, the progression of the activities over time (eg, grooming of children), the use of threats, the types of disclosure, and why children might recant is best prepared to obtain a complete medical history of the events surrounding the abuse. This knowledge and the requisite skills necessary to obtain the history of the alleged inappropriate contact are essential. Medical professionals must be as adept at obtaining and documenting the history as they are at choosing the appropriate test for sexually transmitted infections (STIs).

Children will present for an examination in a variety of ways. A parent may call after a clear disclosure or concerning statement made by a child, seeing changes in the behavior of the child, or having been told of behavioral signs by a relative, friend, or schoolteacher. The presentation of a child who has experienced sexual abuse is unlike that involving other acute pediatric diseases. Children who have experienced sexual abuse do not typically disclose their experiences or demonstrate behavioral signs and symptoms immediately after an episode of sexual contact.[17–23] As a result of the delay in disclosure, children are not typically identified as having physical findings that support their disclosures of abuse. Children who disclose shortly after a sexually inappropriate contact are more likely to have experienced force and/or restraint and are more likely to demonstrate acute signs of injury. Children presenting with acute injuries involving extragenital and anogenital sites are the least difficult to diagnose. Most children are sexually abused by individuals who have ready access to them and are known, loved, and trusted by the child.[21,22,24]

When children are engaged in sexual activities, the individual initiating the contact tends not to have a desire to harm the child physically, differentiating sexual abuse of prepubertal children from rape, where there is forced sexual intercourse. This is also in contrast to child physical abuse, in which there may have been some intent to harm the child physically.[21] Most children who are physically maltreated have cutaneous or other manifestations of their abuse that suggest a non-accidental etiology. In sexual abuse, the perpetrator's pathologic but effective strategy is to engage the child with as little discomfort as possible, which increases the likelihood of engaging the child again in the inappropriate contact. Although most children are not physically injured during sexual abuse, the individual engaging the child in the activities demonstrates a callous indifference to the emotional effect of the activities. Thus, it is essential to understand the contextual framework in which children are engaged and maintained in sexual activities[9,21,22,25] and, when a disclosure of sexual abuse has been made, to respond appropriately, including the completion of a thorough medical evaluation. The medical professional's diagnostic assessment is based on historical and behavioral details that, at times, are supported by confirmatory physical findings, forensic evidence, and/or STIs.

Medical History

The cornerstone of evaluating any medical problem is the medical history. The history determines how the medical professional will proceed with the examination and the scope of testing required. It is therefore expected that children being seen by a medical professional for concerns of sexual abuse will have a complete medical history obtained. Without a complete history, the ability to reach an appropriate diagnosis and treatment plan is limited. The child's history helps the medical professional to understand the child's experience, including the context and time frame of the event(s). To obtain a complete history, the medical professional should be familiar with the relevant mental health and social work literature on child sexual abuse. With this knowledge, medical professionals will understand how children are engaged and maintained in sexually inappropriate activities and begin to appreciate the clinical expression of their experience.[21,22,26–32]

A complete medical history should be obtained from the child's non-offending caregiver, including birth, family, surgical, developmental, hospitalization, medication, behavioral, and mental health history. It is important to recognize that the adult providing the history may have been unaware of the specific symptoms that the child may have had related to the sexual contact. Therefore, for verbal children, the medical professional is encouraged to meet with the child to assess factors from the history that can guide and add to the understanding of the child's experiences. This can include specific symptoms related to gastrointestinal (GI) and genitourinary (GU) systems but should also include behavioral symptoms such as sleep, appetite, worries, and depressive symptoms.[33] The medical professional should consider using standard screens to assess for behavioral difficulties as recommended by the American Academy of Pediatrics (AAP) in the primary care setting.

Statements made by the child spontaneously or elicited through non-leading questions must be preserved verbatim and documented with context. The medical professional is not expected to complete the role of a forensic interviewer (see Chapter 9, Taking Forensically Sound Histories in Cases of Alleged Sexual Abuse) but instead is expected to meet and talk with the child to assist with identifying the treatment plan. The idiosyncratic statements of children provide the best insight into the child's experience and can assist with understanding the child's experience of the abuse. The medical history obtained from the child may provide great insight into the spectrum of a child's experience and the potential for diagnosing an injury, STI, and/or mental health condition. Child protection and/or law enforcement may have conducted an initial interview of the child before referring the child for diagnosis and treatment of the alleged sexual contact. The medical professional should focus the medical history on whether the child has been physically injured as a result of the alleged contact and significantly affected by the trauma of the abuse and on obtaining historical details of signs and symptoms specific to the contact. Some of these details are obtained from the review of systems and medical history given by the accompanying parent.

The medical record should include verbatim documentation of questions asked and the exact responses of the child. Observations of the child's affect and behavior during the medical history are extremely important and may assist in formulating a clinical assessment. Mental health professionals are best equipped to interpret subtle changes in affect and behavior. However, the medical professional should know when and how to assist with prioritizing referrals to mental health for children who have experienced abuse and consider employing standard developmental and/or behavioral screens as for general pediatric practice.

At times it may be difficult to take a history from a child about sexually inappropriate experiences. The ability to listen to children talk about their experiences is not intuitive but, rather, a developed skill. The medical professional must appear empathic but neutral when obtaining a history. As children talk, they also observe the medical professional's reaction to what they have to say. If the medical professional appears uncomfortable listening or is insensitive to the child's needs, the child may simply stop talking. Therefore, it is critical that the medical professional is nonjudgmental and facilitating while keeping in mind that the questions posed must be presented in a non-leading manner. For older children, the medical professional should meet with the child outside the presence of the caregiver to obtain a complete medical history prior to the physical examination.

Although medical professionals consider the sexual abuse of children abhorrent, a child experiencing inappropriate contact by someone they love and trust may view the activity quite differently, particularly when the activity is presented in a "playful" or "loving" context. Children's responses to these experiences may be neutral, positive, or negative, depending on how the activities were represented to the child.[34] A child may still care about the caregiver despite the nature of the abuse. Therefore, the medical professional should not automatically presume that the child was psychologically damaged, embarrassed, or hurt by the experience and maintain neutrality during the assessment.[21,34] Young children are most likely to express confusion, excitement, or ambivalence and may be less likely to understand the inappropriateness and implications of the experiences.

When obtaining a history, it is important to understand that children who experience abuse have special emotional needs. Because of their abuse, some children may be overly friendly or familiar with the professional, while others may have difficulty developing rapport and trust with the examining medical professional. Other children may not appear different from a child who has not experienced abuse. The examiner should remain unhurried, nonjudgmental, and empathic so the child will be more likely to view the medical professional as understanding and will, therefore, be more likely to share the details of the events and the accompanying affective associations.

The purpose of the medical history is to gather information as well as impart information in the form of therapeutic messages. These messages also assist in relaying to the child that the medical professional understands what the child has experienced. For example, it is important for children to understand that they were incapable of consenting in an informed manner to the sexual contact that they have experienced. Many children who have been repeatedly engaged in an activity and received rewards for participating have difficulty in accepting that they are not responsible for having "allowed" the contact to happen. Unfortunately, such feelings may be reinforced when the child discloses abuse and the non-offending parent responds by saying, "Why did you let him do it?" or "Why didn't you stop him?" or "Why didn't you tell me sooner?" Such responses make the child feel responsible for what has happened. When children are engaged in sexual activities, they are not given choices and are incapable of consenting to sexual activities. Children also are not empowered to stop the activities in which they are engaged.

Another important message to impart is that the child did the right thing by telling and that he or she did not do anything wrong. This concept, coupled with a statement that this type of thing happens to a lot of children, helps decrease the sense of stigmatization, embarrassment, and isolation commonly seen after sexually inappropriate contact.

Children who have experienced abuse have experienced the abuse of power and authority.[21,22] As a result, they may continue to behave, even after disclosure, in a manner reflective of their sense of powerlessness and remain at high risk for future abuse.[27,35] Thus, it is important to begin to empower children after their disclosure. This process can begin by simply asking children what they want to happen now that they have disclosed their abuse. Children must be given the opportunity to begin to make choices that are in their best interests. Children frequently are fearful of the consequences of disclosure because of the overt or implicit threats used by the perpetrator to maintain secrecy. Secrecy permits the abuse to recur and removes accountability by the perpetrator.[21,22,35] Most children who purposefully disclose do so simply because they want the abuse to stop. Children generally cannot conceive of the cascade of events that is precipitated by their disclosures. They cannot anticipate that their disclosure may result in the prosecution of a family member, foster care placement for themselves, and possible abandonment by their non-offending parent. Children should be encouraged to ask questions and be assured that they will be supported through the ensuing process. The medical professional should not make promises about future actions that are outside their control, such as whether someone will be arrested or placed in jail.

Before proceeding with the history, the medical professional should review the interviews completed by CPS and law enforcement. If available, reviews of these interviews will assist the medical professional with understanding the developmental abilities of the child, which will assist in determining the scope of the medical history to be conducted. Children should be spoken to as soon after disclosure as possible because early statements are generally more spontaneous.[36] Limiting the number of people talking about the allegations of abuse is important. However, this should not negate the need for a medical professional to speak to a child. A medical professional has a different role in that there is a need to meet with a child and understand how to interpret physical examination findings and symptoms and ensure a comprehensive plan of care that addresses the child's well-being. In addition to reviewing the details of all prior interviews and obtaining information about worries or concerns with the child, it is important to address the parental response since disclosure and to record any observations that the non-offending caregiver may have made. The non-offending parent can provide a wealth of information about the child's medical history and change in daily habits, as well as any behavioral changes and the child's statements that contributed to the suspicion that the child may have been abused. Additionally, the non-offending parent can assist with understanding any changes to information previously obtained, due to changes in the child's environment since the disclosure.

At the onset of the history taking, the child and parent may be seen together, but then each should be seen independently to address individual concerns or worries. Many times, children and adolescents have unanticipated and unrealistic worries or concerns about their bodies as a result of what they have experienced. Addressing these issues is essential in identifying the possibility of an altered body image resulting from abuse. Prepubertal children frequently express idiosyncratic concerns about their bodies and may worry that they could have a disease or be pregnant in the absence of a rational explanation for their concern.[21,35] It is important to let children know that no worry or question is silly or uninformed.

The young child must view the medical professional as both nonthreatening and empathic if he or she is to separate from the parent. Every effort must be made by the medical professional to create an environment in which the child will feel safe and understood. The medical professional's history-taking style must be modified to meet the needs of the varying ages and developmental levels of children.

The history should focus primarily on the specifics of what the child experienced and the context in which the alleged contact occurred. The child's history of the experience helps guide the medical professional to ensure appropriate examination and assessment of treatment and medication needs, including, but not limited to STIs, concern for injury, and specific symptoms and types of contact. Children are told that the purpose of the examination is to make sure they are physically OK and to address any worries or concerns they may have about their bodies because of what happened.

Some children find it difficult to verbalize their experiences. Using anatomical drawings, paper and crayons, or anatomically detailed dolls may facilitate articulating or demonstrating the child's experience.[37–39] Children use a variety of terms to describe their private parts. The terms a particular child uses for genital and anal anatomy need to be determined and may be obtained by the non-offending caregiver prior to the meeting with the child. If the child appears embarrassed, give the child permission to use his or her own words by telling the child that you have heard all kinds of names, some of which are silly and some of which are embarrassing to say, and that they will not be in trouble for using those names in the medical office. Some children prefer writing the name down or whispering the name of their private parts.

Box 10.1 lists elements the medical history should address.

BOX 10.1
Elements of the Medical History Related to Sexual Abuse

The medical professional responsible for taking the medical history should obtain information from the patient or caregiver about

- How access to the child was achieved
- How the sexual interaction was represented to the child to engage the child in the activity(s)
- Progression of the activity(s) over time
- What rewards, threats, bribery, coercion, and/or intimidation was used to maintain the child in the activity(s) over time
- Where the contact occurred
- The frequency of contact
- The child's description of how he or she felt when engaged in the contact
- Specific details of what the child experienced and any discomfort associated with the events, including observations by the child with regard to bleeding, bruises, or ejaculate
- Circumstances surrounding either accidental or purposeful disclosure
- To whom the disclosure was made and the response of that individual
- Whether any liquids or pills were provided to the child that altered the child's state of consciousness
- What the child would like to happen now that the disclosure has occurred

Adapted with permission from Sgroi SM. *Handbook of Clinical Intervention in Child Sexual Abuse*. Lexington, MA: Lexington Books; 1982 and MacFarlane K, Kerbs S. Techniques for interviewing and evidence gathering. In: MacFarlane K, ed. *Sexual Abuse of Young Children*. New York, NY: The Guilford Press; 1987.

Depending on the child's developmental level and emotional preparedness to discuss what he or she has experienced, the level of detail of the experience will vary. The medical professional should view the child's experience as a puzzle, gathering as many pieces as possible to glean the most accurate and complete picture. When questions are posed, they should be simple, unambiguous, and non-leading. Questions are of value only when they are not suggestive of the answer. Complex questions have the potential to confuse the child and, thus, the child's response will be more difficult to interpret. Make sure the child understands the questions and feels free to ask for clarification if he or she does not understand. By using an open-ended style that progresses from general questioning to more specific areas, it is easier for the child to talk about the experience.[21,40–44] See Chapter 9, Taking Forensically Sound Histories in Cases of Alleged Sexual Abuse, for more information.

To achieve effective communication with children who have experienced sexual abuse, the medical professional must (a) identify and overcome the child's fears and perceived consequences of the experience and subsequent disclosure; (b) understand the coping strategies children use as a defense pattern; (c) appreciate that children provide the details of their experience in a fragmentary manner and may repress specific memories of their experience; (d) recognize that, depending on developmental age, children will have varying abilities to communicate the frequency or time frame in which they experienced the contact; and (e) become adept at providing options for children to answer questions in the most truthful and least-threatening manner.[41,45–48] It is important that medical professional talk to children when they present for care after identification of sexual abuse.

Unique Characteristics of Boys Who Experience Sexual Abuse

Surprisingly little literature exists on medical aspects of boys who experience sexual abuse. Numerous studies have estimated the prevalence rates of boys experiencing sexual abuse as between 4% and 76%.[25,49,50] Some researchers believe that the prevalence of sexual abuse of boys is similar to that of girls, but boys are less likely to disclose their abuse. Boys seem to be less likely to disclose because of anxiety that the abuse may reflect on their sexual identity, perceived threat to "manliness" by inability to stop abuse, and fear. The frequently cited prevalence of experiencing sexual abuse for girls is 1 in 4 and for boys is approximately 1 in 6. There is little doubt that the sexual abuse experienced by boys is under-recognized and underreported, and boys are less likely to receive services.

Boys most commonly experience abuse by males. Male perpetrators are likely to use threats and force to engage boys in sexual acts if coercion and deceit are insufficient. Boys younger than 13 years are most vulnerable to abuse by extrafamilial perpetrators and strangers, whereas children aged 6 years and younger are more likely to experience abuse by family members. Regardless of the child's age, vulnerability increases with any physical or developmental disability. There is an increased vulnerability for boys whose family circumstances involve one parent, separation, divorce, remarriage with blended families, and parental substance abuse. Although less common, boys may be abused by females. Perpetrators often include family members such as mothers, adolescent siblings, and female caregivers. Boys who experience sexually inappropriate contact frequently act out their victimization by engaging other children in sexual activities as well.[51] With ready access to the internet and social media, young adolescents are being exposed to pornography that, when combined with curiosity about emerging sexuality, results in many boys acting out with younger siblings whom they have easy access to and control over.[14,52] Boys, just as girls, are likely to try to push out of their minds these kinds of experiences and fail to disclose in part because of fear but also to protect the perpetrator when the perpetrator is a family member.

Young boys who have experienced sexual abuse are frequently identified because they sexually act out, which not uncommonly includes engaging peers or other children in reciprocal genital touching, oral-genital activities, and genital to anal contact. Parents tend to minimize these behaviors when discovered and may intuitively respond in a punitive manner, thinking that admonition will cease the behaviors. When the age differential between the actors is less than 5 years, the concern is focused on who initiated the activity and where the behavior was learned. Parents and some professionals may view these interactions among age peers as normal and curious interactions. The more intrusive and adultlike the sexual interactions are, the more likely that they emanate from exposure to sexually inappropriate materials, sexual contact, or both.[53]

Just as in girls who have experienced sexual abuse, the medical history is key to understanding the context in which the boy was engaged in the activities, the progression of the interactions, the use of threats, and insight into whether the child experienced physical discomfort associated with the activities and the reasons for disclosure. Two factors that increase the likelihood of physical residua to the sexual contact are a significant age differential between the boy and perpetrator and the use of force and restraint. When children experience anal trauma, there is the potential to develop a fecal retentive disorder, but this disorder on its own is not diagnostic of sexual abuse. If there are signs or symptoms present referable to either the GU or GI systems, there should be an attempt to determine whether those signs and symptoms have any temporal relationship to the alleged contact.

Boys are less likely to disclose their experience of sexual abuse than girls and, thus, are more likely to present long after the last contact, when any injuries they may have incurred have healed. There are no published studies on the frequency of genital trauma in boys. Sporadic case reports generally describe unusual injuries to the penis such as degloving, amputation, and lacerations secondary to an object. Boys can acquire STIs and may have stigmata of such on examination. Oral findings of trauma may be observed secondary to forced fellatio as tears of the labial frenulum and petechiae on the soft and hard palate in both boys and girls.[54]

The dynamics of sexual abuse of boys are not dissimilar to that of girls. Boys also experience engagement generally by someone they know and trust, and the progression of abuse follows the classic sequence of engagement, sexual interaction, secrecy, disclosure, and recantation.

Physical Examination

Setting and Timing

All children alleged to have been sexually abused should have a complete head-to-toe examination, even if the last alleged contact was months or years before and the child, parent, and/or investigators believe the child is fine. The child may feel more comfortable disclosing concerns to a medical professional that he or she has not shared with parents or investigators. The history may reveal that the child has an altered body image or feels that his or her body may have been injured in some nondescript way. If these concerns are present and addressed, the examination has the potential to have considerable therapeutic value, even if there are no concerning anogenital abnormalities or findings concerning for acute or chronic signs of injury or STIs. The purpose of the physical examination is not only to diagnose and treat any "abnormality" as a result of the contact but, of equal importance, to reassure "normality," which may help the child achieve a sense of physical intactness.

The disclosure of abuse precipitates a crisis for the family. Non-offending parents frequently want an immediate answer as to whether the child's statements are true. Child protective services, law enforcement, and parents may believe that the physical examination will confirm the contact; thus, they seek an immediate examination, usually by visiting their primary care medical professional. They also may decide to go to their local emergency department on their own or per the primary care medical professional's instructions.

Unless the contact occurred recently, the emergency department generally is the least appropriate environment for the first encounter.[40,55,56]

Medical professionals with knowledge of child sexual abuse should help determine the most appropriate time and place for an examination. It is of paramount importance to establish the timing of the last abusive encounter so the medical professional can determine the urgency of conducting the medical examination.

Because most children do not disclose abuse immediately, the need for a forensic evidence collection kit (FEK) and the diagnosis of acute GU infections, STIs, and/or trauma are not usually the primary consideration. Consequently, most examinations can be scheduled for an outpatient assessment after the initial CPS or law enforcement intervention.

Acute genital and anal injuries are infrequent, but when they do occur, an immediate examination is indicated.[57] When there is a need for use of a FEK, each component must be performed by personnel who are skilled in the collection and preservation of each component. (See Chapter 13, The Role of Forensic Materials in Sexual Abuse and Assault.) Under most circumstances, the child can identify the perpetrator. When appropriate to conduct an acute sexual assault examination with a FEK, information derived from performing this forensic evaluation can be helpful in confirming contact and an individual's identity.

Typically, when children present for examination after an alleged inappropriate sexual experience, either nonspecific findings or no residua of the contact is evident. When no acute signs of injury are present, the medical professional must determine whether any chronic changes in genital or anal anatomy are present. The medical professional should note that even among children who experience repeated events of penetration, most will lack definitive evidence of penetration on the examination of their external genital structures.[58] The retrospective interpretation of changes in anal and genital anatomy and the inherent difficulties of such an assessment are discussed later in this chapter. As a rule, if the last episode of alleged contact occurred within 72 hours, an examination should be done immediately to identify and treat residua of the contact. Every effort should be made to see that the acute examination is conducted by someone with the appropriate skills and photodocumentation capabilities to avoid the child being subjected to a repeat examination.

When more than 72 hours have passed since the last contact, the primary focus of CPS and law enforcement should be the initial coordinated interview. Once this is completed, the child can be referred for a medical examination followed by an assessment of the effect on mental health of the contact and the development of a therapeutic plan.

Concurrently, CPS will be assessing the non-offending parent and/or caregiver to determine if the safety of the child can be ensured.

Preparation of the Child

Children who have experienced sexual abuse have been deceived, betrayed, and coerced into sexual contact. A chaperone is recommended for the examination, as would be expected for the anorectal, genital, or breast examination in a child without concerns for sexual abuse.[59] These children may have considerable difficulty in developing trust. Completion of a thorough examination depends on the ability of the medical professional to anticipate and address the child's anxiety and fears. Because these children have already experienced the abuse of power and authority, they should never experience the same by coercion and deceit, or the forced abduction of their legs, by a "helping medical professional." A forced examination of an uncooperative child is universally unsuccessful and results only in a more frightened and less trusting child who is more difficult to examine in the future. If it appears that the child is unlikely to cooperate and there is no medically urgent indication for the examination, the examination should be rescheduled to a time when the child may be more receptive and a trusting and informed caregiver is present to support the child. When the presenting signs and symptoms suggest a need for an immediate examination and the child cannot cooperate, sedation and/or examination under anesthesia is appropriate.[60]

When children are fearful, there is usually an underlying basis that can be readily identified. Young children are most fearful of needles, being hurt, or the unknown. Components of the abuse may be remembered during the physical examination. Each of these issues is addressed differently depending on the child's age.[34] The purpose of the examination should be explained, telling the child how the examination will proceed and reassuring the child that he or she can ask questions at any point if there is something that the child does not understand. Wherever appropriate, the child is given choices, which assists him or her in achieving a sense of control. Young children may prefer sitting in their caregiver's lap rather than being positioned on the examination table. In many hospital outpatient settings, trained child life/therapeutic recreational specialists can be used for support or distraction during examinations.

It also is important to address parental anxiety. The most common fear that parents express about the genital examination is that their young child will undergo an adult speculum and bimanual examination.

Reassuring parents that their prepubertal child will not have this type of examination relieves parental anxiety and enables the parents to be supportive, comforting, and attentive to the child's needs during the examination. If possible, written material should be provided to the caregiver(s) before the examination that anticipates and answers frequently asked questions about the medical examination. This information also may decrease anticipatory anxiety on the part of parents and, in turn, reduce the child's anxiety.[61]

Examination of the anogenital region should occur only in the context of a complete physical examination. When children are engaged in sexual activities, the contact is focused on their anogenital region. Implicitly, the message to the child who undergoes a head-to-toe examination is that all parts of his or her body are important. The examination of the genitalia and anus requires a significant amount of time. The anogenital examination should not be the first component of the physical but, rather, a part of the natural progression of the head-to-toe examination.

Extragenital signs of trauma, although less frequently present, are detected during a complete examination. Children who have experienced abuse may have had their general medical needs neglected, and the examination, along with a complete review of systems and medical history, serves to address overall health needs and identify previously unsuspected medical, dental, and/or mental health problems.

Examination Positions for Girls

Over the past 25 years, a profusion of medical literature has described the optimal manner in which to conduct a genital examination of the prepubertal child in a way that is both child sensitive and ensures complete visualization.[62–67] The optimal examination position(s), combined with a variety of techniques, allows a full appreciation of the nuances of typical genital anatomy and the tissue changes that may reflect residua to trauma.

The position in which a child is most comfortable, most cooperative, and least embarrassed is the position that should be used initially. Frequently, a combination of the supine frog-leg and knee-chest positions maximizes observation of the hymenal membrane and structures of the vaginal vestibule.[63] Small children are most likely to be comfortable when examined in the supine frog-leg position on the examination table or while being held in the caregiver's lap (Figure 10.1). All children should wear a gown and be draped to protect their sense of privacy. Very young children are curious and may prefer not to be encumbered by a gown.

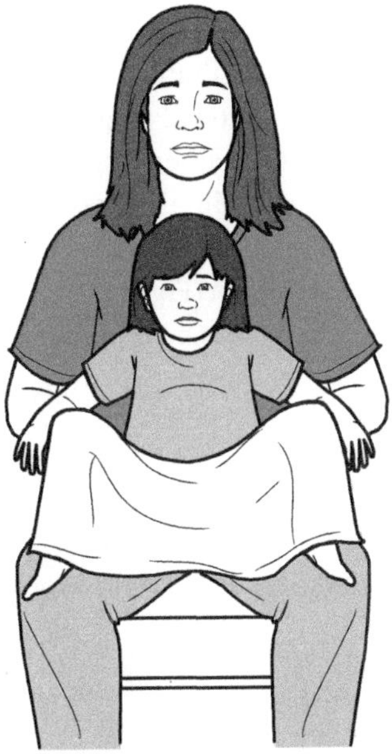

FIGURE 10.1
Prepubertal child positioned in the lap of an accompanying adult for genital and anal examination.

In the recumbent supine position, the child sits like a frog with her legs in full abduction and the feet in apposition. When using the separation technique, place the first and second fingers at the 10- and 2-o'clock positions, exerting gentle pressure until the labia separate and the hymenal membrane is visualized. With this technique, little or no tension is placed on the hymenal membrane (Figure 10.2).

With the child in the frog-leg position, visualization of the structures of the vaginal vestibule is achieved with the use of labial separation with or without traction. The traction technique affords improved visualization of the hymenal orifice.[66] Traction is most valuable in children who have redundant hymenal membrane tissue because the mucosal surface's cohesive forces tend to obscure full visualization of the orifice. When using labial traction (Figure 10.3), grasp the labia between the thumb and index finger of each hand and exert gentle traction in the posterolateral direction. Steady tension may be necessary to overcome cohesive forces of a moist hymenal membrane, allowing the orifice to be visible. When a child is examined in the knee-chest position, the appearance of the hymen may be quite different. For example, a membrane edge that appears as folded over, narrow, and rounded in the frog-leg position may appear wider, thinner, and more delineated than previously observed in the knee-chest position. This change in appearance can be attributed to the effect of gravity, which allows the anterior vaginal wall to fall forward and any redundant tissue in the inferior quadrants of the hymen to thin out. The prone knee-chest position has the advantage of facilitating visualization of the cervix if the hymenal orifice is of sufficient diameter and the patient is relaxed.[64]

The prone knee-chest position (Figure 10.4) is somewhat awkward for all but the youngest children. One approach to preparing the child

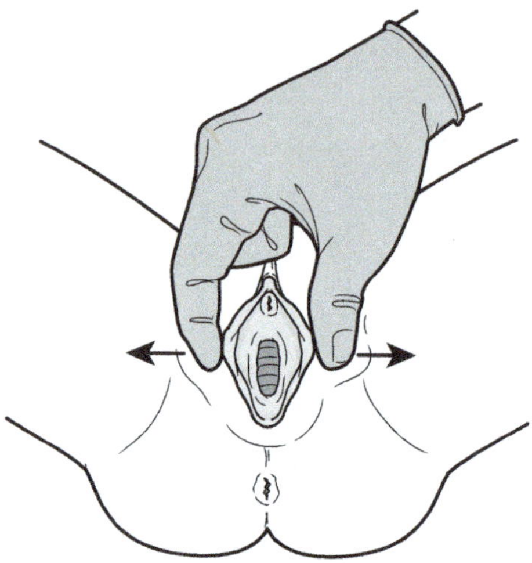

FIGURE 10.2
Visualization of the structures of the vaginal vestibule assisted by placement of the fingers to separate labia, in the supine frog-leg position.

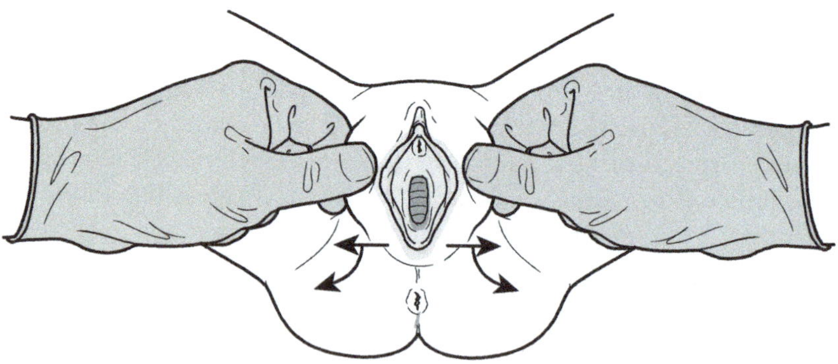

FIGURE 10.3
Lateral and posterior traction of labia further facilitates visualization of structures of the vaginal vestibule, in the supine frog-leg position.

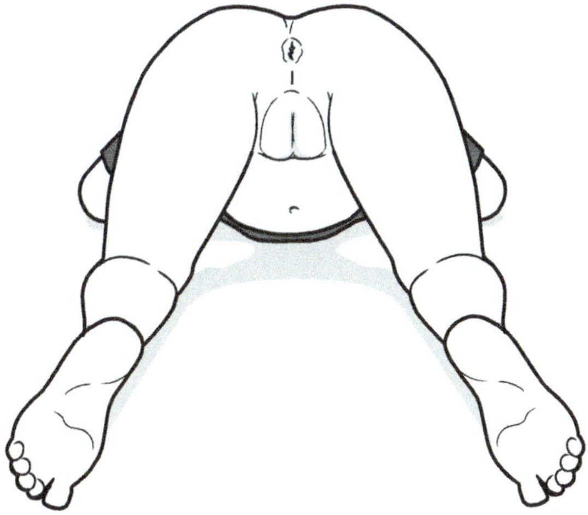

FIGURE 10.4
Knee-chest position for genital examination of the prepubertal child to supplement the supine frog-leg position.

for a knee-chest examination is to ask if she has seen how babies sleep on their tummies with their behinds up in the air. Explain to the child that this is the position that you want her to be in and have the accompanying adult assist in positioning the child. While the child is in this position, the medical professional places the thumbs on the buttocks at the 10- and 2-o'clock positions and gently elevates the buttocks in a lateral and superior direction (Figure 10.5). The prone knee-chest position may not be necessary if the examiner is confident that complete visualization of all the tissues has been achieved in the supine frog-leg position. One caveat is that if there seems to be an abnormal finding observed when the child is in the frog-leg position, it should be confirmed in the knee-chest position as well. Attempts should be made for confirmation by other means, such as by using saline to float the tissues, when children are unable to participate in the knee-chest position.

Other variables that may account for a changing appearance of the hymenal orifice are the state of relaxation and degree of labial traction and separation.[63,66,68] McCann et al[66] observed that the prone knee-chest position and the supine traction technique proved superior to the supine separation technique for visualizing the hymenal membrane and its orifice. Maximal anteroposterior hymenal orifice diameters were obtained in the prone knee-chest position. Maximal transverse horizontal diameters were obtained in the supine position with traction. Variability in measurements due to differences in the state of relaxation occur

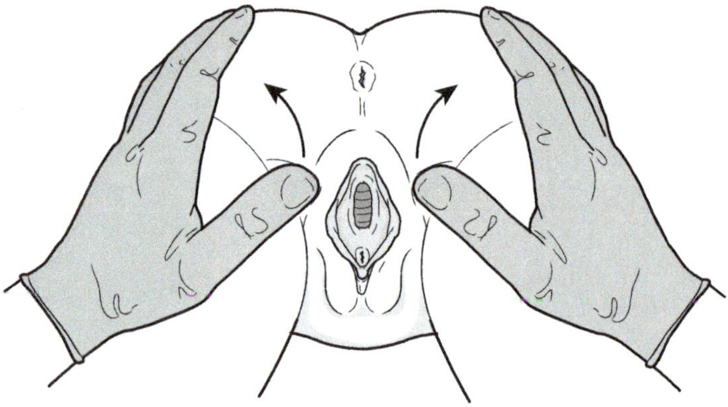

FIGURE 10.5
Visualization of the structures of the vaginal vestibule while in the knee-chest position is facilitated by superior and lateral traction, as noted by hand placement.

because the hymenal membrane is attached laterally to the vaginal wall. When the pubococcygeal muscles are tense, the vestibule is contracted, and the orifice may appear small; when relaxed, the orifice appears more dilated. The addition of labial traction provides another variable in measuring the maximal orifice diameter. The greater the traction, the larger the orifice might appear.

The lithotomy position also can be used for examining the older prepubertal girl. Once the patient is in the appropriate position for the examination, every effort must be made to minimize any discomfort.

Generally, the examination of the prepubertal child is principally an external visualization facilitated by varying techniques of separation, traction, and positioning. Using instrumentation on prepubertal children is rarely necessary. Use of a nasal speculum, as described in standard texts, is awkward and of limited value.[69] Vaginal specula are reserved for prepubertal children who require an examination under anesthesia when there is a concern for internal injuries following an acute assault. Even removal of the most commonly found foreign body (toilet paper) can generally be achieved without a speculum or anesthesia using a simple irrigation technique. Children may be fearful of being touched by a cotton swab because of a previous experience with throat cultures. Due to the current recommendation to use nucleic acid amplification tests when testing for possible infection with *Neisseria gonorrhea* and/or *Chlamydia trachomatis* instead of culture, the use of a cotton swab may not be indicated.[70] If needed for additional specimen collection, a few simple steps can minimize the potential for causing discomfort. All visualization should be done before attempting any touching with cotton swabs. The non-estrogenized hymenal membrane is very sensitive, and direct touch will cause discomfort. A urethral swab moistened with sterile non-bacteriostatic saline before use will further reduce the chances of discomfort if the hymen is touched. Large cotton swabs are more likely to cause discomfort and should be avoided in prepubertal children.

Examination of the Anus

The anus can be readily visualized in the prone or supine knee-chest position. The prone knee-chest position may be uncomfortable for any child who has experienced anal penetration. Thus, the left lateral decubitus (lateral knee-chest) or supine frog-leg with legs flexed onto the abdomen (supine knee-chest) is the best position for examining either the male or female anus (Figure 10.6).

The anal and perianal tissues are carefully examined for acute and healed signs of trauma. Acute signs of trauma may be evident as superficial abrasions and chafing of the anal verge and the tissues that form the gluteal cleft. Perianal redness is frequently observed in children who have and have not experienced abuse and, thus, is a nonspecific finding. The specificity of erythema increases when associated with other signs of trauma and confirms that there is a timely relationship between the alleged contact and the observed finding. When examining the anal verge tissues with the anus in a dependent position, it should

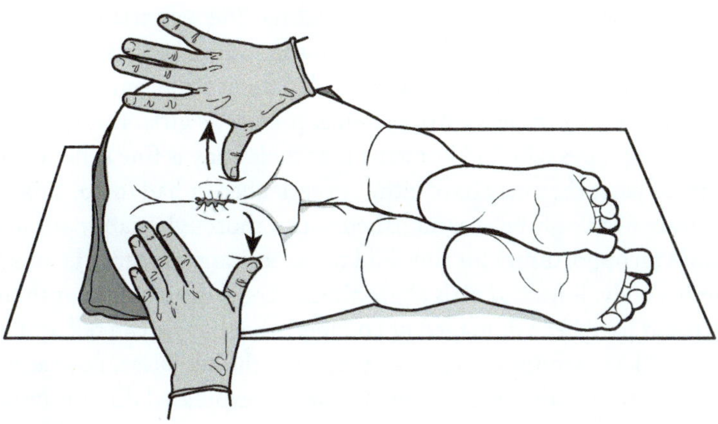

FIGURE 10.6
Hand placement for separation of the buttocks to view external anal tissues with the child in the left lateral decubitus position.

be anticipated that the longer the tissues are examined in this position the greater the likelihood that there will be dependent pooling of blood in the venous plexus surrounding in the perianal area, creating a bluish coloration to the tissue that can be quite dramatic and may be misinterpreted as bruising. If this is observed, the examiner simply touches the anal verge, resulting in contraction of the sphincter, which should then result in the disappearance of the "bruising."

The anal sphincter is anatomically designed to contract and pass stool on a routine basis. Children can pass, by parental description, surprisingly large-diameter stools without problems. Anal fissures can be seen following passage of a large-diameter stool, as commonly associated with constipation. Fissures can also be the result of the introduction of a foreign body, such as a finger, penis, or other object. Anal fissures are a nonspecific finding of superficial mucosal trauma. The specificity of a fissure increases with a corroborating history.

An anoscope can be introduced into the most distal portion of the rectosigmoid for visualization of the pectinate line. If there is a concern for internal blunt force trauma beyond the rectosigmoid, the examination should be completed with sigmoidoscopy under anesthesia. The probability of finding extensive internal injuries when there are no external anal verge signs of trauma is minimal and, thus, sigmoidoscopy is rarely indicated, except when acute blunt force anal penetrating trauma is suspected.

Examination of Male Genitalia

Boys benefit, just as girls do, from a genital examination conducted as part of a head-to-toe physical examination. The potentially embarrassing nature of a genital examination should be acknowledged and the examination should proceed with patience and sensitivity, affording boys the same level of personal privacy as girls. Following the examination, boys will find knowing that their body is fine is beneficial in spite of what they may have either experienced or had to do. This reassurance can only be accomplished with a thorough examination that provides an opportunity for the child to express any concerns he has about his body. Boys and girls share similar concerns of whether their body could have been damaged or changed, that people can tell, or that they could have acquired an STI as a result of the activities. Boys and their parents may also be concerned, whether expressed directly or not, that because of their experience their sexual identity has been changed or affected. The medical professional should encourage the parent and the child, when developmentally appropriate, to discuss any concerns or worries they have about the effect of the abuse. The medical professional can assist with assurance that just because there was coercion into an activity they could not consent to does not mean their sexual identity has been affected.

Improving Visualization and Documentation

Once a child is comfortable and positioned for the examination, supplemental lighting, filters, and magnification can assist in optimizing visualization of all the details of the genital and anal tissues. Adequate lighting is a prerequisite to a thorough examination and any photographic or video documentation that should follow. Several inexpensive light sources, such as gooseneck lamps, halogen procedure lights, and handheld devices, can be used, although they are usually inadequate to ensure the consistent results that can be achieved by a light source attached to a colposcope or a fiberoptic scope with video capabilities. Moreover, the light created by inexpensive sources is insufficient for adequate photodocumentation.[71]

The genital and anal tissues of prepubertal children are best examined with the use of magnification. Although this task can be achieved with a handheld lens or the magnifying capabilities of an otoscope or ophthalmoscope, none of these methods are satisfactory. The least optimal choice is the otoscope or ophthalmoscope, in part because of a limited angle of view, a small lens, and a short working distance required between the child's genitalia and the examiner.

The colposcope, designed to view the cervix, vagina, and vulva for signs of disease, is an instrument that provides an excellent light source with multiple or variable magnification capabilities, and for most examiners it is the instrument of choice. An alternative to the traditional colposcope is the fiber-optic scope that incorporates an excellent light source, variable magnification, and a wide angle of view. Most fiber-optic scopes are a far less expensive alternative to the traditional colposcope. See Chapter 25, Photodocumentation, for more information.

A colposcope generally provides between 4- and 30-fold magnification, depending on the manufacturer.[72] The most useful range is between 4 × and 15 × magnification. Above 15 × magnifications, both the angle of view and depth of the field are minimal. A colposcope equipped with an intraocular scale assists in obtaining the dimensions of specific abnormal findings. Colposcopes have built-in, red-free filters that cast a green light, enhancing the appearance of the vascular pattern and the mucosa. A filter assists in the recognition of superficial abrasions of the mucosa of the vestibule and interruptions in the vascular pattern. Scar tissue also may be more apparent because its avascular appearance contrasts with the surrounding vascularized tissues.

Before photographing a child, explain that the only person who can take a picture of the child with his or her clothing off is a doctor, with a trusted caregiver present who has given permission. Reassure the child that the photograph will represent only a small part of his or her body and that no one can identify him or her from the photograph. Ask the investigators and the child if anyone has ever taken a picture of the child with his or her clothing off. This question may uncover previously unsuspected pornography. Further questioning may include, "Have you ever seen any pictures of people with their clothing off?" and "Were any of the people in the photograph children?" Show the children the camera, whether handheld or attached to a colposcope, and allow them to take a picture of their names and identifying information, such as date of birth and visit, if they so desire. Always respect the child's desire not to be photographed if expressed or sensed. With the advent of the internet, there has been unfortunate and unprecedented access to pornography by young children and adolescents.

Anatomy and Terminology

Familiarity with genital and anal anatomy and knowledge of descriptive terminology assist medical professionals in enhancing their level of comfort in examining the child who has experienced sexual abuse and providing documentation in the medical record. The medical record must accurately reflect all the nuances of the child's genital and anal anatomy in clear and descriptive terms. Before the American Professional Society on the Abuse of Children consensus statement on terminology in the medical evaluation of sexual abuse, there was some inconsistency in the way findings were interpreted and described. It is important that medical professionals involved in examining children speak from a common lexicon and describe normal and abnormal anatomical variations that exist from one child to the next by using the same terminology (figures 10.7 and 10.8). When documenting findings, the description should be as specific as possible, and a term such as *normal genitalia* is of little descriptive value. The term *normal* does not take into account that the genitalia have many components, and the appearance of normal varies from child to child. Vulva, pudenda, and perineum also lack specificity and are of limited value. For example, *vulva* or *pudendum femininum* is a term

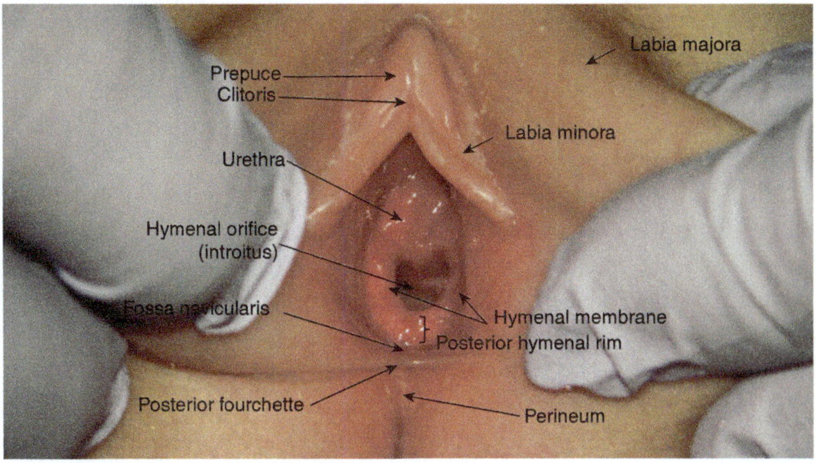

FIGURE 10.7
Genital anatomy of the normal prepubertal girl.

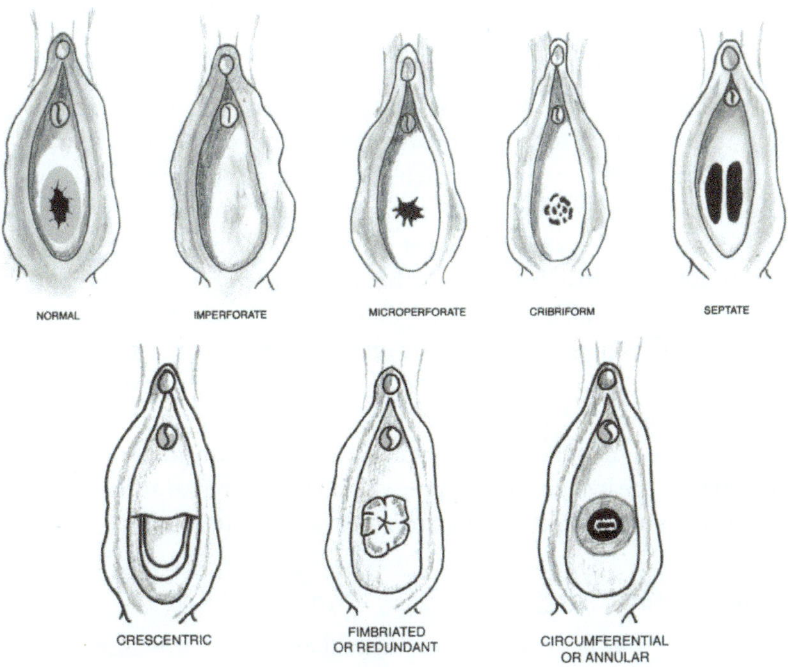

FIGURE 10.8
Anatomical variations of the hymen.

that includes all the components of the external visible genital structures, encompassing the mons pubis, labia majora and minora, clitoris, vestibule of the vagina, bulb of the vestibule, Skene and Bartholin glands, and vaginal orifice. The perineum is the area between the thighs bounded by the vulva and anus in girls and scrotum and anus in boys.[73–77]

When the labia are separated, the vaginal vestibule can be visualized. The vestibule of the vagina encompasses the area bordered laterally by the labia minora, the clitoris superiorly, and the fourchette posteriorly. Within the vestibule there are 6 perforations: urethra, periurethral ducts or Skene glands, vaginal orifice, and greater vestibular ducts or Bartholin glands.[75,76] The vaginal orifice is the perforation of the hymenal membrane.

The hymenal membrane is recessed in the vestibule, protecting it from direct trauma; hence the implausibility of injury to the membrane from athletic activity such as bicycling, horseback riding, or gymnastics. The common misconception that athletic activities result in injuries to the hymen has no scientific support. The rare impaling injury, when it occurs, is readily differentiated from trauma resulting from the direct and premeditated introduction of a foreign body such as a digit or a penis into the vagina.

The internal surface of the hymenal membrane marks the beginning of the vagina. The hymenal membrane is attached laterally to the walls of the vagina and posteriorly to the floor of the vagina. The concave area between the posterior attachment of the hymen and the fourchette is the fossa navicularis. The posterior joining of the labia minora forms the fourchette. The labia majora are described in most texts as joining posteriorly to form the posterior commissure; however, other authors describe them as not joining but tapering off anterolaterally into the perineum.[73–75]

Another anatomically vague term is *introitus*. Introitus is a generic term defined as the entrance to a canal or space.[77] The term *introital diameter* has been used as a synonym for the opening in the hymen typically referred to as the *vaginal orifice*.[78] To avoid confusion of terms, the opening in the hymenal membrane should be referred to as the *hymenal membrane orifice* or *vaginal orifice* rather than introitus.

Hymenal Membrane

As stated by Ira S. Wile, "The most insignificant anatomical structure of the female without an analog in the male has assumed a social importance at variance with its almost neutral physiologic value or its potential influence upon health."[79] This vestigial remnant has merited mythological, psychological, sociological, and now an amazing degree of medical notoriety as medical professionals begin to take a 21st century look at this tissue.

Much of the assessment of child sexual abuse has been focused on the appearance of the hymenal membrane orifice. Law enforcement, social workers, and parents may want to know if the hymen is intact or broken, as if it were either impenetrable or a piece of china. The legal and medical definitions of *penetration* differ. The medical definition of penetration is "the passing into the deeper tissues or into a cavity."[77] From a strictly medical perspective, penetration with regard to the female genitalia implies the introduction of an object between the labia, through the hymenal orifice, and into the posterior portion of the vagina. As previously cited, children frequently state that an object was placed inside of them when corroborating evidence is not present. Most penetration of children is akin to the legal definition, which is "the insertion of the male part into the female parts to however slight an extent; and by which insertion the offense is complete without proof of an emission."[80] Certainly, any genital-to-genital or genital-to-anal contact is inappropriate, regardless of the depth of penetration. In most jurisdictions, the legal definition of penetration is "between the labia no matter how so slight." Many medical professionals believe that the determination as to whether a child has been sexually abused will be answered by the mere examination of the hymen alone. In support of this desire to know, there is a volume of literature describing the appearance of the hymenal membrane in terms of its normative state and changes due to injury.[9,22,65,81]

Hymenal Development

Embryologically, "the hymen develops as a result of the advancement of mesenchyme into the epithelial mass at the junction of the pelvic part of the urogenital sinus and the vaginal plate."[82] The external surface of the hymen is covered by urogenital sinus epithelium. Cells derived from the vagina cover the inner aspect of the hymen. The degree of vascularity and the amount of connective tissue between the epithelial layers vary considerably. The membrane is innervated and, in the prepubertal child, the hymen can be exquisitely sensitive to touch.

Many misconceptions concerning the hymen have developed over the years. The origin of these misconceptions is difficult to trace. One misconception is the existence of an entity known as congenital absence of the hymen. Children may occasionally be referred because the child "does not appear to have a hymen" or is thought to have been "born without a hymen." Absence of the hymen cannot and does not exist on an embryologic basis as a sole congenital anomaly. It may be absent in the presence of other major urogenital anomalies, of which the least significant concern is the presence or absence of the hymen. If the GU tract is normally developed, the hymen is present. In a 1904 discussion concerning malformations of the hymen, Gelhor[83] noted, "Total absence of hymen, reports of which are found in older literature, have not been observed by modern authors, while not denying the possibility, consider this phenomenon exceedingly rare." Jenny et al[81] examined 1,311 female newborns, all of whom had hymens.

Genital trauma can alter the appearance of the prepubertal and pubertal child's hymen in a variety of ways. In adult women, remnants of the hymenal membrane are referred to as *carunculae hymenales.* Microscopically, these carunculae are compact mounds of elastic and connective tissue that have lost their papillae.[83] Carunculae hymenales do not exist in prepubertal children.

Appearance of the Hymen

The appearance of the hymenal membrane is quite variable. Some aspects of the membrane, such as the orifice configuration and the transverse and horizontal diameters, are easily described and measured. Other characteristics, such as thickness and the degree of elasticity or distensibility, which also are quite variable, present problems for objective quantification. Whenever the hymen and the hymenal tissues are described in the medical record, it is important to be as specific as possible concerning the character of the hymen and to avoid inaccurate and nondescriptive terms, such as *marital, broken, virginal,* or *intact.*

Many nonmedical professionals have the perception that the hymen is an impermeable membrane, and any opening is abnormal. An imperforate hymen is the only anatomical variant of hymenal configurations in which no opening is present. Distal vaginal atresia can be confused with imperforate hymen. Classically, the imperforate hymen is diagnosed in puberty when the amenorrheic girl presents with a midline abdominal mass and blue-domed appearance of the hymen.[84] Before puberty, the imperforate hymen results in the formation of a mucocolpos. Other configurations of the hymenal membrane orifice are annular, crescentic, fimbriated, septate, or cribriform.

For an *annular* orifice to exist, hymenal membrane tissue must be present circumferentially. The orifice itself can be placed either centrally or ventrally. When the orifice appears *crescentic,* hymenal membrane tissue is not evident between approximately the 11- and 1-o'clock positions; the superior edge of the hymenal membrane interdigitates with the vaginal walls laterally, leaving a posterior rim of tissue that is variable in its width. When a band of hymenal membrane traverses an annular orifice, creating 2 openings, it is referred to as *septate.* This configuration is much different, however, from a septum of the vagina that extends posteriorly and divides the vaginal canal and may be associated with other congenital anomalies. When multiple openings are present in the membrane, the term *cribriform* is used, which means "like a sieve."[77] A hymenal membrane orifice with multiple fingerlike projections on the edge of the membrane is referred to as *fimbriated.* These fingers most likely represent papillary excrescences.[82,83] These projections frequently overlap, obscuring the orifice unless considerable labial separation and traction are applied. The degree of tautness of the membrane bridging the vaginal canal is variable and is dependent on the degree of relaxation of the patient when the membrane is examined. The terms *redundant* or *folded* also have been used to describe the membrane when it is not taut. The membrane's edge may have congenital clefts, external hymenal ridges, tags, bumps, or cysts. Supporting structures called *pubourethral, pubovaginal,* or *pubococcygeal* ligaments may be visible. Pubourethral ligaments, sometimes referred to as *periurethral supporting bands,* are most commonly seen and become more apparent with labial traction.[63] Hymenal tags,[85] longitudinal intravaginal columns (columnae rugarum),[73,86] and anterior clefts can be seen and alone do not support a diagnosis of penetrating trauma. Initial research completed by Berenson et al[80] did not identify posterior clefts, further supporting concerns of most experts that interruptions in the integrity of the membrane's edge observed posteriorly are of post-traumatic etiology.

The unestrogenized tissues of the hymenal membrane and the vestibular aspects of the labia minora and fossa are vascular and can appear diffusely reddened. Redness is nonspecific and, without knowledge of the premorbid appearance of the genitalia, it is difficult to determine whether the redness is due to increased vascularity and secondary to trauma unless it is accompanied by signs of injury. Retrospective interpretation of changes in vascular patterns of the vestibular tissues without other stigmata and/or a history of genital trauma should be approached with caution. Traction can create midline blanching. Thus, before interpreting a midline avascular area as scar tissue, the examiner must be sure that traction is not creating the observed finding. The frequency of congenital midline avascular interruptions of the external surface of the membrane or fossa is unknown. The vascular pattern of the external surface of the hymenal membrane and fossa is most commonly described as *reticular, fine lacy,* and *symmetrical.* An interruption in the vascular pattern of the fossa that is interpreted as scar tissue should be accompanied by a history of significant trauma. Small 1- to 2-mm, ovoid translucent elevations that may be observed in the fossa generally represent lymphoid follicles and should be readily differentiated from vesicles or cysts.[87] The study by McCann et al[66] of genital findings in prepubertal children who had not experienced abuse further elucidated a spectrum of normal variants.[88]

Another characteristic of the hymenal membrane that has resulted in much interpretive debate is the hymenal orifice's transverse diameter measurement.[2,62,77,89–91] Early reference to the significance of a specific hymenal orifice diameter that, if exceeded, was strongly suggestive of sexual abuse has been problematic. One author noted, "The findings presented indicate that in the absence of known perineal injury, the discovery of an enlarged vaginal opening (greater than 4 mm) correlates 3 out of 4 incidents to positive sexual abuse history given by the child."[2] This criterion alone cannot be considered evidence of sexual abuse. Subsequent commentary by Paradise[91] on the predictive accuracy of interpreting orifice diameters illustrates the limitations of a single measurement: "Most medical providers would be relieved to have a single specific test for sexual abuse. Until we have this test, an overemphasis on minute changes in the diameter of the hymenal opening will result in a number of children being identified as victims of sexual abuse, whereas a majority of sexual abuse victims with normal hymenal measurements will remain unidentified."

Medical professionals are frequently asked to make a statement as to whether an object has been placed through a given hymenal orifice into the vagina. Measurements obtained during an examination have low predictive value and may not be helpful in determining whether penetration has occurred. Clinically, the routine measurement of the anteroposterior and trans-hymenal orifice diameter may be of limited value. Obtaining a maximal transverse and vertical diameter can be difficult because of the significant variability of the diameter depending on the examination position, degree of traction, and state of relaxation of the child (figures 10.9–10.11). Measurements alone are of limited value, however, because of the wide variability of "normal."

Children frequently state that a given object was placed inside them, and yet there may be no confirmatory physical findings. The ability to differentiate "in" from "on" is a developmental task for which limited normative data exist. Children feeling pressure between the labia and over the fourchette and the periurethral/clitoral hood region may perceive an object, such as a penis, as being placed inside. This form of genital-to-genital contact is referred to as *vulvar coitus*. When vulvar coitus occurs, trauma to the fourchette, medial aspects of the labia, and the periurethral area may be obvious without signs of injury to the hymen, due to the recessed location of the hymen. Genital-to-genital contact in the context

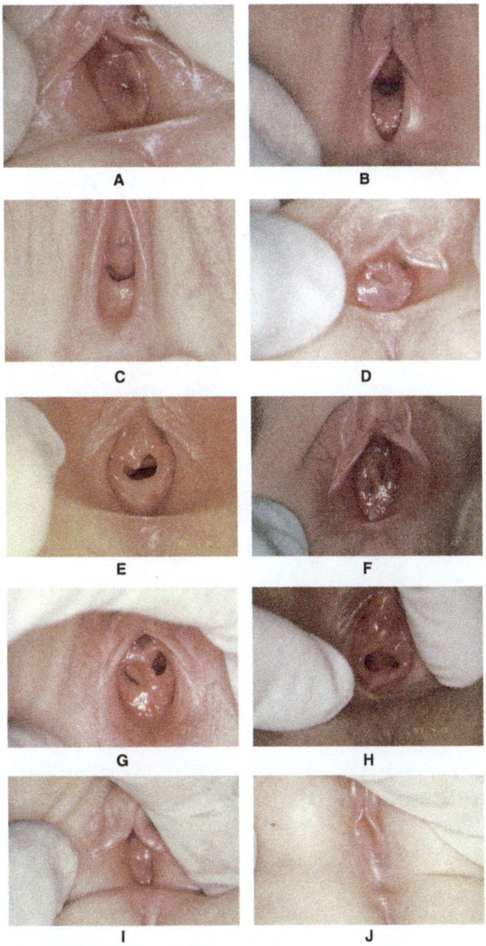

FIGURE 10.9

Normal prepubertal anatomical variations. A, A 15-month-old girl has flared configuration to the annular orifice. Note thickened normal variation of the membrane. B, A 4-year-old girl has a crescentic orifice with thin, sharply demarcated edge. External surface of the membrane has a lacy vascular pattern. Slight blanching in the fourchette results from traction. C, A 7½-year-old girl with a crescentic orifice. The membrane has a less translucent and thicker appearance. Urethral meatus is apparent. D, A 2-year-old girl has a superior and eccentrically oriented annular orifice. External surface of the membrane is translucent. Labial traction is necessary to visualize the orifice. E, A 9-year-old girl has a prominent hymenal membrane projection of tissue at the 11-o'clock position with a small bump at the 5-o'clock position. Projection and bump may have been previously attached, forming a septum. F, A 5-year-old girl has a septum of the hymen, resulting in 2 orifices. Cohesive characteristics of moist tissue might obscure the presence of 2 orifices if traction is not used. G, A 5-year-old girl has a vaginal septum that bisects the annular orifice. Associated upper genital tract anomalies must be considered. H, A 6-year-old girl has a prominent hymenal tag prolapsing from the vagina through the orifice and onto the external surface of the membrane. I, A 2-year-old girl has no observable hymenal orifice with labial separation, traction, or positioning. J, A 4½-year-old girl has acquired labial agglutination that obscures examination of structures of the vaginal vestibule. Small anterior separation of labia minora allows urine to escape.

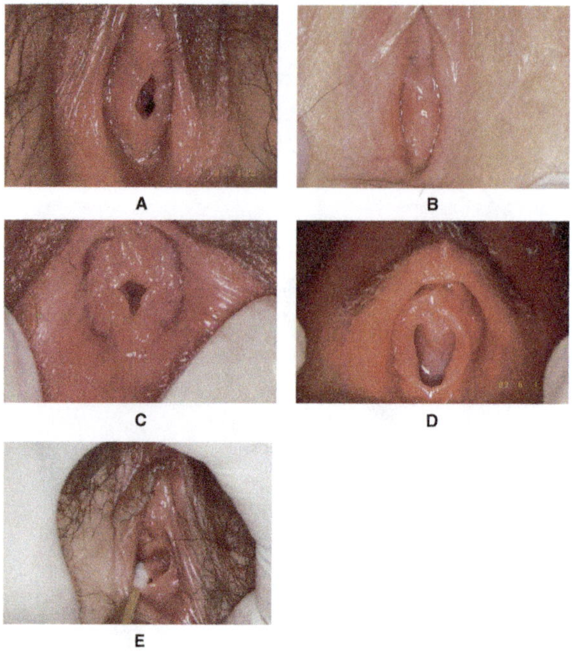

FIGURE 10.10

Normal pubertal anatomical variations. (Note: All pubertal children were examined in lithotomy position unless otherwise noted.) A, A 12-year-old girl has an annular-configured orifice with minimal redundancy of tissue. Hormonal influence of puberty results in thickened, pinkish coloration, obscuring prepubertal vascular pattern. B, A 9-year-old girl has redundant tissue surrounding an anteriorly placed orifice. Tanner stage 1, pubic hair estrogen effect of early puberty, is evident. C, A 12-year-old girl with Tanner stage 3 anatomy. Multiple congenital clefts circumferentially lead to fimbriated or "frilly" appearance of hymen. Note that clefts do not extend to the vaginal wall. D, An 11-year-old with Tanner stage 3 anatomy. Note the flared appearance of the annular orifice but no interruptions in the edge circumferentially. Elasticity of tissues is sufficient to admit a foreign body, such as a digit, without residua as alleged. E, A 14-year-old girl with Tanner stage 4 anatomy. Prominent intravaginal longitudinal ridge (columnae rugarum) is attached to the internal surface of the membrane. When ridge attaches to membrane, it may result in the appearance of a bump on the external surface. Intravaginal ridges and small transverse ridges (rugae vaginalis) are normal anatomical structures.

of vulvar coitus does not necessarily result in trauma to the vestibular structures. If injury does occur, it is most likely to be superficial and heal without residua. A digit placed between the labia also may be perceived as being inside without findings of penetration through the orifice. In genital fondling, penetration of a finger is generally limited to the vestibule itself.

In prepubertal children, the hymen can vary in appearance from thick and presumably elastic to thin and nonelastic. The extent to which the hymen is distensible in the prepubertal child is difficult to quantify clinically. Muram[92] studied the relation between specific sexual acts and genital findings in cases in which the perpetrators admitted to the sexual contact. Specific findings of hymenal vaginal tears were found in 60% of

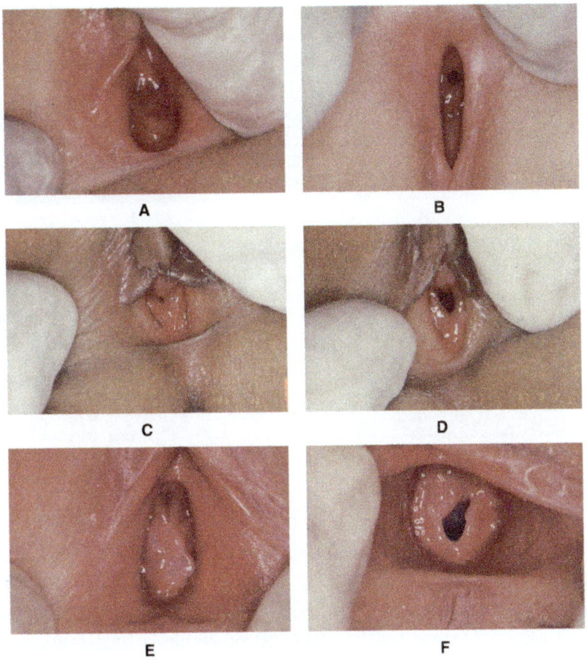

FIGURE 10.11
Variability of appearance of genital tissues because of positional changes and relaxation. A, A 4-year-old girl in whom the hymenal orifice was not visualized with labial separation and traction in the supine frog-leg position because of redundant hymenal membrane tissue surrounding the orifice. This observation requires examination in the prone knee-chest position for improved visualization. B, Same patient as in Figure 10.11A, examined in the knee-chest position. Note how gravity has resulted in redundant anterior tissue falling forward, allowing visualization of the annular orifice. C, A 4-year-old with a minute orifice visualized with labial separation. D, Same patient as in Figure 10.11C, but note the different appearance of the orifice now that the child is relaxed. E, A 9-year-old with Tanner stage 2 anatomy. With redundant estrogenized tissue, labial separation alone is insufficient to visualize hymenal orifice. F, Same patient as in Figure 10.11E viewed with labial traction, which affords complete visualization of the hymenal orifice edge circumferentially. When labial traction is exerted, superficial tears of the fourchette may occur, particularly in prepubertal children.

the girls when the offender had admitted to vaginal penetration, contrasted to 23% when penetration was denied. Normal-appearing genital tissues or nonspecific findings were present in 39% of those who had experienced abuse when penetration was admitted. A *hymenal vaginal tear* is defined as a laceration of the hymen extending to the posterior vaginal wall. An interruption in the integrity of the edge of the hymenal membrane extending to the floor of the vagina is specific to traumatic penetration. McCann et al[66] studied the genital anatomy of 114 carefully selected girls who had not experienced abuse and ranged in age from 10 months to 10 years. This study emphasized the frequency of normal or acquired genital findings that are not the result of abuse and the effect of examination technique and position on the varying appearance of a particular finding (Figure 10.12).

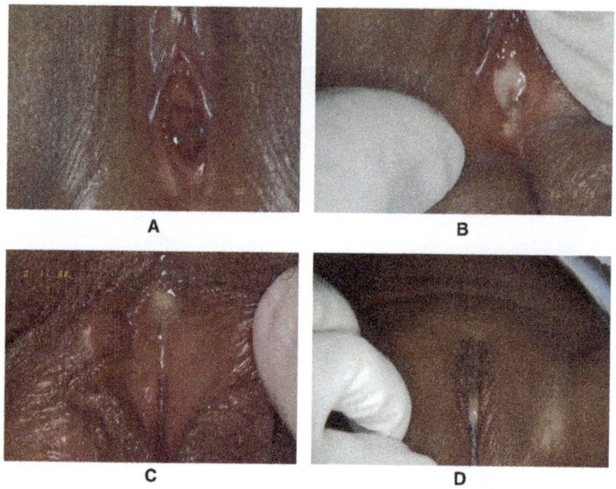

FIGURE 10.12

Miscellaneous. A, A 5-year-old girl has erythema of the tissues of the vestibule. She had persistent vaginal discharge for 4 months and intermittent vaginal bleeding. B, Same patient as in Figure 10.12A after irrigation of vagina with sterile water removed the tissue paper that was the nidus for persistent infection. C, A 4-year-old girl in whom the labial agglutination line is translucent. Agglutination obscures the appearance of the vaginal vestibule. D, A 4-year-old girl with labial agglutination that is thickened and was present longer than that in the patient in Figure 10.12C. This child experienced genital fondling, and this agglutination may be the postinflammatory residual to this contact.

Findings of erythema of the vestibular tissues, periurethral bands, lymphoid follicles, urethral dilatation, labial adhesions, posterior fourchette midline avascular areas, friability of the fourchette, tags, notches, mounds and projections, and intravaginal columns and transverse ridges are common normal variants. When an intravaginal column buttresses against the hymenal membrane edge, it may appear as a bump or mound on the edge of the hymen. Hymenal mounds or bumps are considered normal variants in any location of the hymen.

If the posterior rim of the hymen is narrow without signs of trauma, the examiner should avoid referring to this finding as *attenuated*. The definition of attenuation is "to make thin."[77] To apply this term correctly, the examiner must know that the posterior rim of the hymen was wider at some previous point in time and has since been narrowed. If the premorbid state is unknown, the examiner should describe the observed finding as a narrow posterior rim and dispense with the term *attenuated*.

The 2013 clinical report of the AAP Committee on Child Abuse and Neglect note the following: "Most sexually abused children have normal anogenital examinations....Even children who have been sexually penetrated often have normal examinations."[40] As such, sexual abuse is rarely diagnosed on the basis of physical examination or laboratory findings. Diagnostic findings in the AAP clinical report deemed concerning are "(1) abrasions or bruising of the genitalia; (2) an acute or healed tear in the posterior aspect of the hymen that extends to or nearly to the base of the hymen; (3) a markedly decreased amount of hymenal tissue or absent hymenal tissue in the posterior aspect; (4) injury to or scarring of the posterior fourchette, fossa navicularis, or hymen; and (5) anal bruising or lacerations." The guidelines further state: "...the presence of semen, sperm or acid phosphatase; a positive culture for *N gonorrhoeae* or *C trachomatis;* or a positive serologic test for syphilis or HIV infection make the diagnosis of sexual abuse a near medical certainty, even in the absence of a positive history, if perinatal transmission has been excluded for the [STIs]."

Whether an acute or healed genital or anal injury is identified, it is incumbent on the medical professional to obtain a complete history of the nature of the injury. When inflicted trauma is suspected, the essential components of the history include (a) the description and type of penetrating object; (b) the degree of discomfort associated with the event, including sensory details; (c) whether the contact occurred one time or more than one time; (d) associated physical symptoms (eg, bleeding, dysuria); (e) whether treatment was sought and received; and (f) the interval of time between the last alleged contact and the time of examination. Key differences in the history of accidental trauma, such as a straddle injury, are that accidental injuries are more commonly observed by a third party, medical attention is sought immediately after the injury, a scene-of-injury visit confirms the plausibility of the injuries and the accompanying history, and the pattern of injury is consistent with the history.[93,94] Of 161 accidental genital injuries reported in the literature, 3.7% involved the hymen. Impaling injuries do not always correspond with dramatic histories, and the resulting injuries can mimic those of sexual abuse.[95] There is no support for the supposition that hymenal injuries are the direct result of masturbation or the use of tampons.[96]

Male Genitalia

When examining the male genitalia, the medical record should document the following: (a) Tanner stage, (b) circumcision status, (c) retractability of foreskin if uncircumcised, (d) appearance of glans and frenulum, (e) urethral discharge, (f) any signs of injury to the glans or shaft of the penis, (g) the location of testes, (h) signs of scrotal trauma, (i) presence of hernias, and (j) inguinal adenopathy.

Injury to the male genitalia may include superficial abrasions to the shaft, petechiae, tears of the frenulum of the glans, bruising, and bite marks. When superficial injuries are present, an accompanying history of fondling, masturbation, and/or oral-genital contact is frequently present. Under most circumstances, there are no residua to these activities. Occasionally, the male genitalia may have evidence of a patterned injury that was the result of physical discipline striking the genitalia but without the genitalia being the target organ from a sexual perspective.

Anal Anatomy

When documenting anal findings, it is important to be as specific as possible when describing normal and abnormal observations (Figure 10.13). The tissue overlying the subcutaneous external anal sphincter is the *anal verge.* The anal verge begins at the most distal portion of the anoderm and extends to the exterior margin of the anal skin. Within the loose connective tissue surrounding the external anal orifice is the external hemorrhoidal plexus of the perianal space. The anoderm extends from the anal verge to the pectinate or dentate line. There is a scalloped appearance to the anoderm at the point in which it interdigitates with the ampulla of the rectum because of the alternating rectal sinuses and columns. The external anal tissue generally has symmetrical, circumferentially radiating folds known as *rugae,* formed by the corrugator cutis ani muscle.[73]

Anal and Perianal Findings

Despite a consensus as to the appropriate descriptive terminology of anal anatomy, disagreement remains regarding the interpretation of anal findings and the frequency with which anal signs are observed. Contributing to the difficulty of interpreting the residua of anal trauma is the unquestionable ability of the external anal sphincter to dilate to

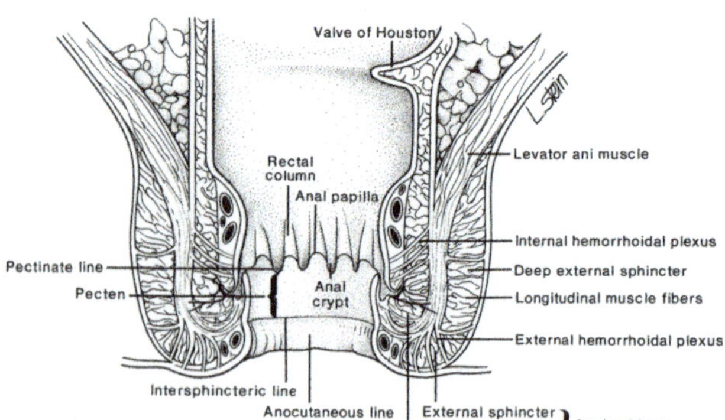

FIGURE 10.13
Cross-section of clinically significant structures of the rectosigmoid and anus.

accommodate a large bolus of fecal matter without injury to the tissues. Therefore, depending on the presence or absence of the following variables, a child may or may not have any residua to the introduction of a foreign body into the anus (Figure 10.14): (a) size of object introduced, (b) presence or absence of force, (c) use of lubricants, (d) degree of "cooperativeness" of child, (e) number of episodes of penetration, and (f) time interval since last alleged contact.

Descriptive studies of diagnostic findings generally are found in limited case report publications.[93,97,98] The literature on anal findings in males is quite limited, and the earlier studies that describe findings reflect considerable variability from study to study regarding frequency. There is not one published series of cases that attempts to systematically correlate the presence of physical findings with the medical history of anal penetration or interpret findings in a manner that correlates with the timing of anal injuries. The anal sphincter by design dilates to allow passage of large-diameter objects on a routine basis without injury to the anoderm or verge. Thus, it is not surprising that objects such as a penis or digit could readily pass into the anorectal canal without significant injury if the perpetrator uses lubrication and avoids the use of force, and when the activities occur in the context of a "cooperative" child. When injuries occur, they will typically be superficial, such as fissures that heal rapidly. Genital injuries occur most commonly as the result of rubbing, pinching, sucking, and biting, and these injuries also are generally superficial and heal without permanent scarring.

Hobbs and Wynne[7] reported that 40% to 50% of boys and girls with a history of anal penetration have abnormalities identified on examination. In the only article in the American literature specific to findings after anal abuse, 66% of 310 prepubertal children had normal-appearing perianal tissues.[97] There has been a paucity of recent medical literature on the residua of anal abuse, with a trend suggesting that, just as in other forms of sexual abuse, diagnostic findings are infrequent. Acute anal injuries are easily recognizable and must be considered in light of the presenting history.

The adult literature concerning descriptive reports of anal injuries in the consenting male homosexual population is limited. No description of chronic sequelae could be found, except an anecdotal notation that "colleagues in genitourinary medicine tell me that even in adults admitting to regular anal intercourse, the anus may appear entirely normal."[98]

Of the physical findings considered to result from chronic anal penetration, the most controversial is the reflexive dilatation of the buttocks with separation. Hobbs and Wynne[99] have confidence in this particular sign and state, "Dilatation over 0.5 cm without the passage

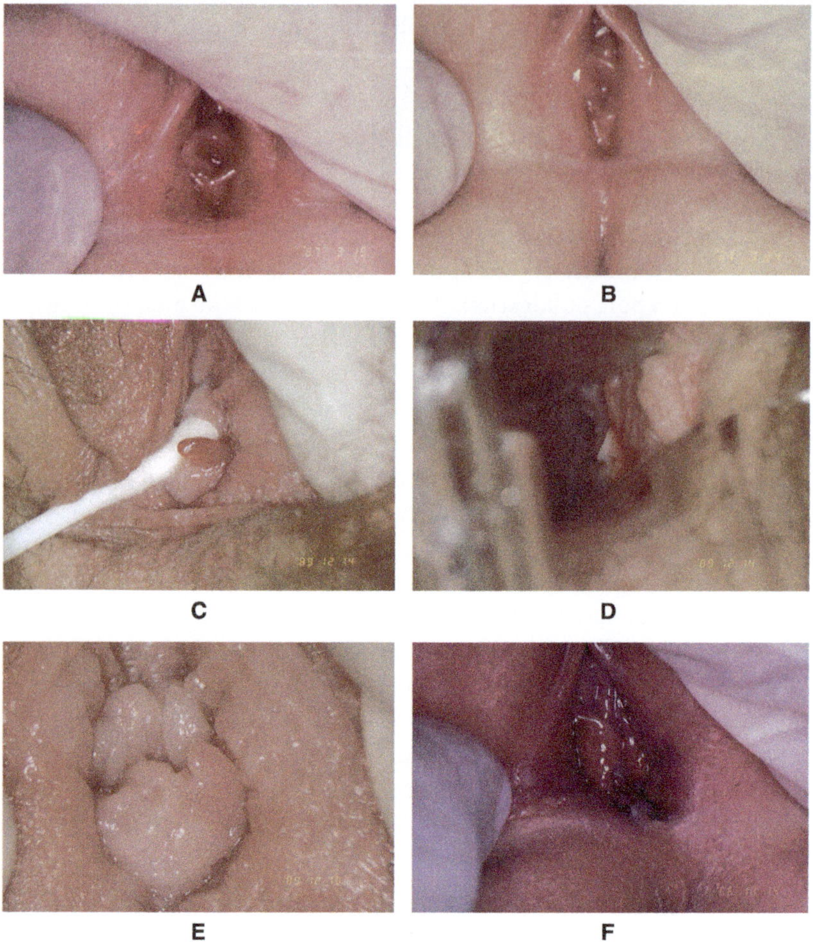

A B C D E F

FIGURE 10.14

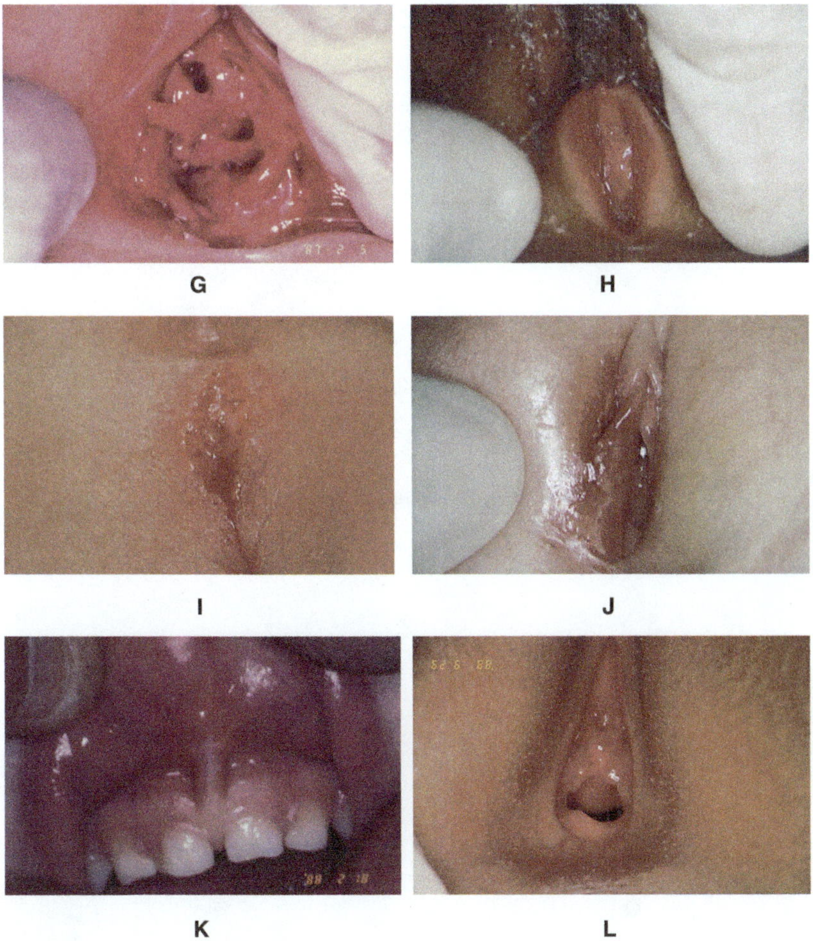

FIGURE 10.14 (*continued*)

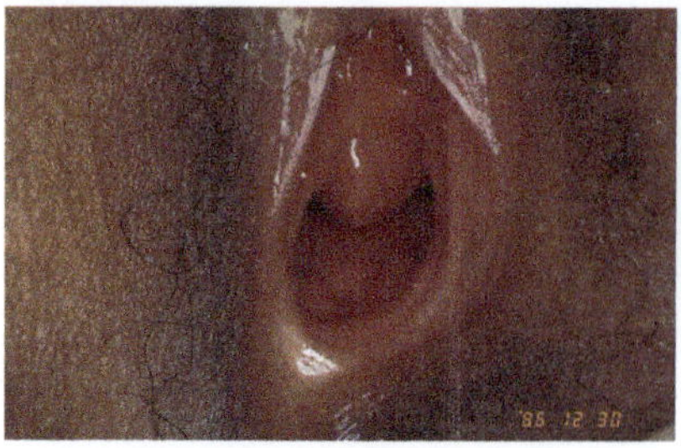

M

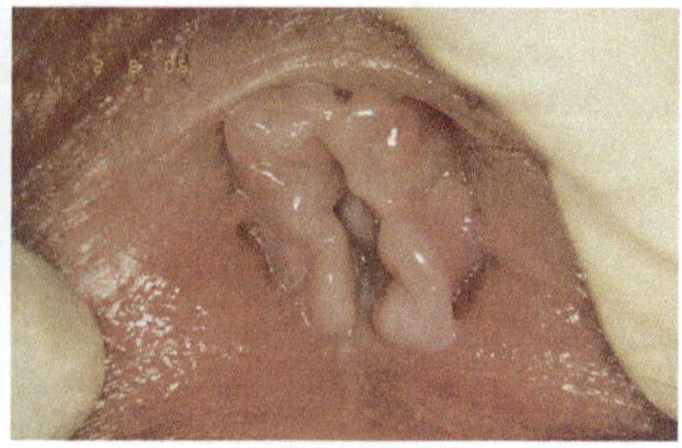

N

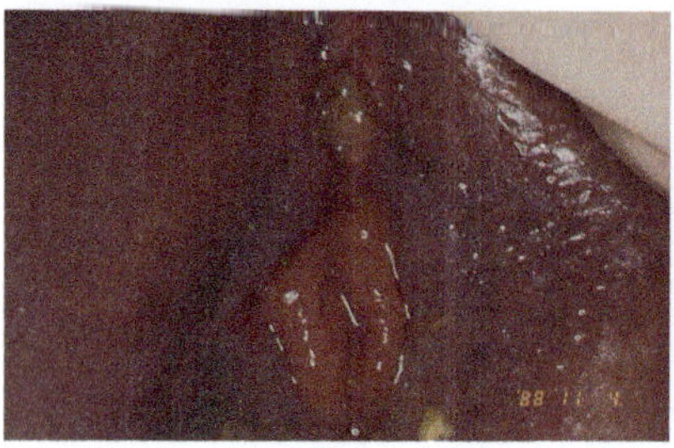

O

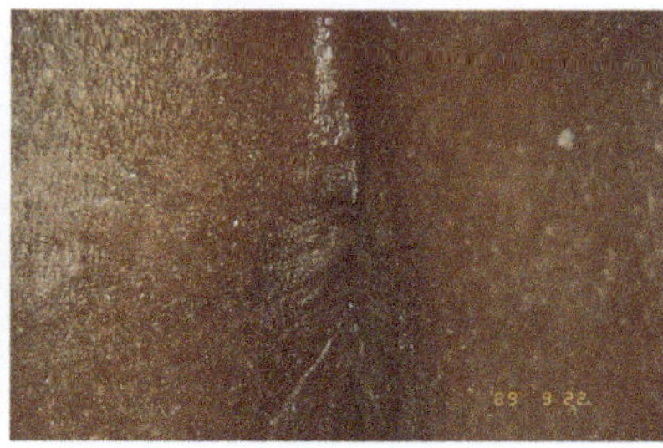

P

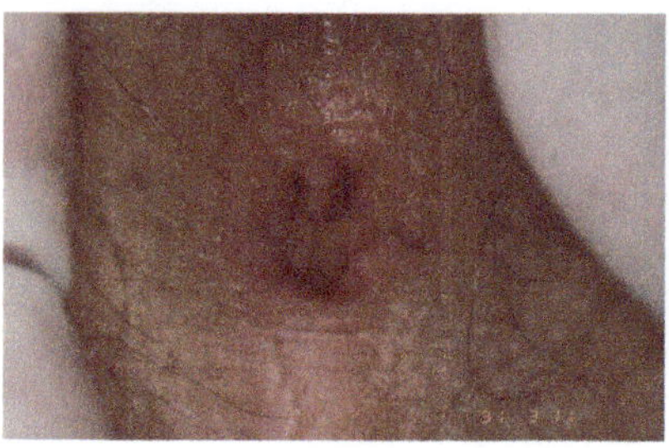

Q

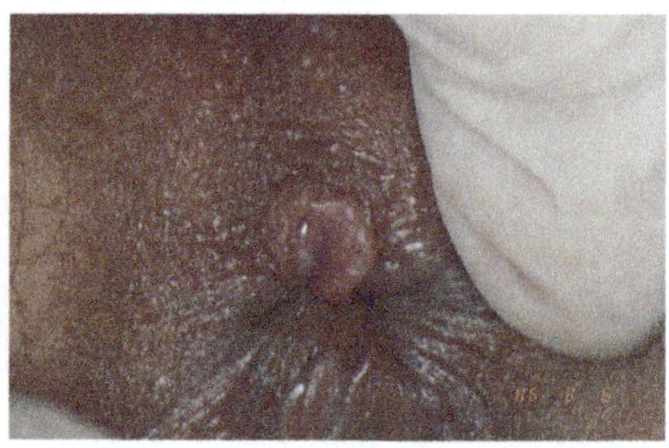

R

FIGURE 10.14 (*continued*)

Acute genital and anal trauma and healed residua. A, A 10-month-old girl has acute hemorrhage into the hymenal membrane and perihymenal tissues after attempted penetration. B, Same patient as in Figure 10.14A, 5 days after acute injury. No residua are apparent because of healing of superficial injuries by regeneration of labile cells. C, A 13-year-old girl has acute hemorrhage into the fimbria of the hymenal membrane after penile penetration of the vagina. D, Same patient as in Figure 10.14C, examined intravaginally with a speculum. Note the acute laceration of the vaginal canal (from the 3- to 5-o'clock position). E, Same patient as in figures 10.14C and 10.14D, 5 days later. Examination demonstrates complete healing of the injury to the membrane as well as the intravaginal mucosal laceration (not illustrated). F, A 19-month-old girl with prominent lacerations to the vaginal wall, membrane, and fourchette 4 days after penile vaginal penetration. Tissue edema and hemorrhage into tissues are evident. G, Same patient as in Figure 10.14F. Follow-up examination demonstrates healed residua to acute genital trauma, illustrating a marked difference from the appearance of acute injuries. Lacerated hymenal membrane remnants and scar tissue distort appearance in an unanticipated manner. Also evident are 2 condylomata the at 7-o'clock position, emphasizing the need for continued follow-up of children at risk for contracting sexually transmitted infections with

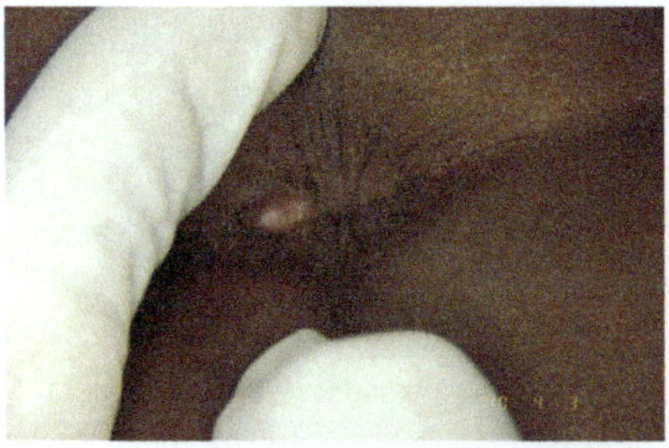

S

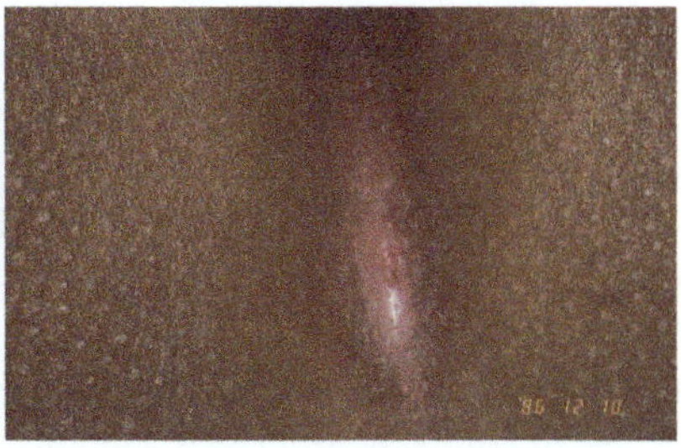

T

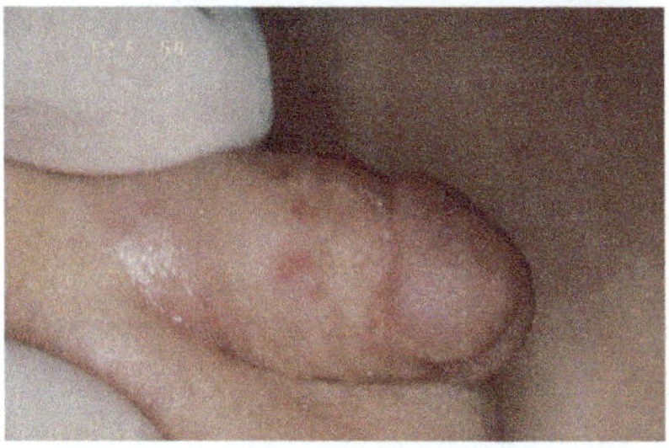

U

FIGURE 10.14 (*continued*)

long incubation periods. H, A 5-year-old girl with erythema and superficial abrasions to the medial aspect of the labia minora after vulvar coitus. Note the lack of signs of penetration through the hymenal orifice. I, A 2-year-old girl with acute laceration of the perineum and anal verge tissue at the 12-o'clock position after attempted penile anal penetration. J, A 6-year-old girl with an acute crush injury to the labia minora and majora after falling on a metal bar of a jungle gym. Note that the injury does not involve the hymenal membrane recessed in the vaginal canal. K, A 2-year-old girl has complete avulsion of the labial frenulum after physical and sexual assault. The mother's fingers elevate the upper lip to reveal residua to the avulsion. The minimal amount of scar tissue demonstrates the difficulty in appreciating how extensive the initial injuries may have been by observing only healed residua. L, A 4-year-old girl has healed interruption in the integrity of the hymenal membrane between the 8- and 10-o'clock positions after painful digital penetration through the orifice. Lymphoid follicles are present in the fossa between the 6- and 7-o'clock positions. M, A 12-year-old girl with Tanner stage 2 anatomy. Extremely narrowed posterior ring appears contiguous with the floor of the vagina. The child experienced repeated penile vaginal penetration. Premorbid appearance of the posterior rim is not observed. N, A 13-year-old girl with Tanner stage 3 anatomy. Healed residua to complete transection of the hymenal membrane at the 6-o'clock position. Scar tissue is evident at the base of the transection in the fossa. O, A 10-month-old girl after surgical repair of complete transection of the external anal sphincter after penile anal penetration. Rectal mucosa prolapsed because of tissue edema and decreased rectal tone. P, Same patient as in Figure 10.14O at final follow-up examination 10 months after acute injury. Note minimal distortion of the rugal pattern. With traction and flattening of verge tissues, a small avascular area remains. Q, A 12½-year-old girl has healed laceration of the anal sphincter at the 10-, 5-, and 7-o'clock positions. Anus remains open without traction. Rectal tone is dramatically diminished, and no reflex constriction occurs. R, A 14-year-old girl has a post-traumatic anal tag, the result of resorbed hematoma of anal verge tissue after penile anal penetration. S, A 4-year-old boy has a hypopigmented area in the anal verge with neovascularity apparent as granulation tissue continues to mature. T, A 3-year-old boy has superficial ulceration of the gluteal crease, which represents residua to the rubbing of the ventral side of a penis between the buttocks. U, A 3-year-old boy has circumferential bite marks to the shaft of the penis.

of wind does not, in our experience, occur in normal children examined as described. The presence of stool visible in the rectum should not discount the significance of the finding." Hobbs and Wynne[99] reported this finding in 42% of children who experienced sexual abuse with anal signs. Other authors have not found reflexive dilatation as prevalent in their series.[67,98,100] In a population of children who had not experienced abuse, McCann and Voris[67] observed that anal sphincter dilation occurred in 49% of children, and the mean anteroposterior diameter of the orifice was 1 cm, with a range of 0.1 to 2.5 cm. On its own, this sign should not be interpreted as abnormal. McCann and Voris[67] observed that a variety of perianal findings seen in children who had experienced abuse also may be seen in children who had not, thus highlighting problems with the sensitivity and specificity of soft tissue findings. Nonspecific findings noted by McCann and Voris included perianal erythema (41%), increased perianal pigmentation (30%), venous congestion (73%), anal dilatation (49%), skin tags (11%), and scars (2%). Also described were congenital smooth areas in 26% of the children. These "smooth fan-shaped areas in the mid-line of the verge, either with or without depressions, appeared to be a congenital anomaly of the superficial division of external sphincter muscle fibers." This particular finding has the potential to be misinterpreted as scar tissue. Once more, a history of injury must be obtained before concluding that scar tissue is present.

Trauma to the anal verge may result in a localized collection of blood distorting the anal verge. After resorption of the hematoma, a small tag of loose skin may remain.[101] The most commonly observed perianal tags are congenital. A prominent extension of the median raphe, a normal variation of anatomy, may extend into the anal verge and appear similar to a tag.

Children have difficulty in determining whether an object has been placed "in" their anorectal canal. Pressure over the external anal verge tissues may cause a slight dilation of the anus and thus be perceived as "in" when, in fact, penetration into the canal per se did not occur. Therefore, reliance on the child's perception of the experience as confirmatory of penetration should be approached with caution until further studies address the accuracy of a child's ability to differentiate "in" from "on" at varying developmental stages.

The most common object to penetrate the anus of a child is a digit. A digit can be readily introduced into the anus repeatedly without discomfort or residua. When reviewing a history of penetration, it is important to determine whether the child had any discomfort associated with the contact or whether there was discomfort following the event, and to record any associated observations. A simple question to ask the child is, "What did it feel like when it happened?" If the child responds that it hurt, clarify whether it was his or her feelings or body that hurt. If the child complained of physical discomfort or pain following anal penetration, the child should be asked to explain how she or he experienced the discomfort and whether she or he observed anything that made the child know she or he was hurt. The child might respond that he or she observed blood when wiping self or on stool with passage of a bowel movement. When there has been trauma to the anoderm, the child may express experiencing a burning sensation with passage of a bowel movement.

When examining the anus for residua to penetration, boys are best examined in the left lateral decubitus position, a position in which they have not experienced the alleged abuse (see Figure 10.6). If a child has a history of chronic abuse, and no acute abnormalities are observed externally, anoscopy will provide little additional information. The digital rectal examination also provides little information to assist the examiner in determining if a child has been anally assaulted. If, however, on anoscopy or digital rectal examination the child provides a spontaneous utterance likening the experience to that of the penetrating event, this valuable disclosure information should be recorded as the child's verbatim statement. If the anus dilates, the presence or absence of stool should be noted. Reflex dilation of the anus with stool in the rectal ampulla is a normal response.

When acute signs of injury to the anal verge tissue are observed, anoscopy is important to identify the presence of lacerations, petechiae, bruising of the anorectal canal, and seminal products. Surprisingly, external signs of trauma may be minimal in patients with significant acute internal injuries to the anorectal canal. Accidental impaling injuries involving the anus and perineum are readily differentiated from sexual assault both in their pattern and the history of their presentation.

Residua of Sexual Contact

Patterns of Trauma

The difficulties associated with the retrospective interpretation of the residua of sexual contact are numerous. Research continues to support that few physical findings represent definitive evidence of sexual assault and repeated episodes of sexual assault do not result in significant changes to the examination.[102] When a child presents with acute injuries, the pattern and extent of the trauma should be documented. The spectrum of acute injury is variable, involving superficial mucosal abrasions and scratches to clear transecting lacerations of genital and anal structures.[103] Superficial injuries and signs of irritation may be subtle and nonspecific. The extent of injury depends on many variables, most significant of which are the degree of force, the object used to inflict the injury, and the nature of the contact, with particular reference to whether penetration occurred.

In genital fondling of the female, the hand is usually placed over the mons pubis and the index and third finger separate the labia and enter the vaginal vestibule. Rubbing of the tissues bordering the vaginal vestibule may acutely demonstrate evidence of erythema, superficially denuded mucosa, abrasions or scratches, and edema of the inner aspects of the labia minora and the periurethral area. Generally, fondling or penetration between the labia results in injuries between the 9- and 3-o'clock positions, with the child supine, and less likely to involve the fourchette or fossa. Most fondling or digital penetration contact does not result in serious trauma, but the forceful introduction of a finger into the vagina can result in significant trauma due to the limited elasticity of the prepubertal hymen.[80]

Depending on the differential between the hymenal orifice size and the penetrating digit, the child may have either no observed injuries from introduction through the orifice or a laceration of the membrane edge. Acute injuries to the hymen should be readily apparent, although injury to the hymenal membrane or fossa as a result of fondling is infrequent.

Children who are fondled and experience trauma to the periurethral area may complain of dysuria after the alleged event. The past medical history should therefore include asking about urogenital symptoms and past diagnoses, including presumed urinary tract infections. Dysuria is specific to irritation or inflammation of the distal urethra. If a history of dysuria is obtained in a non-leading and non-suggestive manner, it is valuable corroborating history of sexual contact and may be admissible in court. In a review of 161 cases of girls who had been sexually abused, 37% provided a history of dysuria directly as a result of the genital touch. All these children answered standard questions that were non-leading and non-suggestive.[104]

Dysuria also can be a posttraumatic event, occurring during vulvar coitus. This form of genital-to-genital contact also may be perceived by the child as penetrating. In vulvar coitus, the shaft of the penis is rubbed between the labia and can result in abrasions and bruising of the inner aspects of the labia minora. The penis can cause trauma to the periurethral/clitoral hood region and the fourchette as well. Because the hymenal membrane is recessed in the vaginal canal, vulvar coitus is not likely to result in injury to the hymenal orifice. Berkowitz et al[105] reported that trauma to the external surface of the hymenal membrane occurring within the context of vulvar coitus resulted in scar tissue, presumably creating a stenosis of a previously larger orifice, creating the appearance of an acquired imperforate hymen. Dysuria also may follow coitus.[106]

When genital-to-anal contact occurs frequently, the dorsal side of the shaft of the penis is rubbed over the external anal verge tissues, causing pressure on the external sphincter, which may be perceived as penetration in the anorectal canal. When the shaft is rubbed between the buttocks over the natal cleft, it may result in superficial abrasions. This activity is commonly referred to by boys as "freaking." When either vulvar coitus or natal cleft rubbing occurs, the individual may ejaculate, and seminal products may be collected from the abdomen, inner thighs, buttocks, and back.

When an object forcefully penetrates the vagina through the hymenal orifice in a young child, residual signs are generally obvious when examined acutely. This type of penetration will most likely result in a laceration to the edge of the membrane that extends to the vaginal floor. Most lacerations are seen between the 5- and 7-o'clock positions with the child supine but can be seen anywhere between the 3- and 9-o'clock positions. Forceful penetration also may result in lacerations to the fossa navicularis and the lateral walls of the vagina and possible perforation of the posterior fornix into the peritoneum.[101,107] Although most lacerations of the hymen stop at the floor of the vagina, some extend through the fossa and fourchette and into the perineal body. This type of injury is readily recognizable, and its full extent must be assessed with the child under anesthesia.

Accidental injuries to the genitalia do occur, and the pattern of trauma and the accompanying history are usually suggestive of its etiology.[108,109] Most accidental injuries are the result of a child falling on a horizontal bar of a bicycle, jungle gym, or the classic picket fence. The horizontal bar usually results in a crush injury of the clitoral hood/labia minora between the bar and the inner aspect of the thigh. This injury is usually unilateral. Picket injuries are more likely to be impaling. Occasionally, the forceful abduction of thighs results in a superficial laceration of the perineum. One report of injury to the genitalia occurred as a result of a seat belt.[110] Masturbation is unlikely to result in any injuries to the genitalia other than localized erythema or superficial abrasions as the result of rubbing. Children do insert objects between the labia, but they rarely do so in a forceful way that would result in injury because of the exquisite sensitivity of the hymenal tissue.

Rubbing of the inner aspects of the labia occurring in the context of vulvar coitus, genital fondling, or possibly masturbation can result in inflammation. Because of the close proximity of the inner aspects of the inflamed labia minora in prepubertal children, the mucosal surfaces may agglutinate. Labial agglutination is an acquired post-inflammatory condition seen only in the prepubertal child and involves the thin, unestrogenized vascular tissues of the inner aspect of the labia minora. The ability to examine the hymenal membrane may be compromised depending on the degree of fusion. The agglutination may extend from the fourchette to the clitoral hood with only a minute opening for urine to escape, creating the appearance of an "absent" vagina. Although labial agglutination is a common finding in young children, its association as a residual to sexual abuse was described only recently.[111–113] Labial agglutination alone, without a history of concerns, does not raise a concern for sexual abuse. Caution should be exercised if agglutination is the only abnormal finding on examination. When agglutination is present, it can be medically dehisced by estrogen cream. "Gentle traction," as described in standard texts, should not be used because it results only in denuded edges that are painful and quickly readhere, making reexamination even more difficult.

Extragenital signs of trauma are infrequent in most cases of child sexual abuse. When they do occur, they usually occur within the context of rape.[114] If a child is forced to perform fellatio on an individual, tears to the labial frenulum and petechiae of the palate may be noted. Injuries reflective of force and restraint may be seen as ligature marks around the wrists and ankles. Bruising of the extremities may appear as grasp marks. Bite marks may be present on the neck, breast, buttocks, or inner thighs.

Retrospective Interpretation

Most children do not present for an examination immediately after their alleged sexual abuse; therefore, few children will have acute signs of injury or evidence to collect.[57] In fact, fewer than 5% of children examined non-acutely are found to have signs of injury to the anogenital area.[115] Thus, the medical professional is required to examine tissues that have healed. Without knowledge of the premorbid appearance of the genital tissues, it is difficult to judge whether a particular finding is the direct result of sexual abuse. Several clinical scenarios can occur. First, the child may be seen long after the last episode of alleged contact, and, thus, only healed residua can be observed. Second, the child may have experienced genital or anal trauma resulting in residua and is being examined during the period of formation of granulation tissue and no obvious acute injury. Third, the child may present when nonspecific findings are present, and the medical professional must correlate the history of the alleged contact and the findings as residual to that contact. Finally, the child may present with acute signs of injury, the least problematic situation to evaluate.

Over the past 25 years, there has been a limited but developing body of literature describing changes to the hymen in the prepubertal child resulting from trauma.[16,67,116–119] The pathology of healing is well understood.[120] These principles of healing have only recently been applied to genital and anal injuries for a prospective look at how acute injuries heal.[116,121] Observations by Finkel[116] on the healing chronology of genital and anal injuries have laid the foundation for our understanding of the retrospective interpretation of changes in genital and anal anatomy. Studies by McCann et al[121] and Heppenstall-Heger et al[122] have continued to elucidate the residua to genital and anal trauma.

Formulating a Conclusion

In formulating a diagnostic assessment, the medical professional must consider (a) historical details, events leading to a disclosure (if available), and behavioral indicators reflective of the contact; (b) symptoms that result from the contact; (c) acute genital/anal injuries and/or chronic residua; (d) forensic evidence; and (e) STIs. The medical assessment only rarely can stand on its own because of the relative infrequency of findings that are diagnostic. The diagnosis will reflect a combination of disclosure evidence, behaviors, medical history, physical examination, and laboratory and evidentiary results. In most states, even if medical professionals are not able to reach a diagnosis of sexual abuse, they are mandated to report suspected child abuse and neglect to the appropriate governmental agencies[40] (Table 10.1).

TABLE 10.1
Guidelines for Making the Decision to Report Sexual Abuse of Children

Data Available				Response	
History	Behavioral Symptoms	Physical Examination	Diagnostic Tests	Level of Concern About Sexual Abuse	Report Decision
Clear statement	Present or absent	Normal or abnormal	Positive or negative	High	Report
None or vague	Present or absent	Normal or nonspecific	Positive test for *Chlamydia trachomatis*, gonorrhea, *Trichomonas vaginalis*, HIV, syphilis, or herpes[a]	High	Report
None or vague	Present or absent	Concerning or diagnostic findings	Negative or positive	High[b]	Report
Vague, or history by parent only	Present or absent	Normal or nonspecific	Negative	Indeterminate	Refer when possible
None	Present	Normal or nonspecific	Negative	Intermediate	Possible report,[c] refer, or follow

[a] If nonsexual transmission is unlikely or excluded.

[b] Confirmed with various examination techniques and/or peer review with expert consultant.

[c] If behaviors are rare/unusual in normal children.

From Jenny C, Crawford-Jakubiak JE; American Academy of Pediatrics Committee on Child Abuse and Neglect. The evaluation of children in the primary care setting when sexual abuse is suspected. *Pediatrics*. 2013;132(2):e558–e567.

Outcomes of Sexual Abuse

Sexual abuse has the potential for profound lifelong adverse effects on a developing child and his or her future children. It is the responsibility of the medical professional to know how to respond and refer to appropriate services. With education and primary prevention, the pediatrician can help to reduce the potential for child sexual abuse.[123,124] The long-term effect of sexual abuse is potentially significant. Children who experience sexual abuse are at risk of running away, being trafficked, or becoming engaged in commercial sexual exploitation, and of developing posttraumatic stress disorder, major depression, anxiety disorders, dissociation, bulimia, sexual dysfunction, and high-risk behaviors such as suicide and substance abuse, among others.[5,125–127] Multiple chronic disease, health risk behaviors, and premature death have been associated with adverse childhood experiences such as child maltreatment, including sexual abuse. It is incumbent on the medical professional to refer all children who have experienced sexual abuse for a comprehensive mental health assessment to determine the effect of this abuse. The treatment plan prepared by the psychologist should include trauma-focused cognitive behavior therapy because it is the treatment of choice for children who have experienced sexual abuse and has been demonstrated to effectively treat posttraumatic stress disorder and many of the behavioral problems that children who have been sexually abused experience. Treatment also reduces the potential for continuing the cycle of sexual abuse and sexually reactive behaviors.[128]

Sexual Abuse Prevention

The evaluation of a child alleged to have been sexually abused is a challenging and emotionally charged issue that requires the medical professional to reach a balanced, objective, and defensible opinion. The medical professional can play an important role in education about and the prevention of sexual abuse as well as recognition, evaluation, and referral. Children and parents would be well served if medical professionals routinely, as a part of annual health supervision visits, spoke to parents and children beginning at the 3-year visit about the importance of personal space and privacy.

Some suggestions for these conversations include

- Begin talking to parents about delivering information on personal space and privacy to their children by 3 years of age.
- Tell parents that they should limit the number of individuals who provide genital, perianal, and bathing care to reduce risk.

- Let parents know the more independence children have for their own genital care, the better.
- Have parents teach their children the appropriate names for their private parts so they have the language to communicate. When supervising bathing in the preschool years, the parent can help with providing appropriate naming of the genitalia by explaining that the parts of their body covered by a bathing suit or their underwear are called *private parts* and the reason they are called that is because they belong to them. A parent can help with establishing rules regarding touching by saying: "Don't forget to wash your vagina/penis and butt, and when you're done let me know and I will help you with your hair. Don't forget to wipe your private parts. Who is allowed to touch your private parts? What do you do if someone touches your private parts?" Over time, when these simple questions are asked, the child will respond by saying, "Mommy/daddy, I know that." Surely just because kids know what is OK and what is not OK does not mean that they are invulnerable or that they can stop someone from touching them inappropriately. However, armed with the information, they may be more likely to see what they are experiencing as inappropriate and disclose sooner rather than later.
- Discourage co-bathing.
- Parents can help explain that they can touch the child's private parts when they are taking a bath or wiping themselves after going to the bathroom. A doctor can touch their private parts when their parents are in the room. Parents can introduce the concept of "OK and not OK" touching and the need to tell if anyone touches their private parts in a context other than providing care. Medical professionals have moved away from "good touch–bad touch," as it was problematic because children do not anticipate being touched in a way that is "bad" by someone they know, love, and trust. Touching in private parts can feel "good" and be confusing to children. If what they experienced is perceived as being "bad," there is the possibility that they may think that they are "bad." Parents and medical professionals can inform children that they need to tell 2 adults right away and they will not get into trouble or be punished if anyone ever touches them or makes them touch someone else's private parts.
- Emphasize that it is never OK to have a "secret," and if anyone tells them to keep a secret or they think they need to keep a secret,

they need to tell 2 adults. Explain how "surprises" can be fine because we find out, but secrets are never OK. All these messages should be delivered at every annual visit. A good time to provide information to the child is just before completion of the genital examination.

- If a child walks into a bedroom or bathroom and the parent needs privacy, he or she should tell the child that he or she needs privacy. Wherever the message of privacy can be reinforced, it should be. Children should be taught to respect siblings' need for privacy.

The science of prevention is still evolving, and there is no body of literature that purports a single message or approach that can be used to simply supply the magic bullet of prevention. We know that children armed with information about personal safety are more likely to develop protective behaviors, enhance potential for disclosure, and experience less self-blame. As in the early development of every area of prevention, "common sense" was used to build a foundation that was then tested and led to the science. Parents want to protect their child against a sexually abusive experience, and when we begin to give parents the language to communicate these concepts, we educate children about this potential risk and empower them to tell. It is the collective responsibility of parents, medical professionals, and our institutions to deliver and reinforce children's right to personal space and privacy. Now it is time for medical professionals to integrate anticipatory guidance into every annual health supervision visit.

References

1. Enos WF, Conrath TB, Byer JC. Forensic evaluation of the sexually abused child. *Pediatrics*. 1986;78(3):385–398 PMID: 3748672
2. Cantwell HB. Vaginal inspection as it relates to child sexual abuse in girls under thirteen. *Child Abuse Negl*. 1983;7(2):171–176 PMID: 6685559 https://doi.org/10.1016/0145-2134(83)90069-8
3. DeJong AR, Emmett GA, Hervada AR. Sexual abuse of children. Sex-, race-, and age-dependent variations. *Am J Dis Child*. 1982;136(2):129–134 PMID: 7064927 https://doi.org/10.1001/archpedi.1982.03970380041010
4. Ellerstein NS, Canavan JW. Sexual abuse of boys. *Am J Dis Child*. 1980;134(3):255–257 PMID: 7361732
5. Elliott DM, Briere J. Posttraumatic stress associated with delayed recall of sexual abuse: a general population study. *J Trauma Stress*. 1995;8(4):629–647 PMID: 8564276 https://doi.org/10.1002/jts.2490080407
6. Giardino A, Finkel MA. *A Practical Guide to the Evaluation of Sexual Abuse in the Prepubertal Child*. Newbury Park, CA: Sage Publications; 1992

7. Hobbs CJ, Wynne JM. Buggery in childhood—a common syndrome of child abuse. *Lancet*. 1986;2(8510):792–796 PMID: 2429126 https://doi.org/10.1016/S0140-6736(86)90310-7
8. Jaffe AC, Dynneson L, ten Bensel RW. Sexual abuse of children. An epidemiologic study. *Am J Dis Child*. 1975;129(6):689–692 PMID: 1155399 https://doi.org/10.1001/archpedi.1975.02120430029008
9. Kempe CH. Sexual abuse, another hidden pediatric problem: the 1977 C. Anderson Aldrich lecture. *Pediatrics*. 1978;62(3):382–389 PMID: 704212
10. Paul DM. The medical examination in sexual offences. *Med Sci Law*. 1975;15(3):154–162 PMID: 1160560 https://doi.org/10.1177/002580247501500302
11. Rimsza ME, Niggemann EH. Medical evaluation of sexually abused children: a review of 311 cases. *Pediatrics*. 1982;69(1):8–14 PMID: 7054766
12. Spencer MJ, Dunklee P. Sexual abuse of boys. *Pediatrics*. 1986;78(1):133–138 PMID: 3725484
13. Tilelli JA, Turek D, Jaffe AC. Sexual abuse of children: clinical findings and implications for management. *N Engl J Med*. 1980;302(6):319–323 PMID: 7350499 https://doi.org/10.1056/NEJM198002073020604
14. Wolak J, Finkelhor D, Mitchell K. Internet-initiated sex crimes against minors: implications for prevention based on findings from a national study. *J Adolesc Health*. 2004;35(5):424.e11–424.e20 PMID: 15488437 https://doi.org/10.1016/j.jadohealth.2004.05.006
15. Finkel MA. Technical conduct of the child sexual abuse medical examination. *Child Abuse Negl*. 1998;22(6):555–566 PMID: 9649895 https://doi.org/10.1016/S0145-2134(98)00026-X
16. Adams JA, Kellogg ND, Farst KJ, et al. Updated guidelines for the medical assessment and care of children who may have been sexually abused. *J Pediatr Adolesc Gynecol*. 2016;29(2):81–87 PMID: 26220352 https://doi.org/10.1016/j.jpag.2015.01.007
17. Burgess AW, Holmstrom LL. Sexual trauma of children and adolescents. *Nurs Clin North Am*. 1975;10(3):551–563 PMID: 1041637
18. Burgess AW, Holmstrom LL. Coping behavior of the rape victim. *Am J Psychiatry*. 1976;133(4):413–418 PMID: 1267040 https://doi.org/10.1176/ajp.133.4.413
19. Finkelhor DH. *Sexually Victimized Children*. New York, NY: The Free Press; 1979
20. Green AH. True and false allegations of sexual abuse in child custody disputes. *J Am Acad Child Psychiatry*. 1986;25(4):449–456 PMID: 3745724 https://doi.org/10.1016/S0002-7138(10)60001-5
21. Sgroi SM. *Handbook of Clinical Intervention in Child Sexual Abuse*. Lexington, MA: Lexington Books; 1982
22. Summit RC. The child sexual abuse accommodation syndrome. *Child Abuse Negl*. 1983;7(2):177–193 PMID: 6605796 https://doi.org/10.1016/0145-2134(83)90070-4
23. Heger A, Ticson L, Velasquez O, Bernier R. Children referred for possible sexual abuse: medical findings in 2384 children. *Child Abuse Negl*. 2002;26(6–7):645–659 PMID: 12201160
24. Kann L, Warren CW, Harris WA, et al; Centers for Disease Control and Prevention. Youth risk behavior surveillance—United States, 1995. *MMWR CDC Surveill Summ*. 1996;45(4):1–84 PMID: 8841032
25. Finkelhor DH, ed. *Child Sexual Abuse: New Theory and Research*. New York, NY: The Free Press; 1984
26. Finkelhor D, Hotaling GT. Sexual abuse in the National Incidence Study of Child Abuse and Neglect: an appraisal. *Child Abuse Negl*. 1984;8(1):23–32 PMID: 6609754 https://doi.org/10.1016/0145-2134(84)90046-2

27. Finkelhor DH, Browne A. Assessing the long-term impact on child sexual abuse: a review and conceptualization. In: Walker LEA, ed. *Handbook on Sexual Abuse of Children—Assessment and Treatment Issues.* New York, NY: Springer; 1988
28. Finkelhor D, Hotaling G, Lewis IA, Smith C. Sexual abuse in a national survey of adult men and women: prevalence, characteristics, and risk factors. *Child Abuse Negl.* 1990;14(1):19–28 PMID: 2310970 https://doi.org/10.1016/0145-2134(90)90077-7
29. Krugman RD. Recognition of sexual abuse in children. *Pediatr Rev.* 1986;8(1):25–30 PMID: 3332329 https://doi.org/10.1542/pir.8-1-25
30. National Center on Child Abuse and Neglect. *Study Findings—Study of National Incidence and Prevalence of Child Abuse and Neglect, 1988.* Washington, DC: US Department of Health and Human Services; 1988
31. Rosenfeld AA. Sexual abuse of children: personal and professional responses. In: Newberger EH, ed. *Child Abuse.* Boston, MA: Little Brown; 1982
32. Vander Mey BJ. The sexual victimization of male children: a review of previous research. *Child Abuse Negl.* 1988;12(1):61–72 PMID: 3284613 https://doi.org/10.1016/0145-2134(88)90008-7
33. DeLago C, Finkel MA, Clarke C, Deblinger E. Urogenital symptoms after sexual abuse vs irritant contact in premenarchal girls. *J Pediatr Adolesc Gynecol.* 2012;25(5):334–339 PMID: 22980412 https://doi.org/10.1016/j.jpag.2012.06.003
34. Lynch L, Faust J. Reduction of distress in children undergoing sexual abuse medical examination. *J Pediatr.* 1998;133(2):296–299 PMID: 9709727 https://doi.org/10.1016/S0022-3476(98)70241-0
35. Finkelhor D, Browne A. The traumatic impact of child sexual abuse: a conceptualization. *Am J Orthopsychiatry.* 1985;55(4):530–541 PMID: 4073225 https://doi.org/10.1111/j.1939-0025.1985.tb02703.x
36. Cronch LE, Viljoen JL, Hansen DJ. Forensic interviewing in child sexual abuse cases: current techniques and future directions. *Aggress Violent Behav.* 2006;11(3):195–207 https://doi.org/10.1016/j.avb.2005.07.009
37. Boat BW, Everson MD. Use of anatomical dolls among professionals in sexual abuse evaluations. *Child Abuse Negl.* 1988;12(2):171–179 PMID: 3395893 https://doi.org/10.1016/0145-2134(88)90025-7
38. Goodwin J. Evaluation and treatment for incest victims and their families: a problem-oriented approach. In: Goodwin J, ed. *Sexual Abuse.* Chicago, IL: Yearbook; 1989
39. White S, Strom GA, Santilli G, Halpin BM. Interviewing young sexual abuse victims with anatomically correct dolls. *Child Abuse Negl.* 1986;10(4):519–529 PMID: 3791029 https://doi.org/10.1016/0145-2134(86)90057-8
40. Jenny C, Crawford-Jakubiak JE; American Academy of Pediatrics Committee on Child Abuse and Neglect. The evaluation of children in the primary care setting when sexual abuse is suspected. *Pediatrics.* 2013;132(2):e558–e567 PMID: 23897912 https://doi.org/10.1542/peds.2013-1741
41. MacFarlane K, Kerbs S. Techniques for interviewing and evidence gathering. In: MacFarlane K, ed. *Sexual Abuse of Young Children.* New York, NY: The Guilford Press; 1987
42. Green HA. Overview of normal psychosexual development. In: Green AH, Schetky DH, eds. *Child Sexual Abuse: A Handbook for Health Care and Legal Professionals.* New York, NY: Brunner Mazel Publishers; 1988
43. Jampole L, Weber MK. An assessment of the behavior of sexually abused and nonsexually abused children with anatomically correct dolls. *Child Abuse Negl.* 1987;11(2):187–192 PMID: 3594279 https://doi.org/10.1016/0145-2134(87)90057-3

44. Long S. Guidelines for treating young children. In: MacFarlane K, ed. *Sexual Abuse of Young Children*. New York, NY: The Guilford Press; 1987
45. Jones DPH, McQuiston M. *Interviewing the Sexually Abused Child*. 2nd ed. Denver, CO: C. Henry Kempe National Center for the Prevention and Treatment of Child Abuse and Neglect; 1986
46. Myers JEB. Role of physician in preserving verbal evidence of child abuse. *J Pediatr*. 1986;109(3):409–411 PMID: 3746528 https://doi.org/10.1016/S0022-3476(86)80108-1
47. Myers JEB. *Legal Issues in Child Abuse and Neglect Practice*. 2nd ed. Thousand Oaks, CA: Sage; 1998:102–152
48. Drummond R, Gall JA. Evaluation of forensic medical history taking from the child in cases of child physical and sexual abuse and neglect. *J Forensic Leg Med*. 2017;46:37–45 PMID: 28122285 https://doi.org/10.1016/j.jflm.2016.12.006
49. Holmes WC, Slap GB. Sexual abuse of boys: definition, prevalence, correlates, sequelae, and management [see comments]. *JAMA*. 1998;280(21):1855–1862 PMID: 9846781 https://doi.org/10.1001/jama.280.21.1855
50. West DJ. Boys and sexual abuse: an English opinion. *Arch Sex Behav*. 1998;27(6):539–559 PMID: 9883304 https://doi.org/10.1023/A:1018717032762
51. Friedrich WN, Urquiza AJ, Beilke RL. Behavior problems in sexually abused young children. *J Pediatr Psychol*. 1986;11(1):47–57 PMID: 3958867 https://doi.org/10.1093/jpepsy/11.1.47
52. Mitchell KJ, Finkelhor D, Wolak J. Protecting youth online: family use of filtering and blocking software. *Child Abuse Negl*. 2005;29(7):753–765 PMID: 16051350 https://doi.org/10.1016/j.chiabu.2004.05.008
53. Kellogg ND; American Academy of Pediatrics Committee on Child Abuse and Neglect. Clinical report—the evaluation of sexual behaviors in children. *Pediatrics*. 2009;124(3):992–998 PMID: 19720674 https://doi.org/10.1542/peds.2009-1692
54. Fisher-Owens SA, Lukefahr JL, Tate AR; American Academy of Pediatrics Section on Oral Health; Committee on Child Abuse and Neglect; American Academy of Pediatric Dentistry Council on Clinical Affairs, Council on Scientific Affairs; Ad Hoc Work Group on Child Abuse and Neglect. Oral and dental aspects of child abuse and neglect. *Pediatrics*. 2017;140(2):e20171487 PMID: 28771417 https://doi.org/10.1542/peds.2017-1487
55. Makoroff KL, Brauley JL, Brandner AM, Myers PA, Shapiro RA. Genital examinations for alleged sexual abuse of prepubertal girls: findings by pediatric emergency medicine physicians compared with child abuse trained physicians. *Child Abuse Negl*. 2002;26(12):1235–1242 PMID: 12464298 https://doi.org/10.1016/S0145-2134(02)00419-2
56. Wright RJ, Wright RO, Farnan L, Isaac NE. Response to child abuse in the pediatric emergency department: need for continued education. *Pediatr Emerg Care*. 1999;15(6):376–382 PMID: 10608320 https://doi.org/10.1097/00006565-199912000-00002
57. Heger A, Ticson L, Velasquez O, Bernier R. Children referred for possible sexual abuse: a comparison of clinical history and medical findings in 2384 children. *Child Abuse Negl*. 2002;26:645–659 PMID: 12201160 https://doi.org/10.1016/S0145-2134(02)00339-3
58. Anderst J, Kellogg N, Jung I. Reports of repetitive penile-genital penetration often have no definitive evidence of penetration. *Pediatrics*. 2009;124(3):e403–e409 PMID: 19661051 https://doi.org/10.1542/peds.2008-3053
59. American Academy of Pediatrics Committee on Practice and Ambulatory Medicine. Use of chaperones during the physical examination of the pediatric patient. *Pediatrics*. 2011;127(5):991–993 PMID: 21518716 https://doi.org/10.1542/peds.2011-0322
60. Parker RI, Mahan RA, Giugliano D, Parker MM. Efficacy and safety of intravenous midazolam and ketamine as sedation for therapeutic and diagnostic procedures in

children [see comments]. *Pediatrics*. 1997;99(3):427–431 PMID: 9041300 https://doi.org/10.1542/peds.99.3.427
61. Finkel MA, Giardino A. *Medical Evaluation of Child Sexual Abuse: A Practical Guide*. Newbury Park, CA: Sage Publications; 2002:81–84
62. Adams JA, Ahmad M, Phillips P. Anogenital findings and hymenal diameter in children referred for sexual abuse examination. *Adolesc Pediatr Gynecol*. 1988;1(2):123–127 https://doi.org/10.1016/S0932-8610(88)80035-5
63. Bays J, Chewning M, Keltner L, Sewell R, Steinberg B, Thomas P. Changes in hymenal anatomy during examination of prepubertal girls for possible sexual abuse. *Adolesc Pediatr Gynecol*. 1990;3(1):42–46 https://doi.org/10.1016/S0932-8610(19)80057-9
64. Emans SJ, Goldstein DP. The gynecologic examination of the prepubertal child with vulvovaginitis: use of the knee-chest position. *Pediatrics*. 1980;65(4):758–760 PMID: 7367082
65. Herman-Giddens ME, Frothingham TE. Prepubertal female genitalia: examination for evidence of sexual abuse. *Pediatrics*. 1987;80(2):203–208 PMID: 3615090
66. McCann J, Wells R, Simon M, Voris J. Genital findings in prepubertal girls selected for nonabuse: a descriptive study. *Pediatrics*. 1990;86(3):428–439 PMID: 2388791
67. McCann J, Voris J. Perianal injuries resulting from sexual abuse: a longitudinal study. *Pediatrics*. 1993;91(2):390–397 PMID: 8424016
68. Paradise JE. The medical evaluation of the sexually abused child. *Pediatr Clin North Am*. 1990;37(4):839–862 PMID: 2199918 https://doi.org/10.1016/S0031-3955(16)36939-5
69. Davies J. Anatomy of the female genital tract. In: Danforth D, ed. *Danforth's Obstetrics and Gynecology*. 6th ed. Philadelphia, PA: Lippincott; 1990
70. Workowski KA, Bolan GA; Centers for Disease Control and Prevention. Sexually transmitted diseases treatment guidelines, 2015. *MMWR Recomm Rep*. 2015;64(RR-03): 1–137 PMID: 26042815
71. Ricci LR. Medical forensic photography of the sexually abused child. *Child Abuse Negl*. 1988;12(3):305–310 PMID: 3167620 https://doi.org/10.1016/0145-2134(88)90043-9
72. Ferris DG, Willner WA, Ho JJ. Colpophotography systems: a review [erratum in *J Fam Pract*. 1992;34:25]. *J Fam Pract*. 1991;33(6):633–639 PMID: 1744608
73. Gray H. *Anatomy of the Human Body*. Philadelphia, PA: Lea & Febiger; 1985
74. MacNaulty AS. *British Medical Dictionary*. Philadelphia, PA: Lippincott; 1961
75. Pritchard JA. Anatomy of the reproductive tract of woman. In: Cunningham FG, MacDonald C, Grant NC, eds. *Williams Obstetrics*. Norwalk, CT: Appleton-Century-Crofts; 1985
76. Sloane E. *Biology of Women*. New York, NY: Wiley and Sons; 1985
77. *Stedman's Medical Dictionary*. Baltimore, MD: Williams and Wilkins; 1990
78. White ST, Ingram DL, Lyna PR. Vaginal introital diameter in the evaluation of sexual abuse. *Child Abuse Negl*. 1989;13(2):217–224 PMID: 2743182 https://doi.org/10.1016/0145-2134(89)90008-2
79. Wile IS. The psychology of the hymen. *J Nerv Ment Dis*. 1937;85(2):143–156 https://doi.org/10.1097/00005053-193702000-00003
80. Berenson AB, Chacko MR, Wiemann CM, Mishaw CO, Friedrich WN, Grady JJ. A case-control study of anatomic changes resulting from sexual abuse. *Am J Obstet Gynecol*. 2000;182(4):820–834 PMID: 10764458 https://doi.org/10.1016/S0002-9378(00)70331-0
81. Jenny C, Kuhns ML, Arakawa F. Hymens in newborn female infants. *Pediatrics*. 1987;80(3):399–400 PMID: 3627892
82. Mahran M, Saleh AM. The microscopic anatomy of hymen. *Anat Rec*. 1964;149(2):313–318 PMID: 14173802 https://doi.org/10.1002/ar.1091490213

83. Gelhor G. Anatomy, pathology and development of the hymen. *Am J Obstet Dis Women Child*. 1904;50:161
84. Deuterman JL, Gabby SL. Imperforate hymen. *Ill Med J*. 1942;82:161
85. Mor N, Merlob P, Reisner SH. Tags and bands of the female external genitalia in the newborn infant. *Clin Pediatr (Phila)*. 1983;22(2):122–124 PMID: 6822016 https://doi.org/10.1177/000992288302200206
86. Berenson A, Heger A, Andrews S. Appearance of the hymen in newborns. *Pediatrics*. 1991;87(4):458–465 PMID: 2011421
87. Merlob P, Bahari C, Liban E, Reisner SH. Cysts of the female external genitalia in the newborn infant. *Am J Obstet Gynecol*. 1978;132(6):607–610 PMID: 568882 https://doi.org/10.1016/0002-9378(78)90851-7
88. Myhre AK, Berntzen K, Bratlid D. Genital anatomy in non-abused preschool girls. *Acta Paediatr*. 2003;92(12):1453–1462 PMID: 14971798 https://doi.org/10.1111/j.1651-2227.2003.tb00831.x
89. Goff CW, Burke KR, Rickenback C, Buebendorf DP. Vaginal opening measurement in prepubertal girls. *Am J Dis Child*. 1989;143(11):1366–1368 PMID: 2816868
90. Heger A, Emans SJ. Introital diameter as the criterion for sexual abuse [comment]. *Pediatrics*. 1990;85(2):222–223 PMID: 2296512
91. Paradise JE. Predictive accuracy and the diagnosis of sexual abuse: a big issue about a little tissue. *Child Abuse Negl*. 1989;13(2):169–176 PMID: 2663118 https://doi.org/10.1016/0145-2134(89)90003-3
92. Muram D. Child sexual abuse: relationship between sexual acts and genital findings. *Child Abuse Negl*. 1989;13(2):211–216 PMID: 2743181 https://doi.org/10.1016/0145-2134(89)90007-0
93. Bond GR, Dowd MD, Landsman I, Rimsza M. Unintentional perineal injury in prepubescent girls: a multicenter, prospective report of 56 girls. *Pediatrics*. 1995;95(5):628–631 PMID: 7724296
94. Kadish HA, Schunk JE, Britton H. Pediatric male rectal and genital trauma: accidental and nonaccidental injuries. *Pediatr Emerg Care*. 1998;14(2):95–98 PMID: 9583387 https://doi.org/10.1097/00006565-199804000-00002
95. Boos SC. Accidental hymenal injury mimicking sexual trauma. *Pediatrics*. 1999;103(6 Pt 1):1287–1290 PMID: 10353944 https://doi.org/10.1542/peds.103.6.1287
96. Emans SJ, Woods ER, Allred EN, Grace E. Hymenal findings in adolescent women: impact of tampon use and consensual sexual activity. *J Pediatr*. 1994;125(1):153–160 PMID: 8021768 https://doi.org/10.1016/S0022-3476(94)70144-X
97. Muram D. Anal and perianal abnormalities in prepubertal victims of sexual abuse. *Am J Obstet Gynecol*. 1989;161(2):278–281 PMID: 2764045 https://doi.org/10.1016/0002-9378(89)90498-5
98. Clayden GS. Reflex anal dilatation associated with severe chronic constipation in children [see comments]. *Arch Dis Child*. 1988;63(7):832–836 PMID: 3415302 https://doi.org/10.1136/adc.63.7.832
99. Hobbs CJ, Wynne JM. Sexual abuse of English boys and girls: the importance of anal examination. *Child Abuse Negl*. 1989;13(2):195–210 PMID: 2743180 https://doi.org/10.1016/0145-2134(89)90006-9
100. Stanton A, Sunderland R. Prevalence of reflex anal dilatation in 200 children [see comments]. *BMJ*. 1989;298(6676):802–803 PMID: 2496861 https://doi.org/10.1136/bmj.298.6676.802
101. Paul DM. The medical examination in sexual offences against children. *Med Sci Law*. 1977;17(4):251–258 PMID: 927088 https://doi.org/10.1177/002580247701700406

102. Biggs M, Stermac LE, Divinsky M. Genital injuries following sexual assault of women with and without prior sexual intercourse experience. *CMAJ*. 1998;159(1):33–37 PMID: 9679484
103. Norvell MK, Benrubi GI, Thompson RJ. Investigation of microtrauma after sexual intercourse. *J Reprod Med*. 1984;29(4):269–271 PMID: 6716372
104. DeLago C, Deblinger E, Schroeder C, Finkel MA. Girls who disclose sexual abuse: urogenital symptoms and signs after genital contact. *Pediatrics*. 2008;122(2):e281–e286 PMID: 18676513 https://doi.org/10.1542/peds.2008-0450
105. Berkowitz CD, Elvik SL, Logan M. A simulated "acquired" imperforate hymen following the genital trauma of sexual abuse. *Clin Pediatr (Phila)*. 1987;26(6):307–309 PMID: 3581642 https://doi.org/10.1177/000992288702600609
106. Macklin M. "Honeymoon cystitis" [letter]. *N Engl J Med*. 1978;298(18):1035 PMID: 643003 https://doi.org/10.1056/NEJM197805042981826
107. Paul DM. "What really did happen to Baby Jane?"—the medical aspects of the investigation of alleged sexual abuse of children. *Med Sci Law*. 1986;26(2):85–102 PMID: 3724400 https://doi.org/10.1177/002580248602600203
108. Dowd MD, Fitzmaurice L, Knapp JF, Mooney D. The interpretation of urogenital findings in children with straddle injuries. *J Pediatr Surg*. 1994;29(1):7–10 PMID: 8120766 https://doi.org/10.1016/0022-3468(94)90513-4
109. Waltzman ML, Shannon M, Bowen AP, Bailey MC. Monkeybar injuries: complications of play. *Pediatrics*. 1999;103(5):e58 PMID: 10224202 https://doi.org/10.1542/peds.103.5.e58
110. Baker RB. Seat belt injury masquerading as sexual abuse [letter]. *Pediatrics*. 1986;77(3):435 PMID:3951927 https://doi.org/10.1542/peds.2011-1430
111. Berkowitz CD. Sexual abuse of children and adolescents. *Adv Pediatr*. 1987;34:275–312 PMID: 3318298
112. Berkowitz CD, Elvik SL, Logan MK. Labial fusion in prepubescent girls: a marker for sexual abuse? *Am J Obstet Gynecol*. 1987;156(1):16–20 PMID: 3026184 https://doi.org/10.1016/0002-9378(87)90195-5
113. McCann J, Voris J, Simon M. Labial adhesions and posterior fourchette injuries in childhood sexual abuse. *Am J Dis Child*. 1988;142(6):659–663 PMID: 3369406 https://doi.org/10.1001/archpedi.1988.02150060093040
114. Brew-Graves E, Morgan L. Injuries and allegations of oral rape: a retrospective review of patients presenting to a London sexual assault referral centre. *J Forensic Leg Med*. 2015;34:155–158 PMID: 26165676 https://doi.org/10.1016/j.jflm.2015.06.004
115. Smith TD, Raman SR, Madigan S, Waldman J, Shouldice M. Anogenital findings in 3569 pediatric examinations for sexual abuse/assault. *J Pediatr Adolesc Gynecol*. 2018;31(2): 79–83 PMID: 29111300 https://doi.org/10.1016/j.jpag.2017.10.006
116. Finkel MA. Anogenital trauma in sexually abused children. *Pediatrics*. 1989;84(2):317–322 PMID: 2748261
117. Kissane JM, ed. Inflammation and healing. In: Kissane JM, ed. *Anderson's Pathology*. 8th ed. St Louis, MO: CV Mosby; 1985
118. Emans SJ, Woods ER, Flagg NT, Freeman A. Genital findings in sexually abused, symptomatic and asymptomatic, girls. *Pediatrics*. 1987;79(5):778–785 PMID: 3575037
119. Lauber AA, Souma ML. Use of toluidine blue for documentation of traumatic intercourse. *Obstet Gynecol*. 1982;60(5):644–648 PMID: 7145256
120. McCann J. The appearance of acute, healing, and healed anogenital trauma. *Child Abuse Negl*. 1998;22(6):605–615 PMID: 9649900 https://doi.org/10.1016/S0145-2134(98)00035-0
121. McCann J, Voris J, Simon M. Genital injuries resulting from sexual abuse: a longitudinal study. *Pediatrics*. 1992;89(2):307–317 PMID: 1734401

122. Heppenstall-Heger A, McConnell G, Ticson L, Guerra L, Lister J, Zaragoza T. Healing patterns in anogenital injuries: a longitudinal study of injuries associated with sexual abuse, accidental injuries, or genital surgery in the preadolescent child. *Pediatrics*. 2003;112(4):829–837 PMID: 14523174 https://doi.org/10.1542/peds.112.4.829
123. Dube SR, Felitti VJ, Dong M, Giles WH, Anda RF. The impact of adverse childhood experiences on health problems: evidence from four birth cohorts dating back to 1900. *Prev Med*. 2003;37(3):268–277 PMID: 12914833 https://doi.org/10.1016/S0091-7435(03)00123-3
124. Felitti VJ, Anda RF, Nordenberg D, et al. Relationship of childhood abuse and household dysfunction to many of the leading causes of death in adults. The Adverse Childhood Experiences (ACE) Study. *Am J Prev Med*. 1998;14(4):245–258 PMID: 9635069 https://doi.org/10.1016/S0749-3797(98)00017-8
125. Boudewyn AC, Liem JH. Childhood sexual abuse as a precursor to depression and self-destructive behavior in adulthood. *J Trauma Stress*. 1995;8(3):445–459 PMID: 7582609 https://doi.org/10.1002/jts.2490080307
126. Brown LK, Kessel SM, Lourie KJ, Ford HH, Lipsitt LP. Influence of sexual abuse on HIV-related attitudes and behaviors in adolescent psychiatric inpatients. *J Am Acad Child Adolesc Psychiatry*. 1997;36(3):316–322 PMID: 9055511 https://doi.org/10.1097/00004583-199703000-00009
127. Wolfe DA, Sas L, Wekerle C. Factors associated with the development of posttraumatic stress disorder among child victims of sexual abuse. *Child Abuse Negl*. 1994;18(1):37–50 PMID: 8124597 https://doi.org/10.1016/0145-2134(94)90094-9
128. National Child Traumatic Stress Network. Trauma treatments. https://www.nctsn.org/treatments-and-practices/trauma-treatments. Accessed January 18, 2019

CHAPTER 11

Medical Management of the Adolescent Who Has Experienced Sexual Abuse or Assault

Sarah A. W. Northrop, MD, FAAP
Department of Pediatrics
Brenner Children's Hospital
Assistant Professor of Pediatrics
Wake Forest School of Medicine
Wake Forest Baptist Health
Winston-Salem, NC

Shalon M. Nienow, MD, FAAP
Medical Clinic Director
Chadwick Center for Children and Families
Rady Children's Hospital—San Diego
Clinical Assistant Professor
Division of Pediatric Emergency Medicine
University of California San Diego
San Diego, CA

Epidemiology of Sexual Abuse and Assault of Adolescents

Sexual abuse definitions vary based on discipline, locality, and legal system employed. The United Nations Children's Fund (UNICEF) describes *child sexual abuse* as "engaging in sexual activities with a child who, according to the relevant provisions of national law, has not reached the legal age for sexual activities; engaging in sexual activities with a child where: use is made of coercion, force or threats; or abuse is made of a recognized position of trust, authority or influence over the child, including within the family; or abuse is made of a particularly vulnerable situation of the child, notably because of a mental or physical disability or a situation of dependence."[1] Child sexual abuse may include contact (eg, fondling, anal/genital penetration, forced oral sex) and noncontact (eg, exhibitionism, voyeurism, exposure to child sexual abuse materials, sexting) acts. It may also include elements of child exploitation such as commercial sexual exploitation.[2] Adolescents may initially experience abuse and assault during their teen years, or they may have experienced long-standing abuse initiated prior to puberty.[3] Many adolescents who were previously sexually abused may still be experiencing the adverse effects of such trauma, even if it has since discontinued.

The prevalence of sexual abuse among adolescents is difficult to assess with accuracy. It is well recognized that many who experience sexual abuse during childhood do not disclose for many years, and often not until adulthood, if they disclose at all.[3,4] True prevalence data would only be possible if all those who experienced sexual abuse could be identified, making underreporting a significant sampling concern. The available data are widely variable, with lifetime prevalence estimates of abuse ranging from 1% to 62%.[5,6] This large disparity is likely related to differences in definitions of what constitutes abuse, the populations assessed, and the techniques employed by studies attempting to obtain such data. Additionally, many studies consist of retrospective accounts of adults, which rely on participant reports of abuse that occurred during childhood. This raises concerns for the accuracy of data that rely heavily on memory of events that occurred many years prior. Among the studies that are available, there is a paucity of information from which the prevalence of abuse occurring specifically during adolescence can be determined. One study conducted among schoolchildren in grades 7 through 12 reported that 1% of the participants were experiencing ongoing abuse.[7] However, this information fails to account for past abuse that may have taken place during the teen years and may represent a significant underestimation of occurrence. Two additional studies report much higher rates. The first, a national telephone survey of US adults, found that 46% of males who had experienced sexual abuse were 11 years or older when the abuse occurred, as were 42% of females who had experienced sexual abuse.[8] The second involved a birth cohort study of New Zealand residents interviewed when they were 18 years old. This research reported that 57% of sexual abuse incidents described occurred when the individual was between the ages of 11 and 16 years.[9] This shows that although the data are sparse, the number of adolescents at risk for sexual abuse is significant.

Teens may experience not just child sexual abuse (acts perpetrated by a person with whom a child cannot otherwise legally consent) but also sexual assault. As defined by the US Department of Justice, *sexual assault* is “any type of sexual contact or behavior that occurs without the explicit consent of the recipient.”[10] This comprises acts such as forced intercourse, forced sodomy, and attempted rape. This also includes when someone is asleep, unconscious, or unable to consent due to impairment from alcohol or drugs. Adolescents are at much greater risk than prepubertal children of experiencing sexual assault in general, especially those committed by a peer or acquaintance[11]; however, the prevalence of sexual assault among adolescents has been studied much less frequently than that of sexual abuse, and primarily in females. Many studies that do report rates of sexual assault in this age group often do so in conjunction with adults.[12,13] Others focus specifically on dating violence.[14] Thus, the findings of these studies likely are an underrepresentation of the actual prevalence of sexual assault among all teens. The few available data report prevalence rates of sexual assault ranging from 3% to 16% in females and from 2% to 3% in males.[14–17] The National Women's Study found that the largest proportion of reported rapes occurred in women between the ages of 11 and 17 years, comprising 32.3% of the sample.[18]

For medical professionals to adequately determine whether sexual abuse has occurred, it is imperative that they understand the consent laws in the locality in which they practice. Age of consent varies by state and is a number designated at or above which a person has the legal capacity to consent to sexual activity. Most states set the legal age of consent between 16 and 18 years. More than 50% of states designate a minimum age below which no one can give legal consent and above which age parameters are provided for the participants. Such close in age exemptions, also known as Romeo and Juliet laws, serve to decriminalize sexual activity between partners who are both below the age of consent or who are within several years of each other in age. A large number of localities also make designations regarding persons in a position of authority, such as coaches, schoolteachers, and parents, to whom consent cannot be given until the age of 18 years.[19] Medical professionals need to familiarize themselves with the consent laws as well as be aware of the mandated reporting laws. These also vary by locality and may affect whether a patient who has experienced sexual assault has the ability to voluntarily withhold reporting to a law enforcement entity.

Risk Factors

Risk factors for the sexual abuse of adolescents, in particular, have not been clearly delineated in the literature but are likely the same as those for all those who experience sexual abuse during childhood. Although sexual abuse occurs across all ethnicities and socioeconomic statuses, several elements have been identified that increase the risk to children. Those include female gender, presence of disabilities, absence of one or both parents, presence of other forms of abuse in the household, and presence of domestic violence and/or substance abuse by caregivers.[20] The most specific risk factor in this population is age. Prior studies have revealed that older age presents an independent risk of sexual abuse, with vulnerability dramatically increasing at age 10 years.[21] Furthermore, there is an anecdotal observation that sexual abuse is often a multigenerational phenomenon within families; however, data to determine the actual rates of such cyclical abuse are lacking. There are multiple theories about why this occurs, including differences in maternal parenting style.[22]

Risk factors for the occurrence of sexual assault have been studied almost exclusively in females. This research has shown that the most consistently identified risk factor is previous childhood abuse, especially sexual abuse.[23,24] Other risk factors include early initiation of sexual activity, multiple sexual partners, and substance use[25,26]; all such behaviors are also found more frequently in those with prior experience of childhood sexual abuse.[23,27,28] Furthermore, teens who have previously experienced sexual assault are more likely to experience subsequent assault events.[24,29,30] Lesbian, gay, bisexual, transgender, and queer/questioning youth have also been shown to be at increased risk for sexual violence and for commercial sexual exploitation (sex trafficking).[31] This may be related to the higher rates of runaway and throwaway issues in this population, which lead to survival sex behaviors.[32] Please refer to Chapter 22, Human Trafficking and Sexual Exploitation via Electronic Media, for a more detailed discussion of this problem.

Data on sexual assault in male teens are lacking because it is likely underreported and understudied. Research suggests that there are many similarities in the risk factors between male and female adolescents who have experienced sexual assault and that the perpetrators of adolescent sexual assault are overwhelmingly male no matter the gender or sexual identity of the person who experiences the assault.[33]

Clinical Presentation

Adolescents who experience sexual abuse or assault may present to the medical professional in several different ways. It is important for medical professionals who work with teen patients to understand that many who have experienced these events will not spontaneously disclose; in fact, they may never have disclosed their sexual abuse or assault to anyone else prior to the health care visit. Often, adolescents will not disclose past sexual abuse or assault because of fears of how disclosure will affect family members or because they may view themselves as partially responsible for the abuse.[34] In most cases of long-standing abuse, overt violence on the part of the perpetrator is absent and patients are progressively "groomed" with a gradual escalation of the intrusiveness of the events. Once patients recognize what has been happening to them, their initial lack of disclosure serves to inhibit current and future opportunities for admission due to feelings of self-blame or fear of not being believed. They may also have feelings of love or dependence toward the perpetrator, further hindering their ability or willingness to make disclosures.[35] Other adolescents do not report their experiences because they do not view the acts as abuse or assault; they may see themselves as willing participants even if they cannot legally provide consent or if violence is involved. This is especially true in acts of intimate partner violence, peer sexual assault, and commercial sexual exploitation (see Chapter 22, Human Trafficking and Sexual Exploitation via Electronic Media).[19]

Given the myriad impediments to disclosure of sexual violence, it is imperative that medical professionals perform routine screening with their adolescent patients. This should be done at every access point in the health system. Box 11.1 provides questions that can be used for screening teen patients. It is essential that medical professionals conduct questioning in a supportive and nonjudgmental fashion. It is also important for screening to be done outside of the presence of any parent or caregiver who may have accompanied the patient to his or her appointment. Assuring teens that the goal of questioning is to ensure overall health and safety can aid in eliciting truthful responses. Screening questions should be asked following discussions of more general health care topics to increase the adolescent's comfort with the health care appointment.

Teens may present emergently to the health care setting with signs and symptoms of a physical assault, acute alcohol or drug intoxication, emotional sequelae of abuse such as self-harm behaviors or suicidality, or consequences of sexual activity such as pregnancy, miscarriage, or sexually transmitted infections (STIs). It is important that medical professionals recognize these manifestations as harbingers of potential abuse and that they screen for it as appropriate.

If patients present to the health care visit with verbalized sexual abuse concerns, they may do so to seek sexual assault nurse examiner services or a "rape kit" following an acute sexual assault, or with a trusted adult who brings them for care following a delayed report. In these cases, the medical professional will need to determine when the last contact occurred. If the teen reports that the last sexual abuse or assault event has taken place within the preceding 4 to 7 days (depending on jurisdiction),[36] DNA forensic evidence collection is warranted. These evaluations are usually conducted in a hospital setting or at a specialized clinic. Medical professionals should familiarize themselves with the resources available for evidence collection in their communities. The patient should be assisted in setting up an appointment for the forensic examination and transportation should be provided or ensured. If patients are being seen after the window for evidence collection, referral to specialized sexual abuse services should be made. This evaluation can take place at any point following the abusive events, regardless of how far removed in time.[37]

Medical professionals also need to ascertain whether the abusive event has previously been reported to investigative entities. If not, a determination of whether the abuse requires a mandated report is essential. Medical professionals should be honest with patients about their duty to report so that adolescents do not feel that there has been a breach of trust if a report must be made. All states require reporting of abuse or assault by persons in a position of authority (eg, teachers, coaches, clergy, counselors, medical professionals). In contrast, most do not require a report if a similar-aged peer commits the assault, if the child is above a certain age. Statutory rape mandates are highly variable.

BOX 11.1
Example of Screening Questions for Sexual Abuse and Sexual Assault Experiences

- Has anyone, male or female, ever tried or succeeded in touching you in a sexual way or having any kind of sexual contact with you that you did not want?
- Have you ever had a sexual experience with someone older or someone who had authority over you, such as a doctor, teacher, minister, therapist, babysitter, or any other older person?
- Have you ever had sexual contact with a relative, such as an uncle, brother, father, grandfather, mother, stepparent, or sister?
- Have you ever had any kind of sexual contact with someone that you did not want because you were asleep, unconscious, or "out of it," such as from using alcohol or drugs?
- Have you ever had someone threaten to hurt you or actually use physical force to make you have any kind of sexual contact with them?
- Have you had any other upsetting sexual experiences that you haven't mentioned yet?

Evaluation of the Adolescent Patient With Experiences of Sexual Abuse or Assault

If patients acknowledge the experience of sexual abuse or assault, additional information should be gathered. Box 11.2 lists follow-up questions that can be asked. A thorough assessment of consensual sexual experiences, menstrual history, and contraceptive use should be done. In addition, medical professionals should inquire about physical and mental health sequelae of abusive experiences. Ongoing safety threats should be addressed immediately. It is imperative that each adolescent be referred for specialized sexual abuse services after all acute medical needs are addressed.

In the case in which a patient presents after an acute sexual assault or concerns of a sexual assault following alcohol or drug toxicity, it is imperative to remember that persons who are under the influence cannot

BOX 11.2
Types of Questions to Be Asked of an Adolescent Patient Who Has a Positive Screening Result for an Experience of Sexual Abuse or Assault

- How many times have you had this type of unwanted sexual contact? Was it only once or more than one time?
- When was the first time this happened? When was the last time?
- Who was the person who did this to you?
- What did the person do to you? Did he or she touch your private parts or other parts of your body? Did he or she put anything in your mouth? Your vagina? Your butt?
- Did he put his penis in your mouth? Your vagina? Your butt?
- Did he or she do anything to make you have sexual contact with him or her? Offer you something if you agreed? Threaten to hurt you or someone you loved? Force you by holding you down or hitting or slapping you?
- Were you drinking alcohol or using any other drugs when this happened?
- Has this person hurt you in any other way, such as slapping you or punching you?
- After this experience, did you have any pain or other physical symptoms?
- Does any other person hurt you in any way?
- Have you told anyone else about this experience?
- Have the police or child protective services been told about this experience?

appropriately consent to a sexual assault examination and that the DNA evidence collection must be withheld until the adolescent is able to give consent. It is also imperative to remember that medical care always takes precedence over DNA forensic evidence collection. Medical care should never be delayed or withheld in favor of evidence collection.

Examination of the Adolescent Who Has Experienced Sexual Abuse or Assault

Examinations of an adolescent who has experienced sexual abuse or assault should be done by persons trained for and comfortable with doing them. They should be undertaken in a sensitive and trauma-informed fashion providing for as much patient autonomy as possible. Patients should never be forced to undergo an examination that they do not want and should be made aware that they can withdraw consent at any time. Those who have experienced abuse and assault often fear that they are permanently injured or scarred, which can lead to significant anxiety prior to and during the examination. Medical professionals should allow the patient to visualize the examination to the best of their ability and should be comfortable addressing concerns about injury, being sure to emphasize normal findings or complete healing as able. A medical chaperone, such as a nurse or certified medical assistant, should always be a part of the genital examination in acute and non-acute settings.

The Acute Sexual Assault Examination

An acute examination is performed within 72 to 168 hours from the last event, as per jurisdictional mandates. The primary focus of this examination is to assess for potential injury, test for and provide prophylactic treatment of STIs and pregnancy, and obtain any available forensic evidence while maintaining chain of custody.[38] An emergent evaluation may also be performed outside of the time frames listed if there are current medical or safety concerns that may be related to the sexual abuse or assault. These include, but are not limited to, pain, bleeding, discharge, suicidal ideation, self-harm behaviors, alcohol or drug intoxication, and/or exploitation. Acute sexual assault examinations are most commonly performed in emergency departments but may also be offered in child advocacy centers, mobile health clinics, college or university student health centers, local health departments, or other community centers. These examinations may be performed by medical professionals with experience with child abuse, sexual assault nurse examiners, or emergency medicine physicians who have completed extra training and who can maintain appropriate chain of custody for forensic evidence.[39] All evaluations include a medical interview and a thorough head-to-toe physical, which includes a focused anogenital examination. A cervical evaluation is not an essential component of a female sexual assault examination unless there is need to determine where bleeding is originating from, so use of a speculum is not always indicated.

It is the standard of care for examinations to be photodocumented using appropriate lighting and magnification.[40,41] This includes taking pictures of any extragenital injuries that may be present as well as anogenital findings both normal and potentially indicative of trauma. Photodocumentation is necessary because it allows for detailed review of physical examination findings without prolonging the examination itself, thereby reducing patient discomfort and anxiety. It also provides a comparison for the follow-up examination so that medical professionals can assess for healing of any acute injury. Furthermore, it allows for ongoing peer review of examination technique and evaluation. Finally, photodocumentation can be an important educational tool for future court proceedings, especially in cases where injury is present.[40,41]

The medical interview is an essential part of any sexual assault evaluation. This should come before any physical examination. For this portion of the assessment, the adolescent patient should be questioned in private using sensitive and open-ended queries whenever possible (see Chapter 9, Taking Forensically Sound Histories in Cases of Alleged Sexual Abuse). The main goal of the interview is to assess the types of contact that occurred to focus evidence collection; for example, documentation of and swabbing of oral to skin contact, or sites where ejaculate was deposited, that might not be readily apparent on visual examination. Statements made by the patient should be documented verbatim in the medical record. It is imperative that medical professionals record exact wording provided by the adolescent, and not their interpretation of statements made. Care should be taken before the examination has started, preferably while the adolescent is still clothed, to fully explain what will happen during the examination and to give the patient the opportunity to ask questions. Establishing a caring, trusting rapport with patients will not only help facilitate disclosure but will also make the examination easier for the medical professional and the patient.

It is important for the medical professional to be familiar with the rape kit and the examination equipment prior to starting the examination.[38] Specimens should be collected according to the rape kit manufacturer's recommendations and in accordance with the type of assault disclosed in the patient's interview. Some adolescents are embarrassed and do not want anyone with them during the examination. Other patients would prefer a support person present. Either scenario is acceptable provided it is in accordance with the patient's wishes. The alleged perpetrator should never be present during any portion of the evaluation. Nonbelieving, non-offending caregivers should also have limited access during the evaluation so as not to influence the patient's disclosure.

Testing for STIs and pregnancy and attainment of swabs for forensic evidence are performed as part of an acute examination. It is important to note that while an acute examination for sexual assault integrates forensic and medical components, the forensic evidence is not part of the medical record, and the medical examination and stabilization of the patient should take precedence over any forensic component. Patients who present for evaluation outside of the window for DNA evidence collection may still benefit from testing and/or treatment of STIs. Sexually transmitted infection testing should include pharyngeal swabs, genital swabs or urine collection, and anal swabs regardless of the types of acts described because disclosure is often not a singular event but a process over time, and not all types of contact are readily described at initial reporting (see Chapter 12, Sexually Transmitted Infections in Child Sexual Abuse).[42]

The Non-acute Examination

Non-acute examinations for sexual abuse or assault can occur at any point following the abusive acts, regardless of the time delay; research supports that most who experience sexual abuse delay disclosure for weeks, months, or years.[43] The delayed examination should be coordinated with a multidisciplinary team so that it is completed following a forensic interview. If there is not an ongoing legal investigation, the assessment can be an isolated comprehensive medical evaluation performed by a trained medical professional.[40] Regardless, identification of physical symptoms that may be related to sexual abuse or psychological consequences of sexual abuse or assault should be addressed.

A non-acute examination is very similar to an acute examination but does not include collection of forensic evidence. A genital examination is performed using a variety of positioning techniques to examine the anogenital structures (please refer to Chapter 10, Medical Evaluation of Suspected Sexual Abuse in Prepubertal Children, for more detailed explanations of examination techniques). Positioning techniques including labial separation and labial traction are often sufficient to fully examine the female genitalia. If healed hymenal injury is found or suspected, a second technique must be employed to confirm this finding. This can be accomplished by use of the prone knee-chest position or with cotton swabs or Foley catheters. Photodocumentation is also important in the non-acute setting for the same reasons as in the acute examination.[40] Sexually transmitted infection testing should also be obtained and should include oral swabs, anal swabs, and genital swabs or urine collection for gonorrhea, chlamydia, and trichomonas, as well as blood testing for HIV, syphilis, and hepatitis.

As in the acute examination, a non-acute examination should incorporate therapeutic components. The adolescent should be actively involved in the evaluation and must consent to the examination. The patient can refuse any or all parts of the examination at any time. The examiner should explain the nature of examination and what they are doing and why during each individual aspect. The overwhelming majority of these examinations do not find injury or evidence of older injury, regardless of the types of sexual acts involved; therefore, examination rooms that allow for the patient and the examiner to simultaneously view images can be very therapeutic to patients who fear that they are somehow marked, scarred, or different. Additionally, for many patients, visualization of the examination provides an element of control. However, if the patient does not wish to watch, care should be taken so that the patient does not have to visualize the images. Different patients will have different needs following sexual abuse or assault; discussing the examination and honoring the wishes of the individual patient can help make the assessment less intrusive and more therapeutic.

Specific physical or mental health concerns related to the abuse should be assessed during the history, including depression, self-harm, anger, suicidality, and somatic symptoms such as difficulty sleeping, headaches, and stomachaches. Many patients who have experienced sexual abuse or assault have varying degrees of self-blame regarding the events, and not every patient will have a supportive or protective caregiver.[44] The medical history is an ideal time to address these concerns and to emphasize the importance of counseling, specifically trauma-focused cognitive behavioral therapy, or other evidence-based modality, in recovery.[45]

Documentation

The medical professional should take careful notes when speaking to the patient about the sexual abuse or assault, documenting the adolescent's history in detail. Notations of any injuries, their exact location and nature, and the patient's explanation for how they occurred should also be made, preferably on a body map. The examiner should also photodocument any nongenital injuries present that may be related to the abuse or assault.

Medical professionals should be careful in the language used when discussing and/or documenting the adolescent's abuse. Words that suggest the history is in doubt, such as "alleges" or "claims," should be avoided. Instead, matter-of-fact, objective language should be used, such as, "Patient reports that her boyfriend forced her to have vaginal intercourse 2 weeks ago." Statements about the perceived truthfulness of the patient's report should also be avoided. The medical professional should not assume that an absence of an emotional response when discussing the abuse or assault suggests that the assault did not occur. Similarly, the presence of delinquent or other problem behaviors by an adolescent does not negate the possibility that he or she experienced sexual abuse or assault. Indeed, these behaviors often are a response to sexual abuse or assault.[46]

Pathophysiology

As previously noted, the most frequent physical examination finding in children who have been sexually abused or assaulted is normal anogenital anatomy. However, there are times when injuries can be seen. This is most likely in cases of acute assault, in which violence is a factor.

Following are illustrations of some possible physical examination findings in acute and non-acute sexual abuse or assault. The most common findings of sexual assault are nongenital injuries.[47] These include bruises, suction hematomas or hickeys, superficial abrasions, grab marks, and slap marks. However, many adolescents who have experienced sexual assault have no physical findings of injury, and it is important to remember that a lack of physical examination findings, genital or nongenital, does not rule out sexual or physical assault.[48,49]

Nongenital Findings

Suction hematomas (Figure 11.1), frequently referred to as hickeys, designate places on the body in which traction on the skin, applied by a mouth, leaves petechial bruising.

Bite marks may be seen in cases of sexual abuse or assault. They can often be seen in conjunction with suction hematomas or with central ecchymosis, which is the result of crush trauma.

Palatal petechiae (Figure 11.2) can be found in penile-oral contact in which the perpetrator's penis forcibly strikes the palate, causing injury. It is important to distinguish this from other causes such as forceful vomiting, streptococcal pharyngitis, and paroxysmal coughing.

Forceful hand grabs can cause *grab marks,* or bruising found on various parts of the body.

Slap marks are petechial bruising that is the result of high velocity impact by a hand. Such marks often appear as an outline of the hand or as parallel linear bruises.

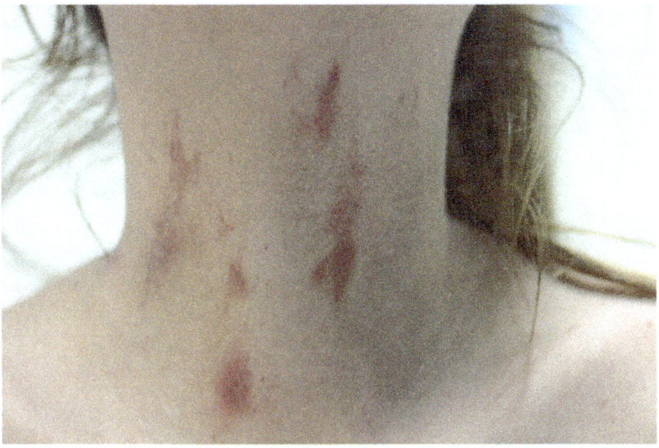

FIGURE 11.1
Suction hematomas.

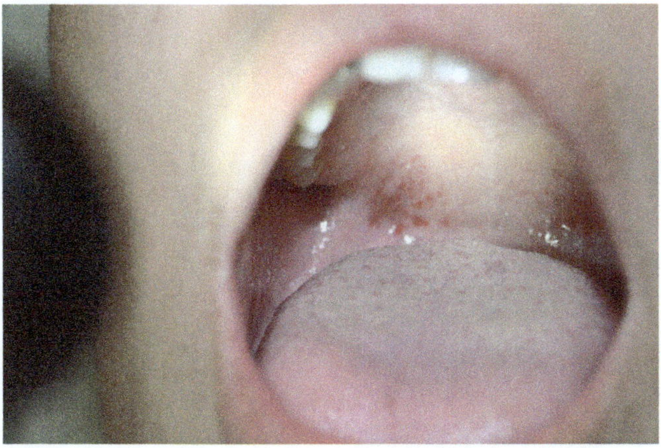

FIGURE 11.2
Palatal petechiae.

Strangulation injury (Figure 11.3) is caused by traction on the skin. Periorbital and postauricular cluster of petechiae, as well as scattered petechiae on the face or neck above the level of compression, may be seen.

Ligature marks (Figure 11.4) are an injury caused by an object being placed tightly around a body part. They may consist merely of bruising or of a combination of bruising, abrasion, and/or laceration.

Tagging is a form of graffiti in which a perpetrator signs his or her name anonymously. It is prevalent in gang culture.

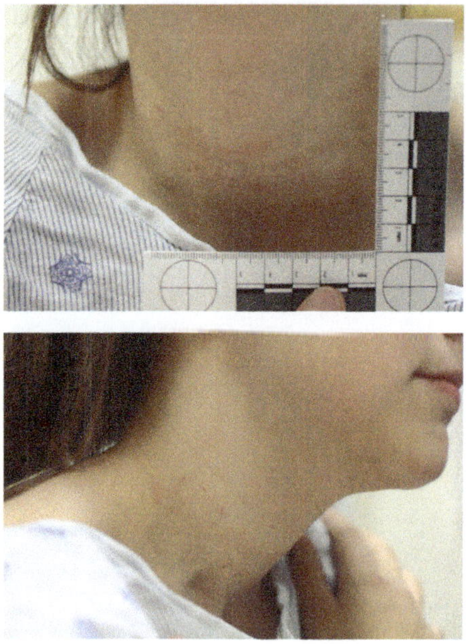

FIGURE 11.3
Strangulation injury.

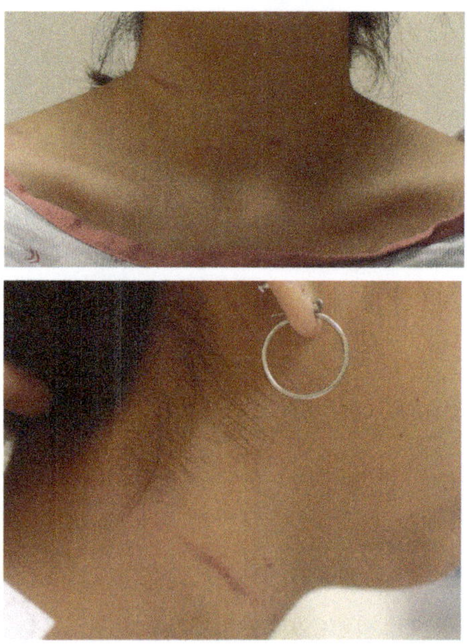

FIGURE 11.4
Ligature marks may appear similar to strangulation injury.

Tattoos or brands (Figure 11.5) are a permanent ink or body disfigurement used frequently in child commercial sexual exploitation for perpetrators to mark their "product."

Genital Injuries

Acute genital injuries include bruising (Figure 11.6), tears (Figure 11.7), and bleeding of various extragenital and intra-genital structures. Non-acute genital injuries include healed hymenal transection (Figure 11.8) and scarring of the genital structures.

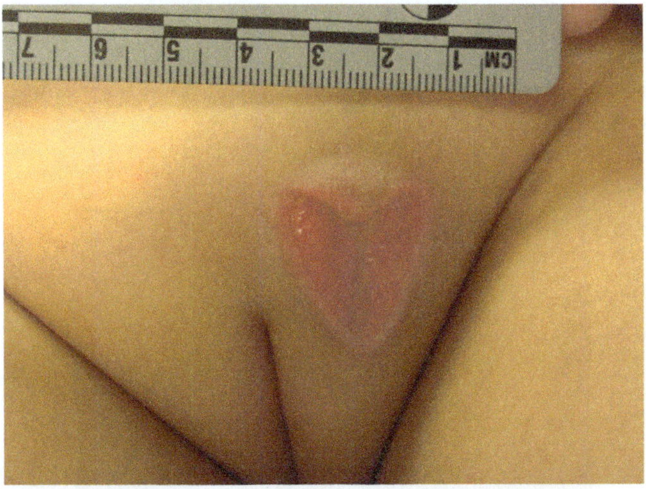

FIGURE 11.5
Example of branding, often used in human trafficking.

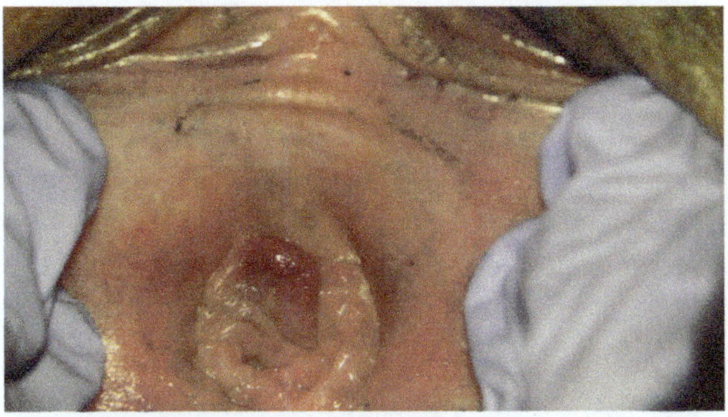

FIGURE 11.6
Bruising of the hymen and vestibule.

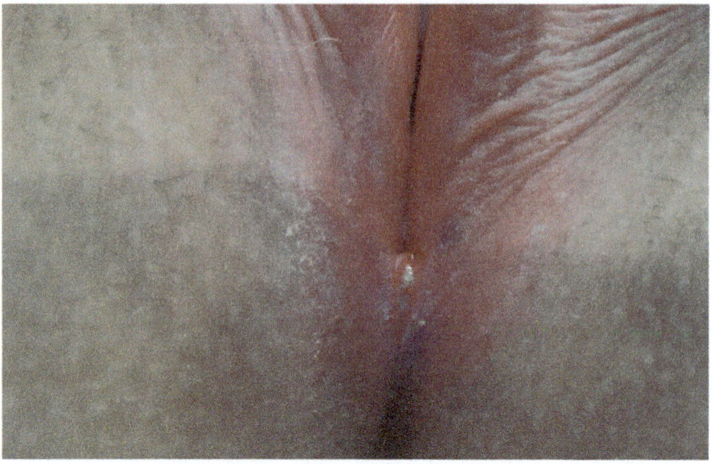

FIGURE 11.7
Perineal tearing and bruising.

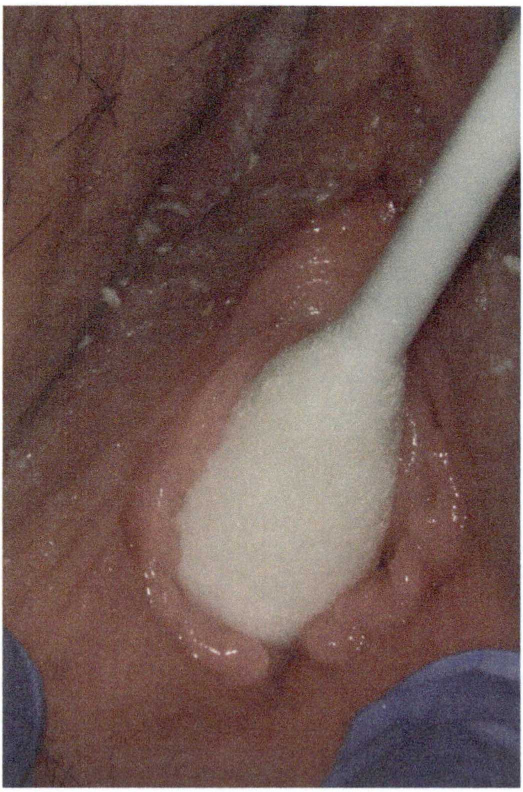

FIGURE 11 .8
Healed hymenal transection.

Anal Injuries

Acute anal injuries include bruising, laceration (Figure 11.9), and bleeding. Non-acute signs may include healing injuries (Figure 11.10) and scarring.

Sexually Transmitted Infections

Chlamydia (Figure 11.11) and/or gonorrhea infection may be found in youth who have been sexually abused or assaulted, as can *Trichomonas* (Figure 11.12), HIV, or syphilis. Coinfection with multiple pathogens is not uncommon in cases of abuse or assault, and comprehensive testing should be completed (see Chapter 12, Sexually Transmitted Infections in Child Sexual Abuse).

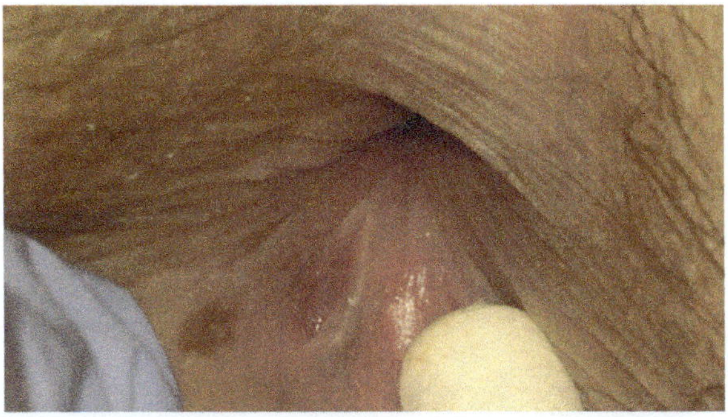

FIGURE 11.9
Acute anal laceration.

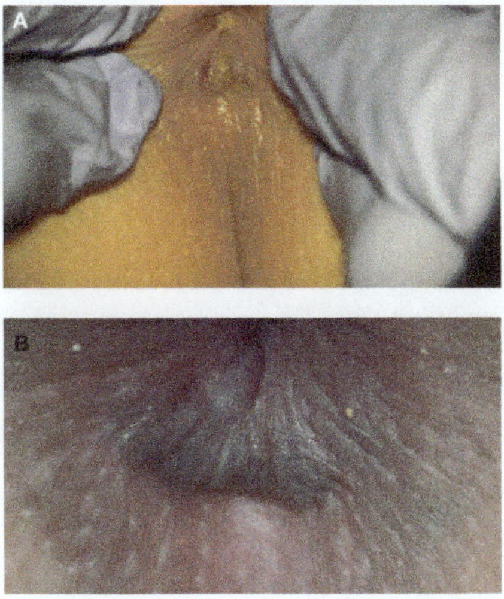

FIGURE 11.10
Healing anal laceration. A, The same patient as in Figure 11.9; B, a different patient.

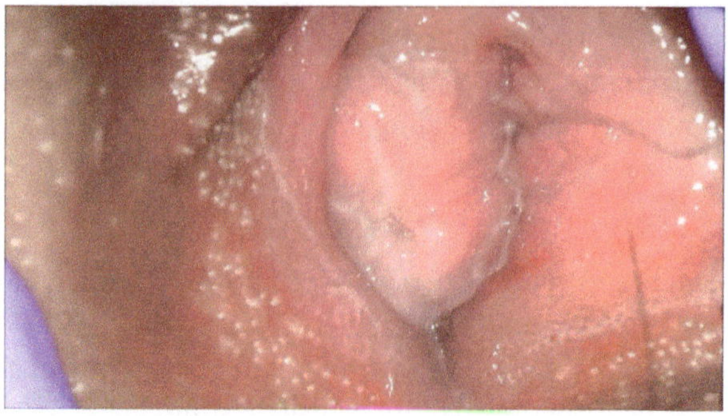

FIGURE 11.11
Chlamydia trachomatis infection.

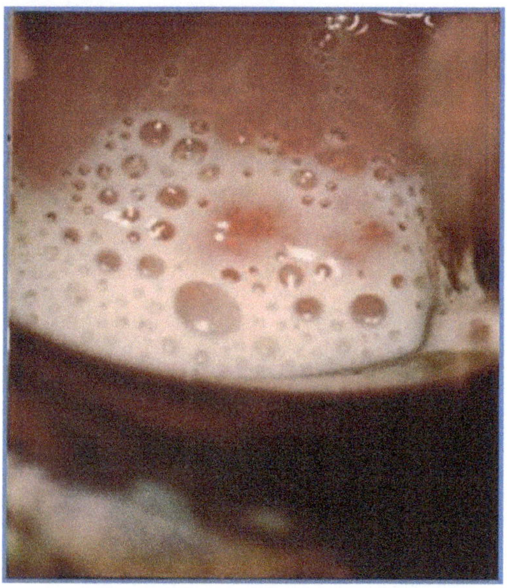

FIGURE 11.12
Trichomonas vaginalis infection. From Nienow SM, Burrell T, Phillips J. Findings in sexual abuse. In: Anderst JD, ed. *Visual Diagnosis of Child Abuse*. 4th ed. Elk Grove Village, IL: American Academy of Pediatrics; 2016.

Possibly Sexually Transmitted Infections

Anogenital Herpes Simplex Virus

Although historically genital herpes was thought to indicate sexual contact, there are nonsexual means of transmission, including autoinoculation and hand-genital transmission in persons with herpetic whitlow. In the absence of a sexual abuse disclosure, this is a nonspecific finding (Figure 11.13).

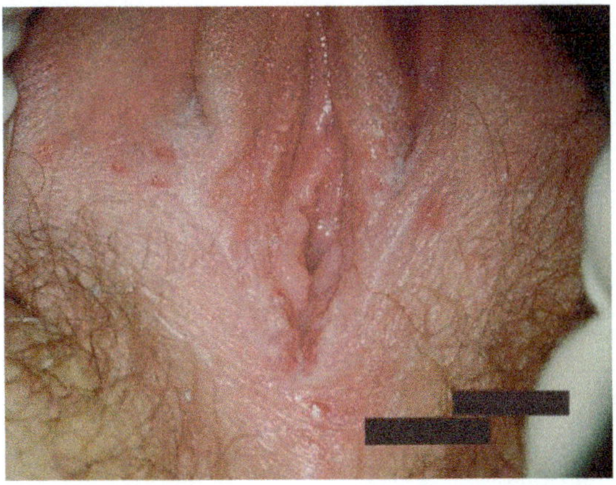

FIGURE 11.13

Herpes simplex virus infection. From Nienow SM, Burrell T, Phillips J. Findings in sexual abuse. In: Anderst JD, ed. *Visual Diagnosis of Child Abuse*. 4th ed. Elk Grove Village, IL: American Academy of Pediatrics; 2016. Courtesy of Shalon M. Nienow, MD.

Anogenital Human Papillomavirus

There are multiple modes of transmission for human papillomaviruses, including congenital infection, autoinoculation, and hand-genital transmission in the course of normal caregiving activities in small children, as well as via sexual contact. In the absence of a sexual abuse or assault disclosure, the presence of this infection is also nonspecific (Figure 11.14).

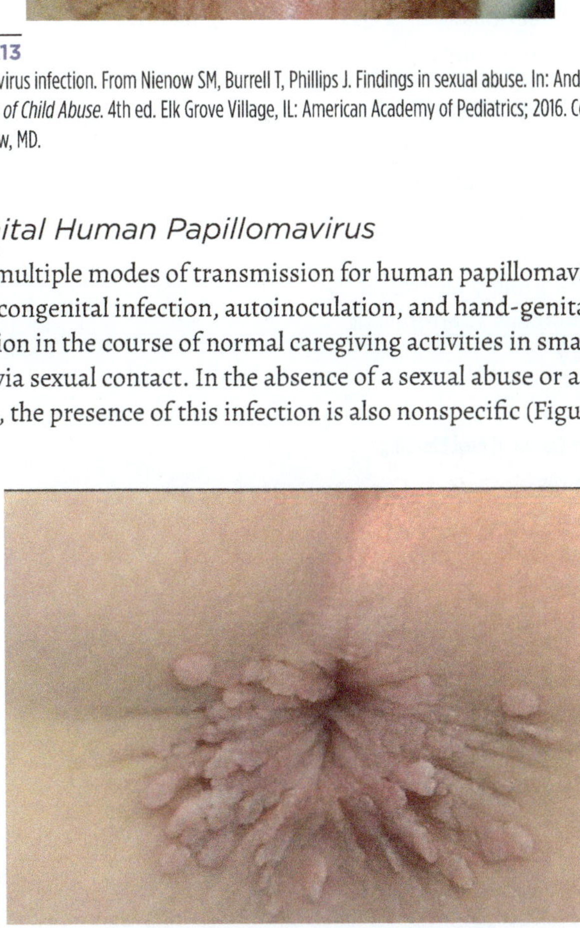

FIGURE 11.14

Anal warts resulting from human papillomavirus infection in an almost 5-year-old boy.
From Nienow SM, Burrell T, Phillips J. Findings in sexual abuse. In: Anderst JD, ed. *Visual Diagnosis of Child Abuse*. 4th ed. Elk Grove Village, IL: American Academy of Pediatrics; 2016. Courtesy of Shalon M. Nienow, MD.

Differential Diagnosis/Mimics

Some physical examination findings can be confused as resulting from reported sexual abuse or assault but may be unrelated entirely (Box 11.3).

If present, nonspecific findings may be related to abusive events. However, because they could have alternate explanations, they are not definitive evidence of abuse. *Anal fissures* (Figure 11.15) are superficial cuts in

BOX 11.3
Findings Unrelated to Sexual Abuse/Assault

Nonsexual Causes of Discharge

Bacterial vaginosis
Candidal infections
Retained foreign body

Non-abusive Causes of Vaginal Bleeding

Consensual sexual activity
Abnormal uterine bleeding
Straddle injury
Vaginal foreign body
Genital tract malignancies
Lichen sclerosus et atrophicus
Pregnancy
Menstruation

Non-abusive Causes of Anal Bleeding

Anal fissures
Hemorrhoids
Inflammatory bowel disease
Infectious colitis
Juvenile polyps

Nonsexual Causes of Anogenital Ulcerations

Aphthous ulcers (ie, Lipschütz ulcers)
Epstein-Barr virus infection
Cytomegalovirus infection
Behçet syndrome
Crohn disease
Pyoderma gangrenosum

Nonsexual Causes of Anogenital Papules

Molluscum contagiosum
Epidermal nevi

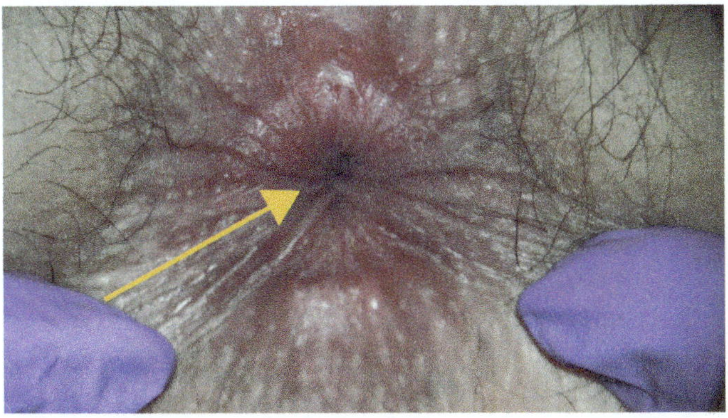

FIGURE 11.15
Anal fissure.

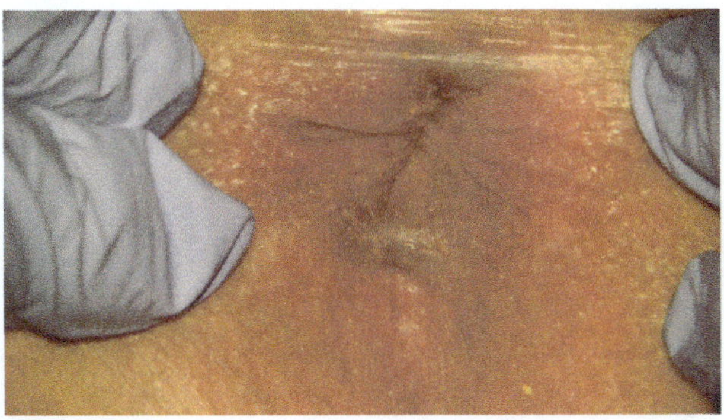

FIGURE 11.16
Anal maceration.

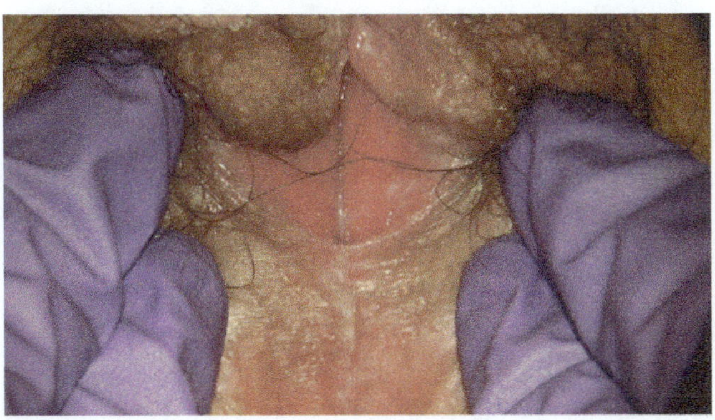

FIGURE 11.17
Labial adhesions.

the epidermal tissue surrounding the anus. They can result from any minor trauma, including passing hard stool. *Perineal maceration* is poor skin condition with superficial softening and breakdown related to prolonged exposure to moisture. This is often seen in females with copious vaginal secretions. Like perineal maceration, *anal maceration* (Figure 11.16) is poor skin condition of the anal tissues that is related to prolonged exposure to moisture. *Labial adhesions* (Figure 11.17) are the result of agglutination of labial tissues from chronic irritation. They are relatively rare in pubertal females but can be seen. Minimal traction may cause them to dehisce and bleed.

Medical Management of the Patient Who Has Experienced Sexual Abuse or Assault

As previously noted, all adolescent patients should have comprehensive STI testing as part of their sexual abuse evaluation. Female patients should also be tested for pregnancy. Any positive STI test result, in the acute setting, may represent prior infection from consensual sexual activity or infected perpetrator secretions. If the adolescent has not been previously sexually active, a positive STI result is definitive evidence of sexual contact and therefore has forensic implications.

Incidence and prevalence rates of STIs among sexually active teens are high, with estimates suggesting that half of all newly acquired infections are found among young people aged 15 to 24 years.[50,51] Based on these numbers and the public health risks involved, it is important for adolescents to be aware of their infectious status so that all sexual partners can be adequately treated as well. This serves to prevent reinfection of patients who are treated for STIs, as well as further transference.

Adolescents who present acutely (within 72–168 hours) after a sexual abuse/assault event should be provided with prophylactic STI treatment after testing is obtained, because compliance with follow-up visits is, in general, poor. Females should be offered emergency contraception, and all teens should be screened for HIV transmission risk and provided with HIV postexposure prophylaxis as necessary. Because adherence to HIV postexposure prophylaxis in teens can be especially poor, attention to follow-up visits by a medical or public health professional is warranted (see Chapter 12, Sexually Transmitted Infections in Child Sexual Abuse).

Appropriate Referrals and Follow-up

At each initial visit, regardless of the acuity of the abuse, patients should be screened for suicidal ideation, self-harming behaviors, signs of anxiety and/or depression, symptoms of trauma, and risk-taking behaviors. If the patient is actively suicidal or homicidal, referral to emergency psychiatric services is warranted. Education on safer sex practices, harm reduction, and responsible decision-making is a crucial aspect of any medical appointment to ensure the ongoing health and safety of the patient. Further, mental health issues such as anxiety, depression, acute stress disorder, and post-traumatic stress disorder (PTSD) are frequent sequelae in those who have experienced sexual abuse or assault.[52,53] Referral to outpatient psychological services should be provided to all adolescents who have experienced sexual abuse or assault, so that they can adequately address the issues stemming from their experiences. All patients should also be given information about community resources for those who have experienced sexual abuse or assault, such as support groups, crisis lines, emergency shelters, crime victim's assistance, legal system advocates, and volunteer opportunities.

Every adolescent who presents following an acute sexual assault should also be provided with a medical follow-up in 6 to 8 weeks. This allows for evaluation of healing of any previously noted injury, ongoing surveillance for STIs, and reassessment of trauma symptoms.

Many male patients who have experienced assault by male perpetrators may become concerned about their sexual identity and orientation. For example, these males may believe that because they experienced physiological arousal during the abuse, they are potentially homosexual. Similarly, boys may be concerned that they were targeted for the abuse because they were perceived as feminine or homosexual. Some adolescents will attempt to overcome these concerns through engaging in excessive sexual activity or by being sexually aggressive.[54,55] Thus, medical professionals working with male adolescents who have experienced sexual abuse or assault should carefully assess for these concerns and reassure the patient that his physiological response to the abuse is not an indicator that he wanted the events to take place. In addition, medical professionals should discuss appropriate sexual behavior with these male patients and refer those engaging in aggressive sexual behavior for appropriate treatment.

Prevention

Sexual abuse and assault are most frequently perpetrated by persons known to and trusted by the patient.[56] Historically, adults have focused education efforts with children on "stranger danger" when, in actuality, this population is of the least risk to them.[57] It is imperative that prevention efforts be initiated early and continued throughout childhood and adolescence.[58] Please see Chapter 10, Medical Evaluation of Suspected

Sexual Abuse in Prepubertal Children, for detailed prevention strategies designed to start in younger age groups.

In children who have previously experienced sexual abuse, there has been shown to be increased risk of later sexual abuse, sexual assault, and/or exploitation.[28] A history of abuse or assault has been associated with a number of increased sexual risk-taking behaviors among adolescents, including having multiple intimate partners, inconsistent use of condoms, early age of sexual debut, adolescent pregnancy, and use of substances before sexual activity. These behaviors may place adolescents in positions that increase the likelihood of further abuse.[23,24] To mitigate the risks of repeat abuse, it is imperative for these adolescents to be engaged in trauma-informed, evidence-based, therapeutic modalities that can help them to deal with the underlying issues driving such sexual risk-taking behaviors.

Adolescents who have experienced sexual abuse or assault have also been found to be more likely to engage in a number of other risk-taking behaviors beyond those related to sexuality. Teens who have experienced sexual abuse or assault report having more suicidal thoughts, are more likely to engage in self-harm behaviors, and are more likely to have made one or multiple suicide attempts compared with peers who have not.[59–61] A sexual abuse history also has been associated with an increased risk of substance misuse, including binge drinking, heavy smoking, and marijuana use.[62,63] There are a number of potential reasons for these associations. First, adolescents who experience sexual violence may come from homes where there are high levels of parental conflict and low levels of parental monitoring, making engagement in these behaviors easier. It may also increase teens' association with other adolescents who are engaging in delinquent behaviors. Additionally, adolescents who have experienced sexual abuse or assault may be experiencing high levels of distress and, thus, could engage in risky behaviors in an attempt to reduce this distress. Therefore, medical professionals should carefully assess if abused adolescents are engaging in such behaviors and discuss treatment options with them for these problems.

In addition to the risk-taking behaviors seen in adolescents who have previously experienced sexual abuse or assault, teens who have never experienced sexual abuse or assault may be engaging in activities that increase their risk of violation. Social media use creates numerous risks due to this age group's limited capacity for self-regulation and susceptibility to peer pressure. Research has shown increases in online expression of sexual experimentation and sexting behaviors.[64] Additionally, teens may engage in these behaviors with people whom they do not know well or have never personally met. Rapidly advancing sexual "talk" with strangers may increase vulnerability to assault when there is a sense of anonymity involved. Also of significant concern is the use of alcohol and/or drugs, which has been shown to precede sexual assault in more than half of patients. Recreational drug and alcohol use is common in teens,[65–67] and perpetrators may take advantage of decreased inhibitions or altered levels of consciousness in which adolescents have an inability to consent. Sexual violence that includes substance use is more likely to be severe, associated with physical injury, and result in completed rape.[68] It is imperative that medical professionals who provide anticipatory guidance to adolescents include risks of sexual assault in discussions of alcohol and drug experimentation.

Sexual dating violence is also a serious issue in adolescence, occurring in 10.6% of students nationwide. It is reported more frequently by females (15.6%) than males (5.4%), as well as by those in earlier grade levels.[69] Sexual dating violence is also associated with other forms of intimate partner violence such as physical aggression, stalking, and verbal abuse. Experiencing these in the young adult years is highly associated with previous adolescent dating violence,[70] either physical or sexual. Therefore, prevention of intimate partner violence during teen years can significantly alter the likelihood of later abuse. Prevention strategies that are shown to reduce the risk of involvement in unsafe relationships include teaching healthy relationship skills, engagement of influential peers and adults, creating protective environments, and supporting survivors to increase safety and reduce harm.[71] In recent years, there has been a significant push to introduce school-based interventions for reduction in sexual and dating violence. These programs include primary and secondary prevention strategies and are being implemented in grade schools as well as on college and university campuses.[72,73] Additionally, primary care medical professionals should screen for the presence of intimate partner and dating violence to offer guidance and provide resources to adolescents who are engaged in such relationships.

Prognosis

The immediate goal of the medical professional is to ensure the safety of the patient. This means contacting appropriate investigative agencies as necessary, especially if abuse is occurring in the home or if caregivers are non-protective. The time frame for reporting varies by jurisdiction, so it is imperative that medical professionals know the reporting guidelines for their area. Adolescents who have ongoing contact with perpetrators or who live with non-protective caregivers are at high risk for recanting any previous disclosures and for continued abusive events. Any patient who is verbalizing or exhibiting signs or symptoms of current suicidal or homicidal ideation should be provided with emergency psychiatric stabilization services.

Long-term outcomes for those who have experienced sexual abuse or assault are dependent on many factors. One of the most important indicators of abuse-specific self-blame and associated trauma symptoms is having a non-believing mother.[44] Conversely, one of the most important factors in positive outcomes for patients is having a supportive family member.[74,75]

To mitigate long-term health and psychological sequelae, it is imperative for those who have experienced sexual abuse or assault to receive evidence-based, trauma-informed services. One of the most well-studied forms of therapy for this population is cognitive behavioral therapy. This modality has been shown to improve PTSD, internalizing, externalizing, and sexually inappropriate behaviors.[20] All patients should be referred to such services as available in their locale. In many areas, a children's advocacy center (CAC) is available to help organize and provide services such as forensic interviews and therapy. A CAC can provide services such as care coordination and multidisciplinary team staffing as the forensic aspect of the case progresses. Advocates may also be available to help walk the patient and family through all steps in the medicolegal process. If not available through the CAC, advocates are often located at rape crisis centers or district attorney offices.

Conclusion

A significant number of adolescents will experience sexual assault or have had previous sexual abuse experiences. This makes it imperative for medical professionals to be able to adequately screen for and treat these conditions. Many teens will not spontaneously disclose incidents of sexual abuse or assault for fear of being blamed, due to family instability, or because of fears related to the consequences of disclosure. In addition, adolescents may not consider their experience to be abusive or may have ambivalent feelings toward the perpetrator. Thus, medical professionals should routinely assess for these events using age-appropriate questions.

Once identified, adolescents who have experienced sexual abuse or assault should be offered testing and treatment of STIs as well as pregnancy testing. If the last abusive event occurred within 72 to 168 hours, forensic evidence should be collected and STI and pregnancy prophylaxis should be offered.

Many adolescents will experience significant psychological sequelae following sexual abuse or assault, such as the development of depression or PTSD. Therefore, medical professionals should screen for the presence of significant psychological distress in all patients who have experienced sexual abuse or assault and make appropriate referrals for further mental health treatment.

Medical professionals also should be aware of the legal issues in working with these adolescents. Medical professionals are mandated reporters of all suspected incidents of childhood sexual abuse. In addition, in most states adolescents are able to consent for testing and treatment of STIs, including HIV, and medical professionals do not need parental permission to provide these services to them. In many states, adolescents who are pregnant may be considered able to give consent for pregnancy treatment and prevention. There are variations in reporting requirements and procedures, in age of consent laws, and differences in what an adolescent can maintain as confidential based on jurisdiction. It is important for medical professionals to be familiar with the laws in their state.

Finally, medical professionals should be aware of potentially difficult issues that may arise when working with adolescents who have experienced sexual abuse or assault. These adolescents engage in more high-risk behaviors and, once having experienced abuse or assault, are at significant risk for further abuse and/or exploitation. Medical professionals should aim to mitigate as many of these risk-taking behaviors as possible, through education, to prevent further harm and/or abuse.

References

1. United Nations Children's Fund. Select child protection definitions. https://www.unicef.org/protection/conceptual_clarity_definitions_-_28_Jan_2010_-_clean_1.doc. Published 2010. Accessed May 28, 2019
2. Leeb RT, Paulozzi L, Melanson C, Simon T, Arias I. *Child Maltreatment Surveillance: Uniform Definitions for Public Health and Recommended Data Elements: Version 1.0*. Atlanta, GA: Centers for Disease Control and Prevention, National Center for Injury Prevention and Control; 2008. https://www.cdc.gov/violenceprevention/pdf/CM_Surveillance-a.pdf. Published January 2008. Accessed May 28, 2019
3. Collin-Vézina D, De La Sablonnière-Griffin M, Palmer AM, Milne L. A preliminary mapping of individual, relational, and social factors that impede disclosure of childhood sexual abuse. *Child Abuse Negl.* 2015;43(suppl C):123–134 PMID: 25846196 https://doi.org/10.1016/j.chiabu.2015.03.010
4. Hanson RF, Resnick HS, Saunders BE, Kilpatrick DG, Best C. Factors related to the reporting of childhood rape. *Child Abuse Negl.* 1999;23(6):559–569 PMID: 10391513 https://doi.org/10.1016/S0145-2134(99)00028-9

5. Finkelhor D, Vanderminden J, Turner H, Hamby S, Shattuck A. Child maltreatment rates assessed in a national household survey of caregivers and youth. *Child Abuse Negl.* 2014;38(9):1421–1435 PMID: 24953383 https://doi.org/10.1016/j.chiabu.2014.05.005
6. Finkelhor D. Current information on the scope and nature of child sexual abuse. *Future Child.* 1994;4(2):31–53 PMID: 7804768 https://doi.org/10.2307/1602522
7. Luster T, Small SA. Sexual abuse history and number of sex partners among female adolescents. *Fam Plann Perspect.* 1997;29(5):204–211 PMID: 9323496 https://doi.org/10.2307/2953396
8. Finkelhor D, Hotaling G, Lewis IA, Smith C. Sexual abuse in a national survey of adult men and women: prevalence, characteristics, and risk factors. *Child Abuse Negl.* 1990;14(1):19–28 PMID: 2310970 https://doi.org/10.1016/0145-2134(90)90077-7
9. Lynskey MT, Fergusson DM. Factors protecting against the development of adjustment difficulties in young adults exposed to childhood sexual abuse. *Child Abuse Negl.* 1997;21(12):1177–1190 PMID: 9429770 https://doi.org/10.1016/S0145-2134(97)00093-8
10. US Department of Justice Office on Violence Against Women. Sexual assault. https://www.justice.gov/ovw/sexual-assault. Accessed May 28, 2019
11. Finkelhor D, Ormrod R, Turner H, Hamby SL. The victimization of children and youth: a comprehensive, national survey. *Child Maltreat.* 2005;10(1):5–25 PMID: 15611323 https://doi.org/10.1177/1077559504271287
12. Morgan RE, Kena G. *Criminal Victimization, 2016: Revised.* Washington, DC: US Department of Justice, Office of Justice Programs, Bureau of Justice Statistics; 2018. https://www.bjs.gov/index.cfm?ty=pbdetail&iid=6166. Accessed May 28, 2019
13. Planty M, Langton L, Krebs C, Berzofsky M, Smiley-McDonald H. Female Victims of Sexual Violence, 1994–2010. Washington, DC: US Department of Justice, Office of Justice Programs, Bureau of Justice Statistics; 2016. https://www.bjs.gov/content/pub/pdf/fvsv9410.pdf. Accessed May 28, 2019
14. Hall ER, Flannery PJ. Prevalence and correlates of sexual assault experiences in adolescents. *Victimology.* 1984;9(3–4):398–406
15. Ackard DM, Neumark-Sztainer D. Date violence and date rape among adolescents: associations with disordered eating behaviors and psychological health. *Child Abuse Negl.* 2002;26(5):455–473 PMID: 12079084 https://doi.org/10.1016/S0145-2134(02)00322-8
16. Raghavan R, Bogart LM, Elliott MN, Vestal KD, Schuster MA. Sexual victimization among a national probability sample of adolescent women. *Perspect Sex Reprod Health.* 2004;36(6):225–232 PMID: 15687080 https://doi.org/10.1363/3622504
17. Ackard DM, Neumark-Sztainer D. Multiple sexual victimizations among adolescent boys and girls: prevalence and associations with eating behaviors and psychological health. *J Child Sex Abuse.* 2003;12(1):17–37 PMID: 16221658 https://doi.org/10.1300/J070v12n01_02
18. Market Opinion Research. *National Women's Study, 1975.* Ann Arbor, MI: Inter-university Consortium for Political and Social Research [distributor]; 2009. https://www.icpsr.umich.edu/icpsrweb/ICPSR/studies/7532/version/2
19. AgeOfConsent.net. United States age of consent map. https://www.ageofconsent.net/states. Accessed May 28, 2019
20. Putnam FW. Ten-year research update review: child sexual abuse. *J Am Acad Child Adolesc Psychiatry.* 2003;42(3):269–278 PMID: 12595779 https://doi.org/10.1097/00004583-200303000-00006
21. Finkelhor D. Epidemiological factors in the clinical identification of child sexual abuse. *Child Abuse Negl.* 1993;17(1):67–70 PMID: 8435788 https://doi.org/10.1016/0145-2134(93)90009-T

22. Lev-Wiesel R. Intergenerational transmission of sexual abuse? Motherhood in the shadow of incest. *J Child Sex Abuse.* 2006;15(2):75–101 PMID: 16702149 https://doi.org/10.1300/J070v15n02_06
23. Fergusson DM, Horwood LJ, Lynskey MT. Childhood sexual abuse, adolescent sexual behaviors and sexual revictimization. *Child Abuse Negl.* 1997;21(8):789–803 PMID: 9280383 https://doi.org/10.1016/S0145-2134(97)00039-2
24. Classen CC, Palesh OG, Aggarwal R. Sexual revictimization: a review of the empirical literature. *Trauma Violence Abuse.* 2005;6(2):103–129 PMID: 15753196 https://doi.org/10.1177/1524838005275087
25. East PL, Hokoda A. Risk and protective factors for sexual and dating violence victimization: a longitudinal, prospective study of Latino and African American adolescents. *J Youth Adolesc.* 2015;44(6):1288–1300 PMID: 25788124 https://doi.org/10.1007/s10964-015-0273-5
26. Abbey A, Ross LT, McDuffie D, McAuslan P. Alcohol and dating risk factors for sexual assault among college women. *Psychol Women Q.* 1996;20(1):147–169 https://doi.org/10.1111/j.1471-6402.1996.tb00669.x
27. Testa M, VanZile-Tamsen C, Livingston JA. Childhood sexual abuse, relationship satisfaction, and sexual risk taking in a community sample of women. *J Consult Clin Psychol.* 2005;73(6):1116–1124 PMID: 16392972 https://doi.org/10.1037/0022-006X.73.6.1116
28. Krahé B, Scheinberger-Olwig R, Waizenhöfer E, Kolpin S. Childhood sexual abuse and revictimization in adolescence. *Child Abuse Negl.* 1999;23(4):383–394 PMID: 10321775 https://doi.org/10.1016/S0145-2134(99)00002-2
29. Rickert VI, Wiemann CM, Vaughan RD, White JW. Rates and risk factors for sexual violence among an ethnically diverse sample of adolescents. *Arch Pediatr Adolesc Med.* 2004;158(12):1132–1139 PMID: 15583097 https://doi.org/10.1001/archpedi.158.12.1132
30. Humphrey JA, White JW. Women's vulnerability to sexual assault from adolescence to young adulthood. *J Adolesc Health.* 2000;27(6):419–424 PMID: 11090744 https://doi.org/10.1016/S1054-139X(00)00168-3
31. Hampton MD, Lieggi M. Commercial sexual exploitation of youth in the United States: a qualitative systematic review. *Trauma Violence Abuse.* 2017:1524838017742168 PMID: 29334030 https://doi.org/10.1177/1524838017742168
32. Greenbaum J, Crawford-Jakubiak JE; American Academy of Pediatrics Committee on Child Abuse and Neglect. Child sex trafficking and commercial sexual exploitation: health care needs of victims. *Pediatrics.* 2015;135(3):566–574 PMID: 25713283 https://doi.org/10.1542/peds.2014-4138
33. Choudhary E, Gunzler D, Tu X, Bossarte RM. Epidemiological characteristics of male sexual assault in a criminological database. *J Interpers Violence.* 2012;27(3):523–546 PMID: 21987510 https://doi.org/10.1177/0886260511421674
34. Goodman-Brown TB, Edelstein RS, Goodman GS, Jones DPH, Gordon DS. Why children tell: a model of children's disclosure of sexual abuse. *Child Abuse Negl.* 2003;27(5): 525–540 PMID: 12718961 https://doi.org/10.1016/S0145-2134(03)00037-1
35. Crisma M, Bascelli E, Paci D, Romito P. Adolescents who experienced sexual abuse: fears, needs and impediments to disclosure. *Child Abuse Negl.* 2004;28(10):1035–1048 PMID: 15519434 https://doi.org/10.1016/j.chiabu.2004.03.015
36. Bechtel K, Podrazik M. Evaluation of the adolescent rape victim. *Pediatr Clin North Am.* 1999;46(4):809–823, xii PMID: 10494258 https://doi.org/10.1016/S0031-3955(05)70153-X
37. Sinal SH. Sexual abuse of children and adolescents. *South Med J.* 1994;87(12):1242–1258 PMID: 7973924 https://doi.org/10.1097/00007611-199412000-00008
38. Poirier MP. Care of the female adolescent rape victim. *Pediatr Emerg Care.* 2002;18(1):53–59 PMID: 11862142 https://doi.org/10.1097/00006565-200202000-00016

39. US Department of Justice Office on Violence Against Women. *A National Protocol for Sexual Assault Medical Forensic Examinations—Adults/Adolescents*. 2nd ed. https://www.ncjrs.gov/pdffiles1/ovw/241903.pdf. Published April 2013. Accessed May 28, 2019
40. Adams JA, Kellogg ND, Farst KJ, et al. Updated guidelines for the medical assessment and care of children who may have been sexually abused. *J Pediatr Adolesc Gynecol*. 2016;29(2):81–87 PMID: 26220352 https://doi.org/10.1016/j.jpag.2015.01.007
41. National Children's Alliance. *National Children's Alliance Standards for Accredited Members*. 2017 ed. http://www.nationalchildrensalliance.org/wp-content/uploads/2015/06/NCA-Standards-for-Accredited-Members-2017.pdf. Accessed May 28, 2019
42. Centers for Disease Control and Prevention. *2015 Sexually Transmitted Diseases Treatment Guidelines*. Sexual assault and abuse and STDs. https://www.cdc.gov/std/tg2015/sexual-assault.htm. Reviewed June 4, 2015. Accessed May 28, 2019
43. Smith DW, Letourneau EJ, Saunders BE, Kilpatrick DG, Resnick HS, Best CL. Delay in disclosure of childhood rape: results from a national survey. *Child Abuse Negl*. 2000;24(2):273–287 PMID: 10695522 https://doi.org/10.1016/S0145-2134(99)00130-1
44. Melville JD, Kellogg ND, Perez N, Lukefahr JL. Assessment for self-blame and trauma symptoms during the medical evaluation of suspected sexual abuse. *Child Abuse Negl*. 2014;38(5):851–857 PMID: 24630439 https://doi.org/10.1016/j.chiabu.2014.01.020
45. Finkel MA, Alexander RA. Conducting the medical history. *J Child Sex Abuse*. 2011;20(5):486–504 PMID: 21970642 https://doi.org/10.1080/10538712.2011.607406
46. Tyler KA. Social and emotional outcomes of childhood sexual abuse: a review of recent research. *Aggress Violent Behav*. 2002;7(6):567–589 https://doi.org/10.1016/S1359-1789(01)00047-7
47. Sugar NF, Fine DN, Eckert LO. Physical injury after sexual assault: findings of a large case series. *Am J Obstet Gynecol*. 2004;190(1):71–76 PMID: 14749638 https://doi.org/10.1016/S0002-9378(03)00912-8
48. Adams JA, Kellogg ND, Moles R. Medical care for children who may have been sexually abused: an update for 2016. *Clin Pediatr Emerg Med*. 2016;17(4):255–263 https://doi.org/10.1016/j.cpem.2016.09.002
49. Kellogg ND, Menard SW, Santos A. Genital anatomy in pregnant adolescents: "normal" does not mean "nothing happened". *Pediatrics*. 2004;113(1 Pt 1):e67–e69 PMID: 14702498 https://doi.org/10.1542/peds.113.1.e67
50. Satterwhite CL, Torrone E, Meites E, et al. Sexually transmitted infections among US women and men: prevalence and incidence estimates, 2008. *Sex Transm Dis*. 2013;40(3):187–193
51. Forhan SE, Gottlieb SL, Sternberg MR, et al. Prevalence of sexually transmitted infections among female adolescents aged 14 to 19 in the United States. *Pediatrics*. 2009;124(6):1505–1512 PMID: 19933728 https://doi.org/10.1542/peds.2009-0674
52. Rees S, Silove D, Chey T, et al. Lifetime prevalence of gender-based violence in women and the relationship with mental disorders and psychosocial function. *JAMA*. 2011;306(5):513–521 PMID: 21813429 https://doi.org/10.1001/jama.2011.1098
53. Faravelli C, Giugni A, Salvatori S, Ricca V. Psychopathology after rape. *Am J Psychiatry*. 2004;161(8):1483–1485 PMID: 15285977 https://doi.org/10.1176/appi.ajp.161.8.1483
54. Holmes WC, Slap GB. Sexual abuse of boys: definition, prevalence, correlates, sequelae, and management. *JAMA*. 1998;280(21):1855–1862 PMID: 9846781 https://doi.org/10.1001/jama.280.21.1855
55. Romano E, De Luca RV. Male sexual abuse: a review of effects, abuse characteristics, and links with later psychological functioning. *Aggress Violent Behav*. 2001;6(1):55–78 https://doi.org/10.1016/S1359-1789(99)00011-7

56. US Office of Justice Programs, Bureau of Justice Statistics. Data collection: National Crime Victimization Survey (NCVS). https://www.bjs.gov/index.cfm?ty=dcdetail&iid=245. Accessed May 28, 2019
57. Babatsikos G. Parents' knowledge, attitudes and practices about preventing child sexual abuse: a literature review. *Child Abuse Rev.* 2010;19(2):107–129 https://doi.org/10.1002/car.1102
58. Davis MK, Gidycz CA. Child sexual abuse prevention programs: a meta-analysis. *J Clin Child Psychol.* 2000;29(2):257–265 PMID: 10802834 https://doi.org/10.1207/S15374424jccp2902_11
59. Bensley LS, Van Eenwyk J, Spieker SJ, Schoder J. Self-reported abuse history and adolescent problem behaviors. I. Antisocial and suicidal behaviors. *J Adolesc Health.* 1999;24(3):163–172 PMID: 10195799 https://doi.org/10.1016/S1054-139X(98)00111-6
60. Martin G, Bergen HA, Richardson AS, Roeger L, Allison S. Sexual abuse and suicidality: gender differences in a large community sample of adolescents. *Child Abuse Negl.* 2004;28(5):491–503 PMID: 15159067 https://doi.org/10.1016/j.chiabu.2003.08.006
61. Wright J, Friedrich W, Cinq-Mars C, Cyr M, McDuff P. Self-destructive and delinquent behaviors of adolescent female victims of child sexual abuse: rates and covariates in clinical and nonclinical samples. *Violence Vict.* 2004;19(6):627–643 PMID: 16004066 https://doi.org/10.1891/vivi.19.6.627.66343
62. Howard DE, Wang MQ. Psychosocial correlates of U.S. adolescents who report a history of forced sexual intercourse. *J Adolesc Health.* 2005;36(5):372–379 PMID: 15837340 https://doi.org/10.1016/j.jadohealth.2004.07.007
63. Champion HLO, Foley KL, DuRant RH, Hensberry R, Altman D, Wolfson M. Adolescent sexual victimization, use of alcohol and other substances, and other health risk behaviors. *J Adolesc Health.* 2004;35(4):321–328 PMID: 15450546 https://doi.org/10.1016/S1054-139X(04)00099-0
64. O'Keeffe GS, Clarke-Pearson K; American Academy of Pediatrics Council on Communications and Media. The impact of social media on children, adolescents, and families. *Pediatrics.* 2011;127(4):800–804 PMID: 21444588 https://doi.org/10.1542/peds.2011-0054
65. Eaton DK, Kann L, Kinchen S, et al; Centers for Disease Control and Prevention (CDC). Youth risk behavior surveillance—United States, 2011. *MMWR Surveill Summ.* 2012;61(4):1–162 PMID: 22673000
66. Johnston LD, O'Malley PM, Miech RA, Bachman JG, Schulenberg JE. *Monitoring the Future National Results on Drug Use: 1975–2013: Overview, Key Findings on Adolescent Drug Use.* Ann Arbor, MI: Institute for Social Research, The University of Michigan; 2014
67. National Institute on Drug Abuse. Monitoring the Future survey: high school and youth trends. https://www.drugabuse.gov/publications/drugfacts/monitoring-future-survey-high-school-youth-trends. Revised December 2018. Accessed May 28, 2019
68. Hall JA, Moore CB. Drug facilitated sexual assault—a review. *J Forensic Leg Med.* 2008;15(5):291–297 PMID: 18511003 https://doi.org/10.1016/j.jflm.2007.12.005
69. Kann L, McManus T, Harris WA, et al. Youth Risk Behavior Surveillance—United States, 2015. *MMWR Surveill Summ.* 2016;65(6):1–174 PMID: 27280474 https://doi.org/10.15585/mmwr.ss6506a1
70. Smith PH, White JW, Holland LJ. A longitudinal perspective on dating violence among adolescent and college-age women. *Am J Public Health.* 2003;93(7):1104–1109 PMID: 12835193 https://doi.org/10.2105/AJPH.93.7.1104
71. Niolon PH, Kearns M, Dills J, et al. *Preventing Intimate Partner Violence Across the Lifespan: A Technical Package of Programs, Policies, and Practices.* Atlanta, GA: National Center for Injury Prevention and Control, Centers for Disease Control and Prevention; 2017

72. De La Rue L, Polanin J, Espelage D, Pigott T. School-based interventions to reduce dating and sexual violence: a systematic review. *Campbell Syst Rev.* 2014;10(7)
73. Dills J, Fowler D, Payne G. *Sexual Violence on Campus: Strategies for Prevention*. Atlanta, GA: National Center for Injury Prevention and Control; 2016
74. Lovett BB. Child sexual abuse disclosure: maternal response and other variables impacting the victim. *Child Adolesc Social Work J.* 2004;21(4):355–371 https://doi.org/10.1023/B:CASW.0000035221.78729.d6
75. Ullman SE. Social reactions to child sexual abuse disclosures: a critical review. *J Child Sex Abuse.* 2003;12(1):89–121 PMID: 16221661 https://doi.org/10.1300/J070v12n01_05

CHAPTER 12

Sexually Transmitted Infections in Child Sexual Abuse

Allan R. De Jong, MD, FAAP
Medical Director
Children at Risk Evaluation (CARE) Program
Nemours/Alfred I. duPont Hospital for Children
Wilmington, DE

Stephanie A. Deutsch, MD, FAAP
Co-Medical Director
Children at Risk Evaluation (CARE) Program
Nemours/Alfred I. duPont Hospital for Children
Wilmington, DE

Introduction

Children and adolescents who have experienced sexual abuse are at risk for acquiring infections prevalent among sexually active adolescents and adults. The infection or colonization may be symptomatic or asymptomatic. Sexually transmitted infections (STIs) are not commonly identified in prepubertal children. Therefore, the presence of an STI in a child should raise concerns for sexual abuse. Some children, however, may acquire STIs through perinatal transmission at birth or through nonsexual contact. Discovery of an STI in a child may prompt an evaluation for child sexual abuse and may be the only physical evidence of sexual abuse in some cases.[1-7]

Adolescents and young adults who are sexually active have the highest rates of STIs, and STIs are more commonly identified in pubertal adolescents than in prepubertal children evaluated for suspected sexual assault or abuse. The presence of an STI in the pubertal adolescent may represent an infection acquired through abuse or prior consensual sexual activity. The risk of acquiring an STI through sexual assault or abuse is directly related to the prevalence of STIs found in the adult and adolescent population.[8–13] Recently, rates of gonorrhea, chlamydia, and syphilis have increased dramatically in the United States among adolescents and adults; more than 2 million cases of STIs were reported in 2016, the highest number reported to date.[14]

The actual risk of acquiring STIs by children who have experienced sexual abuse is unknown. Several studies suggest rates of STIs among prepubertal children evaluated for sexual abuse are low, approximately 5%.[1,9,11,13] In a recent prospective multicenter study of children aged 0 to 13 years,[13] one or more STIs were identified in 8.2% of 485 girls and no STIs in 51 boys; among girls, the genitourinary prevalence was 3.1% for *Chlamydia trachomatis* via nucleic acid amplification testing (NAAT) and 3.3% for *Neisseria gonorrhoeae*. *Trichomonas vaginalis* was detected by wet mount among 5.9% of symptomatic children (5 of 85), and herpes simplex virus type 2 (HSV-2) antibody was identified in 2.5%; 5 of 12 (42%) of children with lesions had positive HSV-2 cultures. Notably, no cases of HIV infection were detected, and syphilis prevalence was 0.3% by serologic testing. Based on the age distribution of this study, at least one-third of the children were likely to be pubertal. In addition, only children evaluated for suspected abuse who were thought to be at risk for STIs based on clinical or historic risk factors were included in the study. Differences in observed frequency of STIs among children studied may be related to many variables: type of sexual contact, age of the child, frequency of the abuse, types of testing performed, regional differences in the prevalence of STIs, and percentage of children screened specifically because of risk factors or symptoms of STI (selective) versus universal screening practices. The incubation periods for the organisms and the timing of the examination after the abuse also critically influence detection.[15–18]

The Centers for Disease Control and Prevention (CDC) suggests a general rule: "The identification of sexually transmissible agents in children beyond the neonatal period strongly suggests sexual abuse."[2,9,16] While this general rule is useful, the strength of the association between STI and child sexual abuse varies from disease to disease (Table 12.1). Specificity for abuse depends in part on the child's age, the specific pathogen identified, and the possibilities of perinatal, fomite, or nonsexual transmission. Children with STIs may be unable or unwilling to disclose sexual abuse, and the absence of a disclosure does not preclude sexual transmission. When no source of the organism is identified, it is not acceptable to conclude that the transmission must have been perinatal or nonsexual. Likewise, the inability to document a specific STI in a possible or suspected perpetrator does not exclude the possibility that this individual was the source of the child's infection.[7]

Despite more widespread clinical use of NAATs for the identification of STIs among children, adolescents, and adults, current CDC guidelines primarily recommend confirmation of infection using high-specificity culture techniques when child sexual abuse is suspected.[16] It is possible upcoming revisions to CDC testing guidelines (anticipated in 2019) will recommend NAAT as the forensic, diagnostic standard, including use at extragenital sites.

TABLE 12.1
Significance of Sexually Transmitted Infections in Children

Sexually Transmitted Infection	Persistence Following Perinatal Transmission	Significance of Relationship to Sexual Contact
Gonorrhea	Up to 1 y	Definitive[a]
Chlamydia trachomatis	Up to 3 y	Definitive[a]
Syphilis	Months to years	Definitive[a]
HIV	Asymptomatic for years	Definitive[b]
Trichomonas vaginalis	Up to 1 y	Definitive
Chancroid	Unlikely to be asymptomatic	Very likely[c]
Granuloma inguinale	Unlikely to be asymptomatic	Very likely[c]
Human papillomavirus	Asymptomatic up to 3 y	Possible[d]
Herpes simplex virus (types 1 and 2)	Symptomatic by 6 wk	Possible[e]
Hepatitis B virus	Asymptomatic for years	Possible
Pubic lice	Symptomatic within 3 wk	Possible
Head/body lice	Symptomatic within 3 wk	Inconclusive
Hepatitis C	Asymptomatic for years	Inconclusive
Molluscum contagiosum	Unknown	Inconclusive
Bacterial vaginosis	Unknown	Inconclusive
Group B streptococci	Unknown	Inconclusive
Genital mycoplasma	Unknown	Inconclusive

[a] Unless there is evidence of perinatal transmission or clearly, reasonably, or independently documented but rare nonsexual transmission.
[b] Unless acquired perinatally or through blood transfusion or contaminated needle.
[c] Rare infection with few data available on children.
[d] Longer asymptomatic time frames in laryngeal papillomas.
[e] Genital location of lesions increase likelihood of abuse.

Infections and Organisms

Children can acquire a variety of STIs through sexual and nonsexual transmission. These infections and organisms are discussed in detail in this chapter; Table 12.2 presents a summary of incubation period, symptoms, and appropriate diagnostic tests.

Gonorrhea

N gonorrhoeae is a small, gram-negative, oxidase-positive, diplococcal bacterium that causes gonorrhea or gonococcal infections. The incubation period is 2 to 7 days. Infections may be associated with symptoms including vaginal discharge (vaginitis), rectal pain, pruritus and discharge (proctitis), and exudative pharyngotonsillitis (pharyngitis). Gonococcal infections of the pharynx and of the rectum, however, are

TABLE 12.2
Incubation, Symptoms, and Diagnostic Tests for Sexually Transmitted Infections in Children

Sexually Transmitted Infection	Incubation	Symptoms	Diagnostic Tests
Gonorrhea	2–7 d	Vaginal discharge in prepubertal girls. Cervical, throat, and rectal infections are typically asymptomatic.	Culture on selective media with confirmation by 2 or more tests; NAAT with confirmation may be used when testing vaginal secretions or urine from girls.
Chlamydia trachomatis (except LGV)	Usually 5–7 d	Vaginal discharge in some prepubertal girls, but most infections of vagina, cervix, throat, and rectum are asymptomatic.	Tissue culture with confirmatory staining with fluorescein-conjugated species-specific antibody; NAAT with confirmation may be used when testing vaginal secretions or urine from girls.
LGV	Usually 10–14 d	Usually single ulcer, papule, pustule, or vesicle with tender inguinal adenopathy; proctocolitis.	Tissue culture; in appropriate clinical setting, NAAT with confirmation (NAAT for *C trachomatis* typically positive but not specific for LGV serovars).
Syphilis	Range 10–90 d; usually 2–4 wk	Primary—usually painless typically single ulcer with slightly raised borders. Secondary—fever and rash, particularly palms and soles, condyloma latum.	Nontreponemal test (RPR or VDRL) confirmed by a positive treponemal test (FTA-ABS or MHA-TP). Treponemal tests may be performed first in some laboratories. Dark field examination of primary lesion.
HIV	6 wk–6 mo	Lymphadenopathy, wasting, opportunistic infections asymptomatic for many years.	Fourth-generation HIV-1/HIV-1 combined antibody/antigen immunoassay; if reactive, HIV-1/HIV-2 antibody differentiation assay.
Trichomonas vaginalis	4–28 d	Vaginal discharge but often asymptomatic.	Microscopy of fresh wet mount secretions, culture on special culture media; data on use of NAAT for detection of *T vaginalis* in children are too limited to inform recommendations, but no evidence suggests that performance of NAAT for detection of *T vaginalis* in children would differ from that in adults.
Chancroid	1–35 d; usually 3–7 d	Single or few shallow, painful ulcers with irregular edges.	Culture recommended by CDC,[16] difficult to obtain.
Granuloma inguinale	Several days to several months	Irregular typically painless ulcers and granulomas, with subcutaneous inguinal swelling.	Tissue smears or biopsy showing Donovan bodies; *Klebsiella granulomatis* culture difficult to obtain.
Human papillomavirus	1 mo–2 y (or longer)	Irregular raised lesions of variable sizes, but infections may be asymptomatic.	Clinical diagnosis, biopsy atypical lesions. Subclinical infection—viral typing by PCR NAAT.

(continued)

TABLE 12.2 (*continued*)

Sexually Transmitted Infection	Incubation	Symptoms	Diagnostic Tests
Herpes simplex virus (types 1 and 2)	2–14 d; usually 2–7 d	Painful vesicles and ulcers. Systemic symptoms common in primary infection.	Tissue culture; PCR swab of lesion; serology not helpful.
Hepatitis B virus	45–160 d	Anorexia, abdominal pain, and jaundice, but sometimes asymptomatic.	Hepatitis B serology.
Pubic lice	2–3 wk to mature	Pruritus, visible lice and nits on pubic hair or eyelashes.	Microscopic identification of lice.
Head/body lice	2–3 wk to mature	Pruritus, visible lice and nits never on eyelashes.	Microscopic identification of lice.
Hepatitis C	2–6 mo	Asymptomatic for years.	Hepatitis C serology.
Molluscum contagiosum	2 wk–6 mo	Small skin-colored papules with central depressed core.	Visual identification of lesions.
Bacterial vaginosis	Variable 7–14 d	Vaginal discharge but may be asymptomatic.	Microscopy showing clue cells, with pH of secretions >4.5 and positive "whiff test" = fishy odor following addition of 10% potassium hydroxide (criteria less helpful in prepubertal child).
Group B streptococci	Variable but typically <1 wk	Typically asymptomatic but may cause vaginal discharge.	Culture.
Mycoplasma genitalium	Unknown (possibly 7–60 d)	Genital pain, abdominal pain, dysuria, vaginal/penile discharge.	Culture recommended by CDC,[16] difficult to obtain; NAAT available in some large medical centers and commercial laboratories, not yet FDA approved for use in United States; no recommendations around NAAT use in children.

Abbreviations: CDC, Centers for Disease Control and Prevention; FDA, US Food and Drug Administration; FTA-ABS, fluorescent treponemal antibody; HIV, human immunodeficiency virus; LGV, lymphogranuloma venereum; MHA-TP, microhemagglutination assay-*Treponema pallidum;* NAAT, nucleic acid amplification test; PCR, polymerase chain reaction; RPR, rapid plasma reagin; VDRL, Venereal Disease Research Laboratories.

typically asymptomatic. If symptoms do occur, they almost always develop within a week of exposure. Vaginal discharge, if left untreated, may turn from purulent to serous and disappear in 2 months. Within 28 weeks of incubation, spontaneous resolution of the infection occurs in 90% of infected children and adults[19–21] (Figure 12.1). Among prepubertal children, genital infections are commonly associated with perineal pain, pruritus, dysuria, or a purulent penile or vaginal discharge, although symptoms may decrease or even resolve within several weeks without treatment. Vaginitis is the most common manifestation of this infection among prepubertal girls,[16] which may be related to thin atrophic non-estrogenized vaginal mucosa being more susceptible to

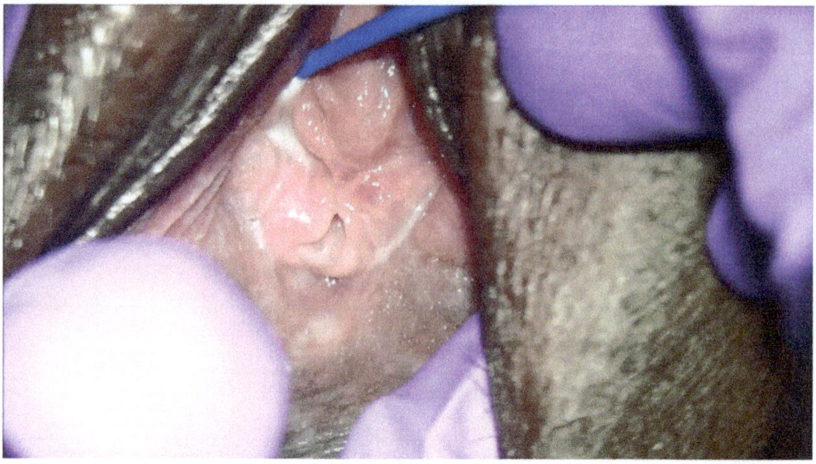

FIGURE 12.1
Seventeen-year-old patient found to have gonorrhea and chlamydia after an acute sexual assault. Patient is also consensually sexually active.
Courtesy of Shalon M. Nienow, MD.

gonococcal vulvovaginitis compared with adolescent or adult mucosal tissue. Adolescents may present with cervical or urethral discharge, but up to one-half of infections in adolescents and adults are asymptomatic. Gonococcal-associated PID after vaginal infection occurs more commonly among adolescents and adults than prepubertal girls.[16] In prepubertal boys the infection may present as asymptomatic pyuria, but symptomatic urethritis is more typical, as it is in adult males.[15,21,22] Concurrent infections with *C trachomatis* are common.[16]

Sexual contact is the most frequent cause of gonococcal infection in infants, children,[16] adolescents, and adults.[23] *N gonorrhoeae* is not part of the normal genital flora.[24–26] While identification of gonorrhea within the immediate neonatal period (birth through the first postnatal month) may represent perinatal transmission, detection of gonorrhea beyond that period is most indicative of contact with infected mucosal secretions. Nonsexual, fomite transmission of gonorrhea in children after the neonatal period, by use of communal baths; sharing of towels, fabric, and rectal thermometers; and caregiver's hands, has been proposed.[27] Gonococci can survive up to 24 hours on fomites (toilet seats, towels) in moist purulent secretions. However, supportive evidence for nonsexual transmission has methodological flaws and lacks rigorous study design.[21,27] Genital, rectal, or pharyngeal gonorrhea infection indicates sexual contact, unless evidence of perinatal transmission or clear, reasonable, and independently documented and rare nonsexual transmission exists.[28]

Current CDC guidelines recommend culture of potentially infected sites as the preferred, diagnostic gold standard for the identification of gonorrhea in children who have experienced sexual abuse, primarily due to its high specificity for medicolegal cases.[9,11,16,28] Culture is recommended specifically for specimens collected from the pharynx and anus in boys and girls, the vagina in girls, and the urethra in boys; cervical specimens are not recommended for prepubertal girls.[16] When culture methods are employed, accurate diagnosis is predicated on use of appropriate selective growth medium (modified Thayer-Martin, Martin-Lewis, or chocolate blood agar–based media) whose antibiotic components suppress endogenous bacteria and fungi present in the anatomical sites sampled.[11] Gram stain morphology is insufficient for diagnosis, because similar bacteria, including *Moraxella catarrhalis, Kingella denitrificans, Neisseria meningitidis, Neisseria lactamica,* and *Neisseria cinerea,* can be misidentified as *N gonorrhoeae*.[11,16,29] Use of multiple confirmatory techniques (biochemical carbohydrate utilization, enzyme substrate, serologic, or nucleic acid testing) is recommended by the CDC guidelines.[2,11,16,29] Follow-up cultures may be unnecessary, but all children diagnosed with gonococcal infections should be tested for *C trachomatis,* syphilis, and HIV.[16] Use of culture techniques presents limitations: many laboratories no longer offer culture-based tests, and risk for false results exists given limited laboratory experience with this historic testing technique.[9] Blood tests for the presence of antibody to the organism are unreliable because of a high false-negative rate among recently infected individuals.[19,20]

The American Academy of Pediatrics (AAP) recommends use of NAAT for the detection of gonorrhea infection among children who are suspected of having experienced sexual abuse.[9,30] Use of NAAT offers several clear advantages over culture, including higher sensitivity and noninvasive testing modality. However, limitations to the accurate detection of *N gonorrhoeae* by use of NAAT exist,[11] primarily related to the gonococcus capacity for genetic variation and recombination, which can affect targets for amplification and lead to false-negative results.[11,31,32] Nucleic acid amplification tests may also demonstrate cross-reactivity with other nongonococcal species and commensals, including *N cinerea, N flavescens, N lactamica, N sicca, N subflava,* and *M catarrhalis,* which may influence interpretation of results.[16,33]

To date, the US Food and Drug Administration (FDA) has not yet approved NAATs for the diagnosis of gonorrheal infections of extragenital sites (oropharynx and anus). However, laboratories may use NAATs for extragenital testing if internal validation of the method used occurs.[9,34] Studies evaluating extragenital testing by NAATs in prepubertal children are limited,[16,35] although literature on adult use is robust.[36–39] Insufficient data exist to guide use of NAATs in children for rectal or pharyngeal specimens, and results should be interpreted with caution.[9,16]

Chlamydial Infections

C trachomatis is a gram-negative, obligate intracellular bacteria. The species include oculo-genital and lymphogranuloma venereum (LGV) biovars. The oculo-genital biovars cause most urogenital infections as well as perinatal conjunctivitis and pneumonia, while LGV biovars are responsible for LGV. Some infected prepubertal girls have a vaginal discharge, but most chlamydial infections do not produce symptoms. The time between sexual contact and onset of vaginal symptoms in children is unknown; whether infections can relapse and how long infections may persist remains unclear. Therefore, it is difficult to determine when an infection was acquired.[21] Untreated chlamydia may be associated with serious complications in adolescents and adults, including pelvic inflammatory disease, ectopic pregnancy, and infertility; however, similar to gonococcal infections, spontaneous resolution also occurs.[40]

The mode of transmission is sexual in chlamydial infections in adolescents and adults, and *C trachomatis* or chlamydial infections are the most frequently diagnosed STI in adolescents and adults.[15] Among infants, perinatal maternal-neonate transmission is common. As many as 50% to 60% of neonates born to infected mothers acquire the infection or colonization, including 14% with subclinical rectal and vaginal colonization. The introduction of widespread screening of pregnant women as part of routine obstetric care has resulted in dramatically decreased rates of perinatally acquired infections among neonates in the United States.[2] Neonatal infections have been documented to persist for 12 months in 35% of colonized newborns, and 1 newborn still had a positive oropharyngeal culture at 28.5 months after birth but was subsequently negative at 3 years.[41,42] Therefore, positive cultures in children 3 years or younger may occasionally represent persistent perinatal infections. The obligate intracellular nature of the bacteria renders fomite transmission less likely, although transmission of ocular infection through nonporous surfaces has been suggested.[43] Genital or rectal chlamydia infection is indicative of sexual contact, unless evidence of perinatal transmission or clear, reasonable, and independently documented and rare nonsexual transmission exists.[20]

Culture techniques continue to be recommended by the CDC for children suspected to have experienced sexual abuse,[16] for specimens collected from the anus in both sexes and from the vagina in girls. Culture also remains the preferred testing method for extragenital sites. Only standard culture systems for the isolation of *C trachomatis* should be used, and when used, isolation of *C trachomatis* should be confirmed by microscopic identification of inclusions by staining with fluorescein-conjugated monoclonal antibody specific for *C trachomatis*. Isolates should be preserved for additional testing. Use of culture to detect chlamydial infections has significant limitations; cellular material must be collected because chlamydiae are obligate intracellular organisms,[44] estimated sensitivity of swabs is low, and recovery of the organism also depends on specimen handling. Enzyme immunoassay (EIA) and direct fluorescence antibody tests are extremely unreliable for vaginal or rectal specimens in children due to cross-reactivity with many common bacteria, including *N gonorrhoeae, Gardnerella vaginalis, Escherichia coli,* gram-negative enteric organisms, and group A and B streptococci.[11] False-positive cultures have been associated with the use of EIA to confirm tissue cultures.[2,45]

Nucleic acid amplification tests are recommended for use by the AAP among children suspected to have experienced sexual abuse,[9] and CDC guidelines indicate NAATs can be used for detection of *C trachomatis* in vaginal specimens or urine from girls.[46] Use of NAAT enhances sensitivity, especially for chlamydia infection, precisely because of the previously described limitations with culture techniques.[28] Limited data are available on the use of NAAT from urine in boys or for extragenital specimens (rectum, oropharynx) in both boys and girls.[16,35]

Nucleic Acid Amplification Tests for Chlamydia trachomatis *and* Neisseria gonorrhoeae

Nucleic acid amplification tests performed on urine specimens with confirmation offer a clear advantage over culture in sensitivity, are less invasive than swabs, reduce patient trauma and discomfort, and should be considered the new forensic standard for diagnosis in children who have experienced sexual abuse.[47] In a large multicenter study that compared use of NAAT urine and genital swabs versus culture for identification of *C trachomatis* and *N gonorrhoeae,* results demonstrated that prevalence of infection among 485 girls was 2.7% for chlamydia and 3.3% for gonorrhea, and the sensitivity of urine NAATs for chlamydia and gonorrhea relative to vaginal culture was 100%. Eight children with chlamydia-positive and 4 with gonorrhea-positive NAATs had negative culture results ($P = 0.018$); 24 of 485 (4.9%) of girls had a positive NAAT for chlamydia or gonorrhea or both, versus 16 of 485 (3.3%) with a positive culture for either, resulting in a 33% increase in children with positive diagnosis.[47]

A recent study described use of NAAT in detection of genital and extragenital gonorrhea and chlamydia infections among children and adolescents assessed for sexual abuse or assault. Of the 1,319 children and adolescents tested, 120 (9.1%) had at least 1 infected site, and more than 75% of those with positive extragenital tests had additional positive tests or anogenital injury. Most with a positive anal (59%) or oral (77%) test did not report the perpetrator's genitals contacted those specific sites. These results suggest that targeted testing based on disclosure may result in under-detection of infection.[35]

However, one major problem inherent in the use of NAATs in prepubertal children is the low prevalence of gonorrhea and chlamydia among children who have experienced sexual abuse. If very few tested patients have the disease, even a highly specific test will yield a substantial number of false positives. The positive predictive value of a test is dependent on the specificity of the test and the prevalence of the disease in the population studied. If the prevalence of gonorrhea or chlamydia in prepubertal children evaluated for sexual abuse is 1%, even if the test has a specificity of 99%, about one-half of the positive tests will be false positives. If the prevalence of either infection is 2%, about one-third of the tests will be false positives. However, clinicians face a dilemma because the false-negative rate is likely to be high for chlamydia cultures, and cultures may not be available in many localities, which leads to concerns about underdiagnosing and undertreating infections in children. This dilemma forces clinicians to consider options. If the major goal is to identify and treat the highest number of prepubertal children who are at risk of having gonorrhea or chlamydia, using NAATs achieves this goal. It also allows testing with minimally invasive urine tests. If the major goal is to identify the child with either infection, using the "gold standard" tests that are accepted proof of sexual contact, cultures are appropriate. If the goal is to have the best assessment of risk of infection and the best evidence, a dual or serial approach is best, such as obtaining both NAATs and cultures at the same time, or initially "screening" with a NAAT and confirming with culture. However, this serial approach poses practical challenges and requires getting the child to return for confirmatory testing, which may be difficult in some settings. Data on adults suggest a confirmatory test using a second NAAT that targets a different genetic sequence may be acceptable.[2,9]

Despite the widespread use of NAATs in clinical practice, acceptance by the medicolegal system of NAATs as a diagnostic standard for child sexual abuse cases remains controversial, and further study is required before changes to practice recommendations are definitive.[48,49] To overcome medicolegal challenges, more than one NAAT assay (2 NAATs that target different genetic sequences) should be used to assure confirmation of a diagnostic result, to ensure legal admissibility in court. It is possible that emerging technologies and upcoming revisions to CDC STI testing guidelines (anticipated in 2019) will recommend use of NAAT over culture routinely among those suspected of having experienced sexual abuse.

Medical professionals need to understand the testing capabilities and limitations of their local or regional laboratories. As a practical matter, there is no access to laboratories performing cultures for gonococcal or chlamydial infections in many localities. Sending a "culture specimen" to a laboratory unable to perform cultures will result in the specimen being rejected and discarded. Sending an improperly packaged sample for NAAT testing may also result in the specimen being rejected. Neither result serves the best interests of the child who presents with suspected sexual abuse or assault. Knowing what tests are available and the proper sample to send allows the medical professional to choose testing of genital, pharyngeal, and anal samples with NAATs that may not be currently FDA approved for these cases, rather than be left with no way to test for infection at all.

Syphilis

Treponema pallidum, the causative organism of syphilis infection, is a thin, motile spirochete that is capable of surviving only briefly outside a host and cannot grow on any known media. Primary lesions or chancres are painless, moist ulcerations with raised borders that may be mistaken for anal fissures or perianal cellulitis. Secondary syphilis may be mistaken for a viral exanthem with a variable skin rash, mucocutaneous lesions, and adenopathy; classic lesions of the palms and soles; or flat-surfaced, raised perineal lesions known as *condylomata lata*.[50–52] Tertiary syphilis occurs years after the primary infection and is characterized by cardiac involvement and gummatous changes of the skin, bone, or viscera. Latent syphilis occurs between the other stages and is characterized by positive syphilis serology in the absence of clinical signs or symptoms of the disease.[16]

There is extensive literature on syphilis in adults, but information on children, except for perinatal transmission, is limited to case reports or small case series. Infections occurring in infancy may have resulted from prenatal exposure, and recent CDC data indicate a resurgence in cases of congenital syphilis in the United States.[14] Primary disease presenting after 4 months of age or secondary disease presenting after the first year after birth should not be considered congenitally acquired. Evaluation of the mode of transmission of syphilis in preschool-aged children is difficult, however.[53] Prepubertal children with primary or secondary stages of syphilis occurring beyond early infancy should be presumed to have experienced sexual abuse.[6,52,54–56] Acquiring syphilis through blood transfusions is rare, and a few cases of facial lesions resulting from nonsexual transmission in children have been reported.[17] Two case reports attribute transmission by kissing from adult relatives with oral syphilis lesions to a 6-year-old girl and a 2½-year-old boy in the absence of disclosure of abuse.[57,58] Fomite transmission is extremely rare, because *T pallidum* is rapidly killed by drying, heat, disinfectant agents, and soaps;

does not survive well outside the human host; and has not been detected in urine, sweat, or milk. Syphilis is indicative of sexual contact unless evidence of perinatal transmission or clear, reasonable, and independently documented and rare nonsexual transmission exists.[16]

Syphilis is detected in 0.0% to 1.8% of those who reported experiencing sexual abuse.[3–5,15,55,56,59,60] Although routine testing of all those who have experienced sexual abuse is usually advisable, the low risk in children who have experienced abuse may support the practice of screening all adolescents but testing only children with a history of genital or perianal lesions, an exanthem, or another STI, or children whose known perpetrator has syphilis infection or who live in high-risk areas for syphilis.[15,55,59] Rising incidence of syphilis infections among certain adult sexually active populations, including males who have sex with males,[16] may result in changed epidemiology of infection among children who have experienced sexual abuse over time. Nontreponemal tests may yield negative results within months of treatment, and all results are negative within 2 years. Treponemal test results usually remain positive for life, but up to one-quarter of individuals with treated primary syphilis will have negative treponemal test results.

Nontreponemal reagin tests, such as the VDRL test and the rapid plasma regain, are commonly used for screening those who have experienced sexual abuse. Specific antibody tests for *T pallidum,* such as the fluorescent treponemal antibody or the microhemagglutination–*T pallidum,* must be done to confirm the screening test. Treponemal EIAs may be used for initial screening and positive test results confirmed with a nontreponemal test, reversing the traditional syphilis screening sequence.[11,16,61] The false-positive rate for both treponemal and nontreponemal test results in the general population is 1% to 2%. False-positive nontreponemal test results are the result of cross-reactivity with 1 of more than 200 nontreponemal antigens. False-positives can occur in numerous conditions, including other spirochetal infections, HIV, infectious mononucleosis, measles, varicella, hepatitis, autoimmune diseases, pregnancy, lymphoma, intravenous drug use, atopic dermatitis, bacterial pneumonias, bacterial endocarditis, and rickettsial infections and after immunizations. False-negative results can occur when very high antibody concentrations inhibit agglutination, known as the *prozone effect.* False-positive treponemal test results can occur in patients with elevated globulins, Lyme disease, leprosy, malaria, infectious mononucleosis, relapsing fever, leptospirosis, and autoimmune disease. False-negative treponemal and nontreponemal test results can occur in HIV infections. Repeat testing is often required because of the long, variable incubation period (10–90 days).[7,50,55]

Human Papillomavirus

Human papillomavirus (HPV) is a DNA virus that infects skin and mucous membranes. More than 150 types of HPV have been identified, with variable tropism for anogenital, oropharyngeal, or cutaneous sites. Anogenital warts are most commonly caused by types 6 and 11 (also types 16, 18, 31, and 35). Cutaneous warts are usually caused by types 1, 2, 3, 4, 7, and 10. Human papillomavirus types 16, 18, 31, and 45 have the highest oncogenic potential. Tropism exhibited by different HPV types is not absolute; cutaneous HPV types have been documented to occur at anogenital sites. Types 6 and 11 are predominant in oropharyngeal infection, primarily laryngeal papillomas or juvenile onset respiratory papillomatosis.[62]

An average incubation period of 2 to 3 months in both non-sexually and sexually acquired HPV infections has been suggested, but the interval from exposure to development of the lesions is extremely variable, possibly ranging from several weeks to several years.[62,63] Most infections are subclinical or latent, and viral transmission may occur from an individual without obvious mucosal or cutaneous lesions. Classic visible lesions characterizing HPV infection, condylomata acuminata, are soft, irregular, multidigitate verrucose growths (Figure 12.2). Other common HPV lesions

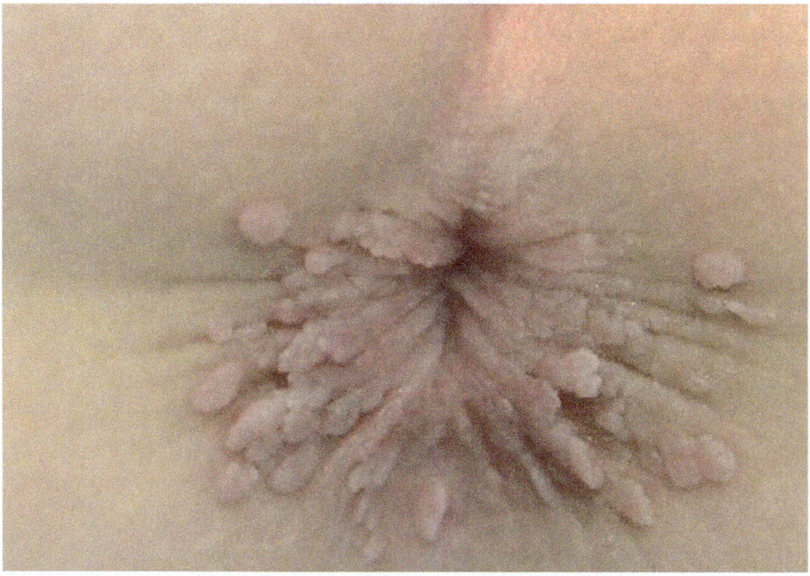

FIGURE 12.2
Anal warts in a 5-year-old boy.
From Nienow SM, Burrell T, Phillips J. Findings in sexual abuse. In: Anderst JD, ed. *Visual Diagnosis of Child Abuse.* 4th ed. Elk Grove Village, IL: American Academy of Pediatrics; 2016. Courtesy of Shalon M. Nienow, MD.

include small, flat, red, violaceous, or pigmented papules on the penile shaft; flat cervical growths; and fine irregularities of the vulvar tissues called *papillomatosis labialis*. While most lesions occur in the perineal area, they can be found on any moist skin areas or mucous membranes. Several levels of the genitourinary tract may be involved simultaneously, and some lesions may be entirely internal, located inside the urethra, vagina, or rectum.[63] Oral lesions and laryngeal lesions may also occur in children, having a similar appearance to the lesions on anogenital mucous membranes. Laryngeal papillomas or juvenile onset recurrent respiratory papillomatosis represent another presentation of HPV infection in children. National data suggest that two-thirds of cases are diagnosed by age 4 years and more than three-quarters of cases are diagnosed before age 7 years.[62] Laryngeal infections are rare: the CDC estimates 2 or fewer cases per 100,000 children younger than 18 years.[64]

Human papillomavirus infections are the most common STI in adolescents and young adults, and prevalence of HPV among sexually active young women as demonstrated by PCR testing ranges from 13% to 80%.[62] While mode of transmission among adults and adolescents is most commonly sexual, infections may be spread by sexual and nonsexual contact; fomite transmission has not been reported. Prenatal transmission, presumably through hematogenous spread, has been reported in a few cases presenting within the first week after birth.[62,65] The role of perinatal transmission remains unclear. The most comprehensive prospective study of infants and toddlers presents a strong argument against perinatal transmission: 74% of the mothers were HPV positive, but fewer than 3% of the infants were positive. Women who were HPV DNA positive were just as likely as HPV DNA–negative women to have HPV DNA–positive infants and toddlers, and the HPV subtypes in infant-mother pairs were not concordant.[66] This study and others suggest that exposure of an infant to HPV during vaginal delivery may be associated with only a low risk of acquiring HPV infection, and nonsexual transmission may occur during activities of normal infant care such as diapering and bathing.[62,67,68] Subclinical HPV infection has been demonstrated by DNA probes and antibody techniques in up to 24% of oral mucosal samples in preschool-aged children,[69] in 52% of oral samples in children 3 to 11 years of age,[70] and in the anal area in 1.2% and genital area in 3% of 5- to 6-year-olds who were reported to have not experienced abuse.[71] Subclinical infection has also been demonstrated in 5% to 33% of children who have experienced sexual abuse.[72–74] Nonsexual transmission of common warts (usually HPV type 2) has been implicated in some of the typical perineal lesions in young children.[65,75–77] However, it cannot be assumed that all perineal HPV are acquired by non-abusive digital genital contact; cutaneous warts could be transferred by autoinoculation or by common acts of sexual abuse such as fondling and digital penetration. Finally, whereas perinatal transmission is considered the etiology of laryngeal papillomatosis in children (and sexual transmission is rarely considered), the etiology of laryngeal papillomas in adults is attributed to sexual contact.[62]

The proportion of HPV infection among children resulting from sexual transmission is also unknown, but the likelihood of sexual contact versus nonsexual contact seems to increase with the age of the children studied. A prospective, multicenter, cross-sectional study conducted among children aged 0 to 13 years who were evaluated for sexual abuse found a genital HPV prevalence of 14% among children with definite, probable, or possible sexual abuse versus only 1% in those with no evidence of child sexual abuse.[30,78] Genital or anal condyloma acuminata in the absence of other indicators of abuse is a finding with no expert consensus on interpretation with respect to sexual contact, although lesions appearing for the first time in a child older than 5 years are considered more likely to be the result of sexual transmission.[28,48]

Diagnosis of HPV is primarily clinical, based on the typical wartlike appearance of the lesions; however, lesions may resemble condyloma lata and cautious interpretation is advisable. Clinical diagnosis is followed occasionally by biopsy and specific HPV viral typing techniques. Qualitative NAAT assays detect viral mRNA from high-risk HPV subtypes. Viral typing could allow comparison of the child's lesions with lesions from individuals with possible contact with the child[79]; however, similar HPV types in a child and an adult contact neither proves the adult was the source nor specifies whether the transmission was sexual or nonsexual. Multiple HPV types may coexist in the same individual, and the high prevalence of subclinical infections further undermines the utility of HPV typing for confirming child sexual abuse.[80]

Every child with anogenital or oral HPV infection, or diagnosed with laryngeal papillomatosis after age 5 years, should have a complete medical evaluation for sexual abuse.[7,28] However, if the history, the child's interview, the physical examination, and tests for other STIs do not support a diagnosis of sexual abuse, the conclusion should be that there was no clear evidence of sexual abuse and the case might represent nonsexual transmission. A referral to child protective services should be considered, although reporting may be deferred in circumstances in which suspicion of sexual abuse is low.

The Advisory Committee on Immunization Practices recommends HPV vaccination be initiated or completed for all children aged 9 years or older who have experienced sexual abuse during the initial evaluation for suspected abuse.[30] Children who have experienced sexual abuse are at high risk for future unsafe sexual practices linked to increased risk of HPV acquisition. While HPV vaccination will not protect against progression of infection already acquired or promote clearance of the infection, vaccination could provide protection against virus subtypes not yet acquired.[30] As a result of broader, more systematic vaccination of children and adolescents that is protective against multiple HPV subtypes, it is possible that the distribution of HPV subtypes responsible for disease manifestation in the future may change.

Trichomoniasis

T vaginalis is 1 of 3 related flagellated protozoans that infect humans. *T vaginalis* is the only clinically important species; the other 2 are primarily nonpathogenic species: *Trichomonas tenax* is normal mouth flora occasionally associated with dental or respiratory disease; *Pentatrichomonas hominis* is normal fecal flora. *P hominis* can survive and multiply at room temperature and survive in feces up to 24 hours. Skilled technicians can differentiate *T vaginalis* from the other species found in fresh vaginal secretions or urine through morphological differences, including the number and location of flagella, the appearance of the undulating membrane, and the characteristic motility pattern. *T vaginalis* must be differentiated from the other species that occasionally will be found in contaminated urine or vaginal secretions, including a structurally related but nonflagellated protozoan, *Dientamoeba fragillis*.[15] *T vaginalis* infections are characterized by a purulent vaginal discharge, although asymptomatic infections can occur. It is unknown how long children can be infected before developing symptoms.[22]

Trichomoniasis and bacterial vaginosis (BV) are the most frequently acquired infections following sexual assault in adult and adolescent females.[8,15,17] Infected mothers may transmit the infection to their neonates during birth, and these infections can persist for up to 1 year. However, the prevalence of *T vaginalis* in vaginally delivered neonates of mothers with documented infection is not known.[15] *T vaginalis* infection is uncommon in prepubertal girls beyond infancy and strongly suggests sexual abuse. Nonsexual transmission is theoretically possible because the organism can survive up to several hours on objects and in wet clothing, mud baths, and warm mineral water, although no cases of proven fomite transmission have been reported in either adults or children.[4,7] Therefore, trichomoniasis infections in prepubertal children beyond the first months after birth are strongly suggestive of sexual abuse.[1,81] *Trichomonas* infections are considered transmitted by sexual contact, unless there is evidence of perinatal transmission or clearly, reasonably, and independently documented but rare nonsexual transmission.[28] Evaluation of a child with *T vaginalis* infection should include an appropriate interview of the child, physical examination, and appropriate testing for other STIs.

Two older studies employing routine testing using wet mount preparations found no cases of *T vaginalis* among prepubertal children who are suspected of having experienced sexual assault.[24,60] Recent studies have described the prevalence of *Trichomonas* among children and adolescents evaluated for child sexual abuse. *Trichomonas* was detected by either wet mount or culture in 4% of 10- to 17-year-old girls with "evidence of hymenal estrogenization" (pubertal girls), of which only 5 of 12 had symptoms of vaginal discharge during examination.[82] Another study described results of *Trichomonas* NAAT testing on 406 urine samples obtained from children 0 to 13 years old who underwent child sexual abuse evaluations and found that 14 (3.4%) were positive by nested PCR assays, of which 6 of 14 samples came from individuals without vaginal discharge.[83] These results suggest that asymptomatic children who have experienced sexual abuse may also be infected and testing for asymptomatic infection may be warranted.[30]

The CDC recommends culture for *T vaginalis* infection and wet mount of a vaginal swab specimen for *T vaginalis* infection as gold standard testing modalities. Wet mount preparations identify only 50% to 65% of cases detectible by specific culture techniques. The sensitivity of cultures and NAATs approaches 95% in adults.[16] Testing for *T vaginalis* should not be limited to girls with vaginal discharge if other indications for vaginal testing exist, because there is some evidence to indicate that asymptomatic children who have experienced sexual abuse might be infected with *T vaginalis* and might benefit from treatment.[9,13] Data on use of NAAT for detection of *T vaginalis* in children are too limited to inform recommendations, but no evidence suggests that performance of NAAT for detection of *T vaginalis* in children would differ from that in adults.[16]

Herpes Simplex Virus Infection

Herpes simplex viruses are enveloped, double-stranded DNA viruses that are neurotrophic and capable of establishing latent and recurrent infections. Herpes simplex virus infection is characterized by painful vesicular or ulcerated lesions involving skin and mucous membranes, but primary infection can be asymptomatic (figures 12.3 and 12.4). The lesions in primary infections, often accompanied by fever, appear after an incubation period of 2 to 20 days (mean 6 days) after exposure. Nonsexual transmission is not well studied, but HSV type 1 (HSV-1) infections are a fairly common childhood infection usually involving only the mouth but occasionally the mouth and genital area simultaneously.[84–87] Herpes simplex virus type 1 infections usually cause

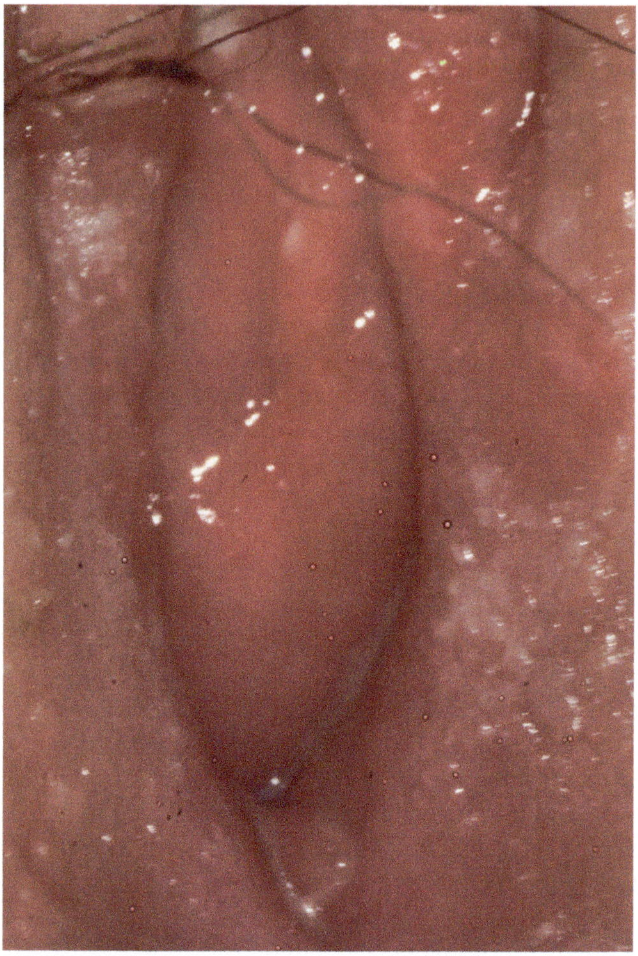

FIGURE 12.3

Herpes infection. This 11-year-old presented to the emergency department with complaints of acute genital pain. She was unable to urinate, defecate, or sit down. Result of human herpesvirus culture of this patient was positive for herpes simplex virus type 2 (human herpesvirus 2). The child had no other sexually transmitted infections and was determined to be HIV negative after completion of her testing cycle. Note the ulcerative lesions at the bases of the labia minora, on either side of the hymen.

From Nienow SM, Burrell T, Phillips J. Findings in sexual abuse. In: Anderst JD, ed. *Visual Diagnosis of Child Abuse*. 4th ed. Elk Grove Village, IL: American Academy of Pediatrics; 2016. Courtesy of Nancy Kellogg, MD.

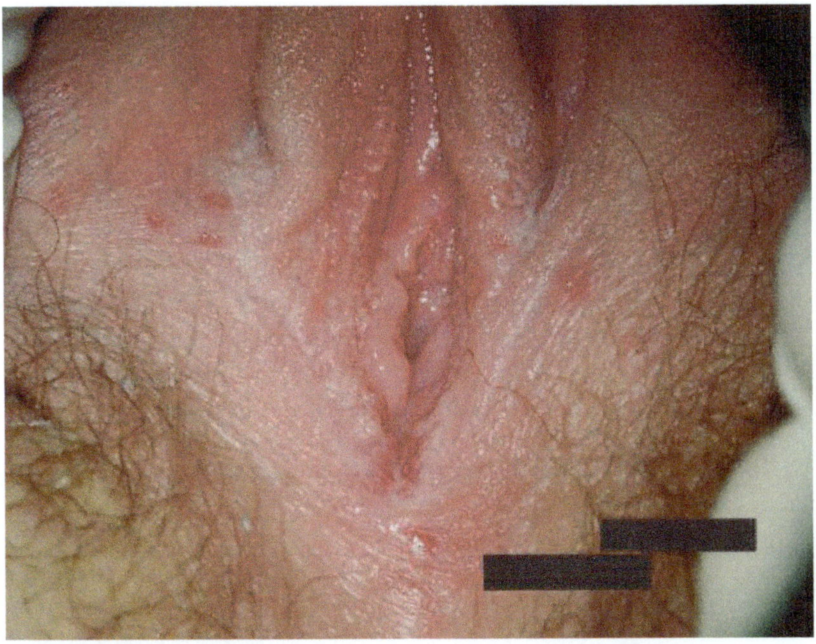

FIGURE 12.4
Herpes infection in a 14-year-old girl. Note the red ulcerated lesions on the medial aspects of her labia minora and in the fossa. Culture results proved these lesions to be herpes simplex virus type 2 (human herpesvirus 2).
Courtesy of Shalon M. Nienow, MD.

oral, labial, ocular, and brain infections, and most HSV-2 infections occur in the genital area or in cutaneous and disseminated neonatal infections. While both may cause recurrent disease, HSV-1 is more likely associated with mouth or lip lesions. Most cases of recurrent genital herpes are caused by HSV-2; therefore, a genital infection with HSV-1 is usually a primary infection because recurrent genital HSV-1 is uncommon. However, HSV-1 or HSV-2 can be found at either location. Historically, less than 20% of herpes genital infections were due to HSV-1, but multiple, more recent studies from around the world have documented HSV-1 as the cause of 33% to 71% of all herpes infections in the genital area. This increasing proportion of genital herpes caused by HSV-1 may be in part due to increased condom use during penile-anal and penile-genital intercourse but lack of condom use in oro-genital sex.[88]

Primary herpes genital infection is seen most frequently among sexually active adolescents and young adults. Genital herpes infections are uncommon in prepubertal children, and sexual abuse has been documented to be the cause in many cases.[4,18,21] In one study of

1,583 children younger than 13 years evaluated for suspected sexual abuse, 2 children (0.1%) had HSV-2 infection, but only 1 gave a history of sexual abuse.[59] However, most of the data on HSV-1 and HSV-2 genital infections in children come from case reports or small case series.[24,84–87,89] These cases include isolated genital infections with either HSV-1 or HSV-2, simultaneous infection of the oral and genital areas with HSV-1 and HSV-2, and one case of isolated perianal HSV-2 infection. A history of sexual contact was present in some cases and absent in others. The actual risk of acquiring the infection through sexual abuse is unknown.[15]

When a child has simultaneous oral and genital infection, or when an infant or toddler has a caregiver with oral lesions, it may be reasonable to conclude that nonsexual transmission of genital lesions due to HSV-1 is the cause. No cases of fomite transmission have been documented, but HSV can survive for up to 4 hours on plastic, rubber, and metal surfaces.[4] The evidence suggests that except for transmission at birth, most HSV-2 genital infections are sexually transmitted.[84,85] Either HSV-1 or HSV-2 infections in the genital area of a child or adolescent should be considered possible evidence of sexual abuse or sexual contact considering the changing epidemiology of HSV infection in the genital area in adolescents and adults. However, diagnosis of HSV-1 or HSV-2 infection in the genital or anal area of a child with no other indicators of sexual abuse is a finding with no expert consensus on interpretation with respect to sexual contact.[28]

Centers for Disease Control and Prevention guidelines recommend that specimens should be obtained from all vesicular or ulcerative genital or perianal lesions and then sent for viral culture or PCR.[16] Although asymptomatic viral shedding is frequent in adults, routine HSV cultures are of little value in asymptomatic children. Culture results of active lesions may be positive in approximately 95% from vesicles but only 70% from ulcerations and 30% from crusted lesions. Culture may distinguish HSV-1 from HSV-2 infection and differentiate between herpes simplex and varicella zoster, which may mimic genital or perianal infection.[90,91] Similar lesions include Lipschütz ulcers and aphthous ulcers and can also be caused by Epstein-Barr virus, influenza virus, coxsackievirus, and mycoplasma infections. While viral culture has remained the standard diagnostic method for isolation of HSV, real-time HSV PCR assays have emerged as a more sensitive method to confirm HSV infection in clinical specimens from genital ulcers or mucocutaneous sites.[11] While this methodology is particularly useful for detecting asymptomatic HSV infection among adults, cost may be a prohibitive factor.

In a study that tested 283 children for HSV-1 and HSV-2 antibodies by serology using a dot blot enzyme assay with monoclonal antibody inhibition for confirmation, antibody to HSV-1 was detected in 45.6% of samples, antibody to HSV-2 was detected in 7 (2.5%) of the samples, and 3 samples had antibody to both. Among cultures obtained from 12 children with compatible lesions, 5 (41.7%) results were positive, but only 1 culture-positive child had HSV-2 antibody.[13] Results suggest that type-specific serology for HSV has poor predictive value for diagnosis of HSV infection in children suspected to be sexually abused, and serology is not routinely warranted.

Bacterial Vaginosis

Bacterial vaginosis seems to be a marker of sexual activity in adults, but children may acquire the infection through sexual or nonsexual contact. Bacterial vaginosis (or nonspecific vaginitis) is a polymicrobial infection resulting from the replacement of *Lactobacillus* species with *G vaginalis*, *Mycoplasma hominis*, *Ureaplasma urealyticum*, and various anaerobic organisms. Although *G vaginalis* is one bacterium that may be involved in this infection, the presence or absence of this organism in a vaginal culture does not prove or disprove the diagnosis. Diagnosis requires both a microscopic examination of the discharge and simple chemical tests (Figure 12.5). The characteristic thin, gray-white to yellow vaginal discharge is examined microscopically for the presence of clue cells, which are epithelial cells with clusters of bacteria adhering to the surface. A "whiff test" is performed by the addition of 10% potassium hydroxide to the vaginal secretions, which results in a fishy or amine aroma in the

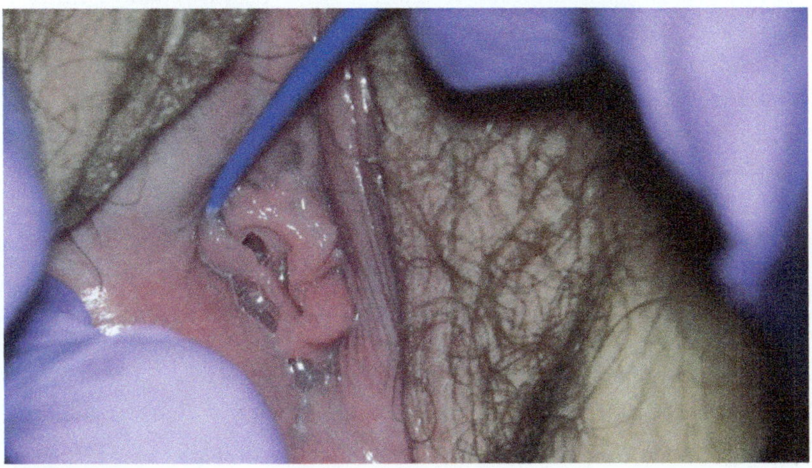

FIGURE 12.5
Bacterial vaginosis.
Courtesy of Shalon M. Nienow, MD.

presence of BV. Bacterial vaginosis is defined as "definite" when both clue cells and a positive whiff test result are found and "possible" when one of the 2 test results is positive.[7,17] A vaginal pH greater than 4.5 is present in pubertal females with the infection, but vaginal pH is not a reliable criterion in younger girls. Gram-stained vaginal smears showing no lactobacilli and predominant gram-negative and gram-variable rods are sensitive and specific for BV in adults.[15]

The infection rate is increased following sexual contact, but this entity may be the most common cause of non-sexually transmitted vaginitis in children and adolescents.[15,92] In a study of 26 girls younger than 14 years with symptomatic vulvovaginitis, the vaginal washings of 9 (35%) had diagnostic test results positive for BV. Only 3 of these girls had a history of sexual abuse.[22,93] The development of a new vaginal discharge following sexual abuse has been associated with BV, but the presence of this infection in a child may be attributed to either sexual or nonsexual transmission.[15,92,93] There is extensive literature on *G vaginalis* and BV in adults. Both the organism and the clinical infection are more prevalent among sexually active individuals, but both are also found in individuals who are not sexually active.

Several studies have compared the prevalence of *G vaginalis* in predominantly premenarcheal girls with and without vaginitis. Two studies of premenarcheal girls with vaginitis reported no positive culture results for *G vaginalis* among 54 and 200 girls, respectively.[26,94] One study found 2 of 50 cases were positive and 0 of 21 controls were positive for GV,[95] and another had no positive cultures for GV in either the 50 cases or 50 controls. Of 59 children cultured for GV, 3 of 8 positives had vaginitis and 8 of 51 negatives had vaginitis. The rate of positive cultures varied by age: 18% in children younger than 3 years, 2.5% in children 3 to 10 years old, and 63% in children 11 to 15 years old.[25]

Some studies have compared the prevalence of *G vaginalis* in cases of sexual abuse and in controls. One study found definite BV in 4 vaginal washings from 31 children, obtained 2 or more weeks after sexual abuse, whose initial test results were negative.[93] None of 23 specimen results from girls who had not experienced abuse were positive. Another study evaluated girls 1 to 11 years of age for *G vaginalis*. Of 137 with highly suspected or known sexual abuse, 14.6% of the results were positive; of 48 girls with genital symptoms but no history of abuse, 4.2% of the results were positive. Of 71 girls with neither a history of abuse or genital symptoms, 4.2% were positive.[96] A study involving girls 1 to 12 years of age found similar prevalence of *G vaginalis* in 3 groups of girls: 191 girls giving a history of sexual abuse or having another STI (5.3% positive), 144 girls evaluated for possible abuse but who gave no history of sexual contact and had no STI (4.9% positive), and 31 controls (6.4%).[97] Another study found *G vaginalis* in 24 of 209 girls who had experienced sexual abuse but in only 1 of 101 controls whose parents denied they were sexually active or sexually abused.[24] Two studies in menarcheal adolescents show higher rates of *G vaginalis* in girls who are sexually active (34% and 60%) compared with girls denying sexual activity (17% and 33%). Clinical BV was equally prevalent among those reporting or denying sexual contact in the one study[92] and was slightly more common among girls with *G vaginalis* than those without *G vaginalis*.[98] Only 2 studies provide data on prepubertal asymptomatic boys: one study found no anogenital culture results positive for *G vaginalis* in 99 boys, while the other found 2 positive anal cultures but no positive genital cultures in 99 boys.[99,100] Review of the literature on children and adolescents with *G vaginalis* and BV suggests both are found in girls with and without a history of sexual abuse or sexual contact, both are more prevalent in individuals who have experienced sexual abuse or who are sexually active than in controls, both are more prevalent in menarcheal than in premenarcheal girls, the *G vaginalis* organism is inconsistently associated with either genital symptoms or clinical BV, and the *G vaginalis* organism is rarely (but occasionally) found in boys who are asymptomatic and have not experienced abuse. Therefore, despite an association with sexual contact in children and adolescents, *G vaginalis* and BV have limited or indeterminate specificity for sexual contact or sexual abuse.

HIV Infection

HIV infection in children and adolescents is a complex, variable disease.[16,101–104] As a retrovirus, HIV carries single-stranded RNA and uses the enzyme reverse transcriptase to copy RNA into DNA and infect host cells of the immune system, CD4 helper T-lymphocyte cells. Once HIV infects a cell, it uses the host cell's machinery to replicate multiple copies of the entire virus, by a process known as reverse transcription. Replicated copies of HIV are released from the host cell and infect other immune cells, fundamentally impairing the body's ability to fight infection.

The potential long-term risk of HIV infection among children who have experienced sexual abuse is unknown, but it would be extremely unlikely for HIV infection to follow a single episode of sexual abuse. Sexual abuse has been implicated in cases of HIV infection,[101,102] although prevalence of infection among those suspected of experiencing abuse is low. One study found an extremely low prevalence (0% [95% CI, 0%–2%]) among children and adolescents aged 0 to 19 years who were evaluated for sexual abuse, despite location in a geographic area with high HIV prevalence.[103] Diagnosis of HIV infection in children should be considered sexually transmitted unless transmission perinatally or through transfusion is documented.[28]

Screening of children who have experienced sexual abuse for HIV infection seems most reasonable if they give a history of vaginal or rectal penetration by multiple perpetrators or an unknown perpetrator or are symptomatic for HIV or any STI, or if the perpetrator is known to have HIV infection, is known to be homosexual or bisexual, or is a known intravenous drug user[15]; high prevalence of HIV infection regionally may also be considered a risk factor. Some experts recommend that all children who have experienced sexual abuse be screened for HIV, recognizing that many positive tests will result because of previously undocumented neonatal transmission. Screening of the perpetrator first, and then screening only a child whose perpetrator was positive for HIV is ideal, but this may not be a legal option in many states. The issue of HIV infection should be addressed with every child and his or her family, and regardless of the decision about testing, appropriate counseling support and follow-up should be provided.[15,88]

Laboratory testing to detect HIV infection is rapidly evolving. Currently, the CDC recommends that initial testing be performed with an antigen/antibody combination (fourth-generation) immunoassay[16,103,104] that detects HIV-1 and HIV-2 antibodies and HIV-1 p24 antigen to screen for established infection with HIV-1 or HIV-2 and for acute HIV-1 infection. Initial testing using a fourth-generation technique detects more acute HIV-1 infections than third-generation antibody immunoassays and identifies established HIV-1 and HIV-2 infections with comparable specificity.[103] If initial immunoassay is repeatedly reactive, supplemental testing (HIV-1/HIV-2 antibody differentiation assay, Western blot, or indirect immunofluorescence assay) should be performed.[16] It is recommended that HIV antigen/antibody testing be repeated at 4 to 6 weeks, 3 months, and 6 months after exposure.[16,105]

Other Sexually Transmitted Infections

Anogenital signs and symptoms can be the result of sexual abuse, but these are common in children who have not experienced abuse as well. Most children presenting with anogenital signs and symptoms in the absence of a verbal disclosure of abuse are unlikely to be diagnosed with either STIs or sexual abuse even after a thorough assessment.[106] Symptoms suggesting urinary tract infections are much more common than actual urinary tract infections in children who have experienced sexual abuse.[107] Information is limited about other STIs and their association with sexual abuse of children. This lack of information is attributed to several factors; many have primarily nonsexual modes of transmission in children, some have a low prevalence among adults, and some are extremely rare in children.[7,15]

Genital Mycoplasmas

Other STIs are considered "emerging" in adults, with limited information on acquisition among children.[16,108] For example, *M hominis*, *Mycoplasma genitalium*, and *U urealyticum* are small pleomorphic bacteria that lack a cell wall. Colonization or asymptomatic infections with the genital mycoplasmas, *M hominis*, *M genitalium*, and *U urealyticum*, strongly correlate with sexual activity in adults. Neither organism is clearly linked to vaginal infections, although they may be present in some cases of BV, but *U urealyticum* and *Mycoplasma* have been increasingly recognized as causes of nongonococcal urethritis in adults.[16,22] Two controlled studies of pharyngeal, anorectal, and vaginal colonization rates in children who had and had not experienced abuse with genital mycoplasmas have been reported.[109,110] In one study, *M hominis* was isolated from the anorectal and vaginal cultures of 23% and 34% of the 47 girls who had experienced abuse, compared with 8% and 17%, respectively, of the 36 controls. *U urealyticum* was isolated from the anorectal and vaginal cultures of 19% and 30% of the girls who had experienced abuse, compared with 3% and 8%, respectively, of 36 controls.[109] The other study showed no significant difference in colonization with genital mycoplasmas between children who had experienced abuse and controls.[110] No association was found between colonization with either organism and the presence of a discharge in these children. In summary, increased colonization has been demonstrated among children who have experienced sexual abuse for both genital mycoplasmas and *U urealyticum*. These organisms should not be considered significant markers for sexual abuse, however, because asymptomatic colonization is also common among children who have not experienced abuse. With the concerns about the increasing role of *M genitalium* as an adult STI, additional inquiry as to its role in children is warranted.[108]

Nucleic acid amplification testing is the preferred method for laboratory detection specifically for *Mycoplasma*, based in part on the limitations of culture technique due to the organism's slow growth. While NAAT is not widely available or approved yet by the FDA for use in the United States, PCR or transcription-mediated amplification techniques for *Mycoplasma* are available in some large medical centers, commercial laboratories, and research settings.[16] Nucleic acid amplification testing of urine, urethral, vaginal, and cervical swabs can be considered.[16]

Ectoparasites

Ectoparasites including *Sarcoptes scabiei* (scabies), *Phthirus pubis* (pubic or "crab" lice), *Pediculus humanus humanus* (body lice), and *Pediculus humanus capitis* (head lice) can be sexually transmitted, but close nonsexual body contact is the predominant mode of transmission in children. Pubic lice is the only species of lice to infest the eyelashes, and in addition to the pubic and perianal hair, it can infest the beard, eyebrows, and axillary hair. Scabies, body lice, and head lice are primarily spread by close body contact in all age groups. Sexual contact is the primary mode of transmission for pubic lice in adolescents and adults, and the possibility of sexual abuse should be considered in children with this ectoparasite.[2,7,16]

Molluscum Contagiosum

Molluscum contagiosum, a poxvirus infection, is transmitted through close body contact. The lesions are dome-shaped, skin-colored papules that often have umbilicated white centers. Occasionally they form larger, clustered lesions that may have multiple umbilications and mimic the appearance of warts. The lesions are typically found on the extremities and trunk in children, but the virus may be self-inoculated through scratching and touching of the perineal skin. It has been linked to sexual activity in adolescents and adults, but nonsexual transmission is common in both children and adults.[7] Molluscum is a finding commonly seen in children who have not experienced abuse and lacks specificity for sexual abuse.

Miscellaneous Enteric Pathogens

Shigellosis, salmonellosis, amoebiasis, giardiasis, and infections with *Campylobacter* species are predominantly caused by nonsexual transmission. These enteric pathogens are also known to be sexually transmitted, primarily among males having sexual contact with males.[2,7]

Viral Hepatitis

Sexual transmission accounts for most hepatitis B virus (HBV) infections in the United States. Homosexuals, bisexuals, and heterosexuals with multiple partners have higher rates of HBV infections. Infants can acquire the infection through vertical transmission, and older children develop HBV primarily through nonsexual contact with infected individuals. Sexual transmission is possible for hepatitis C virus (HCV), but the very low prevalence of infection among sexual partners of individuals with chronic HCV infection suggests the risk of sexual transmission is limited. Men who have sex with men and individuals with HIV infection are at increased risk of HCV transmission. Most cases of HCV infections in children result from perinatal transmission, and in adults result from exposure to infected blood.[2,16] Baseline serologic testing for HBV is recommended by the CDC for those who have experienced sexual abuse, but there is no consensus on HCV testing.[10,16] Accurate interpretation of HBV serology is critical to assess the likelihood of acquisition of infection from sexual contact.

Hepatitis B surface antigen (HBsAg) is present in both acute and chronic infection, whereas the presence of hepatitis B core antigen (IgM anti-HBc) is diagnostic of acute or recently acquired HBV infection. Antibody to HBsAg is produced after a resolved infection and is the only HBV antibody marker present after vaccination. The presence of HBsAg and total anti-HBc, with a negative test result for IgM anti-HBc, indicates chronic HBV infection. The presence of anti-HBc alone might indicate acute, resolved, or chronic infection or a false-positive result.[16] Hepatitis B vaccine is recommended by the CDC for children who have experienced sexual abuse at the time of assault evaluation if not previously immunized, whereas hepatitis B immune globulin is recommended as adjuvant therapy to hepatitis B vaccination if the perpetrator is known to be hepatitis B positive.[16] If screening for HCV is desired, testing should include an FDA-cleared test for antibody to HCV, followed by confirmatory testing using a NAAT to detect HCV RNA.[16]

Lymphogranuloma Venereum, Chancroid, and Granuloma Inguinale

Lymphogranuloma venereum, chancroid, and granuloma inguinale are uncommon STIs in the United States. In 2016, the CDC received reports of only 7 cases of chancroid. Granuloma inguinale is considered rare, and no current data are available.[14] The prevalence of LGV in the United States is unknown, because tests to differentiate LGV from non-LGV *C trachomatis* are not widely available. All 3 diseases are likely to be underdiagnosed and underreported. Children can acquire LGV through sexual contact, but accidental inoculation may occur through contact with drainage from ulcers or buboes (abscesses). Lymphogranuloma venereum, caused by *C trachomatis* biovars or serotypes L1, L2, and L3, is a systemic infection that is associated with ulcers and granulomas, inguinal and perianal abscesses, and proctocolitis. Lymphogranuloma venereum may be becoming better recognized among adults, particularly in males. Chancroid is caused by *Haemophilus ducreyi,* a gram-negative coccobacillus, with sexual contact its only known route of transmission. Granuloma inguinale is caused by *Klebsiella granulomatis,* an intracellular gram-negative bacillus, and is rare outside of the tropics.[22] This organism is not highly contagious; however, it can be transmitted sexually, through close nonsexual contact, and through fomites.

Group B β-hemolytic Streptococci

Group B β-hemolytic streptococci (GBS) colonize the genital tract of between 5% and 40% of postpubertal women, and neonates may develop severe infections through vertical transmission. The organism is also a known colonizer of the anogenital area of children and a possible pathogen for vulvovaginitis in children, adolescents, and adults.[111] In a study of the normal vaginal flora of girls 2 months to 15 years of age, colonization with GBS was found in 23% of girls 2 to 35 months of age, 16% of girls 3 to 10 years of age, and 20% of girls 11 to 15 years of age. Multiple site colonization (vaginal, anal, pharyngeal) was common in the youngest group, and 2-site colonization (vaginal, anal) was common in the oldest group. In girls 3 to 10 years of age, vaginal and anal colonization were 4% each, and pharyngeal colonization was 14%.[112] One study of childhood vulvovaginitis showed that 5% of controls but no symptomatic girls had GBS, and in another study, 2% of both cases and controls had GBS.[95,113] Group B streptococci commonly colonize the anogenital tract of females of all ages and occasionally are found in symptomatic females with vulvovaginitis. There are no clear data to link either symptomatic or asymptomatic GBS with sexual abuse considering the significant rate of colonization in all age groups.

Recommended Sexually Transmitted Infection Testing of Children Who Are Suspected of Having Experienced Sexual Abuse or Assault

Prepubertal Children

The CDC does not recommend STI testing of all children who are suspected of having experienced sexual abuse.[9,16,30] The decision to test for STIs should be made on an individual basis, weighing the risk of infection against the additional discomfort of obtaining specimens from a young child. Criteria for screening for STI include historical and physical parameters associated with increased risk of infection (Box 12.1). The CDC recommends selected, high-risk children who have experienced sexual abuse be tested for gonorrhea, chlamydia, syphilis, HIV, and hepatitis B. In girls, vaginal secretions should be evaluated for trichomoniasis and BV. Children should be assessed for warts or lesions and any ulcers or vesicles cultured for herpes. Follow-up testing for STIs is also recommended by the CDC[16] (Box 12.2). Follow-up testing has been shown to increase detection of STIs in children and adolescents who have recently experienced abuse.[114]

Pubertal Adolescents and Adults

Routine STI testing of pubertal adolescents and adults who are suspected of having experienced sexual abuse is generally warranted (Box 12.3). Among sexually active adolescents and adults who have high prevalence of STIs, post-assault STI testing may identify previously acquired STIs,

BOX 12.1
Selection Criteria for Testing Children and Adolescents Who Have Experienced Sexual Abuse for Sexually Transmitted Infections[a]

Historical

History of penetration or evidence of recent or healed penetrative injury to the genitals, anus, or oropharynx

Abuse by a stranger

Perpetrator has known STI or has high risk for STI

Sibling or another child in household has known STI

Abuse by multiple perpetrators

Prior consenting sexual contact

History of genital discharge, signs or symptoms of an STI, or already diagnosed with an STI

Physical

Sexual maturity rating/Tanner stage 3 or greater

Genital discharge present

Genital/oral/anal injury present (recent or healed)

Presence of specific STI lesions (ulcers, warts)

General

Child or parent requests STI testing

High prevalence of STIs in child's community

Abbreviation: STI, sexually transmitted infection.

[a] Data supporting criteria from girls primarily; limited data available from boys.

Criteria adapted from Workowski KA, Bolan GA; Centers for Disease Control and Prevention. Sexually transmitted diseases treatment guidelines, 2015. *MMWR Recomm Rep*. 2015;64(RR-03):1–137; Seña AC, Hsu KK, Kellogg N, et al. Sexual assault and sexually transmitted infections in adults, adolescents, and children. *Clin Infect Dis*. 2015;61(Suppl 8):S856–S864; and Jenny C, Crawford-Jakubiak JE; American Academy of Pediatrics Committee on Child Abuse and Neglect. The evaluation of children in the primary care setting when sexual abuse is suspected. *Pediatrics*. 2013;132(2):e558–e567.

incubating STI infection from the assault, or, in some cases, pathogens in the ejaculate that may or may not result in infection. Some evaluators do not routinely test adolescents and adults whom they are routinely treating with prophylactic antibiotics because of concerns that information about a previously acquired STI may undermine the credibility of the victim. This approach may negatively affect the public health response to reporting, assessing, and treating sexual contacts for infection, while ignoring the fact that identification and treatment of STIs following an assault in adolescents and adults is more important from a psychological and medical standpoint rather than from an evidentiary perspective.

Sexually transmitted infections may be diagnosed in children evaluated for sexual abuse who have not made a disclosure of abuse. For both prepubertal

BOX 12.2
Centers for Disease Control and Prevention–Recommended Sexually Transmitted Infection Testing for Prepubertal Children Evaluated for Suspected Sexual Abuse

Routine testing is not recommended. The following tests for STI should be performed on selected, high-risk children who have experienced sexual abuse:

1. Gonococcal (gonorrhea) cultures from pharyngeal, anal, and urethral (boys) or vaginal (girls) sites. Vaginal or urine NAATs for girls, with confirmation.
2. Chlamydial cultures from vaginal and anal sites in girls and anal and urethral sites in symptomatic boys. Vaginal or urine NAATs for girls, with confirmation.
3. Blood sample for immediate serology for syphilis, HIV, hepatitis B, and preserved for subsequent analysis.
4. Examination for anogenital warts or ulcerative lesions and cultures sent for herpes if ulcers are present.
5. For girls, culture or wet mount of vaginal secretions for microscopic examination for *Trichomonas* and tests for bacterial vaginosis; data insufficient to recommend use of NAATs for children.
6. Follow-up evaluation approximately 2 weeks after last exposure can be considered.
7. Six weeks and 3 months later, recommend repeating all serologic tests.
8. For prepubertal girls presenting with vaginal discharge, add routine bacterial cultures because they may have non-sexually transmitted rather than sexually transmitted pathogens.

Abbreviations: HIV, human immunodeficiency virus; NAAT, nucleic acid amplification test; STI, sexually transmitted infection.

From Workowski KA, Bolan GA; Centers for Disease Control and Prevention. Sexually transmitted diseases treatment guidelines, 2015. *MMWR Recomm Rep.* 2015;64 (RR-03):1–137.

BOX 12.3
Centers for Disease Control and Prevention–Recommended Sexually Transmitted Infection Evaluation for Adolescents and Adults Who Have Experienced Acute Sexual Assault

1. NAATs for gonorrhea and chlamydia from all sites of penetration or attempted penetration.
2. NAATs from a urine or vaginal specimen or point-of-care testing (ie, DNA probes) from a vaginal specimen for *Trichomonas vaginalis*.
3. Point-of-care testing and/or wet mount with measurement of vaginal pH and potassium hydroxide application for the "whiff test" from vaginal secretions should be done for evidence of BV and candidiasis, especially if vaginal discharge, malodor, or itching is present.
4. Blood sample for serologic testing for syphilis, HIV, and hepatitis B. (**Note:** Hepatitis C serology is not recommended routinely by the CDC 2015 STI guidelines[16] but is recommended by the 2016 CDC

(continued)

BOX 12.3 (*continued*)

"Updated Guidelines for Antiretroviral Postexposure Prophylaxis After Sexual, Injection Drug Use, or Other Nonoccupational Exposure to HIV"[105] and others.[10])

5. Repeat testing should be considered at a 2-week follow-up.
6. Four to 6 weeks and 3 months later, repeat syphilis serology; 6 weeks, 3 months, and 6 months later, repeat HIV serology. For those receiving postexposure prophylaxis for HIV, repeat hepatitis B and hepatitis C serology at 6 months.[105]
7. Follow-up examination at 1–2 months should be considered to reevaluate for development of anogenital warts.

Abbreviations: BV, bacterial vaginosis; CDC, Centers for Disease Control and Prevention; HIV, human immunodeficiency virus; NAAT, nucleic acid amplification test; STI, sexually transmitted infection.

children and adolescents who have experienced sexual abuse, reliance on report of symptoms or types of disclosed sexual contact to determine need for testing and sites of testing may result in under-detection of STIs.[35]

Sexually Transmitted Infection Treatment

Prophylactic Antibiotic Therapy

Prophylactic antibiotic therapy for children who have experienced sexual abuse is a controversial subject, but routine prophylaxis is not generally recommended.[1,2,7,16,17,21,22,30,60] Routine prophylaxis with an antibiotic that covers chlamydia, gonorrhea, trichomoniasis, and BV is commonly offered to adolescents and adults presenting with recent sexual contact (Table 12.3). If the individual was not immunized for hepatitis B, the CDC recommends a first dose of vaccine, with follow-up doses to be given 1 to 2 months and 4 to 6 months after the initial dose.[16]

Postexposure prophylaxis (PEP) for HIV is controversial in people of all ages who are suspected of having experienced sexual abuse. HIV prophylaxis has been shown to be effective for perinatal transmission and occupational needlestick exposures, but there are few data on the efficacy of HIV prophylaxis for nonoccupational exposures. The CDC recommends considering the use of PEP for HIV in sexual abuse or assault cases when the perpetrator is known to be HIV infected, multiple perpetrators are involved, the exposure event presents a substantial risk of transmission (eg, oral, anal, or vaginal penetration or trauma; ejaculation occurring on a mucous membrane; mucosal lesions present), local HIV prevalence is high, and treatment can be initiated within 72 hours.[10,16,30] If the perpetrator's HIV status is unknown, PEP should be considered on a case-by-case basis. If there is "negligible exposure risk," HIV PEP is not recommended. Health care

TABLE 12.3

Centers for Disease Control and Prevention–Recommended Prophylaxis for Adolescents and Adults Who Have Experienced Acute Sexual Assault[a]

Drug	Dosage
Ceftriaxone	250 mg intramuscularly in a single dose
	Plus
Metronidazole or tinidazole	2 g orally in a single dose
	Plus
Azithromycin	1 g orally in a single dose
OR	
Doxycycline	100 mg orally twice a day for 7 d
Hepatitis B vaccine	If not previously immunized, give initial dose and schedule follow-up doses 1–2 mo and 4–6 mo after first dose.
HBIG	Recommended as adjunct to hepatitis B immunization if perpetrator known to be hepatitis B positive.
HPV vaccination	Prophylaxis (initiation or series completion) should be considered among age-eligible adolescents/adults (females 9–26 y, males 9–21 y).
HIV PEP	Generally recommended if adolescent/adult presents for evaluation $\leq$ 72 h postexposure and perpetrator known to be HIV positive or have significant exposure risk.[b] May also be considered, on a case-by-case basis, if the perpetrator HIV status is unknown. For adolescents and adults presenting with "negligible exposure risk" or presenting > 72 h postexposure, PEP is not recommended.

Abbreviations: HBIG, hepatitis B immune globulin; HIV, human immunodeficiency virus; HPV, human papillomavirus; PEP, postexposure prophylaxis.

[a] This is empiric therapy for gonorrhea, chlamydia, incubating syphilis, trichomoniasis, and bacterial vaginosis. Routine prophylaxis is not recommended for prepubertal children. HIV prophylaxis is controversial. Discuss risk of HIV and HIV prophylaxis, including toxicity and unknown efficacy. Consultation with HIV specialist is recommended if prophylaxis is to be given.

[b] Significant exposure risk: high local/community geographic prevalence of HIV infection; multiple perpetrators; likelihood of ejaculation of mucous membrane contact; mucosal lesions present; oral, vaginal, or anal trauma or penetration.

Derived from Workowski KA, Bolan GA; Centers for Disease Control and Prevention. Sexually transmitted diseases treatment guidelines, 2015. *MMWR Recomm Rep*. 2015;64(RR-03):1–137; and Centers for Disease Control and Prevention. Updated guidelines for antiretroviral postexposure prophylaxis after sexual, injection drug use, or other nonoccupational exposure to HIV—United States, 2016. https://www.cdc.gov/hiv/pdf/programresources/cdc-hiv-npep-guidelines.pdf. Published 2016. Accessed August 7, 2019.

professionals should discuss the risk of the person who has experienced sexual abuse acquiring HIV; the potential benefits of PEP, yet its unknown efficacy in this setting; and known toxicity with the patient and his or her parents in the case of children. Most experts advise a highly active antiretroviral therapy, a 3-drug combination of 2 nucleoside analog reverse transcriptase inhibitors, plus 1 protease inhibitor for child and adolescent PEP.[105] The 3-drug regimens have been shown to be more likely to suppress virus replication, but multiple drug regimens are likely to increase potential toxicity and decrease compliance with the required 28-day PEP course. Clinicians involved in acute sexual abuse evaluations of children and adolescents should establish a protocol that includes the approach to PEP discussion, immediate availability of a 3- to 7-day starter kit of the PEP drugs, and a follow-up in consultation with a pediatric infectious disease specialist.[10,16,30,105]

Specific Therapy for Documented Infections

Appropriate treatment regimens are shown in Table 12.4. Ceftriaxone is the preferred treatment of proctitis, pharyngitis, and vaginal or urethral gonococcal infections and is effective in treating gonorrhea

TABLE 12.4
Guidelines for Treatment of Sexually Transmitted Infections in Children and Adolescents According to Organism

Preferred regimens are listed. For more information about other acceptable regimens and diseases not included, see the Centers for Disease Control and Prevention (CDC) 2015 sexually transmitted diseases treatment guidelines and updates on the CDC website.		
Organisms/Diagnoses	**Treatment of Adolescent**	**Treatment of Child**
Neisseria gonorrhoeae Uncomplicated infections of the cervix, vagina, urethra, rectum, pharynx	Ceftriaxone, 250 mg, IM, in a single dose **OR** cefixime, 400 mg, orally, in a single dose **PLUS** Azithromycin, 1 g, orally, in a single dose	**Children < 45 kg** Ceftriaxone, 25–50 mg/kg, IM, in a single dose, not to exceed 125 mg **Children ≥ 45 kg** Treat with adolescent medication dosages.
Chlamydia trachomatis	Azithromycin, 1 g, orally, in a single dose **OR** Doxycycline, 100 mg, orally, twice a day for 7 d	Erythromycin base or ethylsuccinate, 50 mg/kg per day, orally, in 4 divided doses (maximum 2 g/d) for 14 d **Children < 45 kg and Younger Than 8 y** Azithromycin 20 mg/kg orally as a single dose **OR** 20 mg/kg orally once daily for 3 d **Children ≥ 45 kg but Younger Than 8 y** Azithromycin, 1 g, orally, in a single dose **Children 8 y or Older** Treat with adolescent medication dosages.
Trichomonas vaginalis	Metronidazole, 2 g, orally, in a single dose **OR** Tinidazole, 2 g, orally, in a single dose	**Children < 45 kg** Metronidazole 15 mg/kg/d divided 3 times daily orally for 7 days, not to exceed 2,000 mg **Children ≥ 45 kg** Treat with adolescent medication dosages.
Syphilis Primary and secondary syphilis	Benzathine penicillin G, 2.4 million units, IM, in a single dose	Benzathine penicillin G, 50,000 units/kg, IM, in a single dose, not to exceed 2.4 million units

Abbreviation: IM, intramuscularly.

and incubating syphilis. Ceftriaxone 250 mg intramuscularly or cefixime 400 mg orally alone are not adequate for treatment because of increasing bacterial resistance and should only be given when combined with azithromycin. Therapy of anogenital warts is complicated, and some clinicians often wait for spontaneous resolution of the lesions. Each therapeutic method is directed toward symptomatic warts. These methods, however, often do not eradicate the infection, prevent recurrences, or decrease infectivity. Most therapeutic methods require administration by a health care professional. Two options are available for patient-applied treatment of HPV lesions: podofilox 0.5% solution or gel, an antimitotic drug, and imiquimod 5% cream, an immune enhancer that stimulates production of interferon and other cytokines. Inflammatory reactions are common but often milder than with other agents. There are no data on the efficacy of cimetidine in genital warts in children. Oral antiviral agents seem to shorten the duration of symptoms and reduce viral shedding in primary HSV infections but have no effect on the risk, frequency, or severity of recurrences. Primary infections may be treated with oral acyclovir, valacyclovir, or famciclovir for 7 to 10 days. These agents also can be effective in reducing the severity and duration of symptoms when used to treat recurrent episodes.[2,16,22]

Conclusion

Children and adolescents who have experienced sexual abuse are at risk for acquiring STIs. Sexually transmitted infections are common among sexually active adolescents but are not commonly identified in prepubertal children. Therefore, the presence of an STI in a child should raise concerns of sexual abuse, and an appropriate evaluation for child sexual abuse should be initiated. Several studies suggest approximately 5% of prepubertal children evaluated for sexual abuse will have an STI. Sexually transmitted infections are more commonly identified in pubertal adolescents than in prepubertal children being evaluated for suspected sexual assault or abuse. The presence of an STI in the pubertal adolescent may represent an infection acquired through the abuse or prior consensual/peer-aged sexual activity. Selective testing and specific treatment of STIs are often warranted in prepubertal children, while routine testing and prophylaxis are typically warranted in adolescents.

Although any STI could be acquired through abusive contact, the strength of the association between STI and child sexual abuse varies from disease to disease. Several factors must be considered when evaluating the strength of association between an STI and child sexual abuse, particularly the age of the child and the specific disease identified. The disease must be diagnosed by using tests that have an acceptable degree of specificity in children. The diagnosis of an STI in a child who is suspected of experiencing sexual abuse has social and legal implications. Missing evidence of an STI in a child may place the child at risk for continued abuse; however, a mistaken diagnosis or mistaken interpretation could lead to inappropriate child protection and criminal interventions.

References

1. Kellogg N; American Academy of Pediatrics Committee on Child Abuse and Neglect. The evaluation of sexual abuse in children. *Pediatrics*. 2005;116(2):506–512 PMID: 16061610 https://doi.org/10.1542/peds.2005-1336
2. Workowski KA, Berman SM; Centers for Disease Control and Prevention. Sexually transmitted diseases treatment guidelines, 2006. *MMWR Recomm Rep*. 2006;55 (RR-11):1–94 PMID: 16888612
3. De Jong AR. Sexually transmitted diseases in sexually abused children. *Sex Transm Dis*. 1986;13(3):123–126 PMID: 3764623 https://doi.org/10.1097/00007435-198607000-00002
4. Neinstein LS, Goldenring J, Carpenter S. Nonsexual transmission of sexually transmitted diseases: an infrequent occurrence. *Pediatrics*. 1984;74(1):67–76 PMID: 6610855
5. White ST, Loda FA, Ingram DL, Pearson A. Sexually transmitted diseases in sexually abused children. *Pediatrics*. 1983;72(1):16–21 PMID: 6688126
6. Hammerschlag MR. Sexually transmitted diseases in sexually abused children: medical and legal implications. *Sex Transm Infect*. 1998;74(3):167–174 PMID: 9849550 https://doi.org/10.1136/sti.74.3.167
7. Finkel MA, De Jong AR. Medical findings in child sexual abuse. In: Reece R, Ludwig S, eds. *Child Abuse: Medical Diagnosis and Management*. 2nd ed. Philadelphia, PA: Lippincott Williams & Wilkins; 2001:207–286
8. Jenny C, Hooton TM, Bowers A, et al. Sexually transmitted diseases in victims of rape. *N Engl J Med*. 1990;322(11):713–716 PMID: 2155389 https://doi.org/10.1056/NEJM199003153221101
9. Jenny C, Crawford-Jakubiak JE; American Academy of Pediatrics Committee on Child Abuse and Neglect. The evaluation of children in the primary care setting when sexual abuse is suspected. *Pediatrics*. 2013;132(2):e558–e567 PMID: 23897912 https://doi.org/10.1542/peds.2013-1741
10. Crawford-Jakubiak JE, Alderman EM, Leventhal JM; American Academy of Pediatrics Committee on Child Abuse and Neglect, Committee on Adolescence. Care of the adolescent after an acute sexual assault. *Pediatrics*. 2017;139(3):e20164243 PMID: 28242861 https://doi.org/10.1542/peds.2016-4243
11. Hammerschlag MR, Guillén CD. Medical and legal implications of testing for sexually transmitted infections in children. *Clin Microbiol Rev*. 2010;23(3):493–506 PMID: 20610820 https://doi.org/10.1128/CMR.00024-09
12. Risser WL, Bortot AT, Benjamins LJ, et al. The epidemiology of sexually transmitted infections in adolescents. *Semin Pediatr Infect Dis*. 2005;16(3):160–167 PMID: 16044389 https://doi.org/10.1053/j.spid.2005.04.004
13. Girardet RG, Lahoti S, Howard LA, et al. Epidemiology of sexually transmitted infections in suspected child victims of sexual assault. *Pediatrics*. 2009;124(1):79–86 PMID: 19564286 https://doi.org/10.1542/peds.2008-2947

14. Centers for Disease Control and Prevention. *Sexually Transmitted Disease Surveillance 2016*. Atlanta, GA: US Dept of Health and Human Services; 2017
15. Hammerschlag MR. The transmissibility of sexually transmitted diseases in sexually abused children. *Child Abuse Negl*. 1998;22(6):623–635 PMID: 9649901 https://doi.org/10.1016/S0145-2134(98)00038-6
16. Workowski KA, Bolan GA; Centers for Disease Control and Prevention. Sexually transmitted diseases treatment guidelines, 2015. *MMWR Recomm Rep*. 2015;64(RR-03):1–137 PMID: 26042815
17. Beck-Sagué CM, Solomon F. Sexually transmitted diseases in abused children and adolescent and adult victims of rape: review of selected literature. *Clin Infect Dis*. 1999;28(suppl 1):S74–S83 PMID: 10028112 https://doi.org/10.1086/514726
18. Woods CR. Sexually transmitted diseases in prepubertal children: mechanisms of transmission, evaluation of sexually abused children, and exclusion of chronic perinatal viral infections. *Semin Pediatr Infect Dis*. 2005;16(4):317–325 PMID: 16210111 https://doi.org/10.1053/j.spid.2005.06.012
19. Alexander WJ, Griffith H, Housch JG, Holmes JR. Infections in sexual contacts and associates of children with gonorrhea. *Sex Transm Dis*. 1984;11(3):156–158 PMID: 6505918 https://doi.org/10.1097/00007435-198407000-00007
20. Folland DS, Burke RE, Hinman AR, Schaffner W. Gonorrhea in preadolescent children: an inquiry into source of infection and mode of transmission. *Pediatrics*. 1977;60(2): 153–156 PMID: 887328
21. Ingram DL. Controversies about the sexual and nonsexual transmission of adult STDs to children. In: Krugman RD, Leventhal JM, eds. *Child Sexual Abuse. Report of the Twenty Second Ross Roundtable on Critical Approaches to Common Pediatric Problems*. Columbus, OH: Ross Laboratories; 1991:14–28
22. Hammerschlag MR. Sexually transmitted diseases in sexually abused children. *Adv Pediatr Infect Dis*. 1988;3:1–18 PMID: 3061389
23. Bump RC, Sachs LA, Buesching WJ III. Sexually transmissible infectious agents in sexually active and virginal asymptomatic adolescent girls. *Pediatrics*. 1986;77(4):488–494 PMID: 3083395
24. Gardner JJ. Comparison of the vaginal flora in sexually abused and nonabused girls. *J Pediatr*. 1992;120(6):872–877 PMID: 1593345 https://doi.org/10.1016/S0022-3476(05)81952-3
25. Hammerschlag MR, Alpert S, Rosner I, et al. Microbiology of the vagina in children: normal and potentially pathogenic organisms. *Pediatrics*. 1978;62(1):57–62 PMID: 98750
26. Paradise JE, Campos JM, Friedman HM, Frishmuth G. Vulvovaginitis in premenarcheal girls: clinical features and diagnostic evaluation. *Pediatrics*. 1982;70(2):193–198 PMID: 7099784
27. Goodyear-Smith F. What is the evidence for non-sexual transmission of gonorrhoea in children after the neonatal period? A systematic review. *J Forensic Leg Med*. 2007;14(8):489–502 PMID: 17961874 https://doi.org/10.1016/j.jflm.2007.04.001
28. Adams JA, Kellogg ND, Farst KJ, et al. Updated guidelines for the medical assessment and care of children who may have been sexually abused. *J Pediatr Adolesc Gynecol*. 2016;29(2):81–87 PMID: 26220352 https://doi.org/10.1016/j.jpag.2015.01.007
29. Whittington WL, Rice RJ, Biddle JW, Knapp JS. Incorrect identification of *Neisseria gonorrhoeae* from infants and children. *Pediatr Infect Dis J*. 1988;7(1):3–10 PMID: 3124073 https://doi.org/10.1097/00006454-198801000-00002
30. Seña AC, Hsu KK, Kellogg N, et al. Sexual assault and sexually transmitted infections in adults, adolescents and children. *Clin Infect Dis*. 2015;61(suppl 8):S856–S864 PMID: 26602623 https://doi.org/10.1093/cid/civ786

31. Ison CA, Bellinger CM, Walker J. Homology of cryptic plasmid of Neisseria gonorrhoeae with plasmids from Neisseria meningitidis and Neisseria lactamica. *J Clin Pathol.* 1986;39(10):1119–1123 PMID: 3097079 https://doi.org/10.1136/jcp.39.10.1119
32. Whiley DM, Garland SM, Harnett G, et al. Exploring "best practice" for nucleic acid detection of Neisseria gonorrhea. *Sex Health.* 2008;5(1):17–23
33. Palmer HM, Mallinson H, Wood RL, Herring AJ. Evaluation of the specificities of five DNA amplification methods for the detection of Neisseria gonorrhoeae. *J Clin Microbiol.* 2003;41(2):835–837 PMID: 12574295 https://doi.org/10.1128/JCM.41.2.835-837.2003
34. US Food and Drug Administration. *Methods. Method Verification and Validation. Version No 1.5.* Vol II. Silver Spring, MD: US Food and Drug Administration; 2003. ORA Laboratory Procedure
35. Kellogg ND, Melville JD, Lukefahr JL, Nienow SM, Russell EL. Genital and extragenital gonorrhea and chlamydia in children and adolescents evaluated for sexual abuse. *Pediatr Emerg Care.* 2018;34(11):761–766 PMID: 28072668
36. Papp, JR, Schachter J, Gaydos CA, Van Der Pol, B. Recommendations for the laboratory-based detection of Chlamydia trachomatis and Neisseria gonorrhoeae—2014. *MMWR.* 2014;63(RR-2):1–19
37. Bachmann LH, Johnson RE, Cheng H, et al. Nucleic acid amplification tests for diagnosis of Neisseria gonorrhoeae and Chlamydia trachomatis rectal infections. *J Clin Microbiol.* 2010;48(5):1827–1832 PMID: 20335410
38. Schachter J, Moncada J, Liska S, Shayevich C, Klausner JD. Nucleic acid amplification tests in the diagnosis of chlamydial and gonococcal infections of the oropharynx and rectum in men who have sex with men. *Sex Transm Dis.* 2008;35(7):637–642 PMID: 18520976
39. Giannini CM, Kim HK, Mortensen J, Mortensen J, Marsolo K, Huppert J. Culture of non-genital sites increases the detection of gonorrhea in women. *J Pediatr Adolesc Gynecol.* 2010;23(4):246–252 PMID: 20434928
40. Geisler WM, Lensing SY, Press CG, Hook EW III. Spontaneous resolution of genital Chlamydia trachomatis infection in women and protection from reinfection. *J Infect Dis.* 2013;207(12):1850–1856 PMID: 23470847 https://doi.org/10.1093/infdis/jit094
41. Schachter J, Grossman M, Sweet RL, Holt J, Jordan C, Bishop E. Prospective study of perinatal transmission of *Chlamydia trachomatis. JAMA.* 1986;255(24):3374–3377 PMID: 3712696 https://doi.org/10.1001/jama.1986.03370240044034
42. Bell TA, Stamm WE, Wang SP, Kuo CC, Holmes KK, Grayston JT. Chronic *Chlamydia trachomatis* infections in infants. *JAMA.* 1992;267(3):400–402 PMID: 1727964 https://doi.org/10.1001/jama.1992.03480030078041
43. Novak KD, Kowalski RP, Karenchak LM, Gordon YJ. Chlamydia trachomatis can be transmitted by a nonporous plastic surface in vitro. *Cornea.* 1995;14(5):523–526 PMID: 8536467 https://doi.org/10.1097/00003226-199509000-00013
44. Hammerschlag MR. Chlamydial infections. *J Pediatr.* 1989;114(5):727–734 PMID: 2654346 https://doi.org/10.1016/S0022-3476(89)80128-3
45. Hammerschlag MR. Appropriate use of nonculture tests for the detection of sexually transmitted diseases in children and adolescents. *Semin Pediatr Infect Dis.* 2003;14(1): 54–59 PMID: 12748923 https://doi.org/10.1053/spid.2003.127218
46. Papp JR, Schachter J, Gaydos C, Van Der Pol B; Centers for Disease Control and Prevention. Recommendations for the laboratory-based detection of Chlamydia trachomatis and Neisseria gonorrhoeae--2014. *MMWR Recomm Rep.* 2014;63(RR-02):1–19 PMID: 24622331
47. Black CM, Driebe EM, Howard LA, et al. Multicenter study of nucleic acid amplification tests for detection of Chlamydia trachomatis and Neisseria gonorrhoeae in children

being evaluated for sexual abuse. *Pediatr Infect Dis J*. 2009;28(7):608–613 PMID: 19451856 https://doi.org/10.1097/INF.0b013e31819b592e
48. Hammerschlag MR, Gaydos CA. Guidelines for the use of molecular biological methods to detect sexually transmitted pathogens in cases of suspected sexual abuse in children. *Methods Mol Biol*. 2012;903:307–317 PMID: 22782828 https://doi.org/10.1007/978-1-61779-937-2_21
49. Hammerschlag MR. Use of nucleic acid amplification tests in investigating child sexual abuse. *Sex Transm Infect*. 2001;77(3):153–154 PMID: 11402219 https://doi.org/10.1136/sti.77.3.153
50. Ginsburg CM. Acquired syphilis in prepubertal children. *Pediatr Infect Dis*. 1983;2(3):232–234 PMID: 6866786 https://doi.org/10.1097/00006454-198305000-00012
51. Goldenring JM. Secondary syphilis in a prepubertal child. Differentiating condylomata lata from condylomata acuminata. *N Y State J Med*. 1989;89(3):180–181 PMID: 2922156
52. Connors JM, Schubert C, Shapiro R. Syphilis or abuse: making the diagnosis and understanding the implications. *Pediatr Emerg Care*. 1998;14(2):139–142 PMID: 9583398 https://doi.org/10.1097/00006565-199804000-00013
53. Christian CW, Lavelle J, Bell LM. Preschoolers with syphilis. *Pediatrics*. 1999;103(1):E4 PMID: 9917484 https://doi.org/10.1542/peds.103.1.e4
54. Argent AC, Lachman PI, Hanslo D, Bass D. Sexually transmitted diseases in children and evidence of sexual abuse. *Child Abuse Negl*. 1995;19(10):1303–1310 PMID: 8556444 https://doi.org/10.1016/0145-2134(95)00082-J
55. Lande MB, Richardson AC, White KC. The role of syphilis serology in the evaluation of suspected sexual abuse. *Pediatr Infect Dis J*. 1992;11(2):125–127 PMID: 1741184
56. Horowitz S, Chadwick DL. Syphilis as a sole indicator of sexual abuse: two cases with no intervention. *Child Abuse Negl*. 1990;14(1):129–132 PMID: 2310968 https://doi.org/10.1016/0145-2134(90)90088-B
57. Oztürk F, Gürses N, Sancak R, Bay A, Baris S. Acquired secondary syphilis in a 6-year-old girl with no history of sexual abuse. *Cutis*. 1998;62(3):150–151 PMID: 9770132
58. Williams J, Radha S, Sundararaj AS. Nonvenereal transmission of venereal syphilis in a child. *Indian J Sex Transm Dis*. 1990;11(1):27–28 PMID: 12284869
59. Ingram DL, Everett VD, Lyna PR, White ST, Rockwell LA. Epidemiology of adult sexually transmitted disease agents in children being evaluated for sexual abuse. *Pediatr Infect Dis J*. 1992;11(11):945–950 PMID: 1454437 https://doi.org/10.1097/00006454-199211110-00008
60. Siegel RM, Schubert CJ, Myers PA, Shapiro RA. The prevalence of sexually transmitted diseases in children and adolescents evaluated for sexual abuse in Cincinnati: rationale for limited STD testing in prepubertal girls. *Pediatrics*. 1995;96(6):1090–1094 PMID: 7491226
61. Centers for Disease Control and Prevention (CDC). Syphilis testing algorithms using treponemal tests for initial screening—four laboratories, New York City, 2005-2006. *MMWR Morb Mortal Wkly Rep*. 2008;57(32):872–875 PMID: 18701877
62. Sinclair KA, Woods CR, Kirse DJ, Sinal SH. Anogenital and respiratory tract human papillomavirus infections among children: age, gender, and potential transmission through sexual abuse. *Pediatrics*. 2005;116(4):815–825 PMID: 16199688 https://doi.org/10.1542/peds.2005-0652
63. De Jong AR, Weiss JC, Brent RL. Condyloma acuminata in children. *Am J Dis Child*. 1982;136(8):704–706 PMID: 6896603
64. National Institute on Deafness and Other Communication Disorders. Recurrent respiratory papillomatosis or laryngeal papillomatosis. NIH Pub No. 10–4214. https://

www.nidcd.nih.gov/health/recurrent-respiratory-papillomatosis. Updated November 28, 2017. Accessed February 4, 2019

65. Obalek S, Misiewicz J, Jablonska S, Favre M, Orth G. Childhood condyloma acuminatum: association with genital and cutaneous human papillomaviruses. *Pediatr Dermatol.* 1993;10(2):101–106 PMID: 8393994 https://doi.org/10.1111/j.1525-1470.1993.tb00031.x
66. Watts DH, Koutsky LA, Holmes KK, et al. Low risk of perinatal transmission of human papillomavirus: results from a prospective cohort study. *Am J Obstet Gynecol.* 1998;178(2):365–373 PMID: 9500501 https://doi.org/10.1016/S0002-9378(98)80027-6
67. Smith EM, Ritchie JM, Yankowitz J, et al. Human papillomavirus prevalence and types in newborns and parents: concordance and modes of transmission. *Sex Transm Dis.* 2004;31(1):57–62 PMID: 14695959 https://doi.org/10.1097/01.OLQ.0000105327.40288.DB
68. Rintala MAM, Grénman SE, Puranen MH, et al. Transmission of high-risk human papillomavirus (HPV) between parents and infant: a prospective study of HPV in families in Finland. *J Clin Microbiol.* 2005;43(1):376–381 PMID: 15634997 https://doi.org/10.1128/JCM.43.1.376-381.2005
69. Jenison SA, Yu XP, Valentine JM, et al. Evidence of prevalent genital-type human papillomavirus infections in adults and children. *J Infect Dis.* 1990;162(1):60–69 PMID: 2162371 https://doi.org/10.1093/infdis/162.1.60
70. Rice PS, Mant C, Cason J, et al. High prevalence of human papillomavirus type 16 infection among children. *J Med Virol.* 2000;61(1):70–75 PMID: 10745235 https://doi.org/10.1002/(SICI)1096-9071(200005)61:1<70::AID-JMV11>3.0.CO;2-Y
71. Myhre AK, Dalen A, Berntzen K, Bratlid D. Anogenital human papillomavirus in nonabused preschool children. *Acta Paediatr.* 2003;92(12):1445–1452 PMID: 14971797 https://doi.org/10.1111/j.1651-2227.2003.tb00830.x
72. Stevens-Simon C, Nelligan D, Breese P, Jenny C, Douglas JM Jr. The prevalence of genital human papillomavirus infections in abused and nonabused preadolescent girls. *Pediatrics.* 2000;106(4):645–649 PMID: 11015503 https://doi.org/10.1542/peds.106.4.645
73. Gutman LT, St Claire K, Herman-Giddens ME, Johnston WW, Phelps WC. Evaluation of sexually abused and nonabused young girls for intravaginal human papillomavirus infection. *Am J Dis Child.* 1992;146(6):694–699 PMID: 1317670 https://doi.org/10.1001/archpedi.1992.02160180052016
74. Siegfried E, Rasnick-Conley J, Cook S, Leonardi C, Monteleone J. Human papillomavirus screening in pediatric victims of sexual abuse. *Pediatrics.* 1998;101(1 Pt 1):43–47 PMID: 9417149 https://doi.org/10.1542/peds.101.1.43
75. Handley J, Hanks E, Armstrong K, et al. Common association of HPV 2 with anogenital warts in prepubertal children. *Pediatr Dermatol.* 1997;14(5):339–343 PMID: 9336800 https://doi.org/10.1111/j.1525-1470.1997.tb00976.x
76. Cohen BA, Honig P, Androphy E. Anogenital warts in children. Clinical and virologic evaluation for sexual abuse. *Arch Dermatol.* 1990;126(12):1575–1580 PMID: 2175163 https://doi.org/10.1001/archderm.1990.01670360039004
77. Boyd AS. Condylomata acuminata in the pediatric population. *Am J Dis Child.* 1990;144(7):817–824 PMID: 2192544
78. Unger ER, Fajman NN, Maloney EM, et al. Anogenital human papillomavirus in sexually abused and nonabused children: a multicenter study. *Pediatrics.* 2011;128(3):e658–e665 PMID: 21844060
79. Rock B, Naghashfar Z, Barnett N, Buscema J, Woodruff JD, Shah K. Genital tract papillomavirus infection in children. *Arch Dermatol.* 1986;122(10):1129–1132 PMID: 3021069 https://doi.org/10.1001/archderm.1986.01660220047012

80. Weaver BA, Feng Q, Holmes KK, et al. Evaluation of genital sites and sampling techniques for detection of human papillomavirus DNA in men. *J Infect Dis*. 2004;189(4): 677–685 PMID: 14767822 https://doi.org/10.1086/381395
81. Jones JG, Yamauchi T, Lambert B. *Trichomonas vaginalis* infestation in sexually abused girls. *Am J Dis Child*. 1985;139(8):846–847 PMID: 3875279 https://doi.org/10.1001/archpedi.1985.02140100108046
82. Gallion HR, Dupree LJ, Scott TA, Arnold DH. Diagnosis of Trichomonas vaginalis in female children and adolescents evaluated for possible sexual abuse: a comparison of the InPouch TV culture method and wet mount microscopy. *J Pediatr Adolesc Gynecol*. 2009;22(5):300–305 PMID: 19576816 https://doi.org/10.1016/j.jpag.2008.12.006
83. Bandea CI, Joseph K, Secor EW, et al. Development of PCR assays for detection of Trichomonas vaginalis in urine specimens. *J Clin Microbiol*. 2013;51(4):1298–1300 PMID: 23390274 https://doi.org/10.1128/JCM.03101-12
84. Gardner M, Jones JG. Genital herpes acquired by sexual abuse of children. *J Pediatr*. 1984;104(2):243–244 PMID: 6694018 https://doi.org/10.1016/S0022-3476(84)81002-1
85. Kaplan KM, Fleisher GR, Paradise JE, Friedman HN. Social relevance of genital herpes simplex in children. *Am J Dis Child*. 1984;138(9):872–874 PMID: 6475878 https://doi.org/10.1001/archpedi.1984.02140470070024
86. Taieb A, Body S, Astar I, du Pasquier P, Maleville J. Clinical epidemiology of symptomatic primary herpetic infection in children. A study of 50 cases. *Acta Paediatr Scand*. 1987;76(1):128–132 PMID: 3031926 https://doi.org/10.1111/j.1651-2227.1987.tb10428.x
87. Schmitt DL, Johnson DW, Henderson FW. Herpes simplex type 1 infections in group day care. *Pediatr Infect Dis J*. 1991;10(10):729–734 PMID: 1658720 https://doi.org/10.1097/00006454-199110000-00002
88. Roberts C. Genital herpes in young adults: changing sexual behaviours, epidemiology and management. *Herpes*. 2005;12(1):10–14 PMID: 16026639
89. Nahmias AJ, Dowdle WR, Naib ZM, Josey WE, Luce CF. Genital infection with *Herpesvirus hominis* types 1 and 2 in children. *Pediatrics*. 1968;42(4):659–666 PMID: 4300687
90. Christian CW, Singer ML, Crawford JE, Durbin D. Perianal herpes zoster presenting as suspected child abuse. *Pediatrics*. 1997;99(4):608–610 PMID: 9093310 https://doi.org/10.1542/peds.99.4.608
91. Simon HK, Steele DW. Varicella: pediatric genital/rectal vesicular lesions of unclear origin. *Ann Emerg Med*. 1995;25(1):111–114 PMID: 7802360 https://doi.org/10.1016/S0196-0644(95)70365-9
92. Bump RC, Buesching WJ III. Bacterial vaginosis in virginal and sexually active adolescent females: evidence against exclusive sexual transmission. *Am J Obstet Gynecol*. 1988;158(4):935–939 PMID: 3259076 https://doi.org/10.1016/0002-9378(88)90097-X
93. Hammerschlag MR, Cummings M, Doraiswamy B, Cox P, McCormack WM. Nonspecific vaginitis following sexual abuse in children. *Pediatrics*. 1985;75(6):1028–1031 PMID: 4000776
94. Pierce AM, Hart CA. Vulvovaginitis: causes and management. *Arch Dis Child*. 1992;67(4):509–512 PMID: 1580682 https://doi.org/10.1136/adc.67.4.509
95. Jaquiery A, Stylianopoulos A, Hogg G, Grover S. Vulvovaginitis: clinical features, aetiology, and microbiology of the genital tract. *Arch Dis Child*. 1999;81(1):64–67 PMID: 10373139 https://doi.org/10.1136/adc.81.1.64
96. Bartley DL, Morgan L, Rimsza ME. *Gardnerella vaginalis* in prepubertal girls. *Am J Dis Child*. 1987;141(9):1014–1017 PMID: 3497575

97. Ingram DL, White ST, Lyna PR, et al. *Gardnerella vaginalis* infection and sexual contact in female children. *Child Abuse Negl*. 1992;16(6):847–853 PMID: 1486513 https://doi.org/10.1016/0145-2134(92)90086-7
98. Shafer MA, Sweet RL, Ohm-Smith MJ, Shalwitz J, Beck A, Schachter J. Microbiology of the lower genital tract in postmenarchal adolescent girls: differences by sexual activity, contraception, and presence of nonspecific vaginitis. *J Pediatr*. 1985;107(6):974–981 PMID: 3877803 https://doi.org/10.1016/S0022-3476(85)80208-0
99. Myhre AK, Bevanger LS, Berntzen K, Bratlid D. Anogenital bacteriology in non-abused preschool children: a descriptive study of the aerobic genital flora and the isolation of anogenital *Gardnerella vaginalis*. *Acta Paediatr*. 2002;91(8):885–891 PMID: 12222710 https://doi.org/10.1111/j.1651-2227.2002.tb02850.x
100. Wahl NG, Castilla MA, Lewis-Abney K. Prevalence of *Gardnerella vaginalis* in prepubertal males. *Arch Pediatr Adolesc Med*. 1998;152(11):1095–1099 PMID: 9811287 https://doi.org/10.1001/archpedi.152.11.1095
101. Gellert GA, Durfee MJ, Berkowitz CD, Higgins KV, Tubiolo VC. Situational and sociodemographic characteristics of children infected with human immunodeficiency virus from pediatric sexual abuse. *Pediatrics*. 1993;91(1):39–44 PMID: 8416504
102. Lindegren ML, Hanson IC, Hammett TA, Beil J, Fleming PL, Ward JW. Sexual abuse of children: intersection with the HIV epidemic. *Pediatrics*. 1998;102(4):E46 PMID: 9755283 https://doi.org/10.1542/peds.102.4.e46
103. Girardet RG, Lemme S, Biason TA, Bolton K, Lahoti S. HIV post-exposure prophylaxis in children and adolescents presenting for reported sexual assault. *Child Abuse Negl*. 2009;33(3):173–178 PMID: 19324415 https://doi.org/10.1016/j.chiabu.2008.05.010
104 Centers for Disease Control and Prevention and Association of Public Health Laboratories. Laboratory testing for the diagnosis of HIV infection: updated recommendations. http://stacks.cdc.gov/view/cdc/23447. Published June 27, 2014. Accessed February 4, 2019
105. Centers for Disease Control and Prevention. Updated guidelines for antiretroviral postexposure prophylaxis after sexual, injection drug use, or other nonoccupational exposure to HIV—United States, 2016. https://www.cdc.gov/hiv/pdf/programresources/cdc-hiv-npep-guidelines.pdf. Published 2016. Accessed February 1, 2019
106. Kellogg ND, Parra JM, Menard S. Children with anogenital symptoms and signs referred for sexual abuse evaluations. *Arch Pediatr Adolesc Med*. 1998;152(7):634–641 PMID: 9667533 https://doi.org/10.1001/archpedi.152.7.634
107. Klevan J, De Jong AR. Urinary tract symptoms and urinary tract infections in sexually abused children. *Am J Dis Child*. 1990;144:242–244 PMID: 2301332
108. Rogstad KE, Wilkinson D, Robinson A. Sexually transmitted infections in children as a marker of child sexual abuse and direction of future research. *Curr Opin Infect Dis*. 2016;29(1):41–44 PMID: 26658657 https://doi.org/10.1097/QCO.0000000000000233
109. Hammerschlag MR, Doraiswamy B, Cox P, Cummings M, McCormack WM. Colonization of sexually abused children with genital mycoplasmas. *Sex Transm Dis*. 1987;14(1):23–25 PMID: 3563830 https://doi.org/10.1097/00007435-198701000-00005
110. Ingram DL, White ST, Lyna P, et al. Ureaplasma urealyticum and large colony mycoplasma colonization in female children and its relationship to sexual contact, age, and race. *Child Abuse Negl*. 1992;16(2):265–272 PMID: 1559174 https://doi.org/10.1016/0145-2134(92)90033-N
111. Clark LR, Atendido M. Group B streptococcal vaginitis in postpubertal adolescent girls. *J Adolesc Health*. 2005;36(5):437–440 PMID: 15837348 https://doi.org/10.1016/j.jadohealth.2004.03.009

112. Hammerschlag MR, Baker CJ, Alpert S, et al. Colonization with group B streptococci in girls under 16 years of age. *Pediatrics*. 1977;60(4):473–476 PMID: 333366
113. Heller RH, Joseph JM, Davis HJ. Vulvovaginitis in the premenarcheal child. *J Pediatr*. 1969;74(3):370–377 PMID: 4974526 https://doi.org/10.1016/S0022-3476(69)80193-9
114. Gavril AR, Kellogg ND, Nair P. Value of follow-up examinations of children and adolescents evaluated for sexual abuse and assault. *Pediatrics*. 2012;129(2):282–289 PMID: 22291113 https://doi.org/10.1542/peds.2011-0804

CHAPTER 13

The Role of Forensic Materials in Sexual Abuse and Assault

Kathi Makoroff, MD, MEd, FAAP
Mayerson Center for Safe and Healthy Children
Cincinnati Children's Hospital Medical Center
Associate Professor
University of Cincinnati College of Medicine
Cincinnati, OH

Jonathan Thackeray, MD, FAAP
Chief Medical Community Health Officer
Department of Medical Affairs
Dayton Children's Hospital
Professor and Vice Chair
Department of Pediatrics
Wright State University Boonshoft School of Medicine
Dayton, OH

Elizabeth Benzinger, PhD
Ohio Bureau of Criminal Investigation
London, OH

Definition and Importance of Forensic Material

In the context of child abuse, the term *forensic* refers to evidence or information that is used in the investigation of a crime. One of the most common scenarios where forensic evaluation is critical involves cases of suspected child sexual abuse. Forensic evidence collection for child sexual abuse may include materials from skin, mucosal membranes, saliva, hair samples, blood samples, and any material found on clothing or linens. Although verbal disclosures and statements and physical examination findings are important, this chapter will focus on the detection and collection of materials from the body or potential crime scene that can be analyzed in the course of a child sexual abuse investigation.

The Effect of Forensic Evidence in Child Sexual Abuse Cases

The identification of forensic evidence in child sexual abuse varies from approximately 3% to 80%, depending on the population studied and laboratory methods used.[1–4] In a review of 500 patients who had experienced sexual assault, Dahlke et al[2] reported forensic evidence identification in only 3% of children younger than 11 years, compared with 36% of young adolescents who were sexually assaulted. Adolescents, for whom sexual assault may be more characteristic of adult rape crimes, may be better able to disclose their experienced abuse and are more likely than prepubertal children to have forensic evidence identified after sexual assault.

The evidence to support the effect of forensic evidence collection on judicial outcomes in cases of pediatric sexual assault, however, is less clear. In a study of 355 sexual assault cases, for example, successful prosecution was associated with younger age (adolescent vs adult) of the person who experienced the assault, the presence of trauma on examination, and weapon use by the assailant.[5] Forensic evidence identification (sperm detection), however, was not associated with conviction. De Jong and Rose[6] reviewed prosecution results for 137 children aged 1 to 16 years who experienced sexual abuse and found that physical or forensic evidence was neither predictive nor essential for conviction. Cases of young children, in fact, had lower rates of felony conviction of the perpetrator, despite higher frequencies of physical findings, in part because the young children were less able than older children to testify about their experiences.[7,8]

Use of multidisciplinary teams (eg, sexual assault response teams) that integrate sexual assault nurse examiners to conduct evidence collection have demonstrated positive outcomes relative to prosecution rates in at least one study. In this study, improved community stakeholder engagement and collaboration were predictive of prosecution success, while decreased allocation of community resources to adolescent sexual assault cases had a significant negative effect on prosecution outcomes.[8] Studies, however, that focus specifically on use of the pediatric sexual assault nurse examiner to conduct forensic evidence collection and subsequent judicial outcomes have produced mixed results.[9–12]

Challenges of Forensic Evidence Collection and Analysis in Child Sexual Abuse Cases

Because of the dynamics and nature of child sexual abuse, opportunities to collect forensic evidence may be less frequent than in cases of sexual abuse of adults. Few children disclose their sexual abuse during the first hours after an assault, when the yield from forensic evidence collection is greatest. For those who are identified shortly after an assault, some are not brought for medical evaluation immediately. Others have already bathed and changed their clothing, which presumably decreases the likelihood of obtaining evidence from physical examination. Furthermore, the abuse may not have involved any exchange of body tissues or secretions, potentially limiting the yield from evidence collection.

Additionally, there are well-described barriers to collection of forensic evidence in the pediatric health care setting, including inadequate training of medical staff, concerns with the time it takes to perform evidence collection, inconsistent payment for services, and perceived and actual stress on the medical professional and the child to complete the evidence collection.[13,14]

Finally, it is important for the medical professional to recognize that there exist several barriers, external to the medical system, that result in completed evidence collection kits never being submitted for testing by law enforcement. Campbell and colleagues identify a "conservative" estimate of as many as 400,000 untested evidence collection kits in US police departments.[14] Regional studies suggest nearly half of evidence collection kits collected in the health care setting are not submitted for further testing.[15]

Timing Considerations

Time since assault is an important factor when deciding whether or not to collect forensic evidence. In cases of acute sexual abuse, physical evidence is lost with time. Eating, drinking, cleansing after defecation and urination, douching, and bathing reduce the amount of evidence material present. Skin cells of the one who experienced the abuse, with the accompanying forensic evidence, are sloughed off the body with physical activity and time. Microbial action and cellular breakdown processes rapidly degrade DNA present in foreign body fluids, such as blood and semen, and the rate of breakdown varies by specimen and from one body part to another. Finally, the constant turnover of cells on mucous membranes serves to add new DNA from the patient to the mix, overwhelming the smaller amount of DNA present from the perpetrator.

Recommendations on timing of evidence collection for children and adolescents vary from one jurisdiction to another. Traditionally, many states recommend that forensic evidence be collected if less than 72 hours have passed since the assault, although some states require evidence collection as far out as 96 hours from the assault. As new technologies develop and the ability to detect DNA (even in the absence of body fluids) is enhanced, however, it is necessary to continue to reexamine the parameters for evidence collection.

For prepubertal children, for example, previous research suggested that swabbing the child's body for evidence was unnecessary after 24 hours. In a study of 273 prepubertal children who underwent forensic evidence collection, no swabs taken from the child's body were positive for spermatozoa or blood more than 13 hours following the assault.[1] More than 90% of children with positive forensic evidence findings were evaluated within 24 hours of assault. Most forensic evidence was found on clothing and linens, although it was collected in only 35% of cases. In a second study of 190 children younger than 13 years who were evaluated within 72 hours of sexual assault, no child younger than 10 years had a positive body swab result for semen or sperm.[16] Another study examined 80 children and adolescents who presented to an emergency department within 72 hours of a reported episode of sexual abuse or assault.[17] Only 3 children (aged < 12 years) had semen recovered from forensic testing. All 3 presented within 24 hours after the reported abuse or assault, and all 3 children had semen recovered from clothing or linen only.

With the emergence of newer technologies to process evidence collection and identify DNA, however, subsequent studies have reported infrequent, but nonetheless important, cases of evidence detection on prepubertal children beyond 24 hours after the reported assault. Thackeray et al reported 3 of 20 positive samples from children younger than 10 years, including 1 positive result for salivary amylase on the thighs 54 hours following an assault.[18] Girardet et al similarly found evidence collection from 3 children younger than 10 years had a positive DNA test from a body swab collected as far out as 95 hours, 1 of which included positive DNA from invasive body swabs collected 35 hours after the assault.[19] Well-designed studies are necessary to continue to inform recommendations for evidence collection for both prepubertal and pubertal children who experience sexual assault.

What is clear is that evidence collection should be performed as soon as possible after a recent assault. The American Academy of Pediatrics currently recommends that "children who have had recent sexual contact involving the exchange of bodily fluids should be immediately referred to a specialized clinic or emergency department capable of collecting evidence using a forensic evidence kit." Most forensic evidence will be collected within the first 24 hours after assault, and the ability to detect evidence decreases rapidly with time, regardless of the age of the child. Clothing and linens must be remembered as an important potential source of forensic evidence in cases of suspected sexual abuse.[13]

Forensic Evidence Collection

Evidence Collection in Cases of Acute Sexual Assault

The roles of the medical professional include assessing the medical and mental health needs of the patient, collecting evidence when indicated, determining the need to report to the proper authorities, and ensuring the patient's safety. Special sensitivity must be used when caring for patients following acute sexual assault; social, cultural, ethnic and religious backgrounds must always be considered.

Although protocols for evidence collection vary between jurisdictions, general guidelines do exist. Using a standardized protocol with specific instructions for proper specimen collection, packaging, labeling, storing, and processing is essential to preserve the physical evidence in suspected cases of sexual or physical abuse. Standardized collection kits with detailed instructions, checklists, collection devices, and containers should be provided (Figure 13.1). In addition, chain of evidence procedures in which each person handling the evidence documents receipt and delivery of specimens should be followed to ensure that the evidence will be admissible in legal proceedings.[20,21]

A medical examination and evidence collection should begin as soon as the patient is medically stable. Examiners should wear gloves at all times, when collecting and handling specimens, to prevent contamination. Specimens should be obtained from all orifices and other areas believed to have been in contact with the perpetrator, including genitals, anus, mouth, and fingers.

Assault histories may not correspond to forensic laboratory findings. For example, the patient may not recall important details due to the effects of drugs and/or alcohol or trauma. Certain acts may not be discussed because of embarrassment. Very young children may not understand the

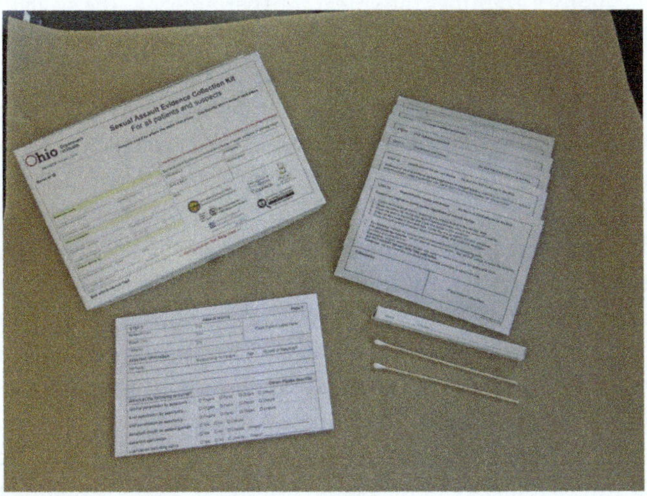

FIGURE 13.1
Example of evidence collection kit.

relationship between the sexual abuse act and the need for the medical evaluation. Thus, evidence collection protocols that advise specimen collection only at the site of the assault may cause key evidence to be missed. Rather, the best evidence collection strategy uses a thorough basic collection protocol that is expanded, rather than limited, by the patient's history.[20,21]

Collecting Samples From the Patient and the Perpetrator

Cotton-tipped swabs are the best collection medium. Calcium alginate culture swabs are not used because the calcium alginate interferes with DNA extraction procedures and renders the collection unusable. Although gauze squares or other wipes are the most efficient way to swab a large area, recovering the DNA from such large pieces of material is technically difficult. In most cases, 2 to 3 swabs are taken from each body site (oral, genital, and anal). Dry swabs are used for wet secretions and saline-moistened swabs for dry sites. All swabs should be completely air-dried for at least 1 hour before labeling and placing in a tube or envelope. To prevent cross-contamination, swabs should not touch one another.

Some forensic laboratories request dry smears of the samples. If so, one of the collected swabs should be used to make a smear by rolling the swab back and forth across a slide in nonoverlapping strokes. The smear is then allowed to dry; it is not stained or fixed, and a coverslip is not used. The forensic laboratory examines the smear for spermatozoa. The swab that is used for the smear is retained. In prepubertal children who may have vaginal openings that do not permit insertion of a cotton swab, all swabs are collected from the external genitalia. In adolescent patients, separate swabs should be collected from the vagina and the cervix. Saliva and DNA left by the perpetrator during any oral-genital contact can be collected from the external genitalia using 2 to 3 additional swabs. Oral swabs should be obtained by swabbing the buccal mucosa and under the tongue.

Anal samples are important to collect in all cases. Due to drainage and/or external deposition of semen, anal swabs are frequently positive in cases of reported vaginal assault. In addition, less DNA from the female is present on the anal swabs, which assists in interpreting mixed DNA profiles. If the patient is unable to cooperate with the collection of internal anal samples, the swabs are collected only from the external anal area. In males, the external surface of the penis is swabbed; swabs should not be inserted into the urethra.

The underwear that the patient wears to the examination is collected in all cases. If underwear has been changed since the assault, advise law enforcement to obtain those garments worn at the time of the assault and include them in the forensic analysis. Underwear frequently contains better semen or saliva evidence than body cavity swabs. When no underwear is worn, the garment closest to the body is treated as underwear. Each item of clothing should be placed in its own brown paper bag. If any of the collected garments are wet, they should be allowed to air-dry prior to placing in a brown paper bag. Plastic bags should not be used because they may lock in moisture and promote the degradation of evidence.

Fingernail scrapings can be obtained by collecting material from under the patient's nails onto a clean piece of paper. A fingernail scraper should be used to scrape the underside of all fingers of one hand with the debris collected onto a paper. The paper should be folded and labeled, and the same procedure should be repeated for the other hand.

Foreign hairs are collected by gently combing head and pubic hair over a sheet of paper or an envelope. Pubic hairs found on genitalia of prepubertal children should be packaged separately and labeled with the exact location from which they were obtained. As classical microscopic hair comparisons have been largely discontinued in forensics, the painful practice of collecting plucked exemplar pubic and head hairs from victims is no longer necessary.

If dried blood is present, a slightly moistened swab can be rubbed over the dried blood to collect the sample and then allowed to air-dry, as is procedure for the rest of the evidence swabs.

Body fluids or DNA foreign to the patient is found in slightly more than half of evidence collection kits. Those cases involving intercourse and possible ejaculation are more likely to yield evidence than those involving acts such as fondling or digital penetration. However, body fluids, tissue, or DNA may also be transferred from the patient to the perpetrator, and it is important to convey this information to police so that timely evidence collections can be made. Collections of assailant clothing, underwear, genital swabbings, hand and finger swabbings, and fingernail scrapings may contain DNA from the victim. No data are available on persistence of evidence on suspects, but the same guidelines used for those who experienced the sexual assault could be applied.

A standardized assault history form (https://tinyurl.com/y35drr68) prompts the collection of information that will assist forensic scientists during the testing of the evidence.

Specimen Preservation

Warm, moist conditions promote microbial destruction of human DNA. All swabs and clothing items should be thoroughly air-dried for at least 1 hour before packaging. It is important that chain of evidence procedures are maintained while the samples are air-drying. Culture tubes are not to be used to store the swabs because the medium in the tubes is designed to promote the growth of microorganisms, which will destroy the DNA. All packaging should be made of paper or light cardboard to permit additional drying. All samples must be labeled with the patient's information, including the collection site, when applicable.

Detecting Foreign Materials on Skin

Monochromatic light sources may help identify foreign materials on a patient's skin. Traditionally, a black light (Wood lamp), which emits wavelengths of approximately 365 nm, has been used to detect specimens not clearly visible to the eye. A Wood lamp can illuminate semen as well as other substances, such as milk, petroleum, lubricating jelly, lotions, and contraceptive foams, but does not adequately differentiate between these various substances. Thus, it may actually make it more difficult to identify semen among the nonbiological fluids.[22,23] One study examined pediatric emergency medicine physician use of a Wood lamp to differentiate between semen applied to skin and other substances typically found on a child's perineal area, such as diaper cream.[24] Physicians had difficulty identifying semen from the other specimens. This further supports the fact that if a Wood lamp is used for substance detection, interpretation of the results should be viewed with caution because the sensitivity and specificity of findings are not very high.

Because different specimens, including biological fluids, hairs, and fibers, illuminate under distinct wavelengths, having the ability to vary the wavelength of light emitted can increase the yield and differentiation of material detection. Therefore, contemporary adjustable alternative light sources are preferable to Wood lamps because they can emit light of wavelengths ranging from 365 to 700 nm and are, thus, more successful at identifying foreign materials on a patient's body.

Semen, for example, hydrolyzes to a clear residue when it dries and may not be readily visible on physical examination. Its peak fluorescence is at a smaller wavelength (approximately 450 nm) than a Wood lamp; thus, an alternative light source that could identify semen at its peak fluorescence would better detect semen residue. Alternative light sources also help differentiate biological fluids by their illumination pattern. For instance, while semen and urine both fluoresce at approximately 450 nm, urine fluoresces homogenously and semen fluoresces irregularly.[23] Additionally, the intensity of the fluorescence of semen diminishes dramatically by 28 hours after application to the skin, yet the fluorescence of urine lasts up to 80 hours.[22]

Besides examining the skin with a Wood lamp or alternative light source, the skin should also be examined under normal white light. Any area of the skin that fluoresces, or any area that appears suspicious as a forensic substance, should be swabbed with a lightly moistened cotton-tipped swab. A gauze pad should not be used because DNA from such large pieces of material is difficult to extract. Because saliva does not fluoresce, blind swabbing of the skin should be done with damp swabs based on the patient's history of oral contact by the perpetrator.

Forensic Toxicology

Drug-facilitated sexual assault (DFSA) involves sexual acts with an individual who has been rendered unable to resist or unable to consent through administration of drugs or alcohol. The same result can be achieved in cases where the person who experiences the assault voluntarily partakes of alcohol or other drugs. The objective of DFSA testing is to determine what substances were present and assess whether the patient would have been capable of giving consent (for those who are legally able to consent).[24]

In a common scenario, the person who experienced the assault may wake up in an unexpected location, with clothing missing or disheveled, with physical injuries, and possibly with memory impairment. The decision whether to collect urine and blood samples for toxicology screening should be based on the assessment of the patient's clinical signs and reported symptoms. Blood and urine samples should be collected as soon as possible; the sooner samples are collected, the more likely substances will be detected. If the suspected ingestion was less than 24 hours before presentation, urine and blood should be collected. If the suspected ingestion was between 24 and 96 hours before presentation, only urine should be collected. Strict chain of custody should always be maintained and documented. The testing available in hospital laboratories is directed at therapeutic levels of drugs and will generally not detect the compounds used for DFSA at the time of testing. Medical examiners' toxicology laboratories are among those capable of confirming very low levels of drugs and their metabolites.

More than 75 different drugs are known to be used for DFSA. The compounds that may be used vary widely and reflect what is available to the perpetrator. Much attention is given to certain compounds, including flunitrazepam (eg, Rohypnol), γ-butyrolactone, γ-hydroxybutyric acid, and ketamine, but many others, including diphenhydramine, are seen. By far the most common drug associated with DFSA is alcohol.[24]

The Forensic Laboratory Toolbox

The specific analysis methods available and approach to testing vary from laboratory to laboratory. However, overall similarity is driven by uniform standards. In the United States, forensic DNA testing is governed by voluntary quality assurance standards (International Organization for Standardization [ISO] 17025) linked to DNA database participation and substantial National Institute of Justice grant funding.[25]

Body Fluid Detection

Frequently, the first step in testing rape kits is the identification of semen or other body fluids. An array of presumptive and confirmatory tests is available for this purpose. Presumptive tests are rapid and relatively sensitive but may give false-positive results, while confirmatory tests are very specific.[26]

Much of the value in testing for body fluids is to identify which samples or clothing areas are best suited for DNA testing. Tests for semen, saliva, blood, urine, and feces exist, but no tests are available for vaginal secretions. The sensitivity of DNA tests exceeds that of body fluid tests, so the failure to identify a body fluid is not necessarily reason to discontinue testing. Additionally, the value added to the investigation by the body fluid test may not warrant the small amount of sample that is consumed in the process.

Semen

Semen contains 3 markers that are used in forensic laboratories. Human seminal fluid contains acid phosphatase activity, which can be detected using a rapid color test. The test is considered presumptive because some bacteria also produce positive results. Prostate-specific antigen (PSA) is the basis of another presumptive test for human semen. Although this test was originally considered to be confirmatory, PSA is now known to be present in some human milk and female urine specimens. The only confirmatory test for semen is microscopic identification of human spermatozoa. Thus, a forensic semen confirmation is not possible in the case of azoospermic individuals.

Saliva

Saliva is another body fluid without a confirmatory test. The presumptive test for saliva relies on the detection of amylase activity. Human saliva and feces contain significantly higher levels of amylase activity than other body fluids such as semen and sweat. The detection of amylase activity relies on hydrolysis of starch and subsequent clearing of the blue color of a starch-iodine complex.

Hair

Hairs are frequently transferred among individuals and between individuals and the environment. Due to the casual nature of hair transfer, hairs may not provide strong evidence of a crime. In the past, hair comparisons were made by microscopically comparing an evidence hair to plucked exemplars from victims and suspects. However, it is now known that hair comparisons are subject to an approximately 10% error rate and have contributed to wrongful convictions. Hairs are now compared using DNA analysis.[27] While hairs present on outer clothing may be explained by casual transfer, those found in underwear or on genital samples may constitute very strong evidence. Still, such findings may have innocuous explanations when the individuals share a household.

Fibers and Other Trace Particles

Fibers shed from clothing, curtains, linen, carpeting, and upholstery are ubiquitous and generally not able to be matched to a specific source. Rarely, fibers and particles such as sawdust, soil, plant debris, or metal filings can provide investigative leads regarding a perpetrator's environment or occupation.[28]

DNA Profiling

Standard forensic DNA testing is based on the detection of length differences at short tandem repeat (STR) loci. Forensically useful STR loci contain tracts of 3-, 4-, or 5-base repeats that are highly variable between individuals. A complete test result is obtainable with an effective sample size consisting of 300 to 600 cells. Such a DNA profile is sufficient to individualize a body fluid sample to one individual to the exclusion of all others. If the sample size is smaller or the DNA is degraded, a comparison might be made but with less power of discrimination. Detailed descriptions of forensic DNA methods are found in other sources.[29]

Autosomal Short Tandem Repeat Loci

The primary tool for DNA profiling is commercially available multiplexes that use polymerase chain reaction (PCR) to detect repeat differences at more than 20 loci across the autosomal chromosomes. The primary commercial products are called GlobalFiler (Thermo Fisher Scientific) and PowerPlex Fusion (Promega). With both products, the DNA is amplified using PCR, tagged with fluorescent dyes for visualization, and size-sorted using capillary gel electrophoresis. The resulting data are processed into charts called *electropherograms*. The ISO 17025 guidelines for forensic laboratories specify the developmental and implementation process for these products. As a result, the products are well-accepted in the legal system and the data are intercomparable.

For samples containing DNA from just one individual, or where mixtures of profiles can be deconvoluted (eg, major/minor, non-patient), an estimate of the frequency of occurrence in the general population is prepared. Rarity estimates for individual loci are prepared by plugging population data into the Hardy-Weinberg law. Relying on non-linkage of the individual loci, these single-locus estimates are then multiplied together to obtain the estimated frequency for the combined profile. When a full profile is obtained, frequency estimates in excess of 1 in several quadrillion are standard—essentially, identity. DNA profiles developed from extremely small amounts of DNA or degraded DNA will have fewer interpretable loci and the resultant frequency estimate will be more common.

Mixtures where the data cannot be deconvoluted have in the past been interpreted by low-power statistical means such as combined probability of inclusion, which estimates the frequency of all possible contributors. More recently, likelihood ratios and probabilistic models that rely on proprietary software are being applied. These more powerful methods permit the interpretation of complex mixtures that previously would have been declared inconclusive. An additional benefit of these programs is the ability to reliably deconvolute mixtures so that individual contributors can be identified.

Y-Short Tandem Repeat Loci

Analysis of STR markers occurring only on the Y chromosome (Y-STRs) is useful for identifying trace amounts of male DNA against an overwhelming background of female DNA. Mixtures of body fluids and, hence, DNA are typical of sexual assault samples. When the amount of DNA from one individual is much greater than that from the other, the interpretation of the minor component is constrained by the ability of the system to detect it. Minor contributors are detectable down to approximately 1 part in 15. Where spermatozoa are present, a differential lysis procedure permits the separation of sperm and epithelial fractions. However, autosomal STR testing of a vaginal sample containing seminal fluid from an azoospermic perpetrator may not permit visualization of the male contributor's profile. For this situation, similar STR multiplexes using loci confined to the Y chromosome can be used to visualize male contributors that are otherwise masked by an overwhelming amount of female DNA. When both perpetrator and patient are male, Y-STR testing does not provide any advantages over standard autosomal STR methods.

The ability of Y-STR analysis to detect trace amounts of male DNA may lead to a question of context when resident male relatives or caregivers are accused.

Since all Y-STR loci are confined to one chromosome, and because they are, by definition, haploid, the amount of data and the mathematical power to calculate frequencies of occurrence rely on a basic counting method. With typical frequency estimates in the thousands, the Y-STR tests do not provide the same power of discrimination as the autosomal STRs. Furthermore, absent occasional mutations, all members of a particular paternal lineage share the same Y-STR profile, making it impossible to distinguish Y-STR profiles of grandfather, father, uncle, son, cousin, and nephew. Due to the low power of discrimination, it is not feasible to search Y-STR profiles in the national database.

Touch DNA

Touch is a term applied to low-level samples in which no body fluid is identified. Typically, this might be a swabbing of a firearm used in a crime or a swabbing of the arm of a patient who experienced sexual assault where she was grabbed by the perpetrator. Any contact from the hand may leave behind DNA from sloughed skin cells and other common contaminants, such as the owner's nasal secretions, saliva, sweat, dander, etc. The same hand might also pick up DNA from persons or objects touched. This type of sample routinely leads to arrests in property crimes. Its use in sexual assault investigations is equally fruitful. Digital penetration cases, typically devoid of semen, rely on blind swabbings of skin areas and clothing approximating hand contact from the perpetrator. The inside surface of underwear often collects substantial touch DNA specimens. Strangulation marks and bruises from restraining are also good sources of DNA.[30]

Perpetrator Identification

Combined DNA Index System

The US Federal Bureau of Investigation Combined DNA Index System (CODIS) is a 3-part national database of DNA profiles. The offender database contains samples from convicted offenders. State legislation determines which felons are eligible and whether felony arrestees and juveniles may be uploaded. The forensic database contains profiles developed from crime scene evidence including rape kits, whether or not the crime is considered solved. All government forensic laboratories upload crime scene DNA profiles to CODIS. DNA profiles from those who experienced the crime are not permitted in CODIS. The final section of the database is made up of profiles from unidentified human remains and reference samples from the relatives of missing persons. CODIS searches are comprehensive and automated and span data from all local, state, and national regions.

As of March 2018, the CODIS database contained more than 16 million offender and arrestee profiles and more than 837,000 crime scene profiles. More than 1 in 3 uploaded crime scene profiles return a match to either a known offender or an evidence profile from a different case. Matches between unsolved cases are frequently instrumental in solving cases because they allow the investigating agencies to pool their leads.[31]

Factors Affecting How Forensic Testing Proceeds and How the Results Are Used in the Legal System

Forensic scientists report the identification of body fluids and make comparisons between DNA exemplars and evidence, but it is the court that determines how well the evidence supports the criminal charges. Because it is not feasible to run every test on every sample, the forensic laboratory uses the case information to choose how to approach the testing.

The most straightforward case scenario is where the perpetrator is a stranger. Because there has been no previous contact, any evidence that identifies the unknown perpetrator will be powerful. Genital samples, which may contain semen or other evidence suggestive of sexual contact, are almost always tested first, but swabbings of skin areas where the perpetrator kissed, licked, or simply touched the skin often provide sufficient DNA for database searching and identification.

Perpetrators who are family friends, relatives, or neighbors have a small opportunity to casually transfer body fluids and hairs to the patient during normal visits. A sneeze or spray from talking could be invoked to explain DNA left on the patient's face and arms. Casual transfer of DNA to genitals and other skin areas normally covered by clothing is a less likely scenario.

Perpetrators who live in the home or are caregivers of the patient pose special interpretation challenges. It is well known that family members have each other's DNA on their clothing and skin. Furthermore, spermatozoa have been demonstrated to withstand washing[32] or even to transfer from one fabric to another in the washing machine.[33] A perpetrator may invoke laundry hamper transfer to explain semen on children's clothing or bedding.

Conclusion

The collection and analysis of forensic evidence in cases of child sexual abuse is challenging and has barriers. The best means of overcoming these barriers is regular communication between community professions—health care, patient advocacy, forensic laboratory, law enforcement, and prosecution. The paramount concern is the welfare of the child, and a comprehensive medical and forensic examination should be performed only after stabilization of the child's health. Evidence collection protocols have been established to delineate appropriate chain of evidence specimen collection techniques, and it is imperative that medical professionals are familiar and proficient in specimen identification, collection, and handling. It is also important to remember that the likelihood of identifying a perpetrator can be maximized not only with a thorough and timely examination but, more importantly, with a comprehensive event history.

References

1. Christian CW, Lavelle JM, De Jong AR, Loiselle J, Brenner L, Joffe M. Forensic evidence findings in prepubertal victims of sexual assault. *Pediatrics*. 2000;106(1 Pt 1):100–104 PMID: 10878156 https://doi.org/10.1542/peds.106.1.100
2. Dahlke MB, Cooke C, Cunnane M, Chawla J, Lau P. Identification of semen in 500 patients seen because of rape. *Am J Clin Pathol*. 1977;68(6):740–746 PMID: 602911 https://doi.org/10.1093/ajcp/68.6.740
3. Enos WF, Conrath TB, Byer JC. Forensic evaluation of the sexually abused child. *Pediatrics*. 1986;78(3):385–398 PMID: 3748672
4. De Jong AR, Rose M. Legal proof of child sexual abuse in the absence of physical evidence. *Pediatrics*. 1991;88(3):506–511 PMID: 1881730
5. Gray-Eurom K, Seaberg DC, Wears RL. The prosecution of sexual assault cases: correlation with forensic evidence. *Ann Emerg Med*. 2002;39(1):39–46 PMID: 11782729 https://doi.org/10.1067/mem.2002.118013
6. De Jong AR, Rose M. Frequency and significance of physical evidence in legally proven cases of child sexual abuse. *Pediatrics*. 1989;84(6):1022–1026 PMID: 2587130
7. Campbell R, Bybee D, Townsend SM, Shaw J, Karim N, Markowitz J. The Impact of sexual assault nurse examiner programs on criminal justice case outcomes: a multisite replication study. *Violence Against Women*. 2014;20(5):607–625 PMID: 24875379 https://doi.org/10.1177/1077801214536286
8. Campbell R, Patterson D, Bybee D. Prosecution of adult sexual assault cases: a longitudinal analysis of the impact of a sexual assault nurse examiner program. *Violence Against Women*. 2012;18(2):223–244 PMID: 22433229 https://doi.org/10.1177/1077801212440158
9. Edinburgh L, Saewyc E, Levitt C. Caring for young adolescent sexual abuse victims in a hospital-based children's advocacy center. *Child Abuse Negl*. 2008;32(12):1119–1126 PMID: 19041133 https://doi.org/10.1016/j.chiabu.2008.05.006
10. Hansen LA, Mikkelsen SJ, Sabroe S, Charles AV. Medical findings and legal outcomes in sexually abused children. *J Forensic Sci*. 2010;55(1):104–109 PMID: 20002274 https://doi.org/10.1111/j.1556-4029.2009.01230.x

11. Patterson D, Campbell R. A comparative study of the prosecution of childhood sexual abuse cases: the contributory role of pediatric Forensic Nurse Examiner (FNE) programs. *J Forensic Nurs*. 2009;5(1):38–45 PMID: 19222688 https://doi.org/10.1111/j.1939-3938.2009.01029.x
12. Hornor G, Thackeray J, Scribano P, Curran S, Benzinger E. Pediatric sexual assault nurse examiner care: trace forensic evidence, ano-genital injury, and judicial outcomes. *J Forensic Nurs*. 2012;8(3):105–111 PMID: 22925125 https://doi.org/10.1111/j.1939-3938.2011.01131.x
13. Jenny C, Crawford-Jakubiak JE; American Academy of Pediatrics Committee on Child Abuse and Neglect. The evaluation of children in the primary care setting when sexual abuse is suspected. *Pediatrics*. 2013;132(2):e558–e567 PMID: 23897912 https://doi.org/10.1542/peds.2013-1741
14. Campbell R, Fehler-Cabral G, Bybee D, Shaw J. Forgotten evidence: a mixed methods study of why sexual assault kits (SAKs) are not submitted for DNA forensic testing. *Law Hum Behav*. 2017;41(5):454–467 PMID: 28661168 https://doi.org/10.1037/lhb0000252
15. Patterson D, Campbell R. The problem of untested sexual assault kits: why are some kits never submitted to a crime laboratory? *J Interpers Violence*. 2012;27(11):2259–2275 PMID: 22258072 https://doi.org/10.1177/0886260511432155
16. Palusci VJ, Cox EO, Shatz EM, Schultze JM. Urgent medical assessment after child sexual abuse. *Child Abuse Negl*. 2006;30(4):367–380 PMID: 16616367 https://doi.org/10.1016/j.chiabu.2005.11.002
17. Young KL, Jones JG, Worthington T, Simpson P, Casey PH. Forensic laboratory evidence in sexually abused children and adolescents. *Arch Pediatr Adolesc Med*. 2006;160(6):585–588 PMID: 16754819 https://doi.org/10.1001/archpedi.160.6.585
18. Thackeray JD, Hornor G, Benzinger EA, Scribano PV. Forensic evidence collection and DNA identification in acute child sexual assault. *Pediatrics*. 2011;128(2):227–232 PMID: 21788217 https://doi.org/10.1542/peds.2010-3498
19. Girardet R, Bolton K, Lahoti S, et al. Collection of forensic evidence from pediatric victims of sexual assault. *Pediatrics*. 2011;128(2):233–238 PMID: 21788219 https://doi.org/10.1542/peds.2010-3037
20. US Department of Justice Office on Violence Against Women. *A National Protocol for Sexual Abuse Medical Forensic Examinations—Pediatric*. https://www.justice.gov/ovw/file/846856. Published April 2016. Accessed May 28, 2019
21. National Institute of Justice. *National Best Practices for Sexual Assault Kits: A Multidisciplinary Approach*. Laurel, MD: US Department of Justice, Office of Justice Programs, National Institute of Justice; 2017. https://www.nij.gov/topics/law-enforcement/investigations/sexual-assault/Pages/national-best-practices-for-sexual-assault-kits.aspx. Accessed May 28, 2019
22. Gabby T, Winkleby MA, Boyce WT, Fisher DL, Lancaster A, Sensabaugh GF. Sexual abuse of children. The detection of semen on skin. *Am J Dis Child*. 1992;146(6):700–703 PMID: 1375806 https://doi.org/10.1001/archpedi.1992.02160180058017
23. Santucci KA, Nelson DG, McQuillen KK, Duffy SJ, Linakis JG. Wood's lamp utility in the identification of semen. *Pediatrics*. 1999;104(6):1342–1344 PMID: 10585986 https://doi.org/10.1542/peds.104.6.1342
24. LeBeau MA, Mozayani A, eds. *Drug-Facilitated Sexual Assault: A Forensic Handbook*. San Diego, CA: Academic Press; 2001
25. US Department of Justice. Advancing justice through DNA technology. https://www.justice.gov/archives/ag/advancing-justice-through-dna-technology-table-contents. Updated March 7, 2017. Accessed May 28, 2019

26. Gaensslen RE, Camp FR; National Institute of Justice. *Sourcebook in Forensic Serology, Immunology, and Biochemistry*. Unit IX. Washington, DC: US Department of Justice, National Institute of Justice; 1983
27. Houck MM, Budowle B. Correlation of microscopic and mitochondrial DNA hair comparisons. *J Forensic Sci*. 2002;47(5):964–967 PMID: 12353582 https://doi.org/10.1520/JFS15515J
28. Waltke H, LaPorte G, Weiss D, Schwarting D, Nguyen M, Scott F. Sexual assault cases: exploring the importance of non-DNA forensic evidence. *NIJ Journal*. https://www.nij.gov/journals/279/Pages/non-dna-evidence-in-sexual-assault-cases.aspx. Published April 2018. Accessed May 28, 2019
29. Butler J. *Fundamentals of DNA Typing*. San Diego, CA: Academic Press; 2009
30. Graham EA, Rutty GN. Investigation into "normal" background DNA on adult necks: implications for DNA profiling of manual strangulation victims. *J Forensic Sci*. 2008;53(5):1074–1082 PMID: 18624892 https://doi.org/10.1111/j.1556-4029.2008.00800.x
31. FBI Laboratory. *National DNA Index System (NDIS) Operational Procedures Manual*. https://www.fbi.gov/file-repository/ndis-operational-procedures-manual.pdf/view. Effective May 1, 2019. Accessed May 28, 2019
32. Brayley-Morris H, Sorrell A, Revoir AP, Meakin GE, Court DS, Morgan RM. *Persistence of DNA from laundered semen stains: implications for child sex trafficking cases. Forensic Sci Int Genet*. 2015;19:165–171 PMID: 26232275 https://doi.org/10.1016/j.fsigen.2015.07.016
33. Noël S, Lagacé K, Rogic A, et al. DNA transfer during laundering may yield complete genetic profiles. *Forensic Sci Int Genet*. 2016;23:240–247 PMID: 27236542 https://doi.org/10.1016/j.fsigen.2016.05.004

PART 3

Neglect

CHAPTER 14

Environmental Neglect and Social Determinants of Health

Wendy G. Lane, MD, MPH, FAAP
Clinical Associate Professor
Department of Epidemiology and Public Health
Department of Pediatrics
University of Maryland School of Medicine
Baltimore, MD

Howard Dubowitz, MD, MS, FAAP
Professor
Department of Pediatrics
University of Maryland School of Medicine
Baltimore, MD

Introduction

Social determinants of health (SDH) are defined by the World Health Organization as "the conditions in which people are born, grow, work, live, and age, and the wider set of forces and systems shaping the conditions of daily life."[1] Social determinants of health lead to disparities in health outcomes through increased risk for illness, decreased access to health care, and fewer opportunities for health promotion and disease prevention. While the World Health Organization has primarily focused on community- and societal-level issues, such as economic and social policies and social and cultural norms, others have also identified individual- and family-level factors that may contribute to poor health.[2,3]

The National Academies of Sciences[4] has stated that SDH should be integral to medical professional education and training to better understand the context of a patient's illness. It is also careful to note that medical professionals should understand a community's issues and needs before identifying and intervening on SDH. The National Academies has noted that action should take place within the context of "well thought-out partnerships" between medical professionals and others in the community.

This topic is not new to child health professionals. Child health has long been viewed in the context of family and community.[5] However, the extent to which pediatricians can and should act for individual children and families in the context of the health encounter has evolved over the past decade. This is due, in part, to the now extensive literature on how SDH contribute to adverse health outcomes. This development is also the result of a small number of interventions that have successfully identified and ameliorated some of the adverse effects of SDH for many children and families. This chapter describes research supporting the relationship between SDH and child maltreatment, some health care–based interventions for addressing SDH, and challenges facing medical professionals, particularly regarding child neglect and the child welfare system.

Relationship Between Social Determinants of Health and Child Maltreatment

There is no doubt that adverse childhood experiences (ACEs) and SDH have short- and long-term physical and mental health consequences, as evidenced by the Centers for Disease Control and Prevention ACEs study, as well as a number of confirmatory studies. Research has also found numerous associations between SDH and child maltreatment, as well as some studies establishing cause and effect. This section reviews some of the more prevalent SDH and their associations with child maltreatment.

Poverty

In 2016, 13.6 million children in the United States lived in poverty, representing 18% of the child population. While children represented 23% of the US population, they accounted for 32.6% of people in poverty.[6] Children living in poverty are more likely to have developmental issues and physical and mental health conditions compared with children not living in poverty. For example, children who are poor are more likely to have asthma, dental caries, language delays, impaired growth, depression, and conduct disorders.[7] In general, families living in poverty have a reduced capacity to provide for the basic needs of their children, including food, shelter, and health care. They may also have high levels of stress that impede their child-rearing and contribute to more reactive discipline methods, such as yelling and corporal punishment. In addition, economic stressors may increase parental conflict, decrease nurturing, and increase harsh discipline.[7,8] Research has shown a strong relationship between poverty and child maltreatment. An Australian study estimated that 27% of child maltreatment in that country was directly attributable to poverty.[7] Several studies have shown temporal associations between poverty and child maltreatment, such as a documented 25% increase in out-of-home placements after welfare payments were decreased in Denmark.[9] In the United States,[10] reported increases in child welfare involvement in one study were associated with home foreclosure. Importantly, several studies have shown reductions in maltreatment when economic circumstances improve.[11,12]

Neighborhood Poverty

Neighborhood poverty has also been directly linked to child maltreatment. Families living in high-poverty neighborhoods have been found to be at increased risk for child maltreatment.[13] In an examination of census tract data from Baltimore, MD, neighborhood poverty was identified as one of the strongest predictors for child maltreatment.[14] In addition, even sharing a border with at least one other poor neighborhood increases the risk for maltreatment,[15] particularly in African American neighborhoods.[16]

Housing Insecurity

Housing insecurity may be defined by a number of factors, including high housing costs in relation to income, poor housing quality, unstable neighborhoods, overcrowding, homelessness, multiple moves in the past year, and difficulty paying rent.[17,18] In 2015, 2.9 million households with children in the United States were considered to have "worst-case" housing needs, defined as renters with incomes below 50% of the area median income who do not receive government housing assistance or who pay more than one-half of their income for rent, live in severely inadequate conditions, or both.[19] Housing insecurity has been associated with poor health, poor growth, and developmental delays in children.[20] Unsafe neighborhoods and inadequate housing can put mental and emotional strains on parents, making it more difficult to cope with daily stressors and children's needs. Multiple studies have examined the effect of frequent moves and housing instability on children, finding higher rates of child maltreatment when compared with families in more stable living situations.[15,21,22] Children living with caregivers in unsafe housing conditions, already at increased risk, are less likely to receive adequate physical care.[22] Housing insecurity is directly associated with neglect and indirectly via maternal stress.[23]

Energy Insecurity

Energy insecurity is closely linked to housing insecurity. Energy insecurity includes threatened or actual utility shutoff or refused delivery of heating fuel, an unheated or uncooled day because of unpaid utility bills, or the use of a cooking stove as a source of heat.[17] Children have an increased skin surface area to mass ratio, which makes them more vulnerable to extreme heat and cold. A 1996 study identified a possible association between energy insecurity and failure to thrive. The authors reported lower weight for age in children going to an emergency department within 3 months following the coldest month of the year than at other times of the year, which is thought to be related to increased caloric needs during winter months due to cold stress and infections.[24]

Food Insecurity

Food insecurity is also closely associated with poverty and may be linked both directly and indirectly to child maltreatment. Severe child hunger has been directly linked to overall poor health in school-aged children, even after controlling for low birth weight, housing status, maternal distress, and stressful life events.[25] Food insecurity may be directly linked to failure to thrive. In one urban pediatric clinic, 27% of food-insecure families of infants acknowledged diluting infant formula, therefore providing inadequate caloric intake.[26] Food insecurity may also be associated with obesity, potentially mediated through maternal depression.[27] In addition to these direct associations, food insecurity is indirectly associated with child maltreatment through several pathways. Parents who are experiencing food insecurity are more likely to be depressed and anxious; these are independent predictors of maltreatment.[28,29] They also express fewer positive parenting behaviors, less sensitivity to infant cues, less responsiveness to infant distress, and less optimal behavior directed at fostering their babies' social and emotional growth compared with parents who are food secure.[27] Similarly, children faced with food insecurity are more likely to exhibit behavioral problems and hyperactivity, increasing their risk for maltreatment.[28–30]

Parental Depression

Parental depression is a frequent problem among mothers and fathers of children seen in pediatric clinics. An estimated 1 in 10 US children are cared for by a mother who is experiencing depression in any given year.[31] Depressed mothers experienced more adversities (eg, poverty, separation or divorce, unemployment, financial difficulties) and had worse functioning. A large representative study of maternal depression in the United States found that only one-half of the mothers experiencing depression received services for their depression. Black and Hispanic mothers who experienced depression were more likely to experience multiple adversities and were less likely to receive services than white mothers who experienced. A large study in the United Kingdom found that by the time a child was 12 years old, 39% of mothers and 21% of fathers had experienced an episode of depression. The highest rates were in the first year postpartum.[32] Parents with a history of depression, younger parents, and those from deprived areas were particularly vulnerable to depression.

Several studies have demonstrated adverse effects of maternal depression on children, including depression, anxiety, and conduct disorder.[33,34] A few studies have also shown consistent associations between postnatal paternal depression and an increased risk of behavioral and emotional problems in children between 3 and 5 years of age.[35–37] One study suggested that the association between depression in fathers during the postnatal period and subsequent child behavior is explained predominantly by family factors, such as depression in the mother and couple conflict.[38] In contrast, the association between maternal depression and child outcomes is better explained by other factors, which might include direct effects of depression on mother-infant interaction. There is also a strong link between maternal depression and child maltreatment.[39] For example, one study found that maternal depression was a significant predictor of a report to child protective services (CPS) in the first 4 years of a child's life.[40] Maternal depression was associated with severe physical abuse, after controlling for sociodemographic factors such as family income, race, and mother's educational level.[39] Another study found that mothers with probable comorbid posttraumatic stress disorder and depression reported greater parenting stress[41] and more psychological aggression toward and physical assaults of their children. The benefits to children of treating maternal depression have been shown. A prospective study of preschoolers' behavior associated with neglect found maternal depression to be strongly predictive of internalizing and externalizing behavior problems.[42]

Parental Substance Use

The number of children in the United States living with at least one parent who uses substances is alarming.[43] Combined 2009 through 2014 data from the National Survey on Drug Use and Health found that 8.7 million children, or 12.5% of children younger than 18 years, lived with at least one parent who used drugs or alcohol.[44] The 2012 National Survey on Drug Use and Health found that an estimated 7.5 million children, or 10.5% of children younger than 18 years, live with at least one parent who uses drugs or alcohol.[45] More than one-third of these children (36%) are younger than 6 years.[46]

Neger and Prinz summarized the literature on the harm to children related to parental substance use.[43] Infants exposed to drugs prenatally have been found to have difficult temperament including irritability, sleep and feeding disturbances, excessive crying, and physical ailments such as gastrointestinal problems, fever, and seizures. Children younger than 3 years are at risk for insecure and disorganized attachment and poor development, especially with regard to speech and language. School-aged children are apt to show aggressive behaviors, have fewer friends, and experience more peer conflict and are at risk for hyperactivity and inattention. Adolescents of parents who use substances show high rates of psychopathology such as depression, anxiety, and substance use. A recent study found that parental substance use was associated with children's hospitalization for somatic and psychiatric conditions.[47] The authors speculated that this may be related to unsafe environment, long-standing stress, and inadequate responses to the child's needs. There is also the likelihood that substance use is associated with ineffective parenting practices, such as coercive parenting styles, less supervision, and harsh punishment.[48,49]

Not surprisingly, parental substance use has been associated with child maltreatment, particularly neglect,[50] as well as increased rates of maltreatment recidivism.[51] In one study, more than 8,000 participants who grew up with 1 or more alcoholic parent were twice as likely to have experienced emotional abuse, physical abuse, sexual abuse, or neglect during childhood as those whose parents were not alcoholics.[52]

Intimate Partner Violence

Intimate partner violence (IPV) is defined as any physical, psychological, or sexual harm committed by a current or former partner or spouse.[53] Intimate partner or domestic violence continues to be a serious problem in the United States and internationally. It is estimated that more than one-third of women (36%) and more than one-quarter of men (29%) in the United States experience rape, physical violence, and/or stalking by an intimate partner in their lifetime.[54,55] Approximately 15.5 million children in the United States are estimated to live in 2-parent households in which IPV has occurred within the previous year,[56] and about 16% have witnessed IPV at least once during their lives.[57]

There is substantial evidence linking children's exposure to IPV with a wide range of serious consequences, including emotional, behavioral, physical, social, and academic problems.[58] Children may become involved in physical altercations, leading to direct injury and the development of violent means of resolving conflict.[59,60] Bair-Merritt and colleagues examined 22 papers reporting associations between children's exposure to IPV and physical health consequences. They concluded that children's exposure to IPV is related to increased adolescent and adult risk-taking behavior (eg, substance use) and is likely related to under-immunization but that there is insufficient evidence to draw conclusions about overall health status, use of health services, breastfeeding practices, and infant weight gain.[60] Some evidence suggests exposure to IPV may also be associated with physical changes in the brain.[61] A meta-analysis reviewed 74 studies that examined longitudinal associations between children's exposure to IPV and adjustment problems.[62] Children exposed to IPV were at risk for externalizing, internalizing, and total adjustment problems, and the association strengthened over time. Associations were also stronger when IPV was conceptualized broadly, including psychological and sexual violence. Child sex, sample type, and whether only the male partner's or both partners' violence was measured did not predict the association between children's exposure to IPV and later adjustment problems. Children exposed to IPV may also exhibit impairment of emotional and cognitive development. Such impairment can have far-reaching implications for children's ability to successfully negotiate school and interpersonal domains and develop into successful adults. A prospective study of 213 adolescents found that exposure to either physical or verbal aggression in adolescence was positively associated with perpetration and experiencing of abuse in adulthood.[63] However, several authors have cautioned that this link may be weak, with many studies having methodological shortcomings such as the lack of prospective longitudinal designs.[58]

Exposure to IPV is also associated with long-term mental health problems[64]; even greater impairment is associated when IPV co-occurs with child maltreatment.[65] Intimate partner violence and child maltreatment frequently co-occur. One review of 31 studies on the overlap of IPV and child maltreatment found co-occurrence rates between 30% and 60% in most of the studies.[66] A review of similar studies found a co-occurrence rate of about 40% with regard to IPV and child physical abuse.[67] This research provided the basis for the American Academy of Pediatrics policy urging pediatricians to help address IPV.[68] However, many children exposed to IPV appear to be resilient. For example, Kitzmann and colleagues found that 37% of children exposed to IPV had outcomes similar to or even better than children who were not exposed to IPV.[69]

Interventions to Address Social Determinants of Health

Several interventions have been developed for addressing SDH within the pediatric primary care setting (Table 14.1). Some common components include identifying risk (and sometimes protective) factors through screening, incorporation of behavioral change strategies, and referrals of families with specific needs to other professionals and/or community-based agencies that provide direct assistance and additional resources. It is clearly important for medical professionals to consider the needs of families they are serving and the resources available in the community.

Given the limited time available for patient visits, more common problems should be prioritized. There are also ethical considerations to screening for problems for which services are not available.

TABLE 14.1
Social Determinants of Health Programs with Web-Based Resources

Program	SDH Items Screened	Additional Resources	Resource Availability
Social needs screening and in-person service navigation—iScreen/FIND[70]	Housing stability and habitability Food security Income security Child care needs Transportation needs Employment needs Legal concerns Medical insurance and other public benefits Adult household members' mental health	Algorithms for program referrals Volunteer training resources	www.bayareahelpdesks.org
Health Leads	**Essential** Food insecurity Housing instability Utility needs Financial resource strain Transportation Exposure to violence **Optional** Child care Employment Health behaviors Social isolation and support Behavioral/mental health	Screening toolkit Social needs roadmap and implementation tools Specific information for CMS AHC grantees	https://healthleadsusa.org

(continued)

TABLE 14.1 (*continued*)

Program	SDH Items Screened	Additional Resources	Resource Availability
Medicolegal partnership	**Core Measures (PRAPARE)** Housing status and stability Employment Income/financial stability Stress Insurance status Transportation Social integration and support **Optional Measures** Incarceration history Safety Intimate partner violence Refugee status	Toolkit for screening implementation and action, including appendix with resources Free EHR templates for commonly used systems, including Epic, eClinicalWorks, Centricity, and NextGen	www.mlpboston.org www.medical-legalpartnership.org PRAPARE Implementation and Action Toolkit (www.nachc.org/research-and-data/prapare/toolkit)
SEEK	Parental depression Major stress Substance abuse Domestic violence Food insecurity Harsh punishment	Video-based trainings Management algorithms Parent handouts	https://www.seekwellbeing.org

Abbreviations: AHC, Accountable Health Communities; CMS, Centers for Medicare & Medicaid Services; EHR, electronic health record; FIND, Family Information & Navigation Desk; PRAPARE, Protocol for Responding to and Assessing Patients' Assets, Risks, and Experiences; SDH, social determinants of health; SEEK, Safe Environment for Every Kid.

Health Leads

Health Leads is a nonprofit organization that trains undergraduate students to volunteer in urban health clinics helping families meet their social needs. The program was developed at Boston Medical Center in 1996 and has since expanded to medical centers around the United States. Families seeking pediatric primary care complete a pre-visit screening form; physicians conduct an initial assessment of needs and make referrals to Health Leads staff. The Health Leads volunteer conducts an in-depth assessment and provides relevant resources to families. The volunteer then provides phone follow-up to the family and updates the physician as needed.[71] The program provides a toolkit for practices to create their own screening questionnaire, identifying essential social needs domains (food insecurity, housing instability, utility needs, financial resource strain, transportation, exposure to violence) and optional social needs domains (child care, employment, health behaviors, social isolation and support, behavioral/mental health). For each topic, one recommended and several additional screening questions are provided, along with references, information about validity and precision, and reading grade level. The program website (https://healthleadsusa.org) includes webinars and additional resources.

WE CARE

The WE CARE (*w*ell-child care visit, *e*valuation, *c*ommunity resources, *a*dvocacy, *r*eferral, *e*ducation) model[72] developed out of the Health Leads program. It consists of a 10-item screening questionnaire, brief provider education, and a family resource book, developed with social work and legal advocate colleagues. Psychosocial issues covered in the questionnaire include education and employment status, food insecurity, homelessness risk, parental depression, parental smoking, household drug use or problem alcohol use, IPV, and child care needs. Families are asked to complete the screening questionnaire before seeing their doctor. Pediatric residents review the questionnaire during the visit and make referrals to resources if the parents request assistance. In a randomized, controlled evaluation of the intervention, parents in the intervention group discussed more family psychosocial topics, were more likely to receive referrals for services, and were more likely to have contacted a community resource compared with parents in the control group.[72] In addition, on multivariable analysis, parents in the intervention group were more likely than control parents to have contacted a community resource. A subsequent cluster randomized trial[73] also found increased use of community resources. In addition, participants in the intervention group were more likely to be employed and to have child care and less likely to be living in a homeless shelter.

Social Needs Screening and In-Person Service Navigation—iScreen/FIND

The iScreen/FIND (Family Information & Navigation Desk) intervention also was developed through Health Leads. It was implemented in primary and urgent care settings at safety net hospitals in San Francisco, CA. The intervention involved trained, volunteer patient navigators who conducted

SDH screening and provided either preprinted handouts with appropriate resources (control group) or additional in-person or telephone follow-up (intervention group). Patient Navigators received training in screening, resources, and motivational interviewing. At 4-month follow-up, intervention families had significantly fewer social needs and significantly better health status.[70]

IHELP

IHELP is an inpatient-based intervention to screen for SDH.[3] Specific domains covered include *i*ncome/health insurance, *h*unger/housing, *e*ducation/ensuring safety (IPV), *l*egal status (immigration), and *p*ower of attorney and guardianship. Residents received a list of screening questions attached to their ID badges. Brief education, including role-playing and attending critique of and feedback to residents about their social histories, was provided. In addition, inpatient rounds on each patient began by asking about IHELP issues. Inpatient social work evaluations were obtained for families with positive screening results. In a post-intervention comparison of inpatient teams using IHELP and control teams, social work consultations were 3 times more frequent, and 78% of families with positive screening results were referred to resources. Follow-up after 21 months found that only 30% of residents continued to use IHELP.

Medicolegal Partnerships

Medicolegal partnerships (MLPs) are programs that place lawyers and legal services within health care settings to address SDH through legal action. Legal services are typically provided by civil legal aid organizations or law schools. Common issues that are addressed include access to health insurance and public benefits, housing conditions, and educational services and accommodations for children with special health care needs. The program began in 1993 at Boston Medical Center, when the chief of pediatrics hired a part-time attorney to address pediatric patients' basic needs, including food, housing, and safety. The program has expanded to nearly 300 health care sites, and a National Center for Medical-Legal Partnership was established at George Washington University in 2006. Each health center selects the SDH for which it wishes to screen. Some focus solely on legal needs that can be addressed by the MLP legal partner, while others take a broader view and screen for other issues that can be addressed by other health center staff, such as social workers or financial counselors.

There has been some critique of MLPs because of lack of routine screening at MLP sites and the absence of a formal screening protocol.[74] To more systematically assess SDH, the National Association of Community Health Centers and several other agencies developed PRAPARE (Protocol for Responding to and Assessing Patients' Assets, Risks, and Experiences), a formal assessment tool, which is now being implemented in many community health centers with MLPs.[75] PRAPARE includes screening questions related to housing, financial stability, stress, employment, and insurance status. Screening questions addressing additional SDH, such as domestic violence and incarceration history, are optional. Screening questions have been incorporated into electronic health record systems at community health centers that participate in MLPs. A number of studies have demonstrated the benefits of MLP programs, including improved health of asthma patients due to improved housing conditions, and improved access to services and decreased barriers to care in children with sickle cell anemia.[76–78]

Project DULCE

Project DULCE (Developmental Understanding and Legal Collaboration for Everyone)[79–81] is a primary care–based intervention focused on infants from birth to 6 months of age that originated at Boston Medical Center. Based on a Strengthening Families protective factors approach,[82] the program builds on 2 previously developed interventions, Healthy Steps[83,84] and MLPs. Healthy Steps is an evidence-based program that embeds a professional with child development expertise into pediatric primary care to educate, support, and refer parents to additional services. The child development professional interacts with families during pediatric and home visits and by telephone. DULCE Family Specialists have postgraduate training in child development and receive training from both Healthy Steps and an MLP. Family Specialists meet with families in the clinic and at their homes and also communicate by phone, email, and text. They conduct child developmental and parental mental health screenings and provide support and referrals to help meet basic needs. They consult with MLP Boston as needed. Decisions about the actual services delivered are made jointly between parents and Family Specialists.

Evaluation by randomized trial demonstrated better immunization rates and fewer emergency department visits for intervention families compared with control families. Intervention families were also more successful in total resource access, including food, energy, telephone, and emergency cash assistance.[81] In 2016, the program expanded to 4 counties in California and one in Vermont (https://dulcenational.org).

SEEK

The Safe Environment for Every Kid (SEEK) model offers a practical, evidence-based approach to help medical professionals address targeted psychosocial risk factors for child maltreatment for families with children aged 0 to 5 years. The targeted problems are parental depression, major stress, substance abuse, domestic violence, food insecurity, and harsh punishment. By helping address these problems, SEEK aims to strengthen families, support parents and parenting, and thereby promote children's health, development, and safety and help prevent child abuse and neglect.

Core components of the SEEK model are 1) training medical professionals to help address the targeted risk factors; 2) the SEEK Parent Questionnaire–R to screen for the problems at selected well-child visits[85–90]; 3) the reflect–empathize–assess–plan (REAP) approach to help medical professionals assess and address problems; 4) principles of motivational interviewing; 5) facilitating referrals to community resources for identified problems; 6) SEEK parent handouts for the targeted problems, customized with local resources; and 7) ideally, a social worker or behavioral health professional.

Evidence Supporting the SEEK Model

Two randomized controlled trials of the SEEK model have been conducted. The first was in pediatric residency primary care ("continuity") clinics serving a very low-income urban population.[91,92] The second was in 18 suburban private pediatric practices serving a mostly middle-income and relatively low-risk population.[93,94]

In both trials, medical professionals demonstrated significant improvement in their level of comfort, perceived competence, and practice behavior with regard to addressing the targeted risk factors. Some of these improvements were sustained for up to 18 to 36 months beyond the initial training.

In the first study, SEEK families benefited by having significantly less child abuse and neglect, assessed in 3 ways: by parental report of how they handled conflict with their child, by review of medical records for instances of abuse or neglect, and by CPS reports. In the second study, SEEK mothers reported less harsh physical punishment and psychological aggression, reasonably considered as child maltreatment, compared with controls. This finding was significant after 12 months as well. The SEEK model did not require additional time, on average, for medical professionals to address psychosocial problems. Cost data were evaluated in the second SEEK study. The SEEK model cost $3.38 per child per year and $210.20 per case of psychological aggression or physical assault averted.[95]

Poverty and Child Maltreatment: When to Refer to Child Protective Services

Child maltreatment and particularly neglect have been clearly linked to poverty.[96–99] The many burdens and stressors associated with poverty, such as food insecurity, living in dangerous neighborhoods, and surrounding drug use, can compromise parents' ability to provide adequate care to their children. Indeed, poverty in the context of the wealthy United States has been considered "societal neglect." Dilemmas may arise when a child's basic needs are not met, primarily due to the family's impoverished circumstances (eg, homelessness). Medical professionals may empathize, consider the situation to be beyond parents' control, and be reasonably reluctant to fault them and refer the family to CPS. How might such circumstances be approached?

Helping alleviate families' economic burdens is invariably a key component of promoting their capacity to care for their children. At a minimum, this involves short-term strategies; preferably, longer-term solutions are found. And, ideally, poverty is addressed at a community or societal level.

Some situations are primarily caused by poverty, such as when a family lacks health insurance and cannot fill a child's prescription, which jeopardizes a child's health. Facilitating health insurance and adherence to the treatment seem to be the first course of action, together with temporary measures such as providing samples of the medication. If, however, the situation persists and a child continues to be harmed or to be at risk of harm despite such efforts, involving CPS may be a last resort or the best way to assist a family and protect a child.

In contrast, many conditions are compounded by poverty, but poverty per se is not the only or main reason explaining the neglect. It is noteworthy that many families living in poverty do manage to adequately care for their children. Consider a parent experiencing substance use disorder and not feeding a child adequately, contributing to that child's failure to thrive. The difficult context may well elicit empathy for the parent, but the neglect needs to be addressed. Such situations often warrant a CPS referral, in addition to other supportive services.

There are also circumstances in which a family is living in poverty but the relationship between poverty and maltreatment is limited. An example is when a father molests his daughter or is emotionally abusive toward his son. It is important not to minimize the abuse or neglect of children in such circumstances. Child protective services must be part of the plan to protect such children.

From a practical standpoint, medical professionals should be knowledgeable about resources in their community so they can refer families when the need arises. Implementing one or more of the programs described in this chapter can help identify families in need before children are significantly affected by poverty. In situations in which children have not been harmed or are not at significant risk of harm, efforts should begin with community referrals. Child protective services should be involved when referrals are not effective, when a child has been harmed, or when a child is at significant risk of harm.

Conclusion

Many individual, family, community, and societal factors may contribute to poor health through increased risk for illness, decreased access to health care, and a reduced opportunity for health promotion and disease prevention. These SDH can seem overwhelming to address in the primary care setting. However, there are a number of resources available that can make it easier to identify and address SDH. Use of these tools has the potential to improve child health and reduce the likelihood of neglect. There will, of course, still be situations in which CPS must be involved, but early intervention may reduce the frequency with which those calls must be made.

References

1. World Health Organization. Social determinants of health. https://www.who.int/topics/social_determinants/en. Accessed February 5, 2019
2. Chung EK, Siegel BS, Garg A, et al. Screening for social determinants of health among children and families living in poverty: a guide for clinicians. *Curr Probl Pediatr Adolesc Health Care*. 2016;46(5):135–153 PMID: 27101890 https://doi.org/10.1016/j.cppeds.2016.02.004
3. Colvin JD, Bettenhausen JL, Anderson-Carpenter KD, et al. Multiple behavior change intervention to improve detection of unmet social needs and resulting resource referrals. *Acad Pediatr*. 2016;16(2):168–174 PMID: 26183003 https://doi.org/10.1016/j.acap.2015.06.001
4. National Academies of Sciences. Engineering, and Medicine. *A Framework for Educating Health Professionals to Address the Social Determinants of Health*. Washington, DC: National Academies Press; 2016
5. Stanton BM, Behrman RE. The field of pediatrics. In: Kliegman RM, Stanton BM, St. Geme JW, Schor NF, eds. Nelson's Textbook of Pediatric. 20th ed. Philadelphia, PA: Elsevier; 2016
6. Semega JL, Fontenot KR, Kollar MA; US Census Bureau. *Current Population Reports P60-259:* Income and Poverty in the United States: 2016. Washington, DC: US Government Printing Office; 2017

7. Pascoe JM, Wood DL, Duffee JH, Kuo A; American Academy of Pediatrics Committee on Psychosocial Aspects of Child and Family Health, Council on Community Pediatrics. Mediators and adverse effects of child poverty in the United States. *Pediatrics*. 2016;137(4):e20160340 PMID: 26962239 https://doi.org/10.1542/peds.2016-0340
8. Doidge JC, Higgins DJ, Delfabbro P, et al. Economic predictors of child maltreatment in an Australian population-based birth cohort. *Child Youth Serv Rev*. 2017;72:14–25 https://doi.org/10.1016/j.childyouth.2016.10.012
9. Wildeman C, Fallesen P. The effect of lowering welfare payment ceilings on children's risk of out-of-home placement. *Child Youth Serv Rev*. 2017;72:82–90 https://doi.org/10.1016/j.childyouth.2016.10.017
10. Berger LM, Collins JM, Font SA, Gjertson L, Slack KS, Smeeding T. Home foreclosure and child protective services involvement. *Pediatrics*. 2015;136(2):299–307 PMID: 26195543 https://doi.org/10.1542/peds.2014-2832
11. Cancian M, Yang M-Y, Slack KS. The effect of additional child support income on the risk of child maltreatment. *Soc Serv Rev*. 2013;87(3):417–437 https://doi.org/10.1086/671929
12. Raissian KM, Bullinger LR. Money matters: does the minimum wage affect child maltreatment rates? *Child Youth Serv Rev*. 2017;72:60–70 https://doi.org/10.1016/j.childyouth.2016.09.033
13. Coulton CJ, Korbin JE, Su M. Neighborhoods and child maltreatment: a multi-level study. *Child Abuse Negl*. 1999;23(11):1019–1040 PMID: 10604060 https://doi.org/10.1016/S0145-2134(99)00076-9
14. Zuravin SJ. The ecology of child abuse and neglect: review of the literature and presentation of data. *Violence Vict*. 1989;4(2):101–120 PMID: 2487128 https://doi.org/10.1891/0886-6708.4.2.101
15. Coulton CJ, Korbin JE, Su M, Chow J. Community level factors and child maltreatment rates. *Child Dev*. 1995;66(5):1262–1276 PMID: 7555215 https://doi.org/10.2307/1131646
16. Korbin JE, Coulton CJ, Chard S, Platt-Houston C, Su M. Impoverishment and child maltreatment in African American and European American neighborhoods. *Dev Psychopathol*. 1998;10(2):215–233 PMID: 9635222 https://doi.org/10.1017/S0954579498001588
17. Children's HealthWatch. http://childrenshealthwatch.org. Accessed February 5, 2019
18. Johnson A, Meckstroth A. Ancillary services to support welfare to work. US Department of Health and Human Services Office of the Assistant Secretary for Planning and Evaluation website. http://aspe.hhs.gov/hsp/isp/ancillary/front.htm. Published June 22, 1998. Accessed February 5, 2019
19. Watson NE, Steffen BL, Martin M, Vandenbroucke DA. *Worst Case Housing Needs: 2017 Report to Congress*. Washington, DC: US Dept of Housing and Urban Development, Office of Policy Development and Research; 2017. https://www.huduser.gov/portal/sites/default/files/pdf/Worst-Case-Housing-Needs.pdf. Published August 2017. Accessed February 5, 2019
20. Cutts DB, Meyers AF, Black MM, et al. US Housing insecurity and the health of very young children. *Am J Public Health*. 2011;101(8):1508–1514 PMID: 21680929 https://doi.org/10.2105/AJPH.2011.300139
21. Deccio G, Horner WC, Wilson D. High-risk neighborhoods and high-risk families: replication research related to the human ecology of child maltreatment. *J Soc Serv Res*. 1994;18(3–4):123–137 https://doi.org/10.1300/J079v18n03_06
22. Ernst JS. Community-level factors and child maltreatment in a suburban county. *Soc Work Res*. 2001;25(3):133–142 https://doi.org/10.1093/swr/25.3.133

23. Warren EJ, Font SA. Housing insecurity, maternal stress, and child maltreatment: an application of the family stress model. *Soc Serv Rev*. 2015;89(1):9–39 https://doi.org/10.1086/680043
24. Frank DA, Roos N, Meyers A, et al. Seasonal variation in weight-for-age in a pediatric emergency room. *Public Health Rep*. 1996;111(4):366–371 PMID: 8711106
25. Weinreb L, Wehler C, Perloff J, et al. Hunger: its impact on children's health and mental health. *Pediatrics*. 2002;110(4):e41 PMID: 12359814 https://doi.org/10.1542/peds.110.4.e41
26. Burkhardt MC, Beck AF, Kahn RS, Klein MD. Are our babies hungry? Food insecurity among infants in urban clinics. *Clin Pediatr (Phila)*. 2012;51(3):238–243 PMID: 22114199 https://doi.org/10.1177/0009922811426767
27. Bronte-Tinkew J, Zaslow M, Capps R, Horowitz A, McNamara M. Food insecurity works through depression, parenting, and infant feeding to influence overweight and health in toddlers. *J Nutr*. 2007;137(9):2160–2165 PMID: 17709458 https://doi.org/10.1093/jn/137.9.2160
28. Whitaker RC, Phillips SM, Orzol SM. Food insecurity and the risks of depression and anxiety in mothers and behavior problems in their preschool-aged children. *Pediatrics*. 2006;118(3):e859–e868 PMID: 16950971 https://doi.org/10.1542/peds.2006-0239
29. Wu Z, Schimmele CM. Food insufficiency and depression. *Sociol Perspect*. 2005;48(4):481–504 https://doi.org/10.1525/sop.2005.48.4.481
30. Murphy JM, Wehler CA, Pagano ME, Little M, Kleinman RE, Jellinek MS. Relationship between hunger and psychosocial functioning in low-income American children. *J Am Acad Child Adolesc Psychiatry*. 1998;37(2):163–170 PMID: 9473912 https://doi.org/10.1097/00004583-199802000-00008
31. Ertel KA, Rich-Edwards JW, Koenen KC. Maternal depression in the United States: nationally representative rates and risks. *J Womens Health (Larchmt)*. 2011;20(11):1609–1617 PMID: 21877915 https://doi.org/10.1089/jwh.2010.2657
32. Davé S, Petersen I, Sherr L, Nazareth I. Incidence of maternal and paternal depression in primary care: a cohort study using a primary care database. *Arch Pediatr Adolesc Med*. 2010;164(11):1038–1044 PMID: 20819960 https://doi.org/10.1001/archpediatrics.2010.184
33. Glasheen C, Richardson GA, Kim KH, Larkby CA, Swartz HA, Day NL. Exposure to maternal pre- and postnatal depression and anxiety symptoms: risk for major depression, anxiety disorders, and conduct disorder in adolescent offspring. *Dev Psychopathol*. 2013;25(4 Pt 1):1045–1063 PMID: 24229548 https://doi.org/10.1017/S0954579413000369
34. Lieb R, Isensee B, Höfler M, Pfister H, Wittchen HU. Parental major depression and the risk of depression and other mental disorders in offspring: a prospective-longitudinal community study. *Arch Gen Psychiatry*. 2002;59(4):365–374 PMID: 11926937 https://doi.org/10.1001/archpsyc.59.4.365
35. Fletcher RJ, Feeman E, Garfield C, Vimpani G. The effects of early paternal depression on children's development. *Med J Aust*. 2011;195(11-12):685–689 PMID: 22171866 https://doi.org/10.5694/mja11.10192
36. Goodman JH. Paternal postpartum depression, its relationship to maternal postpartum depression, and implications for family health. *J Adv Nurs*. 2004;45(1):26–35 PMID: 14675298 https://doi.org/10.1046/j.1365-2648.2003.02857.x
37. Ramchandani P, Stein A, Evans J, O'Connor TG; ALSPAC study team. Paternal depression in the postnatal period and child development: a prospective population study. *Lancet*. 2005;365(9478):2201–2205 PMID: 15978928 https://doi.org/10.1016/S0140-6736(05)66778-5
38. Gutierrez-Galve L, Stein A, Hanington L, Heron J, Ramchandani P. Paternal depression in the postnatal period and child development: mediators and moderators. *Pediatrics*. 2015;135(2):e339–e347 PMID: 25560437 https://doi.org/10.1542/peds.2014-2411

39. Windham AM, Rosenberg L, Fuddy L, McFarlane E, Sia C, Duggan AK. Risk of mother-reported child abuse in the first 3 years of life. *Child Abuse Negl.* 2004;28(6):645–667 PMID: 15193853 https://doi.org/10.1016/j.chiabu.2004.01.003
40. Kotch JB, Browne DC, Dufort V, Winsor J, Catellier D. Predicting child maltreatment in the first 4 years of life from characteristics assessed in the neonatal period. *Child Abuse Negl.* 1999;23(4):305–319 PMID: 10321769 https://doi.org/10.1016/S0145-2134(99)00003-4
41. Chemtob CM, Gudiño OG, Laraque D. Maternal posttraumatic stress disorder and depression in pediatric primary care: association with child maltreatment and frequency of child exposure to traumatic events. *JAMA Pediatr.* 2013;167(11):1011–1018 PMID: 23999612 https://doi.org/10.1001/jamapediatrics.2013.2218
42. Dubowitz H, Papas MA, Black MM, Starr RH Jr. Child neglect: outcomes in high-risk urban preschoolers. *Pediatrics.* 2002;109(6):1100–1107 PMID: 12042549 https://doi.org/10.1542/peds.109.6.1100
43. Neger EN, Prinz RJ. Interventions to address parenting and parental substance abuse: conceptual and methodological considerations. *Clin Psychol Rev.* 2015;39:71–82 PMID: 25939033 https://doi.org/10.1016/j.cpr.2015.04.004
44. Lipari RN, Van Horn SL. Children living with parents who have a substance use disorder. *The CBHSQ Report.* Rockville, MD: Center for Behavioral Health Statistics and Quality, Substance Abuse and Mental Health Services Administration; August 24, 2017. https://www.samhsa.gov/data/sites/default/files/report_3223/ShortReport-3223.html. Accessed February 5, 2019
45. Substance Abuse Mental Health Services Administration. *Results from the 2011 National Survey on Drug Use and Health: Summary of National Findings.* Rockville, MD: Substance Abuse and Mental Health Services Administration; 2012:SMA14–SMA4863
46. Appleyard K, Berlin LJ, Rosanbalm KD, Dodge KA. Preventing early child maltreatment: implications from a longitudinal study of maternal abuse history, substance use problems, and offspring victimization. *Prev Sci.* 2011;12(2):139–149 PMID: 21240556 https://doi.org/10.1007/s11121-010-0193-2
47. Raitasalo K, Holmila M. Parental substance abuse and risks to children's safety, health and psychological development. *Drugs Educ Prev Policy.* 2017;24(1):17–22 https://doi.org/10.1080/09687637.2016.1232371
48. Kandel DB. Parenting styles, drug use, and children's adjustment in families of young adults. *J Marriage Fam.* 1990;52(1):183–196 https://doi.org/10.2307/352849
49. Ondersma SJ. Predictors of neglect within low-SES families: the importance of substance abuse. *Am J Orthopsychiatry.* 2002;72(3):383–391 PMID: 15792050 https://doi.org/10.1037/0002-9432.72.3.383
50. Wekerle C, Wall A-M, Leung E, Trocmé N. Cumulative stress and substantiated maltreatment: the importance of caregiver vulnerability and adult partner violence. *Child Abuse Negl.* 2007;31(4):427–443 PMID: 17445887 https://doi.org/10.1016/j.chiabu.2007.03.001
51. Connell CM, Bergeron N, Katz KH, Saunders L, Tebes JK. Re-referral to child protective services: the influence of child, family, and case characteristics on risk status. *Child Abuse Negl.* 2007;31(5):573–588 PMID: 17537504 https://doi.org/10.1016/j.chiabu.2006.12.004
52. Dube SR, Anda RF, Felitti VJ, Croft JB, Edwards VJ, Giles WH. Growing up with parental alcohol abuse: exposure to childhood abuse, neglect, and household dysfunction. *Child Abuse Negl.* 2001;25(12):1627–1640 PMID: 11814159 https://doi.org/10.1016/S0145-2134(01)00293-9
53. Centers for Disease Control and Prevention. Violence prevention. Intimate partner violence. https://www.cdc.gov/violenceprevention/intimatepartnerviolence/index.html. Updated October 23, 2018. Accessed February 5, 2019

54. Widom CS, Czaja S, Dutton MA. Child abuse and neglect and intimate partner violence victimization and perpetration: a prospective investigation. *Child Abuse Negl.* 2014;38(4):650–663 PMID: 24325940 https://doi.org/10.1016/j.chiabu.2013.11.004
55. Black MC, Basile KC, Breiding MJ, et al. *The National Intimate Partner and Sexual Violence Survey (NISVS): 2010 Summary Report.* Atlanta, GA: National Center for Injury Prevention and Control, Centers for Disease Control and Prevention; 2011. https://www.cdc.gov/violenceprevention/pdf/nisvs_report2010-a.pdf. Accessed February 5, 2019
56. McDonald R, Jouriles EN, Ramisetty-Mikler S, Caetano R, Green CE. Estimating the number of American children living in partner-violent families. *J Fam Psychol.* 2006;20(1):137–142 PMID: 16569098 https://doi.org/10.1037/0893-3200.20.1.137
57. Finkelhor D, Turner HA, Shattuck A, Hamby SL. Prevalence of childhood exposure to violence, crime, and abuse: results from the national survey of children's exposure to violence. *JAMA Pediatr.* 2015;169(8):746–754 PMID: 26121291 https://doi.org/10.1001/jamapediatrics.2015.0676
58. McTavish JR, MacGregor JC, Wathen CN, MacMillan HL. Children's exposure to intimate partner violence: an overview. *Int Rev Psychiatry.* 2016;28(5):504–518 PMID: 27414209 https://doi.org/10.1080/09540261.2016.1205001
59. Ehrensaft MK, Cohen P, Brown J, Smailes E, Chen H, Johnson JG. Intergenerational transmission of partner violence: a 20-year prospective study. *J Consult Clin Psychol.* 2003;71(4):741–753 PMID: 12924679 https://doi.org/10.1037/0022-006X.71.4.741
60. Bair-Merritt MH, Blackstone M, Feudtner C. Physical health outcomes of childhood exposure to intimate partner violence: a systematic review. *Pediatrics.* 2006;117(2): e278–e290 PMID: 16452335 https://doi.org/10.1542/peds.2005-1473
61. Choi J, Jeong B, Polcari A, Rohan ML, Teicher MH. Reduced fractional anisotropy in the visual limbic pathway of young adults witnessing domestic violence in childhood. *Neuroimage.* 2012;59(2):1071–1079 PMID: 21985907 https://doi.org/10.1016/j.neuroimage.2011.09.033
62. Vu NL, Jouriles EN, McDonald R, Rosenfield D. Children's exposure to intimate partner violence: a meta-analysis of longitudinal associations with child adjustment problems. *Clin Psychol Rev.* 2016;46:25–33 PMID: 27136293 https://doi.org/10.1016/j.cpr.2016.04.003
63. Cui M, Durtschi JA, Donnellan MB, Lorenz FO, Conger RD. Intergenerational transmission of relationship aggression: a prospective longitudinal study. *J Fam Psychol.* 2010;24(6):688–697 PMID: 21171767 https://doi.org/10.1037/a0021675
64. Koverola C, Morahan N. Children exposed to domestic violence. In: Green-Hernandez C, Singleton JK, Aronzon SZ, eds. *Primary Care Pediatrics.* Philadelphia, PA: Lippincott; 2001
65. Higgins DJ, McCabe MP. Multiple forms of child abuse and neglect: adult retrospective reports. *Aggress Violent Behav.* 2001;6(6):547–578 https://doi.org/10.1016/S1359-1789(00)00030-6
66. Edleson JL. The overlap between child maltreatment and woman battering. *Violence Against Women.* 1999;5(2):134–154 https://doi.org/10.1177/107780129952003
67. Appel AE, Holden GW. The co-occurrence of spouse and physical child abuse: a review and appraisal. *J Fam Psychol.* 1998;12(4):578–599 https://doi.org/10.1037/0893-3200.12.4.578
68. Thackeray JD, Hibbard R, Dowd MD; American Academy of Pediatrics Committee on Child Abuse and Neglect, Committee on Injury, Violence, and Poison Prevention. Intimate partner violence: the role of the pediatrician. *Pediatrics.* 2010;125(5):1094–1100 PMID: 20421260 https://doi.org/10.1542/peds.2010-0451

69. Kitzmann KM, Gaylord NK, Holt AR, Kenny ED. Child witnesses to domestic violence: a meta-analytic review. *J Consult Clin Psychol*. 2003;71(2):339–352 PMID: 12699028 https://doi.org/10.1037/0022-006X.71.2.339
70. Gottlieb LM, Hessler D, Long D, et al. Effects of social needs screening and in-person service navigation on child health: a randomized clinical trial. *JAMA Pediatr*. 2016;170(11):e162521 PMID: 27599265 https://doi.org/10.1001/jamapediatrics.2016.2521
71. Garg A, Marino M, Vikani AR, Solomon BS. Addressing families' unmet social needs within pediatric primary care: the health leads model. *Clin Pediatr (Phila)*. 2012;51(12):1191–1193 PMID: 22387923 https://doi.org/10.1177/0009922812437930
72. Garg A, Butz AM, Dworkin PH, Lewis RA, Thompson RE, Serwint JR. Improving the management of family psychosocial problems at low-income children's well-child care visits: the WE CARE Project. *Pediatrics*. 2007;120(3):547–558 PMID: 17766528 https://doi.org/10.1542/peds.2007-0398
73. Garg A, Toy S, Tripodis Y, Silverstein M, Freeman E. Addressing social determinants of health at well child care visits: a cluster RCT. *Pediatrics*. 2015;135(2):e296–e304 PMID: 25560448 https://doi.org/10.1542/peds.2014-2888
74. Theiss J, Regenstein M. Facing the need: screening practices for the social determinants of health. *J Law Med Ethics*. 2017;45(3):431–441 https://doi.org/10.1177/1073110517737543
75. Williamson A, Trott J, Regenstein M. *Health Center-Based Medical-Legal Partnerships: Where They Are, How They Work, and How They Are Funded*. Washington, DC: National Center for Medical-Legal Partnership; 2018. https://medical-legalpartnership.org/mlp-resources/health-center-mlps. Accessed February 5, 2019
76. Klein MD, Beck AF, Henize AW, Parrish DS, Fink EE, Kahn RS. Doctors and lawyers collaborating to HeLP children--outcomes from a successful partnership between professions. *J Health Care Poor Underserved*. 2013;24(3):1063–1073 PMID: 23974381 https://doi.org/10.1353/hpu.2013.0147
77. O'Sullivan MM, Brandfield J, Hoskote SS, et al. Environmental improvements brought by the legal interventions in the homes of poorly controlled inner-city adult asthmatic patients: a proof-of-concept study. *J Asthma*. 2012;49(9):911–917 PMID: 23020301 https://doi.org/10.3109/02770903.2012.724131
78. Pettignano R, Caley SB, Bliss LR. Medical-legal partnership: impact on patients with sickle cell disease. *Pediatrics*. 2011;128(6):e1482–e1488 PMID: 22084325 https://doi.org/10.1542/peds.2011-0082
79. Sege R, Kaplan-Sanoff M, Morton SJ, et al. Project DULCE: strengthening families through enhanced primary care. *Zero to Three*. 2014;35(1):10–18
80. Sege R, Morakinyo G, Eugenio J. *Project DULCE: Developmental Understanding & Legal Collaboration for Everyone Final Report. September 2010–December 2013*. https://www.cssp.org/reform/early-childhood/qic-ec/Final-Report-Project-Dulce-Boston-MA.pdf. Published December 31, 2013. Accessed February 7, 2018
81. Sege R, Preer G, Morton SJ, et al. Medical-legal strategies to improve infant health care: a randomized trial. *Pediatrics*. 2015;136(1):97–106 PMID: 26034248 https://doi.org/10.1542/peds.2014-2955
82. Horton C. *Strengthening Families through Early Care and Intervention. Washington, D.C.: Center for the Study of Social Policy*. https://cssp.org/reform/strengthening-families/resources/body/LiteratureReview.pdf. Published September 2003. Accessed February 7, 2018
83. Minkovitz CS, Hughart N, Strobino D, et al. A practice-based intervention to enhance quality of care in the first 3 years of life: the Healthy Steps for Young Children Program. *JAMA*. 2003;290(23):3081–3091 PMID: 14679271 https://doi.org/10.1001/jama.290.23.3081

84. Zuckerman B, Parker S, Kaplan-Sanoff M, Augustyn M, Barth MC. Healthy Steps: a case study of innovation in pediatric practice. *Pediatrics*. 2004;114(3):820–826 PMID: 15342859 https://doi.org/10.1542/peds.2003-0999-L
85. Dubowitz H, Feigelman S, Lane W, et al. Screening for depression in an urban pediatric primary care clinic. *Pediatrics*. 2007;119(3):435–443 PMID: 17332195 https://doi.org/10.1542/peds.2006-2010
86. Dubowitz H, Prescott L, Feigelman S, Lane W, Kim J. Screening for intimate partner violence in a pediatric primary care clinic. *Pediatrics*. 2008;121(1):e85–e91 PMID: 18166548 https://doi.org/10.1542/peds.2007-0904
87. Feigelman S, Dubowitz H, Lane W, et al. Screening for harsh punishment in a pediatric primary care clinic. *Child Abuse Negl*. 2009;33(5):269–277 PMID: 19477005 https://doi.org/10.1016/j.chiabu.2008.09.011
88. Kim J, Dubowitz H, Hudson-Martin E, Lane W. Comparison of 3 data collection methods for gathering sensitive and less sensitive information. *Ambul Pediatr*. 2008;8(4):255–260 PMID: 18644548 https://doi.org/10.1016/j.ambp.2008.03.033
89. Lane WG, Dubowitz H, Feigelman S, et al. Screening for parental substance abuse in pediatric primary care. *Ambul Pediatr*. 2007;7(6):458–462 PMID: 17996841 https://doi.org/10.1016/j.ambp.2007.07.007
90. Lane WG, Dubowitz H, Feigelman S, Poole G. The effectiveness of food insecurity screening in pediatric primary care. *Int J Child Health Nutr*. 2014;3(3):130–138 PMID: 28649292 https://doi.org/10.6000/1929-4247.2014.03.03.3
91. Dubowitz H, Feigelman S, Lane W, Kim J. Pediatric primary care to help prevent child maltreatment: the Safe Environment for Every Kid (SEEK) Model. *Pediatrics*. 2009;123(3):858–864 PMID: 19255014 https://doi.org/10.1542/peds.2008-1376
92. Feigelman S, Dubowitz H, Lane W, Grube L, Kim J. Training pediatric residents in a primary care clinic to help address psychosocial problems and prevent child maltreatment. *Acad Pediatr*. 2011;11(6):474–480 PMID: 21959095 https://doi.org/10.1016/j.acap.2011.07.005
93. Dubowitz H, Lane WG, Semiatin JN, Magder LS. The SEEK model of pediatric primary care: can child maltreatment be prevented in a low-risk population? *Acad Pediatr*. 2012;12(4):259–268 PMID: 22658954 https://doi.org/10.1016/j.acap.2012.03.005
94. Dubowitz H, Lane WG, Semiatin JN, Magder LS, Venepally M, Jans M. The safe environment for every kid model: impact on pediatric primary care professionals. *Pediatrics*. 2011;127(4):e962–e970 PMID: 21444590 https://doi.org/10.1542/peds.2010-1845
95. Lane WG, Dubowitz H, Frick K, et al. The Safe Environment for Every Kid (SEEK) program: a cost-effectiveness analysis. Paper presented at: 139th Annual Meeting of the American Public Health Association; November 2011; Washington, DC
96. Eckenrode J, Smith EG, McCarthy ME, Dineen M. Income inequality and child maltreatment in the United States. *Pediatrics*. 2014;133(3):454–461 PMID: 24515511 https://doi.org/10.1542/peds.2013-1707
97. Jonson-Reid M, Drake B, Zhou P. Neglect subtypes, race, and poverty: individual, family, and service characteristics. *Child Maltreat*. 2013;18(1):30–41 PMID: 23109353 https://doi.org/10.1177/1077559512462452
98. Lefebvre R, Fallon B, Van Wert M, Filippelli J. Examining the relationship between economic hardship and child maltreatment using data from the Ontario Incidence Study of Reported Child Abuse and Neglect-2013 (OIS-2013). *Behav Sci (Basel)*. 2017;7(1):E6 PMID: 28208690 https://doi.org/10.3390/bs7010006
99. Maguire-Jack K, Font SA. Community and individual risk factors for physical child abuse and child neglect: variations by poverty status. *Child Maltreat*. 2017;22(3):215–226 PMID: 28595465 https://doi.org/10.1177/1077559517711806

CHAPTER 15

Supervisory Neglect

François M. Luyet, MD
Clinical Assistant Professor of Pediatrics
University of Wisconsin School of Medicine and Public Health
University of Wisconsin Child Protection Program
University of Wisconsin American Family Children's Hospital
Madison, WI

Barbara L. Knox, MD, FAAP
Professor of Pediatrics
University of Wisconsin School of Medicine and Public Health
Medical Director, University of Wisconsin Child Protection Program
University of Wisconsin American Family Children's Hospital
Madison, WI

Definitions

According to Straus and Kantor, "[N]eglect is a behavior by a caregiver that constitutes a failure to act in ways that are presumed by the culture of a society to be necessary to meet the developmental needs of a child, and which are the responsibility of the caregiver to provide."[1] *Supervision* is a term used to describe the process of a person having responsibility for another person. Historically, lack of adequate child supervision has fallen under the category of physical neglect.[2] However, this form is so complex that it merits its own category. The definition of *supervisory neglect* varies in the literature, as some authors focus more on what the parent/caregiver does and others focus more on the effect on the child. This is discussed at length by Coohey,[3] who concludes that supervisory neglect is "the failure of a parent or caretaker to provide the child with adequate protection from harmful people or situations."

Coohey[3] defined 5 main types of supervisory neglect (Box 15.1).

BOX 15.1
Definitions for Types of Supervision Problems

1. *Did not watch child closely enough:* The parent was near the child, but the parent did not know exactly where the child was, whom he or she was with, or what he or she was doing; or did not check up on him or her often enough.
2. *Inadequate substitute child care*
   a. Left alone: The parent temporarily left the child alone without a caretaker and was not nearby.
   b. Left with suitable caretaker but without consent or adequate planning: The parent temporarily left the child with or sent the child to a person who was able to adequately care for the child but without proper planning or consent.
   c. Refused custody or abandoned: The parent permanently refused to take care of the child.
   d. Left with unsuitable caretaker, not a child abuser: The parent temporarily left the child with a person who was not able to adequately care for the child. Unsuitable caretakers include a person who was too young, used alcohol or drugs, had a mental health problem, was inattentive, or was inappropriate (eg, stranger).
3. *Failure to protect child from a third party*
   a. Left with unsuitable caretaker—child abuser: The parent temporarily left the child with an alleged or known child sexual or physical abuser.
   b. Exposed to child abuser: The parent exposed the child to an alleged or known child sexual or physical abuser or put the child at risk of being exposed to future abuse.
   c. Exposed to domestic violence: The parent exposed the child to battering or put the child at risk of being exposed to future battering.
   d. Exposed to person engaged in an illegal or inappropriate activity: The parent exposed the child to a person engaged in an illegal or inappropriate activity or put the child at risk of being exposed to this person in the future. These persons include someone who was using alcohol or drugs; selling drugs, guns, or pornography; having sex in front of the children; or engaging in another illegal or inappropriate activity.
4. *Allowed, encouraged, or forced a child to engage in a harmful activity:* The parent knew the child was engaged in an illegal or other harmful activity and did not try to stop it. These activities include a child who was using alcohol or drugs, not attending school, coming home late, staying out all night, or engaging in another illegal or harmful activity (eg, prostitution).
5. *Drove recklessly or while intoxicated/impaired:* The parent drove recklessly or while intoxicated with the child in or on a motor vehicle.

From Coohey C. Defining and classifying supervisory neglect. *Child Maltreat.* 2003; 8(2):145–156.

Epidemiology

Neglect is the most common form of child maltreatment, and more than half of cases of child neglect are due to inadequate supervision.[4] A 2001 report estimated that 30% to 40% of maltreatment deaths are caused by neglect.[5] Neglect, alone or combined with other forms or abuse, is involved in 74% of child maltreatment deaths.[6] These deaths occurred as a result of infant abandonment, starvation, medical neglect, drowning, home fires, being left alone in cars, and firearms.

Risk Factors

According to Berkowitz, an increased risk of death due to neglect is attributed to circumstances related to the child, the parents, the family, and the community.[5] Berkowitz also reported that preterm birth, low birth weight, and developmental disabilities are among the child risk factors.[5] Risk factors associated with parents include limited parenting skills, substance abuse, mental illness, developmental disabilities of the parent, and illiteracy.[5] Common family risk factors are larger families, absence of an extended family, social isolation, and multiple stressors (eg, homelessness, unemployment, imprisonment).[5] Risk factors may also originate in the community or neighborhood, including low educational resources and inadequate access to child care and transportation.[5] Basic safety education can prevent situations in which no one understands that there is a supervision problem or takes responsibility for it.[7] Affordable child care and transportation decrease the likelihood that single parents will leave their children alone and unsupervised.[4] Supervisory neglect is more likely to be long lasting if the mother's partner is not the father of her child(ren) or has a drug, alcohol, or mental health problem.[7]

Supervisory neglect implies an omission behavior or failure to act, often brought about by factors that may or may not directly be controlled by the responsible caregiver.[8] Poverty is the most important of these risk factors. According to Pelton, poverty-associated factors such as unemployment, run-down and crowded housing, food stress, and lack of recreation opportunities induce stressful situations that facilitate abuse and neglect.[9] Families experiencing poverty may have supervisory challenges due to poor access to safe products and resources, as well as life stresses.[8] In a longitudinal study, supervisory neglect was associated with difficulty obtaining child care, moving from a safe to an unsafe neighborhood, maternal exposure to domestic violence, and maternal physical health problems.[10]

Evaluation

An evaluation for supervisory neglect should consider 3 sets of factors: the child, the caregiver, and the specific incident.

Child factors include the child's age, developmental level, and physical and mental ability to make decisions and care for or protect himself or herself. Higher rates of physical harm are found among children with mental health issues such as depression, anxiety, and/or social withdrawal; attention-deficit/hyperactivity disorder; self-harming behavior; substance use; intellectual/developmental disabilities; and aggressive behavior.[11]

Caregiver factors include the caregiver's physical and mental ability to make decisions and care for and protect the child, the caregiver's possible involvement in substance or alcohol use, and the caregiver's accessibility and number of children he or she is responsible for, as well as the involvement of the caregiver in previous incidents of neglect or abuse. This also includes mental health problems and domestic violence.

According to Coohey, "[W]hen the caretaker and child are in the same location but the child is not supervised closely enough, parental drug and/or alcohol problems or poor mental health is a contributing factor in 2/3 of the cases."[12] Children who are left with inadequate caregivers are more likely to be harmed than children left alone or children who are not supervised closely enough by their parent.[12] One-third of these children are also physically or sexually assaulted.[12]

Incident factors include the type of activities the child was involved in while unsupervised, the potential danger to the child in an environmental context, how often and how long the child was inadequately supervised, the time of day, and the weather conditions.[13] When there is no evidence of child injury, it is particularly important to take into account the social context (eg, poverty, neighborhood, family structure) as well as cultural differences in child-rearing practices.[14,15] For instance, in lower-income countries, and especially in rural areas, many children are left under the supervision of other children, which places them at higher risk of injuries.[16] The lack of documented harm does not rule out supervisory neglect. In a Canadian study of 12,705 cases classified as supervisory neglect by the child welfare system, there was no documented evidence of physical child injury in 96% of cases.[11] When no harm to the child is documented, a referral to family support services may be more appropriate than a child welfare investigation. In the evaluation of supervisory neglect, assessing what meets a minimal standard of parenting as defined by state law remains subjective, particularly if the situation is complicated by socioeconomic and/or cultural factors. However, acknowledgment of cultural differences shouldn't prevent the recognition of a child in need of protection; some cultural practices are harmless, but others can be highly detrimental (eg, female genital mutilation).[17] Often, the identification of supervisory neglect ends up being a subjective decision.[8]

Consequences

The long-term consequences of supervisory neglect have rarely been studied. It is hard to differentiate the effects of a chronic lack of supervision from its multiple risk factors, such as poverty, parental psychopathology, substance use, homelessness, and family breakup. Child neglect in general has frequent, severe, adverse long-term consequences on children's cognitive, socioemotional, and behavioral development. Neglect occurring early in life is particularly detrimental. According to Hildyard and Wolfe, severe cognitive and academic deficits, social withdrawal, limited peer interactions, and symptoms of depression and anxiety are more frequently found in children who have experienced neglect when compared with children who have experienced physical abuse.[18] For older children (fifth grade and above), studies have implicated a lack of supervision (especially if associated with general neglect and insensitive discipline) in the future development of aggressive or antisocial behavior and association with deviant peers.[19]

Situations in Which Supervisory Neglect Is Frequently Implicated

Child Left Home Alone or With an Inadequate Substitute Caregiver

Case Example

A mother left her 4-year-old, 2-year-old, and 8-month-old alone in an urban apartment at night while she went to get cigarettes at the local convenience store. The 4-year-old reported waking up and getting scared by a blinking red light in the apartment. She reported that she went outside to look for her mother and the door automatically locked behind her. She was found alone crying on a busy street by an unrelated adult at 2:00 am. She suffered psychological trauma from this event. The case was substantiated as supervisory neglect because all the children were at serious risk of harm. The children were taken into custody by child protective services after the mother was located and found to be under the influence of street drugs.

One of the most important factors for serious risk of harm to minor children is being left home alone or with an inadequate substitute caregiver. There is no current standard for the age when a child can be left home alone. Factors used to evaluate a child's readiness to be in an unsupervised situation include the child's age, developmental level, emotional readiness, ability to use a phone or other method of obtaining emergency assistance, and comfort with the situation. Infants and very young children are at times left unattended in a home while the parent or caregiver leaves for extended periods. Other parents will leave a child home alone at night after bedtime while the parents are working. Additionally, minor children come to the attention of child protective services (CPS) and/or law enforcement after they are found alone while the parent(s) are reported to be out drinking or partying. Coohey reported that most children who were left home alone were in a household consisting of a single mother.[12] Mothers in this study justified leaving the child home despite acknowledging that it was wrong by reporting that it happened only once, was a short amount of time, or was someone else's fault.[12] In a survey of US adults who were asked the minimum age at which a child could safely stay home alone, the average response was 13 years of age.[20] The literature reports that for children left home alone at 3 years, there is a higher risk of psychotic behavior and conduct disorder at age 17.[20]

Coohey notes that children left with an inadequate caregiver are at greatest risk of being harmed.[12] Additionally, parents who leave children with an inadequate caregiver are reported to have more resources and fewer impairments when compared with parents who leave children home alone.[12]

Some states have legislation or CPS rules for an age requirement that must be met for a child to be left home alone. Medical professionals should be aware of individual state laws on this subject. When discussing recommendations with a parent about when to start leaving a child home alone, it is important to recommend trial runs to ease the child into the situation and to lengthen the time left home alone sequentially during those trial runs. It is also important to set up regular check-in times with the child or check-in routines. Having a trusted neighbor available is also of help in these situations.

Drowning

Case Example

A mother left her 4-year-old son, who had autism spectrum disorder, in the bathtub along with her 18-month-old daughter. She reported the 2 were splashing in the tub, with the tub one-third full of water, when she left them to work in the kitchen. The father was in another room studying. The mother reported that when she returned to the bathroom, she found her 18-month-old floating face down in the bathtub. Emergency medical services personnel were called and the child was taken by ambulance to

(continued)

Case Example (*continued*)

the hospital, where she was later pronounced brain dead and supportive care was withdrawn. The father was reported to have been using marijuana. The case was determined by child welfare to be drowning due to supervisory neglect leading to great bodily harm/death to the child.

According to the Centers for Disease Control and Prevention (CDC), from 2005 to 2014, there were an average of 3,536 fatal unintentional drownings annually in the United States—about 10 deaths per day.[21] About 1 in 5 people who die from drowning are children 14 years and younger.[21] For every child who dies from drowning, another 5 children receive emergency department (ED) care for nonfatal submersion injuries.[21] Nonfatal drowning injuries can cause severe brain damage that may result in long-term disabilities such as memory problems, learning disabilities, and permanent loss of basic functioning.[22,23]

Age is strongly associated with the circumstances of drowning. Infant drownings most often occur in bathtubs,[24,25] either when they are left unattended or as the result of abusive injury. Swimming pools are the most common location for toddlers' drowning.[25] Teenagers frequently drown in natural bodies of water while intoxicated or engaging in risk-taking behavior.[25] Szpilman et al reported that additional drowning risk factors are male sex, alcohol use, low income, poor education, and rural residency.[24] According to Bain et al, children and adults with epilepsy drown at a rate nearly 10 times greater than the general population.[26] Most deaths in people with epilepsy occur in the bathtub.[26] Additionally, children with autism spectrum disorder are at increased risk.

A lack of direct supervision is implicated in most cases of childhood drowning. Another risk factor is the lack of barriers around swimming pools. The proper use of life jackets[27] and children's swimming ability are protective factors. The American Academy of Pediatrics recommends that every child should learn how to swim.[28,29]

Supervisory neglect should be considered in cases of child drowning or near drowning. However, a decision by medical professionals to diagnose a drowning event as child neglect can be problematic. Fatal drowning cases involving possible neglect can be emotionally difficult for the medical staff because the practitioner's primary concern is to address the family guilt and grief. Thus, cases are often not reported to CPS unless a prior CPS report is recognized, social work is involved, or consideration of neglect is documented in the medical record. Supervisory neglect should be addressed in these cases, because it is important to protect other children in the family.[30]

Medical professionals should counsel families on water safety, including safe monitoring of infants and young children during bathing, swimming, and all recreational water activities. Children younger than 5 years are the highest-risk age group for drowning events when left unsupervised near water.

The medical professional should report a drowning or near drowning event to CPS or law enforcement for supervisory neglect when the child is showing symptoms from the event or it is a child fatality case. If the child is brought for care after a reported near drowning event, is monitored by the medical facility, and shows no symptoms, the medical professional can use his or her discretion in deciding if the case rises to the level of reporting. Generally, if the child exhibits no symptoms, it is likely that the caregiver did demonstrate supervision that prevented a symptomatic near drowning or fatal drowning event. Despite a parent's efforts, a child might slip in a bathtub or get into a pool, but a parent who is adequately supervising the child will be there and get the child out promptly. When the caregiver is not present, the child can die within 4 to 5 minutes.

Fire

According to Istre and colleagues, the rates of injuries and deaths from house fires are greatest in the elderly and young children, low-income populations, minorities, and those who live in houses without functioning smoke detectors.[31] Although child deaths in house fires are generally considered a tragic accident, a 10-year review of all such fatalities concluded that they were largely due to poor supervision or related to the activities of adults in the home.[32] According to Squires and Busuttil, approximately 30% of fires resulting in child fatalities can be attributed to the actions of children, such as playing with matches or cigarette lighters; coal or electric fires; or flammable liquids. Another 30% of fire-related child fatalities occurred in fires resulting from inebriation, usually of a parent. Squires and Busuttil concluded, "Children are being killed in house fires because their parents and caregivers are neglecting their duty to ensure the child's well-being."[32] In a study by Istre and colleagues of residential fire-related deaths and injuries among children, fire play (ie, children playing with matches or lighters) accounted for 42% of all injuries, as well as 62% of deaths, in children 0 to 4 years of age and 94% of deaths from apartment and mobile home fires.[33] Because there was no adequate supervision, smoke alarms were not effective in preventing deaths or injuries when fire play was involved.[33] A study involving child fatalities in house fires found that in 29 out of 34 cases, children had been left alone by their parents.[34]

The possibility of homicide shouldn't be overlooked. In Squire and Busuttil's study, 10 of 168 child deaths in house fires either were homicide involving a parent or the result of a fire ignited deliberately by an adult.[32]

Cigarette smoking is also an important causal factor in house fires. In a 2001 study, 5.5% of house fires were caused directly by smoking and 4.5% by children playing with fire, which is greatly facilitated by the presence of smoking paraphernalia, such as matches and lighters, in the home.[31]

Pediatricians play an important role in anticipatory guidance for families to understand the risks of fire and death for children in residential dwellings, especially when cigarette lighters and other flammable objects are left within reach of minors. Guiding parents on leaving children in the care of a responsible adult if they (as caregivers) are impaired also helps ameliorate the risk of injury from fires.

Burns

An estimated 10% to 20% of pediatric burns are a result of maltreatment, and 50% to 90% of these are secondary to neglect.[35,36] Recently, a screening tool has been developed to detect burns secondary to maltreatment, the BuRN Tool. It focuses on the following key features: 1) previous CPS or social service involvement; 2) age younger than 5 years; 3) concern about supervision; 4) concern about inappropriate explanation; 5) severity of injury; 6) scald burn located on the back, buttock, groin, or scalp; 7) symmetry of a scald burn; and 8) non-scald burn. A subsequent study confirmed that this screening tool was beneficial when used in an ED setting.[37]

In a recent retrospective chart review of 408 pediatric burns, 84.8% were accidental, 7.8% were found to be inflicted, and 7.4% were attributed to neglect.[35] In this study, several features helped to distinguish characteristics of neglectful types of burns, including inaccurate histories, delay in care, and location and severity of scald burns.

Leaving cigarette lighters, grill fire starters, matches, and other flammable implements within the reach of children puts them at serious risk of harm for burn injuries and house fires and could constitute supervisory neglect.

Falls

Case Example

A parent left an 18-month-old upstairs in a bedroom with the window open while she went to get laundry in the basement. The mother heard a scream and came running upstairs. She found the window without the screen in it. She reported looking out the window and found her child on the ground outside lying in the gravel. The child sustained a linear parietal skull fracture and facial/scalp lacerations. She also had a small subdural hemorrhage associated with the fracture. The case was reported for evaluation of supervisory neglect.

Falls are the most common type of unintentional injury in the home, accounting for more than 1.5 million children's medical visits each year in the United States.[38] Falls are more common among boys than girls, infants and preschool-aged children are at higher risk than older children, and the poor are disproportionally affected.[38]

Building design is often implicated in falls from windows and balconies. When balcony rails are spaced more than 10 cm apart, or when the window is situated within 60 cm of the floor, the risk of falls markedly increases.[39] Fall prevention includes reducing the use of baby walkers; installation of stair gates, window locks, or windows with limited openings; and avoiding the placement of furniture near windows and balconies. In New York, NY, in 1976, a public health campaign to inform the community about the hazards of windows and distribution of free window guards resulted in a marked reduction of unintentional window falls.[40]

Supervision and vigilance by parents and caregivers in preventing childhood falls has been recommended in the medical literature for centuries.[41] Although neglect can undoubtedly be responsible for many falls from heights, it is not clear how often a lack of supervision is implicated in such occurrences. In a 2005 study of 90 cases of children falling from windows, there was a total absence of supervision in one case, and a minor was in charge of supervision in 2 cases.[42] Similarly, in Texas, an adult was reported to be supervising the child in 97% of falls from windows or balconies.[39] However, a recent study indicated a much higher rate of supervisory neglect: 45.7% of fall victims were alone at the time of the mishap.[41] It is also important to assess if the caregiver had knowledge of the risk beforehand.

Pediatricians should consider making a report of supervisory neglect to CPS or law enforcement when a child falls from a window. Medical professionals should use clinical judgment in assessing whether to report other types of falls, such as stairwell falls. It is important to report cases in which the parent or caregiver was impaired when such an incident occurred. A home safety checklist should be encouraged to assess whether other hazards might be present and can be prevented.

Child Left Alone in the Car/Hyperthermia

According to Zonfrillo et al, between 1990 and 2014, 3,115 US children were injured from being left unattended in hot vehicles; 729 of these injuries resulted in death.[43] On average, 38 children die each year of hyperthermia related to being left unattended in a car, most younger

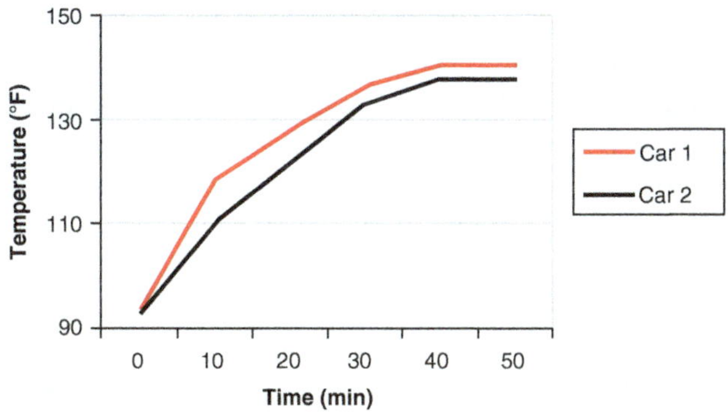

Car 1: Dark blue, windows closed
Car 2: Light gray, windows open approximately 1.5 inches

FIGURE 15.1

Increase in interior car temperature by minutes in the sun, New Orleans, July 1995.

From Gibbs LI, Lawrence DW, Kohn MA. Heat exposure in an enclosed automobile. *J La State Med Soc.* 1995;147(12):545–546.

than 2 years.[44] Death from hyperthermia occurs most often when a child is left alone in a parked car. It also happens if a child is napping in a hot dwelling or sleeping under heavy blankets.[45] In these cases, those who experience hyperthermia are primarily infants or very young children.[45]

In a parked car, the temperature can reach high levels quickly. Krous et al reported that with an outside temperature of 36.8°C (98.2°F), the temperature in a car in direct sunlight reaches between 51°C (123.8°F) and 67°C (152.6°F) within 15 minutes of closing the doors.[45] On average, temperatures increase 1.7°C to 1.9°C every 5 minutes.[45] Within 60 minutes, vehicles have reached peak temperatures, regardless of whether windows are closed or cracked open.[46] (See Figure 15.1.)

In an analysis of 231 fatalities, Booth and colleagues report that the elapsed time between when a child was last known alive and when he or she was found dead or dying inside a vehicle averaged 4.6 hours, with a range of 0.25 to 16 hours.[46] Lack of adequate supervision was most commonly cited as the cause for the event; most victims were simply "forgotten" inside the vehicle.[46,47] This could be explained on the basis of stress-induced memory impairment.[47] However, in a few cases, the caregiver was determined to be intentionally negligent during the investigation and the manner of death was classified as homicide.[46]

Autopsies on the deceased found that intrathoracic petechiae suggesting terminal gasping are the most consistent postmortem finding.[48] Signs of dehydration can be found in roughly half of the deceased.[48]

In cases of fatal hyperthermia, the ambient and body temperatures should be documented as well as the vehicle's exposure to direct sunlight, the car's type and color, and the position of the doors and windows relative to the deceased.[45] When a child who has died of hyperthermia is found in bed, a description of the child's clothing, the type and amount of bedding, and other items found in the bed, such as pillows and stuffed toys, should be documented.[45]

Other mishaps have been described when small children are left unsupervised in a parked car; in the United States, over a 25-year period, 61 strangulation deaths occurred due to closing of an electric power window on the child's neck.[43] Also, fatal accidents have occurred when children released the emergency brake and the car started to roll.[49]

Frostbite

Case Example

A 2-year-old girl woke up at night, got the front door of the home open, and went outside. The temperature with wind chill factor was -37.2°C (-35°F). The child was found in the morning huddling under the car. She suffered severe frostbite of her face and extremities and required amputation of multiple fingers and toes. Both parents were found to have been impaired by illegal drugs and alcohol the night this incident occurred. The case was substantiated as supervisory neglect leading to great bodily harm.

Infants and young children are more sensitive to hypothermia and frostbite because of their large surface area relative to body volume. Boles et al define *frostbite* as tissue damage occurring when the human body is exposed to temperatures below the freezing point.[50] In children, frostbite injuries begin at temperatures below -6°C (21.2°F); the risk of tissue loss increases at temperatures below -23°C (-9.4°F).[50] Frostbite can be classified as superficial or deep. Superficial injuries present with erythema, edema, and vesiculation.[51] Deep frostbite presents with hemorrhagic blisters resulting in hard eschar and leading to necrosis and tissue loss.[51] In small children, the hands are more commonly involved than the feet because toddlers tend to lose their mittens.

In a recent Canadian review of 47 pediatric patients with frostbite, it was found that two-thirds of younger children were unsupervised, whereas alcohol intoxication was a common cause of frostbite in adolescents.[50] Symptoms of depression were found in 32% of adolescents.[50] Eleven of the 47 patients needed a surgical procedure, 9 of whom required amputation of at least 1 digit.[50]

Poulakidas et al reported 3 cases of toddlers who were exposed to temperature extremes without protective hand coverage and developed severe frostbite of their hands. They stated, "Parents were not aware of the seriousness of frostbite injury in the growing child, and the necessity of gloves in protecting children's hands in the colder climates. The mothers were either walking to or waiting for buses to ride to their destinations with the children, losing gloves along the way. Exposure lasted from 30–60 minutes."[52]

Frostbite injury in children can lead to premature fusion of the epiphyseal cartilage with long-term sequela including abnormal growth, deformity, and possibly amputation of the phalanges.[53]

If patients present within 48 hours of cold exposure, the toes, digits, and hands may be revitalized enough to either avoid amputation or decrease the loss of tissue. Therefore, medical attention should be sought within 1 to 2 days when frostbite is suspected. Negative pressure wound therapy has been used in several adult frostbite patients, who successfully avoided the need for amputation or skin grafting. Recently, Poulakidas et al used negative pressure wound therapy with good results on 3 toddlers.[52]

Close supervision of infants and toddlers is mandatory during cold spells to avoid frostbite or death from hypothermia.

Firearms

Approximately 1,300 children die each year from firearm-related injuries in the United States.[54] Most of these deaths resulted from homicide or suicide, 4% were unintentional, and 1% were of undetermined origin.[55] Dowd and colleagues report that in 2010, 15,576 US children and adolescents were treated in EDs for nonfatal firearm-related injuries. Rates of nonfatal firearm injury are nearly 3 times higher among adolescents aged 15 to 19 years than among the population as a whole.[55]

Whereas firearm-related homicides and suicides are more likely to involve teenagers, a review of 277 unintentional pediatric gun injury events showed that half of those who were injured or killed were younger than 13 years. Most of these injuries occurred at home, involved family guns, and could have been prevented by adults taking responsibility for minimizing child access to and secure storage of firearms.[56] The possibility of child neglect should be examined as a potential contributing factor to the occurrence of firearm injury. In a random digit dial interview conducted with 5,801 California adolescents, 5% of respondents reported that they had handled a gun without adult knowledge or supervision.[57] Although many studies report "unintentional" gun-related deaths, it is important to understand that unintentional does not mean that a case is not neglect.

There is good evidence that access to guns increases the number of suicides, homicides, and injuries, as well as serious unintentional injury and death. There is a 3-fold increase in the risk of homicide and a 5-fold increase in the risk of suicide when a gun is stored in the home.[55] Firearms are found in 33% to 40% of American households with children.[58] For those who have guns in the home, the most effective measures for reducing firearm injuries involve practices of safe storage. In a 2006 study of gun-owning Americans with children younger than 18 years, 21.7% stored a gun loaded, 31.5% stored a gun unlocked, and 8.3% stored at least 1 gun unlocked and loaded.[59] There was not much improvement over the next 10 years; in a 2015 survey of gun-owning households with children, Azrael et al estimated that only 30% of gun owners stored their guns unloaded and locked.[60] The other 70% of owners stored at least 1 gun loaded and/or unlocked.[60]

Firearm-related accidents are most prevalent in young white children living in states with lenient gun laws.[54,61,62] Firearm safety education programs directed at children have been shown to be ineffective.[55,63] Thus, prevention of firearm-related injuries and deaths in children rests mainly on preventing unsupervised children's access to guns. Failure to safely store guns in the home or control children's access to loaded and/or unlocked guns should be considered reportable as supervisory neglect.

It is important for medical professionals to advocate for gun safety legislation. In Florida, it is a law that parents are responsible if children get access to guns. The parents can go to jail in such cases. Also, gun injuries are required to be reported by EDs to law enforcement. Law enforcement should cross-report these cases to CPS to ensure safety of all children in the home. Pediatricians can assist in advocating for this multidisciplinary teaming for local and state jurisdictions.

Non-powder firearms, such as paintball guns, ball bearing (BB) guns, pellet guns, or air rifles, are marketed to a young audience and are often considered toys. Parents who do not allow their children to have these guns and parents whose children had been injured by such guns tend to view BB and pellet guns as significantly more dangerous than parents who allow their children to possess these "toys."[64]

Over a 10-year period in the United States, there were 55,060 estimated ED visits primarily occurring in younger children (aged 6–12 years) for non-powder firearms–related eye injuries.[65] Many of these children had visual acuity worse than 20/50 after initial treatment, and most had no eye protection.[66]

Drug and/or Alcohol Ingestion and Poisoning

Exposures to potential ingestions and poisons in children younger than 6 years result in 40,000 ED visits, 3,000 hospital admissions, and more than 100 deaths annually in the United States.[67] In 2013, there were

59,000 ED visits for unsupervised pediatric medication exposures.[68] In a review of 928 cases of poisonings by Wood et al, the most common source was household products (41%), followed by nonnarcotic prescription drugs (29%), over-the-counter drugs (20%), prescription narcotics/sedatives (7%), and ethanol, illicit drugs, and other substances (≤1% each).[69] Supervisory neglect was responsible for a large subset of these events. Neglect was more likely to be diagnosed in cases of poisoning with drugs of abuse; all illicit drug poisonings and 44% of ethanol poisonings were referred to CPS.[69] However, an average of 160 cases of intentional child poisonings per year are reported to American poison control centers.[70]

It is critical to evaluate infants with altered mental status for deliberate addition of alcohol or drugs to formula, which has been used by some parents and caregivers as a means to quiet a child. Pediatric patients presenting with altered mental status should be evaluated for possible poisoning with cannabis or other drugs of abuse.[71] Since the legalization of marijuana in 2014 in Colorado, the number of cases of marijuana exposure in young children (average 2 years of age) has doubled.[72]

Acute alcohol intoxication is common in adolescents,[73] but there are only isolated case reports for children of younger ages.[74,75] It is unclear if supervisory neglect was a factor in these cases.

Infants and toddlers in homes with access to drugs such as cocaine, opiates, or other stimulants are at risk for accidental ingestions. An impaired caregiver cannot adequately supervise the safety of children for whom they are responsible. See Chapter 16, Drug-Endangered Children, for more information.

A child who has previously experienced a poisoning event is more likely to experience another one.[76] A study of 1,943 potentially toxic ingestions in children younger than 6 years found that 30% reported a prior poison exposure.[77] Parental education certainly has a role in preventing recurrence of toxic ingestion,[78] but the possibility of supervisory neglect needs to be addressed. Therefore, even if the parents report poisoning as accidental, a thorough history must be obtained, including timeline of symptoms, description of home environment, developmental history, and history of prior ingestions. Also, a complete physical examination looking for signs of physical abuse and neglect must be performed.[69]

Medical professionals should report cases of ingestion of substances by a child to CPS if the child exhibits symptoms from the ingestion or if there are safety concerns that could prevent discharge home (eg, parent seems unconcerned, parent is not receptive to counseling on prevention of recurrent ingestion, parent appears under the influence or impaired by drugs or alcohol). If the parent is showing concern about a possible (not proven) ingestion, reporting may not be needed if no other risk factors are present. Emergency care settings may have social work or case managers who can help with an initial assessment and in determining need to report to CPS. Intervention and assistance to the family via a home visit and additional discussion on safety and prevention may be necessary and helpful.

Unsafe Sleep

In cases of sudden unexplained infant death, unintentional asphyxia due to overlaying by a parent is often difficult to ascertain and relies on parental reporting. (This topic is described in detail in Chapter 24, SIDS, SUID, and the Child Fatality Review Team Approach to Unexpected Childhood Death.) While unsafe sleep may constitute supervisory neglect, attributing the fatality to this may be difficult in many instances. Medical professionals must therefore work collaboratively with other disciplines, using established death investigation protocols that can help in making this assessment and decision to report.

Traffic-Related Injuries

Traffic-related injuries are the leading cause of fatality among children in the United States.[79] This includes motor vehicle collisions and motor-pedestrian collisions.

Motor-Pedestrian Collisions

According to Ma and colleagues, pedestrians are 1.5 times more likely than vehicle passengers to die in a traffic collision, with the highest mortality among toddlers.[80] Children 5 to 9 years old, boys, and children in lower socioeconomic classes are at higher risk of pedestrian injury.[80]

Parental supervision is essential in protecting children from pedestrian injury risk.[81] In a study of 142 children aged 5 to 12 years treated for pedestrian injury, 64% of those treated were unsupervised at the time of injury and 20 of the 51 supervisors were teenagers.[82]

Parents should be educated that children younger than 9 years should not cross streets without adult supervision.[83] Some parents overestimate their children's understanding of pedestrian safety and allow their children to walk alone on streets, despite recognizing the limitations of child pedestrian skills in general. They may also not take time to demonstrate safe pedestrian skills to their children.[79]

Motor Vehicle Collisions

Motor vehicle crashes remain the leading cause of injury-related death in children aged 1 to 17 years.[84] According to the CDC, 9,182 US children aged 0 to 12 years died in motor vehicle crashes between 2002 and 2011.[85] Child safety seats reduce the risk of fatal injury by 71% for infants and 54% for toddlers in passenger cars. Forty-six percent of the fatally injured children younger than 5 years were completely unrestrained.[86] The lowest compliance with restraint use is in the 4- to 8-year age group, with most children prematurely graduated to seat belts alone.[87]

Hazards facing children in motor vehicles are related to parents driving at excessive speed, when sleep deprived, while under the influence, or while using their cell phone. Speed and/or alcohol or drug use have been determined to be the most important predisposing factors in road crashes. In the United States, there were more than 32,000 crash deaths in 2013, and drunk driving contributed to more than 10,000 of these deaths.[88] A recent study estimated that a 10% reduction in adult per capita alcohol consumption was associated with a 3% reduction in child mortality from overall injuries and road traffic injuries.[89]

Bicycle Accidents

According to the CDC, more than 1,000 bicyclists died in the United States in 2015, and there were almost 467,000 bicycle-related injuries.[21] In a recent case-control study, the use of a protective helmet was associated with up to a 74% reduction in risk of head injury in bicycle collisions with motor vehicles; the reduction in risk increased with the severity of the potential injury.[90] With enactment of laws mandating the use of helmets for young bicyclists, the proportion of children using a helmet has more than doubled. However, a national survey reported that only 48% of children aged 5 to 14 years wore bicycle helmets when riding, and older children were particularly resistant to helmet use.[91] In evaluating bicycle-related injuries related to lack of helmet use for supervisory neglect, one must consider individual state laws. The United States does not have a federal law mandating helmet use.

All-Terrain Vehicles

In 2000, the American Academy of Pediatrics recommended that the use of all-terrain vehicles (ATVs) be restricted to those older than 16 years and to off-road use only and to disallow passengers.[92] Helmets, eye protection, and sturdy shoes should be worn.[92] However, in 2007, children younger than 16 years accounted for 40,000 (26%) of the 150,990 ED visits for ATV-related injuries.[93] Children between the ages of 10 and 17 years have the highest death rate among all ATV users.[94] Severe neurologic, multi-organ torso and extremity injuries with long-term disability are linked with ATV-related injuries.[95] Allowing children younger than 16 years to ride on an ATV could be considered reportable neglect.[95] However, when analyzing individual cases of ATV-related child injury for concern of supervisory neglect, medical professionals should have knowledge of individual state laws regarding ATV use, because these vary from state to state. In most cases in which a diagnosis of supervisory neglect has been made in conjunction with ATV use, the parent or caregiver either was not present or adequately watching the child or was impaired by drug or alcohol use, and bodily harm or significant risk of harm to the child resulted.

Witnessing Intimate Partner Violence

Children's exposure to intimate partner violence is recognized as a type of violence exposure with outcomes similar to physical, sexual, and emotional abuse.[96] It is now recognized that the mere awareness of potential violence between caregivers, and not just witnessing the violent acts, can result in harmful outcomes for a child.[97] Medical professionals should know the mandated reporting requirements as they relate to childhood exposure to intimate partner violence in the state(s) in which they practice. There could be variation in how to report intimate partner violence exposure, for example, as neglect, emotional maltreatment, or imminent risk of harm. This topic is addressed in detail in Chapter 21, Interpersonal Violence.

Child Abandonment

Child abandonment occurs when a parent or caregiver leaves a child without sufficient regard for the child's welfare. An epidemiological study of discarded infants and infanticide found an incidence of 2.1 in 100,000 over 16 years in North Carolina.[98] Sherr et al reported on 124 abandoned babies over a 7-year period. Newborns (≤1 week old) accounted for 96 (77.4%) of these cases, and they were less likely to survive than older babies.[99] According to Mariano et al, about 2.5% of all homicide arrests in the United States are for parents who have killed their children.[100] This amounts to an average of about 500 filicide arrests each year.[100] Asphyxia by smothering, drowning, and exposure (abandonment) are the most common causes of death.[101] An attempt to hide the body almost always occurs.[101]

"Safe haven" laws exist to allow women to drop a newborn at a safe location without fear of facing criminal charges. Unless a case of abandonment is encompassed under state-specific safe haven legislation, this action would constitute supervisory neglect.

Children abandoned by their parents are at risk of having a lower IQ (average 70 for institutionalized vs 80 for foster children vs 100 for children who have not been abandoned), delay in language development, major attachment problems, lower brain volumes, and a 50% risk of a psychiatric diagnosis by 5 years of age.[102,103]

Fatal Neglect

Child neglect without associated physical abuse constitutes one-third to nearly two-thirds of all child maltreatment fatalities.[84,104] The failure to properly supervise and attend to children is the largest contributor to neglect-related deaths.[4]

Fatalities due to neglect alone affect predominantly young children. In a review of 372 such cases, 56% of the deceased were younger than 2 years and 90% were younger than 5 years.[104] Fatalities were attributed to 3 main categories of neglect: lack of adequate supervision (61%); failure to attend the child's basic needs such as food, shelter, and clothing (7.8%); and medical neglect (9.7%).[104] The main causes of death from supervisory neglect were drowning, smoke exposure, suffocation, head trauma (falls), and unintentional gunshots. Biological parents were the caregivers in most cases.[104]

In another review of 115 deaths due to child maltreatment, 51 (44.4%) were determined to be related to inadequate caregiver supervision.[105] Of those, 53% were related to lack of supervision in a hazardous environment, 33% were related to general supervisory neglect, and 14% were related to inappropriate substitute care.[105] Most deaths were caused by drowning or smoke inhalation.[105] As compared with fatal cases due to failure to attend the child's basic needs, deaths related to supervisory neglect were more likely to involve slightly older children (4 years vs 2 years) who lived in homes with higher numbers of children (3 vs 2) and who were looked after by a biological relative.[105]

Child Fatality Review

In many cases of child fatality, it might be difficult to determine the exact mechanism leading to death. For instance, burns might be accidental, secondary to poor supervision, or inflicted; starvation may be deliberately inflicted, secondary to neglect, or a consequence of poverty or medical illiteracy. Child fatality review (CFR), the systematic evaluation of individual child deaths by a multidisciplinary team, is an essential operation in trying to understand the processes leading to a fatal outcome.

Tracking and reviewing infant deaths can reveal what changes are needed to prevent future fatalities. For instance, a hospital receiving feedback from the local CFR about infants who had been discharged from their nursery and then died due to unsafe sleep environments was able to improve its existing safe sleep program.[106] This was followed by a decrease in the average death rate due to sudden unexplained infant death, from 1.08 infants per 1,000 births to 0.48 infants per 1,000 births, after complete intervention.[107] On a regional level, systematic CFR has become a powerful tool in reducing preventable child deaths through the implementation of prevention strategies.[108] However, reporting of the death of children is subject to potential bias.[109] For instance, investigators are less likely to examine for physical and sexual abuse among middle class children when reporting child death. Also, there are stark differences between individual sites with regard to data completeness and quality and consistency of the procedures performed postmortem. This leads to issues regarding quality of the reports and death diagnosis certainty.[109] In the same cases, different CFR panels often reach different conclusions, especially in cases of child neglect.[110]

Conclusion

The scenarios presented in this chapter are offered as a reflective starting point for medical professionals. A universally accepted definition of supervisory neglect is difficult to attain, given the community-specific, societal, and cultural differences that influence how adults parent and raise children. Even with this recognition, the determination of what constitutes reportable supervisory neglect can be a challenge. As with any form of child maltreatment, prevention begins with education of the parents and the child's caregivers.

So what can medical professionals do?

- Review supervision of the child with the parents at every health supervision visit and encourage sharing the same information with all caregivers of the child.
- Know the reporting requirements for the state in which you practice and understand the recommendations for when supervisory neglect reports should be made to CPS or law enforcement.

- Recommend medication lockboxes and secure firearm storage for all households to prevent childhood ingestions and firearm-related injuries.
- Collaborate as medical experts with local and state agencies, public health agencies, and CFR teams to advocate for education on injury prevention, safe sleep, and childhood safety.

References

1. Straus MA, Kantor GK. Definition and measurement of neglectful behavior: some principles and guidelines. *Child Abuse Negl*. 2005;29(1):19–29 PMID: 15664423 https://doi.org/10.1016/j.chiabu.2004.08.005
2. American Professional Society on the Abuse of Children. Practice guidelines: challenges in the evaluation of child neglect. https://docs.wixstatic.com/ugd/4700a8_f0c7bccba0a14627831cf4e8a0b1bbb8.pdf. Published 2008. Accessed February 14, 2019
3. Coohey C. Defining and classifying supervisory neglect. *Child Maltreat*. 2003;8(2):145–156 PMID: 12735717 https://doi.org/10.1177/1077559502250786
4. Mennen FE, Kim K, Sang J, Trickett PK. Child neglect: definition and identification of youth's experiences in official reports of maltreatment. *Child Abuse Negl*. 2010;34(9):647–658 PMID: 20643482 https://doi.org/10.1016/j.chiabu.2010.02.007
5. Berkowitz CD. Fatal child neglect. *Adv Pediatr*. 2001;48:331–361 PMID: 11480762
6. US Department of Health and Human Services, Administration for Children and Families, Children's Bureau. Child maltreatment. https://www.acf.hhs.gov/cb/research-data-technology/statistics-research/child-maltreatment. Reviewed January 28, 2019. Accessed February 14, 2019
7. Coohey C, Zhang Y. The role of men in chronic supervisory neglect. *Child Maltreat*. 2006;11(1):27–33 PMID: 16382089 https://doi.org/10.1177/1077559505283548
8. Scott D, Higgins D, Franklin R. The role of supervisory neglect in childhood injury. CFCA Paper No. 8. Australian Institute of Family Studies website. https://aifs.gov.au/cfca/publications/role-supervisory-neglect-childhood-injury. Published September 2012. Accessed February 14, 2019
9. Pelton LH. Child abuse and neglect: the myth of classlessness. *Am J Orthopsychiatry*. 1978;48(4):608–617 PMID: 707612 https://doi.org/10.1111/j.1939-0025.1978.tb02565.x
10. Yang M-Y, Maguire-Jack K. Predictors of basic needs and supervisory neglect: evidence from the Illinois Families Study. *Child Youth Serv Rev*. 2016;67:20–26 https://doi.org/10.1016/j.childyouth.2016.05.017
11. Ruiz-Casares M, Trocmé N, Fallon B. Supervisory neglect and risk of harm. Evidence from the Canadian Child Welfare System. *Child Abuse Negl*. 2012;36(6):471–480 PMID: 22770635 https://doi.org/10.1016/j.chiabu.2012.03.005
12. Coohey C. The nature of parental supervisory neglect. *Child Welfare*. 2008;87(4):55–77 PMID: 19391467
13. Hymel KP; American Academy of Pediatrics Committee on Child Abuse and Neglect. When is lack of supervision neglect? *Pediatrics*. 2006;118(3):1296–1298 PMID: 16951030 https://doi.org/10.1542/peds.2006-1780
14. Nadan Y, Spilsbury JC, Korbin JE. Culture and context in understanding child maltreatment: contributions of intersectionality and neighborhood-based research. *Child Abuse Negl*. 2015;41:40–48 PMID: 25466427 https://doi.org/10.1016/j.chiabu.2014.10.021

15. Raman S, Hodes D. Cultural issues in child maltreatment. *J Paediatr Child Health*. 2012;48(1):30–37 PMID: 22040215 https://doi.org/10.1111/j.1440-1754.2011.02184.x
16. Ruiz-Casares M, Nazif-Muñoz JI. Non-adult child supervision practices in Lao People's Democratic Republic. *Child Abuse Negl*. 2018;84:217–228 PMID: 30118971 https://doi.org/10.1016/j.chiabu.2018.08.001
17. Koramoa J, Lynch MA, Kinnair D. A continuum of child-rearing: responding to traditional practices. *Child Abuse Rev*. 2002;11(6):415–421 https://doi.org/10.1002/car.766
18. Hildyard KL, Wolfe DA. Child neglect: developmental issues and outcomes. *Child Abuse Negl*. 2002;26(6-7):679–695 PMID: 12201162 https://doi.org/10.1016/S0145-2134(02)00341-1
19. Knutson JF, DeGarmo D, Koeppl G, Reid JB. Care neglect, supervisory neglect, and harsh parenting in the development of children's aggression: a replication and extension. *Child Maltreat*. 2005;10(2):92–107 PMID: 15798006 https://doi.org/10.1177/1077559504273684
20. Mack KA, Dellinger A, West BA. Adult opinions about the age at which children can be left home alone, bathe alone, or bike alone: Second Injury Control and Risk Survey (ICARIS-2). *J Safety Res*. 2012;43(3):223–226 PMID: 22974688 https://doi.org/10.1016/j.jsr.2012.06.001
21. Centers for Disease Control and Prevention, National Center for Injury Prevention and Control. Welcome to WISQARS. http://www.cdc.gov/injury/wisqars. Reviewed January 18, 2019. Accessed February 14, 2019
22. Cummings P, Quan L. Trends in unintentional drowning: the role of alcohol and medical care. *JAMA*. 1999;281(23):2198–2202 PMID: 10376572 https://doi.org/10.1001/jama.281.23.2198
23. Spack L, Gedeit R, Splaingard M, Havens PL. Failure of aggressive therapy to alter outcome in pediatric near-drowning. *Pediatr Emerg Care*. 1997;13(2):98–102 PMID: 9127416 https://doi.org/10.1097/00006565-199704000-00004
24. Szpilman D, Bierens JJ, Handley AJ, Orlowski JP. Drowning. *N Engl J Med*. 2012;366(22):2102–2110 PMID: 22646632 https://doi.org/10.1056/NEJMra1013317
25. Meyer RJ, Theodorou AA, Berg RA. Childhood drowning. *Pediatr Rev*. 2006;27(5):163–168 PMID: 16651273 https://doi.org/10.1542/pir.27-5-163
26. Bain E, Keller AE, Jordan H, et al. Drowning in epilepsy: a population-based case series. *Epilepsy Res*. 2018;145:123–126 PMID: 29957568 https://doi.org/10.1016/j.eplepsyres.2018.06.010
27. Peden AE, Demant D, Hagger MS, Hamilton K. Personal, social, and environmental factors associated with lifejacket wear in adults and children: a systematic literature review. *PLoS One*. 2018;13(5):e0196421 PMID: 29718971 https://doi.org/10.1371/journal.pone.0196421
28. Conover K, Romero S. Drowning prevention in pediatrics. *Pediatr Ann*. 2018;47(3):e112–e117 PMID: 29538784 https://doi.org/10.3928/19382359-20180220-02
29. Pharr J, Irwin C, Layne T, Irwin R. Predictors of swimming ability among children and adolescents in the United States. *Sports (Basel)*. 2018;6(1):E17 PMID: 29910321
30. Feldman KW, Monastersky C, Feldman GK. When is childhood drowning neglect? *Child Abuse Negl*. 1993;17(3):329–336 PMID: 8330219 https://doi.org/10.1016/0145-2134(93)90055-A
31. Istre GR, McCoy MA, Osborn L, Barnard JJ, Bolton A. Deaths and injuries from house fires. *N Engl J Med*. 2001;344(25):1911–1916 PMID: 11419429 https://doi.org/10.1056/NEJM200106213442506
32. Squires T, Busuttil A. Child fatalities in Scottish house fires 1980-1990: a case of child neglect? *Child Abuse Negl*. 1995;19(7):865–873 PMID: 7583744 https://doi.org/10.1016/0145-2134(95)00050-I

33. Istre GR, McCoy M, Carlin DK, McClain J. Residential fire related deaths and injuries among children: fireplay, smoke alarms, and prevention. *Inj Prev*. 2002;8(2):128–132 PMID: 12120831 https://doi.org/10.1136/ip.8.2.128
34. Fornes P, Lecomte D, Imbert M, Lambert P, Baud FJ, Julien H. An analysis of the factors implicated in fire deaths in children. *J Clin Forensic Med*. 1994;1(2):79–82 PMID: 16371271 https://doi.org/10.1016/1353-1131(94)90004-3
35. Collier ZJ, Ramaiah V, Glick JC, Gottlieb LJA. A 6-year case-control study of the presentation and clinical sequelae for noninflicted, negligent, and inflicted pediatric burns. *J Burn Care Res*. 2017;38(1):e101–e124 PMID: 28009699 https://doi.org/10.1097/BCR.0000000000000408
36. Mullen S, Begley R, Roberts Z, Kemp AM. Fifteen-minute consultation. Childhood burns: inflicted, neglect or accidental. *Arch Dis Child Educ Pract Ed*. 2018;edpract-2018-315167 PMID: 29934360 https://doi.org/10.1136/archdischild-2018-315167
37. Mullen S, Quinn-Scoggins HD, Nuttall D, Kemp AM. Qualitative analysis of clinician experience in utilising the BuRN Tool (Burns Risk assessment for Neglect or abuse Tool) in clinical practice. *Burns*. 2018;44(7):1759–1766 PMID: 30075971 https://doi.org/10.1016/j.burns.2018.03.013
38. Kendrick D, Watson MC, Mulvaney CA, et al. Preventing childhood falls at home: meta-analysis and meta-regression. *Am J Prev Med*. 2008;35(4):370–379 PMID: 18779031 https://doi.org/10.1016/j.amepre.2008.06.038
39. Istre GR, McCoy MA, Stowe M, et al. Childhood injuries due to falls from apartment balconies and windows. *Inj Prev*. 2003;9(4):349–352 PMID: 14693898 https://doi.org/10.1136/ip.9.4.349
40. Spiegel CN, Lindaman FC. Children can't fly: a program to prevent childhood morbidity and mortality from window falls. 1977. *Inj Prev*. 1995;1(3):194–198 PMID: 9346026 https://doi.org/10.1136/ip.1.3.194
41. Grivna M, Al-Marzouqi HM, Al-Ali MR, Al-Saadi NN, Abu-Zidan FM. Pediatric falls from windows and balconies: incidents and risk factors as reported by newspapers in the United Arab Emirates. *World J Emerg Surg*. 2017;12(1):45 PMID: 29046710 https://doi.org/10.1186/s13017-017-0156-z
42. Vish NL, Powell EC, Wiltsek D, Sheehan KM. Pediatric window falls: not just a problem for children in high rises. *Inj Prev*. 2005;11(5):300–303 PMID: 16203839 https://doi.org/10.1136/ip.2005.008664
43. Zonfrillo MR, Ramsay ML, Fennell JE, Andreasen A. Unintentional non-traffic injury and fatal events: threats to children in and around vehicles. *Traffic Inj Prev*. 2018;19(2):184–188 PMID: 28933560 https://doi.org/10.1080/15389588.2017.1369053
44. Dowd MD. Vehicular hyperthermia—a highly preventable and potentially fatal problem. *Pediatr Ann*. 2018;47(3):e88–e90 PMID: 29538778 https://doi.org/10.3928/19382359-20180220-04
45. Krous HF, Nadeau JM, Fukumoto RI, Blackbourne BD, Byard RW. Environmental hyperthermic infant and early childhood death: circumstances, pathologic changes, and manner of death. *Am J Forensic Med Pathol*. 2001;22(4):374–382 PMID: 11764905 https://doi.org/10.1097/00000433-200112000-00008
46. Booth JN III, Davis GG, Waterbor J, McGwin G Jr. Hyperthermia deaths among children in parked vehicles: an analysis of 231 fatalities in the United States, 1999-2007. *Forensic Sci Med Pathol*. 2010;6(2):99–105 PMID: 20204546 https://doi.org/10.1007/s12024-010-9149-x
47. Ferrara P, Vena F, Caporale O, et al. Children left unattended in parked vehicles: a focus on recent Italian cases and a review of literature. *Ital J Pediatr*. 2013;39(1):71 PMID: 24195780 https://doi.org/10.1186/1824-7288-39-71

48. Adato B, Dubnov-Raz G, Gips H, Heled Y, Epstein Y. Fatal heat stroke in children found in parked cars: autopsy findings. *Eur J Pediatr*. 2016;175(9):1249–1252 PMID: 27438022 https://doi.org/10.1007/s00431-016-2751-5
49. Hassall IB. Small children left alone in parked cars. *N Z Med J*. 1983;96(723):25 PMID: 6571752
50. Boles R, Gawaziuk JP, Cristall N, Logsetty S. Pediatric frostbite: a 10-year single-center retrospective study. *Burns*. 2018;44(7):1844–1850 PMID: 30072195 https://doi.org/10.1016/j.burns.2018.04.002
51. Murphy JV, Banwell PE, Roberts AH, McGrouther DA. Frostbite: pathogenesis and treatment. *J Trauma*. 2000;48(1):171–178 PMID: 10647591 https://doi.org/10.1097/00005373-200001000-00036
52. Poulakidas SJ, Kowal-Vern A, Atty C. Pediatric frostbite treated by negative pressure wound therapy. *J Burn Care Res*. 2016;37(5):e489–e492 PMID: 26284629 https://doi.org/10.1097/BCR.0000000000000284
53. Crouch C, Smith WL. Long term sequelae of frostbite. *Pediatr Radiol*. 1990;20(5):365–366 PMID: 2349021 https://doi.org/10.1007/BF02013182
54. Fowler KA, Dahlberg LL, Haileyesus T, Gutierrez C, Bacon S. Childhood firearm injuries in the United States. *Pediatrics*. 2017;140(1):e20163486. PMID: 28630118 https://doi.org/10.1542/peds.2016-3486
55. Dowd MD, Sege RD; American Academy of Pediatrics Council on Injury, Violence, and Poison Prevention Executive Committee. Firearm-related injuries affecting the pediatric population. *Pediatrics*. 2012;130(5):e1416–e1423 PMID: 23080412 https://doi.org/10.1542/peds.2012-2481
56. Faulkenberry JG, Schaechter J. Reporting on pediatric unintentional firearm injury—who's responsible. *J Trauma Acute Care Surg*. 2015;79(3 suppl 1):S2–S8 PMID: 26308117 https://doi.org/10.1097/TA.0000000000000676
57. Miller M, Hemenway D. Unsupervised firearm handling by California adolescents. *Inj Prev*. 2004;10(3):163–168 PMID: 15178673 https://doi.org/10.1136/ip.2004.005447
58. Grossman DC, Mueller BA, Riedy C, et al. Gun storage practices and risk of youth suicide and unintentional firearm injuries. *JAMA*. 2005;293(6):707–714 PMID: 15701912 https://doi.org/10.1001/jama.293.6.707
59. Johnson RM, Miller M, Vriniotis M, Azrael D, Hemenway D. Are household firearms stored less safely in homes with adolescents? Analysis of a national random sample of parents. *Arch Pediatr Adolesc Med*. 2006;160(8):788–792 PMID: 16894076 https://doi.org/10.1001/archpedi.160.8.788
60. Azrael D, Cohen J, Salhi C, Miller M. Firearm storage in gun-owning households with children: results of a 2015 national survey. *J Urban Health*. 2018;95(3):295–304 PMID: 29748766 https://doi.org/10.1007/s11524-018-0261-7
61. Hamilton EC, Miller CC III, Cox CS Jr, Lally KP, Austin MT. Variability of child access prevention laws and pediatric firearm injuries. *J Trauma Acute Care Surg*. 2018;84(4):613–619 PMID: 29283962 https://doi.org/10.1097/TA.0000000000001786
62. Tseng J, Nuño M, Lewis AV, Srour M, Margulies DR, Alban RF. Firearm legislation, gun violence, and mortality in children and young adults: a retrospective cohort study of 27,566 children in the USA. *Int J Surg*. 2018;57:30–34 PMID: 30071359 https://doi.org/10.1016/j.ijsu.2018.07.010
63. Holly C, Porter S, Kamienski M, Lim A. School-Based and Community-Based Gun Safety Educational Strategies for Injury Prevention. *Health Promot Pract*. 2018:1524839918774571 PMID: 29745263

64. Damore DT, Ramundo ML, Hanna JP, Dayan PS. Parental attitudes toward BB and pellet guns. *Clin Pediatr (Phila)*. 2000;39(5):281–284 PMID: 10826075 https://doi.org/10.1177/000992280003900504
65. Dandu KV, Carniol ET, Sanghvi S, Baredes S, Eloy JAA. A 10-year analysis of head and neck injuries involving nonpowder firearms. *Otolaryngol Head Neck Surg*. 2017;156(5):853–856 PMID: 28457218 https://doi.org/10.1177/0194599817695546
66. Lee R, Fredrick D. Pediatric eye injuries due to nonpowder guns in the United States, 2002-2012. *J AAPOS*. 2015;19(2):163–8.e1 PMID: 25818283 https://doi.org/10.1016/j.jaapos.2015.01.010
67. Bronstein AC, Spyker DA, Cantilena LR Jr, Green JL, Rumack BH, Giffin SL. 2009 annual report of the American Association of Poison Control Centers' National Poison Data System (NPDS): 27th annual report. *Clin Toxicol (Phila)*. 2010;48(10):979–1178 PMID: 21192756 https://doi.org/10.3109/15563650.2010.543906
68. Lovegrove MC, Weidle NJ, Budnitz DS. Trends in emergency department visits for unsupervised pediatric medication exposures, 2004-2013. *Pediatrics*. 2015;136(4):e821–e829 PMID: 26347435 https://doi.org/10.1542/peds.2015-2092
69. Wood JN, Pecker LH, Russo ME, Henretig F, Christian CW. Evaluation and referral for child maltreatment in pediatric poisoning victims. *Child Abuse Negl*. 2012;36(4):362–369 PMID: 22571909 https://doi.org/10.1016/j.chiabu.2012.01.001
70. Yin S. Malicious use of pharmaceuticals in children. *J Pediatr*. 2010;157(5):832–6.e1 PMID: 20650468 https://doi.org/10.1016/j.jpeds.2010.05.040
71. Thomas AA, Mazor S. Unintentional marijuana exposure presenting as altered mental status in the pediatric emergency department: a case series. *J Emerg Med*. 2017;53(6):e119–e123 PMID: 28987305 https://doi.org/10.1016/j.jemermed.2017.08.007
72. Wang GS, Le Lait MC, Deakyne SJ, Bronstein AC, Bajaj L, Roosevelt G. Unintentional pediatric exposures to marijuana in Colorado, 2009-2015. *JAMA Pediatr*. 2016;170(9):e160971 PMID: 27454910 https://doi.org/10.1001/jamapediatrics.2016.0971
73. Bitunjac K, Saraga M. Alcohol intoxication in pediatric age: ten-year retrospective study. *Croat Med J*. 2009;50(2):151–156 PMID: 19399948 https://doi.org/10.3325/cmj.2009.50.151
74. Hon KL, Leung AK, Cheung E, Lee B, Tsang MM, Torres AR. An overview of exposure to ethanol-containing substances and ethanol intoxication in children based on three illustrated cases. *Drugs Context*. 2018;7:212512 PMID: 29344053 https://doi.org/10.7573/dic.212512
75. Minera G, Robinson E. Accidental acute alcohol intoxication in infants: review and case report. *J Emerg Med*. 2014;47(5):524–526 PMID: 25216537 https://doi.org/10.1016/j.jemermed.2014.06.032
76. Pélissier F, Claudet I, Pélissier-Alicot AL, Franchitto N. Parental cannabis abuse and accidental intoxications in children: prevention by detecting neglectful situations and at-risk families. *Pediatr Emerg Care*. 2014;30(12):862–866 PMID: 25407034 https://doi.org/10.1097/PEC.0000000000000288
77. Litovitz TL, Flagler SL, Manoguerra AS, Veltri JC, Wright L. Recurrent poisonings among paediatric poisoning victims. *Med Toxicol*. 1989;4(5):381–386 PMID: 2811675 https://doi.org/10.1007/BF03259919
78. Demorest RA, Posner JC, Osterhoudt KC, Henretig FM. Poisoning prevention education during emergency department visits for childhood poisoning. *Pediatr Emerg Care*. 2004;20(5):281–284 PMID: 15123897 https://doi.org/10.1097/01.pec.0000125654.20443.33
79. Schwebel DC, Davis AL, O'Neal EE. Child pedestrian injury: a review of behavioral risks and preventive strategies. *Am J Lifestyle Med*. 2012;6(4):292–302 PMID: 23066380 https://doi.org/10.1177/0885066611404876

80. Ma P, Hussain N, Abbe M. An examination of traffic-related traumatic injuries among children at a Level-1 pediatric trauma center, 2005–2014. *J Trauma Acute Care Surg.* 2017;83(5S Suppl 2):S233–S239 PMID: 28697022
81. Barton BK, Schwebel DC. The roles of age, gender, inhibitory control, and parental supervision in children's pedestrian safety. *J Pediatr Psychol.* 2007;32(5):517–526 PMID: 17442691 https://doi.org/10.1093/jpepsy/jsm014
82. Wills KE, Tanz RR, Christoffel K, et al. Supervision in childhood injury cases: a reliable taxonomy. *Accid Anal Prev.* 1997;29(1):133–137 PMID: 9110047 https://doi.org/10.1016/S0001-4575(96)00057-7
83. Cross D, Stevenson M, Hall M, et al. Child pedestrian injury prevention project: student results. *Prev Med.* 2000;30(3):179–187 PMID: 10684740 https://doi.org/10.1006/pmed.1999.0622
84. Centers for Disease Control and Prevention. Underlying cause of death 1999–2017. https://wonder.cdc.gov/wonder/help/ucd.html. Reviewed December 6, 2018. Accessed February 14, 2019
85. Sauber-Schatz EK, West BA, Bergen G; Centers for Disease Control and Prevention. Vital signs: restraint use and motor vehicle occupant death rates among children aged 0-12 years—United States, 2002-2011. *MMWR Morb Mortal Wkly Rep.* 2014;63(5):113–118 PMID: 24500292
86. Truong WH, Hill BW, Cole PA. Automobile safety in children: a review of North American evidence and recommendations. *J Am Acad Orthop Surg.* 2013;21(6):323–331 PMID: 23728957
87. Winston FK, Durbin DR, Kallan MJ, Moll EK. The danger of premature graduation to seat belts for young children. *Pediatrics.* 2000;105(6):1179–1183 PMID: 10835054 https://doi.org/10.1542/peds.105.6.1179
88. Centers for Disease Control and Prevention. Vital signs. Motor vehicle crash deaths: how is the US doing? https://www.cdc.gov/vitalsigns/motor-vehicle-safety/infographic.html. Reviewed July 6, 2016. Accessed February 14, 2019
89. Laslett AM, Jiang H, Chikritzhs T. Child injury deaths linked with adult alcohol consumption: a time series analysis. *Drug Alcohol Depend.* 2018;185:360–366 PMID: 29524873 https://doi.org/10.1016/j.drugalcdep.2017.11.024
90. Bambach MR, Mitchell RJ, Grzebieta RH, Olivier J. The effectiveness of helmets in bicycle collisions with motor vehicles: a case-control study. *Accid Anal Prev.* 2013;53:78–88 PMID: 23377086 https://doi.org/10.1016/j.aap.2013.01.005
91. Dellinger AM, Kresnow MJ. Bicycle helmet use among children in the United States: the effects of legislation, personal and household factors. *J Safety Res.* 2010;41(4):375–380 PMID: 20846554 https://doi.org/10.1016/j.jsr.2010.05.003
92. American Academy of Pediatrics Committee on Injury and Poison Prevention. All-terrain vehicle injury prevention: two-, three-, and four-wheeled unlicensed motor vehicles. *Pediatrics.* 2000;105(6):1352–1354 PMID: 10835081 https://doi.org/10.1542/peds.105.6.1352
93. Greenberg BSSC, Shah CC. All-terrain vehicle use by children: a form of child neglect? *Pediatr Radiol.* 2009;39(7):657–658 PMID: 19381622 https://doi.org/10.1007/s00247-009-1258-x
94. Jinnah H, Stoneman Z. Age- and gender-based patterns in youth all-terrain vehicle (ATV) riding behaviors. *J Agromed.* 2016;21(2):163–170 PMID: 26786819 https://doi.org/10.1080/1059924X.2016.1141736
95. Shah CC, Ramakrishnaiah RH, Bhutta ST, Parnell-Beasley DN, Greenberg BS. Imaging findings in 512 children following all-terrain vehicle injuries. *Pediatr Radiol.* 2009;39(7):677–684 PMID: 19308368 https://doi.org/10.1007/s00247-009-1213-x

96. McTavish JR, MacGregor JC, Wathen CN, MacMillan HL. Children's exposure to intimate partner violence: an overview. *Int Rev Psychiatry*. 2016;28(5):504–518 PMID: 27414209 https://doi.org/10.1080/09540261.2016.1205001
97. MacMillan HL, Wathen CN. Children's exposure to intimate partner violence. *Child Adolesc Psychiatr Clin N Am*. 2014;23(2):295–308, viii–ix PMID: 24656581 https://doi.org/10.1016/j.chc.2013.12.008
98. Herman-Giddens ME, Smith JB, Mittal M, Carlson M, Butts JD. Newborns killed or left to die by a parent: a population-based study. *JAMA*. 2003;289(11):1425–1429 PMID: 12636466 https://doi.org/10.1001/jama.289.11.1425
99. Sherr L, Mueller J, Fox Z. Abandoned babies in the UK—a review utilizing media reports. *Child Care Health Dev*. 2009;35(3):419–430 PMID: 19397605 https://doi.org/10.1111/j.1365-2214.2009.00952.x
100. Mariano TY, Chan HC, Myers WC. Toward a more holistic understanding of filicide: a multidisciplinary analysis of 32 years of U.S. arrest data. *Forensic Sci Int*. 2014;236:46–53 PMID: 24529774 https://doi.org/10.1016/j.forsciint.2013.12.019
101. Meyer CL. *Mothers Who Kill Their Children*. New York, NY: New York University Press; 2001
102. Hamilton-Giachritsis C, Browne K. Forgotten children? An update on young children in institutions across Europe. *Early Hum Dev*. 2012;88(12):911–914 PMID: 23058300 https://doi.org/10.1016/j.earlhumdev.2012.09.018
103. Nelson CA III, Fox NA, Zeanah CH Jr. Anguish of the abandoned child. *Sci Am*. 2013;308(4):62–67 PMID: 23539791 https://doi.org/10.1038/scientificamerican0413-62
104. Welch GL, Bonner BL. Fatal child neglect: characteristics, causation, and strategies for prevention. *Child Abuse Negl*. 2013;37(10):745–752 PMID: 23876861 https://doi.org/10.1016/j.chiabu.2013.05.008
105. Damashek A, Drass S, Bonner BL. Child maltreatment fatalities related to inadequate caregiver supervision. *J Interpers Violence*. 2014;29(11):1987–2001 PMID: 24861819 https://doi.org/10.1177/0886260513515951
106. Kuhlmann S, Ahlers-Schmidt CR. The use of the child fatality review committee to contribute to a longitudinal quality improvement project on safe sleep. *Hosp Pediatr*. 2018;8(8):504–505 PMID: 30026249 https://doi.org/10.1542/hpeds.2018-0097
107. Krugman SD, Cumpsty-Fowler CJ. A hospital-based initiative to reduce postdischarge sudden unexpected infant deaths. *Hosp Pediatr*. 2018;8(8):443–449 PMID: 30026250 https://doi.org/10.1542/hpeds.2017-0211
108. American Academy of Pediatrics Committee on Child Abuse and Neglect; Committee on Injury, Violence, and Poison Prevention; Council on Community Pediatrics. Child fatality review. *Pediatrics*. 2010;126(3):592–596 PMID: 20805149
109. Posey BM, Neuilly MA. A fatal review: exploring how children's deaths are reported in the United States. *Child Abuse Negl*. 2017;72:433–445 PMID: 28918234 https://doi.org/10.1016/j.chiabu.2017.09.005
110. Parrish JW, Schnitzer PG, Lanier P, Shanahan ME, Daniels JL, Marshall SW. Classification of maltreatment-related mortality by Child Death Review teams: how reliable are they? *Child Abuse Negl*. 2017;67:362–370 PMID: 28365427 https://doi.org/10.1016/j.chiabu.2017.03.003

CHAPTER 16

Drug-Endangered Children

Karen Farst, MD, MPH, FAAP
Associate Professor and Section Chief for Children at Risk
Department of Pediatrics
University of Arkansas for Medical Sciences
Little Rock, AR

Kathryn Wells, MD, FAAP
Associate Professor and Section Head for Child Abuse and Neglect
Department of Pediatrics
University of Colorado School of Medicine
Aurora, CO

Introduction

Substance use by caregivers creates an intersection of risks for adverse events for newborns, infants, and children. These risks include opportunities for direct harm from exposure to the drug or drug manufacturing process and indirect harm from exposure to the effects that substance use can have on a caregiver and the co-occurring issues surrounding substance use. The pediatric medical professional should be prepared to

- Recognize different settings in which newborns, infants, and children could be drug endangered.
- Perform a physical and laboratory assessment of a drug-endangered child.
- Develop a management plan for risk assessment and coordinated care when a child is identified as drug endangered.
- Advocate for a local, state, and national response to drug-endangered children that is based on provision of services for family preservation within a public health model.

Case Presentation

A newborn of a 28-year-old gravida 5, para 3 mother who presented to the emergency department (ED) in active labor with vaginal bleeding tests positive for amphetamines and marijuana by urine immunoassay screening. The mother did not seek prenatal care during pregnancy. She smokes 3 to 4 cigarettes daily and denies substance use or alcohol intake during pregnancy. However, she was agitated and had slurred speech on presentation to the ED. Following vaginal delivery, the neonate is estimated at 38 weeks' gestation by examination, and birth weight is appropriate for gestational age. Apgar score at 1 minute was 5 with notable poor respiratory effort, low heart rate, and acrocyanosis. After 30 seconds of positive pressure ventilation, the patient has good respiratory effort, normal heart rate, and no cyanosis. Initial physical examination on admission to the term nursery shows no abnormalities. The following issues will need to be assessed or considered by the medical professional:

- Medical issues to anticipate in the postnatal course
- Usefulness of additional drug testing in the neonate
- Need for mandated reporting to child welfare services in the state
- Assessment of the mother's need for services for addiction disorder
- Assessment for concomitant psychosocial stressors in the mother's life
- Safety disposition or follow-up plan following discharge from the nursery
- Health and safety of other children in the mother's care

Recognition

Definition

A *drug-endangered newborn, infant, or child* is one who is at risk of experiencing physical or emotional harm as a result of exposure to use, possession, manufacturing, cultivation, or distribution of illegal drugs.[1] The use of illegal drugs may also interfere with the caregiver's ability to parent and provide a safe and nurturing environment for a newborn, infant, or child in his or her care. Newborns, infants, and toddlers have higher risks for exposure to drugs in their environments due to their close proximity to adult caregivers; higher resting respiratory rates, which can facilitate exposure from airborne toxins; and hand-to-mouth behaviors, which can facilitate exposure from ingestion.[2] Young children have been found to be more likely to test positive from drug exposure compared with older children from the same home.[3]

The settings that can result in newborns, infants, or children becoming drug endangered overlap and contain opportunities for direct and indirect risk of harm to the child. These are illustrated in Figure 16.1 and include

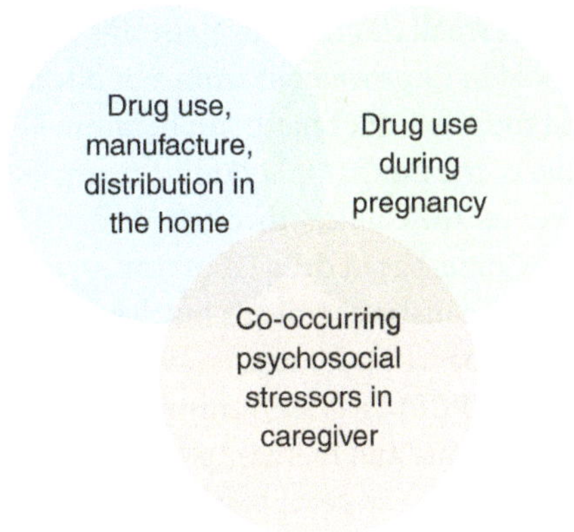

FIGURE 16.1
Areas of risks for drug-endangered infants and children.

- Drug use, manufacture, and/or distribution by caregivers in the home
- Drug use during pregnancy
- Co-occurring psychosocial issues in the life of the caregiver, including, but not limited to, interpersonal violence, undiagnosed or undertreated mental health issues, and prior history of child maltreatment in the home

Drug Use, Manufacture, and/or Distribution by Caregivers in the Home

The most common substances affecting drug-endangered children can be broken down into those that produce stimulant or depressant effects on the central nervous system (CNS). Cocaine and methamphetamine are CNS stimulants with strong addictive potential due to the powerful high associated with their use. These drugs can be injected, snorted, smoked, ingested, or inserted in the vagina or rectum to produce the desired effect. Methamphetamine gained popularity in the 1990s when "recipes" became available to produce the drug from over-the-counter decongestant medications and other household chemicals.[4,5] Homes where methamphetamine was being produced became a source of injury to children from issues such as caustic ingestions and explosions as well as public health crises from the contamination of the home and surrounding property.[6] Young children removed from these homes have been found to test positive for the drug itself from passive exposure.[3,7]

Policy and legislation restricting the over-the-counter sale of common cold medicines that can be used to manufacture methamphetamine have reduced the number of small clandestine meth labs in the United States. While this has resulted in improvement from a public health standpoint, it has not decreased the amount of methamphetamine being distributed for use because most of the methamphetamine being used in the United States continues to enter the country through Mexico.[4,8] While cocaine is not manufactured in home-based drug laboratories, children can still be exposed to the drug and caustic chemicals involved in "freebasing" and "cutting" the drug in preparation for use.

Use of phencyclidine (PCP) as a CNS stimulant declined in the United States in the 1980s as cocaine and methamphetamine became popular. It is regaining popularity for use in combination with other substances, such as marijuana. For children, toxicity can result in ataxia, hallucination, and impaired motor skills.[9]

Drugs considered CNS depressants include opiates/opioids, benzodiazepines, barbiturates, and cannabinoids. The opiate/opioid class of drugs includes heroin as well as controlled prescription medications such as hydrocodone, oxycodone, and fentanyl. According to the Centers for Disease Control and Prevention (CDC), the rate of deaths from overdose of heroin and opioid pain relievers has increased by 200% since 2000.[10] Between 1999 and 2010, the amount of prescription opioids sold to pharmacies, hospitals, and doctors' offices nearly quadrupled even though studies of pain management in the United States showed that the overall pain patients were reporting during this period was not increasing.

Benzodiazepines are another class of prescription medication with CNS sedation effects that have an addictive potential. They are commonly prescribed for issues such as anxiety and insomnia. Appropriate use is short-term and on an as-needed basis. When used on a regular basis, dependence develops and risk for adverse events from overdosage increases. Benzodiazepine misuse commonly co-occurs with stimulant drugs such as methamphetamine and cocaine because the sedating properties can ease the ill feelings following a stimulant high. Concurrent usage of benzodiazepines and opioids is not only on the rise but is associated with an increased risk for opioid overdose compared with those who use opioids without benzodiazepines.[11] Similar to opiates/opioids, prescription numbers, amount of medications per prescription, and adverse events from benzodiazepine overdosage are on the increase.[12]

As the misuse of prescription medications continues to increase, so does the opportunity for children to be harmed by ingestion of these medications. Opioids and sedative-hypnotics such as benzodiazepines are the most common classes of pharmaceutical agents involved with overall ingestions and those that lead to fatality in young children.[13]

While some exposures and ingestions of illicit or pharmaceutical substances could likely be prevented by increased supervision, these events are typically unintentional. When encountering a child with a toxidrome concerning for ingestion, the medical professional should be aware of the potential for intentional poisoning, which would present an even greater risk to the child's health and safety if he or she was to return to the home with the same caregivers. The most commonly reported categories involved in intentional or malicious poisoning include analgesics; stimulants or street drugs; sedatives, hypnotics, and antipsychotics; cough and cold preparations; and ethanol.[14] In cases of malicious poisonings, history of ingestion may be lacking. Presentations with unusual metabolic, gastrointestinal, or CNS findings may indicate intentional poisoning and necessitate expanded toxicological testing (see Drug Testing section later in this chapter).[15]

Marijuana continues to be the most commonly used illicit drug in the United States. While it remains illegal by federal law, many states have made it possible to access marijuana for specific medical purposes and some have legalized it for recreational use.[4] While the health effects of marijuana use are commonly discussed as being similar to nicotine, medical professionals should be aware of several caveats pertaining to children living with caregivers who use marijuana.

- Potency of tetrahydrocannabinol (THC) has more than doubled since the mid-1990s.
- Marijuana is often used concurrently with other illicit drugs to ease the uncomfortable physical symptoms following a high. Since it is lipophilic, the window of detection in urine is longer than it is for other drugs. Therefore, when a caregiver tests positive for marijuana and negative for other illicit drugs, it does not necessarily mean that the caregiver is solely using marijuana.
- Regular, habitual usage of marijuana impairs reaction time, cognition, and judgment.
- Regions where marijuana has been legalized have been affected by an increase in adverse events from ingestion of marijuana products as well as an increase in severity of marijuana-related ingestions in young children.[16,17]

Drug Use During Pregnancy

Drug use during pregnancy has been a worldwide problem throughout all societies since ancient times.[18] While many still view addiction as a moral failure and personal choice, medical professionals play a critical role in educating affected families and the public that drug use is a chronic relapsing disease that requires medical care to manage. The increased understanding that virtually all substances of use and abuse cross the placenta and reach the fetus has elevated the health care focus on the issue. Historically, a distinction was made between legal and illegal drugs, but with increasing legalization of recreational marijuana, the growing misuse of opioids, and the expanding understanding of the effect of alcohol on the fetus, the conversation is shifting to a public health concern related more to risk and effect than primarily legal or child welfare intervention. Despite this, child welfare involvement often occurs because drug use can adversely affect the parents' ability to safely care for their children. Child welfare trends appear to demonstrate that younger children comprise a larger percentage of out-of-home care, which is believed to be at least in part related to prenatal substance use. Medical professionals have an increasing opportunity to be involved in not only the prevention, identification, and treatment of newborns who have been exposed to drugs but also policy issues affecting them and their families.

Issues related to drug use during pregnancy are complicated. A pregnant woman using drugs is usually a woman with an addiction who got pregnant and who sincerely wants a healthy baby. She is often consumed with guilt about her substance use and is accustomed to disrespect but grateful to anyone who treats her with respect and dignity. She is often very sensitive to signs of withdrawal, which is important to consider if she will be caring for an infant who may show such signs. Pregnancy can be a strong incentive to discontinue substance use and begin recovery, but it is also accompanied by added stress and is a very short time to change behavior, social life, and relationships, as is often necessary. Behavior change in general is difficult and compounded by everyday life stresses as well as the extreme stresses of poverty, when present, although substance use disorder affects all socioeconomic groups. It may involve many failed attempts, relapses, and false starts with commitment that appears to vary from moment to moment. In addressing addiction, it is important to identify the motivations for use and address appropriate alternative interventions.

Few data exist on the extent of the problem and the best approaches to address it. Women may be reluctant to disclose their substance use during pregnancy due to fear of criminal prosecution or child welfare involvement. This could reduce their use of medical and treatment resources. However, prevention or early identification and intervention are important to reduce risks to the mother and infant as well as to enhance outcomes. Women who are pregnant or contemplating pregnancy should be encouraged to discontinue drug and alcohol use and should be counseled about the potential risks and ramifications of using substances during pregnancy, including health consequences and child welfare involvement. Child welfare involvement is often portrayed as a punitive or negative event. In reality, it can result in positive change for the mother and her child by providing the motivation, accountability, structure, and support needed to get a mother into substance use treatment that may not have occurred if left to the mother's initiative.

Medical professionals play a critical role in addressing these complex issues along the continuum of care for the mother and infant. Addiction is a chronic, relapsing biological and behavioral disorder, so policies that deter women from seeking prenatal care should be discouraged because they are contrary to the health and welfare of the mother and fetus.[19]

Epidemiology and Prevalence

Prevalence estimates vary widely and are difficult to clearly and consistently establish. There are many reasons why it is difficult to get a clear picture of incidence, but it is believed that the number of cases is underestimated due to the social stigma it creates for mothers and families, fear of criminal prosecution or child welfare involvement, unreliability of mothers' self-reports, limitations of toxicology testing techniques, and lack of uniformity in hospital policies and procedures for screening, testing, and referral for services.

The best data are likely derived from the Substance Abuse and Mental Health Services Administration National Survey on Drug Use and Health, which regularly provides information on trends in drug use, including those related to pregnant women. This annual survey provides national and state-level data, combined in 2-year epochs, on the use of alcohol, tobacco, and illicit drugs in a sample of more than 67,000 noninstitutionalized individuals older than 12 years. Data from the 2013 survey that specifically measured rates in pregnant women indicated that the rate of illicit drug use among pregnant women aged 15 to 44 years was 5.4%, compared with 11.4% among women in this age group who were not pregnant. The rate of illicit drug use among pregnant women aged 15 to 17 years was 14.6%; 8.6% among women aged 18 to 25 years; and 3.2% among women aged 26 to 44 years.[20] In general, pregnant women use alcohol and other drugs less than nonpregnant women of the same age, with the exception of pregnant teens aged 15 to 17 years, who use alcohol and other drugs more than nonpregnant teens. While most women achieve some level of abstinence during pregnancy, the net rate of abstinence in one study[21] was only 24% because of the high likelihood of postpartum relapse. The lowest rates of abstinence during pregnancy are in smoking,[22] which may be related to women substituting smoking for illicit drug or alcohol use due to the perception of reduced risk as well as the greater social acceptance[23] of smoking. Therefore, smoking status is a known predictor of illicit drug use in pregnancy.[24] The decrease in drug use throughout pregnancy is often followed by a rebound increase during the 6 months to 1 year after delivery.

Pathophysiology and Outcomes

The effects of drug exposure on the mother and baby during the prenatal period vary widely. It is difficult to study fully the effect on the mother-infant dyad due to the limitations of such research and the common confounding variables such as frequent polysubstance use, psychosocial factors, and socioeconomic and environmental variables like poverty and violence. The direct effect of maternal drug use on the fetus in the prenatal period is also difficult to fully determine due to co-occurring issues. Polysubstance use is common, so the effect of a specific drug may be difficult to isolate. Additionally, other variables may play a role, including poor maternal physical and mental health, timing and amount of the exposure, and frequency and method of use. Documentation of drug use during pregnancy is usually based on self-report. If toxicological testing is undertaken, it has limitations. Due to the passive diffusion of most drugs across the placenta, the fetus is exposed and at risk. During fetal growth, the organs are undergoing growth and differentiation, and exposure may result in disruptions affecting several areas. Exposure during the embryonic stage of pregnancy can result in structural or birth defects. During the remainder of the pregnancy, nutrition delivered to the fetus can be affected by placental insufficiency or inadequate maternal intake, resulting in poor growth.

Advances in brain imaging have contributed to the understanding of the effects of prenatal drug exposure on the developing human brain.[25] Brain growth begins early in gestation and continues into the postnatal period, creating different windows of vulnerability prenatally and postnatally. Therefore, drug exposure can affect brain organization and cause alterations in neurotransmitters and their receptors. Studies reveal that outcomes can improve if exposure is reduced or eliminated at some time during the pregnancy.

There are a wide range of possible clinical presentations in the newborn related to prenatal drug exposure. It is important to consider the risks for newborns who have been exposed to drugs in the context of many factors in the newborn's environment that may place them at risk, such as dysfunctional parenting, unstable and chaotic home environments, and frequent polysubstance use in the mother. Prenatal drug exposure increases risk for fetal loss or death, placental insufficiency and abruption, preterm delivery, and toxemia. Fetal growth can be affected, and the exposed fetus is at risk for premature delivery and associated complications, physical dependence, and/or withdrawal. Tobacco has the greatest effect on preterm delivery and low birth weight.[26] Prenatal drug exposure increases infant mortality through several means, including associated risks of preterm birth and related complications and positional overlay, and has been linked to an increased risk of sudden unexplained infant death (SUID). Table 16.1 lists common clinical presentations for newborns of mothers who used drugs during pregnancy.

Long-term effects are subtle but measurable, with the best studies controlling for other issues than can adversely affect neurodevelopmental outcomes.[18] Children who were prenatally exposed to drugs may go on to develop disruptive behaviors such as oppositional defiant disorder, mood and anxiety disorders, low self-esteem, and perceived lack of control over their environment. They are more likely to show gaps in problem-solving skills, self-regulation, memory, and the ability to remain attentive. The prenatally exposed child may demonstrate impaired intellectual and academic achievement and cognitive problems such as delayed language development, poor memory, and inability to learn from mistakes.[27] Prenatal exposure to alcohol creates the greatest risk for effects on growth, cognition, behavior, language, and achievement throughout life. Affected children may go on to demonstrate school problems and employment failure as well as behavioral, mental health, and drug use problems. These children are at greater risk for impaired attachment and maltreatment, often resulting in child welfare involvement, and may be at higher risk of developing their own drug use problems. While prenatal exposure to drugs increases the risk of behavior problems in adolescence, studies have shown that protective factors at individual, family, and societal levels may attenuate some of the detrimental effects.[28]

Management

Assessment and intervention for prenatal drug exposure should begin prior to pregnancy and continue throughout the newborn period. Pediatric medical professionals have great opportunity for involvement throughout this continuum. See Box 16.1 for 5 points of intervention that have been described[29] for drug-exposed newborns: prepregnancy, prenatal, birth, postnatal, and throughout childhood.

Pregnancy and motherhood are times of increased motivation because motherhood is often the only legitimate social role valued by women who are dependent on drugs. Most women in treatment are very concerned about how their drug use has affected their children. Ideally, the mother's health history during pregnancy and delivery should include serial screening for substance use, including alcohol, tobacco,

TABLE 16.1
Possible Clinical Presentations Related to Prenatal Substance Exposure

	Alcohol	Nicotine/Tobacco	Marijuana/THC	Opiates	Cocaine	Methamphetamine
Effect on fetal growth	• Effect on growth must be present to diagnose FASD. • Associated with even moderate levels of exposure.	• Low birth weight and IUGR • Directly proportional to number of cigarettes smoked • Appears to resolve by 24 mo of age	• Studies limited • May be associated with low birth weight/small for gestational age	• Reported but many confounding variables • Low birth weight due to symmetric IUGR or preterm birth • Microcephaly	• Effect on intrauterine growth demonstrated/small for gestational age • Decreased head circumference	• Studies limited • Independent effect on fetal growth demonstrated
Congenital anomalies	• Multiple anomalies described throughout the literature • FASD	Weak data for association with oral facial clefts	No clear teratogenic effect	No clear teratogenic effect	Original reports not confirmed	Studies limited
Withdrawal	One study reporting withdrawal symptoms, but not confirmed in longitudinal studies	• No clear withdrawal described • Abnormal newborn behavior consistent with drug toxicity	• No clear withdrawal • Abnormal newborn behavior	NAS	Early reports but not substantiated	No prospective studies available
Neurobehavior in newborn	• Poor habituation and low levels of arousal • Motor abnormalities	Impaired orientation and autonomic regulation and abnormalities of muscle tone	Increased startle and tremors	• Abnormal neurobehavior related to NAS/withdrawal • Subacute/delayed withdrawal	• Irritability and lability of state • Decreased behavioral and autonomic regulation • Poor alertness and orientation	Abnormal neurobehavioral patterns including poor movement quality, decreased arousal, and increased stress

(continued)

TABLE 16.1 *(continued)*

	Alcohol	Nicotine/Tobacco	Marijuana/THC	Opiates	Cocaine	Methamphetamine
Long-term effects	• Significant attention problems from childhood through adulthood • Lower IQ scores • Poorer memory and executive functioning skills • Impaired development and use of language • Variety of significant academic and school problems, primarily deficits in reading and math skills	• Impulsivity and attention problems • Associated with hyperactivity and negative and externalizing behaviors through childhood and into adulthood • Possible abnormalities in learning and memory • Slightly lower IQ scores • Poor language development • Poorer performance on arithmetic and spelling tasks • Increased probability of tobacco use • Experimentation with drugs among adolescents	• Inattention and impulsivity in toddlers • Memory and perceptual problems in older children • Associated with deficits in problem-solving skills that require sustained attention and visual memory, analysis, and integration • Subtle deficits in learning and memory • Associated with academic underachievement, especially in reading and spelling • Associated with behavioral problems	• Hyperactivity and short attention span • Improved developmental scores with appropriate medical and environmental controls	• Some reports of problems, possibly moderated by other risks, such as attention difficulties and oppositional/defiant behavior • Does not predict overall development or IQ scores • Alterations in executive functioning including visual-motor ability, attention, and working memory • Association with subtle language delays	• Possible association with externalizing behaviors and peer problems • Possible association with lower IQ scores

Abbreviations: FASD, fetal alcohol spectrum disorder; IUGR, intrauterine growth retardation; NAS, neonatal abstinence syndrome; THC, tetrahydrocannabinol.

BOX 16.1
Five Points of Intervention for Drug-Exposed Newborns

Prepregnancy

Increase awareness (eg, billboards, points of sale).

Integrate prevention and education into the public education system.

Standardize information about newborns who have been exposed to substances into the training curricula for professionals who serve women.

Counsel any women of childbearing age to decrease/discontinue use of substances and/or to adequately use contraception.

Prenatal

Increase use of available treatment programs for pregnant women.

Develop guidelines and standards of care for medical professionals.

Implement universal baseline and ongoing screening using standardized tools and scripting.

Enhance referral networks.

Consider universal baseline and periodic ongoing testing.

Implement multidisciplinary planning around birth options for women who are incarcerated.

Improve access to treatment and prenatal health care for pregnant women identified through criminal justice, child welfare, behavioral health, and community systems.

Birth

Universal screening for alcohol and drug use using standardized tools and scripts.

Testing of mothers and newborns for clearly defined indications.

Referral to child welfare as indicated or required by law.

Postnatal

Implement a clear plan for follow-up care and transfer of information at time of discharge.

Establish follow-up care for the newborn in a medical home, including an appointment within 48–72 hours.

Initiate developmental screening and indicated referrals.

Monitor and support maternal medical and mental health, including postpartum depression screening.

Obtain consents for sharing information between medical professionals to integrate services.

Educate and support caregivers, families, and all service providers.

Counsel caregivers about breastfeeding and the importance of a sober caregiver at all times.

(*continued*)

BOX 16.1 *(continued)*

Throughout Childhood

Educate, support, and provide linkages for families of children with increased needs due to substance exposures.

Monitor development and ensure indicated interventions.

Collaborate with education system to assist in understanding and addressing effects.

Support and provide prevention programming for these children and youth at risk of future substance use.

Communicate across systems and integrate care strategies.

Support the whole family in sustaining long-term recovery.

marijuana, and illicit drugs, and the communication of any concerns to the medical professional. Questions for the mother such as, "In the time prior to finding out you were pregnant, what drugs or alcohol did you use, including prescription medications, tobacco, and marijuana?" can be helpful in obtaining maternal substance use history. Hospitals should have well-developed policies related to screening and testing of newborns for prenatal exposures, ideally based on defined risk factors. Newborns should receive medical interventions as indicated based on symptoms and clinical findings including close monitoring of feeding and attachment. For newborns who are identified as being prenatally exposed to substances, social assessment should be undertaken in the health care setting and may include referral to child welfare for additional safety assessment and support services. Additionally, medical professionals should be aware of local and state laws and policies addressing reporting to child welfare.

Birth outcomes for women and neonates are drastically better when the woman has received drug use treatment and prenatal care during her pregnancy. Pregnant women have varying and complex needs, so drug use treatment must be tailored to a woman's individual needs. A treatment program should provide adequate support services and resources, focus on helping a woman to have a safer pregnancy and healthy baby, and offer encouragement and training for mothers to improve parenting skills to ensure that their babies receive appropriate interventions and supports. Brief interventions, particularly using motivational interviewing, have been shown to reduce prenatal substance use. Drug use treatment of adults with addiction disorders may include behavioral counseling, cognitive behavioral therapy (CBT), motivational interviewing, and contingency management with financial incentives.[30] Drug use treatment must also address related issues such as underlying depression and other mental health conditions, intimate partner violence, health issues such as HIV/AIDS and disability, low income, unemployment, and inadequate or unsafe housing because recovery will only be successful to the extent that the issues that precipitate the drug use are also ameliorated. Barriers to successful treatment and recovery must be removed. This may include removing barriers to attendance by allowing children to accompany the parent(s) and providing for transportation, addressing children's emotional and behavioral problems by providing therapeutic child care, children's social skills training, and drug use education for the children. Other parent support services should be provided as well, such as parenting classes, home visitation, and job skills training.

The potential effects of drugs on the newborn's brain should be considered when discussing breastfeeding, balancing risk and benefit. Breastfeeding is an important intervention in newborns who were exposed to opioids prenatally because it is the only available intervention demonstrated to reduce NAS severity in newborns exposed to opioids.[31] For other substances, additional studies and consensus are needed, but generally, use of illicit drugs while breastfeeding should be discouraged.[32]

Drug-exposed newborns may benefit from many services for which pediatric medical professionals can be instrumental in advocating. The development of a clear, comprehensive, and supportive plan of safe care for the newborn through structured discharge planning is perhaps the most critical intervention for the drug-exposed newborn. A well-planned warm handoff to the pediatric medical home ensures the best potential for integrated support for the newborn and mother, whether or not child welfare is involved. In cases in which the involvement of child welfare is necessitated, the pediatric medical professional can approach the family in a transparent, supportive, and empathetic way and demonstrate willingness to engage with the family for the ongoing care of the child. It is also helpful to have the caregiver sign consent to share information among the medical team, support services, and child welfare services (if involved) so communication can be optimized.

On hospital discharge, newborns who have been exposed to drugs may face additional challenges for which the health care community can play a critical role in support. Population-based analyses have demonstrated that infants born to mothers with a substance use disorder are at a significantly greater risk for adverse health outcomes in the perinatal period and are also more likely to be rehospitalized in the first year after birth.[33] The care of these high-risk newborns in a medical home can assist in minimizing challenges related to disrupted parental care and early dysfunctional mother-baby interactions.[34] It is critical for caregivers to understand normal newborn/infant development and growth as well as potential challenges drug-exposed newborns may face to reduce risk of frustration related to unrealistic expectations, a known risk factor for child abuse. The pediatric medical professional should be aware that decreased drug use during pregnancy is frequently offset by increased use after delivery, which is important because this is a time when newborn/infant needs are high and maternal bonding is critical for infant development. Women may cease breastfeeding early to restart smoking, alcohol intake, or other drug use. There may be other environmental risks, such as intimate partner violence or a chaotic home environment. Secondhand tobacco smoke is associated with increased risk of respiratory and ear infections, sudden infant death syndrome or SUID, behavioral dysfunction, and cognitive impairment.[35] Other substances have also been linked to an increased risk of infant death through positional overlay as well as SUID.

Alcohol Exposure

Alcohol deserves special consideration due to its social acceptance and the frequency of use as well as the high risk to the newborn. The CDC reports that approximately half of US women of childbearing age admit to alcohol consumption within the past month, with use ranging from sporadic to 15% reporting binge drinking. Most women are able to cut down or discontinue alcohol use during pregnancy, but there is no known safe amount of alcohol exposure for the fetus. The detrimental effects of prenatal alcohol exposure on the fetus are well documented.[36] Fetal alcohol spectrum disorder (FASD) is a general term that encompasses the range of adverse effects associated with prenatal alcohol exposure. It is the most common preventable cause of nongenetic intellectual disability. Effects range in severity depending on the timing and amount of exposure. The greatest risk for alcohol-related birth outcomes is for exposures that occur in the first trimester.[37] The American Academy of Pediatrics (AAP) published a clinical report on fetal alcohol spectrum disorder in 2015, which underscored that alcohol-related birth defects and related developmental disabilities are completely preventable, that no amount of alcohol intake during pregnancy is considered to be safe, that the effects appear to be dose related, and that the neurocognitive and behavioral problems resulting from prenatal alcohol exposure are lifelong.[36] Updated diagnostic guidelines based on a thorough review of the literature were released in 2016.[38] These guidelines address the precise definition of documented prenatal alcohol exposure; neurobehavioral criteria for diagnosis of FASD, partial fetal alcohol syndrome, and alcohol-related neurodevelopmental disorder; revised diagnostic criteria for alcohol-related birth defects; an updated comprehensive research dysmorphology scoring system; and a new lip/philtrum guide for the white population. The goal of these new guidelines is to assist in the accurate diagnosis of newborns, infants, and children prenatally exposed to alcohol. Studies have revealed a high rate of missed or misdiagnosis of FASD in children and youth in foster and adoptive care, leading to inadequate interventions and services.[39]

Pediatric medical professionals play an important role in the early recognition of, intervention in, and support for services for children with FASD. Early diagnosis, especially before 6 years of age, along with early intervention correlates with improved outcomes.[40] Delayed or inaccurate diagnoses may lead to higher incidence of secondary disabilities and higher need for special education services.[41] Pediatric medical professionals are encouraged to consider FASD when evaluating children with developmental concerns, behavioral problems, and school failure, especially children in foster care. These children need a pediatric medical home in which necessary medical, behavioral, social, and educational services can be provided and coordinated.[42]

Opioid Exposure

Opioids create unique challenges when considering prenatal exposures and risk due to their rapidly increasing use, potential for addiction in the user, and risk of withdrawal in the exposed newborn.

There are several important features that create additional challenges for prenatal opioid use. Opioids are small lipophilic molecular weight compounds that readily cross placental and blood-brain barriers. Active or passive maternal detoxification is associated with increased risk of fetal distress and loss, so the management goal is to optimize prenatal care and general maternal physical and mental health and reduce potential withdrawal in the newborn. At this time, methadone maintenance for the mother as a part of a treatment program is the standard of care. This allows for transition from illicit opioid use to medically managed opioid maintenance therapy. This approach decreases maternal and neonatal morbidity by providing superior relapse prevention, reduced risk-taking behavior, enhanced compliance with prenatal care, and better neonatal outcome rates. Maintenance programs with methadone for pregnant women are beneficial because they can sustain opioid concentrations in the mother and fetus in ranges that minimize opioid craving, suppress abstinence symptomatology, block heroin-induced euphoria, and prevent fetal stress. The disadvantages of such programs are that the achievement of successful detoxification after delivery is extremely unlikely and the newborn will likely have a more severe and prolonged course of NAS compared with prenatal heroin exposure. However, the newborn is usually normally grown, and most adverse maternal factors are eliminated.

Buprenorphine is gaining popularity for use during pregnancy, although some studies suggest treatment retention rates are inferior to methadone with flexibly delivered and low fixed doses but equally effective with fixed medium or high doses. Newborns of mothers treated with buprenorphine appear to have minimal to mild withdrawal that is of shorter duration, requiring lower medication intervention and shorter hospital stays.[43] Further, buprenorphine has been shown to be as safe as methadone for treatment of pregnant women who are dependent on opioids. Medication-assisted treatment programs are most effective when combined with a formal treatment program that includes contingency management. Medication-assisted withdrawal is less optimal because it is associated with a high relapse rate and some evidence suggests increased fetal morbidity and mortality rates.

Neonatal abstinence syndrome (NAS) was first described by Finnegan in the 1970s. Symptoms include sweating, sneezing, yawning, lacrimation, hyperpyrexia, tachypnea, hyperpnea, respiratory alkalosis, irritability, increased muscle tone and activity, abnormal suck or poor feeding, diarrhea, tremors, and seizures. It has been shown to affect anywhere from 45% to 94% of newborns exposed to opioids in utero, including methadone and buprenorphine, and results in significant neonatal morbidity and health care utilization.[44] Preterm newborns may be at lower risk with less severe/prolonged courses of withdrawal. Severity depends on the drug, maternal drug history (including timing of most recent use), maternal metabolism, net transfer of drugs across the placenta, placental metabolism, newborn metabolism and excretion, and maternal use of other drugs that may increase the severity and duration of the withdrawal. Withdrawal often manifests within 24 hours of birth for a neonate exposed to heroin but can be delayed until 24 to 72 hours after birth when the exposure is heroin. Withdrawal symptoms may last anywhere from 2 to 3 weeks to 4 to 6 months and potentially as long as 1 year. Subacute withdrawal symptoms include restlessness, agitation, irritability, and poor socialization.

Scoring systems specific to NAS are available to monitor severity of symptoms and response to treatment. The Finnegan Neonatal Abstinence Scoring System has been used to guide the management of newborns with NAS since it was developed in the mid-1970s. However, despite its broad use and acceptance, it has never been validated.[44] Recently, concerns have been raised that it may lead to unnecessary opioid treatment of newborns with NAS because the scoring system does not focus on how the exhaustive list of symptoms scored affect the newborn's ability to function. Due to these concerns, a new approach to assessing newborns by focusing on their ability to function regardless of the number of withdrawal symptoms was developed. This method, entitled the Eat, Sleep, Console approach, which was developed and tested at Yale University, demonstrated a significant decrease in the use of morphine for the management of newborns with NAS, resulting in substantial reductions in lengths of stay.[45]

Treatment of newborns exhibiting NAS often requires hospitalization and medication. In the AAP clinical report on neonatal drug withdrawal, a 2-tiered approach to treatment is recommended, beginning with the use of nonpharmacologic interventions, followed by opioids and other medications only if these measures fail.[44] Nonpharmacologic support includes minimizing environmental stimuli, promoting adequate sleep and rest, and providing sufficient caloric intake to establish weight gain. Medication therapy may be indicated with the primary goal being to relieve moderate to severe signs of NAS and to prevent complications such as fever, weight loss, and seizures. However, the optimal threshold for implementation of pharmacologic treatment has not been established and unnecessary treatment will prolong the drug exposure and duration of the hospitalization. Most physicians use an opioid such as morphine or methadone as their drug of first choice, but there are growing efforts to maximize nonpharmacologic interventions whenever possible.[46] These interventions, which include encouraging skin-to-skin contact, better breastfeeding training, and giving mothers a comfortable, private place to bond with their newborns, can reduce the need for intensive care.

Marijuana

Addressing marijuana use during pregnancy has become more challenging due to the growing legalization of medicinal and recreational use of the drug as well as rapidly increasing potency of THC and methods of ingestion of the drug. Marijuana remains the most commonly used illicit drug during pregnancy and is particularly problematic because many marijuana users believe it is relatively safe to use during pregnancy.[47] Delta-9-THC, the active psychogenic component of marijuana, is a small, highly lipophilic molecule that is rapidly distributed to the brain and fat and also crosses the placenta to the fetus and into human milk. While the effect of cannabinoids on the fetus is not fully known, animal studies demonstrate that endocannabinoids play important roles in brain development, including affecting neurotransmitter systems as well as neuronal proliferation, migration, differentiation, and survival. Studies in humans reveal that cannabinoid receptors develop as early as 14 weeks of gestation and increase rapidly in density throughout gestation.[48]

Although studies exploring the effects of marijuana use during pregnancy and breastfeeding are limited by confounding variables, there are growing concerns related to impaired neurodevelopment of the prenatally exposed newborn, resulting in hyperactivity, poor cognitive function, and changes in dopaminergic receptors.[49,50] There is moderate evidence that maternal use of marijuana during pregnancy is associated with decreased cognitive function, decreased IQ scores, attention problems, decreased growth, and decreased academic ability in exposed offspring.[51] Additionally, the level of THC is much higher in the drug that is currently being used than was studied previously in the 1980s, raising additional concerns about risk.[49] Therefore, the American College of Obstetricians and Gynecologists (ACOG) recommends that women who are pregnant or contemplating pregnancy should be encouraged to discontinue drug use.[52] Additionally, ACOG recommends that marijuana use should be avoided during pregnancy and pregnant women should be counseled about the potential risks of use during pregnancy. Because marijuana is not regulated or evaluated by the US Food and Drug Administration, there are no approved indications, contraindications, safety precautions, or recommendations for its use during pregnancy and lactation.[52]

Co-occurring Psychosocial Issues in the Life of the Caregiver

Drug use in a caregiver rarely occurs in a vacuum. There are often co-occurring issues that can adversely affect the health and safety of children in the home.[27,53–57]

- Drug use is often part of an underlying mental health issue (undiagnosed or undertreated).
- Interpersonal violence occurring in the home.
- Exposure to other caregivers/adults in the home who may also have drug use issues.
- Drug use is often intergenerational, so caregivers often lack a strong support system and had poor parenting role models.
- Risk for other forms of abuse or neglect, including injuries resulting from lack of supervision.
- Impaired bonding and attachment between caregiver and child due to the impact of drug use on the caregiver and/or separation from a parent during incarceration.
- Addiction issues increase risk of poverty.

The interplay of these overlapping risks poses a challenge for designing effective prevention and treatment strategies. These issues have been shown to individually have a detrimental effect on the trajectory of the child's physical and emotional well-being. Unfortunately, as these adverse childhood experiences accumulate during infancy and childhood, the negative effect on adult physical health and well-being increases in exponential increments.[58]

Assessment

Physical Assessment

The medical evaluation of infants or children from homes where they have been exposed to the use, manufacturing, or distribution of drugs focuses on an overall assessment of their health and identification of unmet care needs.[1,59] If the child presents from the scene of an active drug laboratory in which there has been an explosion or chemical spill onto the child, or if the child has a chemical odor, decontamination by removing the child's clothing and assisting with a warm soap and water bath in a private setting would be appropriate. Medical professionals should be aware of the potential for secondary exposure during the decontamination process, taking care to dispose of contaminated clothing appropriately and protect their own clothing from exposure. If the child does not have acute need for decontamination, a soap and water bath or shower can be offered in a more private setting once the medical and safety evaluation is completed. Specific medical indications of distress, such as burns, caustic ingestions, and/or respiratory distress, should be addressed with typical trauma and/or pediatric care approaches.

History of exposure to a drug-endangered environment should prompt the medical professional to be alert for possible co-occurring abuse and issues related to caregiver neglect.[8,59] The infant or child should have a complete head-to-toe examination, looking for cutaneous injury, evaluation of appropriateness of growth parameters, developmental screening, and dental evaluation. Laboratory and radiological testing should be guided by the child's presenting symptoms.[60] A low threshold for skeletal survey in children younger than 2 years is appropriate due to the co-occurrence of interpersonal violence in caregivers with substance use issues. Children who are developmentally able to participate in conversations should be asked about sexual abuse in a developmentally appropriate and non-leading manner. Many children from drug-endangered homes have witnessed multiple forms of trauma and benefit from referral for assessment for trauma-focused CBT if developmentally appropriate.[61]

Drug Testing

Drug testing in infants and children is often used as a tool to guide medical treatment and identify children at risk from factors related to substance use by their caregivers.[3,7] The indications for performing drug testing in infants and children could include physical findings in the child, illness or injury potentially related to abuse and/or neglect, behavioral indicators by the caregivers, or historical information of substance use, manufacture, or distribution within the home. The objective indicator(s) that relates to concern for the patient's health and/or safety should be documented when ordering drug testing in infants and children.[62,63] If the drug test is being ordered for a purpose other than to assist with the management of the health and safety of the child, separate informed consent may be needed. Each medical professional should be familiar with his or her hospital or clinic policies for drug testing and discuss with the legal department if needed. Professionals should also be aware of state-specific mandated reporting laws regarding drug exposure in the antenatal period and later in childhood. Professionals practicing in states that mandate reporting of positive drug tests in infants and children to child protective services for an assessment should be prepared to explain the objective indications and "special need" for administering drug tests to infants and children from a health and safety standpoint. This is in contrast to ordering drug testing for the express purpose of involving the criminal justice system, which is not a component of medical care.[64]

There are many options for drug testing in children, including urine, blood, saliva, hair, and nails.[9] In newborns, testing options also include meconium and umbilical cord tissue.[65,66] The medical professional should be aware of the drug exposure time represented in each of the possible testing matrices. Blood, saliva, and urine typically reflect recent use (hours to days). Urine may have a slightly longer window of exposure compared with blood and saliva due to the excretion of metabolized by-products of the parent form of the drug. For regular use of lipophilic drugs such as marijuana, urine testing results may be positive up to 1 month after last use.[9,67]

Hair, nails, meconium, and umbilical cord tissue are typically considered matrices to demonstrate non-acute drug exposure (weeks to months). Meconium formation begins between the 12th and 16th week of gestation. It is composed of ingested amniotic fluid, bile, and intestinal epithelial cells. Meconium typically remains in the bowel until it is passed during the first several days following delivery. It can be passed in utero, creating risk for meconium aspiration at delivery and decreasing its availability for use as a testing matrix in the postnatal period. Meconium has been found to have higher sensitivity than urine in detecting drug use during pregnancy due to its longer window of detection. However, recent exposure (days) can be reflected in meconium sampling as evidenced by postnatal medications being detected in meconium when collection does not occur immediately following birth. Use of umbilical cord tissue as a testing matrix is growing in popularity due to its relative ease of collection compared with meconium. Studies using meconium and umbilical cord tissue to assess for in utero drug exposure have shown comparable rates of detection. Evaluation of paired samples of meconium and umbilical cord tissue from the same patients suggest umbilical cord tissue test sensitivity is lower compared with meconium testing.[65]

Incorporation of drugs into hair is a complex process. Drugs can enter from the body's circulation through the capillary supply to the follicle, through deposition by sweat and/or sebum onto growing or mature hair, or by contamination from the environment to the external hair shaft. Depending on the testing methodology of the specific laboratory, a positive hair drug testing result could reflect a variety of exposure possibilities. Pretest washing of a hair sample to remove drug residue from the surface of the hair shaft is typical when the purpose of the hair test is to determine if an individual is actively using drugs. Some drug testing companies omit the pretest washing step for hair testing in children because the purpose of the test is to evaluate for exposure to a drug-endangered environment. In these cases, the test result could be positive if drug is detected on the surface of the hair shaft or is present in the hair shaft after being transferred to the hair follicle from the systemic circulation and growing out in the hair shaft.[67] Either of these situations would still indicate an environment of risk for the child.[2]

Laboratories performing hair and other confirmatory drug tests may report a quantified level of drug in the hair sample in addition to the lowest level of detection for the specific drug. Use of the quantified level to make assumptions on frequency, duration, or extent of drug exposure should be approached with great caution. There are several factors influencing the amount of drug that may be present in a sample of hair.

- Drugs have different incorporation rates into hair based on affinity to hair melanin and lipophilicity.
- Hair follicle development begins in the 10th week of gestation with active hair growth by the 20th week. The highest rate of hair growth occurs in the last trimester of pregnancy. Hair growth is asynchronous following delivery, and the average growth rate of 1 cm/month does not start until after the first year after birth. Even after the first year, hair growth rates vary in children.
- If hair drug testing is being performed without the prewash step (allowing for detection of environmental exposure), the timing of

when the hair sample is collected can affect the likelihood that the hair will test positive as well as the amount of drug quantified in the hair. This is especially true for children in homes where drugs have been manufactured by a method leading to aerosolization of drug residue or subjected to heavy drug smoke in an enclosed area.

Screening Versus Confirmatory Drug Testing

One of the core clinical issues for medical professionals is an understanding of the difference between screening and confirmatory testing. Initial or screening testing is often performed by immunoassay. This widely available methodology with high test sensitivity offers a platform to test for multiple substances in one sample with rapid results.[9] Because this methodology does not directly identify the particular drug, these tests can be limited by false-positive results because other substances with structural similarities could also cause a positive immunoassay result. Table 16.2 has a partial list of substances known to have the potential to cause a false-positive result on an immunoassay test. Confirmatory testing is designed to have high test specificity. This is achieved by using methodology of gas or liquid chromatography with mass spectroscopy to directly identify the specific chemical structure of the drug of interest.[68] Confirmation testing is limited by increased time and expense to obtain results as compared with immunoassay testing because these tests require specialized equipment and expertise. Confirmation test results are often reported with a quantified level of drug detected in the sample. This level can be used to compare to the established level of detection for the specific drug. Use of quantified levels to determine frequency or amount of exposure is an imprecise practice due to the variabilities of how different drugs are taken up following exposure, variations in metabolism rates of drugs in children, and uncertainties in frequency and timing of exposure incidents.[67]

False-negative immunoassay test results could occur if the urine sample is adulterated. Techniques could include submitting urine from another person or animal as substitute or diluting or concentrating the urine by ingesting water or hypertonic fluids prior to test collection. Adulteration of a urine sample should be suspected if the urine pH is less than 3 or greater than 11 or if the urine specific gravity is less than 1.002 or greater than 1.030. A urine creatinine level of less than 20 mg/dL would also be representative of dilute urine. A urine creatinine level of less than 5 mg/dL or urine specific gravity of less than 1.001 is not consistent with human urine.[9] False-negative urine immunoassay test results are also possible if the immunoassay excludes the parent drug or metabolite of the drug of interest from the testing protocol.

TABLE 16.2
Common Metabolites and Potentials for False-positive/False-negative Immunoassay Results for Selected Illicit Substances

Drug Category	Drug Class/Names (*Common Street Names*)[a]	Common Metabolites[b]	Possible False-positive Immunoassay Screen[c]	Possible False-negative Immunoassay Screen[d]
CNS stimulants	Methamphetamine (*speed, crank, chalk, others; ice = crystal meth*)	Amphetamine	Bupropion Ephedrine Methylphenidate Phenylephrine Promethazine Pseudoephedrine Ranitidine Trazadone	Synthetic cathinone ("bath salts")
	Amphetamine (*uppers, speed, others*)	Alpha-hydroxyamphetamine norephedrine		
	MDMA (*ecstasy, molly*)	MDA MDEA		
	Cocaine (*coke; crack = crystal cocaine; snow = powder cocaine*)	Benzoylecgonine Norcocaine Ecgonine methyl ester Cocaethylene (from crack)	Amoxicillin Coca tea Topical anesthetics	
	PCP (*angel dust, wack*)	PPC	Dextromethorphan Diphenhydramine Ibuprofen Ketamine Tramadol Venlafaxine	

(*continued*)

TABLE 16.2 (*continued*)

Drug Category	Drug Class/Names (*Common Street Names*)[a]	Common Metabolites[b]	Possible False-positive Immunoassay Screen[c]	Possible False-negative Immunoassay Screen[d]
CNS depressants	Opiates Codeine (*cody, others*) Morphine (*white lady, Miss Emma, M, others*)	Codeine → di-hydrocodeine and hydrocodone Morphine → hydromorphone and normorphine	Dextromethorphan Diphenhydramine Poppy seeds Quinine Rifampin Verapamil	Opiate immunoassay only targets morphine and codeine (and metabolites)
	Semisynthetic opioids Heroin (*dope, junk, others*) Hydrocodone (*Vicodin, Lorcet, others*) Hydromorphone (*Dilaudid*) Oxycodone (*Percocet, Roxicet, others*) Oxymorphone (*Opana*)	Heroin → 6-MAM and morphine Hydrocodone Hydromorphone (primary drug or metabolite of hydrocodone) Oxycodone Oxymorphone (primary drug or metabolite of oxycodone)		May not be detected on standard opiate immunoassay (test dependent)
	Synthetic opioids	Methadone (*wafer*) Fentanyl (*China white*) Tramadol (*Ultram*) Meperidine (*Demerol*) — Synthetic opioids do not metabolize to morphine or codeine		Will not be detected on standard opiate immunoassay

(*continued*)

TABLE 17.2 (*continued*)

Drug Category	Drug Class/Names (*Common Street Names*)[a]	Common Metabolites[b]		Possible False-positive Immunoassay Screen[c]	Possible False-negative Immunoassay Screen[d]
	Cannabinoids (*marijuana, weed, joint, Mary Jane, others*)	Delta-9-THC Dronabinol (synthetic)	9-carboxylic acid THC	Ibuprofen/Naprosyn Promethazine Proton pump inhibitors	Synthetic cannabinoids (eg, K2, Spice)
	Barbiturates (*barbs, goofballs, reds, others*)	Phenobarbital Butalbital Secobarbital	p-hydroxyphenobarbital Isobutyl-barbituric acid p-hydroxysecobarbital		
	Benzodiazepines (*benzos, downers, roofies, others*)	Diazepam⟶nordiazepam⟶oxazepam Temazepam (primary drug or metabolite of diazepam) Alprazolam⟶hydroxyalprazolam Clonazepam⟶7-aminoclonazepam Midazolam⟶hydroxymidazolam Lorazepam⟶lorazepam glucuronide		Sertraline Oxaprozin	Most standard immunoassay screens for "benzodiazepines" focus only on diazepam metabolites Flunitrazepam (Rohypnol) and others associated with drug-facilitated assault such as GHB and ketamine (*special K*)

Abbreviations: arrows, metabolism pathways; CNS, central nervous system; GHB, gamma-hydroxybutyrate; MAM, monoacetylmorphine; MDA, methylenedioxyamphetamine; MDEA, methylenedioxyethylamphetamine; MDMA, methylenedioxymethamphetamine; PCP, phencyclidine; PPC, 4-phenyl-4-piperidinylcyclohexanol; THC, tetrahydrocannabinol.

[a] A more extensive list of commercial and street drug names can be found at https://www.drugabuse.gov/drugs-abuse/commonly-abused-drugs-charts (updated July 2018; accessed July 12, 2019).

[b] Common active metabolites listed. Not a complete list of metabolites.

[c] Common substances known to cross-react on immunoassay. Not a complete list.

[d] Common clinically relevant scenarios for false-negative results.

Special Considerations

- Comprehensive urine drug testing is available through many reference laboratories. This type of test allows for expanded testing for common prescription and over-the-counter substances and can be especially helpful in the evaluation of ingestions of unknown substances and in drug-facilitated sexual assaults.[69]
- "Designer" drugs such as synthetic cannabinoids and/or cathinone are difficult to regulate, as designers continually make minor changes to the chemical structure to keep the substance from falling within the category of legally defined illicit substances.[9,70,71]
- The presence of metabolites in a drug test result does not necessarily infer systemic exposure. The drug manufacturing and "cutting" for use can introduce impurities because there are no quality control processes as there are in pharmaceutical manufacturing. For hair testing, the tissues around the hair follicle contain enzymes that have potential to metabolize parent drug into metabolite.[67] Some metabolites, such as benzoylecgonine from cocaine, can metabolize in vitro with exposure to air and moisture. See Table 16.2 for a list of common metabolites associated with drugs of abuse.

Management

Whether as a part of the transition of mother and newborn from delivery to discharge or on identification of a drug-endangered older child, the pediatric medical professional plays an important role in ensuring the needs of the infant or child are met. Pediatric medical professionals have a unique opportunity to identify and engage with families affected by substance use, in relation to their frequency and context of contact and their trusted role. The complex issues related to drug-endangered children often require the collaborative efforts of multiple agencies. Comprehensive services and collaborative relationships should be provided along a continuum of prevention, intervention, and treatment from prepregnancy through childhood. Pediatric medical professionals can play a role in the entire continuum delivered at the different developmental stages in the life of the child and family. Education and treatment are critical, and no single agency can deliver all of these.

Identifying families at risk begins with obtaining a detailed social history to include drug and alcohol use. When obtaining a social history, it is helpful to use a nonjudgmental manner and include questions about drug use in the normal course of obtaining health history. Generally, parents are motivated to provide necessary information to provide the best care possible for their infant or child. It is also helpful to inquire during infant health supervision visits about how feedings are progressing, using this as an opportunity to educate the parents about the transmission of drugs to the infant through human milk. This also creates an opportunity to engage in a broader discussion related to drug use and parenting and associated risks. Several tools are available to assist medical professionals in including drug use screening in their routine care.[27,72] Screening for signs of other psychosocial distress in the family is also important because intimate partner violence and co-occurring parental psychopathology are also common in families struggling with drug use issues and can compound the levels of internalizing and externalizing behaviors exhibited by drug-endangered children compared with their peers.[53,56]

The health care system plays an invaluable role in identifying potential resources and services for drug-endangered children and their families, such as home visitation or other community-based services, case management, specialized clinics, and indicated developmental follow-up and services. Specific programs to consider are nurse home visitation programs, early childhood intervention, and 0 to 3 developmental services. Pediatric medical professionals should also consider assessment for evidence-based mental health interventions for children affected by exposure to violence, such as parent-child interaction therapy and trauma-focused CBT.[73]

Advocacy

The pediatric medical professional has a powerful voice in advocating for the welfare of children at the local, state, regional, and national levels. Using this position to represent the health care perspective along the continuum of needs for these vulnerable children can influence critical policies and responses to these challenging situations. Pediatric medical professionals can engage in a multitude of ways.

Pediatric medical professionals often function within team-based settings. Medical professionals caring for newborns who have been exposed to drugs should collaborate with obstetric professionals to enhance early identification through prenatal screening and referrals to services, as well as increase information sharing among prenatal and postnatal medical professionals, to best inform the care of the drug-exposed newborn. Additionally, they can provide valuable input on case management services and interventions of other involved agencies such as child welfare and substance use treatment professionals. Pediatric medical professionals and other involved professionals are tasked with weighing the safety of the child with the parent's addiction, and related risks and information shared by the health care team may provide valuable insight and guidance to other agencies such as child welfare and the courts, which may include participation in child welfare case staffing or court hearings.

Pediatric medical professionals are powerful educators for the children and families they care for as well as other professionals and policy makers. Key approaches are using a public health approach and the concept that addiction is a chronic relapsing disease rather than a moral failing. Pediatric medical professionals can play an important role in advocating for collaborative regional and state responses to drug-endangered children, such as the expansion of resources that can provide important support to affected mothers and their children. Such resources may include mental health resources (for parents and children), early childhood intervention, home visiting programs, and health department activities, as well as advocating that Medicaid pays for substance use screening.

Pediatric medical professionals can advocate for streamlining points of access for substance use treatment and expanding treatment facilities that accept pregnant women and can also house their children. Advocating for a public health approach to this challenging issue may be most important because many in medical and legal systems believe that addicted women are not just harming themselves but also another life, resulting in some jurisdictions making it a crime to use drugs during pregnancy. In some states, laws originally drafted to protect women from domestic violence are used to prosecute them instead. Medical professionals can also work closely with child welfare agencies to ensure that their policies and procedures are supported by best practice and grounded in public health.

The AAP Committee on Substance Use and Prevention published a policy statement, "A Public Health Response to Opioid Use in Pregnancy," which advocates for **a health care approach, rather than a punitive one, to address the rapidly growing issue of opioid use during pregnancy.** This should include a focus on prevention of unintended pregnancies, universal screening for alcohol and other drug use in women of childbearing age, knowledge and informed consent for drug testing and reporting, and improved access to appropriate necessary prenatal care.[74] The Association of State and Territorial Health Officials has published a report with recommendations for policies and practices to advance knowledge for prevention and best practices of care for children with NAS.[75] One example of specialized need in this area is the need to increase the number of physicians who are trained to administer medication-assisted treatment (a combination of prescription medications and addiction counseling) to pregnant women.

In addition to legislative advocacy and input on policies relating to drug use in pregnancy, **pediatric medical professionals can play a powerful role in providing legislative and policy advocacy on other issues** that affect drug-endangered children. Advocating and providing education on the judicious and appropriate prescribing of benzodiazepines and opiates is needed to reduce the number of people who misuse or overdose on these substances.[10,11] Legalization of marijuana, ranging from use for approved medical conditions to recreational use, is occurring in a growing number of states. The AAP offers guidance to medical professionals who may find themselves involved in discussions concerning legislative action or policy development addressing the potential legalization of marijuana in a 2015 policy statement, "The Impact of Marijuana Policies on Youth: Clinical, Research, and Legal Update."[76]

While advocates of legalization of marijuana characterize recreational use of the drug as being no greater public health risk than "social" alcohol use, pediatric medical professionals should be prepared to be a voice for the unintended consequences of marijuana legalization on children. This can include[16,76]

- Increased use of a substance with addictive potential by youth, which has been shown to increase the likelihood of developing drug dependence and addiction issues in adulthood.
- Impaired motor control, coordination, and reaction time even with short-term use. Unlike alcohol, there are no established normal limits of what constitutes impairment for activities such as safely operating machinery or a vehicle.
- Impaired short-term memory and judgment along with decreased attention span and problem-solving with long-term use. This could not only negatively affect academic achievement of affected youth but also puts more children at risk for injury and neglect by affected caregivers.
- Increased unintentional ingestions in young children with increase in hospitalizations and deaths.

Case Summary

Returning to the case presented at the beginning of the chapter, the case questions can now be addressed.

Medical Issues to Anticipate in the Postnatal Course

This newborn was born at term but had a low initial Apgar score. The mother had no prenatal care and presented with vaginal bleeding, which could predispose the newborn to sequelae of a hypoxic-ischemic event. While amphetamines/methamphetamine and marijuana can result in alterations in normal physiologic state of a newborn (eg, irritable, jittery, fussy), the medical professional should be aware that the newborn may have been exposed to other drugs in utero and be alert for signs of NAS. For long-term outcomes, the patient should be followed regularly by a primary care medical professional who can assess growth and development on a continuum.

Usefulness of Additional Drug Testing in the Neonate

The urine sample that tested positive on screening immunoassay for amphetamines and THC should be sent for confirmatory testing to ensure it is not a false-positive result. Urine drug testing most accurately reflects drug use in the days leading up to delivery (acute exposures). The medical professional could consider expanding the window of detection of drug use in pregnancy by ordering testing from a matrix such as meconium or umbilical cord tissue. The results could be important in the development of a plan for the patient's health and safety, because the mother denies substance use and the results of the urine confirmation testing will take some time to return.

Need for Mandated Reporting to Child Welfare Services in the State

Medical professionals should be familiar with the mandated reporting statutes of the state(s) in which they practice. All state child welfare agencies are required to have a response to newborns who have been exposed to illicit drugs in utero, but the reporting requirements and response vary by state.

Assessment of the Mother's Need for Services for Addiction Disorder, Assessment for Concomitant Psychosocial Stressors in the Mother's Life, and Safety Disposition or Follow-up Plan Following Discharge From the Nursery

This patient's mother presented with an altered mental status and had not sought prenatal care. She should be assessed not only for the need for substance use treatment but also for other co-occurring psychosocial stressors, such as undiagnosed or undertreated mental health issues and the presence of interpersonal violence in her relationships. If the interaction between mother and baby or mother and staff raises concern that the mother may not be able to safely and appropriately care for the newborn following discharge, a report to child welfare services should be considered. If presence of a positive urine drug test result has already triggered a mandated report to child welfare, it would be helpful if child welfare personnel would visit the patient's home to ensure there is an appropriate setting and resources for the care of a newborn. Hospital staff should communicate anticipated discharge date and information to the primary care medical professional and child welfare staff (if involved) to ensure plan of care and follow-up needs are known.

Health and Safety of Other Children in the Mother's Care

The mother was listed as a gravida 5, now para 4, which would indicate that there may be other children in her care. It would be appropriate to assess the health and welfare of other children in the mother's care by history, child welfare intervention, and/or home health or nursing visitation, because substance use disorders in caregivers increase the risk for adverse events related to abuse and neglect of children in the home.

Conclusion

Pediatric medical professionals will encounter newborns, infants, and children affected by substance use by their caregivers in a multitude of practice settings. The response to this issue requires an individual assessment of risk for the patient through physical and laboratory assessment. It also requires being prepared to recognize and formulate a management plan related to concomitant safety risks associated with the exposure as a participant in a multidisciplinary response. Due to the intersecting issues of pediatric and adult health as well as child welfare and policy or legislative issues surrounding the topic, pediatric medical professionals are in a unique position to advocate for a supportive, rather than punitive, response when a newborn, infant, or child is identified as drug endangered.

References

1. National Alliance for Drug Endangered Children. https://www.nationaldec.org. Accessed February 20, 2019
2. Wang X, Drummer OH. Review: interpretation of drug presence in the hair of children. *Forensic Sci Int*. 2015;257:458–472 PMID: 26610304 https://doi.org/10.1016/j.forsciint.2015.10.028

3. Farst K, Reading Meyer JA, Mac Bird T, James L, Robbins JM. Hair drug testing of children suspected of exposure to the manufacture of methamphetamine. *J Forensic Leg Med*. 2011;18(3):110–114 PMID: 21420647 https://doi.org/10.1016/j.jflm.2011.01.013
4. US Drug Enforcement Administration. *2017 National Drug Threat Assessment*. https://www.dea.gov/documents/2017/10/01/2017-national-drug-threat-assessment. Accessed February 20, 2019
5. Massa N, Ludemann JP. Pediatric caustic ingestion and parental cocaine abuse. *Int J Pediatr Otorhinolaryngol*. 2004;68(12):1513–1517 PMID: 15533563 https://doi.org/10.1016/j.ijporl.2004.07.003
6. Farst K, Duncan JM, Moss M, Ray RM, Kokoska E, James LP. Methamphetamine exposure presenting as caustic ingestions in children. *Ann Emerg Med*. 2007;49(3):341–343 PMID: 17141141 https://doi.org/10.1016/j.annemergmed.2006.05.020
7. Grant P, Bell K, Stewart D, Paulson J, Rogers K. Evidence of methamphetamine exposure in children removed from clandestine methamphetamine laboratories. *Pediatr Emerg Care*. 2010;26(1):10–14 PMID: 20042914 https://doi.org/10.1097/PEC.0b013e3181c33085
8. Messina N, Jeter K, Marinelli-Casey P, West K, Rawson R. Children exposed to methamphetamine use and manufacture. *Child Abuse Negl*. 2014;38(11):1872–1883 PMID: 17383002 https://doi.org/10.1016/j.chiabu.2006.06.009
9. Moeller KE, Kissack JC, Atayee RS, Lee KC. Clinical interpretation of urine drug tests: what clinicians need to know about urine drug screens. *Mayo Clin Proc*. 2017;92(5):774–796 PMID: 28325505 https://doi.org/10.1016/j.mayocp.2016.12.007
10. Centers for Disease Control and Prevention. Opioid overdose. https://www.cdc.gov/drugoverdose/index.html. Updated October 29, 2018. Accessed February 20, 2019
11. Sun EC, Dixit A, Humphreys K, Darnall BD, Baker LC, Mackey S. Association between concurrent use of prescription opioids and benzodiazepines and overdose: retrospective analysis. *BMJ*. 2017;356:j760 PMID: 28292769 https://doi.org/10.1136/bmj.j760
12. Bachhuber MA, Hennessy S, Cunningham CO, Starrels JL. Increasing benzodiazepine prescriptions and overdose mortality in the United States, 1996-2013. *Am J Public Health*. 2016;106(4):686–688 PMID: 26890165 https://doi.org/10.2105/AJPH.2016.303061
13. Bond GR, Woodward RW, Ho M. The growing impact of pediatric pharmaceutical poisoning. *J Pediatr*. 2012;160(2):265–270.e1
14. Yin S. Malicious use of pharmaceuticals in children. *J Pediatr*. 2010;157(5):832–836.e1
15. Hines E. Child abuse by poisoning. *Clin Pediatr Emerg Med*. 2016;17(4):296–301 https://doi.org/10.1016/j.cpem.2016.10.003
16. Claudet I, Mouvier S, Labadie M, et al; Marie-Jeanne Study Group. Unintentional cannabis intoxication in toddlers. *Pediatrics*. 2017;140(3):e20170017 PMID: 28808073 https://doi.org/10.1542/peds.2017-0017
17. Wang GS, Roosevelt G, Heard K. Pediatric marijuana exposures in a medical marijuana state. *JAMA Pediatr*. 2013;167(7):630–633 PMID: 23712626 https://doi.org/10.1001/jamapediatrics.2013.140
18. Behnke M, Smith VC; American Academy of Pediatrics Committee on Substance Abuse and Committee on Fetus and Newborn. Prenatal substance abuse: short- and long-term effects on the exposed fetus. *Pediatrics*. 2013;131(3):e1009–e1024 PMID: 23439891 https://doi.org/10.1542/peds.2012-3931
19. American College of Obstetricians and Gynecologists Committee on Health Care for Underserved Women. AGOG Committee Opinion No. 473: substance abuse reporting and pregnancy: the role of the obstetrician-gynecologist. *Obstet Gynecol*. 2011;117(1):200–201 PMID: 21173672 https://doi.org/10.1097/AOG.0b013e31820a6216

20. Substance Abuse and Mental Health Services Administration. *Results from the 2013 National Survey on Drug Use and Health: Summary of National Findings*. NSDUH Series H-48, HHS Publication No. (SMA) 14-4863. Rockville, MD: Substance Abuse and Mental Health Services Administration; 2014. https://www.samhsa.gov/data/sites/default/files/NSDUHresultsPDFWHTML2013/Web/NSDUHresults2013.pdf. Published September 2014. Accessed February 20, 2019
21. Ebrahim SH, Gfroerer J. Pregnancy-related substance use in the United States during 1996-1998. *Obstet Gynecol*. 2003;101(2):374–379 PMID: 12576263
22. Forray A, Merry B, Lin H, Ruger JP, Yonkers KA. Perinatal substance use: a prospective evaluation of abstinence and relapse. *Drug Alcohol Depend*. 2015;150:147–155 PMID: 25772437 https://doi.org/10.1016/j.drugalcdep.2015.02.027
23. Moore DG, Turner JD, Parrott AC, et al. During pregnancy, recreational drug-using women stop taking ecstasy (3,4-methylenedioxy-N-methylamphetamine) and reduce alcohol consumption, but continue to smoke tobacco and cannabis: initial findings from the Development and Infancy Study. *J Psychopharmacol*. 2010;24(9):1403–1410 PMID: 19939863 https://doi.org/10.1177/0269881109348165
24. Yonkers KA, Gotman N, Kershaw T, Forray A, Howell HB, Rounsaville BJ. Screening for prenatal substance use: development of the Substance Use Risk Profile-Pregnancy scale. *Obstet Gynecol*. 2010;116(4):827–833 PMID: 20859145 https://doi.org/10.1097/AOG.0b013e3181ed8290
25. Derauf C, Kekatpure M, Neyzi N, Lester B, Kosofsky B. Neuroimaging of children following prenatal drug exposure. *Semin Cell Dev Biol*. 2009;20(4):441–454 PMID: 19560049 https://doi.org/10.1016/j.semcdb.2009.03.001
26. Janisse JJ, Bailey BA, Ager J, Sokol RJ. Alcohol, tobacco, cocaine, and marijuana use: relative contributions to preterm delivery and fetal growth restriction. *Subst Abuse*. 2014;35(1):60–67
27. Smith VC, Wilson CR; American Academy of Pediatrics Committee on Substance Use and Prevention. Families affected by parental substance use. *Pediatrics*. 2016;138(2):e20161575 PMID: 27432847 https://doi.org/10.1542/peds.2016-1575
28. Bada HS, Bann CM, Whitaker TM, et al. Protective factors can mitigate behavior problems after prenatal cocaine and other drug exposures. *Pediatrics*. 2012;130(6):e1479–e1488 PMID: 23184114 https://doi.org/10.1542/peds.2011-3306
29. Young NK, Gardner S, Otero C, et al. *Substance-Exposed Infants: State Responses to the Problem*. HHS Pub No. (SMA) 09-4369. Rockville, MD: Substance Abuse and Mental Health Services Administration; 2009. https://www.ncsacw.samhsa.gov/files/Substance-Exposed-Infants.pdf. Accessed February 20, 2019
30. Chamberlain C, O'Mara-Eves A, Porter J, et al. Psychosocial interventions for supporting women to stop smoking in pregnancy. *Cochrane Database Syst Rev*. 2017;2:CD001055 PMID: 28196405 https://doi.org/10.1002/14651858.CD001055.pub4
31. Welle-Strand GK, Skurtveit S, Jansson LM, Bakstad B, Bjarkø L, Ravndal E. Breastfeeding reduces the need for withdrawal treatment in opioid-exposed infants. *Acta Paediatr*. 2013;102(11):1060–1066 PMID: 23909865 https://doi.org/10.1111/apa.12378
32. Sachs HC; American Academy of Pediatrics Committee on Drugs. The transfer of drugs and therapeutics into human breast milk: an update on selected topics. *Pediatrics*. 2013;132(3):e796–e809 PMID: 23979084 https://doi.org/10.1542/peds.2013-1985
33. Hwang SS, Diop H, Liu CL, et al. Maternal substance use disorders and infant outcomes in the first year of life among Massachusetts singletons, 2003–2010. *J Pediatr*. 2017;191:69–75 PMID: 29050752 https://doi.org/10.1016/j.jpeds.2017.08.045

34. Mansoor E, Morrow CE, Accornero VH, et al. Longitudinal effects of prenatal cocaine use on mother-child interactions at ages 3 and 5 years. *J Dev Behav Pediatr*. 2012;33(1):32–41 PMID: 22157442 https://doi.org/10.1097/DBP.0b013e31823968ab
35. DiFranza JR, Aligne CA, Weitzman M. Prenatal and postnatal environmental tobacco smoke exposure and children's health. *Pediatrics*. 2004;113(4)(suppl):1007–1015 PMID:15060193
36. Williams JF, Smith VC; American Academy of Pediatrics Committee on Substance Abuse. Fetal alcohol spectrum disorders. *Pediatrics*. 2015;136(5):e1395–e1406 PMID: 26482673 https://doi.org/10.1542/peds.2015-3113
37. Nykjaer C, Alwan NA, Greenwood DC, et al. Maternal alcohol intake prior to and during pregnancy and risk of adverse birth outcomes: evidence from a British cohort. *J Epidemiol Community Health*. 2014;68(6):542–549 PMID: 24616351 https://doi.org/10.1136/jech-2013-202934
38. Hoyme HE, Kalberg WO, Elliott AJ, et al. Updated clinical guidelines for diagnosing fetal alcohol spectrum disorders. *Pediatrics*. 2016;138(2):e20154256 PMID: 27464676 https://doi.org/10.1542/peds.2015-4256
39. Chasnoff IJ, Wells AM, King L. Misdiagnosis and missed diagnoses in foster and adopted children with prenatal alcohol exposure. *Pediatrics*. 2015;135(2):264–270 PMID: 25583914 https://doi.org/10.1542/peds.2014-2171
40. Streissguth AP, Bookstein FL, Barr HM, Sampson PD, O'Malley K, Young JK. Risk factors for adverse life outcomes in fetal alcohol syndrome and fetal alcohol effects. *J Dev Behav Pediatr*. 2004;25(4):228–238 PMID: 15308923 https://doi.org/10.1097/00004703-200408000-00002
41. Autti-Rämö I. Twelve-year follow-up of children exposed to alcohol in utero. *Dev Med Child Neurol*. 2000;42(6):406–411 PMID: 10875527 https://doi.org/10.1017/S0012162200000748
42. Gahagan S, Sharpe TT, Brimacombe M, et al. Pediatricians' knowledge, training, and experience in the care of children with fetal alcohol syndrome. *Pediatrics*. 2006;118(3):e657–e668 PMID: 16950957 https://doi.org/10.1542/peds.2005-0516
43. Jones HE, Kaltenbach K, Heil SH, et al. Neonatal abstinence syndrome after methadone or buprenorphine exposure. *N Engl J Med*. 2010;363(24):2320–2331 PMID: 21142534 https://doi.org/10.1056/NEJMoa1005359
44. Hudak ML, Tan RC; American Academy of Pediatrics Committee on Drugs and Committee on Fetus and Newborn. Neonatal drug withdrawal. *Pediatrics*. 2012;129(2):e540–e560 PMID: 22291123 https://doi.org/10.1542/peds.2011-3212
45. Grossman MR, Lipshaw MJ, Osborn RR, Berkwitt AK. A novel approach to assessing infants with neonatal abstinence syndrome. *Hosp Pediatr*. 2018;8(1):1–6 PMID: 29263121 https://doi.org/10.1542/hpeds.2017-0128
46. Grossman MR, Berkwitt AK, Osborn RR, et al. An initiative to improve the quality of care of infants with neonatal abstinence syndrome. *Pediatrics*. 2017;139(6):e20163360 PMID: 28562267 https://doi.org/10.1542/peds.2016-3360
47. Mark K, Gryczynski J, Axenfeld E, Schwartz RP, Terplan M. Pregnant women's current and intended cannabis use in relation to their views toward legalization and knowledge of potential harm. *J Addict Med*. 2017;11(3):211–216 PMID: 28252456 https://doi.org/10.1097/ADM.0000000000000299
48. Mato S, Del Olmo E, Pazos A. Ontogenetic development of cannabinoid receptor expression and signal transduction functionality in the human brain. *Eur J Neurosci*. 2003;17(9):1747–1754 PMID: 12752773 https://doi.org/10.1046/j.1460-9568.2003.02599.x

49. Metz TD, Stickrath EH. Marijuana use in pregnancy and lactation: a review of the evidence. *Am J Obstet Gynecol*. 2015;213(6):761–778 PMID: 25986032 https://doi.org/10.1016/j.ajog.2015.05.025
50. Jaques SC, Kingsbury A, Henshcke P, et al. Cannabis, the pregnant woman and her child: weeding out the myths. *J Perinatol*. 2014;34(6):417–424 PMID: 24457255 https://doi.org/10.1038/jp.2013.180
51. Foo T; Colorado Department of Public Health and Environment. Marijuana use during pregnancy and breastfeeding: systematic literature review. https://localtvkdvr.files.wordpress.com/2016/02/2014-marijuana-use-during-pregnancy-and-breastfeeding.pdf. Approved January 12, 2015. Accessed February 20, 2019
52. American College of Obstetricians and Gynecologists Committee on Obstetric Practice. Committee Opinion No. 722: marijuana use during pregnancy and lactation. *Obstet Gynecol*. 2017;130(4):e205–e209 PMID: 28937574 https://doi.org/10.1097/AOG.0000000000002354
53. US Department of Health and Human Services Administration for Children and Families; Administration on Children, Youth, and Families; Children's Bureau; Office on Child Abuse and Neglect. Protecting children in families affected by substance use disorders. Child abuse and neglect user manual series. https://www.childwelfare.gov/pubPDFs/substanceuse.pdf. Published 2009. Accessed February 20, 2019
54. Substance Abuse and Mental Health Services Administration Center for Substance Abuse Treatment. Substance abuse treatment and domestic violence. Treatment Improvement Protocol Series No. 25. Rockville, MD: Substance Abuse and Mental Health Services Administration; 1997. https://www.ncbi.nlm.nih.gov/books/NBK64437. Accessed February 20, 2019
55. Center on the Developing Child, Harvard University. Serve and return. https://developingchild.harvard.edu/science/key-concepts/serve-and-return. Accessed February 20, 2019
56. Solis JM, Shadur JM, Burns AR, Hussong AM. Understanding the diverse needs of children whose parents abuse substances. *Curr Drug Abuse Rev*. 2012;5(2):135–147 PMID: 22455509 https://doi.org/10.2174/1874473711205020135
57. Wells K. Substance abuse and child maltreatment. *Pediatr Clin North Am*. 2009;56(2):345–362 PMID: 19358920 https://doi.org/10.1016/j.pcl.2009.01.006
58. Centers for Disease Control and Prevention. Violence prevention. Adverse childhood experiences (ACEs). https://www.cdc.gov/violenceprevention/acestudy/index.html. Reviewed April 1, 2016. Accessed February 20, 2019
59. Connell-Carrick K. Methamphetamine and the changing face of child welfare: practice principles for child welfare workers. *Child Welfare*. 2007;86(3):125–144 PMID: 17722684
60. Shukla RK, Bell K, Maier EA, Newton DC. Forensic evaluations of drug endangered children: "My house caught on fire; my cat jumped out the window." *Child Youth Serv Rev*. 2016;67:67–75 https://doi.org/10.1016/j.childyouth.2016.05.018
61. Altshuler SJ, Cleverly-Thomas A. What do we know about drug-endangered children when they are first placed into care? *Child Welfare*. 2011;90(3):45–68 PMID:22403900
62. Farst KJ, Valentine JL, Hall RW. Drug testing for newborn exposure to illicit substances in pregnancy: pitfalls and pearls. *Int J Pediatr*. 2011;2011:951616 PMID: 21785611 https://doi.org/10.1155/2011/951616
63. Kwong TC, Ryan RM; National Academy of Clinical Biochemistry. Detection of intrauterine illicit drug exposure by newborn drug testing. *Clin Chem*. 1997;43(1):235–242 PMID: 8990259

64. Bornstein BH. Pregnancy, drug testing, and the fourth amendment: legal and behavioral implications. *J Fam Psychol*. 2003;17(2):220–228 PMID: 12828018 https://doi.org/10.1037/0893-3200.17.2.220
65. Colby JM. Comparison of umbilical cord tissue and meconium for the confirmation of in utero drug exposure. *Clin Biochem*. 2017;50(13-14):784–790 PMID: 28288850 https://doi.org/10.1016/j.clinbiochem.2017.03.006
66. Lozano J, García-Algar O, Vall O, de la Torre R, Scaravelli G, Pichini S. Biological matrices for the evaluation of in utero exposure to drugs of abuse. *Ther Drug Monit*. 2007;29(6):711–734 PMID: 18043469 https://doi.org/10.1097/FTD.0b013e31815c14ce
67. White RM. Drugs in hair. Part I. Metabolisms of major drug classes. *Forensic Sci Rev*. 2017;29(1):23–55 PMID: 28119266
68. Nelson ZJ, Stellpflug SJ, Engebretsen KM. What can a urine drug screening immunoassay really tell us? *J Pharm Pract*. 2016;29(5):516–526 PMID: 25917168 https://doi.org/10.1177/0897190015579611
69. Farst K, Bolden BB. Substance-exposed infants and children: forensic approach. *Clin Pediatr Emerg Med*. 2012;13(3):221–228 https://doi.org/10.1016/j.cpem.2012.06.003
70. Palamar JJ, Barratt MJ, Coney L, Martins SS. Synthetic cannabinoid use among high school seniors. *Pediatrics*. 2017;140(4):e20171330 PMID: 28893851 https://doi.org/10.1542/peds.2017-1330
71. Petrie M, Lynch KL, Ekins S, et al. Cross-reactivity studies and predictive modeling of "bath salts" and other amphetamine-type stimulants with amphetamine screening immunoassays. *Clin Toxicol (Phila)*. 2013;51(2):83–91 PMID: 23387345 https://doi.org/10.3109/15563650.2013.768344
72. Anthony EK, Austin MJ, Cormier DR. Early detection of prenatal substance exposure and the role of child welfare. *Child Youth Serv Rev*. 2010;32(1):6–12 https://doi.org/10.1016/j.childyouth.2009.06.006
73. National Child Traumatic Stress Network. Trauma treatments. http://www.nctsn.org/resources/topics/treatments-that-work/promising-practices. Accessed February 20, 2019
74. Patrick SW, Schiff DM; American Academy of Pediatrics Committee on Substance Use and Prevention. A public health response to opioid use in pregnancy. *Pediatrics*. 2017;139(3):e20164070 PMID: 28219965 https://doi.org/10.1542/peds.2016-4070
75. Association of State and Territorial Health Officials (ASTHO). Neonatal abstinence syndrome: how states can help advance the knowledge base for primary prevention and best practices of care. http://www.astho.org/Prevention/NAS-Neonatal-Abstinence-Report. Published 2014. Accessed February 20, 2019
76. American Academy of Pediatrics Committee on Substance Abuse and Committee on Adolescence. The impact of marijuana policies on youth: clinical, research, and legal update. *Pediatrics*. 2015;135(3):584–587 PMID: 25624383 https://doi.org/10.1542/peds.2014-4146

CHAPTER 17

Failure to Thrive

Sarah Passmore, DO, FAAP
Department of Pediatrics
University of Oklahoma
Tulsa, OK

Deborah Lowen, MD, FAAP
Associate Professor of Pediatrics
Vanderbilt University School of Medicine
Director, Center for Child Protection & Well-Being
Vanderbilt University Medical Center
Nashville, TN

Introduction

In the broadest sense, *failure to thrive* (FTT) refers to a child who isn't growing as expected, or a child whose weight is significantly lower than the reference ranges for his or her age and gender.[1] Failure to thrive can be due to numerous causes and can range from mild to severe. Although FTT is more common among infants from low-income families with limited resources, it can be found in all segments of the population.[2] Failure to thrive is often an imprecise diagnostic term and can be frustrating and confusing for the medical professional to evaluate and treat. The differential diagnosis is long, and children don't always respond to treatment as quickly or easily as medical professionals and caregivers would like.

This chapter addresses FTT as it pertains to high-income countries, and not the severe malnutrition that occurs in low-income countries. Reviews of malnutrition in developing countries have reported significant long-term deficits in growth, intelligence, academic performance, and work capacity.[3]

Malnutrition is defined by the World Health Organization (WHO) as deficiencies, excesses, or imbalances in a person's intake of energy and/or nutrients and includes undernutrition and obesity.[4] Underweight malnutrition not only jeopardizes a child's growth but may also impair immunocompetence and undermine cognitive and socio-affective competence.[1,5–10]

Children with severe cases of FTT may need inpatient treatment, but less severe cases can usually be managed as outpatients. Failure to thrive is often managed successfully in specialized, interdisciplinary clinics,[11] but milder cases can be managed by primary care medical professionals.

Definition

The term FTT was first used in 1899 to describe an infant with decreased growth after being weaned off the breast.[12] Since that time there has been no consensus on how FTT is defined, and other terms such as *slow growth, growth failure,* and *failure to gain weight,* among other similar expressions, have been used. It has been suggested that the term FTT is outdated, too broad, or pejorative. However, because it is still commonly used, FTT will be used throughout this chapter with the understanding that other terms have been suggested to replace it.

There are several issues to keep in mind when using the FTT label. First, although FTT usually refers to the physical growth of the child, it is important to note that these children often have developmental and/or emotional delays as well. Second, FTT is a symptom and not a diagnosis; multiple diagnoses can cause FTT, including medical/biological, social, economic, and emotional causes. However, the main cause for the poor growth—regardless of underlying diagnosis—is malnutrition.

Anthropometric indices using growth charts are necessary to identify FTT. The American Academy of Pediatrics identifies a child as failing to thrive if the child's weight is more than 2 SDs below the mean for age and sex, or if the weight curve has crossed more than 2 major percentile lines on a standard growth chart after having achieved a previously stable pattern.[13]

The 2 major growth charts used in the United States are the WHO and Centers for Disease Control and Prevention (CDC) growth charts. The WHO growth charts are used for ages 0 to 2 years. WHO chart standards establish growth of breastfed infants as the norm for growth. They provide a better description of physiologic growth of infancy. The CDC growth charts are used for children older than 2 years. These charts are based on references on how typical children in the United States grow during a specific period and can be used for children up to age 19 years. For children aged 2 to 5 years, the methods used to create both sets of charts are similar.[14] The cutoff values to define typical growth for both sets of charts are statistical constructs not based on health outcome data. Some children classified as underweight on the CDC charts may be classified as typical weight on the WHO charts. Meyers and colleagues showed that children who fell under this category still had a higher risk of adverse health outcomes than children who were not low weight-for-age on the CDC charts.[15]

Some medical professionals base their diagnosis on a single measure of weight-for-age or weight-for-height below the fifth or third percentile; others base their diagnosis on a deceleration in growth over time.[16] Using multiple weights when available, though, can lead to a more accurate diagnosis and identify potential causes.

Traditionally, FTT was dichotomized into "organic" FTT, in which the child's growth failure was ascribed to a major medical illness, and "nonorganic" FTT, which was attributed primarily to psychological neglect or "maternal deprivation."[17–20] This simplistic dichotomous conceptualization of FTT is obsolete[20] and represents the opposite ends of a spectrum. Children often have a combination of different factors contributing to poor growth. Children with an underlying medical condition can be difficult to care for and feed. Children who have experienced neglect may have poor appetites or other medical problems that contribute to poor weight gain. Regardless, in all cases of "nonorganic" FTT, and in many cases of "organic" FTT, the cause of growth failure is malnutrition.[19,21–24]

Overall, FTT can still be an imprecise diagnosis.[25] A child who is proportional (weight-for-height approximates the 50th percentile) and gaining weight along the fifth percentile with respect to weight- and height-for-age, and who has no health or nutritional problems, may be small but normal. In contrast, a child whose rate of growth is below expectations may be of concern, even if none of the growth indices have dropped below the fifth percentile. Deceleration in the rate of growth is a good indicator of growth problems but requires multiple measures over time and relatively sophisticated interpretation.[26]

Prevalence

The known prevalence of FTT is likely an underrepresentation of actual cases because many children do not receive medical attention for their growth failure and up to 50% may not be identified.[16] Failure to thrive is traditionally identified as being found in 3% to 5% of the population in high-income countries.[27] In the United States it may occur in up to 10% of children in primary care and 5% who are hospitalized.[28] Approximately 80% of children with FTT present before 18 months of age.[29]

Etiology and Risk Factors

The ultimate cause of poor growth in children with FTT is inadequate calories for the metabolic needs of the child. This can be due to inadequate intake, increased consumption of calories, and/or increased output (Box 17.1). Most children with FTT do not have an underlying medical condition; instead, they simply are not being fed enough calories. Of children referred to a tertiary pediatric gastroenterology clinic for FTT evaluation, 89% were found to have "nonorganic" causes for their FTT.[30] Children with FTT are also frequently referred for endocrinology evaluation, despite the fact that endocrine causes of FTT are rare; in one study, 51.5% of referred children had purely nutritional deficiency.[31]

Causes and risk factors for FTT are different based on the age of onset. Within the first few weeks after birth, FTT seems to involve biological causes due to specific vulnerabilities of the infant, including intrauterine growth retardation (IUGR), in combination with sociodemographic risk factors. When looking at early detection of slow weight gain in the first 6 to 8 weeks after birth, McDougall et al found an association with slow feeding, weak sucking, consumption of small quantities of milk, and refusal of

BOX 17.1
Categories of Failure to Thrive

Inadequate Caloric Intake

Poor Quality or Caloric Content

Breastfeeding problems: poor latch, poor letdown, inadequate milk supply

Formula problems: incorrect preparation, inadequate supply

Poor nutritional content: excess juice or water, unusual diets, fixed beliefs regarding food allergies or intolerance

Grazing

Inadequate quantities of food given because of poverty, food insecurity, neglect, or purposeful withholding of food

Medical child abuse (formerly known as Munchausen syndrome by proxy)

Feeding Difficulties

Oral-motor dysfunction

Neurological impairment

Gastroesophageal reflux ± esophagitis

Esophageal strictures

Vascular rings/slings

Poor dentition

Anorexia from various causes

Parent-child conflict: temperament, autonomy struggles

Inadequate Absorption and/or Excess Losses

Persistent vomiting

Pyloric stenosis

Central nervous system disease

Gastrointestinal obstruction

Rumination

Psychogenic vomiting

(continued)

BOX 17.1 (*continued*)

Gastrointestinal Disease

Celiac disease
Cystic fibrosis
Protein allergies
Lactose intolerance
Infection: giardiasis, *Salmonella, Clostridium difficile*
Liver disease
Short gut

Increased Caloric Requirements

Cardiorespiratory disease
Congenital heart disease
Acquired heart disease
Chronic lung disease
Cystic fibrosis
Obstructive sleep apnea

Chronic Infection

HIV/AIDS
Tuberculosis
Urinary tract infection

Defective Utilization

Inborn errors of metabolism
Diabetes mellitus
Congenital adrenal hyperplasia

Other

Malignancy
Hyperthyroidism
Excess activity

Reprinted from Lowen D. Failure to thrive. In: Jenny C, ed. *Child Abuse and Neglect: Diagnosis, Treatment and Evidence*. 1st ed. St Louis, MO: Saunders, Elsevier; 2011:547–562, copyright 2011, with permission from Elsevier.

human milk regardless of the age, education, or economic circumstances of the mother.[32] From the first weeks after birth until 6 months of age, FTT may reflect the adverse effects of congenital disorders. Most of this early FTT appears temporary, as the infants show later catch-up growth. After 6 months of age, FTT often represents feeding problems in otherwise healthy children.[33] These feeding problems are often psychosocial in origin.

Psychosocial Causes and Risk Factors

Poverty

Although FTT may occur in all segments of the population, it most often occurs in the context of poverty.[34,35] In some samples, as many as 10% of young American children in low-income families meet criteria for FTT.[36] By definition, the federal poverty level ($25,750 for an average family of 4 in 2019),[37] defined as 3 times the cost of a minimally nutritious diet,[38] implies an income level inadequate for meeting children's needs for shelter, clothing, and food.[35] Indeed, children living in families with incomes up to 185% of the federal poverty level are considered at nutritional risk.[39,40] In addition to an insufficient budget for food purchases, economically disadvantaged families often lack access to supermarkets and may live in homes lacking adequate food storage and preparation facilities.[41–43] A recent study has shown that food stamp benefits are inadequate for purchasing even a marginally healthful diet, even if the family is receiving the maximum allotment.[44]

There are several mechanisms whereby poverty may increase children's vulnerability to FTT. Poverty can affect children directly through lack of food, health care, and adequate educational opportunities and indirectly through increased family stress, which may interfere with parents' ability to provide nutritious meals on a regular basis or in a responsive style. Food insecurity has been associated with increased hospitalizations and parental perceptions of poor health among infants[45] and with developmental, academic, and learning problems among school-aged children.[46] To minimize the temptation to scapegoat families in clinical assessment and intervention, it is important to recognize that FTT often reflects economic conditions and changes in social policy that are far beyond the control of individual parents or medical professionals.[47,48] Children also experience FTT in homes of any social class in cases of parent-child interactive disorders, parental psychopathology, family dysfunction, or organic pathology, as is discussed in the Other Risk Factors section. The effect of such problems on children's health increases dramatically in the context of poverty.

The highly successful Special Supplemental Nutrition Program for Women, Infants, and Children (WIC) is estimated by the US Department of Agriculture to reach only 81% of all eligible women, infants, and children, whereas school breakfast is available to only about 1 in 4 children who receive school lunch.[49–51] Although WIC food packages have been updated and improved over the years, they are intended as only a supplement to the other food provided in the household. For some children in certain age groups receiving WIC, and many pregnant and postpartum mothers, the combination of WIC food and other food available in the household is insufficient to provide adequate nutrients.[52,53] Even with simultaneous participation in multiple programs (food stamps,

WIC, school meals), many low-income families are unable to obtain enough food to avoid frequent episodes of food insecurity and hunger and the chronic mild to moderate undernutrition that ensues.[54,55]

Other Risk Factors

In addition to lower socioeconomic levels, families of infants with FTT have been identified as having higher family stress, less available extended family for help with child-rearing, and greater social isolation than comparison groups.[56–60] All of these factors could affect the family members' capacities to mobilize caregiving resources on behalf of the child. Relationship patterns also may be strained in some families of infants with FTT. Drotar and Eckerle[61] found that mothers of infants with FTT reported less supportive and cohesive family relationships than did families of infants showing adequate growth. The quality of family relationships and organization may affect the timing, frequency, and consistency of reinforcement for feeding patterns, which ultimately may be reflected in the child's growth and health.[62] Additional psychosocial risk factors include an overreliance on liquids for nutrition, nutritional information deficit, ineffective feeding practices, negative maternal-child interaction, and maternal depression.[63]

Medical child abuse (formerly called Munchausen syndrome by proxy and sometimes referred to as caregiver-fabricated illness in a child) may be suspected in children with FTT based on specific clinical characteristics, including a history of pregnancy complications or preterm birth, especially if the history is found to be an exaggeration or falsification of birth history. In addition, caregivers may provide history that the child has a large number of allergies, in particular unusual allergies (eg, soap, beeswax, paprika, ravioli, most fruits, ranch dressing, multiple food types), or intestinal pseudo-obstruction. They are more likely to have multisystem involvement and to have undergone medical procedures. These children are likely to be referred to a multidisciplinary feeding team, but caregivers were more likely to have refused services.[64] Early identification of these children can prevent long-term adverse outcomes, including complications from unnecessary medical procedures and hospitalizations. Child protective services (CPS) will need to be involved in these cases to aid in protecting these children. See Chapter 20, Medical Child Abuse, for a discussion of this particular type of child maltreatment.

Child Characteristics

The Avon Longitudinal Study of Parents and Children found that in infants up to 8 weeks old, risk factors for FTT included feeding problems or illness or admission to the hospital. In particular, weak sucking and difficulty feeding, but not vomiting, dribbling, or refusing foods, correlated with FTT.

The same infant factors applied for breastfed and bottle-fed infants.[65] Most of these infants had good catch-up growth after 8 weeks. However, from 8 weeks to 9 months of age, growth faltering was 3 to 4 times more common than in the younger infant age group. Infant illness was not associated with growth faltering in the older group, but maternal height, parity, ethnicity, breastfeeding after 6 months of age, feeding slowly, and taking small quantities all were factors associated with poor growth in this cohort.

A possible reason for the differences in the age groups is related to an infant's development. The instinct for feeding is inherent at birth and, as infants transition to solid foods starting at around 6 months of age, feeding becomes more of a learned behavior. In older children, problems such as picky eating, slow eating, pocketing food, tantrums at mealtimes, and food struggles can stress parent-child interactions.

Hunger and satiety are guided by internal regulatory processes. Poor appetite, observed sometimes as early as the first 6 weeks after birth[66]; delayed or dysfunctional oral-motor development[67]; and deficient signaling of needs during mealtimes may contribute to FTT. Once a child begins to demonstrate deficient growth and nutrition, whatever the specific cause, the child's irritability and inconsistent social responsiveness may engender feelings of helplessness among parents as well as beliefs that the child is physically limited or ill.

Sensory processing disorders and developmental delays are common in infants and children showing poor growth. Yi et al found that sensory processing problems involving tactile, vestibular, and oral sensations were more common in toddlers with "nonorganic" FTT and feeding problems than with a control group. These authors also demonstrated that the toddlers' sensory processing difficulties were related to delayed cognitive, motor, and expressive language development.[68] Children's physical and temperamental characteristics may contribute to the development of FTT by presenting parents with child-rearing challenges that exceed their economic and psychosocial resources.[1,21,69] Among some children, the behavior problems associated with feeding are part of their overall temperament, including irritability, apathy, and generalized inactivity or overactivity.[70–72] Pollitt and Leibel[73] suggested that lethargic, listless infant behavior might evoke less responsive behavior from parents and contribute to FTT.[67,74,75] Preterm birth, low birth weight, and early childhood illness impose additional caregiving burdens on parents and may heighten the risk for FTT.[76]

Parental Characteristics

Although early clinical studies reported that mothers of children with FTT often had serious psychopathology,[77] controlled studies that have compared mothers of children with FTT with mothers of children showing adequate growth—adjusted for socioeconomic status—have found either no differences in psychopathology[70,78] or no higher rates of affective and personality disorders.[57,79,80] However, in individual cases, parental mood disturbances and/or adjustment problems that do not meet the criteria for a formal psychiatric diagnosis may affect the quality of parent-child interactions and interfere with the effectiveness of early intervention on the behavior and development of children who fail to thrive.[81] In a prospective study, Altemeier et al[82] found that mothers of children who eventually developed FTT reported more problematic childhoods than did mothers whose children grew adequately. Maternal reports of being abused as a child correlated positively with subsequent FTT in their offspring. Conversely, maternal perceptions of a happy childhood, that they were loved as a child, and that their parents were pleased with them correlated negatively with their child's development of FTT.[82] Benoit et al[78] found that more mothers of infants with FTT were classified as insecure in their attachment relationships to their own mothers compared with mothers of infants who grew at an average rate. Lack of resolution of mourning over the loss of a loved one was found in more mothers in the FTT group compared with controls. Mothers of children with FTT have reported high rates of physical abuse as children and as adults.[78,83] Such psychological vulnerabilities in parental emotional resources could contribute to the development of less adaptive parent-child relationship patterns.[79,80,84–87]

Parent-Child Interaction

Parent-child interaction is important in the process of feeding, and this interaction is central in the establishment of a healthy dyadic relationship between parent and child.[88] Impairments in this interaction may play a role in FTT. In some studies, infants who have mild to moderate FTT have fewer positive mealtime interactions than controls.[89] The infants who were failing to thrive appeared to be in a less positive relationship with their caregivers during mealtimes than the control group did. The parents of the control group scored higher on anticipation, autonomy, and responsiveness (ie, less maternal interaction with weight-faltering group). This difference does not necessarily mean that the infants who are failing to thrive are doing so because of the decreased positive interactions but could mean the decreased positive interactions are in response to the FTT.

Families help children build expectations around food and mealtimes. If there is a disruption in the communication between parents and children, mealtimes may become a setting for battles over food. *Feeding styles* refer to behavioral patterns between parents and children that occur during meals: responsive, controlling, indulgent, and uninvolved.[90] Low maternal responsivity, insensitivity to cues, and poor problem-solving skills have been reported between children with FTT and their mothers observed during mealtime and playtime.[91–93] Children involved in mealtime control struggles with their mothers at age 36 months have been shown to manifest other, more general behavior problems.[94] Under optimal circumstances, the communication between parents and children is clear because each adapts to the signals of the other and to the demands of the situation. Having a child who does not grow can be stressful and threaten a parent's sense of competence and ability to communicate with the child. Parent-child interaction breaks down if communication is distorted and marked by signals that lack clarity, misperceptions of signals, inconsistent responses, or responses that are not in keeping with the signals.

Biological Causes and Risk Factors

Medical causes of FTT are less common than psychosocial causes but always must be considered when evaluating children with poor growth.[95] Table 17.1 lists medical causes of poor growth by system.

TABLE 17.1
Medical Causes of Poor Growth by System[28,30,31,95]

System	Differential Diagnosis
Infectious	Frequent acute infections, chronic infection (HIV infection, AIDS, TB, chronic UTI)
Endocrine	Diabetes mellitus, hypothyroidism, constitutional or familial short stature, growth hormone deficiency, Cushing disease
Renal	Renal tubular acidosis
Cardiac	Congenital heart disease
Genetic	Inborn errors of metabolism, glycogen storage diseases, Turner syndrome, Down syndrome, Pierre Robin sequence
Gastrointestinal	History of low birth weight, GERD, celiac disease, cow's milk protein intolerance, post-enteritis enteropathy, inflammatory bowel disease, pancreatic cholestasis, disaccharidase deficiency, biliary atresia
Pulmonology	Cystic fibrosis, chronic lung disease due to preterm birth
Hematologic/oncologic	Malignancy, iron deficiency anemia
Neurologic	Malignancy, iron deficiency anemia
Ear/nose/throat	Cleft palate
Environmental	Increased lead levels leading to anorexia, constipation, or abdominal pain

Abbreviations: AIDS, acquired immunodeficiency syndrome; GERD, gastroesophageal reflux disease; HIV, human immunodeficiency virus; TB, tuberculosis; UTI, urinary tract infection.

Evaluation

A meticulous history and thorough physical examination will point to the cause of FTT in most cases, because illnesses, psychosocial issues, or combinations of both severe enough to limit growth will usually be identified. Boxes 17.2 through 17.6 detail the important components of the medical history by age group, many of which are discussed in the following sections.

BOX 17.2
Historical Factors in the Prenatal Period to Be Considered in an Evaluation of Failure to Thrive

Prenatal History

Biological Factors

Mother's medical history
Mother's obstetric history
Prenatal care obtained
Infections and illnesses during pregnancy
Medical problems with the pregnancy (eg, preterm labor, bleeding, oligohydramnios or polyhydramnios)
Intrauterine growth retardation
Trauma (intentional or accidental)
Medications used during pregnancy
Alcohol and cigarette use during pregnancy
Illicit substance use during pregnancy
Maternal weight gain during pregnancy

Psychosocial Factors

Planned versus unplanned pregnancy
If unplanned, reaction of mother and father
Timing and consistency of prenatal care
Type and amount of social support
Maternal mental illness before and/or during pregnancy
Stressors during pregnancy
Intimate partner violence
Preparations for baby

Reprinted from Lowen D. Failure to thrive. In: Jenny C, ed. *Child Abuse and Neglect: Diagnosis, Treatment and Evidence*. 1st ed. St Louis, MO: Saunders, Elsevier; 2011:547-562, copyright 2011, with permission from Elsevier.

BOX 17.3
Historical Factors About the Child's Birth to Be Considered in an Evaluation of Failure to Thrive

Birth

Biological Factors

Gestational age

Mode of delivery

Complications of delivery

Weight, length, and head circumference

Large, appropriate, or small for gestational age

Dysmorphic appearance or congenital malformations

Psychosocial Factors

Maternal complications of delivery

Maternal perception of delivery

Father's or partner's reaction to birth of baby

Reprinted from Lowen D. Failure to thrive. In: Jenny C, ed. *Child Abuse and Neglect: Diagnosis, Treatment and Evidence.* 1st ed. St Louis, MO: Saunders, Elsevier; 2011:547–562, copyright 2011, with permission from Elsevier.

BOX 17.4
Historical Factors About the Neonatal Period to Be Considered in an Evaluation of Failure to Thrive

Neonatal Course in the Hospital Nursery and Immediately After Discharge

Biological Factors

Breastfeeding or bottle-feeding

Success of initial feedings

Trouble with latching (if breastfeeding)

Weak or strong suck

Availability of lactation support

Medical problems during initial few days

Need for medical tests during nursery stay

Total amount of weight loss during nursery stay

Length of hospitalization

Need for repeat testing after discharge

First follow-up appointment after discharge

Medical problems and weight at first follow-up appointment

(continued)

BOX 17.4 (*continued*)

Psychosocial Factors

Time for and limitations of maternal bonding

Quality of maternal bonding

Mother's perception of newborn's health

Type and amount of social support during and immediately after hospitalization

Acceptance of education while in the hospital

Maternal length of hospitalization

Appropriate baby supplies in the home

Compliance with and reaction to home visitor after discharge (where available)

Reprinted from Lowen D. Failure to thrive. In: Jenny C, ed. *Child Abuse and Neglect: Diagnosis, Treatment and Evidence*. 1st ed. St Louis, MO: Saunders, Elsevier; 2011:547–562, copyright 2011, with permission from Elsevier.

BOX 17.5
Historical Factors About First Months After Birth to Be Considered in an Evaluation of Failure to Thrive

After the Neonatal Period, in the First Several Months After Birth

Biological Factors

Frequency and source of routine medical care

Growth measurements

Immunization status

Medical illnesses

Hospitalizations

Medications

Allergies—medications, food, other

Surgeries

Injuries, including bruises on infants

Feeding issues—vigorous or difficult feeder

Breastfeeding

- Milk letdown
- Sense of fullness/emptying
- Frequency and duration of feedings
- Maternal observation of baby swallowing
- Maternal diet and medical problems while breastfeeding

(*continued*)

BOX 17.5 (*continued*)

Formula feeding

- Type
- Method of mixing (concentration)
- Frequency and quantity of feedings

Other intake in first few months of life, such as

- Water
- Juice
- Tea
- Soda
- Cereal

Sleep schedule

Baby's temperament

Developmental milestones

Use of complementary or integrative medicines

Psychosocial Factors

Provision of baby care, especially feeding

Maternal sleep deprivation

Postpartum depression or other mental illness

Type and amount of social support

Availability of respite for mother

Involvement of father and/or other intimate partner

Intimate partner violence

Financial resources, including money for baby supplies

Enrollment in governmental aid programs

Parental reaction to fussing/crying

Who lives with the baby

Reactions of others in the home to the baby

Parental employment

Use of child care or babysitting

Caregiver perception of weight gain and general appearance

Dietary beliefs of family—food constraints, dangerous foods

Adequate housing, refrigeration, cooking facilities

BOX 17.6
Historical Factors About Toddler Age Group to Be Considered in an Evaluation of Failure to Thrive

From the First Several Months After Birth Through Toddler Period

Biological Factors

Frequency and source of routine medical care
Growth measurements
Immunization status
Medical illnesses
Hospitalizations
Medications
Allergies—medications, food, other
Surgeries
Injuries, including bruises on infants
Feeding issues—picky eater
Breastfeeding

- Frequency and duration of feedings
- Maternal diet and medical problems while breastfeeding

Formula feeding

- Type
- Method of mixing (concentration)
- Frequency and quantity of feedings

Age solids introduced
Tolerance of baby food, solid foods
Tolerance of different textures
Age switched to whole milk
Tolerance of cow's milk
Vitamin or mineral supplements
Sleep schedule
Child's temperament
Developmental milestones
Use of alternative or complementary medicines
Pica
Where and when fed

Psychosocial Factors

Who feeds the baby
Parental sleep deprivation
Postpartum depression or other mental illness
Type and amount of social support

(continued)

BOX 17.6 (*continued*)

Availability of respite for mother
Involvement of father and/or other intimate partner
Intimate partner violence
Financial resources, including money for baby supplies
Enrollment in governmental aid programs
Parental reaction to fussing/crying
Who lives with the child
Reactions of others in the home to the child
Parental employment
Use of child care or babysitting
Caregiver perception of weight gain and general appearance
Dietary beliefs of family—food constraints, dangerous foods
Adequate housing, refrigeration, cooking facilities

Prenatal and Perinatal History

The medical assessment of a child who is not thriving should include a detailed assessment of the child's prenatal and perinatal history by interview and, when possible, by review of neonatal records. This approach not only elucidates potential biological risks to growth but also may be helpful in identifying ongoing psychosocial risk factors that are concurrently influencing postnatal growth. Low birth weight is a major predictor of later referral for FTT. In several clinical series, 10% to 40% of children hospitalized for FTT without a major medical diagnosis had a birth weight less than 2,500 g, compared with 7% of the general population at the time those studies were done.[17,21,96–98] In controlled studies of FTT that excluded infants with birth weights less than 2,500 g from the definition of FTT, infants later diagnosed with FTT still had lower birth weights than those who grew normally.[73]

To evaluate accurately the effect of perinatal risk factors on later growth, a detailed history should be obtained. It is critical to ascertain not only the child's birth weight but also gestational age, length, and head circumference at birth. Such data will identify preterm birth as well as various patterns of IUGR that have prognostic implications for later growth.

Size at birth reflects the duration and rate of growth during gestation. Infants whose rate of intrauterine growth is depressed are at risk for postnatal growth failure, regardless of gestational age. *Intrauterine growth retardation* is conventionally defined as birth weight less than the 10th percentile for gestational age. The degree of risk for poor growth postnatally after IUGR is not uniform, varying with the cause of the IUGR and the pattern of relative deficit in length, weight, or head circumference at birth. It must be stated that infants with poor growth after IUGR may not fail to gain weight enough to cross growth percentile lines but, instead, may simply remain at a low percentile. In such a situation, the label of FTT would be inaccurate.

Infants with symmetrical IUGR whose weight, length, and head circumference are proportionately depressed at birth carry a relatively poor prognosis for later growth and development. A symmetrical pattern of IUGR should alert the medical professional to the possibility of chromosomal abnormalities, intrauterine infections, or prenatal teratogen exposure. For this reason, children with symmetrical IUGR should be carefully scrutinized for dysmorphic features that may provide clues to syndrome diagnosis. Exposure to anticonvulsants, including hydantoin and valproate sodium, may be associated with symmetrical IUGR and dysmorphic features.[99]

The best prognosis for postnatal growth pertains to infants with asymmetrical IUGR, whose weight at birth is disproportionately more depressed than their length or head circumference. Such infants are at risk for FTT because they are often behaviorally difficult.[100] With enhanced postnatal nutrition, however, they can manifest significant catch-up growth in the first 6 to 8 months after birth so that later growth trajectories may be within the reference range.[100,101] For such infants, early identification of growth failure and intensive nutritional and environmental intervention are critical because the potential for catch-up growth to repair the intrauterine deficit is maximal in the first 6 months after birth.[102,103] Infants with a history of IUGR usually catch up in growth by 2 years of age, but approximately 10% to 15% will have persistent short stature in childhood.[104]

Prenatal exposure to legal and illegal psychoactive substances during pregnancy often contributes to symmetrical IUGR, but the prognostic implications for later growth, particularly somatic growth, are variable.[105] Because the issue of prenatal substance exposure and later growth potential is often raised in CPS cases, it warrants discussion in some detail.

Preterm Birth

Children born prematurely may be inappropriately labeled as FTT if the percentiles used for assessing growth parameters are not corrected for gestational age. A statistically significant difference in growth percentiles will be found without such correction in head circumference until

18 months' postnatal age, in weight until 24 months' postnatal age, and in length until 40 months' postnatal age.[106] Even after such correction, infants with very low birth weights (<1,501 g) may remain smaller than infants born at term for at least the first 3 years after birth.[107] In these children, the distribution of mean height, weight, and head circumference corrected for gestational age is shifted downward relative to the reference ranges so that the proportion of children with attained weight or height below the fifth percentile is increased.[107] The rate of growth of such infants, however, should be the same as that of term infants of the same corrected age.[107,108] Moreover, weight-for-length should be proportional despite somewhat lower fat stores.[109] Although the field lacks clear guidelines, preterm neonates born before 34 weeks' gestational age generally should be fed a formula for preterm neonates until they weigh at least 2,000 g, and then an enriched "post-discharge formula" that is higher in calories and micronutrients per ounce than that designed for term neonates. Such enriched formulas are more expensive than formula for term neonates and may be difficult for economically stressed families to afford unless the family receives a physician's prescription to WIC. In general, these post-discharge formulas should be continued until 9 to 12 months' corrected age or minimally until the baby's weight-for-length is maintained above the 25th percentile.[110]

Children who were born preterm who show depressed weight-for-height or whose growth progressively deviates from a channel parallel to the reference ranges should be assessed carefully for potentially correctable (and sometimes iatrogenic) causes of growth failure. These causes may include inappropriate feeding practices for corrected age, such as early discontinuation of post-discharge formula or initiation of solid feedings at 6 months' postnatal age for an infant born at 28 weeks' gestational age whose corrected age is only 3 months. In addition, the neurologic, gastrointestinal, and cardiorespiratory sequelae of preterm birth, as well as the behavioral disorganization characteristic of some preterm neonates, may all contribute to postnatal malnutrition. Growth difficulties should not be discounted in such children on the grounds that they were "born small." In addition to affecting the neonate's behavior or physical growth potential directly, preterm birth and low birth weight also may act indirectly to increase the risk of growth failure by intensifying family stress and requiring early separation between parents and child for neonatal intensive care.

Past Medical History

Almost all severe and chronic childhood illnesses can cause growth failure. The mechanisms of such failure are multiple: enzymatic, metabolic, and endocrine in some cases, but also nutritional and psychosocial.[111,112]

Chronic physical problems that necessitate procedures such as gastrostomy or nasogastric feedings may impede the development of normal feeding patterns.

Hospitalization should not be regarded as a diagnostic test for chronic illness.[113] It was previously thought that children who experienced a depriving environment ("nonorganic" FTT) would grow in the hospital, whereas children with serious medical illnesses ("organic" FTT) would not. In fact, a positive growth response to hospitalization poorly differentiates major organic illness from environmental risk because children with such illness and children who were not receiving an appropriate diet will grow if given adequate caloric intake.[114] Children with chronic illness who do well in the hospital usually have complex technical, psychosocial, and nutritional needs that can be met by multiple shifts of highly trained medical personnel but may overwhelm parents who are not receiving adequate caregiving support at home. Conversely, unless the hospital provides specialized milieu therapy, which is usually not available on general pediatric wards, children with severe interactive feeding disorders or depression may deteriorate in the hospital because separation from primary attachment figures and multiple caregivers may exacerbate their affective and behavioral feeding difficulties. Children who are simply underfed do well in any setting when adequate calories are offered. Thus, response to hospitalization often cannot be used to identify the cause of FTT.

The list of medical conditions presenting as FTT is relatively circumscribed and, as mentioned previously, often these conditions are identified during the history, physical examination, and/or review of systems. In a series of children hospitalized for FTT of unknown origin, the most common previously undiagnosed illnesses were gastrointestinal, including chronic nonspecific diarrhea, celiac disease, food allergies, gastroesophageal reflux, cystic fibrosis, and lactose intolerance.[20,115–118] Immigrant children and children attending congregate child care or living in homeless shelters should be evaluated for giardiasis and enteric pathogens if they have gastrointestinal symptoms such as diarrhea or abdominal pain, because these are common causes of malabsorption and growth failure.[119,120] Outside the gastrointestinal system, medical professionals should consider urinary tract infections and renal tubular acidosis as potentially clinically silent contributors to FTT. Subtle neurologic dysfunction manifested as fine and oral-motor dysfunction also should be considered and evaluated by direct observation.[74]

Both overdiagnosis and underdiagnosis of "food allergy" can contribute to FTT.[121] In 1995 the European Academy of Allergy and Clinical Immunology created a standard terminology by which to assign a patient's reaction to a food.[122] Only those reactions that are the consequence of an immune response (immunoglobulin [Ig] E mediated) to a food or food additive are formally considered to be food allergies,[123,124] whereas a non–IgE-mediated immune reaction is classified as *adverse food reactions* or *food sensitivity*.[123,125] An exceedingly restrictive diet based on an imprecise or factitious diagnosis of food allergy may present as FTT.[121] It is crucial that the cause of an apparent adverse reaction to a food be aggressively sought. Whereas negative skin tests are 95% accurate, positive tests are only 50% accurate and must be confirmed by history or a food challenge.[123] It may take as long as 14 days to see a clinical response to an elimination diet. A double-blind, placebo-controlled food challenge is the criterion (gold) standard for food allergy diagnosis but may not always be practical in primary care settings.[126] Alternative or additional methods, such as radioallergosorbent tests, may be easier to obtain.[119,126] The physician should be aware that *Helicobacter pylori*, other infections, and celiac disease may be manifested by the same symptoms as food allergies.[119,123,125,127,128] Conversely, 30% of atopic dermatitis in young children is triggered by food allergy, so that evaluation for food allergy should be considered in any child with FTT and eczema. Because children often "outgrow" their adverse reaction to a food by age 3 years, such evaluations should be repeated periodically so that the child's diet does not remain unnecessarily restricted.[123,126,129]

Infection with HIV is another potential cause of FTT that may be clinically silent, depending on the degree of immune suppression. This diagnosis should be considered particularly in children whose mothers have a history of illicit psychoactive substance use, have had multiple sexual partners, or who are sexual partners of substance-abusing or bisexual men. The diagnosis also must be ruled out in children of immigrants from areas where heterosexual transmission of HIV is endemic and when the child or mother, or her sexual partner, has had a blood transfusion.[130]

In addition to medical illnesses that may cause growth failure, medical professionals must be alert to the medical complications of the malnutrition itself, particularly recurring infections and lead poisoning. Malnutrition severe enough to produce growth failure also impairs immunocompetence, particularly cell-mediated immunity and the production of complement and secretory IgA.[131–133] Recurring otitis media and gastrointestinal and respiratory illnesses are more common among children who fail to thrive than among well-nourished children of the same age.[96,134–136] Children who fail to thrive are often trapped in an infection-malnutrition cycle, in which illness causes decreases in a child's appetite and intake, while nutrient requirements increase as a result of fever, diarrhea, and vomiting. The additional malnutrition leaves the child increasingly vulnerable to more severe and prolonged infections, causing ever worsening growth.

Elevated lead levels correlate with impaired growth, even in the 5- to 35-mg/dL range.[137] Here, too, a negative cycle develops. Nutritional deficiencies of iron and calcium enhance the absorption of lead and other heavy metals.[138] As lead levels rise, constipation, abdominal pain, and anorexia occur, leading to even less adequate dietary intake.[139] In one study, 16% of children with FTT had lead levels high enough to warrant chelation.[140]

Nutritional History

Of obvious importance in the evaluation of FTT is a detailed nutritional history, even in the face of a documented medical condition that can cause growth failure itself. The assessment should focus not only on current feeding practices but also on the development of feeding since birth. In some children, feeding struggles and growth failure begin with the introduction of solid foods at age 5 to 7 months. Thus, comparison of the lifelong feeding history with the growth curve can provide diagnostic clues to the etiology of a child's FTT.

Medical professionals should ascertain when, where, how, and by whom the child is fed, as well as what the child is fed and why. Comprehensive assessment of feeding problems requires a combination of methods such as structured interviews with primary caregivers and direct observation of the child's response to feeding in multiple situations. Caregivers should be asked to complete an oral or written checklist of possible behavioral feeding problems (eg, spitting out food, tantrums during meals, food refusal), to supply a few days of food-intake records, and to indicate how the parents have tried to manage the child's problems.[141–143] A food-intake diary should include not only when and by whom the child was fed but also what and how much liquid the child drank, in what location the child was fed (eg, kitchen table, high chair, couch, stroller, lap of caregiver, floor), and any issues encountered during the feeding. This information often elucidates inconsistencies in feedings that may be contributing to the problem.

In addition to how the child is fed, the medical professional must ascertain what the child is fed and why. The family's level of nutritional knowledge and dietary beliefs should be assessed. American parents and children are continually bombarded with nutritional misinformation from commercial sources urging them to spend their scant food resources on heavily sweetened or salted foods of low nutritional quality.[144–146] Certain groups of parents, particularly adolescents and those who are intellectually limited, illiterate, or unable to speak English, are particularly likely to lack adequate information on nutritionally sound feeding practices. Immigrants are at risk unless they are able to obtain culturally appropriate foods. Most ethnic diets are adequate, but when traditional foods are unavailable, immigrants may not know what to select from the foods available in American markets. Parents may also restrict food intake due to unusual dietary beliefs or from excessive fear of obesity, diabetes, or cardiovascular disease.[147]

Parents seeking to prevent obesity or cardiovascular disease also may inadvertently cause their toddlers to fail to thrive by overzealous enforcement of a low-fat diet appropriate for adults but not for growing children.[147] Restricted diets imposed because of actual or presumed food allergies often are not adequately supplemented with alternate sources of calories and micronutrients, with consequent nutritional deficiencies.[148] Lastly, families of all types may receive inaccurate and inappropriate nutritional information from friends and social media.

For infants who are breastfed or bottle-fed, determining the quantity taken by the infant with each feeding and the frequency of the feedings is necessary. Breastfed infants may be weighed immediately before and immediately after a breastfeeding session, without changing clothes, to determine how many grams were taken in. For both bottle-fed and breastfed infants, caregivers should be asked if they can hear the baby sucking and swallowing and if the infant dribbles while feeding, coughs, or spits the liquid out. Caregivers who are formula feeding must be asked exactly how they obtain the formula and if they can afford it. It is critical to ask how the formula is mixed to determine the caloric concentration. Medical professionals should never assume that an infant, however young, is not being given water or other liquids in addition to the formula or human milk and, therefore, should ask directly about this. In addition, caregivers should be directly queried about "stretching" the formula or expressed milk by diluting it to make it last longer.

The family's economic resources for food purchase, food storage, and food preparation must be tactfully ascertained. A 24-hour dietary recall and/or 7-day diet diary are essential in determining the quality and quantity of the child's diet. Common findings among children with FTT include excessive intake of juice, water, tea, or carbonated and sweetened beverages, which depress appetite but provide few nutrients. In addition, fruit juices high in fructose or sorbitol have been associated with malabsorption and osmotic diarrhea in some cases of FTT.[148,149] Low-income families may have particular difficulties in meeting the needs of children with increased nutritional needs (eg, children born preterm; children with significant heart or lung disease) or those with restricted and, therefore, more expensive diets, as in the cases of multiple food allergies, lactose intolerance, or gluten-sensitive enteropathy.[125,150]

Family History

A detailed family history should be obtained and should include maternal and paternal sides of the family. Issues of importance include consanguinity, recurrent miscarriage or stillbirth, developmental delay, atopy, HIV risk, alcoholism and other substance use, psychiatric diagnoses, and familial illnesses such as cystic fibrosis, celiac disease, inflammatory bowel disease, or lactose intolerance. Height of both parents should be ascertained, as well as parents' history of growth delay in childhood and timing of puberty. A familial pattern of short stature, or constitutional delay of growth, may relieve the medical professional and the family of the need for extensive workup if the child is short but not underweight for height.[151,152] Reference ranges exist for correcting height percentiles for midparental height by using the National Center for Health Statistics (NCHS) grids.[152] It is critical, however, to assess whether the parents themselves were malnourished as children, as may be the case among immigrant and low-income families. In such cases, the parents' short stature does not provide an accurate indication of the child's genetic growth potential.[153] Moreover, an experience of severe childhood deprivation may influence the parents' caregiving practices.[154]

A detailed family history may uncover significant psychosocial stressors. A chronically ill grandparent or sibling may divert the family's caregiving energies from the child who fails to thrive; FTT has been described in siblings of children with leukemia.[155] A family history of serious mental illness, intergenerational substance abuse, or developmental impairment also may be present.[18] Detailed family history may also reveal a parental history of an eating disorder in childhood or adolescence, including a history of anorexia nervosa diagnosis.[156,157]

Psychosocial History

A detailed psychosocial history is critical in the evaluation of FTT to help determine etiology, possible barriers to treatment, and the effects of malnutrition on the child's psychological functioning. Typical details, such as determining with whom the child lives and who provides care for the child, are just the starting points of a good psychosocial evaluation in an FTT evaluation. The type and quality of family relationships, the presence or absence of supportive caregivers, child care issues, education, employment, and financial stability are all critical pieces of the FTT diagnostic and treatment puzzle.

The quality of relationships within the family, including the relationships and interactions of other family members with the child, can have an important influence on the child who fails to thrive. For this reason, focused and sensitive clinical assessments are needed to assess family feeding and cultural practices, routines and organization, finances, the quality of maternal relationships with other family members, and family members' perceptions of the causes, influences, and consequences of the child's FTT.[61,158] Clinical interviews are especially useful in helping family members share their ideas about what may be influencing the child's feeding, physical growth, and development and to provide a context in which to observe fathers' and other family members' interactions with their children.[61,158] Because parents' appraisal of their child's temperament, such as "passive," "difficult," or "demanding," may influence their interactions with the child, it also is instructive to assess parents' perceptions of the child's need for interaction and nurturance. Multiple and/or inconsistent caregivers can lead to difficulties with feeding; in older infants and children, it can lead to food refusal.

Parental beliefs about food, children's size and health, nutritional needs, and family mealtime patterns may contribute to children's growth by influencing the availability of foods and the feeding atmosphere.[159] Approximately one-third of families of children with FTT do not recognize that their child has a growth problem.[160] Such failures even occur in cachectic children in whom the malnutrition is obvious; it is always important to ask the caregivers' perspectives without making assumptions, no matter how severe the situation may be. Parents who do not believe that their child is experiencing a problem are unlikely to adhere to treatment plans and, depending on the severity of the malnutrition, may be indicative of medical neglect.

It is necessary to assess aspects of the family environment (relationships, resources, and parent-child interaction) that would be expected to influence the child's response to medical and psychological intervention. Given the effect of parent-child relationships on child development, observations of the parents' interactions with the child in a range of situations (eg, feeding, teaching the child a skill, free play) provide a useful method of assessment.[161,162] Observing the caregiver feeding the child can give invaluable insights into the parent-child relationship and each participant's relationship with feedings and mealtime. The patterns of parent-child relationships associated with FTT are complex and heterogeneous.[89,141,142,163–165] Deficient stimulation is one typical pattern; conflict and parental reinforcement of deviant behavior is another.[89,141,142]

A wide range of psychological functions, including intellectual and socioemotional development, may be affected by growth deficiency, malnutrition, and associated risk factors and should be documented in a comprehensive assessment approach.[89,166] Psychological assessment is best construed as a continuing process that begins with an initial or baseline assessment at the time the child's growth deficiency is first noticed and includes sequential assessments of the child's short- and longer-term responses to intervention.[165] One important purpose of assessment is to document the functional effect of the child's malnutrition and associated risk factors on cognitive, motor, and socioemotional development and behavior. The second is to monitor the effects of treatment. These detailed evaluations may be beyond the scope of a primary care medical professional and necessitate involvement of appropriate multidisciplinary services, including psychology, specialists in behavior and development, and ancillary services such as physical or occupational therapy.

Review of Systems

A very thorough review of systems must be obtained, including determining if the child is currently ill. Positives and negatives on the review of systems can indicate a medical cause for the FTT or at least point to an organ system as an area of concern. In addition, effects of the malnutrition may become evident. A current illness may also explain temporary growth failure and may provide guidance on the timing of additional medical workup and treatment plans.

Physical Examination

Early detection of faltering growth can aid in faster treatment and improved outcomes. Children with early deceleration in weight gain more than −0.85 SDs between the 2- to 4-month or 4- to 6-month interval are at increased risk of reaching underweight status by 24 months of age. Identification of these children at a younger age allows the medical professional to start a closer assessment to identify feeding concerns and unmet nutritional needs and may prevent the slowing of growth later.[166]

The physical examination of the child who fails to thrive has 3 goals: (1) identification of medical illness, (2) recognition of syndromes that alter growth, and (3) documentation of the effects of malnutrition. Some findings may be nonspecific and require evaluation by laboratory assessment. For example, hepatic enlargement may be seen with primary malnutrition, AIDS, or underlying liver disease.

The following should be included in the physical examination and clearly documented:

- General: affect, interaction, absence of subcutaneous fat stores, poor muscle mass, loose skinfolds
- Vital signs: hypertension or hypotension, tachycardia or bradycardia, tachypnea, hypothermia, hypoxia (by pulse oximetry)
- Head, eyes, ears, nose, throat: hair quality, hair loss, positional plagiocephaly, dysmorphic facies, scleral icterus, cleft palate (including submucosal), poor dentition, tonsillar hypertrophy, thyroid masses
- Chest: increased work of breathing, rales or wheezes, clubbing
- Cardiac: pathologic murmur, poor peripheral perfusion, cyanosis
- Abdomen: hepatomegaly, abdominal mass, ascites
- Genitourinary and anus: anomalies, anal fistulae, signs of trauma
- Skin: skin rashes, poor hygiene, decreased turgor, scars, bruises
- Neurological: hypertonia or hypotonia, hyperreflexia, poor suck, uncoordinated swallow, developmental delay[167]

Growth Measurements

Serial anthropometric criteria should be used to determine if a child has FTT, because plotting a child's growth over time gives more information than a single point on a chart. There are multiple different criteria to determine if a child has FTT: weight deceleration crossing 2 major percentile lines, weight-for-age less than 5th percentile, weight less than 75% of median weight-for-age, and/or weight less than 75% of median weight-for-length.

Continuous variables, such as height and weight, are distributed along a bell-shaped curve, also known in statistical terms as the *normal distribution*. The total area under the curve includes 100% of the analyzed population values. Smaller children are distributed to the left and larger children to the right of the mean value for that population, located at the center of the curve. The SD, or *z* score, is obtained by subtracting the mean value of the reference population from the observed value and dividing by the SD of the reference population.[106]

Children referred for FTT evaluation must be measured in a standard fashion by trained personnel using the same scale at each measurement, according to published protocols for obtaining accurate and reproducible anthropometric measurements.[1,26,168,169] In 2006, WHO released updated charts with data on 6 countries using breastfeeding as the biologic norm.[170] The 2000 CDC charts include formula-fed infants, reflecting norms for heavier children.[171] The WHO Global Database on Child Growth and Malnutrition uses a range within 2 SD below and above the mean as the standard measure for identifying children with typical growth. These limits correspond to the 2.3rd or 97.7th percentiles rather than to the fifth and 95th percentiles, as in many older growth charts. A cutoff point of >2 SD below the mean is used to identify children with short stature (ie, low height-for-age), low weight-for-age, or low weight- and low height-for-age.[106] There are special growth charts for very preterm neonates.[107] Another option is to use standard growth charts and correct for preterm birth. There are also standardized growth charts for specific conditions, including trisomy 21, Prader-Willi syndrome, Turner syndrome, and achondroplasia, among others.

Infants should be weighed naked, and young children should wear underwear only; weight should be obtained on a properly calibrated scale. For follow-up over time, it is important to use the same scale each time. Length should be measured with the child recumbent for children aged 2 years and younger. Between ages 2 and 3 years children can be measured either recumbent or standing. For children older than 3 years, standing height is measured. When measuring height using a wall stadiometer, the child faces away from the wall, with heels together and back straight. The head, shoulders, buttocks, and heels should contact the wall with the child looking straight ahead. It is inadequate to lay an infant on paper and mark the head and foot with a pen, then measure with a ruler; a stadiometer with inflexible head and foot boards will give a more accurate measurement.

Weight-for-age is commonly used in pediatric clinics to track children's growth and is an excellent indicator of changes in weight over time.[172] However, weight-for-age may be difficult to interpret because it does not account for variations in height.[173] When a child's weight-for-age is low, it may not be clear whether the primary problem is low weight, short stature, or a combination. Weight-for-height (weight plotted by height regardless of age) reflects body proportionality. The update of the growth charts by the NCHS in 2000 included body mass index (BMI) for children older than 2 years (BMI = weight in kilograms/height in centimeters squared) and provides an assessment of weight-for-height in these older children. These growth charts are available online at www.cdc.gov/growthcharts. By international consensus, the NCHS growth charts serve currently as the references for evaluating growth in young children regardless of ethnic or racial background.[36] These growth charts eliminate the discontinuity between recumbent length and standing height and provide percentile lines above and beyond the fifth and 95th percentiles.[174] It is important to note that despite their accepted use, these references include an unknown number of ill and deprived children and, thus, may be imprecise tools for identifying aberrant growth.[36] WHO has developed standards for expected growth from a multiethnic, multinational sample restricted to healthy, initially breastfed children, and growth charts are now available at www.who.int/childgrowth/standards/en/.

Low weight-for-height, or wasting, is often an early and/or acute sign of malnutrition and may reflect low caloric intake. This measurement can help identify children who need more immediate treatment. Chronic malnutrition may result in decelerated skeletal growth, indicated by low height-for-age in addition to low weight-for-age, and is called *stunting*. In this situation, the weight-for-height may be in the reference range and the child could appear somewhat proportional, although small overall. Thus, weight-for-height and height-for-age provide a nonredundant, comprehensive picture of growth.[173,175] When constitutional, endocrine, and genetic factors can be ruled out, depressed height-for-age is considered a manifestation of the cumulative effects of chronic malnutrition.[136] Children at highest risk are those for whom both weight-for-height and height-for-age are depressed, indicating acute malnutrition superimposed on a chronic problem.

Weight-for-age, weight-for-height, and height-for-age can be expressed as percentile scores, SD scores, or percentage of median scores. Percentile scores are commonly used clinically because they are relatively easy to interpret, but they are less useful when describing variations at the extremes (eg, less than fifth percentile). SD scores (*z* scores) are commonly used for analyses because they can be used to characterize extremes and facilitate comparisons across ages.[173] Percentage of median scores are often used to describe change and are calculated by dividing the child's weight (or height) by the median expected weight (or height) (50th percentile) based on the child's chronological (or corrected for preterm birth) age.

A useful clinical technique, initially devised by Kaplowitz and Webb,[151] Waterlow,[136] and Gomez et al[176] is to categorize the child's malnutrition as first (mild), second (moderate), or third (severe) degree based on the child's weight-for-age, height-for-age, and weight-for-height percentage of median. Children with third-degree malnutrition (weight-for-age <60% of median, or weight-for-height <70% of median) are in acute danger of severe morbidity and possible mortality from their malnutrition and should usually be hospitalized. At present, the standard NCHS growth charts are cross-sectional for monitoring weight gain over time and, therefore, do not fully illustrate the magnitude of changes in a child's weight relative to height.[26]

When analyzing the growth chart, abrupt changes in rates of growth should be carefully evaluated. For instance, if a 12-month-old was growing normally until 4 months of age and then began falling off the growth curve, determining what changes occurred in the infant or family at that time may help point to an etiology. For example, did the infant have a significant illness? Did a caregiver leave the family? Did financial resources change?

Laboratory and Radiology Workup

Most children with FTT do not require an extensive laboratory or radiology workup. Laboratory and imaging rarely change the diagnosis or management of children with FTT unless there is a clinical suspicion based on history and physical examination.[30] Thus, laboratory evaluation should be restrained and guided by history and the findings of the physical examination. For example, a child who has no symptoms of cardiorespiratory distress or heart murmur does not need an electrocardiogram. Basic laboratory studies should be used to identify derangements caused by malnutrition and to rule out the potentially occult diseases previously discussed.[97]

All children should have a complete blood cell count, assessment of lead and free erythrocyte protoporphyrin levels (in mobile infants and older children), urinalysis, albumin, and comprehensive chemistry panel. Thyroid function can be included because of the detrimental effects of hypothyroidism on brain development in infancy. Iron deficiency is a common finding. Other testing should be guided by the history and physical examination, such as checking liver functions in those with hepatomegaly or jaundice, anti-tissue transglutaminase or anti-endomysial antibodies if celiac disease is suspected, echocardiogram if a pathologic murmur is present, or chromosomal analysis if a genetic syndrome is of concern.

In children with severe anthropometric deficits, prealbumin and albumin levels are important to assess protein status. A depressed alkaline phosphatase value suggests zinc deficiency; an elevated level, especially if associated with a depressed phosphorous value, is suggestive of rickets.[177] Human immunodeficiency virus testing, sweat test, and stool assessments for *Giardia* or other parasites should be performed in epidemiologically at-risk populations, including children with recent travel to or emigration from endemic areas.[130,134,178] Radioallergosorbent or skin testing for food allergies should be considered in children with FTT and atopic dermatitis, as well as for those with a history of rash, urticaria, or recurring vomiting and diarrhea after ingestion of selected foods.

In a child with FTT who has vomiting not explained by food allergies and unresponsive to empiric management, radiographic or endoscopic studies, or pH probe, may be indicated to rule out anatomical abnormalities, gastroesophageal reflux, and esophagitis, particularly among children with neurologic impairments and unexplained respiratory symptoms.[152]

For short children with weight proportionate to height, bone-age radiographic studies are helpful in distinguishing those who are constitutionally short (bone age equals chronological age and is greater than height age) from those with growth hormone or thyroid deficiencies or stunting due to chronic malnutrition (bone age equals height age and is less than chronological age).[112,179]

A child younger than 2 years with any findings concerning for inflicted injury needs to have a skeletal survey performed; this should also be done for those in whom medical neglect is a consideration.

Observation of Parent-Child Interaction

Analysis of a child's feeding skills or problems is ideally performed via observation of a feeding or meal, which will also provide valuable insight into the interactions between parent and child. Parents may bring food the child likes, or the clinic or hospital may provide age-appropriate food (eg, baby food, microwavable meals, applesauce, pudding, crackers, milk); observing an infant bottle-feeding or breastfeeding also provides valuable information. Video recording the feeding observation may assist families in recognizing their own strengths and weaknesses. Parental interactions with and response to their children during mealtimes should be assessed to determine the interrelationship among specific child problem behaviors, parental responses, and antecedent cues. Rating systems, such as the Behavioral Pediatrics Feeding Assessment Scale, are useful in characterizing the interaction between the parent and child.[180] In some cases, supplementing a clinic or hospital feeding observation with a home-based feeding observation will elucidate not only interactive or mechanical feeding difficulties but also the material conditions of the home and family routines.[181]

Additional Testing

Standardized infant assessment tests provide objective information about the infant's strengths and weaknesses in intellectual and motor functioning.[165,182,183] Assessments are useful to determine children's eligibility for early intervention services. In addition, cognitive assessment data can be used to develop a program of stimulation that can be incorporated into a plan for home intervention. Sequential assessments of cognitive and motor development are especially helpful to document progress in test performance after initial nutritional or psychological intervention and to plan additional interventions.[158]

Intellectual assessment can be a productive means of involving the parents of children with FTT in their child's treatment planning.[158] Observing their child's assessment helps parents appreciate the nature of their children's developmental strengths and weaknesses. When parents have observed the developmental testing, it is also easier and more productive to discuss the pattern of their child's intellectual strengths and deficits with them. If parents are invited to discuss their child's development and participate in the evaluation, they may be less defensive about the overall evaluative process.

In evaluating the child's development, the medical professional should pay careful attention to the potential effects of the infant's nutritional state on his or her response to test items. Infants who have experienced nutritional and/or stimulus deprivation are often withdrawn, which may severely limit their capacity to respond, at least initially.[7] Intellectual tests given shortly after referral may underestimate intellectual potential and, therefore, should not be used for prognostic purposes.

Treatment

One of the first steps in treatment of children experiencing FTT is to determine if they require hospitalization for evaluation and/or treatment. Most children who are failing to thrive can be treated as outpatients, but some will need to be admitted to the hospital. The need for hospitalization depends on the severity of the malnutrition, the presence and severity of dehydration, the presence of significant medical conditions that also need treatment, if there is a concern about possible refeeding syndrome, and if compliance is a concern. If the safety of the child is a concern, hospitalization provides a safe environment to monitor feeding and weight gain. Those children for whom outpatient treatment has failed also qualify for hospitalizations, because the multiple disciplines that can aid in the diagnosis and treatment are often more readily available in the hospital setting.

The clinical management of FTT, especially for those children not requiring hospitalization, should be approached as a chronic condition often requiring long-term multidisciplinary follow-up, with exacerbations and remissions expected. Of the children treated as outpatients, the more severe situations are ideally treated in interdisciplinary specialty clinics, but the primary care medical professional can manage a large proportion of the cases of these children, with involvement of a nutritionist and other consultants as needed.

Successful intervention often requires active team involvement of a pediatric health care clinician, a pediatric nutritionist, a pediatric psychologist, and a social worker, with other professionals available as needed. In many centers, the availability of interdisciplinary outpatient clinics for the diagnosis and management of FTT has greatly reduced the need for hospitalization.[184] Interdisciplinary programs are ideal for treating feeding difficulties. An occupational therapist, speech therapist, nutritionist, psychologist, and physician working together can help prevent feeding difficulties from becoming FTT and treat children who have FTT. Parental education programs can help facilitate the development of functional feeding in young children.[185] Referral for specialized, interdisciplinary outpatient assessment should be considered for any child who has not responded to 2 or 3 months of intensive management in a primary care setting. Children with more severe developmental delay or poorer intellectual ability are more likely to be referred to specialist care.[27]

The initial focus of interdisciplinary management is assessment of the child and family for purposes of planning treatment. Subsequently, the focus concerns intervention and ongoing monitoring of the child's progress. In an optimal team approach, professionals interact frequently and directly with the family and with each other, ideally in the context of scheduled clinic visits and case conferences. In addition, regular home visits by one or several of these professionals are effective to gather diagnostic information and provide ongoing support and guidance for the family.[21,186]

Outpatient Treatment

In the outpatient setting, parent education is a primary component in treatment. As previously mentioned, other disciplines may be necessary to help the child and family, including social work, nutrition, lactation, psychology, and rehabilitation services such as speech, physical, and/or occupational therapy.

Interdisciplinary teams can improve outcomes. Bithoney et al[114] evaluated a multidisciplinary team treatment approach including comprehensive assessment and treatment planning. This team included pediatricians, a pediatric nurse practitioner, a child development specialist, a pediatric gastroenterologist, and a social worker who delivered treatments including intensive case management and follow-up use of calorie-dense formulas and, when appropriate, referral for developmental stimulation, behavior modification (for eating disorders), visiting nurse, or homemaker services. Analysis of physical growth outcomes over a 6-month follow-up indicated that children with FTT who received the comprehensive, multidisciplinary team approach grew better than children with comparable physical growth deficits who received a typical management approach in a pediatric primary care clinic.[116] However, although involvement of an interdisciplinary team is ideal, it may not be available in all areas or be sustainable as a separate clinic. Reasons for lack of sustainability include low referral numbers, less-severe cases being referred, and loss to follow-up.[64]

For infants who are exclusively breastfed, ensuring a good latch, improving feeding techniques, and increasing feeding frequency will help increase milk production and feeding. A lactation consultant can aid in this evaluation and education. A breast pump may be necessary to aid in increase of milk production. Mothers can breastfeed their infant and use a breast pump after each feed. Young infants will need to be followed closely with twice-weekly and sometimes daily weight checks to ensure they are beginning to gain weight and are not becoming dehydrated. If these techniques do not improve feeding and growth, formula supplementation may be necessary. Families may be concerned that this will wean the infant from breastfeeding, but these techniques, when followed consistently, can maintain breastfeeding in most infants.[187]

Mildly and moderately malnourished children may be offered food ad-lib while calorie counts are maintained. Once a baseline of spontaneous intake is established, preferred foods may be enriched to bring dietary intake to catch-up levels. Children must be seen more frequently by the pediatric medical professional than is dictated by routine health management schedules to monitor their growth and development in response to interventions. Weekly visits are often necessary at the beginning of diagnosis and treatment. Meticulous management of concurrent illness is essential, as is enlisting and coordinating assessments in as many disciplines as necessary. Lead poisoning, if identified, should be treated according to standard protocols,[188] as should any other identified comorbidities, such as vitamin deficiencies.

The medical professional must take an aggressive stance to interrupt the infection-malnutrition cycle. The child needs to receive all immunizations, including the annual influenza vaccine. Recurring otitis media or sinusitis is an indication for otolaryngology referral. In addition, for each episode of acute illness, the medical professional should provide specific instruction about appropriate diet during and after the illness to try to maintain and repair nutritional status. A child should never receive a clear liquid diet for more than 24 hours.[118]

Serious deficits in age-appropriate feeding behavior, such as chewing, self-feeding, use of utensils, swallowing, or sucking, may benefit from intensive behavioral training or occupational therapy programs using procedures such as shaping, fading, and modeling to teach novel behaviors (eg, chewing for a child who has had prolonged pureed feedings) or to enhance adaptive feeding responses.[141,142,189] Disruptive behaviors, such as tantrums, expelling food, selective food refusal, attempting to leave the table or high chair, throwing food, whining, or crying, may improve after application of learning treatment methods such as extinction and time-out and the contingent application of reinforcers, such as parental attention.[190] Inappropriate parental responses, such as coaxing, threatening, or "giving in" to the child's demands by terminating the meal or allowing the child to eat only preferred items, reinforce these maladaptive behaviors and should be modified.[158]

Inpatient Treatment

As mentioned previously, hospitalization is indicated for children who are severely malnourished, children who are dehydrated, those with serious concurrent infections or chronic medical conditions, and those whose safety is in question, or if the specialized coordination of disciplines or diagnostic procedures is necessary and can be assembled most efficiently inside the hospital. Children hospitalized for FTT often have complex chronic medical conditions; many such children are also at risk for readmission for the same diagnosis within 6 months of their initial hospitalization.[191]

Children requiring inpatient treatment may be dehydrated enough to require intravenous (IV) fluids. The IV fluids should be discontinued as soon as the child is rehydrated to better encourage and monitor oral intake and weight gain. In addition, children who are severely malnourished must be monitored closely for the development of refeeding syndrome. *Refeeding syndrome* is caused by metabolic and fluid derangements that can occur when nutrition is reintroduced, even at quantities considered normal for age without additional caloric supplementation. If high food intakes are provided at the beginning of nutritional resuscitation, these children may develop vomiting, diarrhea, and circulatory decompensation.[192,193] Therefore, in the first several days of hospitalization of children who are severely malnourished, their vital signs need to be monitored closely and they require frequent laboratory evaluation specifically for potassium, phosphate, and magnesium levels. Intravenous supplementation of these electrolytes may be required.

Hospitalization also provides opportunities to observe and monitor parent-child interactions, not only around feeding issues but also throughout the day. Close monitoring of the child's intake and output allows determination of the accuracy of parental reports. In addition, inpatient observation can answer such questions as the amount and quality of parental nurturing, the child's response to redirection, and the parental response to a tired and stressed child.

Nutritional Goals of Treatment

The goal of nutritional intervention in FTT is to achieve catch-up growth (ie, growth at a rate for age that is faster than reference so the child's relative deficit of body size is restored). If the child with an established growth deficit simply resumes growth at the reference rate for age, relative deficits persist compared with children of the same age who have always grown normally. To assess whether catch-up growth is occurring, the medical professional must be aware of age-specific changes in reference growth rates, as summarized by Guo et al[174]: in the first 3 months after birth median weight gain averages 26 to 31 g/d; from 3 to 6 months, 17 to 18 g/d; from 6 to 9 months, 12 to 13 g/d; from 9 to 12 months, 9 g/d; and from 12 months onward, 7 to 9 g/d. A goal for catch-up growth may be as much as 2 to 3 times the average rate of weight gain for corrected age. Thus, a 1-year-old who is gaining 30 g/d is showing excellent catch-up growth, whereas a 1-month-old who also is gaining 30 g/d is growing at only the reference rate for age and will not repair existing deficits. The goal for catch-up growth must be continually revised as the child grows and matures.

To achieve catch-up growth, the underweight child must receive nutrients in excess of the typical age-specific requirements of the recommended dietary allowance (RDA).[194] Daily caloric needs for catch-up growth in calories per kilogram can be estimated as follows: kilocalories per kilogram = 120 kcal/kg × median weight for current height / current weight (kg).[192] In most cases, according to this calculation, children require 1.5 to 2 times the expected intake for their age to achieve optimal catch-up growth.[22,192,195] Protein intake should be enhanced in similar proportions to permit maximal growth.[192]

Nutritional rehabilitation must address the child's needs for micronutrients as well as calories and protein. Iron deficiency, with or without associated anemia, may be seen in children presenting with FTT.[1] Vitamin D–deficiency rickets also has been described.[177] Even among children whose micronutrient stores are adequate at initial presentation with FTT, the demand of rapid tissue synthesis during catch-up growth may produce nutritional deficiencies. Even if zinc status cannot be measured, zinc supplementation should be provided to meet the RDA because such supplementation has been shown to decrease the energy cost of weight gain.[163,196,197] A multivitamin supplement containing the RDA for all vitamins, as well as iron and zinc, should be prescribed routinely for children with FTT during nutritional rehabilitation, with additional supplementation of iron or vitamin D to therapeutic levels in children with iron deficiency or rickets.[198] Use of a once-a-day vitamin supplement also is useful to reduce pressure on caregivers to ensure that their child is receiving a completely balanced diet. Caregivers will no longer have to worry about whether their child is eating green beans or other low-calorie vegetables as a source of vitamins and can focus on ensuring adequate intake of minerals, fiber, calories, and protein.

In general, it is difficult, if not impossible, for a child to eat twice the normal volume of food to obtain the nutrient levels necessary for catch-up growth. In these cases, the child's usual diet must be fortified to increase nutrient density (eg, providing formula of 24–30 cal/oz rather than the standard 19–20 cal/oz). Commercially available shakes with up to 30 cal/oz can be used as a supplementation in older children. For those children receiving governmental support such as WIC, there is another commercially available instant breakfast product, sold in the cereal section of grocery stores, that provides the same number of calories, vitamins, and minerals when mixed with whole milk. Some families find it more economical to purchase this product and continue to receive the food package from WIC. Detailed protocols for other methods of dietary supplementation have been published elsewhere.[195] The participation of an experienced pediatric nutritionist is critical in developing a dietary regimen appropriate for each child.

Depending on the severity of initial deficit, 2 days to 2 weeks may be required to initiate catch-up growth.[22] Children who are experiencing less severe malnourishment should be monitored frequently as outpatients during this phase. Accelerated growth must then be maintained for 4 to 9 months to restore a child's weight-for-height.[22,194] After initial stabilization and commencement of weight gain, biweekly to monthly outpatient visits for weight checks, adjustment of diet, monitoring of feeding practices and behavior, and treatment of concurrent medical problems are essential. The frequency of these visits depends on the child's age, the severity of the malnutrition, other illnesses, and the psychosocial issues. Intake and rates of growth spontaneously decelerate toward reference levels for age as deficits are replenished. Because weight is restored more rapidly than height, caregivers may become alarmed that the child is becoming overweight. They should be reassured that the catch-up growth in height lags behind that in weight by several months, but balance will occur if dietary treatment is not prematurely terminated.[114,184,199] However, growth and feeding patterns should be monitored closely to ensure that families are not adopting maladaptive patterns that may lead to overweight.

Family Considerations in Treatment

After stabilization of any acute medical problems and nutritional deficits, the next priority revolves around the family. Issues such as unstable housing, financial barriers to food acquisition, child care instability, and intimate partner violence all require urgent attention. Social work support to mobilize community resources is invaluable in addressing these issues. Intervention also includes attention to the family dynamics around food, including mealtime routines and developmentally appropriate expectations and opportunities for children. For example, as infants acquire the ability to pick up food (during months 6–12 after birth), encouraging them to self-feed keeps their attention during meals and builds confidence and competence. Because children learn to eat by modeling from others, family members should eat with children. Mealtime and snack time routines enable children to anticipate when they will be eating and to avoid anxiety associated with hunger. Children need to eat frequently but should not graze or eat continuously throughout the day. Parents are responsible for establishing mealtime routines and determining what and when food will be offered.[200] Children are responsible for determining how much they will eat. When children refuse to eat, parents should calmly terminate the meal rather than engaging in conflict, bribery, or force-feeding and offer another feeding at the next scheduled time (during the day, usually no more than 2.5 hours after the previous feeding).

Eligibility and referral to early intervention or Head Start programs is often indicated to enhance the child's level of cognitive, motor, and social development and to reduce the risk for developmental problems in later life.[201] Children who have developmental disabilities in addition to FTT may be eligible for Supplemental Security Income (SSI) payments, which are frequently higher than those usually provided by Temporary Assistance to Needy Families. However, SSI standards for disability are strict and can be difficult to meet. Impoverished families should receive help in applying for these benefits. Moreover, whenever possible, services that supplement and structure the efforts of the primary caregiver, such as visiting nurses, trained homemakers, or respite child care, can be helpful and should be considered. Various forms of mental health intervention, ranging from behavior modification of feeding problems to medication for a severely depressed parent to multigenerational family therapy, may be needed. Even after nutritional resuscitation has been achieved, families and children should be offered periodic reassessment as the child reaches school age to ensure early identification of behavioral or psychoeducational problems, which may require specialized educational services.

Enhancing Parental Participation in Assessment and Treatment Planning

Parents of children who are failing to thrive may be uncomfortable or even uncooperative with the assessment process and treatment recommendations. There are multiple potential explanations for this, including embarrassment, fear of being blamed, mental illness, unusual beliefs, and concern about CPS, among others. Performing the evaluation in an objective manner without any indication of blame is the first step in partnering with them. It is helpful to assess parental thoughts and beliefs about the etiology, effects, and appropriate treatment of their child. Asking parents about their specific concerns regarding their child's problems may enhance their acceptance of assessment and, eventually, of an intervention plan. In addition, parents are more likely to accept a psychological or behavioral explanation of FTT if it is linked to their child's temperament, behavior, or sensitivities. For example, management of meals, food selection, or caloric requirements can be interpreted as ways that parents can meet their child's special needs.[158] Informing parents that their child may be especially sensitive to stress or events in family life also provides a rationale to evaluate the effect of family routines or parental relationships on the child's growth and nutrition.

Open discussion of alternatives for treatment is usually more productive than engaging in debates about what may have caused FTT. Focusing on what parents can do to help the child in the future, rather than what they may have done in the past, emphasizes the positive opportunity parents now have to help their child.[202] Parents are more likely to accept recommendations for treatment if they feel that their opinions concerning their child's condition and treatment are respected and understood. For this reason, involving parents in the treatment process by asking their opinions, listening to their concerns, and providing opportunity for expression of anger and frustration can be effective. If agreeable to the parents, involving other family members (eg, grandparents, supportive relatives, child care providers) in the assessment and discussion of treatment recommendations can help to mobilize support within the family.

As mentioned previously, video recordings made of mealtimes are often an effective part of the intervention and may facilitate parental involvement in the process. The therapeutic use of video recorded interactions has been effective in promoting interactive behavior with adolescent mothers[203] and caregivers who are intellectually limited or burdened with multiple stressors.[203–206] Repeated video recording becomes familiar to families if it is incorporated into routine clinical evaluation and intervention procedures. One objective of incorporating the recording into intervention is to help parents recognize how important they are to their child and to enhance the value of the child to them. Parents of children with FTT may feel frustrated, guilty, and disappointed with their child's poor growth. These feelings can be exacerbated by medical professionlas who either encourage parents to get more calories into their child without addressing the problems associated with low weight gain or who blame parents when their child does not gain weight. Effective medical professionals look for examples of strengths in the parent-child relationship, including parental responsivity, such as acknowledging the child who looks to the parent for guidance, cues, or reactions. This strategy emphasizes the parent's importance in the partnership and helps the parent develop a sense of efficacy in improving the relationship.

Viewing interaction on video also helps parents see the relationship from the child's perspective. They see how the child communicates internal signals of hunger and satiety and reacts to a smile or to a criticism from the parent. For example, some children signal satiety by throwing food or turning the bowl upside down. Recognizing the child's perspective is a critical step in intervention because it helps parents understand that children are influenced not only by internal regulatory processes but also by the behavior of others. By watching themselves interacting with their child, parents learn to differentiate successful from unsuccessful strategies. Parents serve as their own models and are empowered by identifying strategies that work for them and their child. By practicing newly acquired skills through repeated video-recorded observations, parents learn to analyze interaction patterns and identify aspects of their own behavior that contribute to feeding problems or success in their children. The medical professional helps the parents gain a better understanding of the feeding partnership and how behavior in one partner influences the entire interaction. Parents practice responsive feeding styles with their child with the goal of improving and clarifying their communication so it is not based on feeding problems.

Another technique that may be beneficial is a home visitation program. Studies on their efficacy are somewhat variable, however. They have been shown to have positive effects on behavior at age 8 years.[207] However, other studies have shown conflicting results.[61,91,207–210] Different enrollment criteria, outcome measurements, and duration of the home visitation program all contribute to this variability. Nonetheless, medical professionals should consider this option in communities in which it is available.

Barriers to Treatment

To avoid overburdening families, medical professionals should set treatment priorities in collaboration with parents. Whenever possible, the first priority should be addressing a problem that is salient to parents, if the child's medical condition is amenable to this. In addition, goals for intervention should fit with the family's resources and understanding of the child's problem. Parents of infants with FTT may have difficulty participating actively and productively in their infant's clinical management for several reasons. The suspicion that they may have contributed, however unwittingly, to their infant's growth deficiency is threatening to most parents. In addition, parents may be so preoccupied with personal, family, or financial stresses that they fail to adhere to recommendations for treatment.[61]

Another reason that parents may have difficulty participating is that their concepts of the etiology and appropriate treatment of their child's growth deficiency may differ substantially from those of medical professionals. For example, in contrast with professional concepts that FTT may relate to parental underfeeding or interactional problems, parents often focus on physical or biological explanations of this problem.[81] Sturm and Drotar[202] noted that maternal attributions of the FTT diagnosis included unspecified physical problems or illnesses (47%), specific physical problems (37%), constitutional problems (10%), and child behavior (7%). Maternal perceptions of the physician's diagnosis most often included specific physical problems or growth difficulty rather than family or interactional problems. These findings suggested that mothers understood FTT predominantly as a physical or medical condition and had difficulty acknowledging the potential role of environmental factors. Parental perceptions that their child's FTT reflects physical rather than environmental problems may help to preserve their self-esteem. In addition, the co-occurrence of FTT with other physical symptoms and parental experiences with their child's hospitalization and extensive medical workup may reinforce their perceptions of the physical origins of FTT.

Differences in parent and medical professional concepts of the etiology and treatment of FTT may engender conflict and frustration and disrupt adherence to psychosocial treatment recommendations.[211] For example, parents who believe strongly that their child's growth deficiency is a physical problem may expect a physical, rather than psychosocial, treatment of this problem and may require more explanation and support than parents who are able or willing to acknowledge the relevant environmental factors. For this reason, among others discussed previously, comprehensive, integrated, interdisciplinary treatment is key, rather than segmented treatment that focuses on singular aspects of the problem, such as medical or nutritional, without attention to family or parent-child interactions.[212]

Child Neglect and Involvement of Child Protective Services

Child neglect is one possible cause of FTT and should always be in the differential diagnosis during the evaluation. In addition, medical professionals should consider neglect as a possible explanation when the treatment plan is unsuccessful. Risk factors for neglect include parental history of being abused as a child, substance abuse, mental illness, attachment issues, intimate partner violence, social isolation, and poverty.[213] The presence of these risk factors does not automatically indicate that the FTT is a result of neglect but, rather, indicate a need for further exploration of this possibility.

When FTT and abuse or neglect co-occur, the behavior and developmental consequences for children are more severe than if either condition occurs separately.[211,214] One study found increased risk of subsequent involvement with protective services in children diagnosed with FTT in the first year after birth.[215] Documenting the family's response to intervention, as well as the child's physical, nutritional, and developmental progress, is helpful in decisions about the need to engage CPS. Unless the child's medical condition or evidence of abusive injury demands immediate notification of CPS, medical professionals should first attempt, using the strategies discussed previously in the Enhancing Parental Participation in Assessment and Treatment Planning section, to fully engage parents in the process.

Referral to CPS does not automatically mean that a child with FTT will be removed from the custody of the current caregivers. In some situations, CPS can mobilize additional services to help these families, in addition to providing monitoring of adherence to treatment recommendations. In other situations, though, the child's condition or the family's issues are too severe and the child needs to be placed in protective custody. Situations that merit such a placement include caregivers who are out-of-control substance users, have physically abused the child, have intentionally withheld available food from the child, or are profoundly psychiatrically or cognitively impaired, and when no other competent caregivers are available within the existing family system.[17,214,216,217] When a child is removed from custody, CPS must be informed that the child's weight gain immediately after placement will depend on the child's age, mental health, and eating issues, as well as on the placement.

Placement must be undertaken with great care because suboptimal foster care only worsens FTT.[218] Because children who fail to thrive usually have multiple special needs requiring visits to many different medical professionals as well as specialized dietary, developmental, and medical management at home, foster parents must not be overburdened with the care of many other young children or children with special needs. Foster parents (whether professional or kinship) require the same intensive multidisciplinary support as biological parents to provide adequate care for a child who is failing to thrive. To avoid deterioration of the child with FTT who is placed in foster care, medical professionals should meet face-to-face with prospective alternate caregivers and educate them on the child's dietary and behavioral regimen, medical problems, and emotional needs. Foster parents and kinship caregivers should have a WIC referral, appropriate nutritional supplements, child care equipment, and health insurance before children are placed in their homes. The professional or kinship foster family must be willing to commit to close cooperation with clinic visits and home-based treatment of the child who fails to thrive. Having a CPS worker bring the child to medical care without the foster or kinship caregivers is ineffective because clinical change can be effected only when medical professionals work directly and closely with the child's primary caregivers.

Discharge From Treatment

Children with a history of FTT can be discharged from a specialty clinic when caregivers demonstrate that they can ensure the child receives adequate intake to maintain weight gain once they have restored some, if not all, of the deficit of weight-for-height. This also entails ensuring that the child is medically stable, caregivers understand the child's feeding cues, the family has the necessary resources in place to assist them and the child, and the family agrees to follow up with their primary medical professional for ongoing monitoring. Discharge from a specialty clinic, as well as a return to the normal periodicity of health supervision visits, require that the child displays age-appropriate weight gain on at least 2 assessments and sometimes more, spaced weeks to months apart (depending on the child's age).

Outcomes

Early studies of outcomes showed that children with FTT had delays in physical and intellectual development. Children with FTT have improvement in their physical growth with intervention in most studies.[219]

However, multiple studies have since looked at cognitive outcomes of FTT and have yielded conflicting results.

Children who experience prolonged malnutrition and/or chronic FTT seem to be at risk for intellectual and motor deficits severe enough to affect their learning potential.[40,61,84,220,221] The severity of developmental impairments varies substantially, however, among preschool and school-aged children with histories of early FTT.[7,220–224] Children who have slow weight gain from birth to 9 months of age are more likely to be developmentally delayed as assessed with a Denver Developmental Screening Test at 6 and 18 months, and children with slow growth at earlier ages had a stronger association with the delays.[225] By school age, most children with a history of FTT have experienced growth recovery,[27,212,222,226] but many continue to have overall smaller stature than age-matched peers. However, these children rarely experienced growth deficits severe enough to be classified as wasted or stunted, which are indicators of more severe malnutrition.[27,222]

Studies of cognitive and academic performance of school-aged children with a history of FTT in infancy recruited from primary care or community sites have demonstrated IQ scores that were up to 4.2 points lower than children with a history of adequate growth.[222,226,227] These findings suggest early FTT may have a small, though potentially important, effect on cognitive performance but not the severe deficits implied by earlier studies that evaluated primarily hospitalized children. The Avon Longitudinal Study of Parents and Children demonstrated that children with a history of FTT in infancy, especially between birth and 8 weeks of age, have a persisting deficit in IQ at 8 years old. Data showed that the relationship between early growth and later IQ is actually linear over the whole range of weight velocities.[66,228]

In contrast, when FTT was examined in the general population rather than exclusively low-income families by Belfort and colleagues, no adverse cognitive effects were identified.[229] Corbett and Drewett showed that relatively simple interventions can improve growth outcomes in FTT, but there is no evidence that the cognitive outcomes are also improved.[27] These findings underscore one of the primary reasons for conflicting data on the cognitive outcome of FTT: confounders such as socioeconomic status, parental intelligence, parental education level, and abuse or neglect also play a role in ultimate cognitive outcome. Other factors include age at which the FTT is diagnosed, severity of the malnutrition, types of intervention, and level of follow-up.

Children with FTT are also at risk for deficits in their socioemotional development. Although no one pattern of behavioral disturbance is associated with FTT, deficits in social responsiveness, affect, activity level, and avoidance of social contact have been noted by many observers.[80,84,86,230–235] Polan et al[79] found that children with FTT consistently demonstrated less positive affect in a range of situations than did normally growing children and that acute and chronic malnutrition were associated with heightened negative affect.

Children with early histories of FTT have a higher incidence of insecure attachments characterized by anxious, avoidant, or disorganized behavior than do children with normal patterns of growth.[236–238] Valenzuela[239] suggested that the negative effects of malnutrition on children's reactivity to stress, coupled with the effect of such behaviors on the responsiveness of caregivers, might result in a vicious cycle that could eventually culminate in the development of a behavioral disorder. Controlled studies of children with early histories of FTT are consistent with this hypothesis, in that they suggest a continuing risk to socioemotional development beyond the point of initial diagnosis of FTT.[240] Areas of particular vulnerability among children with early histories of FTT and malnutrition include the ability to contain impulses and to organize their behavior.[5,6,23,89,220,231,241–244] These issues are yet another reason that involvement of a multidisciplinary team is ideal in the evaluation and treatment of children with FTT.

The consequences of FTT may extend into adulthood. Hoddinott et al found that being "stunted" at 2 years of age was associated not only with lower test performance but also a lower household per capita expenditure and increased probability of living in poverty. Women were younger at age of first childbirth and had a higher number of pregnancies. Interestingly, there was little relationship between stunting and adult physical health in this study.[245] A Finnish study found that adults who were born small and showed slower weight gain from 0 to 6 months of age were more hostile as adults. The association was not explained by other confounders in their study.[246]

Therefore, although the literature is somewhat conflicting, FTT during infancy and childhood certainly poses risks for long-term growth and development. This issue needs further study to clarify many of these findings. However, what is clear is that these children deserve close follow-up and early treatment of any identified issues, even after growth rate has been restored.

Conclusion

For children whose growth deviates from the norm, a thorough FTT evaluation is necessary. Rather than using the outdated and overly simplistic "organic versus inorganic" classification scheme, medical professionals must carefully consider medical, psychologic, and social issues and the interplay of each. Partnering with families and having a multidisciplinary approach are keys to a revealing evaluation and effective treatment. Hospitalization may be indicated, and, in some cases, notification of CPS may be necessary. The goal of treatment is not only restoration of typical growth but also helping each child truly thrive, by striving to maximize each child's growth, intellectual capabilities, and emotional development.

References

1. Bithoney WG, Rathbun JM. *Developmental-Behavioral Pediatrics*. Philadelphia, PA: WB Saunders; 1983
2. Karp RJ. *Malnourished Children in the United States: Caught in the Cycle of Poverty*. New York, NY: Springer Publishing Company; 1993
3. Grantham-McGregor S. A review of studies of the effect of severe malnutrition on mental development. *J Nutr*. 1995;125(8)(suppl):2233S–2238S PMID: 7542705 https://doi.org/10.1093/jn/125.suppl_8.2233S
4. World Health Organization. What is malnutrition? http://www.who.int/features/qa/malnutrition/en. Published July 8, 2016. Accessed April 5, 2019
5. Barrett DE, Radke-Yarrow M, Klein RE. Chronic malnutrition and child behavior: effects of early caloric supplementation on social and emotional functioning at school age. *Dev Psychol*. 1982;18(4):541–556 https://doi.org/10.1037/0012-1649.18.4.541
6. Barrett DE, Frank DA. *The Effects of Undernutrition on Children's Behavior*. New York, NY: Gordon Breach; 1987
7. Chase HP, Martin HP. Undernutrition and child development. *N Engl J Med*. 1970;282(17):933–939 PMID: 5436028 https://doi.org/10.1056/NEJM197004232821701
8. Dobbing J. Infant nutrition and later achievement. *Nutr Rev*. 1984;42(1):1–7 PMID: 6199699 https://doi.org/10.1111/j.1753-4887.1984.tb02233.x
9. Drotar D. *Failure to Thrive*. New York, NY: Guilford; 1988
10. Frank DA, Allen D, Brown JL. Primary prevention of failure to thrive: social policy and implications. In: Drotar D, ed. *New Directions in Failure to Thrive*. New York, NY: Plenum Press; 1985 https://doi.org/10.1007/978-1-4684-5095-8_22
11. Bithoney WG, McJunkin J, Michalek J, Snyder J, Egan H, Epstein D. The effect of a multidisciplinary team approach on weight gain in nonorganic failure-to-thrive children. *J Dev Behav Pediatr*. 1991;12(4):254–258 PMID: 1939681 https://doi.org/10.1097/00004703-199108000-00007
12. Al Nofal A, Schwenk WF. Growth failure in children: a symptom or a disease? *Nutr Clin Pract*. 2013;28(6):651–658 PMID: 24170580 https://doi.org/10.1177/0884533613506015
13. American Academy of Pediatrics Committee on Nutrition. *Pediatric Nutrition Handbook*. 5th ed. Elk Grove Village, IL: American Academy of Pediatrics; 2004
14. Centers for Disease Control and Prevention. CDC growth charts: United States. Introduction. https://www.cdc.gov/growthcharts/background.htm. Reviewed August 4, 2009. Accessed April 5, 2019
15. Meyers A, Joyce K, Coleman SM, et al. Health of children classified as underweight by CDC reference but normal by WHO standard. *Pediatrics*. 2013;131(7):e1780–e1787 PMID: 23690515
16. Wright CM. Identification and management of failure to thrive: a community perspective. *Arch Dis Child*. 2000;82(1):5–9 PMID: 10630901 https://doi.org/10.1136/adc.82.1.5
17. Bullard DM Jr, Glaser HH, Heagarty MC, Pivchik EC. Failure to thrive in the "neglected" child. *Am J Orthopsychiatry*. 1967;37(4):680–690 PMID: 6033422 https://doi.org/10.1111/j.1939-0025.1967.tb00509.x

18. Coleman RW, Provence S. Environmental retardation (hospitalism) in infants living in families. *Pediatrics*. 1957;19(2):285–292 PMID: 13400604
19. Goldbloom RB. Failure to thrive. *Pediatr Clin North Am*. 1982;29(1):151–166 PMID: 6276853 https://doi.org/10.1016/S0031-3955(16)34114-1
20. Sills RH. Failure to thrive. The role of clinical and laboratory evaluation. *Am J Dis Child*. 1978;132(10):967–969 PMID: 717305 https://doi.org/10.1001/archpedi.1978.02120350031003
21. Frank DA, Zeisel SH. Failure to thrive. *Pediatr Clin North Am*. 1988;35(6):1187–1206 PMID: 3059294 https://doi.org/10.1016/S0031-3955(16)36578-6
22. Casey PH, Arnold WC. Compensatory growth in infants with severe failure to thrive. *South Med J*. 1985;78(9):1057–1060 PMID: 4035431 https://doi.org/10.1097/00007611-198509000-00008
23. Frank DA. Malnutrition and child behavior: a view from the bedside. In: Brozek P, ed. *Malnutrition and Behavior*. Lausanne, Switzerland: Nestle Foundation; 1984
24. Whitten CF, Pettit MG, Fischhoff J. Evidence that growth failure from maternal deprivation is secondary to undereating. *JAMA*. 1969;209(11):1675–1682 PMID: 5820163 https://doi.org/10.1001/jama.1969.03160240031007
25. Casey PH. Failure to thrive. In: Levine M, Carey W, Crocker A, eds. *Developmental Behavioral Pediatrics*. Vol 2. Philadelphia, PA: WB Saunders; 1992:375–383
26. Wright CM, Matthews JNS, Waterston A, Aynsley-Green A. What is a normal rate of weight gain in infancy? *Acta Paediatr*. 1994;83(4):351–356 PMID: 8025388 https://doi.org/10.1111/j.1651-2227.1994.tb18118.x
27. Corbett SS, Drewett RF. To what extent is failure to thrive in infancy associated with poorer cognitive development? A review and meta-analysis. *Journal of Child Psychology and Psychiatry*. 2004;45(3):641–654 PMID: 15055382
28. Homan GJ. Failure to thrive: a practical guide. *Am Fam Physician*. 2016;94(4):295–299 PMID: 27548594
29. Cole SZ, Lanham JS. Failure to thrive: an update. *Am Fam Physician*. 2011;83(7):829–834 PMID: 21524049
30. Larson-Nath CM, Goday PS. Failure to thrive: a prospective study in a pediatric gastroenterology clinic. *J Pediatr Gastroenterol Nutr*. 2016;62(6):907–913 PMID: 26720767
31. Daniel M, Kleis L, Cemeroglu AP. Etiology of failure to thrive in infants and toddlers referred to a pediatric endocrinology outpatient clinic. *Clin Pediatr (Phila)*. 2008;47(8):762–765 PMID: 18467671 https://doi.org/10.1177/0009922808316989
32. McDougall P, Drewett RF, Hungin AP, Wright CM. The detection of early weight faltering at the 6-8-week check and its association with family factors, feeding and behavioural development. *Arch Dis Child*. 2009;94(7):549–552 PMID: 19052031 https://doi.org/10.1136/adc.2008.139063
33. Olsen EM, Skovgaard AM, Weile B, Petersen J, Jørgensen T. Risk factors for weight faltering in infancy according to age at onset. *Paediatr Perinat Epidemiol*. 2010;24(4):370–382 PMID: 20618727
34. Jones DY, Nesheim MC, Habicht JP. Influences in child growth associated with poverty in the 1970's: an examination of HANESI and HANESII, cross-sectional US national surveys. *Am J Clin Nutr*. 1985;42(4):714–724 PMID: 4050732 https://doi.org/10.1093/ajcn/42.4.714
35. Brown JL, Pizer HF. *Living Hungry in America*. New York, NY: Macmillan; 1987
36. Garza C, de Onis M. Rationale for developing a new international growth reference. *Food Nutr Bull*. 2004;25(1)(suppl):S5–S14 PMID: 15069915 https://doi.org/10.1177/15648265040251S102

37. US Department of Health and Human Services, Office of the Assistant Secretary for Planning and Evaluation. Poverty guidelines. https://aspe.hhs.gov/poverty-guidelines. Revised January 11, 2019. Accessed May 31, 2019
38. US Census Bureau. Poverty. https://www.census.gov/topics/income-poverty/poverty.html. Accessed April 5, 2019
39. Dalaker J, Naifeh M. Poverty in the United States: 1997. Washington, DC: US Government Printing Office; 1998. Current Population Reports, Series P60–201
40. Silver J, DiLorenzo P, Zukoski M, Ross PE, Amster BJ, Schlegel D. Starting young: improving the health and developmental outcomes of infants and toddlers in the child welfare system. *Child Welfare*. 1999;78(1):148–165 PMID: 9919642
41. Blumberg SJ, Bialostosky K, Hamilton WL, Briefel RR. The effectiveness of a short form of the Household Food Security Scale. *Am J Public Health*. 1999;89(8):1231–1234 PMID: 10432912 https://doi.org/10.2105/AJPH.89.8.1231
42. Bickel G, Carlson S, Nord M. *Household Food Security in the United States, 1995–1998*. Washington, DC: US Department of Agriculture Food and Nutrition Services and Economic Research Service; 1999
43. Wehler C. *Community Childhood Hunger Identification Project: A Survey of Childhood Hunger in the United States*. Washington, DC: Food Action Research Center; 1991
44. Breen AB, Cahill R, de Cuba SE, Cook J, Chilton M. The Real Cost of a Healthy Diet: 2011. Philadelphia, PA: Center for Hunger-Free Communities; 2011. http://www.centerforhungerfreecommunities.org/sites/default/files/pdfs/RCOHD_Report2011-FINAL.pdf. Accessed April 5, 2019
45. Cook JT, Frank DA, Levenson SM, et al. Child food insecurity increases risks posed by household food insecurity to young children's health. *J Nutr*. 2006;136(4):1073–1076 PMID: 16549481 https://doi.org/10.1093/jn/136.4.1073
46. Jyoti DF, Frongillo EA, Jones SJ. Food insecurity affects school children's academic performance, weight gain, and social skills. *J Nutr*. 2005;135(12):2831–2839 PMID: 16317128 https://doi.org/10.1093/jn/135.12.2831
47. Huston AC, McLoyd VC, Coll CG. Children and poverty: issues in contemporary research. *Child Dev*. 1994;65(2):275–282 PMID: 7516847 https://doi.org/10.1111/j.1467-8624.1994.tb00750.x
48. Katon W, Kleinman A. Doctor-patient negotiation and other social science strategies in patient care. In: Eisenberg L, Kleinman A, eds. *The Relevance of Social Science for Medicine*. Dordrecht, Holland: Reidel Press; 1981 https://doi.org/10.1007/978-94-009-8379-3_12
49. Center on Budget and Policy Priorities. *WIC Newsletter 1991*. 1992; Vol. 12
50. Garbarino J. The stress of being a poor child in America. *Child Adolesc Psychiatr Clin N Am*. 1998;7(1):105–119, ix PMID: 9894082 https://doi.org/10.1016/S1056-4993(18)30262-1
51. Wiecha JL, Palombo R. Multiple program participation: comparison of nutrition and food assistance program benefits with food costs in Boston, Massachusetts. *Am J Public Health*. 1989;79(5):591–594 PMID: 2705593 https://doi.org/10.2105/AJPH.79.5.591
52. Primus W, Rawlings L, Larin K. *The Initial Impacts of Welfare Reform on the Incomes of Single-Mother Families*. Washington, DC: Center on Budget and Policy Priorities; 1999
53. Kramer-LeBlanc CS, Mardis A, Gerrior S. *Review of the Nutritional Status of WIC Participants*. Washington, DC: USDA Center for Nutrition Policy and Promotion; 1999
54. Castner L, Rosso R. Characteristics of Food Stamp Households: Fiscal Year 1998. *Report Submitted to the US Department of Agriculture*. Washington, DC: Mathematica Policy Research, Inc; 2000. https://fns-prod.azureedge.net/sites/default/files/char98.pdf. Accessed April 5, 2019

55. Garbarino J, Sherman D. High-risk neighborhoods and high-risk families: the human ecology of child maltreatment. *Child Dev*. 1980;51(1):188–198 PMID: 7363733 https://doi.org/10.2307/1129606
56. Kotelchuck M. Nonorganic failure to thrive: the status of interactional and environmental theories. In: Camp B, ed. *Advances in Behavioral Pediatrics*. Greenwich, UK: Jai Press; 1980
57. Kotelchuck M, Newberger EH. Failure to thrive: a controlled study of familial characteristics. *J Am Acad Child Psychiatry*. 1983;22(4):322–328 PMID: 6875125 https://doi.org/10.1016/S0002-7138(09)60666-X
58. Bithoney WG, Newberger EH. Child and family attributes of failure-to-thrive. *J Dev Behav Pediatr*. 1987;8(1):32–36 PMID: 3818963 https://doi.org/10.1097/00004703-198702000-00007
59. Kanawati AA, McLaren DS. Failure to thrive, in Lebanon. II. An investigation of the causes. *Acta Paediatr Scand*. 1973;62(6):571–576 PMID: 4203100 https://doi.org/10.1111/j.1651-2227.1973.tb17067.x
60. Skuse D, Reilly S, Wolke D. Psychosocial adversity and growth during infancy. *Eur J Clin Nutr*. 1994;48(suppl 1):S113–S130 PMID: 8005080
61. Drotar D, Eckerle D. The family environment in nonorganic failure to thrive: a controlled study. *J Pediatr Psychol*. 1989;14(2):245–257 PMID: 2754575 https://doi.org/10.1093/jpepsy/14.2.245
62. Drotar D, Sturm LA. Parental influences in nonorganic failure to thrive: implications for management. *Int Ment Health J*. 1987;8:37–45
63. Atalay A, McCord M. Characteristics of failure to thrive in a referral population: implications for treatment. *Clin Pediatr (Phila)*. 2012;51(3):219–225 PMID: 21997145 https://doi.org/10.1177/0009922811421001
64. Mash C, Frazier T, Nowacki A, Worley S, Goldfarb J. Development of a risk-stratification tool for medical child abuse in failure to thrive. *Pediatrics*. 2011;128(6):e1467–e1473 PMID: 22123876 https://doi.org/10.1542/peds.2011-1080
65. Emond A, Drewett R, Blair P, Emmett P. Postnatal factors associated with failure to thrive in term infants in the Avon Longitudinal Study of Parents and Children. *Arch Dis Child*. 2007;92(2):115–119 PMID: 16905563 https://doi.org/10.1136/adc.2005.091496
66. Wright CM, Parkinson KN, Drewett RF. How does maternal and child feeding behavior relate to weight gain and failure to thrive? Data from a prospective birth cohort. *Pediatrics*. 2006;117(4):1262–1269 PMID: 16585323 https://doi.org/10.1542/peds.2005-1215
67. Mathisen B, Skuse D, Wolke D, Reilly S. Oral-motor dysfunction and failure to thrive among inner-city infants. *Dev Med Child Neurol*. 1989;31(3):293–302 PMID: 2753237 https://doi.org/10.1111/j.1469-8749.1989.tb03998.x
68. Yi SH, Joung YS, Choe YH, Kim EH, Kwon JY. Sensory processing difficulties in toddlers with nonorganic failure-to-thrive and feeding problems. *J Pediatr Gastroenterol Nutr*. 2015;60(6):819–824 PMID: 25564810
69. Kelly C, Ricciardelli LA, Clarke JD. Problem eating attitudes and behaviors in young children. *Int J Eat Disord*. 1999;25(3):281–286 PMID: 10191992 https://doi.org/10.1002/(SICI)1098-108X(199904)25:3<281::AID-EAT5>3.0.CO;2-T
70. Singer LT, Song LY, Hill BP, Jaffe AC. Stress and depression in mothers of failure-to-thrive children. *J Pediatr Psychol*. 1990;15(6):711–720 PMID: 2283576 https://doi.org/10.1093/jpepsy/15.6.711
71. Black MM, Hutcheson JJ, Dubowitz H, Starr RH, Berenson-Howard J. The roots of competence: mother-child interaction among low income, urban, African American families. *Appl Dev Psychol*. 1996;17(3):367–391 https://doi.org/10.1016/S0193-3973(96)90032-5

72. Wolke D, Skuse D, Mathisen B. Behavioral style in failure-to-thrive infants: a preliminary communication. *J Pediatr Psychol*. 1990;15(2):237–254 PMID: 2374078 https://doi.org/10.1093/jpepsy/15.2.237
73. Pollitt E, Leibel R. Biological and social correlates of failure to thrive. In: Greene L, Johnson E, eds. *Social and Biological Predictions of Nutritional Status, Physical Growth, and Neurological Development*. New York, NY: Academic Press; 1980
74. Reilly SM, Skuse DH, Wolke D, Stevenson J. Oral-motor dysfunction in children who fail to thrive: organic or non-organic? *Dev Med Child Neurol*. 1999;41(2):115–122 PMID: 10075097 https://doi.org/10.1017/S0012162299000225
75. Riordan MM, Iwata BA, Wohl MK, Finney JW. Behavioral treatment of food refusal and selectivity in developmentally disabled children. *Appl Res Ment Retard*. 1980;1(1-2):95–112 PMID: 6175281 https://doi.org/10.1016/0270-3092(80)90019-3
76. Shapiro V, Fraiberg S, Adelson E. Infant-parent psychotherapy on behalf of a child in a critical nutritional state. *Psychoanal Study Child*. 1976;31(1):461–491 PMID: 981450 https://doi.org/10.1080/00797308.1976.11822325
77. Elmer E. Failure to thrive: role of the mother. *Pediatrics*. 1960;25:717–725 PMID: 13820080
78. Benoit D, Zeanah CH, Barton ML. Maternal attachment disturbance in failure to thrive. *Infant Ment Health J*. 1989;10(3):185–202 https://doi.org/10.1002/1097-0355(198923)10:3<185::AID-IMHJ2280100306>3.0.CO;2-0
79. Polan HJ, Leon A, Kaplan MD, Kessler DB, Stern DN, Ward MJ. Disturbances of affect expression in failure-to-thrive. *J Am Acad Child Adolesc Psychiatry*. 1991;30(6):897–903 PMID: 1757438 https://doi.org/10.1097/00004583-199111000-00006
80. Pollitt E, Eichler AW, Chan CK. Psychosocial development and behavior of mothers of failure-to-thrive children. *Am J Orthopsychiatry*. 1975;45(4):525–537 PMID: 1180336 https://doi.org/10.1111/j.1939-0025.1975.tb01183.x
81. Hutcheson JJ, Black MM, Talley M, et al. Risk status and home intervention among children with failure-to-thrive: follow-up at age 4. *J Pediatr Psychol*. 1997;22(5):651–668 PMID: 9383928 https://doi.org/10.1093/jpepsy/22.5.651
82. Altemeier WA III, O'Connor SM, Sherrod KB, Vietze PM. Prospective study of antecedents for nonorganic failure to thrive. *J Pediatr*. 1985;106(3):360–365 PMID: 3973773 https://doi.org/10.1016/S0022-3476(85)80657-0
83. Weston JA, Colloton M, Halsey S, et al. A legacy of violence in nonorganic failure to thrive. *Child Abuse Negl*. 1993;17(6):709–714 PMID: 8287284 https://doi.org/10.1016/S0145-2134(08)80002-6
84. Drotar D, Eckerle D, Satola J, Pallotta J, Wyatt B. Maternal interactional behavior with nonorganic failure-to-thrive infants: a case comparison study. *Child Abuse Negl*. 1990;14(1):41–51 PMID:2310972 https://doi.org/10.1016/0145-2134(90)90079-9
85. Drotar D, Sturm LA. The role of parent-practitioner communication in the management of non-organic failure to thrive. *Fam Syst Med*. 1988;6(3):42–51 https://doi.org/10.1037/h0089746
86. Powell GF, Low JF, Speers MA. Behavior as a diagnostic aid in failure-to-thrive. *J Dev Behav Pediatr*. 1987;8(1):18–24 PMID: 3818960 https://doi.org/10.1097/00004703-198702000-00005
87. Ramey CT. Nutrition, response-contingent stimulation and the maternal deprivation syndrome: results of an early intervention program. *Mer Palm Q*. 1975;21:45–53
88. Chatoor I. Feeding and eating disorders of infancy and early childhood. In: *Comprehensive Textbook of Psychiatry*. Vol VII. Baltimore, MD: Williams and Wilkins; 2000:2704–2710
89. Robertson J, Puckering C, Parkinson K, Corlett L, Wright C. Mother-child feeding interactions in children with and without weight faltering; nested case control study. *Appetite*. 2011;56(3):753–759 PMID: 21396417 https://doi.org/10.1016/j.appet.2011.02.016

90. Faith MS, Scanlon KS, Birch LL, Francis LA, Sherry B. Parent-child feeding strategies and their relationships to child eating and weight status. *Obes Res*. 2004;12(11):1711–1722 PMID: 15601964 https://doi.org/10.1038/oby.2004.212
91. Black MM, Hutcheson JJ, Dubowitz H, Berenson-Howard J. Parenting style and developmental status among children with nonorganic failure to thrive. *J Pediatr Psychol*. 1994;19(6):689–707 PMID: 7830212 https://doi.org/10.1093/jpepsy/19.6.689
92. Hutcheson JJ, Black MM, Starr RH Jr. Developmental differences in interactional characteristics of mothers and their children with failure to thrive. *J Pediatr Psychol*. 1993;18(4):453–466 PMID: 7692030 https://doi.org/10.1093/jpepsy/18.4.453
93. Robinson JR, Drotar D, Boutry M. Problem-solving abilities among mothers of infants with failure to thrive. *J Pediatr Psychol*. 2001;26(1):21–32 PMID: 11145729 https://doi.org/10.1093/jpepsy/26.1.21
94. Lewinsohn PM, Holm-Denoma JM, Gau JM, et al. Problematic eating and feeding behaviors of 36-month-old children. *Int J Eat Disord*. 2005;38(3):208–219 PMID:16211627 https://doi.org/10.1002/eat.20175
95. American Academy of Pediatrics Committee on Nutrition. Failure to thrive. In: Kleinman R, Greer F, eds. *Pediatric Nutrition*. 7th ed. Elk Grove Village, IL: American Academy of Pediatrics; 2014
96. Shaheen E, Alexander D, Truskowsky M, Barbero GJ. Failure to thrive—a retrospective profile. *Clin Pediatr (Phila)*. 1968;7(5):255–261 PMID: 5648331 https://doi.org/10.1177/000992286800700505
97. Hawford JT. Growth problems in children: an approach to evaluation and therapy. In: Moss A, ed. *Pediatric Update*. New York, NY: Elsevier; 1979
98. Oates RK, Yu JS. Children with non-organic failure to thrive. A community problem. *Med J Aust*. 1971;2(4):199–203 PMID: 5093862
99. Hanson JW, Smith DW. The fetal hydantoin syndrome. *J Pediatr*. 1975;87(2):285–290 PMID: 50428 https://doi.org/10.1016/S0022-3476(75)80604-4
100. Als H, Tronick E, Adamson L, Brazelton TB. The behavior of the full-term but underweight newborn infant. *Dev Med Child Neurol*. 1976;18(5):590–602 PMID: 976613 https://doi.org/10.1111/j.1469-8749.1976.tb04205.x
101. Villar J, Smeriglio V, Martorell R, Brown CH, Klein RE. Heterogeneous growth and mental development of intrauterine growth-retarded infants during the first 3 years of life. *Pediatrics*. 1984;74(5):783–791 PMID:6493873
102. Hediger ML, Overpeck MD, Maurer KR, Kuczmarski RJ, McGlynn A, Davis WW. Growth of infants and young children born small or large for gestational age: findings from the Third National Health and Nutrition Examination Survey. *Arch Pediatr Adolesc Med*. 1998;152(12):1225–1231 PMID: 9856434 https://doi.org/10.1001/archpedi.152.12.1225
103. Ounsted M, Moar V, Scott A. Growth in the first four years: II. Diversity within groups of small-for-dates and large-for-dates babies. *Early Hum Dev*. 1982;7(1):29–39 PMID: 7173098 https://doi.org/10.1016/0378-3782(82)90005-6
104. Rogol AD, Hayden GF. Etiologies and early diagnosis of short stature and growth failure in children and adolescents. *J Pediatr*. 2014;164(5 Suppl):S1–S14.e6 PMID: 24731744
105. Frank DA, Wong F. Effects of prenatal exposures to alcohol, tobacco, and other drugs. In: Kessler D, Dawson P, eds. *Failure to Thrive and Pediatric Under-nutrition: A Transdisciplinary Approach*. Baltimore, MD: Paul H. Brookes Publishing; 1999
106. Brandt I. Growth dynamics of low birthweight infants with emphasis on the prenatal period. In: Falkner F, Tanner J, eds. *Human Growth, Neurobiology and Nutrition*. New York, NY: Plenum Press; 1979
107. Casey PH, Kraemer HC, Bernbaum J, Yogman MW, Sells JC. Growth status and growth rates of a varied sample of low birth weight, preterm infants: a longitudinal cohort

from birth to three years of age. *J Pediatr*. 1991;119(4):599–605 PMID: 1919893 https://doi.org/10.1016/S0022-3476(05)82414-X

108. Karniski W, Blair C, Vitucci JS. The illusion of catch-up growth in premature infants. Use of the growth index and age correction. *Am J Dis Child*. 1987;141(5):520–526 PMID: 3578164 https://doi.org/10.1001/archpedi.1987.04460050062031
109. Georgieff MK, Mills MM, Zempel CE, Chang PN. Catch-up growth, muscle and fat accretion, and body proportionality of infants one year after newborn intensive care. *J Pediatr*. 1989;114(2):288–292 PMID: 2915289 https://doi.org/10.1016/S0022-3476(89)80799-1
110. Nieman L. Follow up nutrition after discharge from the neonatal intensive care unit. *Building Block for Life*. 2006;29:1–8
111. Kappy MS. Regulation of growth in children with chronic illness. Therapeutic implications for the year 2000. *Am J Dis Child*. 1987;141(5):489–493 PMID: 3578158 https://doi.org/10.1001/archpedi.1987.04460050031025
112. Phillip M, Hershkovitz E, Rosenblum H, et al. Serum insulin-like growth factors I and II are not affected by undernutrition in children with nonorganic failure to thrive. *Horm Res*. 1998;49(2):76–79 PMID: 9485175 https://doi.org/10.1159/000023130
113. Fryer GE Jr. The efficacy of hospitalization of nonorganic failure-to-thrive children: a meta-analysis. *Child Abuse Negl*. 1988;12(3):375–381 PMID: 3048580 https://doi.org/10.1016/0145-2134(88)90050-6
114. Bithoney WG, McJunkin J, Michalek J, Egan H, Snyder J, Munier A. Prospective evaluation of weight gain in both nonorganic and organic failure-to-thrive children: an outpatient trial of a multidisciplinary team intervention strategy. *J Dev Behav Pediatr*. 1989;10(1):27–31 PMID: 2925865 https://doi.org/10.1097/00004703-198902000-00006
115. Berwick DM, Levy JC, Kleinerman R. Failure to thrive: diagnostic yield of hospitalisation. *Arch Dis Child*. 1982;57(5):347–351 PMID: 6807215 https://doi.org/10.1136/adc.57.5.347
116. Fleisher DR. Comprehensive management of infants with gastroesophageal reflux and failure to thrive. *Curr Probl Pediatr*. 1995;25(8):247–253 PMID: 8529429 https://doi.org/10.1016/S0045-9380(06)80020-4
117. Herr TM, Cook PR, Highfill G. In vitro testing in pediatric food allergy. *Otolaryngol Head Neck Surg*. 1999;120(2):233–237 PMID: 9949358 https://doi.org/10.1016/S0194-5998(99)70412-2
118. Homer C, Ludwig S. Categorization of etiology of failure to thrive. *Am J Dis Child*. 1981;135(9):848–851 PMID: 7282664 https://doi.org/10.1001/archpedi.1981.02130330058019
119. Sullivan PB. Nutritional management of acute diarrhea. *Nutrition*. 1998;14(10):758–762 PMID: 9785356 https://doi.org/10.1016/S0899-9007(98)00078-1
120. Gupta MC, Urrutia JJ. Effect of periodic antiascaris and antigiardia treatment on nutritional status of preschool children. *Am J Clin Nutr*. 1982;36(1):79–86 PMID: 7091037 https://doi.org/10.1093/ajcn/36.1.79
121. Roesler TA, Barry P, Bock SA. Exposure to passive cigarette smoking and child development. *Ann N Y Acad Sci*. 1994;148:1150–1155
122. Hattevig G, Sigurs N, Kjellman B. Effects of maternal dietary avoidance during lactation on allergy in children at 10 years of age. *Acta Paediatr*. 1999;88(1):7–12 PMID: 10090539 https://doi.org/10.1111/j.1651-2227.1999.tb01259.x
123. James JM, Burks AW. Food hypersensitivity in children. *Curr Opin Pediatr*. 1994;6(6): 661–667 PMID: 7849811 https://doi.org/10.1097/00008480-199412000-00009
124. Kulig M, Bergmann R, Niggemann B, Burow G, Wahn U. Prediction of sensitization to inhalant allergens in childhood: evaluating family history, atopic dermatitis and sensitization to food allergens. The MAS Study Group. Multicentre Allergy Study. *Clin Exp Allergy*. 1998;28(11):1397–1403 PMID: 9824413 https://doi.org/10.1046/j.1365-2222.1998.00439.x

125. Kaila M, Salo MK, Isolauri E. Fatty acids in substitute formulas for cow's milk allergy. *Allergy*. 1999;54(1):74–77 https://doi.org/10.1034/j.1398-9995.1999.00816.x
126. Niggemann B, Sielaff B, Beyer K, Binder C, Wahn U. Outcome of double-blind, placebo-controlled food challenge tests in 107 children with atopic dermatitis. *Clin Exp Allergy*. 1999;29(1):91–96 PMID: 10051707 https://doi.org/10.1046/j.1365-2222.1999.00454.x
127. Järvinen KM, Juntunen-Backman K, Suomalainen H. Relation between weak HLA-DR expression on human breast milk macrophages and cow milk allergy (CMA) in suckling infants. *Pediatr Res*. 1999;45(1):76–81 PMID: 9890612 https://doi.org/10.1203/00006450-199901000-00013
128. Krämer U, Heinrich J, Wjst M, Wichmann HE. Age of entry to day nursery and allergy in later childhood. *Lancet*. 1999;353(9151):450–454 PMID: 9989715 https://doi.org/10.1016/S0140-6736(98)06329-6
129. Salvioli GP, Faldella G, Alessandroni R, Marchiani E, Grandolfo ME, Novello F. Prevention of allergies of infants: breast-feeding and special formulas. Influence on the response to immunization. *Acta Biomed Ateneo Parmense*. 1997;68(suppl 1):21–27 PMID: 10021713
130. Barbour SD. Acquired immunodeficiency syndrome of childhood. *Pediatr Clin North Am*. 1987;34(1):247–268 PMID: 3543826 https://doi.org/10.1016/S0031-3955(16)36192-2
131. American Academy of Pediatrics Committee on Infectious Diseases. *Red Book: 2006 Report of the Committee on Infectious Diseases*. 27th ed. Elk Grove Village, IL: American Academy of Pediatrics; 2006:405–410
132. Chevalier P, Sevilla R, Sejas E, Zalles L, Belmonte G, Parent G. Immune recovery of malnourished children takes longer than nutritional recovery: implications for treatment and discharge. *J Trop Pediatr*. 1998;44(5):304–307 PMID: 9819496 https://doi.org/10.1093/tropej/44.5.304
133. McLaren DS. Vitamin A deficiency disorders. *J Indian Med Assoc*. 1999;97(8):320–323 PMID: 10643184
134. Mitchell WG, Gorrell RW, Greenberg RA. Failure-to-thrive: a study in a primary care setting. Epidemiology and follow-up. *Pediatrics*. 1980;65(5):971–977 PMID: 7367142
135. Suskind RM. Malnutrition and the immune response. In: Suskind R, ed. *Textbook of Pediatric Nutrition*. New York, NY: Raven Press; 1981
136. Waterlow JC. Classification and definition of protein-calorie malnutrition. *BMJ*. 1972;3(5826):566–569 PMID: 4627051 https://doi.org/10.1136/bmj.3.5826.566
137. Schwartz J, Angle C, Pitcher H. Relationship between childhood blood lead levels and stature. *Pediatrics*. 1986;77(3):281–288 PMID: 3951909
138. Mahaffey KR, Annest JL, Roberts J, Murphy RS. National estimates of blood lead levels: United States, 1976-1980: association with selected demographic and socioeconomic factors. *N Engl J Med*. 1982;307(10):573–579 PMID: 7110203 https://doi.org/10.1056/NEJM198209023071001
139. Centers for Disease Control and Prevention. *Preventing Lead Poisoning in Young Children: A Statement by the Centers for Disease Control and Prevention*. Atlanta, GA: US Department of Health and Human Services; 1991
140. Bithoney WG. Elevated lead levels in children with nonorganic failure to thrive. *Pediatrics*. 1986;78(5):891–895 PMID: 2429250
141. Linscheid TR. Disturbances of eating and feeding. In: Magrab P, ed. *Psychological Management of Pediatric Problems*. Baltimore, MD: University Park Press; 1978
142. Linscheid TR, Rasnake LK. Behavioral approaches to the treatment of failure to thrive. In: Drotar D, ed. *New Directions in Failure to Thrive: Implications for Research and Practice*. New York, NY: Plenum Press; 1985 https://doi.org/10.1007/978-1-4684-5095-8_18

143. McJunkin JE, Bithoney WG, McCormick MC. Errors in formula concentration in an outpatient population. *J Pediatr*. 1987;111(6 Pt 1):848–850 PMID: 3681549 https://doi.org/10.1016/S0022-3476(87)80201-9
144. Faine MP, Oberg D. Snacking and oral health habits of Washington state WIC children and their caregivers. *ASDC J Dent Child*. 1994;61(5-6):350–355 PMID: 7897005
145. Siener K, Rothman D, Farrar J. Soft drink logos on baby bottles: do they influence what is fed to children? *ASDC J Dent Child*. 1997;64(1):55–60 PMID: 9096820
146. Sherman A. *Extreme Child Poverty Rises Sharply in 1997*. Washington, DC: Children's Defense Fund; 1999
147. Pugliese MT, Weyman-Daum M, Moses N, Lifshitz F. Parental health beliefs as a cause of nonorganic failure to thrive. *Pediatrics*. 1987;80(2):175–182 PMID: 3615087
148. Cole CR, Rising R, Lifshitz F. Consequences of incomplete carbohydrate absorption from fruit juice consumption in infants. *Arch Pediatr Adolesc Med*. 1999;153(10):1098–1102 PMID: 10520620 https://doi.org/10.1001/archpedi.153.10.1098
149. Smith MM, Lifshitz F. Excess fruit juice consumption as a contributing factor in nonorganic failure to thrive. *Pediatrics*. 1994;93(3):438–443 PMID: 8115203
150. Maldonado J, Gil A, Narbona E, Molina JA. Special formulas in infant nutrition: a review. *Early Hum Dev*. 1998;53(suppl):S23–S32 PMID: 10102652 https://doi.org/10.1016/S0378-3782(98)00062-0
151. Kaplowitz P, Webb J. Diagnostic evaluation of short children with height 3 SD or more below the mean. *Clin Pediatr (Phila)*. 1994;33(9):530–535 PMID: 8001321 https://doi.org/10.1177/000992289403300904
152. Hillemeier AC. Gastroesophageal reflux. Diagnostic and therapeutic approaches. *Pediatr Clin North Am*. 1996;43(1):197–212 PMID: 8596680 https://doi.org/10.1016/S0031-3955(05)70402-8
153. Frisancho AR, Cole PE, Klayman JE. Greater contribution to secular trend among offspring of short parents. *Hum Biol*. 1977;49(1):51–60 PMID: 844841
154. Fraiberg S, Adelson E, Shapiro V. Ghosts in the nursery. A psychoanalytic approach to the problems of impaired infant-mother relationships. *J Am Acad Child Psychiatry*. 1975;14(3):387–421 PMID: 1141566 https://doi.org/10.1016/S0002-7138(09)61442-4
155. Lansky SB, Stephenson L, Weller E, Cairns GF Jr, Cairns NU. Failure to thrive during infancy in siblings of pediatric cancer patients. *Am J Pediatr Hematol Oncol*. 1982;4(4):361–366 PMID: 6820237 https://doi.org/10.1097/00043426-198224000-00002
156. Agras S, Hammer L, McNicholas F. A prospective study of the influence of eating-disordered mothers on their children. *Int J Eat Disord*. 1999;25(3):253–262 PMID: 10191989 https://doi.org/10.1002/(SICI)1098-108X(199904)25:3<253:AID-EAT2>3.0.CO;2-Z
157. Russell GF, Treasure J, Eisler I. Mothers with anorexia nervosa who underfeed their children: their recognition and management. *Psychol Med*. 1998;28(1):93–108 PMID: 9483686 https://doi.org/10.1017/S003329179700603X
158. Drotar D, Wilson F, Sturm LA. Parent intervention in failure to thrive. In: Schaefer C, Briesmeister J, eds. *Handbook of Parent Training: Parents as Cotherapists for Children's Behavioral Problems*. New York, NY: Wiley; 1989
159. Costanzo PR, Woody EZ. Domain-specific parenting styles and their impact on child's development of particular deviance: the example of obesity. *J Soc Clin Psychol*. 1985;3(4):425–445 https://doi.org/10.1521/jscp.1985.3.4.425
160. Ayoub CC, Milner JS. Failure to thrive: parental indicators, types, and outcomes. *Child Abuse Negl*. 1985;9(4):491–499 PMID: 4084828 https://doi.org/10.1016/0145-2134(85)90058-4
161. Alfasi G. A failure-to-thrive infant at play: applications of microanalysis. *J Pediatr Psychol*. 1982;7(2):111–123 PMID: 7108691 https://doi.org/10.1093/jpepsy/7.2.111

162. Polan HJ, Ward MJ. Role of the mother's touch in failure to thrive: a preliminary investigation. *J Am Acad Child Adolesc Psychiatry*. 1994;33(8):1098–1105 PMID: 7982860 https://doi.org/10.1097/00004583-199410000-00005
163. Casey PH. Failure to thrive: a reconceptualization. *J Dev Behav Pediatr*. 1983;4(1):63–66 PMID: 6187776 https://doi.org/10.1097/00004703-198303000-00012
164. Ramey CT, Hieger L, Klisz D. Synchronous reinforcement of vocal responses in failure-to-thrive infants. *Child Dev*. 1972;43(4):1449–1455 PMID: 4643780 https://doi.org/10.2307/1127533
165. Drotar D, Malone CA, Negray J. Intellectual assessment of young children with environmentally based failure to thrive. *Child Abuse Negl*. 1980;4(1):23–31 https://doi.org/10.1016/0145-2134(80)90030-7
166. Ross ES, Krebs NF, Shroyer AL, Dickinson LM, Barrett PH, Johnson SL. Early growth faltering in healthy term infants predicts longitudinal growth. *Early Hum Dev*. 2009;85(9):583–588 PMID: 19608359 https://doi.org/10.1016/j.earlhumdev.2009.06.004
167. Lowen D. Failure to thrive. In: Jenny C, ed. *Child Abuse and Neglect: Diagnosis, Treatment and Evidence*. 1st ed. St Louis, MO: Saunders, Elsevier; 2011:547–562
168. Solomons NW. Assessment of nutritional status: functional indicators of pediatric nutriture. *Pediatr Clin North Am*. 1985;32(2):319–334 PMID: 3887303 https://doi.org/10.1016/S0031-3955(16)34789-7
169. Graitcer PL, Gentry EM. Measuring children: one reference for all. *Lancet*. 1981;2(8241):297–299 PMID: 6114335 https://doi.org/10.1016/S0140-6736(81)90538-9
170. World Health Organization. The WHO child growth standards. http://www.who.int/childgrowth/standards/en. Accessed April 5, 2019
171. Centers for Disease Control and Prevention. CDC growth charts. https://www.cdc.gov/growthcharts/cdc_charts.htm. Reviewed December 7, 2016. Accessed April 5, 2019
172. Kielmann AA, McCord C. Weight-for-age as an index of risk of death in children. *Lancet*. 1978;1(8076):1247–1250 PMID: 78007 https://doi.org/10.1016/S0140-6736(78)92478-9
173. Waterlow JC, Buzina R, Keller W, Lane JM, Nichaman MZ, Tanner JM. The presentation and use of height and weight data for comparing the nutritional status of groups of children under the age of 10 years. *Bull World Health Organ*. 1977;55(4):489–498 PMID: 304391
174. Guo SM, Roche AF, Fomon SJ, et al. Reference data on gains in weight and length during the first two years of life. *J Pediatr*. 1991;119(3):355–362 PMID: 1880646 https://doi.org/10.1016/S0022-3476(05)82045-1
175. Sherry B. Epidemiology of inadequate growth. In: Kessler D, Dawson P, eds. *Failure to Thrive and Pediatric Under-nutrition*. Baltimore, MD: Paul H. Brookes Publishing Company; 1999:19–36
176. Gomez F, Galvan RR, Cravioto J, Frenk S. Malnutrition in infancy and childhood, with special reference to kwashiorkor. *Adv Pediatr*. 1955;7:131–169 PMID: 14349775
177. Bergstrom WH. Twenty ways to get rickets in the 1990s. *Contemp Pediatr*. 1991;(8):88–93
178. Atwood WJ, Berger JR, Kaderman R, Tornatore CS, Major EO. Human immunodeficiency virus type 1 infection of the brain. *Clin Microbiol Rev*. 1993;6(4):339–366 PMID: 8269391 https://doi.org/10.1128/CMR.6.4.339
179. Orbak Z, Akin Y, Varoğlu E, Tan H. Serum thyroid hormone and thyroid gland weight measurements in protein-energy malnutrition. *J Pediatr Endocrinol Metab*. 1998;11(6):719–724 PMID: 9829226 https://doi.org/10.1515/JPEM.1998.11.6.719
180. Crist W, Napier-Phillips A. Mealtime behaviors of young children: a comparison of normative and clinical data. *J Dev Behav Pediatr*. 2001;22(5):279–286 PMID: 11718230 https://doi.org/10.1097/00004703-200110000-00001
181. Pollitt E. Failure to thrive: socioeconomic, dietary intake and mother-child interaction data. *Fed Proc*. 1975;34(7):1593–1597 PMID: 1132524

182. Drotar D, Malone CA, Negray J. Environmentally based failure to thrive and children's intellectual development. *J Child Psychol Psychiatry*. 1980;10:236–247
183. Bayley N. *Bayley Scales of Infant Development Manual*. 2nd ed. San Antonio, TX: Psychological Corporation; 1993
184. Peterson KE, Washington J, Rathbun JM. Team management of failure to thrive. *J Am Diet Assoc*. 1984;84(7):810–815 PMID: 6736509
185. Owen C, Ziebell L, Lessard C, Churcher E, Bourget V, Villenueve H. Interprofessional group intervention for parents of children age 3 and younger with feeding difficulties: pilot program evaluation. *Nutr Clin Pract*. 2012;27(1):129–135 PMID: 22307496 https://doi.org/10.1177/0884533611430231
186. Black MM, Dubowitz H, Hutcheson J, Berenson-Howard J, Starr RH Jr. A randomized clinical trial of home intervention for children with failure to thrive. *Pediatrics*. 1995;95(6):807–814 PMID: 7539121
187. Hren I, Mis NF, Brecelj J, et al. Effects of formula supplementation in breast-fed infants with failure to thrive. *Pediatr Int*. 2009;51(3):346–351 PMID: 19419499 https://doi.org/10.1111/j.1442-200X.2008.02732.x
188. Van Dyke DC, Mackay L, Ziaylek EN. Management of severe feeding dysfunction in children with fetal alcohol syndrome. *Clin Pediatr (Phila)*. 1982;21(6):336–339. PMID: 6804149 PMID: 6804149 https://doi.org/10.1177/000992288202100603
189. Heptinstall E, Puckering C, Skuse D, Start K, Zur-Szpiro S, Dowdney L. Nutrition and mealtime behaviour in families of growth-retarded children. *Hum Nutr Appl Nutr*. 1987;41(6):390–402 PMID: 3436837
190. Rathbun JM, Peterson KE. Nutrition in failure to thrive. In: Grank R, ed. *Pediatric Nutrition*. Boston, MA: Butterworth; 1987
191. Puls HT, Hall M, Bettenhausen J, et al. Failure to thrive hospitalizations and risk factors for readmission to children's hospitals. *Hosp Pediatr*. 2016;6(8):468–475 PMID: 27439432 https://doi.org/10.1542/hpeds.2015-0248
192. MacLean WC. Protein-energy malnutrition. In: Grand R, Sutphen J, Dietz W, eds. *Pediatric Nutrition*. Boston, MA: Butterworth; 1987
193. Viteri F. Primary protein-calorie malnutrition. In: Suskind R, ed. *Textbook of Pediatric Nutrition*. New York, NY: Raven Press; 1981
194. Morales E, Craig LD, MacLean WC Jr. Dietary management of malnourished children with a new enteral feeding. *J Am Diet Assoc*. 1991;91(10):1233–1238 PMID: 1918741
195. Black MM, Teti LO. Promoting mealtime communication between adolescent mothers and their infants through videotape. *Pediatrics*. 1997;99(3):432–437 PMID: 9041301 https://doi.org/10.1542/peds.99.3.432
196. Black MM. Zinc deficiency and child development. *Am J Clin Nutr*. 1998;68(2)(suppl):464S–469S PMID: 9701161 https://doi.org/10.1093/ajcn/68.2.464S
197. Walravens PA, Hambidge KM, Koepfer DM. Zinc supplementation in infants with a nutritional pattern of failure to thrive: a double-blind, controlled study. *Pediatrics*. 1989;83(4):532–538 PMID: 2927993
198. Doherty CP, Sarkar MA, Shakur MS, Ling SC, Elton RA, Cutting WA. Zinc and rehabilitation from severe protein-energy malnutrition: higher-dose regimens are associated with increased mortality. *Am J Clin Nutr*. 1998;68(3):742–748 PMID: 9734756 https://doi.org/10.1093/ajcn/68.3.742
199. Black MM, Krishnakumar A. Predicting longitudinal growth curves of height and weight using ecological factors for children with and without early growth deficiency. *J Nutr*. 1999;129(2S)(suppl):539S–543S PMID: 10064327 https://doi.org/10.1093/jn/129.2.539S
200. Satter E. *How to Get Your Kid to Eat... But Not Too Much*. New York, NY: Bull Publishing; 1987

201. Grantham-McGregor S, Schofield W, Powell C. Development of severely malnourished children who received psychosocial stimulation: six-year follow-up. *Pediatrics*. 1987;79(2):247–254 PMID:3808797
202. Sturm L, Drotar D. Maternal attributions of etiology in nonorganic failure to thrive. *Fam Syst Med*. 1991;9(1):53–63 https://doi.org/10.1037/h0089369
203. McDonough SC. Interaction guidance: understanding and treating early infant-caregiver relationship disturbances. In: Zeanah CH, ed. *Handbook of Infant Mental Health*. New York, NY: The Guilford Press; 1993:414–426
204. McDonough SC. Promoting positive early parent-infant relationships through interaction guidance. *Child Adolesc Psychiatr Clin N Am*. 1995;4(3):661–672 https://doi.org/10.1016/S1056-4993(18)30426-7
205. Koniak-Griffin D, Verzemnieks I, Cahill D. Using videotape instruction and feedback to improve adolescents' mothering behaviors. *J Adolesc Health*. 1992;13(7):570–575 PMID: 1345129 https://doi.org/10.1016/1054-139X(92)90370-Q
206. Wolke D, Skuse D. The management of infant feeding problems. In: Cooper P, Stein A, eds. *Feeding Problems and Eating Disorders in Children and Adolescents*. Chur, Switzerland: Harwood Academic Publishers; 1992:27–59
207. Black MM, Dubowitz H, Krishnakumar A, Starr RH Jr. Early intervention and recovery among children with failure to thrive: follow-up at age 8. *Pediatrics*. 2007;120(1):59–69 PMID: 17606562 https://doi.org/10.1542/peds.2006-1657
208. Haynes CF, Cutler C, Gray J, Kempe RS. Hospitalized cases of nonorganic failure to thrive: the scope of the problem and short-term lay health visitor intervention. *Child Abuse Negl*. 1984;8(2):229–242 PMID: 6539644 https://doi.org/10.1016/0145-2134(84)90012-7
209. Wright CM, Callum J, Birks E, Jarvis S. Effect of community based management in failure to thrive: randomised controlled trial. *BMJ*. 1998;317(7158):571–574 PMID: 9721113 https://doi.org/10.1136/bmj.317.7158.571
210. Raynor P, Rudolf MC, Cooper K, Marchant P, Cottrell D, Blair M. A randomised controlled trial of specialist health visitor intervention for failure to thrive. *Arch Dis Child*. 1999;80(6):500–506 PMID: 10331996 https://doi.org/10.1136/adc.80.6.500
211. Kerr MA, Black MM, Krishnakumar A. Failure-to-thrive, maltreatment and the behavior and development of 6-year-old children from low-income, urban families: a cumulative risk model. *Child Abuse Negl*. 2000;24(5):587–598 PMID: 10819092 https://doi.org/10.1016/S0145-2134(00)00126-5
212. Black M, Feigelman S, Cureton P. Evaluation and treatment of children with failure to thrive: an interdisciplinary perspective. *J Clin Outcomes Manag*. 1999;6:60–73
213. Block RW, Krebs NF; American Academy of Pediatrics Committee on Child Abuse and Neglect and Committee on Nutrition. Failure to thrive as a manifestation of child neglect. *Pediatrics*. 2005;116(5):1234–1237 PMID: 16264015 https://doi.org/10.1542/peds.2005-2032
214. Mackner LM, Starr RH Jr, Black MM. The cumulative effect of neglect and failure to thrive on cognitive functioning. *Child Abuse Negl*. 1997;21(7):691–700 PMID: 9238552 https://doi.org/10.1016/S0145-2134(97)00029-X
215. Skuse DH, Gill D, Reilly S, Wolke D, Lynch MA. Failure to thrive and the risk of child abuse: a prospective population survey. *J Med Screen*. 1995;2(3):145–149 PMID: 8536184 https://doi.org/10.1177/096914139500200309
216. Goldson E, Cadol RV, Fitch MJ, Umlauf HJ Jr. Nonaccidental trauma and failure to thrive. *Am J Dis Child*. 1976;130(5):490–492 PMID: 1274899 https://doi.org/10.1001/archpedi.1976.02120060036007
217. Koel BS. Failure to thrive and fatal injury as a continuum. *Am J Dis Child*. 1969;118(4):565–567 PMID: 5820598

218. Wyatt DT, Simms MD, Horwitz SM. Widespread growth retardation and variable growth recovery in foster children in the first year after initial placement. *Arch Pediatr Adolesc Med*. 1997;151(8):813–816 PMID: 9265884 https://doi.org/10.1001/archpedi.1997.02170450063010
219. Cunningham CF, McLaughlin M. Nutrition. In: Kessler D, Dawson P, eds. *Failure to Thrive and Pediatric Under-nutrition*. Baltimore, MD: Paul H. Brookes Publishing Co; 1999:99–119
220. Galler JR, Ramsey F, Solimano G. The influence of early malnutrition on subsequent behavioral development III. Learning disabilities as a sequel to malnutrition. *Pediatr Res*. 1984;18(4):309–313 PMID: 6718088 https://doi.org/10.1203/00006450-198404000-00001
221. Singer LT, Fagan JF III. Cognitive development in the failure-to-thrive infant: a three-year longitudinal study. *J Pediatr Psychol*. 1984;9(3):363–383 PMID: 6502402 https://doi.org/10.1093/jpepsy/9.3.363
222. Drewett RF, Corbett SS, Wright CM. Cognitive and educational attainments at school age of children who failed to thrive in infancy: a population-based study. *J Child Psychol Psychiatry*. 1999;40(4):551–561 PMID: 10357162 https://doi.org/10.1111/1469-7610.00473
223. Ashem B, Janes MD. Deleterious effects of chronic undernutrition on cognitive abilities. *J Child Psychol Psychiatry*. 1978;19(1):23–31 PMID: 621227 https://doi.org/10.1111/j.1469-7610.1978.tb01748.x
224. Skuse DH. Non-organic failure to thrive: a reappraisal. *Arch Dis Child*. 1985;60(2):173–178 PMID: 3883912 https://doi.org/10.1136/adc.60.2.173
225. Drewett R, Emond A, Blair P, Emmett P. The importance of slow weight gain in the first 2 months in identifying children who fail to thrive. *J Reprod Infant Psychol*. 2005;23(4):309–317 https://doi.org/10.1080/02646830500273160
226. Rudolf MC, Logan S. What is the long term outcome for children who fail to thrive? A systematic review. *Arch Dis Child*. 2005;90(9):925–931 PMID: 15890695 https://doi.org/10.1136/adc.2004.050179
227. Mackner LM, Black MM, Starr RH Jr. Cognitive development of children in poverty with failure to thrive: a prospective study through age 6. *J Child Psychol Psychiatry*. 2003;44(5):743–751 PMID: 12831118 https://doi.org/10.1111/1469-7610.00160
228. Emond AM, Blair PS, Emmett PM, Drewett RF. Weight faltering in infancy and IQ levels at 8 years in the Avon Longitudinal Study of Parents and Children. *Pediatrics*. 2007;120(4):e1051–e1058 PMID: 17908725 https://doi.org/10.1542/peds.2006-2295
229. Belfort MB, Rifas-Shiman SL, Rich-Edwards JW, Kleinman KP, Oken E, Gillman MW. Infant growth and child cognition at 3 years of age. *Pediatrics*. 2008;122(3):e689–e695 PMID: 18762504
230. Ramey CT, Yeates KO, Short EJ. The plasticity of intellectual development: insights from preventive intervention. *Child Dev*. 1984;55(5):1913–1925 PMID: 6510061 https://doi.org/10.2307/1129938
231. Drotar D. Behavioral diagnosis in nonorganic failure-to-thrive: a critique and suggested approach to psychological assessment. *J Dev Behav Pediatr*. 1989;10(1):48–55 PMID: 2647790 https://doi.org/10.1097/00004703-198902000-00010
232. Chavez A, Martinez C. Consequences of insufficient nutrition on child character and behavior. In: Levitsky D, ed. *Malnutrition, Environment, and Behavior*. New York, NY: Cornell University Press; 1979
233. Drotar D, Sturm L. Personality development, problem solving, and behavior problems among preschool children with early histories of nonorganic failure-to-thrive: a controlled study. *J Dev Behav Pediatr*. 1992;13(4):266–273 PMID: 1506465 https://doi.org/10.1097/00004703-199208000-00005

234. Gaensbauer TJ, Sands K. Distorted affective communications in abused/neglected infants and their potential impact on caretakers. *J Am Acad Child Psychiatry*. 1979;18(2):236–250 PMID: 447957 https://doi.org/10.1016/S0002-7138(09)61039-6
235. Powell GF, Brasel JA, Blizzard RM. Emotional deprivation and growth retardation simulating idiopathic hypopituitarism. I. Clinical evaluation of the syndrome. *N Engl J Med*. 1967;276(23):1271–1278 PMID: 6024346 https://doi.org/10.1056/NEJM196706082762301
236. Crittenden PM. Nonorganic failure to thrive: deprivation or distortion. *Int Ment Health J*. 1987;8:51–64
237. Gordon AH, Jameson JC. Infant-mother attachment in patients with nonorganic failure to thrive syndrome. *J Am Acad Child Psychiatry*. 1979;18(2):251–259 PMID: 447958 https://doi.org/10.1016/S0002-7138(09)61040-2
238. Gilmour J, Skuse D. A case-comparison study of the characteristics of children with a short stature syndrome induced by stress (hyperphagic short stature) and a consecutive series of unaffected "stressed" children. *J Child Psychol Psychiatry*. 1999;40(6):969–978 PMID: 10509891 https://doi.org/10.1111/1469-7610.00514
239. Valenzuela M. Attachment in chronically underweight young children. *Child Dev*. 1990;61(6):1984–1996 PMID: 2128048 https://doi.org/10.2307/1130852
240. Drotar D, Sturm L. Prediction of intellectual development in young children with early histories of nonorganic failure-to-thrive. *J Pediatr Psychol*. 1988;13(2):281–296 PMID: 3171820 https://doi.org/10.1093/jpepsy/13.2.281
241. Galler JR, Ramsey F, Solimano G. A follow-up study of the effects of early malnutrition on subsequent development. II. Fine motor skills in adolescence. *Pediatr Res*. 1985;19(6):524–527 PMID: 3925427 https://doi.org/10.1203/00006450-198506000-00004
242. Galler JR, Ramsey F, Solimano G, Lowell WE, Mason E. The influence of early malnutrition on subsequent behavioral development. I. Degree of impairment in intellectual performance. *J Am Acad Child Psychiatry*. 1983;22(1):8–15 PMID: 6402542 https://doi.org/10.1097/00004583-198301000-00002
243. Galler JR, Ramsey F, Solimano G, Lowell WE. The influence of early malnutrition on subsequent behavioral development. II. Classroom behavior. *J Am Acad Child Psychiatry*. 1983;22(1):16–22 PMID: 6402541 https://doi.org/10.1097/00004583-198301000-00003
244. Galler JR, Ramsey F, Solimano G. Influence of early malnutrition on subsequent behavioral development. V. Child's behavior at home. *J Am Acad Child Psychiatry*. 1985;24(1):58–64 PMID: 3968347 https://doi.org/10.1016/S0002-7138(09)60410-6
245. Hoddinott J, Behrman JR, Maluccio JA, et al. Adult consequences of growth failure in early childhood. *Am J Clin Nutr*. 2013;98(5):1170–1178 PMID: 24004889 https://doi.org/10.3945/ajcn.113.064584
246. Rikkönen K, Pesonen AK, Heinonen K, et al. Infant growth and hostility in adult life. *Psychosom Med*. 2008;70(3):306–313 PMID: 18378874 https://doi.org/10.1097/PSY.0b013e3181651638

CHAPTER 18

Medical Neglect and Obesity

Emily Killough, MD, FAAP
Child Abuse Pediatrician
Division of Child Adversity and Resilience
Children's Mercy Kansas City
Assistant Professor of Pediatrics
Division of Child Abuse and Neglect
UMKC School of Medicine
Kansas City, MO

Brooke Sweeney, MD, FAAP
Medical Director, Weight Management Services
Children's Mercy Kansas City
Clinical Assistant Professor of Pediatrics
UMKC School of Medicine
Kansas City, MO

Sarah E. Hampl, MD, FAAP
General Pediatrics and Weight Management
Center for Children's Healthy Lifestyles and Nutrition
Children's Mercy Kansas City
Professor of Pediatrics
UMKC School of Medicine
Kansas City, MO

Amy R. Beck, PhD
Weight Management Program
Center for Children's Healthy Lifestyles and Nutrition
Children's Mercy Kansas City
Associate Professor of Pediatrics
UMKC School of Medicine
Kansas City, MO

Introduction

Childhood obesity is a national epidemic, with more than 1 of 3 US children and teens having a body mass index (BMI) that meets criteria for overweight or obesity.[1] Rates of childhood obesity in the US have tripled in the past 30 years, paralleling the increases seen in the adult population.[1] Obesity was recognized as a disease by the American Medical Association in 2013,[2] and increasing evidence points to a complex interweave of biological, behavioral, familial, and environmental factors leading to the development and persistence of obesity in children. Children who have obesity are found to have clinically significant medical and psychosocial comorbidities, some of which can be disabling, life-threatening, or life limiting as they age into adulthood. This chapter examines the relationship between obesity and medical neglect.

Background

Definitions, Demographics, and Risk Factors

Body mass index percentile (weight in kilograms/height in meters squared compared with national gender- and age-based references) is generally accepted to be the best population- and health care–level indicator of excess weight in children aged 2 years and older. A child or teen who is considered to have overweight has a BMI between the 85th and 94th percentile for age and gender, while a child or teen with a BMI at or above the 95th percentile is considered to have obesity. Together, 18.5% of children and teens aged 2 to 19 years have obesity.[3] A classification system presented in the last several years[4,5] attempts to better depict the weight status of the approximately 6% of youth who have extreme or severe obesity.[1] Youth with severe obesity have more prevalent and severe comorbidities, and their progress over time and in weight management is difficult to see on standard BMI growth curves. This new classification system suggests that obesity be considered using BMI percent above the 95th percentile, with class I obesity extending from the 95th percentile to less than 120% of the 95th percentile, class II severe obesity encompassing 120% to 140% of the 95th percentile, and class III severe obesity extending to greater than 140% above the 95th percentile[5] (Table 18.1). Demographic-, gender-, and age-based variables influence the prevalence of obesity and severe obesity. Hispanic youth have the highest rates of obesity (21.9%), while non-Hispanic black youth have the highest rates of severe obesity (8.6%). Females have slightly higher rates of obesity and severe obesity (17.1%, 5.9%) than do males (16.9%, 5.7%). Twelve- to 19-year-olds have the highest rates of obesity (20.5%), followed by 6- to 11-year-olds (17.5%) and 2- to 5-year-olds (8.9%).[1]

The multifactorial etiology of obesity includes other elements that might be overlooked but can have significant effect on risk of obesity, including the conditions where children live, learn, work, and play,

TABLE 18.1
Classification of Severe Childhood Obesity[4,5]

Childhood Obesity Class	Percent Above the 95th Percentile BMI	Correlation With Adult Obesity Classification
I	95–120	I
II	120–<140 or BMI ≥35	II
III	≥140 or BMI ≥40	III

Abbreviation: BMI, body mass index.

otherwise known as the *social determinants of health*,[6,7] as well as adverse or traumatic experiences. A considerable social determinant is the economic environment within which the child and family reside. Economics can influence *food security*, or the reliable access to enough safe and nutritious food that meets dietary needs and food preferences for an active and healthy life.[8] Economics can influence access to a community with affordable housing and amenities in which a child and family can reliably and comfortably remain safe, sleep well, prepare meals, spend time outside, and be transported from place to place. Economics influences the tax base with which a school is funded and, thus, the meals provided by the school for a child to eat. Economics influences insurance coverage and consistent access to quality health care. Intergenerational economics can often be related to caregiver health literacy and health knowledge, from which decisions that will affect a child are made.

Another considerable determinant is the social and cultural environment surrounding a child and family. Social and cultural norms can influence health beliefs, food preferences and preparation, and perceptions of body size and weight. Across all environments, there is risk of adverse or traumatic experiences. These experiences can include, but are not limited to, physical, sexual, and emotional abuse or neglect; exposure to intimate partner violence; caregivers with mental health problems; incarcerated caregivers; community violence; bullying and victimization; racism; disasters; terrorism; refugee status; and medical trauma.[9] It is well established that adverse or traumatic experiences can be related to poor health outcomes, including obesity. Although not yet definitive, there are likely theoretical pathways through which this relationship exists. These pathways are primarily conceptualized as dysregulation of psychological, behavioral, neurobiological, and physiological systems.[10] Psychological pathways can run through depression and attention-deficit/hyperactivity disorder (ADHD), discussed later in this chapter as interwoven with obesity.[10,11] Posttraumatic stress disorder has been identified as connected with obesity, possibly even causal.[12] Some individuals have also reported feeling more protected and less vulnerable to harm with extra weight.[10] Behaviorally, changes in eating and activity, particularly disordered behaviors, are thought to be a connection between adverse or traumatic experiences and obesity.[10,13,14] Neurobiological and physiological pathways will be discussed in the Psychosocial Comorbidities section.

Consequences of Childhood Obesity

Medical Comorbidities

Excess weight may follow children and teens into adulthood; not surprisingly, this risk increases with the child's age. Longitudinal studies have revealed that obesity in young children tracks into later childhood[15,16] and obesity in later childhood tracks into adulthood[17]; children who have severe obesity are more likely to become adults with severe obesity.[18] Cohorts with obesity and certain comorbidities, such as hypertension and hyperlipidemia, have been longitudinally followed, leading researchers to state that these comorbidities "seamlessly track into adulthood" along with obesity. Common medical comorbidities include hypertension, hyperlipidemia or dyslipidemia, elevated liver enzymes, prediabetes, and sleep-disordered breathing.[19] Less common comorbidities, such as pseudotumor cerebri (idiopathic intracranial hypertension [IIH]) or slipped capital femoral epiphysis, may have acute consequences necessitating urgent medical or surgical intervention.[19] While some comorbidities and their consequences do not fully manifest until adulthood, others can rapidly progress and pose serious risk to health, resulting in disability, morbidity, and mortality in childhood. Among these are obstructive sleep apnea (OSA), which may lead to cognitive deficits; hypertension and cardiac biventricular hypertrophy[20] or left ventricular hypertrophy and other markers of cardiovascular damage[21]; type 2 diabetes mellitus (T2DM), which may lead to early-onset end-stage renal disease and coronary heart disease[22]; and nonalcoholic fatty liver disease (NAFLD) leading to liver failure.[23]

Psychosocial Comorbidities

The disease of obesity also has many related psychosocial factors. Five of the most common factors are impaired executive functioning, depression, suicidal ideation, weight-based discrimination and maltreatment, and poor quality of life. Each of these factors can individually have significant effects on development and maintenance of obesity, although it is not uncommon for more than 1 psychosocial factor to be present.

Executive function, or self-regulation, is the ability to monitor and modulate cognition, emotion, and behavior to accomplish one's goal and/or to adapt to the cognitive and social demands of specific situations.[24] Nearly 30% of children and adolescents have clinically significant executive function impairments, and the complex relationship is hypothesized to be bidirectional.[25] Furthermore, executive function impairments are commonly, although not always, related to ADHD. Attention-deficit/hyperactivity disorder that is unmedicated may be a risk factor for development of overweight.[26] Hypothesized reasons for this risk include the effect of impulsive behavior and impaired executive functioning, as well as biological links such as decreased dopamine (a neuromodulator in the motivational/reward processing system), in both conditions.[26–28] Additionally, ADHD is highly heritable,[29] and it is common for children with ADHD to have at least 1 parent with the condition, likely affecting the treatment trajectory of the child's impairment and obesity status.

Depression and obesity are also interconnected by complex models involving biological and behavioral pathways.[30,31] Diagnostic criteria for depression include changes in appetite or weight status and reduction in activity level, both of which can be directly tied to obesity. Additionally, the experience of having obesity may be so negative as to trigger a depressed mood and suicidal ideation. From the biological perspective, links between both diseases may travel through the hypothalamic-pituitary-adrenal axis.[31] Risk of suicide is independently related to depression and ADHD.[32,33] Compared with adolescents of a healthy weight, having a weight problem—and being accurately aware of the problem—is associated with significantly increased risk of suicidal ideation. However, it is not related to suicide attempts.[34]

Weight-based discrimination and maltreatment develop from *weight bias and stigma*, or the inclination to form negative and unreasonable judgments, attitudes, stereotypes, and assumptions about an individual's character, skills, and abilities based on his or her weight.[35,36] This experience is prevalent in the pediatric obesity population. In fact, by adolescence, weight-based discrimination and maltreatment are more prevalent than discrimination and maltreatment due to race, religion, or any other disability category.[37] Additionally, youth who have obesity experience this type of treatment in multiple settings from multiple individuals, including peers, family members, and teachers.[38] Unfortunately, this experience is also not uncommon within the health care setting. It is well established within current literature that weight bias and stigma is prevalent among medical professionals.[39] These attitudes can negatively affect outcomes of patients with obesity via professional-patient communication, medical professional treatment decision-making, and patient reluctance to attend appointments for medically necessary care.[40,41]

Unsurprisingly, youth who have obesity have a lower health-related quality of life than do children of a healthy weight. In fact, youth with obesity have impairments in daily functioning across physical, social, emotional, and academic domains equivalent to youth with cancer.[42]

Challenges in Childhood Obesity Identification and Management

Lack of parental awareness of children's excess weight status, medical professionals' reluctance to address obesity, and beliefs about futility of treatment efforts combine to make discussions of obesity a challenge in the primary care setting.[43,44] The presence of weight bias among medical professionals may influence concerned parents' willingness to raise the issue.[45] Both parents and medical professionals may be reluctant to acknowledge obesity as a disease, with implications to current and future health that must be addressed. Other medical professional-level barriers to obesity care mirror similar barriers to recognition of medical neglect, including lack of awareness of the family's health literacy, cultural views, and parenting styles, as well as ineffective communication skills.[46] However, pediatric medical professionals are trusted sources of guidance about obesity prevention in the eyes of parents,[47] and the multiple health supervision visits recommended, particularly in early childhood, make these visits prime opportunities for obesity prevention, detection, and intervention. Additionally, evidence-based, family-centered approaches and implementation resources are available to use in discussing obesity, including motivational interviewing,[48] person-first language (ie, "the child who has obesity" versus "the obese child") to avoid labeling the child,[45] and an approach in working with the family that affirms and incorporates their strengths to set achievable goals.[49]

Pathophysiology

Much debate has occurred over time about the causes and treatment of obesity. The discussion of obesity as a disease dates back hundreds of years, as described in the Obesity Society exploration of the definition of disease and obesity as a disease in 2008.[50] The society concluded that defining obesity as a disease "encourage[s] more high-quality caring professionals to view treating the obese patient as a vocation worthy of effort and respect; and [reduces] the stigma and discrimination heaped on many obese persons."[50] In 2012, the American Association of Clinical Endocrinologists released its position paper on obesity as a disease,[51] and in 2013, the American Medical Association passed a resolution officially defining obesity "as a multi-metabolic and hormonal disease state including impaired functioning of appetite [regulation], abnormal energy [balance], endocrine dysfunction including elevated leptin levels and insulin resistance, infertility, dysregulated adipokine signaling, abnormal endothelial function and blood pressure elevation, nonalcoholic fatty liver disease, dyslipidemia, and systemic and adipose tissue inflammation...."[52] Adipose tissue is the body's largest endocrine organ and not simply a storage depot for excess energy.

Adipose releases a myriad of hormones and interacts with regulating systems throughout the body. Once a certain level of adipose tissue is established, efforts to force the body to reverse the process of increasing adipose tissue meet strong resistance, especially those treatments addressing only one aspect of the disease (ie, the external environment including calorie excess, activity deficit, and behavioral contributors).[53,54] As calories are restricted, the internal physiology adjusts metabolism to conserve energy and maintain homeostasis, resulting in stable or even continued increase in weight.[55]

Typical treatments of weight loss are only or primarily focused on changes in the external environment with lifestyle modification and/or behavioral therapy, which may not address the internal physiological environment.[53] When obesity is severe (≥120% of the 95th percentile or BMI ≥35 in adults and adolescents 15 years and older), successful sustained weight loss will require treatment of the external environment and the internal physiology. The treatments specifically targeting internal physiology for weight loss are medications, devices, and bariatric surgery. One challenge for children who have severe obesity is that there are fewer certified pediatric obesity medicine specialists and fewer available advanced treatments to address the internal physiology. Families with a child who has severe obesity may be viewed incorrectly as "medically nonadherent" to treatments recommended for obesity, when the more accurate evaluation may be that the family has, in fact, attempted to implement recommendations and found them either not possible to implement (eg, due to increased hunger and food seeking with calorie restriction) or ineffective in bringing about change in the weight trajectory. When families have attempted change and have not been successful, this sets up a cycle of increased frustration, decreased trust in medical recommendations, and feelings of futility for implementing future recommendations.

Pathophysiological Effects of Adverse and Traumatic Experiences

Neurobiological and physiological pathways link adverse or traumatic experiences with obesity. The proposed pathways converge on the systemic dysregulation triggered by stress, particularly severe, chronic, or toxic stress.[10] In early childhood, toxic stress can create architectural changes in the brain across various areas, such as the amygdala, hippocampus, and prefrontal cortex. Changes in these areas can have permanent effects on future ability to physiologically regulate stress.[56–58] Furthermore, each of these areas is part of the reward/motivation system,[31] which, when impaired, can contribute to obesity development. Across all ages, the stress response involves activation of the sympathetic nervous system and the hypothalamic-pituitary-adrenal axis. However, this response varies based on the type of stress, namely acute versus chronic. *Acute* stressors may enhance immune function, but *chronic* stress appears to over-activate the immune system, triggering increased peripheral and central inflammation, particularly neuroinflammation. Inflammation is increasingly recognized as having a role in the onset and progression of many chronic diseases, including obesity and related cardiovascular and psychological diseases such as depression.[59] The pathway of the inflammation's contribution to obesity etiology may travel through the gut microbiota, which also has been indicated as having a role in obesity development and/or maintenance.[10,60] Lastly, stress has been demonstrated to enhance the response of ghrelin, a hormone that stimulates hunger.[10]

Evaluation and Treatment of Children With Obesity

Medical Evaluation

History

Evaluation of children who have obesity is critical to identify contributors to excess weight gain, potential secondary causes of obesity, and comorbidities and complications of the excess adiposity. Secondary causes can include genetic disorders, genetic syndromes, endocrine disorders, neurologic disorders, hypothalamic causes, or psychological disorders, or a drug-induced etiology.[61] Children with overweight and obesity have increased risk of adiposity-related comorbidities.[61–63] Even the young child with obesity already has evidence of abnormalities including cardiometabolic changes, insulin resistance, pulmonary disease, sleep disorders, orthopedic complications, cognitive delays, and behavioral problems.[64] Comorbidities having severe effects in childhood and influencing the indication for earlier bariatric surgery in class II severe obesity include hyperlipidemia, hypertension, T2DM, insulin resistance, depressed health-related quality of life, gastroesophageal reflux disease, OSA, NAFLD, orthopedic disease, and IIH.[62] Class III severe obesity is a severe risk factor alone and, therefore, an indication for bariatric surgery.[62]

For all children who have overweight or obesity, medical evaluation includes a thorough review of family history, including others with severe obesity or weight loss surgery or using medications or supplements for weight loss; birth history, including gestational diabetes, initial weight gain, difficulty gaining weight, or need for tube feedings; cardiovascular or respiratory challenges; infections; frequent antibiotic or steroid use; and social history. Past medical history should be elicited, including ADHD or attention concerns, anxiety, depression, intellectual or genetic diagnoses, physical limitations or disabilities, and previous hospitalizations or surgeries.

Review of weight gain patterns from birth to the present should be performed, noting infant weight gain and weight-for-length, times of change in BMI percentile, current stage of obesity, and how long that BMI percentile has been stable within 10 percentile points. Many children, while having obesity, will have maintained their BMI percentile curve for a long time. More concerning are children who are still increasing and crossing BMI percentile lines over time. Children staying between the percentile lines are likely already making a good effort in healthy changes, even if absolute weight is increasing.

Review of current and past medications for those potentially causing weight gain or difficulty with weight loss should be performed (Box 18.1); steroids, antihistamines, atypical antipsychotics and other psychotropic medications, β-blockers, insulin, and gabapentin and other seizure medications are major influences. A history of use of other medications, supplements, or over-the-counter foods or medications tried by the patient or family members for weight loss should be sought. A detailed history of previous weight loss attempts, methods, timing, and results should be elicited. It is important to determine what families have heard or been told from other medical professionals about the diagnosis of obesity and comorbidities, what they needed to do, and how this information was conveyed in the past to understand previous experiences

BOX 18.1
Medications Promoting Weight Gain

Antidepressants
- Tricyclic: trazadone, nortriptyline, amitriptyline
- Selective serotonin reuptake inhibitors: paroxetine, citalopram, escitalopram
- Mirtazapine, venlafaxine

Atypical antipsychotics: clozapine, olanzapine, quetiapine, risperidone, aripiprazole

Lithium

Antiepileptics: gabapentin, valproic acid

Antihistamines

Glucocorticoids

Medroxyprogesterone intramuscular contraceptive

Insulin, sulfonylureas

β-blockers: propranolol, metoprolol, atenolol

Tamoxifen, highly active antiretroviral therapy

with weight loss and other medical professionals. As mentioned earlier, many families will have experienced judgment and weight bias from other medical professionals as they attempted to implement changes in the past and will be resistant to further weight loss efforts due to these previous experiences. A discussion of the current efforts, what the parent thinks needs to be done at this time for the child's weight and health, and possible next steps they are ready for should then ensue.

Eliciting sleep patterns and symptoms, including screening for OSA, is also essential. Review of systems can focus on weight-related conditions, including recurrent illnesses; asthma and allergic symptoms; exercise tolerance; chest pain; headaches; musculoskeletal pain; visual changes; neurologic symptoms; skin changes such as acanthosis, hidradenitis, or yeast infections in skinfolds; hirsutism; pubertal development including gynecomastia, buried penis, concern for advanced puberty, menarche, symptoms, and regularity of menstrual cycles; gastrointestinal symptoms including reflux, vomiting, eating to vomiting or purging behaviors, diarrhea, or constipation; and incontinence of stool or urine during the day or night.

Current diet and activity, including routines, location of meals, and sedentary time are all important to assess. Detailed questioning, which will be discussed later in the chapter, should be performed regarding hunger and satiety cues, sneaking, eating to the point of discomfort or vomiting, night eating, late-night eating (ie, getting up from bed to eat), time between meals and snacks, cravings, pickiness/food selectivity, and child responses to previous attempts to make healthy changes.

Physical Examination, Laboratory Workup, and Other Evaluation

The physical examination should be comprehensive but especially focused on obesity comorbidities. The neurologic examination should include evaluation for papilledema. The cardiorespiratory examination should evaluate for difficulty breathing or noisy breathing, neck length and circumference, and cardiovascular and pulmonary systems examined for hypertension or murmurs, including those worsening with increased intrathoracic pressure, suggesting hypertrophic cardiomyopathy or other cardiac anomaly and hypertension. Liver size and presence of tenderness should be evaluated. Pubertal staging with breast and genital examination should be performed in boys and girls, as well as skin examination for acanthosis nigricans, skinfolds with yeast, or hidradenitis in axilla. Musculoskeletal examination should focus on gait, balance, hip and knee pain and range of motion, pes planus, and ability to sit and stand from the floor.

Laboratory examination to evaluate for additional concerns or comorbidities can include complete blood cell count and iron studies, glucose, hemoglobin A_{1c}, fasting lipid panel, liver function panel, vitamin B_{12}, 25-hydroxyvitamin D, folate, thiamine, thyroid-stimulating hormone and free thyroxine, and genetic testing when indicated. For clinical treatment, less laboratory evaluation is completed, but when considering referral for medical neglect, more detailed characterization of the internal physiology is helpful.

Additional beneficial testing can include a 6-minute walk or step test for physical condition and exercise prescription development, sleep study, indirect calorimetry for basal metabolic rate and calorie needs at rest to develop medical nutrition plan, and dual-energy x-ray absorptiometry scan for percent body fat to accurately determine fat and muscle mass and monitor progress. Many mobile phones have step counter apps, so looking at the health app on the child's phone can also give a baseline step count for the time the child is walking while he or she has the phone, with monthly and yearly averages. Additional screening for children with picky eating or limited food choices can include a food frequency log or a detailed 3-day diet log.

Psychosocial and Behavioral Evaluation

A thorough psychosocial and behavioral evaluation of a child with obesity involves assessment across multiple domains.[65] Assessment of motivation or readiness to change includes learning why change is desired from the child's, caregiver's, and family members' perspectives; how they perceive success or failure in previous attempts; how they think this would affect their lives in the future; and how committed they are to change. Assessment of the environments that the child, caregiver, and family members live within includes asking about home, school, and social (eg, peer) environments. This includes asking about experiences of weight-based discrimination and maltreatment, as well as risky behaviors, such as drug or alcohol use and sexual activity. It also includes asking about financial challenges and food insecurity. Furthermore, understanding how family members manage daily routines, how caregiving roles are fulfilled, and how members of a family communicate and connect emotionally with each other is beneficial information for supporting realistic change behaviors. It is crucial to ask about history of weight gain, particularly what the child, caregiver, and family members believe is the reason for weight gain, family history of weight problems, and feeding history and practices. This includes assessment of disordered eating (eg, restriction, binging, compensatory behaviors such as purging, chewing and spitting, food rules) or dysregulated eating habits (eg, emotional, boredom, impulsive, nighttime, picky, sneaking), as well as what the division of responsibility is in meal preparation and feeding. This information can be gathered via food recalls or food diaries, as well as objective questionnaires. Building on this, understanding of cultural components, such as cultural views of body and weight, as well as food preparation and the meaning of food, provides additional context. Lastly, screening for frequently encountered psychiatric conditions (eg, depression, ADHD, anxiety, history of psychological trauma/posttraumatic stress disorder, eating disorders) and developmental conditions (eg, autism spectrum disorder, intellectual disability), as well as health-related quality of life, is imperative.[65] Ideally, screening takes place through objective measures and clinical interview.

Medical Treatment

The treatment of overweight and obesity is described as a staged approach (Table 18.2). Stage 1 treatment (primary care) is performed in the primary care office and is recommended for all children, particularly those with overweight to class I obesity, by the Endocrine Society as well as by an expert committee including representatives from the American Academy of Pediatrics (AAP) and 14 other professional organizations.[63,66] Basic healthy lifestyle treatment is reinforced for children with overweight and obesity as well as for all children, regardless of weight status. The typical teaching includes a basic healthy diet following the MyPlate model with age-appropriate portions, 5 or more servings of fruits and vegetables daily, minimizing or eliminating sugar-containing beverages including juice, engaging in less than 2 hours of screen time in those 2 years and older, and 60 minutes of vigorous physical activity daily.[63,64]

Stage 2 (primary care plus) can also be implemented in primary care and should be used if no improvement in BMI is seen within 3 to 6 months of starting stage 1 treatment. This stage has more structured dietary recommendations, including optimizing the diet to include lower energy density foods (eg, healthy snacks of fruit, vegetable, and proteins), no additional calories from beverages, drinking water, 3 servings of dairy, and no juice or soda; limiting to 1 artificially sweetened beverage or food per day; limiting treats to every other day or less and working with the family on calorie content of treats depending on diet recommended and severity of obesity; maintaining a regular sleep schedule; limiting screen time to 1 hour or less per day; and getting a minimum of 60 minute of vigorous activity daily (increasing to 2 hours 3–4 times per week for those with more severe obesity). Referral to a dietitian is a component in this stage. Monthly contact is recommended for 3 to 6 months by the Expert Exchange Workgroup on Childhood Obesity.[64] This stage is also ideally suited to affect change in BMI for children with overweight and class I obesity. If not seeing improvement of BMI, or if BMI enters the range of severe obesity (passing 120% of the 95th percentile), the Expert Exchange Workgroup recommends advancement to stage 3 (multidisciplinary

Table 18.2
Treatment by Obesity Severity[53,62,63]

	85%–94% Overweight	95%–120% Class I Obesity	120%–140% Class II Severe Obesity	140%–160%[a] Class III Severe Obesity	160%–180%[a] Class III Severe Obesity	180%–200%[a] Class III Severe Obesity	>200%[a] Class III Severe Obesity
Stages of treatment	Stage 1 Primary care	Stage 2 Primary care plus, with additional support from a person with increased knowledge/ interest in healthy lifestyle change	Stage 3 Multidisciplinary team: dietitian, activity, and behavioral health specialist; medication optimization	Stage 4 Advanced intensive therapy with combination of extremely structured dietary regimens, pharmacotherapy, intensive behavioral assessment and treatment, and bariatric surgery			
Treatment recommended	Lifestyle, optimize meds	Lifestyle, optimize meds, add pharmacotherapy	Lifestyle, optimize meds, add pharmacotherapy; surgery if comorbidity	Lifestyle, optimize meds, add surgery, pharmacotherapy to support surgery preparation		Past optimal BMI for surgery May need to lose weight before surgery is safe if BMI is >60	

Abbreviation: BMI, body mass index.

[a] Actual BMI for children >140th percentile ranges from a BMI ≥27 in a 6-year-old to a BMI ≥40 in a 15-year-old.

team).[64] This level of treatment can be offered in some primary care offices, but the hallmark is having all disciplines represented (behavioral counselor, registered dietitian, and exercise specialist, in addition to a medical professional trained in treatment of obesity). Treatment is weekly for the first 8 to 12 weeks and then monthly. This treatment is typically for those with class I obesity or class II severe obesity (95th percentile–140% of the 95th percentile). These treatments are also used for children with class III severe obesity, but these children would likely also need advanced physiological treatments to bring about effective weight loss. Stage 4 treatment, advanced intensive therapy with combination of extremely structured dietary regimens, pharmacotherapy, intensive behavioral assessment and treatment, and bariatric surgery, is ideally implemented in a pediatric weight management center with the previously mentioned multidisciplinary team, with the addition of a psychologist and pediatric bariatric surgeon. This stage is ideal for all children with class II or III severe obesity (BMI ≥120% of the 95th percentile or BMI ≥35, whichever is lower). In addition to stage 3 treatment recommendations, extremely structured dietary regimens, medications, and bariatric surgery are offered in stage 4 treatment.[61,63]

Pharmacotherapy for weight loss is in the early development phase for children who have obesity. Tertiary care weight management specialists often use the approach to optimize current medications and treatments to ensure minimization of medications causing weight gain, changing to medications that tend to promote weight loss where possible, and adding medications to counteract weight gain effects of other medications. Additional diagnoses should be evaluated to ensure optimal treatment and minimize medications causing weight gain. Common culprits are inadequate treatment of asthma or allergies resulting in oral steroid dosing or frequent use of oral antihistamines, T2DM on sliding scale with high doses of insulin, behavior or sleep concerns managed with antihistamines, partially treated ADHD with impulsivity and rebound hunger in the afternoon or evening, blood pressure or headaches treated with β-blockers, and atypical antipsychotic medications for any diagnosis.

Untreated ADHD can be a cause of weight gain or difficulty losing weight. The impairments associated with ADHD can make maintaining a healthy diet, choosing healthy foods, and being able to limit food intake and choices near impossible.[26] Treatment of ADHD is often an essential missing piece in weight management treatment. Untreated depression and anxiety also often make adherence to recommended lifestyle changes difficult. Bupropion and selective serotonin reuptake inhibitors can be good choices and can support weight loss. Of note, some patients will respond to a selective serotonin reuptake inhibitor by gaining weight, while others will experience weight stability or weight loss. Metformin is a useful adjunct for children with polycystic ovarian syndrome, insulin resistance, or prediabetes. Emerging evidence also exists for the use of metformin and/or topiramate to assist with counteracting the weight gain effect of atypical antipsychotic medications.[67,68] Any advanced therapy, including medication, surgery, or device, can support a child and family to be better able to adhere to the recommended healthy eating plan, by treating the internal physiology driving weight gain. Typical targets of pharmacotherapy are to decrease hunger, improve satiety, or improve focus and attention to the healthy lifestyle plan.

Updated pediatric guidelines released by the American Society for Metabolic and Bariatric Surgery recommend evaluating children sooner for bariatric surgery, with a BMI between 35 and 45 being optimal to allow return to a reference-range BMI after surgery. Additionally, in children younger than 15 years, the BMI percentage of the 95th percentile should be used instead of BMI.[62]

The American Society for Metabolic and Bariatric Surgery guidelines state that candidates for bariatric surgery are children 10 years and older with BMI greater than or equal to 120% of the 95th percentile or BMI greater than or equal to 35, whichever is lower, and an additional comorbidity of hyperlipidemia, hypertension, T2DM, insulin resistance, depressed health-related quality of life, gastroesophageal reflux disease, OSA, NAFLD, orthopedic disease, or IIH; or children with a BMI greater than or equal to 140% of the 95th percentile or above.[62]

Psychosocial and Behavioral Treatment

Typical psychosocial and behavioral interventions to support weight loss fall within 3 general categories: supporting implementation of evidence-based behaviors (eg, reducing sugar-sweetened beverages, reducing screen time), reducing psychosocial/mental health barriers (eg, addressing depression through therapy or referrals, helping address bullying at school, helping secure transportation to appointments), and increasing caregiver/family capacity for family-based change. Family support is a beneficial component of facilitating change,[69] and a crucial element of support is making changes together as a family.[70] Family-based change also can reduce the risk of a child with obesity experiencing weight-based maltreatment in the home environment, because the child is not singled out.[38] Thus, teaching caregivers about *modeling*—how children are more likely to do what they see instead of what they are told—is important.

Another element of healthy family support is increasing caregiver capacity for effective parenting. This is because some behavioral changes that may be recommended can be vast departures from the current functioning of the family, and to implement them requires effective parenting skills. For example, if a child has typically been allowed to have 6 hours of screen time daily, reducing that to the recommended 2-hour limit is not likely to be preferred by the child and could be challenging for an unskilled caregiver to implement. Teaching caregivers strategies for limit setting can help increase the likelihood that the recommendation will be enacted. There are common challenges that, if left unaddressed, can impede caregiver efficacy. These include caregiver history of obesity and weight problems or mental health problems and lack of resources (eg, transportation, financial, health insurance, personal support).[71]

Trauma-Informed Care

The primary perspective to keep in mind while conducting any evaluation or providing any medical or psychosocial/behavioral recommendations is the trauma-informed perspective. A *trauma-informed perspective* necessitates being sensitive to the reasons why a child, caregiver, or family may do particular things.[72,73] People rarely do things without reason, and behaviors, regardless of how atypical or harmful they may seem, typically serve a function. A behavior that manifests as maladaptive may be carried over from when it was adaptive in another situation. The trauma-informed perspective requires medical professionals to seek to understand the function of behaviors in the context of a person's history. For example, a child who is eating impulsively in the absence of hunger may have a history of food insecurity; it may have been adaptive to eat whenever food was available. A rule of thumb when providing trauma-informed care is not thinking, "What is wrong with you?" but rather, "What has happened to you?" or "What is your story?" Further, given the association of adversity and trauma with obesity, as well as the independent prevalence rates of adverse or traumatic experiences and obesity, it is especially important to hold this perspective universally. This type of care and perspective can minimize the blaming of the child, caregiver, or family for what may seem like nonadherence or resistance. Not defaulting to blame can foster more collaborative problem-solving with a child, caregiver, or family, likely improving the relationship among them. This approach is also less likely to result in the child, caregiver, or family experiencing weight-based discrimination or maltreatment in the health care setting, which, as stated earlier in the chapter, can be a predictor of poor outcomes.

Measuring Treatment Progress

When measuring progress in treatment of obesity, the Expert Committee describes ideal desired weight loss by age and stage of treatment.[63] However, for children with obesity, especially those who have severe obesity, an inability to lose weight based on these targets may be due not to lack of adherence to external treatments but to lack of treatment of internal physiological drivers of increased weight. If adequate weight loss is not achieved, it is likely the child needs advanced therapy, including possible pharmacotherapy and/or bariatric surgery, from a stage 4 tertiary care weight management program. For this evaluation, the child would need to see a team of obesity specialists at an adolescent bariatric center.

As seen in the adult literature, the most effective treatments for weight loss are multicomponent, with the inclusion of external treatments and internal physiological treatments. This could include using more than 1 medication, intensive dietary regimens, exercise, and behavioral treatment all at the same time. Finally, optimal management of comorbidities, namely sleep and OSA, orthopedic concerns, asthma and allergies, and depression, anxiety, and ADHD, is also essential for successful induction of weight loss and maintenance of weight loss over time.

Medical Neglect

According to a 2016 report from the US Children's Bureau of the Administration for Children and Families, data collected from the National Child Abuse and Neglect Data System showed that nationally in the United States, 2.2% of children who experienced maltreatment experienced medical neglect, although these data are from only 41 states reporting, and in other states, medical neglect may be combined under neglect.[74] *Medical neglect* is generally defined as failure of a caregiver to seek or provide necessary medical care, which may take 1 of 2 forms: delay in or failure to seek medical care for obvious signs of illness, or failure to adhere to medical and/or treatment recommendations once medical care is sought.[46,75] In 2007, the AAP published a clinical report with guidelines for pediatricians regarding the recognition of medical neglect and recommended responses, graded from least to most intrusive.[46] However, there are no published disease-specific guidelines for the management or reporting of medical neglect, which likely results in inconsistent practices across medical specialties.

Two recent studies aimed to describe cohorts of children reported to child protective services (CPS) for medical neglect from 2 individual medical institutions in attempts to better characterize this population of children.[76,77] Fortin and colleagues described that children reported for medical neglect most commonly have chronic medical conditions and recommended development of improved interventions targeted to the specific underlying diagnoses.[76] A similar study by Parmeter et al also showed that most cases reported to CPS involved children with chronic medical conditions and caregivers who were not adherent to medical recommendations.[77]

Referral to CPS for medical neglect should be considered in cases when other interventions are not available or have not been successful.[46] Additionally, if caregivers are consistently non-adherent to treatment recommendations, a report may be indicated.[78] If a child is being harmed or is at risk of serious and/or imminent harm or death as a result of the lack of medical care or caregiver's failure to follow treatment recommendations a report should be made.

There are no studies examining the relationship between CPS involvement and improved health outcomes in cases of pediatric obesity. There has been an attempt to examine if and when childhood obesity constitutes medical neglect.[79] One suggested approach is to view pediatric obesity as a spectrum of risk, stratified from low risk of harm to very high risk based on the presence of comorbid conditions such as diabetes, sleep apnea, and NAFLD. Using this framework, the diagnosis of medical neglect and referral to CPS would be more likely in patients with more severe obesity because, as the comorbid conditions progress in severity, the risk for premature death and, therefore, risk of imminent harm or actual harm from obesity and obesity-related conditions also increases.[79] Additionally, in children who have obesity of any severity, if there are concerns for or disclosures of other types of child maltreatment, including physical, sexual, or emotional abuse, a referral to CPS is warranted.

There has also been some controversy surrounding the issue of involvement of CPS with children who have obesity.[80–82] Much of the debate is framed by the question of childhood obesity occurring as the result of neglectful parenting and neglectful supervision.[83] As discussed in this chapter, recent research has advanced knowledge of the pathophysiology of obesity and the interplay between trauma and the development of obesity. Establishing obesity as a complex, multifactorial, chronic medical disease provides the cognitive framework for considering the issue of neglect as related to obesity as medical neglect rather than neglectful parenting or neglectful supervision.

Initial Approach

Childhood obesity alone should not result in a concern for neglect or a report to CPS.[78,79,81] Medical professionals caring for children who have severe childhood obesity should ensure that the patient has been referred to a treatment center with a stage 3 to 4 pediatric weight management program, preferably with medical professionals with obesity medicine certification. Given the complex and multifactorial nature of severe obesity, significant change is unlikely to occur with appointment-based counseling in a primary care setting targeting only lifestyle changes. A more intensive, comprehensive treatment program that includes physicians, dietitians, and psychologists is recommended by the overweight and obesity Expert Committee.[63] Even with comprehensive treatment, failure to reduce weight alone is not necessarily an indication for CPS involvement because outcomes for weight management programs are mixed.[79,81]

As previously mentioned, certain comorbidities of obesity may have more immediate and serious consequences than others, making treatment of the comorbidity and obesity more urgent. If concerns arise for nonadherence to medical recommendations for treatment of pediatric obesity and related conditions, the medical professional should first explore if the family, caregiver, and/or patient are experiencing any barriers to obtaining the recommended care. Concerns may include, but are not limited to, consistent failure to attend medical and/or behavioral health appointments, initiate recommended lifestyle changes, take recommended medications or other treatments, or have additional testing/evaluations performed. Barriers to accessing medical care are multiple and may include access to insurance coverage, financial concerns, social anxiety, history of weight-based discrimination in the health care setting, limited transportation, limited English proficiency, limited literacy, intellectual disability, caregiver mental health, and resource-poor geographic areas. Once barriers are explored, resources should be provided, as able, to help the family or caregiver address any barriers to care. Use of a multidisciplinary team, including a social worker, may be helpful in providing appropriate community referrals.[46]

It is also vitally important for the medical professional to ensure that the family understands the treatment plan and recommendations. Medical professionals should recognize the family as a partner in the decision-making process and involve the patient and caregiver(s) in the development of the treatment plan.[46] Successful management of medical neglect frequently involves addressing communication difficulties and resource issues.[77] There may be specific cases in which there are concerns for medical neglect and the medical professional is not able to explore and/or address a family's barriers to seeking medical care; in these instances, a report to CPS may be indicated as a way to access additional community resources and help address potential barriers to following medical recommendations.

Care Contract

If concerns about nonadherence to medical recommendations persist once a medical professional and/or team of multidisciplinary professionals has attempted to identify and address barriers to accessing care and following medical or treatment recommendations and has attempted to address any other communication difficulties, it may be necessary to work with the family to develop a written contract.[46] In cases of concern for medical neglect related to pediatric obesity, a care contract could include the following categories and recommendations:

- Responsibilities of the weight management clinic, which may involve scheduling appointments, working with the family to develop and track goals, calling or contacting the family to provide reminders and/or encouragement, and providing specific resources
- Responsibilities of the patient, which may include keeping a log of eating and activity, following meal and activity plans developed with the medical team, practicing skills, asking for support, and, when applicable, taking prescribed medications or wearing a continuous positive airway pressure mask at night
- Responsibilities of the parent/caregiver, which may include arranging for transportation, calling to cancel or reschedule appointments when needed, participating in physical activity with the patient, providing encouragement and praise for the patient, picking up medications from the pharmacy, and attending other clinic appointments

Medical professionals, the patient, and caregivers should all sign and date the care contract; each person should be provided a copy of the agreed-on plan; and the plan should be unique to each patient and reflect his or her individual needs and care environment.

Reporting to Child Protective Services

Medical professionals may be hesitant to report abuse and neglect due to negative experiences such as ineffectiveness of prior state interventions and the effect on their relationship with the patient following a report.[84] In the 2007 AAP clinical report, it is recommended that several factors be considered when formulating a diagnosis of medical neglect:

- The child has been harmed or is at significant risk of harm due to lack of medical care or nonadherence to medical recommendations.
- The recommended medical care offers significant benefit to the child and the benefit is greater than the associated morbidity.

- Access to medical care can be demonstrated and the available care was not used.
- The caregiver understands the medical/treatment recommendations that have been provided.[46]

When a child is being harmed or is at risk of harm due to lack of medical care, a report to CPS is indicated. Successful management of medical neglect by CPS requires that the CPS worker understands the child's medical condition as well as the specific necessary treatment and goals. It may be necessary for the medical professional to have close and ongoing communication with the CPS worker and his or her supervisor to ensure that all parties involved understand the medical recommendations. Child protective services are mandated by law to ensure that reasonable efforts have been made to ensure family autonomy; while many medical professionals fear that a referral to CPS will lead to removal of a child from the home environment, this is typically seen as a last resort. In many communities, CPS may have access to additional resources and services that might not otherwise be available for the family.[46] Child protective services may also be able to provide a more comprehensive assessment of the role of the home environment and other comorbidities in the home, including caregiver mental health, substance use, and parenting abilities, and other forms of concurrent child maltreatment.[85]

Best Practices for Multidisciplinary Collaboration

Once CPS is involved, communication with the medical team is imperative to ensure that the CPS worker understands the risk to the patient when obesity and obesity-related conditions are untreated. Medical professionals should communicate the rationale behind the medical necessity of treatment and the severity of the risk of harm with CPS.[78] Child protective services will typically initially pursue less invasive interventions, such as providing community resources and behavioral interventions and/or providing in-home services. It may be helpful for the medical team to provide CPS with the care contract signed by the involved medical professionals, patient, and caregivers, if one has been developed, to use as a framework to assist with goal setting and objectives for any CPS-recommended interventions, such as in-home services.

Additionally, it can be burdensome and challenging for a CPS worker to use or understand medical records to support the concern for medical neglect for documentation. The involved medical professionals should consider providing CPS with a document or letter of concern summarizing the patient's applicable medical history, the treatment plan, and adherence or lack of adherence to the treatment plan by the patient and caregivers.

The summary document should conclude with the medical professionals' assessment and diagnoses, including diagnosis of medical neglect, when indicated, and recommendations. The discussion of the diagnoses can include the specifics regarding the harm that the patient has experienced or the patient's risk of harm from lack of adherence to the treatment plan. Recommendations for the patient should be outlined, which may include regular visits with the medical, nutritional, and behavioral health team; in-home interventions, including medications and equipment; and measurable process and outcome measures that will show adherence to the treatment plan. Child protective services could be invited to hospital or clinic care team meetings, and medical professionals could, likewise, attend CPS meetings with the family.

Using this type of collaborative and coordinated response may help CPS to provide a more effective intervention for the family. Child protective services may also be able to help the medical team to develop more appropriate and/or effective lifestyle changes with an improved understanding of the home environment and family culture and suggest alternative approaches that may work better for a specific family given its individual strengths, cultures, and beliefs. If a medical professional is having challenges communicating effectively with CPS, one suggested approach is to request to speak with a worker's supervisor or request an in-person collaborative meeting at which information about the patient's specific needs can be exchanged.

Family/Juvenile Court Referral

In cases in which a family is not willing to cooperate with CPS or participate in provided services, a referral to family/juvenile court may be necessary. Child protective services will typically exhaust all less invasive alternatives before considering removal of a child from a home environment, given the additional psychological trauma that is associated with removal.[46,78,79] In the 2009 article by Varness and colleagues, guidelines are proposed for indications for removal from the home in cases of pediatric obesity and medical neglect. These guidelines state that removal should be considered when there is a high likelihood of serious imminent harm, there is a reasonable likelihood that state intervention will result in effective treatment, and there are no alternative options for addressing the problem.[79]

It is important to note that out-of-home placement is not the only option for family/juvenile court professionals; another approach could be to take the child into state custody but recommend appropriate placement with the child's parents/caregivers with ongoing court oversight. Using this method, the child can remain in the home, preventing additional psychological trauma, but adherence to the recommended medical treatment plan may be court ordered and monitored closely. All involved professionals should be aware that the long-term effect on weight control, medical comorbidities, and/or psychological outcomes after CPS involvement, including removal from the home, is unknown in cases of childhood obesity.

Legal Perspective

While the law may vary somewhat in different states, in general, most states mandate that prior to removal of a child from a home environment, the state must show imminent danger to the child's health or safety, determine if it is in the best interest of the child's welfare to remain or be removed from the home, and make reasonable efforts to prevent removal.[86] States typically view removal of a child from a home as the last option after reasonable efforts to prevent removal have been refused or have failed.

The court has a long history of restricting parental rights in cases of medical neglect when a child is at risk of imminent harm. But, to date, the approach to pediatric obesity in courts has been inconsistent.[86] In recent years, some state courts have taken action in cases of severe pediatric obesity, most commonly in cases where the child has had numerous associated medical conditions in addition to pediatric obesity and the parents/caregivers have repeatedly failed to address the child's obesity-related medical needs. A recent legal publication by Garrahan and Eichner recommends that courts should "apply the standard of medical neglect to instances of morbid childhood obesity."[86]

Case Study

A 13-year-old boy with a history of untreated hypothyroidism for 3 years presented to a new primary care medical professional and was referred for weight management treatment to a stage 3 pediatric tertiary care weight management clinic. At his initial visit in weight management, he weighed more than 400 pounds, his BMI was greater than 60, and he had hypothyroidism, depression, and elevated blood pressure. The team did an evaluation and recommended coordination of care with a local dietitian and counselor as well as primary care and regular follow-up. He was not seen again for 2 years and presented at age 15 years with a weight gain of 100 pounds and a BMI greater than 75. Over the next 2 years, he was seen 4 times in weight management and yet continued to gain weight. He was evaluated by sleep specialists and cardiologists in the office but did not return for his sleep study or further cardiac testing due to weight-based discrimination at these subspecialty visits and fear of getting the tests done. He re-presented at 17 years old, weighing more than 600 pounds and with a BMI greater than 85 from primary care medical professional measurements. He had not completed a recommended sleep study, reported he was sleeping in a recliner due to not being able to breathe well, and had foot pain and possible swelling; his last thyrotropin (ie, thyroid-stimulating hormone) level measurement 2 months prior was elevated at 12 mIU/mL. He had been seen in the remote past for counseling but was not receiving current mental health treatment. He and his mother continued to identify depression as a problem and a contributing factor to weight gain because of stress eating. He had experienced significant bullying at school related to his obesity and other complications of his weight (including the odor caused by untreated yeast in his skinfolds). As a result, he had been out of school for the last 2 school years.

He was not a candidate for bariatric surgery at the time of reevaluation due to the continued weight gain, minimal progress on intensive healthy lifestyle changes, lack of treatment of his depression, untreated hypothyroidism, and undiagnosed cardiopulmonary status. With intensive medical treatment and a therapeutic environment, he could improve his health and prepare to have bariatric surgery over the next 6 to 12 months, which could be lifesaving for him.

The use of a medical neglect plan, including a summary letter of concern, enabled the treatment team to confidently move forward and address the significant needs of this patient. A referral was made to CPS, and the resulting collaboration provided a level of authority and assurance in planning patient care that could not have happened otherwise. A significant component of this was the role of CPS to create accountability for the family and motivation toward adherence. As the family began to hesitantly reengage with care, this allowed the medical team to focus on enhanced relationship repair, which successfully improved the relationship among the team, patient, and family. From this improved relationship, patient and family engagement increased, and as engagement increased, the patient's outcome improved significantly. Ultimately, engagement and adherence continued without the need for intervention or accountability from CPS.

Conclusion

Obesity is a disease that, in most cases, is chronic and may also have acute consequences. Fundamentals of CPS involvement and medical neglect that apply to all chronic conditions should also apply to children who have obesity. Medical professionals should consider referring children with severe obesity to tertiary care weight management centers with multidisciplinary treatment teams to deliver advanced medical and psychological treatments. It may be useful for medical professionals to create a process map to guide when to consider use of a care contract and familiarize colleagues and staff with CPS and the collaboration required in cases of medical neglect.

References

1. Ogden CL, Carroll MD, Lawman HG, et al. Trends in obesity prevalence among children and adolescents in the United States, 1988–1994 through 2013–2014. *JAMA*. 2016;315(21):2292–2299 PMID: 27272581 https://doi.org/10.1001/jama.2016.6361
2. American Medical News. What's next now that the AMA has declared obesity a disease? http://www.amednews.com/article/20130701/house/130709952/1/. Published July 1, 2013. Accessed April 10, 2019
3. Hales CM, Fryar CD, Carroll MD, Freedman DS, Ogden CL. Trends in obesity and severe obesity prevalence in US youth and adults by sex and age, 2007–2008 to 2015–2016. *JAMA*. 2018;319(16):1723–1725 PMID: 29570750 https://doi.org/10.1001/jama.2018.3060
4. Flegal KM, Wei R, Ogden CL, Freedman DS, Johnson CL, Curtin LR. Characterizing extreme values of body mass index-for-age by using the 2000 Centers for Disease Control and Prevention growth charts. *Am J Clin Nutr*. 2009;90(5):1314–1320 PMID: 19776142 https://doi.org/10.3945/ajcn.2009.28335
5. Gulati AK, Kaplan DW, Daniels SR. Clinical tracking of severely obese children: a new growth chart. *Pediatrics*. 2012;130(6):1136–1140 PMID: 23129082 https://doi.org/10.1542/peds.2012-0596
6. Centers for Disease Control and Prevention. Social determinants of health: know what affects health. CDC research on SDOH. https://www.cdc.gov/socialdeterminants. Reviewed January 29, 2018. Accessed April 10, 2019
7. Office of Disease Prevention and Health Promotion. Social determinants of health. HealthyPeople.gov website. https://www.healthypeople.gov/2020/topics-objectives/topic/social-determinants-of-health. Accessed April 10, 2019
8. International Food Policy Research Institute. Food security. http://www.ifpri.org/topic/food-security. Accessed April 10, 2019
9. National Child Traumatic Stress Network. Trauma types. https://www.nctsn.org/what-is-child-trauma/trauma-types. Accessed April 10, 2019
10. Mason SM, Bryn Austin S, Bakalar JL, et al. Child maltreatment's heavy toll: the need for trauma-informed obesity prevention. *Am J Prev Med*. 2016;50(5):646–649 PMID: 26689978 https://doi.org/10.1016/j.amepre.2015.11.004
11. Brown NM, Brown SN, Briggs RD, Germán M, Belamarich PF, Oyeku SO. Associations between adverse childhood experiences and ADHD diagnosis and severity. *Acad Pediatr*. 2017;17(4):349–355 PMID: 28477799 https://doi.org/10.1016/j.acap.2016.08.013
12. Kubzansky LD, Bordelois P, Jun HJ, et al. The weight of traumatic stress: a prospective study of posttraumatic stress disorder symptoms and weight status in women. *JAMA Psychiatry*. 2014;71(1):44–51 PMID: 24258147 https://doi.org/10.1001/jamapsychiatry.2013.2798
13. Puhl RM. Clinical implications of obesity stigma. Yale Rudd Center for Food Policy and Obesity website. http://www.uconnruddcenter.org/files/Pdfs/Clinical_Implications_of_Obesity_Stigma_Presentation_2013.pdf. Accessed April 10, 2019

14. Puhl RM. Pediatric obesity and bullying: implications for patients, providers and clinical practice. Yale Rudd Center for Food Policy and Obesity website. http://www.uconnruddcenter.org/files/Pdfs/Implictions_for_Patients_Providers_Clinical_Presentation_2013.pdf. Accessed April 10, 2019
15. Nader PR, O'Brien M, Houts R, et al; National Institute of Child Health and Human Development Early Child Care Research Network. Identifying risk for obesity in early childhood. *Pediatrics*. 2006;118(3):e594–e601 PMID: 16950951 https://doi.org/10.1542/peds.2005-2801
16. Woo Baidal JA, Locks LM, Cheng ER, Blake-Lamb TL, Perkins ME, Taveras EM. Risk factors for childhood obesity in the first 1,000 days: a systematic review. *Am J Prev Med*. 2016;50(6):761–779 PMID: 26916261 https://doi.org/10.1016/j.amepre.2015.11.012
17. Simmonds M, Llewellyn A, Owen CG, Woolacott N. Predicting adult obesity from childhood obesity: a systematic review and meta-analysis. *Obes Rev*. 2016;17(2):95–107 PMID: 26696565 https://doi.org/10.1111/obr.12334
18. Freedman DS, Mei Z, Srinivasan SR, Berenson GS, Dietz WH. Cardiovascular risk factors and excess adiposity among overweight children and adolescents: the Bogalusa Heart Study. *J Pediatr*. 2007;150(1):12–17.e2 PMID: 17188605 https://doi.org/10.1016/j.jpeds.2006.08.042
19. Santos M, Pont S, Estrada E. Childhood obesity related co-morbidities: identification and treatment. In: Hassink SG, Hampl SE, eds. *Clinical Care of the Child with Obesity: A Learner's and Teacher's Guide*. New York, NY: McGraw-Hill Education; 2016:chap 13
20. Marcus CL, Brooks LJ, Davidson Ward S, et al. Diagnosis and management of childhood obstructive sleep apnea syndrome. *Pediatrics*. 2012;130(3):e714–e755 PMID: 22926176 https://doi.org/10.1542/peds.2012-1672
21. Flynn JT, Kaelber DC, Baker-Smith CM, et al; Subcommittee on Screening and Management of High Blood Pressure in Children. Clinical practice guideline for screening and management of high blood pressure in children and adolescents. *Pediatrics*. 2017;140(3):e20171904 PMID: 28827377 https://doi.org/10.1542/peds.2017-1904
22. Rhodes ET, Prosser LA, Hoerger TJ, Lieu T, Ludwig DS, Laffel LM. Estimated morbidity and mortality in adolescents and young adults diagnosed with type 2 diabetes mellitus. *Diabet Med*. 2012;29(4):453–463 PMID: 22150528 https://doi.org/10.1111/j.1464-5491.2011.03542.x
23. Vos MB, Abrams SH, Barlow SE, et al. NASPGHAN clinical practice guideline for the diagnosis and treatment of nonalcoholic fatty liver disease in children: recommendations from the Expert Committee on NAFLD (ECON) and the North American Society of Pediatric Gastroenterology, Hepatology and Nutrition (NASPGHAN). *J Pediatr Gastroenterol Nutr*. 2017;64(2):319–334 PMID: 28107283 https://doi.org/10.1097/MPG.0000000000001482
24. Berger A. *Self-Regulation: Brain, Cognition, and Development*. Washington, DC: American Psychological Association; 2011:4 https://doi.org/10.1037/12327-000
25. Gowey MA, Lim CS, Dutton GR, Silverstein JH, Dumont-Driscoll MC, Janicke DM. Executive function and dysregulated eating behaviors in pediatric obesity. *J Pediatr Psychol*. 2018;43(8):834–845 PMID: 28595362 https://doi.org/10.1093/jpepsy/jsx091
26. Schwartz BS, Bailey-Davis L, Bandeen-Roche K, et al. Attention deficit disorder, stimulant use, and childhood body mass index trajectory. *Pediatrics*. 2014;133(4):668–676 PMID: 24639278 https://doi.org/10.1542/peds.2013-3427
27. Kim EJ, Kwon HJ, Ha M, et al. Relationship among attention-deficit hyperactivity disorder, dietary behaviours and obesity. *Child Care Health Dev*. 2014;40(5):698–705 PMID: 24438547 https://doi.org/10.1111/cch.12129

28. Carnell S, Gibson C, Benson L, Ochner CN, Geliebter A. Neuroimaging and obesity: current knowledge and future directions. *Obes Rev*. 2012;13(1):43–56 PMID: 21902800 https://doi.org/10.1111/j.1467-789X.2011.00927.x
29. Dark C, Homman-Ludiye J, Bryson-Richardson RJ. The role of ADHD associated genes in neurodevelopment. *Dev Biol*. 2018;438(2):69–83 PMID: 29608877 https://doi.org/10.1016/j.ydbio.2018.03.023
30. Pervanidou P, Bastaki D, Chouliaras G, et al. Circadian cortisol profiles, anxiety and depressive symptomatology, and body mass index in a clinical population of obese children. *Stress*. 2013;16(1):34–43 PMID: 22545868 https://doi.org/10.3109/10253890.2012.689040
31. Jauch-Chara K, Oltmanns KM. Obesity--a neuropsychological disease? Systematic review and neuropsychological model. *Prog Neurobiol*. 2014;114:84–101 PMID: 24394671 https://doi.org/10.1016/j.pneurobio.2013.12.001
32. Fawcett J. Depressive disorders. In: Simon RI, Hales RE, eds. *Suicide Assessment and Management*. 2nd ed. Washington, DC: American Psychiatric Publishing; 2012:109–121
33. Allely CS. The association of ADHD symptoms to self-harm behaviours: a systematic PRISMA review. *BMC Psychiatry*. 2014;14(1):133 PMID: 24884622 https://doi.org/10.1186/1471-244X-14-133
34. Zeller MH, Reiter-Purtill J, Jenkins TM, Ratcliff MB. Adolescent suicidal behavior across the excess weight status spectrum. *Obesity (Silver Spring)*. 2013;21(5):1039–1045 PMID: 23784908 https://doi.org/10.1002/oby.20084
35. Washington RL. Childhood obesity: issues of weight bias. *Prev Chronic Dis*. 2011;8(5):A94 PMID: 21843424 http://www.cdc.gov/pcd/issues/2011/sep/10_0281.htm. Accessed April 10, 2019
36. UCONN Rudd Center for Food Policy and Obesity. Weight bias and stigma: theories of weight bias. http://www.uconnruddcenter.org/weight-bias-stigma-theories-of-weight-bias. Accessed April 10, 2019
37. Puhl RM, Luedicke J, Heuer C. Weight-based victimization toward overweight adolescents: observations and reactions of peers. *J Sch Health*. 2011;81(11):696–703 PMID: 21972990 https://doi.org/10.1111/j.1746-1561.2011.00646.x
38. Puhl RM, Peterson JL, Luedicke J. Weight-based victimization: bullying experiences of weight loss treatment-seeking youth. *Pediatrics*. 2013;131(1):e1–e9 PMID: 23266918 https://doi.org/10.1542/peds.2012-1106
39. Budd GM, Mariotti M, Graff D, Falkenstein K. Health care professionals' attitudes about obesity: an integrative review. *Appl Nurs Res*. 2011;24(3):127–137 PMID: 20974067 https://doi.org/10.1016/j.apnr.2009.05.001
40. Puhl RM, Phelan SM, Nadglowski J, Kyle TK. Overcoming weight bias in the management of patients with diabetes and obesity. *Clin Diabetes*. 2016;34(1):44–50 PMID: 26807008
41. Phelan SM, Burgess DJ, Yeazel MW, Hellerstedt WL, Griffin JM, van Ryn M. Impact of weight bias and stigma on quality of care and outcomes for patients with obesity. *Obes Rev*. 2015;16(4):319–326 PMID: 25752756 https://doi.org/10.1111/obr.12266
42. Schwimmer JB, Burwinkle TM, Varni JW. Health-related quality of life of severely obese children and adolescents. *JAMA*. 2003;289(14):1813–1819 PMID: 12684360 https://doi.org/10.1001/jama.289.14.1813
43. Lundahl A, Kidwell KM, Nelson TD. Parental underestimates of child weight: a meta-analysis. *Pediatrics*. 2014;133(3):e689–e703 PMID: 24488736 https://doi.org/10.1542/peds.2013-2690
44. Klein JD, Sesselberg TS, Johnson MS, et al. Adoption of body mass index guidelines for screening and counseling in pediatric practice. *Pediatrics*. 2010;125(2):265–272 PMID: 20083518 https://doi.org/10.1542/peds.2008-2985

45. Pont SJ, Puhl R, Cook SR, Slusser W; American Academy of Pediatrics Section on Obesity; The Obesity Society. Stigma experienced by children and adolescents with obesity. *Pediatrics*. 2017;140(6):e20173034 PMID: 29158228 https://doi.org/10.1542/peds.2017-3034
46. Jenny C; American Academy of Pediatrics Committee on Child Abuse and Neglect. Recognizing and responding to medical neglect. *Pediatrics*. 2007;120(6):1385–1389 PMID: 18055690 https://doi.org/10.1542/peds.2007-2903
47. Hernandez RG, Cheng TL, Serwint JR. Parents' healthy weight perceptions and preferences regarding obesity counseling in preschoolers: pediatricians matter. *Clin Pediatr (Phila)*. 2010;49(8):790–798 PMID: 20522610 https://doi.org/10.1177/0009922810368288
48. American Academy of Pediatrics Institute for Healthy Childhood Weight. Featured resources. https://ihcw.aap.org/resources/Pages/default.aspx. Accessed April 10, 2019
49. American Academy of Pediatrics. Strength based approach: healthy active living for families implementation guide. https://www.aap.org/en-us/advocacy-and-policy/aap-health-initiatives/HALF-Implementation-Guide/communicating-with-families/Pages/Strength-Based-Approach.aspx. Accessed April 10, 2019
50. Allison DB, Downey M, Atkinson RL, et al. Obesity as a disease: a white paper on evidence and arguments commissioned by the Council of the Obesity Society. *Obesity (Silver Spring)*. 2008;16(6):1161–1177 PMID: 18464753
51. Mechanick JI, Garber AJ, Handelsman Y, Garvey WT. American Association of Clinical Endocrinologists' position statement on obesity and obesity medicine. *Endocr Pract*. 2012;18(5):642–648 PMID: 23047927
52. American Medical Association House of Delegates. Recognition of obesity as a disease. Resolution 420 (A-13). https://www.ama-assn.org/sites/ama-assn.org/files/corp/media-browser/public/hod/a13-reference-committee-reports_0.pdf. Adopted 2013. Accessed April 9, 2019
53. Kelly AS, Fox CK, Rudser KD, Gross AC, Ryder JR. Pediatric obesity pharmacotherapy: current state of the field, review of the literature and clinical trial considerations. *Int J Obes*. 2016;40(7):1043–1050 PMID: 27113643 https://doi.org/10.1038/ijo.2016.69
54. Ochner CN, Tsai AG, Kushner RF, Wadden TA. Treating obesity seriously: when recommendations for lifestyle change confront biological adaptations. *Lancet Diabetes Endocrinol*. 2015;3(4):232–234 PMID: 25682354 https://doi.org/10.1016/S2213-8587(15)00009-1
55. MacLean PS, Bergouignan A, Cornier MA, Jackman MR. Biology's response to dieting: the impetus for weight regain. *Am J Physiol Regul Integr Comp Physiol*. 2011;301(3):R581–R600 PMID: 21677272 https://doi.org/10.1152/ajpregu.00755.2010
56. Shonkoff JP, Garner AS, Siegel BS, et al; American Academy of Pediatrics Committee on Psychosocial Aspects of Child and Family Health; Committee on Early Childhood, Adoption, and Dependent Care; and Section on Developmental and Behavioral Pediatrics. The lifelong effects of early childhood adversity and toxic stress. *Pediatrics*. 2012;129(1):e232–e246 PMID: 22201156 https://doi.org/10.1542/peds.2011-2663
57. Juster RP, McEwen BS, Lupien SJ. Allostatic load biomarkers of chronic stress and impact on health and cognition. *Neurosci Biobehav Rev*. 2010;35(1):2–16 PMID: 19822172 https://doi.org/10.1016/j.neubiorev.2009.10.002
58. McEwen BS, Gianaros PJ. Central role of the brain in stress and adaptation: links to socioeconomic status, health, and disease. *Ann N Y Acad Sci*. 2010;1186(1):190–222 PMID: 20201874 https://doi.org/10.1111/j.1749-6632.2009.05331.x
59. Liu Y-Z, Wang Y-X, Jiang C-L. Inflammation: the common pathway of stress-related diseases. *Front Hum Neurosci*. 2017;11:316 PMID: 28676747 https://doi.org/10.3389/fnhum.2017.00316

60. Maruvada P, Leone V, Kaplan LM, Chang EB. The human microbiome and obesity: moving beyond associations. *Cell Host Microbe*. 2017;22(5):589–599 PMID: 29120742 https://doi.org/10.1016/j.chom.2017.10.005
61. Kumar S, Kelly AS. Review of childhood obesity: from epidemiology, etiology, and comorbidities to clinical assessment and treatment. *Mayo Clin Proc*. 2017;92(2):251–265 PMID: 28065514 https://doi.org/10.1016/j.mayocp.2016.09.017
62. Pratt JSA, Browne A, Browne NT, et al. ASMBS pediatric metabolic and bariatric surgery guidelines, 2018. *Surg Obes Relat Dis*. 2018;14(7):882–901 PMID: 30077361 https://doi.org/10.1016/j.soard.2018.03.019
63. Barlow SE; Expert Committee. Expert committee recommendations regarding the prevention, assessment, and treatment of child and adolescent overweight and obesity: summary report. *Pediatrics*. 2007;120(suppl 4):S164–S192 PMID: 18055651 https://doi.org/10.1542/peds.2007-2329C
64. Mirza N, Phan TL, Tester J, et al. A narrative review of medical and genetic risk factors among children age 5 and younger with severe obesity. *Child Obes*. 2018;14(7):443–452 PMID: 29791184 https://doi.org/10.1089/chi.2017.0350
65. Lenders CM, Gorman K, Lim-Miller A, Puklin S, Pratt J. Practical approaches to the treatment of severe pediatric obesity. *Pediatr Clin North Am*. 2011;58(6):1425–1438, x–xi PMID: 22093860 https://doi.org/10.1016/j.pcl.2011.09.013
66. Styne DM, Arslanian SA, Connor EL, et al. Pediatric obesity—assessment, treatment, and prevention: an Endocrine Society clinical practice guideline. *J Clin Endocrinol Metab*. 2017;102(3):709–757 PMID: 28359099
67. Anagnostou E, Aman MG, Handen BL, et al. Metformin for treatment of overweight induced by atypical antipsychotic medication in young people with autism spectrum disorder: a randomized clinical trial. *JAMA Psychiatry*. 2016;73(9):928–937 PMID: 27556593 https://doi.org/10.1001/jamapsychiatry.2016.1232
68. Wink LK, Adams R, Pedapati EV, et al. Brief report: metformin for antipsychotic-induced weight gain in youth with autism spectrum disorder. *J Autism Dev Disord*. 2017;47(7): 2290–2294 PMID: 28447303 https://doi.org/10.1007/s10803-017-3132-2
69. Zeller MH, Hunsaker S, Mikhail C, et al; TeenView Study Group and in collaboration with the Teen-LABS Consortium. Family factors that characterize adolescents with severe obesity and their role in weight loss surgery outcomes. *Obesity (Silver Spring)*. 2016;24(12):2562–2569 PMID: 27753228 https://doi.org/10.1002/oby.21676
70. Wilfley DE, Saelens BE, Stein RI, et al. Dose, content, and mediators of family-based treatment for childhood obesity: a multisite randomized clinical trial. *JAMA Pediatr*. 2017;171(12):1151–1159 PMID: 29084318 https://doi.org/10.1001/jamapediatrics.2017.2960
71. Hampl S, Demeule M, Eneli I, et al. Parent perspectives on attrition from tertiary care pediatric weight management programs. *Clin Pediatr (Phila)*. 2013;52(6):513–519 PMID: 23539682 https://doi.org/10.1177/0009922813482515
72. Substance Abuse and Mental Health Services Administration. Trauma. https://www.integration.samhsa.gov/clinical-practice/trauma-informed. Accessed June 5,2019
73. Green BL, Saunders PA, Power E, et al. Trauma-informed medical care: CME communication training for primary care providers. *Fam Med*. 2015;47(1):7–14 PMID: 25646872
74. US Department of Health and Human Services; Administration for Children and Families; Administration on Children, Youth and Families; Children's Bureau. *Child Maltreatment 2016*. https://www.acf.hhs.gov/cb/resource/child-maltreatment-2016. Reviewed January 7, 2019. Accessed April 10, 2019

75. Dubowitz H, Giardino A, Gustavson E. Child neglect: guidance for pediatricians. *Pediatr Rev*. 2000;21(4):111–116 PMID: 10756173 https://doi.org/10.1542/pir.21-4-111
76. Fortin K, Kwon S, Pierce MC. Characteristics of children reported to child protective services for medical neglect. *Hosp Pediatr*. 2016;6(4):204–210 PMID: 26931563 https://doi.org/10.1542/hpeds.2015-0151
77. Parmeter J, Tzioumi D, Woolfenden S. Medical neglect at a tertiary paediatric hospital. *Child Abuse Negl*. 2018;77:134–143 PMID: 29353717 https://doi.org/10.1016/j.chiabu.2018.01.004
78. Gray J, Cadieux A, Sweeney B, et al. Medical neglect and pediatric obesity: insights from tertiary care obesity treatment programs. *Child Health Care*. 2017;46(3):246–264 https://doi.org/10.1080/02739615.2016.1163488
79. Varness T, Allen DB, Carrel AL, Fost N. Childhood obesity and medical neglect. *Pediatrics*. 2009;123(1):399–406 PMID: 19117907 https://doi.org/10.1542/peds.2008-0712
80. Murtagh L, Ludwig DS. State intervention in life-threatening childhood obesity. *JAMA*. 2011;306(2):206–207 PMID: 21750301 https://doi.org/10.1001/jama.2011.903
81. Viner RM, Roche E, Maguire SA, Nicholls DE. Childhood protection and obesity: framework for practice. BMJ. 2010;341:c3074 PMID: 20634344
82. Alexander SM, Baur LA, Magnusson R, Tobin B. When does severe childhood obesity become a child protection issue? *Med J Aust*. 2009;190(3):136–139 PMID:19203311
83. Knutson JF, Taber SM, Murray AJ, Valles NL, Koeppl G. The role of care neglect and supervisory neglect in childhood obesity in a disadvantaged sample. *J Pediatr Psychol*. 2010;35(5):523–532 PMID: 19996153 https://doi.org/10.1093/jpepsy/jsp115
84. Flaherty EG, Sege R, Binns HJ, Mattson CL, Christoffel KK; Pediatric Practice Research Group. Health care providers' experience reporting child abuse in the primary care setting. *Arch Pediatr Adolesc Med*. 2000;154(5):489–493 PMID: 10807301 https://doi.org/10.1001/archpedi.154.5.489
85. Harper NS. Neglect: failure to thrive and obesity. *Pediatr Clin North Am*. 2014;61(5):937–957 PMID: 25242707 https://doi.org/10.1016/j.pcl.2014.06.006
86. Garrahan SM, Eichner AW. Tipping the scale: a place for childhood obesity in the evolving legal framework of child abuse and neglect. *Yale J Health Policy Law Ethics*. 2012;12(2):336–370 PMID: 23175918

PART 4

Other Forms of Maltreatment

CHAPTER 19

Psychological Maltreatment

Shelly D. Martin, MD
Child Abuse Pediatrician
Brooke Army Medical Center
San Antonio, TX
Associate Clinical Professor of Pediatrics
Uniformed Services University of the Health Sciences
Bethesda, MD

Katherine Snyder, MD, MPH, FAAP
Department of Pediatrics
Dell Medical School
University of Texas at Austin
Austin, TX

The view(s) expressed herein are those of the author(s) and do not reflect the official policy or position of Brooke Army Medical Center, the US Army Medical Department, the US Army Office of the Surgeon General, the Department of the Army, the Department of the Air Force and Department of Defense, or the US government.

Case Scenarios

A 5-year-old boy has nocturnal enuresis; as punishment, his father makes him wear diapers to school.

A 2-year-old girl falls from a chair; her mother provides no consolation to her and ignores her attempts to seek comfort.

An 11-year-old boy is made to duct tape his 6-year-old sister's hands together as punishment.

A 13-year-old girl is repeatedly told she is "stupid" by her parents, and they describe her that way to others.

A 7-year-old boy is locked in a closet for many hours as punishment.

Psychological maltreatment is a form of child abuse that is difficult to define. It goes by many terms: psychological maltreatment, psychological abuse, emotional abuse, and emotional neglect. This chapter will use *psychological maltreatment,* as was used in the American Academy of Pediatrics (AAP) clinical report of that name.[1] The 5 case scenarios in the box each describe a different form of psychological maltreatment. By the end of this chapter, it should be clear what form of maltreatment is described in each.

Although there is no universally agreed-on definition, the AAP defines psychological maltreatment as a "repeated pattern of parental behavior that is likely to be interpreted by a child that he or she is unloved, unwanted, or serves only instrumental purposes and/or that severely undermines the child's development and socialization."[1] This definition focuses on the behavior of the caregiver, not the effect on the child, and generally requires the behavior to be repetitive over time. Many actions that, in repetition, would qualify as psychological maltreatment would not qualify if they occurred once in isolation. It is often the pattern of behavior and parent-child interaction that rises to the level of abuse. While a single event, if terrifying, could rise to the level of psychological maltreatment, such as witnessing domestic violence or acts involving firearms, it is typically the repetitive nature of the dysfunctional parent-child interactions that rises to the level of psychological maltreatment.

Psychological maltreatment can include acts of omission and commission, can be verbal and nonverbal, and can be active or passive.[2] There is current consensus that actual harm to the child is not required and potential harm is sufficient for a diagnosis of psychological maltreatment.[1,2] Table 19.1 categorizes various types of caregiver behaviors that are often described as psychological maltreatment.

TABLE 19.1
Types of Psychological Maltreatment

Category	Example Behaviors
Spurning	Belittling, degrading, shaming, or ridiculing a child; singling out a child to criticize or punish; humiliating a child in public
Terrorizing	Committing life-threatening acts; making a child feel unsafe; setting unrealistic expectations with threat of loss, harm, or danger if they are not met; threatening or perpetrating violence against a child or child's loved ones or objects
Isolating	Confining, placing unreasonable limitations on freedom of movement or social interactions
Exploiting/corrupting	Modeling, permitting, or encouraging antisocial or developmentally inappropriate behavior; encouraging or coercing abandonment of developmentally appropriate autonomy; restricting or interfering with cognitive development
Neglecting mental health/medical/educational needs	Ignoring, preventing, or failing to provide treatments or services for emotional, behavioral, physical, or educational needs or problems
Witnessing intimate partner violence	

Adapted from Kairys SW, Johnson CF; American Academy of Pediatrics Committee on Child Abuse and Neglect. The psychological maltreatment of children—technical report. *Pediatrics.* 2002;109(4):e68.

An important concern is the lack of consensus across legal and child protective jurisdictions as to how psychological maltreatment is defined and handled. There is no consensus as to the criteria needed to substantiate a child protective services investigation for psychological abuse or neglect. Some states have a low threshold for identifying psychological maltreatment, and the potential for harm is sufficient. Other states require a child to have a psychiatric diagnosis for the case to be substantiated. Because there is wide variation between the extremes, a unified approach is lacking.

Part of the difficulty stems from differentiating psychological maltreatment from suboptimal parenting.[2] There is no agreement on when poor parenting reaches an egregious level. Those asked to determine when behaviors cross the line have their own set of biases, based on how they were raised, personal experiences, and how they parent their children. Over-pressuring children is a good example. Many parents expect their children to do their homework, study for examinations, and do their best to live up to their potential. However, some parents are overbearing, and their children have to study to exclusion of other activities. Less than perfect grades are not acceptable. The children feel pressure to succeed and have a fear of failure. Failure equates to the disappointment of the parents or even punishment. It can be difficult to determine when the line between encouraging children to succeed and pushing too hard is crossed.

Psychological maltreatment can stand alone as the only form of child maltreatment, or it can coexist with other forms of maltreatment, including physical abuse, sexual abuse, or neglect. In many cases, multiple forms of maltreatment coexist. For example, a child who experiences sexual abuse has emotional sequelae. There is often no investigation of the emotional component of the abuse to determine whether it is sufficient to stand as its own form of abuse.

Given the lack of a universal definition, psychological maltreatment is an underreported form of maltreatment. Per the US Department of Health and Human Services report on child maltreatment, in 2016, 5.6% of victimized children were psychologically maltreated, with more than half of these children experiencing multiple types of child maltreatment. This is down from 2015, when the total percentage of victimized children was 6.2%.[3] However, large population-based studies in the United States and United Kingdom showed that 8% to 9% of women and about 4% of men reported experiencing severe emotional abuse as a child.[4]

Risk Factors

While psychological maltreatment can occur in families with a wide array of characteristics, the risk increases when there are additional stressors in the home or life of the caregiver. Common risk factors include alcohol use, substance use, learning disabilities, psychological illness, family dysfunction, intimate partner violence, and lack of other adult support within the home.[2] Parents who are inexperienced or whose child is unplanned are also at higher risk of perpetrating psychological maltreatment.[5] Interestingly, other risk factors cited as playing a role, such as poor self-esteem, poor social skills, lack of empathy, and the caregiver's poorly attached relationship to their own caregiver as a child,[5] are all potential outcomes of psychological maltreatment as a young child.

Intimate Partner Violence

Intimate partner violence, an important subset of psychological maltreatment, is discussed in detail in Chapter 21, Interpersonal Violence. It is also a risk factor for additional forms of child maltreatment. Childhood exposure to domestic violence has been shown to have serious consequences to a child's emotional stability and mental health. There are physical risks to the child as well, but in many cases the child is not physically harmed. Studies estimate that direct abuse to the child occurs in 30% to 60% of homes where intimate partner violence is perpetrated.[6] Children may exhibit internalizing behaviors, such as anxiety, depression, withdrawal, and somatic complaints.[6] Others are more prone to externalizing behaviors that include aggression, attention problems, and noncompliance with rules.[6] Children who witness aggression and violent behavior in the home may become aggressive with others and have problems establishing normal relationships. Learning aggression at an early age and modeling parent behavior can lead to the child perpetuating intimate partner violence as an adult, thus continuing the cycle of violence. Children exposed to intimate partner violence can have difficulty concentrating, which affects cognitive function and academic performance. Children often worry about what happens at home even when they are not there. Although they are powerless to stop the violence, they feel a responsibility and feel they are at fault.

McFarlane and colleagues found that children 6 to 18 years old of mothers who experienced abuse exhibit significantly more internalizing, externalizing, and overall behavior problems than children not exposed to violence.[7] A careful assessment of children exposed to intimate partner violence should be completed with a focus on the type of exposure (eg, use of weapons and/or strangulation, hearing violence, witnessing violence) and how it affects them.

Assessment

It is important to assess children thoroughly when psychological maltreatment is suspected. In the office visit, the parents and the child should be evaluated. Talking to both parents can help the medical professional to understand their perspective and context regarding concerning behaviors. Talking to the child is important to evaluate what the child is experiencing and how he or she is affected by the behavior. Ideally, the child and the parents/caregivers should be evaluated independently of each other. Because both the home environment and the child vary in each case, there is no one way children exhibit signs of psychological maltreatment. Box 19.1 gives examples of how children might present when psychological maltreatment is occurring.

These behaviors could be associated with other underlying issues or disorders as well but are noted to occur with psychological maltreatment. Psychological maltreatment may disrupt child development in domains including cognitive (eg, school achievement, self-evaluations, frequent use of dissociation), social (eg, early attachments, peer relationships, aggression, withdrawal), emotional (eg, self-esteem, anxiety, depression), and physical (eg, failure to thrive, short stature).

BOX 19.1
Behavioral Responses to Psychological Maltreatment by Age

9 to 24 Months

Anxiously attached to caregiver, decline in intellectual function

24 to 42 Months

Noncompliant, unhappy, lacking in persistence, displaying little positive affect, and scoring lower on developmental testing than peers who have not experienced abuse

Preschool

Negativistic, impulsive, highly dependent on teachers, nervous, displays self-abusive behavior

Elementary School

Ranked by teachers to be low in peer acceptance and overall emotional health, more aggressive than peers, performs worse on achievement tests

Teen Years

Higher number of social problems, more delinquent, more aggressive, more suicidal than peers; most have at least 2 psychiatric disorders

Reprinted from Campbell AM, Hibbard R. More than words: the emotional maltreatment of children. Pediatr Clin North Am. 2014;61(5):959-970, copyright 2014, with permission from Elsevier.

Parent behaviors are also an important consideration when doing an evaluation for psychological maltreatment. Among parent and caregiver behaviors concerning for psychological maltreatment are insensitivity to the child's needs; rejection of the child's attention; frightening, threatening, or insulting behavior toward the child; calling the child "bad" or "evil"; lack of interest or concern when talking about the child; and responding emotionally or inconsistently to the child.[2]

When a concern for psychological maltreatment is present, a full evaluation in the medical office is warranted. There should be a discussion with the parents, without the child present, about the home situation and possible risk factors, discipline tactics, and general perceptions about the parent-child relationship. A useful approach to assessing how the parents feel about or view the child is to ask a few general questions, such as

- What is the best thing about your child?
- What is the most frustrating thing about your child?
- What do you like most about your child?
- What do you not like about your child?
- What is one thing you would change about your child if you could?

The medical professional should ask the parents to describe the child while paying attention to the adjectives and phrases used. Additionally, asking questions to assess for behaviors noted in Box 19.1 could also be helpful. Attention should be paid to the parent-child interactions in the office to evaluate how the parents interact, or do not interact, with the child through the use of the parents' verbal and body language.

If old enough, the child should be interviewed without the parents present. The child should be asked about home life, discipline, and interaction with his or her parents as well as life at school. Asking about likes and dislikes at home can be a useful tool. Trying to understand the parent-child relationship from the perspective of the child is important. Does the child feel loved, wanted, and valuable? The child should be asked how he or she feels about the parents. Talking to the child about what happens at home and how that affects him or her is needed not only to make sure the child is appropriately diagnosed and referred to counseling but to evaluate the effect on the child. This information may also be important to child protective services staff when investigating concerns for psychological maltreatment. Document anything said by parent or child and any relational dynamic and behaviors between them, using quotations when possible.[1] Finally, it is important to do a full medical assessment of the child, including assessing overall health, growth, and development, and to look for signs of physical or sexual abuse.

Not all children who experience psychological maltreatment are affected in the same way; the severity, chronicity, and intensity of the maltreatment all contribute to the effect(s) on the child. The resilience of the child, other support networks such as extended family and friends, and participation in out-of-home activities can mitigate the effect of psychological maltreatment on the child. The key point is to define the behaviors in the home to determine if they are concerning for maltreatment and evaluating the mental health needs of the child.

Reporting Psychological Maltreatment

It can be difficult for the medical professional to determine when concerns of psychological maltreatment rise to a level that warrants a report to child protective services. Medical professionals are mandated reporters, and a report is indicated when the suspicion of maltreatment is present, but specifically when to make the report can be a challenging decision. The AAP clinical report provides a good example of this difficulty. A child whose parents' less than amicable relationship spills over into issues of custody or accessibility to the child places the child at risk of psychological harm. The child's pediatrician can provide education as to the potential harm to this child and monitor the situation. If there is no improvement, therapy and/or reporting to child protective services is warranted.[1]

A multidisciplinary approach is needed for the assessment of psychological maltreatment concerns. Medical professionals should work together with investigators to define behavior that meets the criteria for maltreatment and to assess the effect on the child. Talking to school personnel, child care providers, coaches, church groups, family members, or others who interact with the child is an important component of a comprehensive evaluation. Sometimes a child, especially a younger child, is not able to fully describe the extent of maltreatment or articulate how he or she feels. Information about the child's behaviors or reactions from others can provide insight. A report to child protective services allows for the multidisciplinary evaluation to be used in full.[2]

Often the child is referred to counseling for needed therapeutic intervention and/or to gather more information about the child and his or her well-being. A full assessment can be difficult when a child is overwhelmed by investigators or fearful of reporting what goes on at home. Establishing a relationship with a counselor can help the child feel more comfortable talking about unpleasant events and discussing how he or she feels. If the parents do not provide the necessary counseling, a report to child protective services for failing to provide mental health care may be justified.

Treatment

Once a medical professional determines there is a concern for psychological maltreatment, treatment options must be considered. Early intervention and treatment are vital. There is limited information available on the efficacy of treatment modalities for children who have been psychologically maltreated. Additionally, many of these treatment modalities also serve as prevention modalities (discussed in the Prevention section). These modalities typically center on a modified cognitive behavioral therapy model or use multiple session interventions tailored toward the parent-child dyadic relationship.[1]

Medical professionals who treat children are often asked to aid the family in identifying and/or engaging in therapeutic services for themselves. While this may not manifest as individualized treatment of the caregiver as a patient, referral to appropriate resources is indicated. Caregivers who are psychologically maltreating their children are often survivors of various forms of child maltreatment themselves and/or have needs relating to psychological health, alcohol or substance use, or intimate partner violence, among others. In developing a treatment plan for the child, consider having appropriate referral resource information for the adult caregivers as well.

Outcomes

Psychological maltreatment affects attachment as well as physical and psychological development. *Attachment* is the emotional tie between a child and a caregiver. This bond provides the lens through which children establish their understanding of safety and relationships with others and themselves.[8] A child's behaviors are signals to his or her external world. How the caregiver responds to these signals teaches the child about the "value, safety and reliability of relationships"[8] and sets the foundation for how his or her communication will develop as well as the child's concept of trust.[8] When a caregiver responds appropriately and sensitively to the child's behaviors and cues in a consistent manner, the child learns that it is safe to express his or her needs and that these needs will be addressed. Conversely, caregivers who are not responsive to their child's behaviors or cues, are not consistent in their response, or are not effective in their response, or who respond inappropriately, teach the child that it is perhaps not safe or useful to express his or her needs and that the world is unstable.[2,8] The neural connections related to executive function and stress regulation are formed early in life. Alterations in how these connections form can have long-term effects on biologic stress responses, including the hypothalamic-pituitary-adrenal axis and the serotonin and dopamine systems.[8] This is a time of great growth and adaptability for the infant brain. The development of the infant brain is predicated on the way it is used and its exposure to stimuli and inputs, or the lack of such.[2,8] If the infant receives consistent and appropriate responses from a caregiver, as well as other forms of healthy, external stimuli, the infant's brain has the best opportunity to develop well. Alternatively, if an infant does not receive consistent and appropriate responses from a caregiver and does not receive other healthy stimuli, particular areas of the brain do not develop adequately and this poor development is "increasingly irreversible with age."[2] Psychological maltreatment in these early, formative years not only alters a child's attachment to his or her caregiver but can significantly alter the architecture of the developing brain, setting the stage for adverse long-term health consequences.

Psychological maltreatment affects early childhood relationships in a negative way and can lead to myriad effects on psychological and physical health as well as on the quality of interpersonal relationships.

Children who have experienced this form of maltreatment can have poor academic performance and memory, decreased ability to learn, and a lower IQ.[2,9] They are also at increased risk of being diagnosed with depression[2,9–11] and dysthymia.[10,12]

Children who experience psychological maltreatment often grow into adults with multiple problems, including health, social, and behavioral problems (tables 19.2 and 19.3).[2] The adult survivors of psychological maltreatment are at increased risk of psychological illness such as mood[17,18] and anxiety[17–19] disorders, personality disorders,[4,5,13,19] eating disorders,[2,22,23] substance use,[5,19] and alcoholism.[19] Additionally, they are at higher risk of poor self-esteem,[2,5] aggressive or violent behavior,[2,5,24] suicidality,[5,11,18,25] somatization,[5,11] dissociation,[11,15,17] obsessive-compulsive disorder,[11] and a decreased ability to effectively manage stress and anxiety.[2] Childhood psychological maltreatment also places adult survivors at increased risk of developing poorly attached and unhealthy relationships with others,[2,20] and, if they become parents, they have difficulty participating in stable and supportive relationships with their children.[2,12]

TABLE 19.2
Health Outcomes and Behavioral Symptoms Associated With Psychological Maltreatment[a]

Population	Psychological Diagnoses	Behavioral Symptoms	Medical Diagnoses
Child/adolescent	Mood disorders Depression[2,5,9–11] Dysthymia[10,12] Anxiety[2,10,13] ADHD[9,10,14,b]	Dissociation[13] Poor memory/concentration[2,10,14] Poor sleep[14] Withdrawal[9,10,14,15] Low self-esteem[2,9] Impulsivity[9] Anger/irritability[2,9,10,14] Suicidality[5,15] PTSD symptoms[15] Intrusive thoughts[9,14] Hypervigilance[2,8] Exaggerated responses[8,14] Sexualized behaviors[4] Somatization[5]	Failure to thrive[5,16] Worsened chronic health problems due to lack of attention to care[8] Short stature[13]
Adult	Mood disorders[17,18] Depression[17–20] Mania Anxiety disorders Obsessive-compulsive disorder[11] PTSD[19] Personality disorders[4,13,19,21] Borderline[5,11,13] Eating disorders[2,5,22,23] Substance use[5,19] Alcoholism[19]	Dissociation[15,17] Self-isolation[5] Poor self-esteem[2,5] Emotional lability[5] Overestimation of threat[2,14] Emotional unresponsiveness[5] Interpersonal sensitivity[20] Poor impulse control[5] Anger issues[5,24] Aggression/violence[2,5,24] Self-mutilation[5] Suicidality[5,11,18,25] Antisocial[5] Dependency[5] Sexual dysfunction[5,13] Somatization[5,11]	Obesity[4] Chronic pain[4] Ischemic heart disease[4] Liver disease[4] Cancer[4] Short stature[13]

Abbreviations: ADHD, attention-deficit/hyperactivity disorder; PTSD, posttraumatic stress disorder.
[a] All listed can be found as an outcome of one or more forms of child maltreatment, including psychological maltreatment.
[b] Symptoms often mimic those of posttraumatic stress.

TABLE 19.3
Associated Interpersonal and Social Outcomes of Psychological Maltreatment

Population	Associated Interpersonal and Social Outcomes
Child/adolescent	Poor academic performance[2,5,10,13,15] Lower IQ[2,9] Poor social competency[9,10] (leads to lack of or poorly attached relationships) Dating violence[15] Delinquency[5,9,10,14]
Adult	Poor stress management[2] Poor social competency[5] Poorly attached relationships[2,20] (including with own children)[12] Delinquency[5] Criminality[5,10,26]

Many of the long-term physical outcomes of psychological maltreatment reported in adults are related to child maltreatment as a whole or relate to other childhood adversities.[4] Limited data are available for the long-term physical outcomes for adults who experienced childhood psychological maltreatment alone without other forms of childhood maltreatment confounding the data.

Prevention

Most available prevention efforts for psychological maltreatment qualify as secondary or tertiary prevention. There is minimal discussion in the literature about primary prevention of psychological maltreatment, although the first level of the Triple P (discussed later in this section) would qualify.

Current prevention efforts can be categorized as *universal* or *individualized*. Universal approaches focus on encouraging parenting skills known to support ideal child development and are delivered on a global, population-based level. The individual forms are targeted to teaching parenting skills in a subgroup of the population[2] and often focus on improving the parent-child dynamics around infant cues and parental responses to those cues.[1]

Most available prevention efforts are aimed at young children, but there are limited resources to prevent psychological maltreatment in the older age groups. Additionally, most successful prevention efforts focus on the concept of "maternal sensitivity,"[1] which is the mother's ability and efficacy of recognizing and correctly interpreting her infant's behavioral cues. While it is known that this is a key component in attachment, it does not address the "sensitivity" of other caregivers, including the father.

The intervention programs that were deemed most successful in preventing child maltreatment as a whole included multiple sessions focusing on behaviors, some of which used real-time assessment of the caregiver-child interactional relationship followed by discussion. This type of intervention improved caregivers' ability to recognize and appropriately interpret their child's behavioral cues, but whether it helps specifically in the prevention of psychological maltreatment is unknown.[1]

The Nurse-Family Partnership (NFP)[1,27] is a well-known and well-researched program that has been shown to aid in preventing child maltreatment as a whole. This is a home nurse visitation program open to first-time mothers of low income. Intervention begins in the prenatal period and extends through the second year after birth. The home visits focus on 3 areas: "1) health-related behaviors during pregnancy and the early years of the child's life; 2) the care parents provided to their children; and 3) maternal personal life-course development (family planning, educational achievement, and participation in the workforce)."[27] Through the course of the program, the home visiting nurse aims to involve additional members of the family, connect the family with needed resources, teach the caregivers how to care for the infant physically and emotionally, and help the mothers define personal goals and plans for achieving them. Since the inception of NFP, various studies have shown it to have multiple benefits, including decreasing home safety hazards, decreasing controlling behaviors by the mother, increasing intellectually stimulating toys and books in the home, decreasing visits to physicians for injuries or ingestions, and decreasing visits to the emergency department.[28] Long-term follow-up of families involved in NFP showed these families have lower levels of child abuse and neglect, less use of welfare, fewer additional pregnancies, and decreased criminality for low-income, unmarried mothers for up to 15 years after the initial intervention.[27]

Another well-known intervention program, the Positive Parenting Program, or Triple P, was developed at the University of Queensland and is aimed at preschool and school-aged children who have disruptive behaviors. The intervention is based on 5 principles: "1) ensuring a safe, engaging environment, 2) promoting a positive learning environment,

3) using assertive discipline, 4) maintaining reasonable expectations, and 5) taking care of oneself as a parent."[29] Triple P aims to prevent "behavioral, emotional, and developmental problems in children" by improving caregivers' competence and confidence in raising their children.[30] The program uses 5 levels of "intervention intensity," with level 1 universally providing parents with helpful information about parenting in various forms of media (eg, messaging on local radio and in local newspapers, newsletters, mass mailing to family homes) and level 5 focusing on an individualized approach to families in which child behavioral issues are ongoing and/or when there are additional forms of stress affecting the family unit. Multiple meta-analyses have noted that involvement in the Triple P improves parenting skills and child behavior, with most of the studies focusing on the level 4 and 5 interventions. The Primary Care Triple P is a level 3 intervention and designed to be a brief, multi-session intervention that can be used in various medical settings, including home visitation. Each session combines use of tip sheets on common preadolescent behavioral and/or developmental challenges and active skills building for the parent to practice. Primary Care Triple P is best used in the infant, toddler, and preschool population when there is one specific behavioral concern without significant background familial dysfunction.[29] This has shown promise in decreasing conduct problems in children.[30] Triple P has also shown preventive effects on substantiated child maltreatment cases, injuries related to child maltreatment, and out-of-home placements related to child maltreatment.[29]

Parent-child interactional therapy (PCIT) is an intervention targeted at caregivers of children 2 to 7 years old that aims to decrease disruptive child behavior by addressing parent-child interactions in real time. Parent-child interactional therapy is composed of child-directed and parent-directed interactions that are monitored via a one-way mirror by a trained therapist who can provide the caregiver real-time feedback or suggestions while the interaction is occurring. The goal is to improve a caregiver's ability to focus on positive reinforcement and minimize attention to a child's disruptive behaviors while the caregiver learns to handle his or her own emotions during challenging interactions with the child.[31] Physically abusive parents who underwent PCIT had fewer additional reports for physical abuse than did parents in the control group, and changes in parental behaviors were shown to continue through the treatment period.[32] Chaffin et al showed that combining PCIT with motivational interviewing helped increase parental retention in parenting programs among parents involved in child welfare services who had low to moderate motivation for participation.[33] Similar results were found when applying these methods in the field and among families with "chronic and severe child welfare histories."[34]

These methodologies aim to intervene at the fundamental level of the caregiver-child relationship to improve the concept of "maternal sensitivity"[1] to the child's behaviors and cues, while also addressing other stresses to the family. While there has been success with these models, they have limitations, including prohibitive selection criteria that leave many family groups without a resource and a lack of availability in rural and urban areas alike. While these programs have been linked to decreasing child maltreatment overall, there is no known program that specifically decreases psychological maltreatment.

The medical professional has the unique opportunity to participate in primary prevention of psychological maltreatment. Medical professionals can model appropriate behaviors including those that relate to emotional responsiveness to the child, intervene when inappropriate behaviors are identified, and provide anticipatory guidance to the family.[5] Possible scenarios encountered include hearing a caregiver call a child names or threaten him or her with some form of harm such as shots, calling the police, and/or being taken to jail. These are opportunities to redirect the conversation and provide education to the family about the negative outcomes associated with these types of behaviors. For example, when a caregiver calls a child "bad," the medical professional has an opportunity to intervene. Explaining that the child is not bad but that the behavior is less than ideal reinforces to the child and caregiver that the behavior is the issue, and not the moral value of the child. This also allows an open discussion with the caregiver about the possible outcomes associated with this type of labeling should it continue. Another form of primary prevention in the clinical setting is the various forms of media including, but not limited to, pamphlets, handouts, and educational public service announcements on television. There is no evidence base, as of yet, to show that these strategies prevent psychological maltreatment, but there is some evidence that these approaches delivered in a population-based format help prevent child maltreatment overall.[1]

Conclusion

Psychological maltreatment is a complex and likely under-identified form of child maltreatment. It often coexists with other forms of child maltreatment but can occur in isolation. Recognizing psychological maltreatment requires an understanding of the various qualifying parental behaviors and how to assess for them in a clinical setting. Table 19.4 revisits the case scenarios from the beginning of the chapter, filling in the type of psychological maltreatment exemplified by each. There are numerous and varied potential short- and long-term physical, psychological, and interpersonal consequences of psychological maltreatment. Early identification is crucial so treatment methodologies can begin decreasing these potential outcomes. While multiple child maltreatment prevention efforts exist and are somewhat successful, no prevention efforts specifically focus on preventing psychological maltreatment.

TABLE 19.4
Examples of Psychological Maltreatment

Case Scenarios	Type of Psychological Maltreatment
A 5-year-old boy has nocturnal enuresis; as punishment, his father makes him wear diapers to school.	Terrorizing
A 2-year-old girl falls from a chair; her mother provides no consolation to her and ignores her attempts to seek comfort.	Denying emotional responsiveness
An 11-year-old boy is made to duct tape his 6-year-old sister's hands together as punishment.	Exploiting/corrupting
A 13-year-old girl is repeatedly told she is "stupid" by her parents, and they describe her that way to others.	Spurning
A 7-year-old boy is locked in a closet for many hours as punishment.	Isolating

References

1. Hibbard R, Barlow J, Macmillan H; American Academy of Pediatrics Committee on Child Abuse and Neglect; and American Academy of Child and Adolescent Psychiatry Child Maltreatment and Violence Committee. Psychological maltreatment. *Pediatrics*. 2012;130(2):372–378 PMID: 22848125 https://doi.org/10.1542/peds.2012-1552
2. Campbell AM, Hibbard R. More than words: the emotional maltreatment of children. *Pediatr Clin North Am*. 2014;61(5):959–970 PMID: 25242708 https://doi.org/10.1016/j.pcl.2014.06.004
3. US Department of Health and Human Services Administration for Children and Families; Administration on Children, Youth and Families; Children's Bureau. *Child Maltreatment 2016*. https://www.acf.hhs.gov/sites/default/files/cb/cm2016.pdf. Accessed April 3, 2019
4. Gilbert R, Widom CS, Browne K, Fergusson D, Webb E, Janson S. Burden and consequences of child maltreatment in high-income countries. *Lancet*. 2009;373(9657):68–81 PMID: 19056114 https://doi.org/10.1016/S0140-6736(08)61706-7
5. Kairys SW, Johnson CF; American Academy of Pediatrics Committee on Child Abuse and Neglect. The psychological maltreatment of children—technical report. *Pediatrics*. 2002;109(4):e68 PMID: 11927741 https://doi.org/10.1542/peds.109.4.e68
6. Thackeray JD, Hibbard R, Dowd MD; American Academy of Pediatrics Committee on Child Abuse and Neglect and Committee on Injury, Violence, and Poison Prevention.

Intimate partner violence: the role of the pediatrician. *Pediatrics*. 2010;125(5):1094–1100 PMID: 20421260 https://doi.org/10.1542/peds.2010-0451

7. McFarlane JM, Groff JY, O'Brien JA, Watson K. Behaviors of children who are exposed and not exposed to intimate partner violence: an analysis of 330 black, white, and Hispanic children. *Pediatrics*. 2003;112(3 Pt 1):e202–e207 PMID: 12949313 https://doi.org/10.1542/peds.112.3.e202
8. Rees CA. Understanding emotional abuse. *Arch Dis Child*. 2010;95(1):59–67 PMID: 20040686 https://doi.org/10.1136/adc.2008.143156
9. Maguire SA, Williams B, Naughton AM, et al. A systematic review of the emotional, behavioural and cognitive features exhibited by school-aged children experiencing neglect or emotional abuse. *Child Care Health Dev*. 2015;41(5):641–653 PMID: 25733080 https://doi.org/10.1111/cch.12227
10. Thompson R, Tabone JK. The impact of early alleged maltreatment on behavioral trajectories. *Child Abuse Negl*. 2010;34(12):907–916 PMID: 21111247 https://doi.org/10.1016/j.chiabu.2010.06.006
11. Bifulco A, Moran PM, Baines R, Bunn A, Stanford K. Exploring psychological abuse in childhood: II. Association with other abuse and adult clinical depression. *Bull Menninger Clin*. 2002;66(3):241–258 PMID: 12448629 https://doi.org/10.1521/bumc.66.3.241.23366
12. Moran PM, Bifulco A, Ball C, Jacobs C, Benaim K. Exploring psychological abuse in childhood: I. Developing a new interview scale. *Bull Menninger Clin*. 2002;66(3):213–240 PMID: 12448628 https://doi.org/10.1521/bumc.66.3.213.23367
13. Thompson AE, Kaplan CA. Responding to concerns about childhood emotional abuse. *Hosp Med*. 1998;59(12):951–954 PMID: 10696360
14. Sege RD, Amaya-Jackson L; American Academy of Pediatrics Committee on Child Abuse and Neglect and Council on Foster Care, Adoption, and Kinship Care; American Academy of Child and Adolescent Psychiatry Committee on Child Maltreatment and Violence; National Center for Child Traumatic Stress. Clinical considerations related to the behavioral manifestations of child maltreatment. *Pediatrics*. 2017;139(4):e1–e13 PMID: 28320870
15. Egeland B. Taking stock: childhood emotional maltreatment and developmental psychopathology. *Child Abuse Negl*. 2009;33(1):22–26 PMID: 19167068 https://doi.org/10.1016/j.chiabu.2008.12.004
16. Iwaniec D. An overview of emotional maltreatment and failure to thrive. *Child Abuse Rev*. 1997;6(5):370–388 https://doi.org/10.1002/(SICI)1099-0852(199712)6:5<370::AID-CAR362>3.0.CO;2-G
17. Ferguson KS, Dacey CM. Anxiety, depression, and dissociation in women health care providers reporting a history of childhood psychological abuse. *Child Abuse Negl*. 1997;21(10):941–952 PMID: 9330795 https://doi.org/10.1016/S0145-2134(97)00055-0
18. Martins CM, Von Werne Baes C, Tofoli SM, Juruena MF. Emotional abuse in childhood is a differential factor for the development of depression in adults. *J Nerv Ment Dis*. 2014;202(11):774–782 PMID: 25268154 https://doi.org/10.1097/NMD.0000000000000202
19. Taillieu TL, Brownridge DA, Sareen J, Afifi TO. Childhood emotional maltreatment and mental disorders: results from a nationally representative adult sample from the United States. *Child Abuse Negl*. 2016;59:1–12 PMID: 27490515 https://doi.org/10.1016/j.chiabu.2016.07.005
20. Riggs SA, Kaminski P. Childhood emotional abuse, adult attachment, and depression as predictors of relational adjustment and psychological aggression. *J Aggress Maltreat Trauma*. 2010;19(1):75–104 https://doi.org/10.1080/10926770903475976

21. Johnson JG, Cohen P, Smailes EM, Skodol AE, Brown J, Oldham JM. Childhood verbal abuse and risk for personality disorders during adolescence and early adulthood. *Compr Psychiatry*. 2001;42(1):16–23 PMID: 11154711 https://doi.org/10.1053/comp.2001.19755
22. Kent A, Waller G. Childhood emotional abuse and eating psychopathology. *Clin Psychol Rev*. 2000;20(7):887–903 PMID: 11057376 https://doi.org/10.1016/S0272-7358(99)00018-5
23. Waller G, Corstorphine E, Mountford V. The role of emotional abuse in the eating disorders: implications for treatment. *Eat Disord*. 2007;15(4):317–331 PMID: 17710569 https://doi.org/10.1080/10640260701454337
24. Allen B. Childhood psychological abuse and adult aggression: the mediating role of self-capacities. *J Interpers Violence*. 2011;26(10):2093–2110 PMID: 20956437 https://doi.org/10.1177/0886260510383035
25. de Araújo RM, Lara DR. More than words: the association of childhood emotional abuse and suicidal behavior. *Eur Psychiatry*. 2016;37:14–21 PMID: 27442978 https://doi.org/10.1016/j.eurpsy.2016.04.002
26. Jung H, Herrenkohl TI, Lee JO, Klika JB, Skinner ML. Effects of physical and emotional child abuse and its chronicity on crime into adulthood. *Violence Vict*. 2015;30(6):1004–1018 PMID: 26439922 https://doi.org/10.1891/0886-6708.VV-D-14-00071
27. Olds DL, Eckenrode J, Henderson CR Jr, et al. Long-term effects of home visitation on maternal life course and child abuse and neglect. Fifteen-year follow-up of a randomized trial. *JAMA*. 1997;278(8):637–643 PMID: 9272895 https://doi.org/10.1001/jama.1997.03550080047038
28. Olds D, Henderson CR Jr, Kitzman H, Cole R. Effects of prenatal and infancy nurse home visitation on surveillance of child maltreatment. *Pediatrics*. 1995;95(3):365–372 PMID: 7862474
29. Prinz RJ, Sanders MR, Shapiro CJ, Whitaker DJ, Lutzker JR. Population-based prevention of child maltreatment: the U.S. Triple P system population trial. *Prev Sci*. 2009;10(1):1–12 PMID: 19160053 https://doi.org/10.1007/s11121-009-0123-3
30. Boyle CL, Sanders MR, Lutzker JR, Prinz RJ, Shapiro C, Whitaker DJ. An analysis of training, generalization, and maintenance effects of Primary Care Triple P for parents of preschool-aged children with disruptive behavior. *Child Psychiatry Hum Dev*. 2010;41(1):114–131 PMID: 19697120 https://doi.org/10.1007/s10578-009-0156-7
31. Thomas R, Zimmer-Gembeck MJ. Accumulating evidence for parent-child interaction therapy in the prevention of child maltreatment. *Child Dev*. 2011;82(1):177–192 PMID: 21291436 https://doi.org/10.1111/j.1467-8624.2010.01548.x
32. Chaffin M, Silovsky JF, Funderburk B, et al. Parent-child interaction therapy with physically abusive parents: efficacy for reducing future abuse reports. *J Consult Clin Psychol*. 2004;72(3):500–510 PMID: 15279533 https://doi.org/10.1037/0022-006X.72.3.500
33. Chaffin M, Valle LA, Funderburk B, et al. A motivational intervention can improve retention in PCIT for low-motivation child welfare clients. *Child Maltreat*. 2009;14(4):356–368 PMID: 19258303 https://doi.org/10.1177/1077559509332263
34. Chaffin M, Funderburk B, Bard D, Valle LA, Gurwitch R. A combined motivation and parent-child interaction therapy package reduces child welfare recidivism in a randomized dismantling field trial. *J Consult Clin Psychol*. 2011;79(1):84–95 PMID: 21171738 https://doi.org/10.1037/a0021227

CHAPTER 20

Medical Child Abuse

Paige Culotta, MD, FAAP
Child Abuse Pediatrician
Children's Hospital of New Orleans
Audrey Hepburn CARE Center
New Orleans, LA

Jonathan Thackeray, MD, FAAP
Chief Medical Community Health Officer
Department of Medical Affairs
Dayton Children's Hospital
Professor and Vice Chair
Department of Pediatrics
Wright State University Boonshoft School of Medicine
Dayton, OH

Medical child abuse (MCA), previously described with a variety of names, including Munchausen syndrome by proxy and pediatric condition falsification disorder, was first coined by Sir Roy Meadow in 1977 to describe "parents who, by falsification, caused their children innumerable harmful hospital procedures."[1] The original name is derived from Munchausen syndrome, a condition of self-inflicted illness in adults. Acknowledging that the key feature of Munchausen syndrome by proxy is the infliction of harm on a child through the actions of the child's caregiver, and that this phenomenon is similar to other forms of child non-accidental injury, Roesler and Jenny first proposed the term *medical child abuse* in 1995. A full argument for abandonment of previous terminology and adoption of MCA is presented in their 2009 textbook, *Medical Child Abuse: Beyond Munchausen Syndrome by Proxy*.[2]

Regardless of the name, in the decades since its initial description, and compared with other forms of child abuse, MCA has proven to be a form of child maltreatment fraught with unique diagnostic and legal challenges, many of which are described in this chapter.

Definition

Medical child abuse has been defined as "child maltreatment caused by a caregiver who falsifies and/or induces a child's illness, leading to unnecessary and potentially harmful medical investigations and/or treatment."[3] *Falsification,* or fabrication, means that an inaccurate history is provided by the caregiver. A mother, for example, may repeatedly report that her child has episodes of stiffening, shaking, or decreased level of consciousness resulting in multiple evaluations for seizures or intracranial conditions. A caregiver may tell a pediatrician that the child has hematuria and bring in a urine sample that she has contaminated with her own menstrual blood, resulting in unnecessary diagnostic testing to determine the etiology of the child's hematuria. *Induction* means that the caregiver's actions (eg, suffocation of the child; administration of medications) result in symptoms or signs in the child, the fact or the extent of which are not proffered by history.

Regardless of whether the caregiver fabricates or induces illness (or both), it is important to understand that in this form of child abuse, the caregiver's actions result in the health care system being used as a vector of the abuse—the proverbial stick with which the child is struck.[1] Similarly, Roesler and Jenny define MCA as occurring when "a child receives unnecessary and harmful or potentially harmful medical care at the instigation of a caretaker."[2] In MCA, illness in a child is persistently and secretly simulated and/or produced by a caregiver, and the child repeatedly is presented for medical assessment and care. This often results in multiple medical procedures, both diagnostic and therapeutic. The definition specifically excludes separate acts of physical abuse, sexual abuse, and nonmedical causes of failure to thrive that are solely the result of nutritional or emotional deprivation.

Epidemiology

Hundreds of cases of MCA have been reported worldwide, although it is likely that most cases of MCA go unreported in the literature. Clearly, MCA is not a culture-specific disorder, nor is it confined to either a socialized or privatized medical system. Determining a precise incidence of this form of abuse, however, is difficult due to varying definitions of MCA used by researchers and the lack of *International Classification of Diseases* coding to identify this disorder, among other concerns. One study in the United Kingdom estimated the combined annual incidence of MCA, non-accidental poisoning, and non-accidental suffocation as at least 2.8 per 100,000 in infants younger than 1 year.[4] Extrapolation of this data to the United States suggests there are between 200 and 600 new cases of MCA per year[5] due to suffocation or intentional poisoning. A separate study conducted in New Zealand, using an entirely different methodology, reported an overall MCA incidence rate of 2 per 100,000 in children younger than 16 years.[6]

The description of characteristics of those who experience MCA is largely limited to case reports, case series, and a few published literature reviews, so how to extrapolate these data to more generalized populations is unclear. What is known from the existing literature is that most of those who experience MCA are infants and toddlers.[4,7,8] Presumably, younger children are more commonly affected because they lack the verbal skills necessary to disclose their abuse and are relatively helpless physically, making them easier to manipulate and assault. In one literature review, boys and girls experienced MCA almost equally, and no special trend was noted as to birth order.[8] It has been observed that while several children in a family may experience MCA sequentially, it is unusual for more than 1 child to experience MCA within any given period,[9] except during relatively brief transition periods.

Although MCA commonly begins in infancy or toddlerhood, there is usually a delay in establishing the correct diagnosis. In 2 case series, the average time from onset of symptoms and signs to diagnosis ranged from 15 to 22 months.[7,8] There are multiple potential reasons for this delay, including that information provided by the caregiver is rarely, if ever, accurate; reported symptoms may never be observed by medical staff; the range of potential symptoms is diverse; a percentage of children experiencing this form of abuse will also have a true medical diagnosis; care is often sought from multiple medical professionals across multiple institutions; and medical professionals do not always agree on the child's diagnosis. The perpetrator of MCA often evades early detection because the reported symptoms and signs seem plausible. Diagnosis and treatment in the field of pediatrics are founded on the development of a trusting relationship between the medical professional and the child's caregiver. Medical professionals depend on the caregiver history to adequately care for the child, often in the absence of any objective evidence. For example, for a child who is vomiting, a diagnosis can be formulated by the medical professional without actually witnessing the child vomit. The perpetrator's history often sounds cogent to the medical professional, bespeaking a serious illness. Although medical professionals are educated to evaluate critically the reliability of a historian, they do not expect that a history may be an elaborate lie.

Throughout training, medical professionals are taught to fully evaluate all symptoms, making a broad differential diagnosis so as not to miss a significant or life-threatening disorder. They are often humbled by more experienced professionals and feel that if a clinical diagnosis cannot be established the fault lies with them, causing them to work harder to figure out the puzzle, rather than considering that a medical diagnosis cannot be established because there is none. There may be a fear that, in assigning the diagnosis of MCA, one may perhaps be missing an important or rare diagnosis that the medical professional has not yet figured out.[10] The diagnosis, of course, may not ever be made by the medical professional at all.

A rare case report describes cessation of MCA not because of medical diagnosis but because the school-aged child identified the abuse inflicted on her and threatened to disclose her mother's actions.[11]

In most cases of MCA described in the literature, the perpetrator of the abuse has been the biological mother.[4,7,8] A recent systematic review of case reports and series published since 1965 identified nearly 800 children who experienced MCA and descriptions of the perpetrators. In this study, nearly all abusers were female (97.6%) and the child's mother (95.6%).[12] As knowledge of MCA grows, however, a wider range of perpetrators, including fathers,[13,14] other relatives,[15,16] babysitters,[17] and nurses,[18] has been described. Why MCA is overwhelmingly a female-perpetrated form of child abuse is not clear, although female patterns of learned behavior and expression of hostility have been proposed. It certainly stands in contrast with other forms of child abuse, such as physical and sexual abuse, in which male perpetrators predominate. In one study, perpetrators of MCA were frequently reported to be in health care-related professions (45.6%), to have had obstetric complications (23.5%), or to have a personal history of childhood maltreatment (30%).[12,19,20] Comorbid psychiatry diagnoses are common and include factitious disorder imposed on self,[12,21] somatization disorder,[21] personality disorder, and depression.[22] It is not to be understood from this that the mother has some kind of disease that renders her incapable of discerning right from wrong, that makes her compulsively perform acts outside her consciousness, or that makes her either the unwilling or unwitting captive of an irresistible impulse. Only rarely is the mother deemed to be psychotic or delusional.[7,8] No evidence whatsoever, in fact, suggests that the perpetrator of MCA is unaware of his or her actions. On the contrary, the planning and organization often involved, the minute attention to secrecy, the fact that the assaults are committed without witnesses, and the carefully woven fabric of lies presented to the medical professional all suggest great awareness.

Clinical Presentation

As stated previously, MCA involves the fabrication and/or induction of illness. In one series of MCA cases, approximately 25% involved fabrication only, 25% involved induction only, and 50% involved both fabrication and induction.[8] Another larger series, however, showed that nearly 60% of illness was induced.[7] In 50% to 95% of cases, depending on the meta-analytic series, the perpetrator continued abusing the child in the hospital,[7,8] often in the most egregious ways,[23] and even in closely monitored settings, such as the pediatric intensive care unit.[24]

The clinical presentations of MCA cover an enormous spectrum, involving hundreds of potential signs and symptoms and every organ system of the body. Common presenting symptoms described include, but certainly are not limited to, apnea, seizures, feeding problems, bleeding, central nervous system depression, diarrhea, vomiting, rash, allergy, and behavioral problems.[7,8] Table 20.1 provides a system-based list of presentations of MCA, but this list should not be considered exhaustive by any means.

It is important to remember that children experiencing MCA may also have genuine chronic disease. How the perpetrator of MCA addresses and reports symptoms of legitimate disease, including falsification of symptoms of legitimate disease and intentional withholding of treatment to exacerbate symptoms, are not well studied.[25,26]

TABLE 20.1
Some Clinical Presentations of Medical Child Abuse[a]

System	Symptom, Sign, or Laboratory Finding
Head, eyes, ears, nose, throat, mouth	Bleeding from ears, nose, throat
	Conjunctivitis
	External otitis
	Hearing/speech impairment
	Nasal excoriation
	Nystagmus
	Orbital cellulitis
	Otorrhea
	Parotitis
	Tooth loss
Respiratory	Apnea and/or brief resolved unexplained event
	Asthma
	Bleeding from upper respiratory tract
	Choking/dyspnea
	Cyanosis (and other color changes including pallor)
	Cystic fibrosis
	Hemoptysis
	Respiratory arrest
	Respiratory infection
	Sleep apnea

(continued)

TABLE 20.1 (*continued*)

System	Symptom, Sign, or Laboratory Finding
Cardiovascular	Cardiomyopathy
	Cardiopulmonary arrest
	Hypertension
	Rhythm abnormalities (including bradycardia, tachycardia, ventricular tachycardia, and others)
	Shock
Gastrointestinal	Abdominal pain
	Anorexia
	Bleeding from nasogastric tube/ileostomy
	Celiac disease
	Chronic intestinal pseudo-obstruction
	Crohn disease
	Diarrhea
	Esophageal burns
	Esophageal perforation
	Feculent vomiting
	Feeding problems
	Gastrointestinal ulceration
	Hematemesis
	Hematochezia or melena
	Hemorrhagic colitis
	Malabsorption syndromes
	Polyphagia
	Pseudomelanosis coli
	Retrograde intussusception
	Vomiting (cyclic or otherwise)
Genitourinary	Bacteriuria
	Hematuria
	Menorrhagia
	Nocturia
	Polydipsia
	Polyuria and/or impaired urinary concentrating ability

(continued)

TABLE 20.1 (*continued*)

System	Symptom, Sign, or Laboratory Finding
Genitourinary (*continued*)	Proteinuria Pyuria Renal failure Urethral stones Urination from umbilical micropenis Urine gravel
Psychiatric	Behavioral/personality disorders (including anxiety, autism spectrum disorder, panic reactions, rage, disorientation, and others) Irritability Psychotic symptoms Sleep disturbances (including prolonged sleep, others)
Neurologic	Ataxia Cerebral palsy Headache Lethargy Seizures Syncope Unconsciousness Weakness
Musculoskeletal	Arthralgia Arthritis Morning stiffness
Developmental	Developmental delay (failure to attain and/or loss of milestones) Hyperactivity Learning/attention disability Tourette syndrome
Skin	Abscesses Burns Eczema Excoriation Rash

(continued)

TABLE 20.1 (*continued*)

System	Symptom, Sign, or Laboratory Finding
Infectious, immune, allergic	Allergies (to food, drugs, others)
	Bacteremia
	Fevers
	Immunodeficiency
	Osteomyelitis
	Septic arthritis
	Sinopulmonary disease
	Soft tissue/skin infection
	Urinary tract infection
Hematologic	Anemia
	Bleeding diathesis
	Bleeding from specific sites (see system)
	Easy bruising
	Leukopenia
Metabolic, endocrine, fluid and electrolyte	Acidosis
	Alkalosis
	Biochemical chaos
	Creatine kinase and aldolase increase
	Cystinosis
	Dehydration
	Diabetes
	Glycosuria
	Hyperglycemia
	Hyperkalemia
	Hypernatremia
	Hypochloremia
	Hypoglycemia
	Hypokalemia
	Hyponatremia
	MELAS (mitochondrial encephalopathy, lactic acidosis, and stroke-like episodes) syndrome

(*continued*)

TABLE 20.1 (*continued*)

System	Symptom, Sign, or Laboratory Finding
Other	Abuse of the child (sexual, physical, other)
	Diaphoresis
	Failure to gain weight or weight loss
	Fatigue
	Foreign-body ingestions
	Hypothermia
	Pain
	Peripheral edema
	Poisonings
	Preterm birth

[a] Including items reportedly observed by mother or actually observed by medical staff.

Evaluation

Failure to diagnose MCA means that a fundamentally healthy child (and, potentially, his or her siblings) is exposed to ongoing abuse and is, therefore, at risk for long-term morbidity or mortality. Conversely, the failure to exclude MCA as a diagnosis may mean that necessary treatment is withheld from an ill child, a family is not offered prognostic information or genetic counseling, or the child is separated from his or her family. The single largest impediment to establishing a diagnosis of MCA is the failure to include it in the differential diagnosis. Once the diagnosis is entertained and a diagnostic strategy designed, the diagnosis is often much easier to assign or exclude.

Once MCA is suspected, confirmation or elimination of the diagnosis may be undertaken through one of a number of strategies, including review of the child's medical records, diagnostic testing, covert video surveillance (CVS), and separation of the child from the suspected perpetrator.

Review of Medical Records

The foundation of the diagnosis of MCA often begins with a thorough review of the child's medical records and reformulation of a differential diagnosis, perhaps by a medical professional independent of the child's care team. As the data are reviewed, it is prudent to use a 3-question framework provided by the American Academy of Pediatrics[3] to help determine if MCA is occurring.

1. Are the history, signs, and symptoms of disease credible?
2. Is the child receiving unnecessary and harmful or potentially harmful medical care?
3. If so, who is instigating the evaluations and treatment?

This strategy, which one may suppose has been implicit in the medical care previously provided, follows from the observation that the pivotal facts, although present in the medical record, are frequently obscured by the sheer volume of information accumulated. In other words, the crucial data to formulate a diagnosis exist but are hidden. Furthermore, the importance of a comprehensive survey of the child's medical presentation may have been repeatedly overshadowed by the immediacy of the crises. Curiously, the more chronic and intractable the child's problem, the less likely it may be that it is given a fresh, comprehensive look. Finally, a sort of colonial system of medical care sometimes evolves, with fragments of the child's condition being parceled out to subspecialists, whose purview extends only to the edge of their organ systems of interest. They accept without question the "fact" of abnormalities in another system. Overview is neglected. The totality of the presentation is lost.

Records review may be the preferred diagnostic strategy, because it is low risk and often definitive. Records review may also be the only diagnostic strategy available when the child is unavailable for evaluation for some reason, when the symptoms and signs of fabrication are long gone, when the child has received medical care at multiple institutions, or when the child is dead. For cases of suspected MCA, records often number hundreds of encounters and thousands of pages, often from myriad medical facilities. A computerized system for data entry, storage, organization, and retrieval is often indispensable, and any number of commercially available database-management systems can be adapted for this purpose.[2] See the Management section later in this chapter for more information on navigating records.

Diagnostic Testing

Although a thorough review of records may be diagnostic of MCA in and of itself, it may be necessary to undertake additional testing to confirm or exclude the diagnosis of MCA. While the decision to conduct additional testing in any circumstance should be made with the utmost caution and consideration of the risks and benefits to the child, it carries additional importance in cases of suspected MCA because diagnostic testing may be the very harm the medical professional is striving to prevent. When used prudently, however, testing may be the key to diagnosis. Testing such as toxicology studies when poisoning is suspected or blood group typing, subtyping, or DNA typing if contamination with exogenous blood is suspected, for example, may be useful in establishing a diagnosis. The medical literature contains some fascinating accounts in which testing has proven the induction and/or fabrication of illness.

- Ipecac poisoning uncovered by finding a postmortem blood sample result that is positive for the alkaloids in ipecac[27] or by toxicological studies in a living child[28,29]
- Factitious bleeding exposed by minor blood group typing of erythrocytes in urine,[30] injection of radiolabeled erythrocytes as comparisons to the child's "bleeding sites,"[31] DNA typing of the bloody towel presented by the parent compared with that of the child's buccal cells,[32] or comparison of the hemoglobin F concentration of an infant's blood to that of the blood stains on the infant's bedclothes[33]
- Use of sweat potassium to identify falsification of a sweat test for cystic fibrosis[34]
- Confirmation of factitious diabetes mellitus using ascorbic acid as a marker for the child's own urine[35]
- Factitious hyperinsulinemic hypoglycemia diagnosed by detection of hypoglycemic agents in the bloodstream[36,37] or simultaneous low C peptide and high insulin levels in a first critical blood sample of a child with hypoglycemia[38–40]

To a great extent, one must choose, or even design, the test depending on the type of MCA that is suspected. The effort to confirm a diagnosis of MCA must be carefully planned and executed. Depending on the situation, this involves proper chain of evidence, preservation of laboratory specimens, and precise coordination with law enforcement and/or social services. The advantage of this diagnostic strategy is that, if positive evidence is uncovered and is reliable, it is more likely to be accepted as definitive, both medically and legally. The disadvantage is that the child is potentially exposed to at least one more unnecessary test. If the test result is negative, it is often not possible to distinguish between absence of abuse, failure to diagnose the abuse, and a false-negative testing result.

Given that a child experiencing MCA may present with a fatal event, the autopsy becomes a critically important investigative tool for determining cause and manner of death. Specifically, evidence of poisoning should be diligently searched for, with the necessary toxicological studies done from vitreous, blood, urine, gastric content, tissue, or other sources. A "routine toxicology study" may be inadequate and may vary depending on the laboratory.[41] Specific requests may be necessary to have certain tests done because they are not routinely included in typical hospital screening tests. For example, although ipecac is no longer recommended as a household staple, intentional ipecac poisoning still occurs. It is useful to know that its alkaloids persist in urine for weeks, whereas they are detectable in blood for only a few hours.[42] Identifying a substance may be more specifically delineated with gas chromatography or mass spectrophotometry. If both serum sodium and urine sodium levels are elevated and the child is not dehydrated, salt poisoning should be suspected. The premortem blood sodium or the postmortem vitreous sodium level may be useful. Postmortem vitreous urea nitrogen is a reliable study and may be useful as a reflection of hydration status. It is interpreted in the context of other renal function studies, in the same way as is blood urea nitrogen. Microbiology studies may be central to determining whether the child experienced inflicted microbial assault. When postmortem microbiology blood sample results are positive, care must be taken to discriminate between those that reflect infection in the child and those that are the result of postmortem blood contamination with bowel, skin, or other organisms. The condition and contents of any lines into the child (eg, central venous catheter, gastrostomy, endotracheal tube, shunt, pacemaker) should be examined closely, and it may be prudent to preserve them. As in a clinical situation, careful attention should be paid to chain of evidence for laboratory specimens and biomedical appliances. Consulting with the laboratory director or toxicologist on selecting the best method to detect suspected agents or drugs often is useful.

The laboratory should be asked to preserve the samples securely, with proper chain of evidence documented, because they may be needed later for repeated studies or other studies not originally considered. As with all young children suspected of having experienced maltreatment, a skeletal survey should be done to look for fractures. Classic physical abuse injuries have been reported in those who experienced MCA.[7]

Covert Video Surveillance

Another diagnostic strategy involves CVS. It is a highly useful, if somewhat controversial, strategy where a video camera with its lens hidden in, for example, what seems to be a sprinkler head or smoke alarm may be installed and linked to a monitoring and recording unit in a nearby room in the hospital. Observation of activities that confirm the diagnosis of MCA have been reported with use of CVS.[23,43–46] One investigator who videotaped mothers smothering their children noted, for example,

> Smothering has been labeled "gentle" battering. We reject this. The video and physiological recordings showed that both children struggled violently until they lost consciousness. Considerable force was used to obstruct their airways, and this force was needed for at least 70 seconds before electroencephalographic changes, probably associated with loss of consciousness, occurred. Interestingly, in both cases a soft garment was used to smother the children and no marks were seen on the lips or around the nose.[23]

The legal, ethical, and logistic aspects of CVS have been well debated with considerations of the patient's and caregiver's right to privacy while in the hospital balanced with the belief that a caregiver's right to privacy is obviated when there is a concern of child abuse.[45,47–55] Some may consider the use of CVS equivalent to other tests undertaken in the usual diagnostic process that do not individually require consent; the general medical consent form signed on behalf of the child at the time of admission to the hospital covers most procedures. Furthermore, child abuse statutes in every state permit the taking of pictures without parental consent if child abuse is suspected. If CVS is considered, a hospital multidisciplinary team should be convened, consisting of medical professionals, security, nursing staff, social work, risk management, and legal representation, to ensure that the plan for CVS is ethically and legally sound. The process of initiating, monitoring, and acting on the findings of CVS requires a coordinated and well-communicated approach among hospital staff. It is also important to remember that, depending on the jurisdiction, initiation of CVS may require the court order of a local judge or magistrate issued on a case-by-case basis.

Separation of Child From Suspected Perpetrator

While obviously a last resort, an additional strategy that may nonetheless be useful in the diagnosis of MCA involves separation of the child from the caregiver. Depending on the clinical scenario, separation of child and caregiver may, in fact, carry significant diagnostic weight. It is important to have a baseline against which to compare the child's subsequent course during separation, whether that separation occurs in a hospital or in a foster or kinship placement. The baseline is the well-documented history of the child's symptoms and signs as provided by the caregiver. Therefore, it is important that the only major change that is made in the child's care during the separation is the presence of the caregiver. Implementing new therapies, adding or removing medications from the child's regimen, or introducing new subspecialty care concurrent to separation of the child from the caregiver may obscure the clinical significance of the separation. It is sometimes the case that the fabrication of illness causes irreversible medical problems, or that the fabrication of illness is piled onto an already existing illness. Only reversible conditions of the child can be expected to improve, and these only to the degree and at a rate that is consonant with the condition itself. The advantage of this diagnostic strategy is that it can be definitive without exposing the child to further risk. The disadvantage is that, if it turns out that it is not MCA, an ill child has been separated unnecessarily and perhaps harmfully from his or her caregiver, and the correct diagnosis has been delayed.

The diagnostic strategies used to detect MCA in its most common presentations are outlined in Table 20.2. Obviously, these diagnostic strategies will not fit every type of suspected event, and one must tailor the diagnostic strategy to the type of perpetration suspected. This effort may involve contacting colleagues in related fields for information or to seek help. Commonly, one must combine various diagnostic strategies. An excellent example of evaluating seizures by Barber and Davis[56] appears in Box 20.1; this comprehensive approach can be adapted to many clinical presentations and scenarios.

TABLE 20.2
Potential Diagnostic Strategies for Medical Child Abuse

Presentation	Abusive Action	Method of Diagnosis
Apnea	Manual suffocation	• Implantable ECG recorder • Diagnosis by exclusion • Observation of pinch marks on nose • Caregiver observed committing act
	Poisoning • Tricyclic antidepressants • Hydrocarbon	• Toxicology (gastric/blood) • Toxicology of IV fluid
Seizures	Poisoning Phenothiazines Hydrocarbons Salt Sulfonylurea Tricyclic antidepressants	• Toxicology/assay of blood, urine, IV fluid, milk • Serum and urine sodium concentrations

(continued)

TABLE 20.2 (*continued*)

Presentation	Abusive Action	Method of Diagnosis
Seizures (*continued*)	Suffocation/carotid sinus pressure	• Caregiver observed committing act • Forensic photos of pressure points
Diarrhea	Phenolphthalein/other laxative poisoning	Stool/diaper positive
	Salt poisoning	Assay of formula/gastric contents
Vomiting	Emetic poisoning	Assay for drug
	Injection of air into gastrostomy tube	Caregiver observed committing act
CNS depression	Drugs • Diphenoxylate and atropine • Insulin • Chloral hydrate • Clonidine • Barbiturates/narcotics • Benzodiazepines • Aspirin • Diphenhydramine • Tricyclic antidepressants • Acetaminophen • Hydrocarbons • Chlordiazepoxide • Phenytoin • Phenobarbital • Carbamazepine	• Assays of blood, gastric contents, urine, IV fluid, hair • Analysis of insulin type • Video surveillance
	Suffocation	See Apnea and Seizures.
Bleeding	Rodenticide (warfarin) poisoning	Toxicology
	Phenolphthalein poisoning	Diapers positive
	Exogenous blood applied	• Blood group antigen profiling; DNA typing • Isotope labeling of erythrocytes
	Exsanguination of child	• Single-blind study • Caregiver observed committing act
	Addition of other substances (paint, cocoa, dyes)	Testing; washing
Rash	Drug poisoning	Assay
	Scratching	Diagnosis of exclusion
	Caustics applied/painting skin	Assay/wash off

(continued)

TABLE 20.2 (*continued*)

Presentation	Abusive Action	Method of Diagnosis
Fever	Contamination with infected material • Materials Saliva Feces Dirt Contaminated water Coffee grounds Vaginal secretions Others • Target tissues Blood Skin Bones Bladder Others	• Caregiver observed committing act • Improper taping of line discovered • Type of organism growing from infected sites • Trial separation • Epidemiology (relative-risk assessment) • Diagnosis by exclusion
	Falsifying temperature Falsifying chart	• Careful charting, rechecking (especially urine for core body temperature) • Duplication (ghost record) of temperature chart in nursing station

Abbreviations: CNS, central nervous system; ECG, electrocardiographic; IV, intravenous.
Adapted with permission from Rosenberg DA. Web of deceit: a literature review of Munchausen syndrome by proxy. *Child Abuse Negl.* 1987; 11(4):547–563, copyright 1987, with permission from Elsevier.

BOX 20.1
Practical Guidelines: How to Avoid Making a False Diagnosis of Epilepsy

- The starting point is a meticulous history supplemented by carefully chosen diagnostic tests.
- Consider first the differential diagnosis of paroxysmal events (gastroesophageal reflux, gratification phenomena, breath-holding attacks, cardiac arrhythmia, syncope, metabolic disturbances, reflex anoxic seizures, and pseudoseizures).
- Look for clinical epilepsy syndromes with typical supporting electroencephalogram (EEG) findings.
- Ask the caregiver to video record "episodes." Most families have the means to do this, and some hospitals may be able to loan equipment.
- Do not start treatment until sure. At a minimum, seek independent corroboration of a parent's history or supportive EEG findings. It is rarely necessary to start anticonvulsant medication immediately, and it is good practice to have EEG information beforehand.

(*continued*)

BOX 20.1 (*continued*)

- Be especially wary of making the diagnosis if the EEG result is normal. Seek confirmation from purported witnesses early on in the course of investigations, preferably an independent third party.
- Beware of the caregiver who uses the threat of harm coming to the child to influence clinical decision-making.
- Consider hospital admission if the reported episodes are frequent. Cessation of episodes during periods of observation is suspicious.
- Actively seek to verify details given by the caregiver regarding seizures or other aspects of history.
- Question discrepancies—children with severe, polymorphic epilepsy do not generally have normal neurodevelopment.
- Take and analyze blood and urine from any child presenting for the first time with a seizure—he or she may have been poisoned. Ensure that the urine is screened for relevant substances, and not just drugs of abuse. Store serum so future quantitative analysis is possible.
- In the sick child, glucose and electrolytes will usually be checked. An electrocardiogram should also be routine; it may provide a clue to poisoning with tricyclics.
- If poisoning is suspected, collect other body fluids (eg, vomitus or fluid from gastric lavage).
- Look for subtle signs of smothering (eg, petechial bruising to the face, nasal bleeding).
- Arrange appropriate supportive investigations, including prolactin levels, raised glucose and white blood cell count (following prolonged generalized seizures), prolonged EEG or video-EEG records, pH studies, or tilt table tests.

Adapted with permission from Barber MA, Davis PM. Fits, faints, or fatal fantasy? Fabricated seizures and child abuse. *Arch Dis Child*. 2002;86(4):230-233, copyright 2002, with permission from BJM Publishing Group Ltd.

Differential Diagnosis

Most children who present persistently for medical care have not experienced MCA. Waring[57] discusses the 2 questions that are asked with any pediatric patient: 1) What is the matter with the patient? and 2) Why is this child being brought for care at this moment?[57] The answer to the first question is taught in medical schools and during residency training, whereas the ability to answer both questions, in Yudkin's words, is "the beginning of real medicine."[58]

Most children have a primary organic illness that accounts for the totality of their presentation, but there are other possibilities that may account for the persistence, such as a child with yet unidentified organic or psychogenic illness, a parent with anxiety ranging from "normal" new parent anxiety to vulnerable child syndrome, or a parent with cognitive delays who requires additional support and education.

Again, it is important to remember that legitimate illness and MCA may coexist. The discovery of a real illness in a child who is persistently brought for medical care does not exclude MCA; nor does the concern for MCA negate sound symptoms of illness. The question then becomes, does this illness reasonably explain the severity, extent, and type of the child's symptoms and signs? Occasionally, the distinction between MCA and pathological doctor shopping, or magnification of a child's real but minimal illness for the parent's own psychological or fiscal gain, may not be clear. For those cases that seem to fall at the edges of the definition of MCA, it is worth remembering that the name applied to the child's circumstances is not so material as a careful assessment of the threatened harm to the child.

Management

There is no "one size fits all" way to manage cases of suspected MCA, although certain universal steps are necessary to guide the clinician and ensure the child's safety.

The importance of engaging a multidisciplinary team early on cannot be overstated. When a concern of possible MCA arises, a child abuse pediatrician or child protection consultation team should be consulted, if available, to review the child's case. Medical professionals who previously treated the child should also be contacted, because children have typically changed medical professionals and hospital systems, or even states, frequently, especially if one of these medical professionals became suspicious of the child's history.[59] Once a review of the case has taken place and all the necessary data have been collected (discussed later in this section), a meeting of all medical professionals involved in the child's care should be initiated, including the primary care medical professional, subspecialists, therapists, social workers, and any others, to discuss confirmation or exclusion of the diagnosis of MCA. Such a meeting must sometimes be convened on an emergency basis, so that the child is not exposed to potential harm.

When available, psychiatrists and/or psychologists should be engaged to participate in evaluation and support of the child. Assigning a psychiatrist for the medical and nursing staff may also serve an important purpose because cases of MCA carry the risk of significant secondary traumatic stress. It is also common that cases of MCA cause polarization of opinions and emotions among the hospital staff, some of whom have worked with the family for years. Perpetrators of MCA are often well liked by hospital staff, who may therefore have difficulty accepting the diagnosis. The sense of betrayal experienced by some staff members can be enormous and painful. Others simply cannot fathom that MCA is possible. Anticipating the need for a mental professional to help all staff with their feelings is good primary prevention. The primary care nurse and the head nurse or supervisor should also be included in the multidisciplinary team. The primary care nurse is often the person who has spent the most time with the child and the family over an extended period and multiple hospitalizations. He or she often has valuable information about a case that may not be known to the others on the team. This individual certainly must be included in any plans that involve diagnostic procedures for MCA. The primary care nurse often becomes responsible for important items such as documentation and chain of evidence of specimens.

Optimally, collection of definitive data to either include or exclude the diagnosis and protection of the child are processes that can occur simultaneously. Realistically, however, this is often not the case. Professionals find themselves poised between weighing the eventual usefulness of these data against the possibility of a child enduring further harm during the data collection process. When further diagnostic procedures place the child in a situation of untenable risk, the protection of the child is always the paramount consideration. Because of legal mandates to report suspected child abuse, the legal burden does not require diagnostic proof. In the absence of diagnostic proof, epidemiological evidence pertaining to the case may be sufficiently compelling. Medical professionals acting in the best interest of a child are protected because they are working in the interest of the child's safety.

Because medical records in cases of suspected MCA often are voluminous, efficient review must be organized prospectively. Otherwise, the result of the records review is a mass of detail from which no trends can be elicited and no conclusions drawn. Therefore, in beginning the records review, one shortly recognizes certain patterns and then formalizes these preliminary observations into questions one asks of the data. For example, in a child with a chief complaint of intractable vomiting, did the child have any documented episodes of vomiting while in the presence of a doctor or nurse? In a child with repeated episodes of apnea, how many episodes, if any, began in the presence of someone other than the caregiver? In a child with recurrent fevers in the hospital, who actually took and charted the temperatures when the child was febrile? Can history provided by the caregiver be verified during the hospitalization, or is it only known by report of that caregiver? Some of these data may not be discernible from written medical records. Gaps or questions in the medical records will also let clinicians know if there are outside hospital physicians who should be contacted for further information, as many of those who experience MCA receive care at multiple medical facilities. This may further complicate the records review due to difficulty obtaining a complete set of records or refusal of the caregiver to release records.

Medical records of siblings should also be reviewed, including autopsy reports and death certificates, if available. It often requires some effort to obtain these records, but they are vital because neither police summaries nor social work records may be sufficient. Review of the parents' medical, educational, and work history, as far as possible from documents, is also important for completeness and insight into the psychosocial situation. In certain situations, one may also have the ability to gain access to outside records if on the basis that they are relevant to continuity of care for the child.

Presentation of the records review to the multidisciplinary team should include a brief chronological review, followed by a review of discrepancies, if any. How does the caregiver's history compare with the observed clinical findings in the child? How do the laboratory test results compare with the given histories (eg, are drug levels continually subtherapeutic or toxic with a history of absolute compliance; does the caregiver report diagnostic abnormalities with normal reports)? It is impossible to list all of the possible questions, but the data will tell the reviewer which questions are important. In reviewing a case of suspected MCA, it is essential to consider and explore all possible organic explanations.

If the team reaches a consensus diagnosis of MCA, or if any medical professional has a suspicion of abuse that rises to the level of mandated reporting as defined by state law, the county department of social services and/or law enforcement should be contacted, often prior to any discussion with the family. A perpetrating caregiver's knowledge that there is a concern for MCA often places the child (or the perpetrator) at further risk for harm. Reporting to child welfare and/or law enforcement prior to confronting a caregiver allows time to ensure the medical concerns are understood and the county is involved in the development of a safety plan, including the possibility of being prepared with a restraining order.

The social worker from the county to which the case has been reported is a pivotal person in assisting with proper management of these cases. Much will depend on the social worker's communication with the medical staff and understanding of the case.

When evaluating the child's safety, it may be prudent to recommend out-of-home placement.[7,10,20] This measure ensures protection of the child and a diagnostic period of separation to see how the child's health fares.

The fact that a caregiver has hitherto only simulated but not produced illness is no guarantee that he or she will not do something more harmful to the child in the future. Confrontation of the parent with the news of the suspected diagnosis does not, in and of itself, ensure safety of the child.[7,20,60] To the contrary, often when caregivers are questioned or the concern of MCA becomes known to them, they will try to prove that the child is actually sick, inducing additional symptoms or escalating current concerns, placing the child in increased danger, even while hospitalized.[10] The reader is cautioned in particular about the dangers of placing the child with a family member or friend. This is always a difficult situation because, for the child, the easiest transition may be to an aunt or grandmother, but in this situation the perpetrator may continue to have access to the child, despite that relative's or friend's promises to the contrary. It is also difficult for close friends or relatives to believe and fully comply with recommendations of social services, which places the child at ongoing risk.

If the child is to remain in the hospital for a period, complete separation from the caregiver (without communication by phone, social media, or email) is ideal to ensure a child's safety and provide clarity to the medical assessment. Even with a skilled supervisor in the child's room, caregiver interference cannot be excluded. If complete separation cannot be achieved, all visits with all family members must be strictly supervised by a medically experienced person to ensure that no one is tampering with the child's medical care. Sometimes the best course of action is to ask the court for a short (ie, 10-day to 2-week) period of hospitalization as a diagnostic trial to determine if the child's symptoms persist. If they do not, concern about MCA is heightened. If they do, ask the court to vacate the order and turn attention to a fresh look for an organic diagnosis. This approach is useful only if the child's symptoms and signs, if induced, would reasonably be expected to abate rather quickly in the absence of ongoing assault.

When presenting a case of MCA to a civil or juvenile court, some strategies of presentation may assist the trier of fact in coming to a conclusion. Despite the many hours spent in reviewing records and making an extensive chronological compilation of the child's medical history, presentation of the information to the court in long, narrative form often only confuses, rather than elucidates, the material. A short summary is often better. Questions may then be asked to clarify or expand on particular events. Graphs and charts, clearly readable and with a single issue to illuminate, often better illustrate a complex issue than a long, verbal narrative. For example, a growth chart may show that the child consistently gains weight in the hospital but loses weight at home, or a child who reportedly never tolerates feedings continues to maintain his or her growth. A histogram may show the number of apnea episodes that originated in the presence of the mother compared with the number that originated in the presence of the nursing staff or grandmother.

Cases typically involve conflicting medical opinions, and the parents usually have medical experts testify on their behalf. These experts may be the reporting physician's colleagues. A clear grasp of the medical and epidemiological evidence and a professional, non-adversarial attitude is always best. The abuser only rarely admits to MCA but, curiously, will more often agree to voluntary services as long as the court is not involved and a dependency petition is not filed. No success with this approach has been reported.[10] Experience has shown that court-ordered intervention is necessary if there is any hope of successful protection of the child.

Once the child is placed out of the home, his or her health status must be monitored and documented closely. Although often it is optimal to have the original doctor or set of doctors involved in the child's ongoing care, this arrangement sometimes is not practical for reasons of geography or temperament. It is prudent to recommend out-of-home placement of siblings because they may become the next to experience MCA if they remain in the home. At a minimum, medical evaluations and review of the siblings' records should be considered. Even if the children are removed permanently and parental rights are terminated, subsequent children born to the mother are at high risk of experiencing MCA. Sometimes no formal method is available by which to keep track of the mother's pregnancies, but every effort must be made to protect future children.

Prevention

The pathogenic role of a health care system that over-investigates and prescribes testing and therapy unnecessarily has been rightly identified as contributing to MCA.[10,61] But this is perhaps too abstract. After all, what is a system other than a collection of people interacting with each other? Medical professionals are some of those people. And they are driven by many things—they see many children with persistent illness, most of which is identifiably organic, some of which follows an expected course, but some of which is peculiar or does not conform tidily to textbook descriptions. They don't expect a false history. In the pediatric world, medical professionals are often dependent on a child's caregiver to provide a history, one which is trusted as being in the best interest of the child. Perpetrators of MCA are able to take advantage of this and betray that trust.

Young medical professionals are worried by the cautionary tales of missed diagnoses that they have absorbed throughout training; seasoned medical professionals are haunted by their own experiences of having missed a timely diagnosis of serious illness, for this is almost universal in a long and busy primary care practice. This often results in medical professionals wanting to dig further, ruling out more obscure diagnoses, to ensure they have not made a mistake.[10] A well-founded fear of litigation pervades the practice of medicine. What used to be known as defensive medicine has now become almost mainstream medicine. There is little time for pondering.

Most medical professionals want to be thorough and helpful. The hierarchy in the medical world places subspecialty opinion above that of the generalist. Indeed, a curious and paradoxical weakness of most, if not all, children's hospitals is the greater likelihood of attributing exotic, but incorrect, organic diagnoses when the real problem is MCA. There is relief at having a consultant label a hitherto inexplicable case with an organic diagnosis, even when the label is doubtful. Large, complex hospital systems with multiple subspecialists and sub-subspecialists make it increasingly difficult to ensure communication between all medical professionals prior to interaction and intervention with a patient, a fact that works to the advantage of perpetrators of MCA and often draws them to these large academic centers.[10] This, and difficulty obtaining records from other institutions in a timely fashion, often contributes to the confusion initiated by these caregivers. These issues seem to persist despite an ever-increasing availability of data sharing through electronic medical records and health information exchanges. It may be that the sheer volume of available information, in fact, is a barrier to the information being reviewed effectively and efficiently.

These realities, combined with the diverse presentations of MCA, has led to the sensible suggestion that the prevention of MCA "might not be from understanding perpetrators better, but from better understanding of doctors and the health system."[62] But how to do this? It is almost impossible to escape the culture of investigation and subspecialty referral; besides which, such a culture sometimes helps a patient. Therefore, perhaps the most practical answer is that MCA should routinely be on the differential diagnosis for *persistent symptoms, signs, and/or tests with incongruence,* just as pneumonia is routinely the differential diagnosis for dyspnea. Every medical professional knows that most possible diagnoses on a differential will be wrong, hopes that one will be right, and realizes that, as the old saying goes, "If you never think of it, you'll never see it." Importantly, and by corollary, you will never exclude it. Warning signs are not diagnoses, just features that could mean one of several possibilities. But it is possible that if a child's presentation does not make sense, it is for a reason.

Furthermore, the widespread use of the internet in recent years has made the diagnosis of MCA even more difficult to establish. A wealth of medical information is available at the touch of one's fingertips, making it less necessary for a perpetrator of MCA to have direct knowledge of the medical field because they can learn online which symptoms correlate with a particular diagnosis. The internet also allows for an online connected presence of those who feel MCA is overdiagnosed or not a legitimate diagnosis at all. Specific medical professionals and institutions may be identified by name with subsequent effect on future diagnoses and reporting of cases. Likewise, social media is playing a greater role in cases of MCA. Caregiver blogs have been used to draw a huge amount of attention to the "sick" child, resulting in significant support, praise, and even monetary funds for the abusing caregiver.[63,64] This brings a new secondary gain to the forefront as well as a new challenge to medical professionals, who may often be unaware of the use of these sources.

Prognosis and Long-term Effects

Little research has been done on the prognosis of MCA. Short-term morbidity for children who experience MCA, by definition, is 100%, much of it related to the diagnostic and therapeutic procedures ordered by the medical professional. Long-term morbidity, defined as pain and/or illness that causes permanent disfigurement or impairment, is harder to assess. It is estimated that approximately 1 in 10 who experience MCA have long-term morbidity as a result of complications of the abuse.[7,8,65] This figure is probably an underestimate, however, and does not include long-term psychological morbidity, which may be considerable.[20]

Older children who experience MCA, whose abuse may have begun years earlier, may adopt the false symptoms and signs as their own.[66] Older children are less likely than young children to have illness induced but are more likely to have falsified reports of symptoms and medical history.[67] Some evidence suggests that these children may go on to develop factitious disorder[68] or some type of personality disorder.[69,70]

It is important to recognize that some children are killed as the end result of the abuse. The most common cause of death in homicidal MCA is likely suffocation, but there are many others, including poisoning with various drugs, inflicted bacterial or fungal sepsis, hypoglycemia, and salt or potassium poisoning. Death rates reported in case series vary from 6% to 33%.[7,8,65] In the largest series to date, apnea was the most commonly repeated symptom that preceded death.[7] Almost all were infants and toddlers, and the causes of death notably featured suffocation and poisoning. Other causes of death have been described,[8] and still others, as yet undescribed, are possible. Children as old as 8 years have been killed in the context of MCA.[7] Furthermore, siblings of victims of MCA tend to die in alarming numbers, often with the misdiagnosis of sudden infant death syndrome, and there is every reason to believe that they died in a homicidal manner.[7,65,71–74]

Abusive deaths may be assigned an incorrect cause and/or manner of death if MCA is not considered in the differential diagnosis. Either the significantly positive clinical history is undiscovered or ignored; a scene investigation is delayed or inadequate; or the autopsy, if performed, has not included all necessary dissections or tests. Child fatality review teams are now common throughout the country and, with their ability for multidisciplinary review, are occasionally discovering cases of MCA that had previously been designated as accidental, natural, or undetermined manner of death.

Conclusion

The clinical presentations of MCA are limited only by the caregiver's ability to fabricate or induce illness. Accordingly, to properly diagnose MCA, medical professionals must first consider it in the differential diagnosis. Pediatric medical professionals, in particular, should remain skeptical and ask more questions when a child's clinical presentation does not match the caregiver history or when unexpected and dramatic turns in a child's clinical progress occur. A coordinated and comprehensive review of information is vital to the diagnosis, occasionally supplemented by other strategies, including diagnostic testing, video surveillance, and even separation from the caregiver.

A child who experiences MCA is at high risk of harm, as are other children in the home. The fact that the perpetrator abruptly desists from the assault does not ensure that the situation is even minimally adequate for the child; nor does it ensure that the abuse will stop permanently. The impetus to harm the child repeatedly generally reflects a lack of empathy so profound as to likely hobble the overall capacity for caregiving.

References

1. Meadow R. Munchausen syndrome by proxy. The hinterland of child abuse. *Lancet.* 1977;2(8033):343–345 PMID: 69945 https://doi.org/10.1016/S0140-6736(77)91497-0
2. Roesler TA, Jenny C. *Medical Child Abuse: Beyond Munchausen Syndrome by Proxy*. Elk Grove Village, IL: American Academy of Pediatrics; 2008
3. Flaherty EG, Macmillan HL; American Academy of Pediatrics Committee on Child Abuse and Neglect. Caregiver-fabricated illness in a child: a manifestation of child maltreatment. *Pediatrics*. 2013;132(3):590–597 PMID: 23979088 https://doi.org/10.1542/peds.2013-2045

4. McClure RJ, Davis PM, Meadow SR, Sibert JR. Epidemiology of Munchausen syndrome by proxy, non-accidental poisoning, and non-accidental suffocation. *Arch Dis Child.* 1996;75(1):57–61 PMID: 8813872 https://doi.org/10.1136/adc.75.1.57
5. Schreier HA. Error in Munchausen by proxy defined. *Pediatrics.* 2004;113(6):1851–1852 PMID: 15173528 https://doi.org/10.1542/peds.113.6.1851
6. Denny SJ, Grant CC, Pinnock R. Epidemiology of Munchausen syndrome by proxy in New Zealand. *J Paediatr Child Health.* 2001;37(3):240–243 PMID: 11468037 https://doi.org/10.1046/j.1440-1754.2001.00651.x
7. Sheridan MS. The deceit continues: an updated literature review of Munchausen syndrome by proxy. *Child Abuse Negl.* 2003;27(4):431–451 PMID: 12686328 https://doi.org/10.1016/S0145-2134(03)00030-9
8. Rosenberg DA. Web of deceit: a literature review of Munchausen syndrome by proxy. *Child Abuse Negl.* 1987;11(4):547–563 PMID: 3322516 https://doi.org/10.1016/0145-2134(87)90081-0
9. Alexander R, Smith W, Stevenson R. Serial Munchausen syndrome by proxy. *Pediatrics.* 1990;86(4):581–585 PMID: 2216624
10. Bass C, Glaser D. Early recognition and management of fabricated or induced illness in children. *Lancet.* 2014;383(9926):1412–1421 PMID: 24612863 https://doi.org/10.1016/S0140-6736(13)62183-2
11. Bryk M, Siegel PT. My mother caused my illness: the story of a survivor of Munchausen by proxy syndrome. *Pediatrics.* 1997;100(1):1–7 PMID: 9200353 https://doi.org/10.1542/peds.100.1.1
12. Yates G, Bass C. The perpetrators of medical child abuse (Munchausen syndrome by proxy)—a systematic review of 796 cases. *Child Abuse Negl.* 2017;72:45–53 PMID: 28750264 https://doi.org/10.1016/j.chiabu.2017.07.008
13. Makar AF, Squier PJ. Munchausen syndrome by proxy: father as a perpetrator. *Pediatrics.* 1990;85(3):370–373 PMID: 2304791
14. Meadow R. Munchausen syndrome by proxy abuse perpetrated by men. *Arch Dis Child.* 1998;78(3):210–216 PMID: 9613349 https://doi.org/10.1136/adc.78.3.210
15. Atoynatan TH, O'Reilly E, Loin L. Munchausen syndrome by proxy. *Child Psychiatry Hum Dev.* 1988;19(1):3–13 PMID: 3229151 https://doi.org/10.1007/BF00713731
16. Lasher LJ, Feldman MD. Celiac disease as a manifestation of Munchausen by proxy. *South Med J.* 2004;97(1):67–69 PMID: 14746426 https://doi.org/10.1097/01.SMJ.0000054603.03615.70
17. Richardson GF. Munchausen syndrome by proxy. *Am Fam Physician.* 1987;36(1):119–123 PMID:3604845
18. Carrell S. Texas nurse found guilty of killing child. *Am Med News.* 1984;1–27
19. Lesnik-Oberstein M. Munchausen syndrome by proxy [letter]. *Child Abuse Negl.* 1986;10(1):133 PMID: 3955423 https://doi.org/10.1016/0145-2134(86)90043-8
20. McGuire TL, Feldman KW. Psychologic morbidity of children subjected to Munchausen syndrome by proxy. *Pediatrics.* 1989;83(2):289–292 PMID: 2913558
21. Bass C, Jones D. Psychopathology of perpetrators of fabricated or induced illness in children: case series. *Br J Psychiatry.* 2011;199(2):113–118 PMID: 21804147 https://doi.org/10.1192/bjp.bp.109.074088
22. Gojer J, Berman T. Postpartum depression and factitious disorder: a new presentation. *Int J Psychiatry Med.* 2000;30(3):287–293 PMID: 11209995 https://doi.org/10.2190/FU9U-JPW1-YR3R-Q819
23. Southall DP, Plunkett MC, Banks MW, Falkov AF, Samuels MP. Covert video recordings of life-threatening child abuse: lessons for child protection. *Pediatrics.* 1997;100(5):735–760 PMID: 9346973 https://doi.org/10.1542/peds.100.5.735

24. Kamerling LB, Black XA, Fiser RT. Munchausen syndrome by proxy in the pediatric intensive care unit: an unusual mechanism. *Pediatr Crit Care Med*. 2002;3(3):305–307 PMID: 12780974 https://doi.org/10.1097/00130478-200207000-00021
25. Masterson J, Dunworth R, Williams N. Extreme illness exaggeration in pediatric patients: a variant of Munchausen's by proxy? *Am J Orthopsychiatry*. 1988;58(2):188–195 PMID: 3369539 https://doi.org/10.1111/j.1939-0025.1988.tb01580.x
26. Meadow R. Neurological and developmental variants of Munchausen syndrome by proxy. *Dev Med Child Neurol*. 1991;33(3):270–272 PMID: 2026283 https://doi.org/10.1111/j.1469-8749.1991.tb05119.x
27. Schneider DJ, Perez A, Knilans TE, Daniels SR, Bove KE, Bonnell H. Clinical and pathologic aspects of cardiomyopathy from ipecac administration in Munchausen's syndrome by proxy. *Pediatrics*. 1996;97(6 Pt 1):902–906 PMID: 8657536
28. Feldman KW, Christopher DM, Opheim KB. Munchausen syndrome/bulimia by proxy: ipecac as a toxin in child abuse. *Child Abuse Negl*. 1989;13(2):257–261 PMID: 2568160 https://doi.org/10.1016/0145-2134(89)90012-4
29. Carter KE, Izsak E, Marlow J. Munchausen syndrome by proxy caused by ipecac poisoning. *Pediatr Emerg Care*. 2006;22(9):655–656 PMID: 16983253 https://doi.org/10.1097/01.pec.0000227871.69309.d7
30. Outwater KM, Lipnick RN, Luban NLC, Ravenscroft K, Ruley EJ. Factitious hematuria: diagnosis by minor blood group typing. *J Pediatr*. 1981;98(1):95–97 PMID: 7452416 https://doi.org/10.1016/S0022-3476(81)80550-1
31. Kurlandsky L, Lukoff JY, Zinkham WH, Brody JP, Kessler RW. Munchausen syndrome by proxy: definition of factitious bleeding in an infant by 51Cr labeling of erythrocytes. *Pediatrics*. 1979;63(2):228–231 PMID: 440813
32. Wenk RE. Molecular evidence of Munchausen syndrome by proxy. *Arch Pathol Lab Med*. 2003;127(1):e36–e37 PMID: 12562293
33. Bolz WE, Brouwer HG, Schoenmakers CH. Measurement of HbF concentration for diagnosing a case of Munchausen by proxy syndrome. *J Pediatr*. 2006;148(1):145–146 PMID: 16423618 https://doi.org/10.1016/j.jpeds.2005.04.020
34. Leonard A, Leal T, Godding V, Villanueva P, Wallemacq P, Lebecque P. Sweat potassium concentration may help to identify falsification of sweat test: a case report. *Clin Biochem*. 2008;41(13):1110–1112 PMID: 18554505 https://doi.org/10.1016/j.clinbiochem.2008.05.006
35. Nading JH, Duval-Arnould B. Factitious diabetes mellitus confirmed by ascorbic acid. *Arch Dis Child*. 1984;59(2):166–167 PMID: 6703767 https://doi.org/10.1136/adc.59.2.166
36. Akın O, Yeşilkaya E, Sari E, et al. A rare reason of hyperinsulinism: Munchausen syndrome by proxy. *Horm Res Paediatr*. 2016;86(6):416–419 PMID: 27221098 https://doi.org/10.1159/000446497
37. Glatstein M, Garcia-Bournissen F, Scolnik D, Koren G, Finkelstein Y. Hypoglycemia in a healthy toddler. *Ther Drug Monit*. 2009;31(2):173–177 PMID: 19142176 https://doi.org/10.1097/FTD.0b013e318197b7d7
38. Edidin DV, Farrell EE, Gould VE. Factitious hyperinsulinemic hypoglycemia in infancy: diagnostic pitfalls. *Clin Pediatr (Phila)*. 2000;39(2):117–119 PMID: 10696550 https://doi.org/10.1177/000992280003900208
39. Giurgea I, Ulinski T, Touati G, et al. Factitious hyperinsulinism leading to pancreatectomy: severe forms of Munchausen syndrome by proxy. *Pediatrics*. 2005;116(1):e145–e148 PMID: 15995015 https://doi.org/10.1542/peds.2004-2331
40. Green RP, Hollander AS, Thevis M, Thomas A, Dietzen DJ. Detection of surreptitious administration of analog insulin to an 8-week-old infant. *Pediatrics*. 2010;125(5):e1236–e1240 PMID: 20385635 https://doi.org/10.1542/peds.2009-2273

41. Osterhoudt KC. A toddler with recurrent episodes of unresponsiveness. *Pediatr Emerg Care*. 2004;20(3):195–197 PMID: 15094582 https://doi.org/10.1097/01.pec.0000117933.65522.da
42. Yamashita M, Yamashita M, Azuma J. Urinary excretion of ipecac alkaloids in human volunteers. *Vet Hum Toxicol*. 2002;44(5):257–259 PMID: 12361104
43. Rosen CL, Frost JD Jr, Bricker T, Tarnow JD, Gillette PC, Dunlavy S. Two siblings with recurrent cardiorespiratory arrest: Munchausen syndrome by proxy or child abuse? *Pediatrics*. 1983;71(5):715–720 PMID: 6835753
44. Southall DP, Stebbens VA, Rees SV, Lang MH, Warner JO, Shinebourne EA. Apnoeic episodes induced by smothering: two cases identified by covert video surveillance. *Br Med J (Clin Res Ed)*. 1987;294(6588):1637–1641 PMID: 3113565 https://doi.org/10.1136/bmj.294.6588.1637
45. Hall DE, Eubanks L, Meyyazhagan LS, Kenney RD, Johnson SC. Evaluation of covert video surveillance in the diagnosis of Munchausen syndrome by proxy: lessons from 41 cases. *Pediatrics*. 2000;105(6):1305–1312 PMID: 10835073 https://doi.org/10.1542/peds.105.6.1305
46. Epstein MA, Markowitz RL, Gallo DM, Holmes JW, Gryboski JD. Munchausen syndrome by proxy: considerations in diagnosis and confirmation by video surveillance. *Pediatrics*. 1987;80(2):220–224 PMID: 3615092
47. Evans D. The investigation of life-threatening child abuse and Munchausen syndrome by proxy. *J Med Ethics*. 1995;21(1):9–13 PMID: 7776355 https://doi.org/10.1136/jme.21.1.9
48. Johnson P, Morley C. Spying on mothers. *Lancet*. 1994;344(8915):132–133 PMID: 7695683 https://doi.org/10.1016/S0140-6736(94)91320-X
49. Feldman MD. Spying on mothers [letter]. *Lancet*. 1994;344(8915):132 PMID: 7912369 https://doi.org/10.1016/S0140-6736(94)91320-X
50. Samuels MP, Southall D. Covert surveillance in Munchausen's syndrome by proxy. Welfare of the child must come first [letter]. *BMJ*. 1994;308(6936):1101–1102 PMID: 8173440
51. Connelly R. Ethical issues in the use of covert video surveillance in the diagnosis of Munchausen syndrome by proxy: the Atlanta study—an ethical challenge for medicine. *HEC Forum*. 2003;15(1):21–41 PMID: 12776375 https://doi.org/10.1023/A:1023287808056
52. Howe EG. Criteria for deceit. *J Clin Ethics*. 2004;15(2):100–110 PMID: 15481161
53. Leuthner SR. Covert video surveillance in pediatric care: the fiduciary relationship with a child. *J Clin Ethics*. 2004;15(2):173–175 PMID: 15481168
54. Vaught W. Parents, lies, and videotape: covert video surveillance in pediatric care. *J Clin Ethics*. 2004;15(2):161–172 PMID: 15481167
55. Flannery MT. First, do no harm: the use of covert video surveillance to detect Munchausen syndrome by proxy—an unethical means of "preventing" child abuse. *Univ Mich J Law Reform*. 1998;32(1):105–194 PMID: 16594102
56. Barber MA, Davis PM. Fits, faints, or fatal fantasy? Fabricated seizures and child abuse. *Arch Dis Child*. 2002;86(4):230–233 PMID: 11919091 https://doi.org/10.1136/adc.86.4.230
57. Waring WW. The persistent parent. *Am J Dis Child*. 1992;146(6):753–756 PMID: 1595634
58. Yudkin S. Six children with coughs. The second diagnosis. *Lancet*. 1961;2(7202):561–563 PMID: 13787551 https://doi.org/10.1016/S0140-6736(61)90519-0
59. Ali SN, Ali AN, Ali MN. Munchausen syndrome by proxy: the overlooked diagnosis. *J Ayub Med Coll Abbottabad*. 2015;27(2):489–491 PMID: 26411148
60. Berg B, Jones DP. Outcome of psychiatric intervention in factitious illness by proxy (Munchausen's syndrome by proxy). *Arch Dis Child*. 1999;81(6):465–472 PMID: 10569958 https://doi.org/10.1136/adc.81.6.465

61. von Hahn L, Harper G, McDaniel SH, Siegel DM, Feldman MD, Libow JA. A case of factitious disorder by proxy: the role of the health-care system, diagnostic dilemmas, and family dynamics. *Harv Rev Psychiatry*. 2001;9(3):124–135 PMID: 11287407 https://doi.org/10.1080/10673220127886
62. Eminson M, Jureidini J. Concerns about research and prevention strategies in Munchausen syndrome by proxy (MSBP) abuse. *Child Abuse Negl*. 2003;27(4):413–420 PMID: 12686326 https://doi.org/10.1016/S0145-2134(03)00028-0
63. Brown AN, Gonzalez GR, Wiester RT, Kelley MC, Feldman KW. Care taker blogs in caregiver fabricated illness in a child: a window on the caretaker's thinking? *Child Abuse Negl*. 2014;38(3):488–497 PMID: 24393290 https://doi.org/10.1016/j.chiabu.2013.12.002
64. McCulloch V, Feldman MD. Munchausen by proxy by Internet. *Child Abuse Negl*. 2011;35(11):965–966 PMID: 22074757 https://doi.org/10.1016/j.chiabu.2011.05.020
65. Meadow R. Suffocation, recurrent apnea, and sudden infant death. *J Pediatr*. 1990;117(3):351–357 PMID: 2391589 https://doi.org/10.1016/S0022-3476(05)81072-8
66. Janofsky JS. Munchausen syndrome in a mother and daughter: an unusual presentation of folie à deux. *J Nerv Ment Dis*. 1986;174(6):368–370 PMID: 3711881 https://doi.org/10.1097/00005053-198606000-00010
67. Awadallah N, Vaughan A, Franco K, Munir F, Sharaby N, Goldfarb J. Munchausen by proxy: a case, chart series, and literature review of older victims. *Child Abuse Negl*. 2005;29(8):931–941 PMID: 16125235 https://doi.org/10.1016/j.chiabu.2004.11.007
68. Conway SP, Pond MN. Munchausen syndrome by proxy abuse: a foundation for adult Munchausen syndrome. *Aust N Z J Psychiatry*. 1995;29(3):504–507 PMID: 8573056 https://doi.org/10.3109/00048679509064961
69. Raymond CA. Munchausen's may occur in younger persons. *JAMA*. 1987;257(24):3332 PMID: 3586257 https://doi.org/10.1001/jama.1987.03390240022007
70. Roth D. How "mild" is mild Munchausen syndrome by proxy? *Isr J Psychiatry Relat Sci*. 1990;27(3):160–167 PMID: 2265997
71. Beal SM, Blundell HK. Recurrence incidence of sudden infant death syndrome. *Arch Dis Child*. 1988;63(8):924–930 PMID: 3415329 https://doi.org/10.1136/adc.63.8.924
72. Bools CN, Neale BA, Meadow SR. Co-morbidity associated with fabricated illness (Munchausen syndrome by proxy). *Arch Dis Child*. 1992;67(1):77–79 PMID: 1739342 https://doi.org/10.1136/adc.67.1.77
73. Meadow R. Recurrent cot death and suffocation [letter]. *Arch Dis Child*. 1989;64(1): 179–180 PMID: 2923474 https://doi.org/10.1136/adc.64.1.179-a
74. Truman TL, Ayoub CC. Considering suffocatory abuse and Munchausen by proxy in the evaluation of children experiencing apparent life-threatening events and sudden infant death syndrome. *Child Maltreat*. 2002;7(2):138–148 PMID: 12020070 https://doi.org/10.1177/1077559502007002006

CHAPTER 21

Interpersonal Violence

Tara L. Harris, MD, MS, FAAP
Assistant Professor of Clinical Pediatrics
Division of Child Protection Programs
Department of Pediatrics
Indiana University School of Medicine
Riley Hospital for Children
Indianapolis, IN

Case Scenarios

A 13-year-old boy presents after being suspended from school for fighting. Conversation with the child alone reveals that he witnesses his mother and her boyfriend engaged in physical fights nightly. He feels helpless and frustrated, which is making him short-tempered at school.

A 5-month-old presents with failure to thrive. Medical evaluation fails to identify an underlying disorder. One-on-one conversation with the mother reveals that the father is domineering and tightly controls their finances. He limits when she is allowed to leave the home and does not allow her to purchase formula. The mother admits to frequently having to add extra water to make the formula supply last when she's running out.

A 10-year-old girl presents for obesity. Her mother reports that the child used to be very active and loved sports. Now she has quit her sports teams, and after school she goes to her room, where she spends her time alone. The girl reluctantly shares that she witnessed a neighbor be shot and killed, and since then she is scared to be outside her home.

An 8-year-old boy presents for fatigue and declining school performance. He discloses that while his mother and father were fighting, his father threw their elderly dog against the wall, killing him. The boy reports frequent nightmares and daytime thought intrusions in which he envisions ways he could have intervened to save the dog.

A 17-year-old girl presents for her yearly physical. She is a high achiever but seems withdrawn and nervous today. She reports that she is currently in a relationship. You ask about sexual activity, to which she reluctantly replies "yes" and begins to cry. On further questioning, she discloses that her boyfriend is very controlling and possessive. He has also been physically harming her and forcing her to perform sexual acts.

Most of this book is focused on direct maltreatment of children by caregivers. This chapter discusses the ways that other forms of violence and abuse can also profoundly affect children, as demonstrated in the scenarios at the beginning of the chapter. Discussions around violence and violence prevention typically center on a particular population (eg, children who experience abuse, adults who experience domestic violence, teens who experience dating violence, animals that experience abuse). To comprehensively address violence in families and develop effective public policy, however, it is imperative to direct attention toward the underlying source and examine how these different forms of violence overlap and interact.[1] Within families, multiple forms of violence often coexist,[2–10] all of which have an effect on children in affected homes. This chapter will explore the elements of family violence and other forms of interpersonal violence and how medical professionals can advocate for safe and healthy families.

Intimate Partner Violence

Epidemiology

Intimate partner violence (IPV) is defined by the Centers for Disease Control and Prevention (CDC) as physical, sexual, or psychological harm, inflicted by a current or former partner or spouse. Intimate partner violence can occur among opposite-sex or same-sex couples, and it can occur in couples who are not sexually intimate.[11] As traditionally described, IPV includes various forms of controlling behavior and abuse (Figure 21.1). It is important for the medical professional to be aware, however, that not all elements will typically be present and not all are required for IPV to be identified. It is also important to acknowledge that some partners who have experienced abuse will not consider themselves "victims"; this does not mean that children in these homes are not harmed by the exposure. Extensive research over recent decades has demonstrated how shockingly common IPV is in the United States and around the world.[9,12–14] In the United States, a national telephone survey of more than 16,000 men and women found that 30% of women and 23% of men had experienced some form of IPV during their lifetime.[13] A subsequent phone survey conducted by the CDC found slightly lower rates, with 27% of women and 11% of men reporting having experienced sexual violence, physical violence, or stalking by an intimate partner; the lower incidence reported in this survey may reflect that psychological abuse was not included.[15]

Females who experience IPV are often the focus of research and policy regarding IPV. For example, the Patient Protection and Affordable Care Act

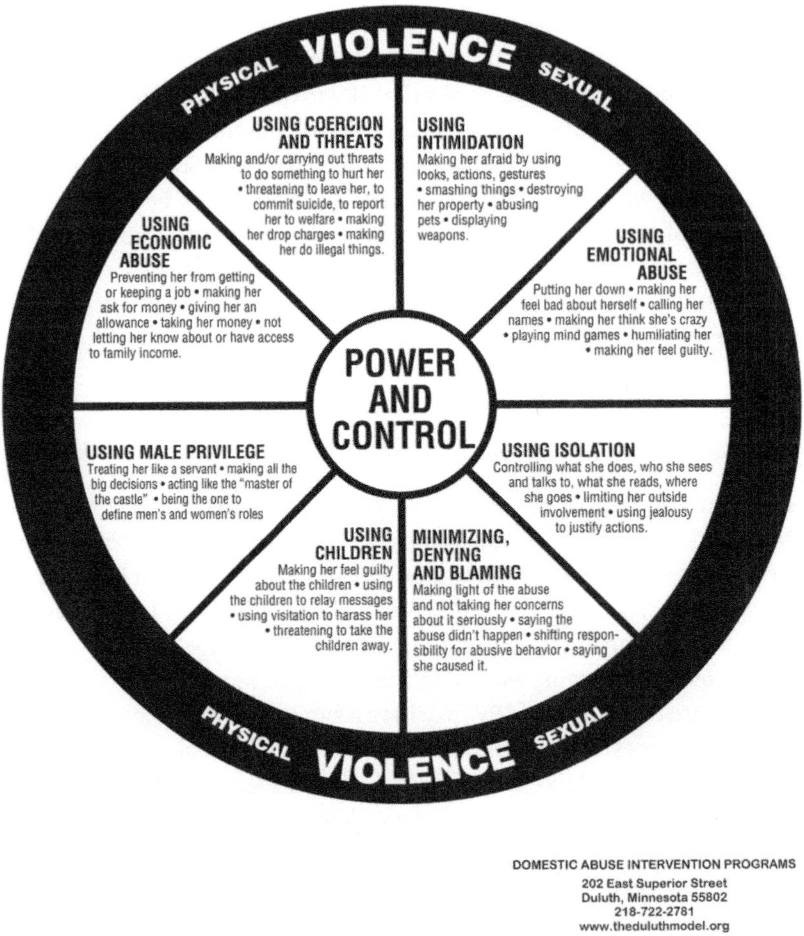

FIGURE 21.1
Power and Control Wheel.
Developed by Domestic Abuse Intervention Programs. Produced and distributed by the National Center on Domestic and Sexual Violence (www.ncdsv.org).

mandates that insurance companies cover the cost of routine screening for IPV at no additional cost to the patient—but only for women. This focus likely stems from the increased physical danger to women and their associated increased likelihood of seeking shelter outside the home. Intimate partner violence is far more likely to be deadly for females than males. More than 40% of women who are murdered in the United States are killed by an intimate partner, compared with 5% among male murder victims.[16] It is important to note, however, that in most families with co-occurring IPV and child abuse, both adult partners act out violently toward each other.[5] And while women may be at greater risk of physical harm, anyone may experience the psychological effect of abuse. Psychological IPV is as strongly correlated as physical IPV to overall negative health outcomes[13] and may have just as much effect on the children in affected homes and on the partner's ability to parent effectively. Some research suggests that witnessing IPV perpetrated by mothers may be *more* predictive of children developing violent tendencies than witnessing IPV perpetrated by fathers.[17] Experts theorize that because female violence is less physically dangerous, that may make it seem more acceptable, leading to more ready acceptance by child witnesses of violent behavior as a norm.

Effect of Intimate Partner Violence on Household Children

According to the 2014 National Survey of Children's Exposure to Violence (NatSCEV), a national telephone survey including more than 4,500 children aged 0–17 years, almost 6% of children had witnessed an assault between their parents in the past year and 25% had witnessed such an assault during their lifetime.[18] Among the oldest group of adolescents, aged 14 to 17 years, the lifetime rate of having witnessed a family assault rose to 32%.[18]

Exposure to any type of IPV may have a significant effect on children in affected homes.[3–6,9,19–23] Children may be affected by seeing and hearing violent events; they may also be affected by events leading up to and following violence.[20] In the course of a violent interaction, children may suffer emotional distress or be inadvertently injured. Some children may attempt to intervene, resulting in violence being redirected toward them. Some abusers may purposely harm or threaten to harm children to manipulate the adult experiencing the abuse.[24]

In addition to physical risks, there are many other ways in which exposure to IPV causes harm to children. Those who experience IPV are at increased risk of depression and other mental health concerns, substance abuse, and chronic disease,[6,13] all of which may impair their ability to parent. Pregnant women who experience IPV also show less consistent prenatal care than unaffected peers, which may result in complications for the pregnancy and, later, the infant.[14] When mothers manifest post-traumatic stress symptoms in response to IPV, their infants and young children often display corresponding trauma symptoms.[25]

Emotional harm is a significant sequela of IPV exposure. Among a group of Spanish IPV survivors, the mothers described that their children always had a reaction to witnessing violence, although it varied from hiding in fear to attempting to intervene, and some children would seem to freeze in shock.[9] Especially after repeated events, behavioral and emotional sequelae are common among children exposed to violence.[4,6,19,20] These can be divided into internalizing versus externalizing behaviors (Box 21.1). *Internalizing behaviors* include anxiety, depression, low self-esteem, and social isolation.[9,12,23] Nightmares and other sleep disturbances are common.[4,9] Some children exposed to IPV develop posttraumatic stress disorder.[3] *Externalizing behaviors* seen among children exposed to IPV include aggression, hyperactivity, delinquency, and other conduct problems.[3,4,12,20,23] Male children and older children are at most risk of developing externalizing behaviors.[20] Their aggressive behaviors may be directed toward other children, back toward parents,[9] or toward their own dating partners, which will be discussed later in this chapter. It is important to note that internalizing and externalizing behaviors are commonly ascribed to other causes (eg, normal development, attention-deficit/hyperactivity disorder [ADHD], conduct disorder). It is, therefore, imperative that when children present with new internalizing or externalizing behaviors, the medical professional must consider whether the symptoms may be a reaction to environmental factors, including exposure to IPV.

Unfortunately, development of negative behaviors by children exposed to IPV often leads to social and academic difficulties. Increased tendency toward bullying and meanness to others disrupts social function and the ability to form and maintain friendships.[3,4,6] Resultant social stress, in addition to difficulty concentrating and missed days of school, all contribute to impaired school performance in many children affected by IPV.[3,4,9]

BOX 21.1
Behavioral Symptoms Among Children Exposed to Intimate Partner Violence

Internalizing Behaviors

Depression
Anxiety
Social withdrawal
Somatic complaints
Sleep disturbance

Externalizing Behaviors

Aggression
Hyperactivity
Rule breaking
Oppositional behavior
Bullying/violence toward peers and dating partners

It is important to note that not all children exposed to IPV will display any externalizing or internalizing manifestations or difficulties with school or social interactions[4,6,12]; therefore, the medical professional must be mindful that if a child is thriving, that does not discount the possibility that he or she is exposed to IPV. It also does not discount the possibility that the child may have long-term psychological effects, increased risk of adopting violent behaviors in the future, or increased risk of other forms of maltreatment.

Association of Intimate Partner Violence With Other Forms of Maltreatment

Exposure to IPV increases a child's risk of experiencing additional forms of violence and abuse. More than one-third of families in which there is violence between adult partners will have co-occurring child maltreatment.[5,8,26] Long-term risk is even higher; by the time they reach age 18 years, more than half of children who had exposure to IPV during their childhood will have experienced at least 1 direct form of maltreatment.[8] Compared with peers from homes without IPV, children who have witnessed IPV are 8 times more likely to experience neglect and 10 times more likely to experience sexual abuse before they reach adulthood.[8] Not surprisingly, IPV is also associated with physical violence directed toward the children. Among children exposed to IPV, almost 1 in 5 have experienced physical abuse in the past year, and 1 in 3 experience physical abuse at some point before they turn 18 years of age.[8] Some studies have estimated the rate of overlap to be much higher, with as many as 70% of children in homes with IPV also being physically abused.[9] When children are exposed to both IPV and maltreatment, they have been shown to have worse outcomes than children exposed to one but not the other.[6,20]

Exposure to IPV increases a child's risk of physical assault not only inside the home but also by others outside the home. Among children who have witnessed IPV, 75% report they have been physically assaulted in the past year (includes assaults by peers and siblings), and 85% experience an assault before they turn 18 years of age.[8] Sadly, being physically assaulted as a child is one of the strongest risk factors for becoming a perpetrator of IPV as an adult,[13] perpetuating the cycle of violence.

An underlying current among all the ways in which IPV affects exposed children is that it causes toxic stress.[4,19,21] The full effects of toxic stress on the developing brain are a topic of active research and are discussed in Chapter 32, Identification of Child Maltreatment, and Chapter 14,

Environmental Neglect and Social Determinants of Health. In the case of IPV, toxic stress may begin to have an effect even before the child is born; more than half of those who experience IPV report that violence either begins or intensifies during their pregnancy.[14] The effect of maternal stress hormones on the developing fetus is an area not yet fully appreciated. Infancy and early childhood are critical periods when considering the effects of toxic stress. While some may presume preverbal children are "too young" to be affected by exposure to violence, very young children may actually be at the greatest long-term risk.[4] Exposure to violence during this period of tremendous brain growth may lead to overdevelopment of the fear-driven limbic system and underdevelopment of the frontal and prefrontal cortex.[21] Elevated cortisol levels may also inhibit hippocampal development, leading to impaired emotional health and learning difficulties.[21]

Clearly, exposure to IPV can present a threat to the well-being of children in a multitude of ways. For pediatric medical professionals, social history is a crucial component of any assessment, because children are reliant on their caregivers to safely nurture their growth, development, and health. While the definition of IPV may refer to adults, the effect it has on children makes it a critical pediatric issue. Intimate partner violence is an important indicator of dysfunction in the home, risk of harm to the child, and risk of other forms of maltreatment. Early intervention is imperative to mitigate the effects on the child in the short term and to prevent the child from becoming the perpetrator of violence toward others as he or she grows into adulthood. Growing up in a home in which there is IPV may lead some children to accept violence as normal and acceptable behavior.[4,6]

Teen Dating Violence

Teen dating violence (TDV) may include physical, psychological, and/or sexual aggression, taking place within the context of an adolescent romantic relationship. Intimate partner violence is closely intertwined with TDV; growing up in a household with IPV makes teens more likely to enter violent relationships, and being in a violent teen relationship makes IPV more likely later in adult relationships.[8,17,27,28] In the 2014 NatSCEV, 2% of children reported dating violence within the past year, and 3.5% reported dating violence during their lifetime.[18] However, NatSCEV includes children aged 0 to 17 years, so these rates are skewed by inclusion of young children, who would not be in dating relationships. Other studies have found rates to be much higher. The Youth Risk Behavior Surveillance System assesses a national sampling of more than 15,000 students in grades 9 through 12 with a lengthy survey. Among respondents to the 2015 Youth Risk Behavior Surveillance survey who reported dating or going out with someone within the past year, 9.6% reported physical dating violence (11.7% of females; 7.4% of males) and 10.6% reported sexual dating violence (15.6% of females; 5.4% of males).[29] Other studies have found TDV (when psychological abuse is included) to be present in up to one-third of adolescent relationships.[30] Teenagers with disabilities appear to be at increased risk compared with their peers.[31]

An element of TDV of emerging significance and prevalence is abuse via technology.[32] This can include emotionally abusive messaging via text or online, surveillance of the teen partner's location and/or who they are with, or coerced sexting. It also may include controlling behavior and isolation, using social media to alienate the victim from friends, family, and/or online supports.

As in violent adult relationships, in many cases there is mutual aggression.[27,33] However, also as found in IPV, women are more likely to be physically harmed or require medical attention as the result of the abuse they experience.[32] Finally, like IPV, TDV is associated with significant comorbidities including depression and suicidal ideation, risk-taking behavior, substance use, anxiety, eating disorders, and other significant mental health concerns.[27,28,31,34–40]

More information about TDV is available through the American Academy of Pediatrics at https://www.aap.org/en-us/advocacy-and-policy/aap-health-initiatives/resilience/Pages/Teen-Dating-Violence.aspx.

Abuse of Companion Animals

Abuse of companion animals is an important, and often overlooked, component of family violence. Violence toward family pets may be a warning sign of other forms of violence in the home, and the abuse of pets may have direct effects on the children and non-offending caregivers. Like children, pets can be used as pawns by an abuser; violence may be directed toward pets to cause distress to other family members and/or to control them.

Among women receiving services for IPV, half to three-quarters report that their partner killed or harmed a pet in their home.[41–46] Abusers target animals that are important to the person who is the focus of the abuse; more than 85% of women report being highly attached to the abused animal and feeling very upset about the abuse.[45] In these homes, two-thirds of children report seeing or hearing abuse of the pets; similar to their mothers, nearly all of the children report being upset about the pet's abuse.[45] Offenders who abuse pets to cause emotional distress to other family members have been shown to be more controlling and at increased risk of especially dangerous forms of violence (eg, marital rape, stalking).[47]

In addition to emotional distress, abuse of pets may also put children at risk of physical harm. Qualitative research suggests that in homes with IPV and pet abuse, the abuse of pets may be triggered by unrealistic expectations (eg, beating a young puppy for having a house-training accident).[44] This scenario raises concern for children in the same environment. Many incidents of child abuse are also triggered by unrealistic expectations (eg, abuse of an infant for crying; abuse of a toddler for toileting accidents). Additionally, children may be injured when they put themselves in harm's way for the sake of a pet; more than half of children in homes with IPV and pet abuse report that they have intervened to try to protect their pet.[45,48] Additionally, children may remain at prolonged risk of physical harm when the non-abusive parent delays leaving the abusive situation due to concerns about the pet's safety and/or lack of a safe place for the pet to go; such delays are reported by 20% to 50% of women receiving IPV services.[41–46]

Risk to dependents in a home appears to be bidirectional. In homes with known abuse of pets, concern should be raised for possible maltreatment of the children. And among homes with substantiated child physical abuse, up to 80% also have abuse of pets.[49] These findings suggest that abuse of children or pets should raise concern and a need to ensure the safety of both.

When pets are abused by children, this too warrants focused assessment and intervention. Exposure to violence in the home, whether IPV or direct maltreatment of the children, has been shown to increase the risk that children will engage in animal cruelty.[7] Childhood abuse of animals is also a predictor of early involvement with the criminal justice system and future violence toward other people—partners, children, and elders.[7] Abuse of pets is a grave warning sign of a need for intervention.

Community Violence

Extensive discussion of violence within the community at large is outside the scope of this chapter; however, awareness of violence within the community where one practices is important for the medical professional. Almost 1 in 5 children witness an assault within their community each year, and before they turn 18 years of age, more than half will have witnessed an assault.[18] Children who have been exposed to violence in their homes seem to be at especially high risk of also being affected by community violence. Of children exposed to IPV, more than 40% report bullying (compared to 20% of controls), almost 50% report emotional bullying (30% among controls), and 70% have experienced a property crime (36% among controls).[8] Experiencing these multiple forms of abuse may amplify the effects of associated toxic stress.

Role of Medical Professional in Screening and Prevention

Clearly, family violence is a complex and multifaceted issue, and, therefore, addressing it demands a complex and multidisciplinary response. The medical professional may play an integral role in this process, because he or she may be the first to identify a problem. While the medical professional cannot address all aspects of family violence, performing screening is a reasonable expectation.

Screening for Intimate Partner Violence

Within the medical community, pediatric medical professionals should encourage adult medical professionals to screen for all forms of IPV, including physical, psychological, and sexual abuse.[13] Screening has been shown to be effective, giving patients an opportunity to disclose and therefore increasing clinicians' awareness when patients are affected.[50] Most obstetricians report that they do targeted screening rather than universal screening.[14] Since this population is at especially high risk and maternal stress hormones may have deleterious effects on the fetus,[3,14,21] universal screening should be encouraged and has been shown to have high levels of acceptability in this patient population.[51] Exposure to violence appears to affect children in a dose-response pattern,[4] so early intervention is critical.

Screening for family violence may also be beneficial in the pediatric setting[19] and has been shown to increase the number of those who have experienced IPV who are identified.[52,53] One study made the notable finding that some new mothers had left their abusive partners after violence during their most recent pregnancy but had not yet taken legal action.[52] Identifying these mothers and their children may be especially important to provide them with extra needed social supports to ensure ongoing safety. As children get older and are developing language comprehension, the medical professional should consider whether screening should be done in written or electronic form or outside of the child's hearing range. All screening should be done with privacy, where others cannot see or hear the responses. Before beginning the screen, it is important to introduce the topic with a normalizing statement (eg, "Because we know violence affects many families in our practice and can affect health, we have a few questions that we ask everyone"). There are several short screening tools available, such as the partner violence screen (Box 21.2).[54–56] If there is a positive response to any screening question, validate the parent's disclosure by thanking the parent for his or her courage to share, letting the parent know he or she is not alone, and reinforcing that abuse is not that parent's fault. It is important that the medical professional use nonjudgmental language and have a plan for immediate response to positive screening responses. Responses will vary based on resources available to the medical professional. If available, a social worker can be valuable in helping the parent think through and plan for safe next steps. If the medical professional does not have social work support, there may be a local IPV advocacy organization that can provide assistance via telephone. For professionals with limited local resources, guidance from national organizations is available (Box 21.3).

Screening for Teen Dating Violence

It is also a good practice for pediatric medical professionals to universally screen teenagers, both male and female, for TDV.[28,57] It is rare for adolescents to spontaneously disclose abuse by dating partners to medical professionals.[32] Screening is, therefore, key to identification of affected teens. Of note, while TDV is a useful term for research and policy purposes, many teenagers in relationships don't consider themselves to be "dating"[32]; medical professionals should be mindful of this when phrasing screening questions or providing prevention

BOX 21.2
Partner Violence Screen

1. Have you been hit, kicked, punched, or otherwise hurt by someone in the past year? If so, by whom?
2. Do you feel safe in your current relationship?
3. Is there a partner from a previous relationship who is making you feel unsafe now?

Source: Feldhaus KM, Koziol-McLain J, Amsbury HL, Norton IM, Lowenstein SR, Abbott JT. Accuracy of 3 brief screening questions for detecting partner violence in the emergency department. *JAMA.* 1997;277(17):1357–1361.

BOX 21.3
Online and Telephone Resources

National Domestic Violence Hotline: 1-800-799-SAFE (7233)

Loveisrespect teen dating abuse helpline: 1-866-331-9474; www.loveisrespect.org

Break the Cycle: www.breakthecycle.org

Futures Without Violence (formerly Family Violence Prevention Fund): www.futureswithoutviolence.org

American Academy of Pediatrics (AAP) Connected Kids violence prevention program: www.aap.org/en-us/advocacy-and-policy/aap-health-initiatives/Pages/Connected-Kids.aspx

AAP The Resilience Project teen dating violence: www.aap.org/en-us/advocacy-and-policy/aap-health-initiatives/resilience/Pages/Teen-Dating-Violence.aspx

Centers for Disease Control and Prevention Essentials for Childhood: https://www.cdc.gov/violenceprevention/childabuseandneglect/essentials.html

US Department of Health and Human Services Agency for Healthcare Research and Quality Intimate Partner Violence Screening: www.ahrq.gov/professionals/prevention-chronic-care/healthier-pregnancy/preventive/partnerviolence.html

US Department of Health and Human Services Child Welfare Information Gateway "Child Witnesses to Domestic Violence": www.childwelfare.gov/topics/systemwide/laws-policies/statutes/witnessdv

American Humane "Understanding the Link Between Animal Abuse and Family Violence" Fact Sheet: www.americanhumane.org/fact-sheet/understanding-the-link-between-animal-abuse-and-family-violence

The Humane Society of the United States Fighting Animal Cruelty and Neglect: https://www.humanesociety.org/all-our-fights/fighting-animal-cruelty-and-neglect

Note: All websites listed were active at time of publication. Additional resources may be found through local or regional advocacy organizations.

messages. For example, the medical professional could ask whether there is anyone the teen is "dating, hanging out with, or hooking up with." Follow-up questions can be broad, including inquiring how that relationship has changed life for the adolescent and whether the adolescent feels safe when he or she is alone with this person. When TDV is identified, there are evidence-based programs aimed at decreasing teens' acceptance of violence within their relationships, including Families for Safe Dates, The Fourth R, and Shifting

Boundaries.[58,59] Effectively intervening when TDV is identified may have profound effects on the likelihood of future violent relationships (both as victim and as perpetrator) for that individual. Another approach that may be especially effective with teenagers is bystander training. Given the importance of peer relationships in adolescents' lives, empowering teenagers to speak out if they witness TDV may be a critical element in prevention efforts.[32,33] Pediatric medical professionals are, therefore, encouraged to deliver dating violence prevention information regardless of whether a screen for TDV has a positive or negative result.[28] Medical professionals should be inclusive in their messaging about violence prevention and reinforce that violence and abuse perpetrated by females is as unacceptable as that perpetrated by males.[17] Medical professionals should also have awareness of dating violence in adolescent same-gender relationships and of specific resources for lesbian, gay, bisexual, transgender, and questioning youth.

Screening for Companion Animal Abuse

Pediatric medical professionals should consider screening for abuse of pets and familiarize themselves with local reporting requirements regarding animal welfare. Screening for pet abuse can easily be combined with rapport building. Asking about the presence of pets is a positive topic for many children. If the child says that the family previously had pets but no longer does, inquiring what happened to those pets may be useful. Asking what happens to the pet when the pet gets in trouble can also provide valuable information about how adults react to frustration in their home. For professionals who desire more structured screening for companion animal abuse, several useful tools are available.[60] While some are lengthy and more tailored toward psychological evaluation, the Physical and Emotional Tormenting Against Animals (PET) Scale is a concise tool that could easily be implemented in the primary care environment (Figure 21.2). This screen is designed to be self-administered and assesses both direct abuse of animals by the child and indirect (witnessed) abuse. When a medical professional becomes aware of abuse of a pet, this must be addressed not only for the sake of the animal but also because this behavior is a red flag for other forms of violence co-occurring in the home.[7] It is also an opportunity to model for the child that abuse is unacceptable and that as a medical professional you will actively advocate for those experiencing abuse.

Please read the following questions and check a box according to *your own experience*. Remember that there are no right or wrong answers; we are interested in what has happened to you or what you have seen. Only you can tell us about it!

Have you ever had any animals at home?

Yes (which______________) No

Sometimes friends enjoy themselves by harming animals. Have you ever seen a friend or a schoolmate hurting an animal in some way?

Never / Hardly ever / Sometimes / Often / Very often

Have you ever bothered animals that you had at home or any other animal? (If you did, please describe how ______________________________________ ______________________________)

Never / Hardly ever / Sometimes / Often / Very often

Have you ever hurt an animal, for example, by kicking them or pulling their tail or hair?

Never / Hardly ever / Sometimes / Often / Very often

Have you ever tormented an animal, for example, by not letting them sleep or by removing their food when eating?

Never / Hardly ever / Sometimes / Often / Very often

Have you ever been cruel to an animal, enjoying yourself by seeing them suffering?

Never / Hardly ever / Sometimes / Often / Very often

Have you ever hit an animal in some way, either with your hands or an object?

Never / Hardly ever / Sometimes / Often / Very often

Sometimes adults also hurt animals. Have you ever seen an adult hurting an animal?

Never / Hardly ever / Sometimes / Often / Very often

Have you ever seen your father hurting an animal?

Never / Hardly ever / Sometimes / Often / Very often

Have you ever seen your mother hurting an animal?

Never / Hardly ever / Sometimes / Often / Very often

FIGURE 21.2

The Physical and Emotional Tormenting Against Animals (PET) Scale.

Adapted from Baldry AC. The development of the PET scale for the measurement of physical and emotional tormenting against animals in adolescents. *Soc Anim.* 2004;12(1):1–17.

Reporting Consideration: Child Protective Services and Law Enforcement

Each medical professional must be familiar with reporting requirements in his or her state, when considering whether or not identification of a particular form of violence in the home warrants a report to child protective services or to law enforcement. When IPV is identified by a pediatric medical professional, whether a report is mandatory may depend on factors including age of the child, relationship to the perpetrator, and whether the child has been present during episodes of violence.[3] Laws specific to each state can be found through its human services/child welfare website or the US Department of Health and Human Services.[61] If the medical professional is caring for an adult who was injured through IPV, depending on local or state laws on domestic violence, additional reporting requirements may apply.

When reporting, the medical professional should discuss this obligation with the non-offending caregiver, to allow him or her the opportunity to create safety plans for both himself or herself and potentially the children before the offender becomes aware of the report.[3] While gun safety is an important topic to address in any primary care practice, it is especially important to address with families affected by IPV. The presence of a gun in a home where there is also history of IPV increases the risk of homicide in that home 20-fold.[62] The medical professional should take caution and consider safety of all parties involved.

The trend within child welfare agencies is to use a comprehensive, strength-based approach when working with families.[2,63] However, it should not be presumed that all child protective services workers have a thorough understanding of, or screen for, IPV, animal abuse, or other forms of violence in the home[22,64]; the medical professional should, therefore, be prepared to offer additional referrals as needed. Medical professionals may worry that involvement of child protective services will automatically entail removal of children from the home and from the non-offending parent, but that may not be the case.[12,23,65,66] The Greenbook and Safe Start initiatives include evidence-based resources for service professionals, and they encourage that in lower severity situations, children remain with their non-offending parent. Ample evidence exists that a secure bond to a stable caregiver is important in ameliorating the effects of exposure to violence.[20] For some children, though, regardless of which parent was the primary offender of IPV, if both parents maltreated the children, removal may be indicated.[5]

Regardless of what legal and/or child protective interventions are made, it is imperative that parents and children in homes where there is violence receive mental health services. When IPV is identified, medical professionals must spend extra time with exposed children as they reach their teen years and discuss safe, healthy relationships, as it is evident they are at significantly increased risk of continuing the cycle of violence by becoming involved in violent dating relationships. Intervening as soon as family violence is identified may be the most effective way to prevent child abuse for current and future generations.[3]

Quick Tips for Medical Professionals

- When children present with behavioral changes, including those that may mimic common disorders like ADHD, depression, or anxiety, consider whether household disruption and/or violence may be the underlying etiology.
- Practice screening for different forms of abuse using nonjudgmental, inclusive phraseology.
- Create a resource sheet with readily available referral information in case IPV, TDV, or companion animal abuse is identified.
- Remember that you are not alone! Responding to family violence requires community effort.

Conclusion

Pediatric medical professionals play an important role in recognizing interpersonal violence between adults in the home because of the serious psychological and sometimes physical consequences for the children. Remembering that families from all backgrounds and people of all ages and sexual orientations can be in a violent relationship is important to identifying situations that require support and help in safety planning.

References

1. Daro D, Edleson JL, Pinderhughes H. Finding common ground in the study of child maltreatment, youth violence, and adult domestic violence. *J Interpers Violence.* 2004;19(3):282–298 PMID: 15005993 https://doi.org/10.1177/0886260503261151
2. Herrenkohl TI, Higgins DJ, Merrick MT, Leeb RT. Positioning a public health framework at the intersection of child maltreatment and intimate partner violence: primary prevention requires working outside existing systems. *Child Abuse Negl.* 2015;48:22–28 PMID: 25979133 https://doi.org/10.1016/j.chiabu.2015.04.013
3. Thackeray JD, Hibbard R, Dowd MD; American Academy of Pediatrics Committee on Child Abuse and Neglect and Committee on Injury, Violence, and Poison Prevention.

Intimate partner violence: the role of the pediatrician. *Pediatrics.* 2010;125(5):1094–1100 PMID: 20421260 https://doi.org/10.1542/peds.2010-0451

4. Howell KH, Barnes SE, Miller LE, Graham-Bermann SA. Developmental variations in the impact of intimate partner violence exposure during childhood. *J Inj Violence Res.* 2016;8(1):43–57 PMID: 26804945
5. Jouriles EN, McDonald R, Slep AM, Heyman RE, Garrido E. Child abuse in the context of domestic violence: prevalence, explanations, and practice implications. *Violence Vict.* 2008;23(2):221–235 PMID: 18624091 https://doi.org/10.1891/0886-6708.23.2.221
6. Kitzmann KM, Gaylord NK, Holt AR, Kenny ED. Child witnesses to domestic violence: a meta-analytic review. *J Consult Clin Psychol.* 2003;71(2):339–352 PMID: 12699028 https://doi.org/10.1037/0022-006X.71.2.339
7. Bright MA, Huq MS, Spencer T, Applebaum JW, Hardt N. Animal cruelty as an indicator of family trauma: using adverse childhood experiences to look beyond child abuse and domestic violence. *Child Abuse Negl.* 2018;76:287–296 PMID: 29175278 https://doi.org/10.1016/j.chiabu.2017.11.011
8. Hamby S, Finkelhor D, Turner H, Ormrod R. The overlap of witnessing partner violence with child maltreatment and other victimizations in a nationally representative survey of youth. *Child Abuse Negl.* 2010;34(10):734–741 PMID: 20850182 https://doi.org/10.1016/j.chiabu.2010.03.001
9. Izaguirre A, Calvete E. Children who are exposed to intimate partner violence: interviewing mothers to understand its impact on children. *Child Abuse Negl.* 2015;48:58–67 PMID: 26009310 https://doi.org/10.1016/j.chiabu.2015.05.002
10. Campbell AM, Thompson SL. The emotional maltreatment of children in domestically violent homes: identifying gaps in education and addressing common misconceptions. The risk of harm to children in domestically violent homes mandates a well-coordinated response. *Child Abuse Negl.* 2015;48:39–49 PMID: 26364914 https://doi.org/10.1016/j.chiabu.2015.08.009
11. Centers for Disease Control and Prevention. Violence prevention. Intimate partner violence. https://www.cdc.gov/violenceprevention/intimatepartnerviolence. Reviewed October 23, 2018. Accessed April 4, 2019
12. Black T, Trocmé N, Fallon B, Maclaurin B. The Canadian child welfare system response to exposure to domestic violence investigations. *Child Abuse Negl.* 2008;32(3):393–404 PMID: 18377986 https://doi.org/10.1016/j.chiabu.2007.10.002
13. Coker AL, Davis KE, Arias I, et al. Physical and mental health effects of intimate partner violence for men and women. *Am J Prev Med.* 2002;23(4):260–268 PMID: 12406480 https://doi.org/10.1016/S0749-3797(02)00514-7
14. Jeanjot I, Barlow P, Rozenberg S. Domestic violence during pregnancy: survey of patients and healthcare providers. *J Womens Health (Larchmt).* 2008;17(4):557–567 PMID: 18447761 https://doi.org/10.1089/jwh.2007.0639
15. Smith SG, Chen J, Basile KC, et al. The National Intimate Partner and Sexual Violence Survey (NISVS): 2010–2012 State Report. Atlanta, GA: National Center for Injury Prevention and Control, Centers for Disease Control and Prevention; 2017. https://www.cdc.gov/violenceprevention/pdf/NISVS-StateReportBook.pdf. Accessed April 4, 2019
16. Cooper A, Smith EL. Homicide trends in the United States, 1980–2008: annual rates for 2009 and 2010. *Patterns Trends.* 2011;NCJ 236018. https://www.bjs.gov/content/pub/pdf/htus8008.pdf. Accessed April 4, 2019
17. Temple JR, Shorey RC, Tortolero SR, Wolfe DA, Stuart GL. Importance of gender and attitudes about violence in the relationship between exposure to interparental violence

and the perpetration of teen dating violence. *Child Abuse Negl.* 2013;37(5):343–352 PMID: 23490056 https://doi.org/10.1016/j.chiabu.2013.02.001
18. Finkelhor D, Turner HA, Shattuck A, Hamby SL. Prevalence of childhood exposure to violence, crime, and abuse: results from the National Survey of Children's Exposure to Violence. *JAMA Pediatr.* 2015;169(8):746–754 PMID: 26121291 https://doi.org/10.1001/jamapediatrics.2015.0676
19. Bair-Merritt M, Zuckerman B, Augustyn M, Cronholm PF. Silent victims—an epidemic of childhood exposure to domestic violence. *N Engl J Med.* 2013;369(18):1673–1675 PMID: 24171514 https://doi.org/10.1056/NEJMp1307643
20. Gonzalez A, MacMillan H, Tanaka M, Jack SM, Tonmyr L. Subtypes of exposure to intimate partner violence within a Canadian child welfare sample: associated risks and child maladjustment. *Child Abuse Negl.* 2014;38(12):1934–1944 PMID: 25455963 https://doi.org/10.1016/j.chiabu.2014.10.007
21. Keeshin BR, Cronholm PF, Strawn JR. Physiologic changes associated with violence and abuse exposure: an examination of related medical conditions. *Trauma Violence Abuse.* 2012;13(1):41–56 PMID: 22186168 https://doi.org/10.1177/1524838011426152
22. Cross TP, Mathews B, Tonmyr L, Scott D, Ouimet C. Child welfare policy and practice on children's exposure to domestic violence. *Child Abuse Negl.* 2012;36(3):210–216 PMID: 22425164 https://doi.org/10.1016/j.chiabu.2011.11.004
23. Ogbonnaya IN, Pohle C. Case outcomes of child welfare-involved families affected by domestic violence: a review of the literature. *Child Youth Serv Rev.* 2013;35(9):1400–1407 https://doi.org/10.1016/j.childyouth.2013.05.014
24. LaLiberte T, Bills J, Shin N, Edleson JL. Child welfare professionals' responses to domestic violence exposure among children. *Child Youth Serv Rev.* 2010;32(12):1640–1647 https://doi.org/10.1016/j.childyouth.2010.06.025
25. Levendosky AA, Bogat GA, Martinez-Torteya C. PTSD symptoms in young children exposed to intimate partner violence. *Violence Against Women.* 2013;19(2):187–201 PMID: 23420836 https://doi.org/10.1177/1077801213476458
26. Appel AE, Holden GW. The co-occurrence of spouse and physical child abuse: a review and appraisal. *J Fam Psychol.* 1998;12(4):578–599 https://doi.org/10.1037/0893-3200.12.4.578
27. Temple JR, Choi HJ, Elmquist J, et al. Psychological abuse, mental health, and acceptance of dating violence among adolescents. *J Adolesc Health.* 2016;59(2):197–202 PMID: 27238840 https://doi.org/10.1016/j.jadohealth.2016.03.034
28. Cutter-Wilson E, Richmond T. Understanding teen dating violence: practical screening and intervention strategies for pediatric and adolescent healthcare providers. *Curr Opin Pediatr.* 2011;23(4):379–383 PMID: 21670679 https://doi.org/10.1097/MOP.0b013e32834875d5
29. Kann L, McManus T, Harris WA, et al. Youth risk behavior surveillance—United States, 2015. *MMWR Surveill Summ.* 2016;65(6):1–174 PMID: 27280474 https://doi.org/10.15585/mmwr.ss6506a1
30. Hickman LJ, Jaycox LH, Aronoff J. Dating violence among adolescents: prevalence, gender distribution, and prevention program effectiveness. *Trauma Violence Abuse.* 2004;5(2):123–142 PMID: 15070553 https://doi.org/10.1177/1524838003262332
31. Mitra M, Mouradian VE, McKenna M. Dating violence and associated health risks among high school students with disabilities. *Matern Child Health J.* 2013;17(6):1088–1094 PMID: 22886316 https://doi.org/10.1007/s10995-012-1091-y
32. Barter C, Stanley N. Inter-personal violence and abuse in adolescent intimate relationships: mental health impact and implications for practice. *Int Rev Psychiatry.* 2016;28(5):485–503 PMID: 27627551 https://doi.org/10.1080/09540261.2016.1215295

33. Reidy DE, Ball B, Houry D, et al. In search of teen dating violence typologies. *J Adolesc Health.* 2016;58(2):202–207 PMID: 26683984 https://doi.org/10.1016/j.jadohealth.2015.09.028
34. Belshaw SH, Siddique JA, Tanner J, Osho GS. The relationship between dating violence and suicidal behaviors in a national sample of adolescents. *Violence Vict.* 2012;27(4):580–591 PMID: 22978076 https://doi.org/10.1891/0886-6708.27.4.580
35. Bonomi AE, Anderson ML, Nemeth J, Rivara FP, Buettner C. History of dating violence and the association with late adolescent health. *BMC Public Health.* 2013;13(1):821 PMID: 24015863 https://doi.org/10.1186/1471-2458-13-821
36. Haynie DL, Farhat T, Brooks-Russell A, Wang J, Barbieri B, Iannotti RJ. Dating violence perpetration and victimization among U.S. adolescents: prevalence, patterns, and associations with health complaints and substance use. *J Adolesc Health.* 2013;53(2):194–201 PMID: 23664626 https://doi.org/10.1016/j.jadohealth.2013.02.008
37. Lormand DK, Markham CM, Peskin MF, et al. Dating violence among urban, minority, middle school youth and associated sexual risk behaviors and substance use. *J Sch Health.* 2013;83(6):415–421 PMID: 23586886 https://doi.org/10.1111/josh.12045
38. van Dulmen MH, Klipfel KM, Mata AD, et al. Cross-lagged effects between intimate partner violence victimization and suicidality from adolescence into adulthood. *J Adolesc Health.* 2012;51(5):510–516 PMID: 23084174 https://doi.org/10.1016/j.jadohealth.2012.02.015
39. Wolitzky-Taylor KB, Ruggiero KJ, Danielson CK, et al. Prevalence and correlates of dating violence in a national sample of adolescents. *J Am Acad Child Adolesc Psychiatry.* 2008;47(7):755–762 PMID: 18520962 https://doi.org/10.1097/CHI.0b013e318172ef5f
40. Cha S, Ihongbe TO, Masho SW. Racial and gender differences in dating violence victimization and disordered eating among U.S. high schools. *J Womens Health (Larchmt).* 2016;25(8):791–800 PMID: 26871758 https://doi.org/10.1089/jwh.2015.5324
41. Ascione FR. Battered women's reports of their partners' and their children's cruelty to animals. *J Emotional Abuse.* 1998;1(1):119–133 https://doi.org/10.1300/J135v01n01_06
42. Faver CA, Strand EB. To leave or to stay? Battered women's concern for vulnerable pets. *J Interpers Violence.* 2003;18(12):1367–1377 PMID: 14678611 https://doi.org/10.1177/0886260503258028
43. Loring M, Bolden-Hines TA. Pet abuse by batterers as a means of coercing battered women into committing illegal behavior. *J Emotional Abuse.* 2004;4(1):27–37 https://doi.org/10.1300/J135v04n01_02
44. Carlisle-Frank P, Frank JM, Nielsen L. Selective battering of the family pet. *Anthrozoos.* 2004;17(1):26–42 https://doi.org/10.2752/089279304786991864
45. Ascione FR, Weber CV, Thompson TM, Heath J, Maruyama M, Hayashi K. Battered pets and domestic violence: animal abuse reported by women experiencing intimate violence and by nonabused women. *Violence Against Women.* 2007;13(4):354–373 PMID: 17420515 https://doi.org/10.1177/1077801207299201
46. Volant AM, Johnson JA, Gullone E, Coleman GJ. The relationship between domestic violence and animal abuse: an Australian study. *J Interpers Violence.* 2008;23(9):1277–1295 PMID: 18326483 https://doi.org/10.1177/0886260508314309
47. Simmons CA, Lehmann P. Exploring the link between pet abuse and controlling behaviors in violent relationships. *J Interpers Violence.* 2007;22(9):1211–1222 PMID: 17704464 https://doi.org/10.1177/0886260507303734
48. McDonald SE, Collins EA, Nicotera N, et al. Children's experiences of companion animal maltreatment in households characterized by intimate partner violence. *Child Abuse Negl.* 2015;50:116–127 PMID: 26520828 https://doi.org/10.1016/j.chiabu.2015.10.005

49. DeViney E, Dickert J, Lockwood R. The care of pets within child abusing families. *Int J Study Anim Probl.* 1983;4:321–329
50. Coker AL, Bethea L, Smith PH, Fadden MK, Brandt HM. Missed opportunities: intimate partner violence in family practice settings. *Prev Med.* 2002;34(4):445–454 PMID: 11914051 https://doi.org/10.1006/pmed.2001.1005
51. Renker PR, Tonkin P. Women's views of prenatal violence screening: acceptability and confidentiality issues. *Obstet Gynecol.* 2006;107(2 Pt 1):348–354 PMID: 16449123 https://doi.org/10.1097/01.AOG.0000195356.90589.c5
52. Siegel RM, Hill TD, Henderson VA, Ernst HM, Boat BW. Screening for domestic violence in the community pediatric setting. *Pediatrics.* 1999;104(4 Pt 1):874–877 PMID: 10506228 https://doi.org/10.1542/peds.104.4.874
53. Parkinson GW, Adams RC, Emerling FG. Maternal domestic violence screening in an office-based pediatric practice. *Pediatrics.* 2001;108(3):E43 PMID: 11533361 https://doi.org/10.1542/peds.108.3.e43
54. Choo EK, Houry DE. Managing intimate partner violence in the emergency department. *Ann Emerg Med.* 2015;65(4):447–451.e1 PMID: 25533139 https://doi.org/10.1016/j.annemergmed.2014.11.004
55. Feldhaus KM, Koziol-McLain J, Amsbury HL, Norton IM, Lowenstein SR, Abbott JT. Accuracy of 3 brief screening questions for detecting partner violence in the emergency department. *JAMA.* 1997;277(17):1357–1361 PMID: 9134940 https://doi.org/10.1001/jama.1997.03540410035027
56. Basile KC, Hertz MF, Back SE. *Intimate Partner Violence and Sexual Violence Victimization Assessment Instruments for use in Healthcare Settings: Version 1.* Atlanta GA: Centers for Disease Control and Prevention, National Center for Injury Prevention and Control; 2007. https://www.cdc.gov/violenceprevention/pdf/ipv/ipvandsvscreening.pdf. Accessed April 4, 2019
57. Wolfe DA, Crooks C, Jaffe P, et al. A school-based program to prevent adolescent dating violence: a cluster randomized trial. *Arch Pediatr Adolesc Med.* 2009;163(8):692–699 PMID: 19652099 https://doi.org/10.1001/archpediatrics.2009.69
58. Foshee VA, McNaughton Reyes HL, Ennett ST, Cance JD, Bauman KE, Bowling JM. Assessing the effects of Families for Safe Dates, a family-based teen dating abuse prevention program. *J Adolesc Health.* 2012;51(4):349–356 PMID: 22999835 https://doi.org/10.1016/j.jadohealth.2011.12.029
59. De Koker P, Mathews C, Zuch M, Bastien S, Mason-Jones AJ. A systematic review of interventions for preventing adolescent intimate partner violence. *J Adolesc Health.* 2014;54(1):3–13 PMID: 24125727 https://doi.org/10.1016/j.jadohealth.2013.08.008
60. Baldry AC. The development of the PET scale for the measurement of physical and emotional tormenting against animals in adolescents. *Soc Anim.* 2004;12(1):1–17 https://doi.org/10.1163/156853004323029513
61. Child Welfare Information Gateway. *Child Witness to Domestic Violence.* Washington, DC: US Department of Health and Human Services, Children's Bureau; 2016. https://www.childwelfare.gov/topics/systemwide/laws-policies/statutes/witnessdv. Accessed April 4, 2019
62. Kellermann AL, Rivara FP, Rushforth NB, et al. Gun ownership as a risk factor for homicide in the home [Erratum appears in *N Engl J Med.* 1998;339(13):928–929; PMID: 9750102]. *N Engl J Med.* 1993;329(15):1084–1091 PMID: 8371731 https://doi.org/10.1056/NEJM199310073291506
63. Edleson JL, Malik NM. Collaborating for family safety: results from the Greenbook multisite evaluation. *J Interpers Violence.* 2008;23(7):871–875 PMID: 18319373 https://doi.org/10.1177/0886260508314850

64. Thackeray JD, Scribano PV, Rhoda D. Domestic violence assessments in the child advocacy center. *Child Abuse Negl.* 2010;34(3):172–182 PMID: 20207001 https://doi.org/10.1016/j.chiabu.2009.10.002
65. English DJ, Edleson JL, Herrick ME. Domestic violence in one state's child protective caseload: a study of differential case dispositions and outcomes. *Child Youth Serv Rev.* 2005;27(11):1183–1201 https://doi.org/10.1016/j.childyouth.2005.04.004
66. Kohl PL, Edleson JL, English DJ, Barth RP. Domestic violence and pathways into child welfare services: findings from the National Survey of Child and Adolescent Well-Being. *Child Youth Serv Rev.* 2005;27(11):1167–1182 https://doi.org/10.1016/j.childyouth.2005.04.003

CHAPTER 22

Human Trafficking and Sexual Exploitation via Electronic Media

Jordan Greenbaum, MD
Institute on Healthcare and Human Trafficking at the Stephanie V. Blank Center for Safe and Healthy Children
Children's Healthcare of Atlanta
Atlanta, GA
International Centre for Missing and Exploited Children
Alexandria, VA

Corey J. Rood, MD, FAAP
Child Abuse Pediatrician
Assistant Professor of Pediatrics
Medical Director, Child Abuse Pediatrics
University of California Irvine
Orange, CA
Medical Director, Child Abuse and Prevention Team
Miller Children's and Women's Hospital
Long Beach, CA

Human Trafficking

Introduction

Human trafficking is not a new phenomenon, but it has gained considerable global attention over the past 20 years. International treaties and national laws typically frame the issue as a legal one, with an emphasis on investigation and prosecution.[1,2] However, given the profound effect of human trafficking on the health and well-being of victims,* families, and populations, as well as the benefits associated with a focus on prevention, there is a growing trend toward adopting a public

* The term *victim* is used in this chapter in its objective, legal sense as indicating a person who has been harmed as a result of some event or action or who has suffered because of someone else's actions. It does not refer to how the person may feel or perceive himself or herself as a result of the event(s) and is not intended to be used to label that person.

health approach to this severe form of exploitation. Studies of children and adults experiencing labor and sex trafficking consistently show a host of adverse health consequences that include traumatic injury associated with physical or sexual assault, sexually and non-sexually transmitted infections (eg, tuberculosis, scabies), substance misuse, pregnancy-associated complications, posttraumatic stress disorder (PTSD), major depression with suicidality, aggression and other behavior problems, somatic symptoms, malnutrition, dental problems, and untreated chronic diseases.[3–14] In one study of suspected and confirmed adolescent victims of sex trafficking, 32% were diagnosed with a sexually transmitted infection (STI) at the time of evaluation[7]; in another, 32% reported a history of pregnancy and 88% reported substance use, with 58% disclosing multidrug use.[6] Edinburgh and colleagues reported that 78% of adolescent victims met *Diagnostic and Statistical Manual of Mental Disorders*, 4th Edition, criteria for PTSD and 50% disclosed a suicide attempt within the past year.[8]

Families of trafficking victims may experience profound changes, including traumatic grief surrounding the disappearance of the victim, shame and ostracism associated with having a child who has been exploited (especially if the child was involved in prostitution), significant debt and worsening poverty, and difficulties integrating the survivor back into the family after the child has undergone complex trauma.[15] Communities may experience traumatic grief over losing children to traffickers and seeing loved ones exploited, as well as social disruption and conflict associated with differing views on how to treat survivors. Population shifts may occur if large numbers of children and youth are trafficked out of a village, changing the economy and social dynamics. Finally, whole societies are affected by human trafficking, as they bear the financial burden of treating physical and psychological adverse consequences experienced by survivors, investigating and prosecuting trafficking offenses, incarcerating offenders, and absorbing the loss of economic productivity by survivors. Even more important is the moral cost of tolerating the exploitation and human rights violations of the vulnerable children and adults in the population.[16]

Definitions

The US federal definition of human trafficking involves 3 components: action, means, and purpose[1,17] (Box 22.1). To fulfill the criteria for human trafficking, one must demonstrate at least 1 factor from each category. *The exception to this is* child sex trafficking, *for which means is not required because those younger than 18 years cannot consent to a commercial sexual act.* Importantly, means involving force, fraud, and coercion must be present for child labor trafficking and all forms of adult trafficking.

BOX 22.1
US Federal Definition of Human Trafficking[1,17]

Action

Recruitment
Harboring
Transporting
Provision
Obtaining
Patronizing (for sex)
Soliciting (for sex)

Means[a]

Force
Fraud
Coercion

Purpose

Labor or services involving

- Commercial sex act (sex act exchanged for something of value)
- Involuntary servitude
- Peonage[b]
- Debt bondage
- Slavery

[a] Means is *not* relevant for sex trafficking of persons younger than 18 years.
[b] *Peonage* refers to any form of unfree labor or wage labor in which a laborer has little control over employment conditions.

However, if a person initially "consents" to exploitation, this consent becomes irrelevant if there is subsequent force, fraud, or coercion.

The definition of human trafficking used by most countries generally refers to the Palermo protocol, which is very similar to the US federal definition.[2] However, unlike the United States, many countries require movement of victims to qualify as human trafficking, although this does not necessarily involve crossing a national border.[18] *Commercial sex acts* can include prostitution (with or without a third party involved in the transaction), production and distribution of child sexual abuse materials (formerly referred to as child pornography),[18] use of a child in a sex-oriented business (eg, strip club), child marriage, forced marriage, and the mail-order bride trade. *Prostitution* may involve children trading sex acts for money, shelter, food, or other survival needs (survival sex) or trading sex for luxury items. Commercial sex may occur in the context of travel and tourism (formerly called sex tourism).[18]

Smuggling is not the same as human trafficking. Smuggling involves the illegal importation of goods or people.[19] While the major element of smuggling involves transportation, that of human trafficking involves exploitation. A 15-year-old boy from El Salvador may pay a "Coyote" to smuggle him across the Texas border. If that smuggler accepts the money, delivers the boy into the United States, and leaves him there, he has committed the act of smuggling. If, on the other hand, he then tells the boy that the youth owes $5,000 for "additional fees" and forces the boy to sell sex or work in a factory to pay back the "debt," he is committing the offense of human trafficking (exploitation using debt bondage).

Epidemiology

While medical professionals, researchers, legislators, donors to anti-trafficking programs, and the lay public seek statistics on the prevalence of human trafficking, reliable estimates are elusive.[20] The criminal nature of the activity, differing definitions of human trafficking, the lack of a centralized database, underreporting by victims, and various methodological challenges in research all preclude an accurate determination of scope.[21–23] Globally, the International Labour Organization and others estimated that 24.9 million people were victims of forced labor in 2016 (including forced labor in the private economy, state-imposed forced labor, and forced sexual exploitation of adult/child commercial sexual exploitation); 18% of these were children (4.5 million). Of the 15.4 million living in a forced marriage, 37% (5.7 million) were children. Approximately 1 million children were victims of commercial sexual exploitation in 2016 (excluding forced marriage).[24] However, as is pointed out by the International Labour Organization, any estimate of prevalence must be accompanied by a clear explanation of the inherent challenges involved and the likely inaccuracies associated with those challenges.

Reliable statistics for numbers of child victims in the United States are similarly unavailable. However, several studies of survival sex among runaway and homeless youth suggest that this form of trafficking is quite common, with studies demonstrating rates of 10% to 50%.[25–27] While males and lesbian, gay, bisexual, transgender, queer/questioning (LGBTQ) youth are clearly victimized,[28–31] they are almost certainly under-recognized and underreported,[32–35] and research tends to focus on female victims.[6,7,36] Reasons for this lack of attention to boys and LGBTQ youth are not entirely clear, although some hypothesize that cultural biases against viewing boys as potentially vulnerable may hinder public perception of the possibility of victimization and preclude boys from disclosing their experiences.[32,34] Homophobia and lack of tolerance for transgender persons may play roles in under-recognition of LGBTQ victims, as may a focus by the public on trafficking by pimps as a major form of exploitation (which, studies suggest, is more common among female victims than male or transgender).[28,30]

Any child or youth may become a victim of sex or labor trafficking, although many victims have one or more vulnerability factors.[37] Consistent with a social-ecological framework,[38] these factors exist at the individual, relationship, community, and societal levels. Histories of running away from home or being thrown out of the home (throwaway), of sexual or other type of abuse, and of involvement in the child protection or juvenile justice systems are very common, as is a history of substance use, LGBTQ status, or membership in another marginalized group.[6,7,25,26,28,39–41] In the United States, most identified victims of sex trafficking are US citizens or legal residents (domestic) and are female, although under-recognition and reporting likely play a role in these statistics. Of confirmed sex trafficking victims identified in the US Human Trafficking Reporting System between January 2008 and June 2010, 84% were domestic and 94% were female. In contrast, of identified labor trafficking victims, fewer than 2% were US citizens or legal residents.[42]

At the relationship level, vulnerability factors include family violence, poverty (a very powerful driver of human trafficking abroad), familial substance abuse, and migration.[21,43–48] Unaccompanied foreign-born minors[49] attempting to enter or stay in the United States are at very high risk of exploitation, given their lack of supervision, cultural and language barriers, limited social support, and limited job skills. Children from communities experiencing natural disasters, such as Hurricane Katrina in 2005 or the earthquake in Nepal in 2015; those subjected to legal and political corruption; communities with increased tourism; and those experiencing major social upheaval and/or violence are at increased risk of human trafficking.[41,43,50–53] Finally, cultural beliefs and practices influence vulnerability to human trafficking at the societal level, with gender bias and violence, the belief that children are the property of parents, and discrimination against certain social, racial, ethnic, religious, or other groups playing major roles. See Box 22.2 for examples of vulnerability.

BOX 22.2
Examples of Vulnerability to Child Trafficking

DL is a 14-year-old Native American girl with a history of sexual abuse by her mother's boyfriend and behavioral problems in school. Her mother is schizophrenic and unemployed. DL runs away from home and is befriended by 2 older males who give her drugs and take her to a motel where other men are waiting to have sex.

Vulnerabilities: young age (adolescent brain development); Native American; history of sexual abuse; poverty; dysfunctional family; sexual objectification of girls

RP is a 15-year-old boy from Guatemala whose family sent him on the "migration trail" to the United States to escape gang violence and poverty in his home town. En route, he encounters a man who offers to help him cross the border for free. RP accepts this offer gratefully, but once in New Mexico, the man tells him he must pay for his trip, as well as fees for food and protection, by working in the fields. The man sells RP to a manager of a farm in Central California, who confiscates RP's identification papers and threatens him with deportation if he does not comply with demands.

Vulnerabilities: poverty, community violence, migration, unaccompanied status, limited resources, lack of immigration papers

Recruitment and Control Tactics

Strategies for recruiting victims for labor or sex trafficking are remarkably similar throughout the world.[30,45,54–56] Youth may be trafficked by a family member, peer, gang member, acquaintance, or stranger.[8,57–60] They may be recruited by another victim.[8] Two very common, and very successful, techniques involve false promises of jobs and false romance, as demonstrated in the following examples:

RM, a 16-year-old girl from Ukraine, is desperate for employment to support her very poor family. An "employment agency" offers her a job as a nanny in America, with a promise that if she borrows the equivalent of US $5,000, the agency will secure her a passport and visa, as well as a job with an affluent American family. She is made to understand that she will be allowed to attend school, will have limited responsibilities, and will be paid very well so that she can pay off her loan within 6 months. She accepts this offer and is brought to Connecticut, where she is forced to work 14-hour days cleaning the house of a wealthy couple, cooking, and caring for 3 children. She is not allowed to leave the house or contact her family, and the woman of the home confiscates her passport and identification. She is repeatedly verbally and physically abused by the mother and sexually assaulted by the father. She is a victim of labor trafficking and sexual exploitation.

LD, a 14-year-old gay boy, faces ostracism by his peers and rejection by his parents due to his sexual orientation. He spends a great deal of time on the internet, searching for men who will accept him and be his friend. In a chat room he meets a 36-year-old man, DS, who appears interested in LD's life and understanding of his troubles. They correspond for several weeks; DS eventually asks LD to send a photograph of himself naked. At this point, LD feels loved and accepted by this man, so he complies. A week later, DS arranges to meet with LD to have sex. LD slips out of the house and meets the man at a motel. They continue to have sex on several more occasions. Then DS begins arriving at the hotel with 2 to 3 other men, who also want to have sex with LD. LD is confused and afraid, but he wants to show his love for DS, so he reluctantly complies. LD is a victim of sex trafficking.

In some cases, children and adolescents may be kidnapped, drugged, or otherwise forcibly obtained by traffickers.[45] In some countries, extremely poor, often rural, families may decide that their only chance of survival involves giving their son or daughter to a person who promises "a better life" for the child and money for the family.[45] They may or may not be aware that their child will be sold as a trafficking victim. Parents in desperate situations during a mass migration may be aware that their child is being exploited in labor; they may offer a daughter in marriage to a man with money or other form of influence, to avoid starvation or eviction.[48] In some cases, a trafficked child's first experience with sexual exploitation or trafficking may be initiated by a potential customer making an offer or by peers teaching them how to "sell sex" to obtain food, shelter, money, drugs, or luxury items.[28,30] In many cases there is no third-party trafficker (pimp) involved in the sexual exploitation.[28] Instead, the trafficker is the customer and the transaction occurs only between victim and buyer.[61] In these cases, the victim may consider himself or herself to be "voluntarily" engaging in transactional sex, but the victim's age precludes legal consent.

Once a child or adult has been recruited into a trafficking or exploitative situation, experiences differ, but violence is common.[3,4,62–65] This may occur at the hands of a buyer of sex, members of law enforcement, strangers, or other victims.[28,55,66,67] Violence also may be used by the trafficker or labor manager to establish and maintain control. Another powerful method of controlling a victim involves establishing trauma bonds. This entails strong emotional attachments that develop between victim and offender when there is a significant imbalance in power and the offender alternates abuse with demonstrations of affection and other positive experiences. The victim feels helpless and hopeless and becomes dependent on, and supportive of, the offender.[68] Traffickers also may control their victims through psychological manipulation, instilling in the child a sense of shame, hopelessness, and humiliation, or pretending to fulfill the youth's need for love and family.

He or she may use blackmail, threats, debt bondage, and other forms of financial control. Some victims are isolated and closely monitored; they may have their travel and identification documents confiscated or be given misinformation about their rights and the laws regarding deportation.[46,55,56] These control mechanisms make it difficult for victims to extricate themselves from their exploitative circumstances. Those children and youth who do not have persons directly overseeing their exploitation may have difficulty leaving "the life" because of feelings of hopelessness, stigma, and shame; lack of education and job skills; discrimination by others; substance dependency; or lack of alternative strategies for survival.[54] The time spent in exploitation varies tremendously and may range from days to years; it may be discontinuous, with multiple episodes of exploitation occurring over time.[54] In one Canadian study of young adult men reporting commercial sexual exploitation (73% began as minors), the average duration of exploitation was 9 years.[54]

Presentation to Medical Services

Medical professionals are in a unique position to encounter human trafficking victims when they present to medical settings for care. Many trafficking victims may present alone and, if asked sensitive, information-gathering questions, may be willing to disclose the current details of their situation and/or take resource information for future reference. Patients and clients, including victims of trafficking, are often willing to disclose medically important history and personal details to medical professionals that they may not otherwise be willing to share. Due to this unique relationship that medical professionals have with their patients and clients, they have a responsibility to recognize the subtle signs, symptoms, and presentations of victims of trafficking when they present to their offices, clinics, inpatient units, and/or emergency departments.

Lederer and Wetzel reported data in 2014 from surveys they conducted with 107 female sex trafficking survivors ranging in age from 14 to 60 years. Nearly 88% of survivors made at least 1 visit to a medical professional during their period of exploitation (Table 22.1). Reasons for seeking care ranged from physical injuries to reproductive health concerns, from issues related to substance abuse to mental health problems. Related to their time as a trafficking victim, just over 67% had at least 1 confirmed STI, 71% became pregnant at least 1 time, 55% of those who became pregnant had at least 1 abortion, and 65% presented alone to a medical professional to discuss birth control.[69]

In 2016, Chisolm-Straker et al showed similar findings in their survey study of 173 US human trafficking survivors of all ages. They found that

TABLE 22.1
Medical Facilities Most Often Frequented by Trafficking Victims

Facility Location	% Presenting (Lederer and Wetzel)[69]	% Presenting (Chisolm-Straker et al)[70]	% Presenting (Goldberg et al)[7]
Any visit to medical care	87.8	68	88
Emergency department	63.3	55.6	63
Planned Parenthood	29.6	NA	NA
Primary care medical professional	22.5	47.8	25
Urgent care clinic	21.4	Combined with emergency	NA
OB-GYN	19.4	25.6	NA
Public health clinic	19.4	NA	NA
Dental	NA	26.5	NA
Other	13.3	13.6	16
Unknown	NA	0.9	NA

Abbreviations: NA, not applicable; OB-GYN, obstetrics-gynecology.

the average ages of first being trafficked were 18.7 years for females and 23.2 years for males.[70] They also found that 68% had sought medical attention during their trafficking victimization.[70]

Goldberg et al[7] did a retrospective chart review of 41 domestic minor sex trafficking (DMST) victims (all younger than 18 years) who presented for medical care to the Aubin Center at Hasbro Children's Hospital, Providence, RI. Of those patients, 88% had presented at least 1 time for medical care in the year prior to their evaluation for domestic minor sex trafficking.

According to multiple studies on minor victims of trafficking, the most common physical complaints reported by survivors include neurological complaints, headaches or migraines, dizziness, severe weight loss, malnutrition, loss of appetite, physical injury, cardiovascular or pulmonary complaint, gastrointestinal complaint, dental problems, and tooth loss. Among those survivors who reported being victims of some form of physical violence, the most often reported incidents were being punched, beaten, kicked, threatened with a weapon, or strangled. These patients presented for the physical complaints primarily and had not disclosed their victimization as the chief complaint.[4,5,7,12,23,69–71]

Common reproductive health issues include violence with sex, unwanted pregnancy from traffickers or buyers, complicated medical or nonmedical abortions, miscarriages, STIs, pelvic inflammatory disease, urinary tract infections, genital and anal trauma from sexual assault or other blunt force trauma, and chronic pelvic pain.[4,5,7,12,23,69–71]

Recommendations of leading medical societies and academies on the routine screening and care for homeless, incarcerated, and refugee populations can be applied to the medical screening and management of minor and young adult victims of human trafficking based on age.[4,23,71–73] With sex trafficking victims controlled by commercial traffickers experiencing, on average, 8 to 13 sexual assaults per day, these victims are exposed to potentially hundreds of unknown individuals over the course of their victimization.[4,7,69,70] Labor trafficking victims may be chronically exposed to the elements, caustic chemicals and poisons, physically demanding working conditions, poor sleeping conditions, and poor nutrition. Overall health concerns may include a significant delay in, or complete lack of, immunizations; cognitive or developmental delays; poor oral hygiene with numerous dental caries; chronic musculoskeletal and neurological pain and fatigue; chronic gastrointestinal, respiratory, or cardiovascular complaints; anemia; vitamin deficiencies; general malnutrition; exposure to liquid or aerosolized chemicals and poisons; and exposure to tuberculosis and other communicable diseases.[4,5,7,12,23,69–71]

Psychological health problems, often linked to extensive physical and psychological trauma, can include PTSD, suicidality, depression, anxiety, eating disorders, shame or guilt, nightmares, and more. Nearly 42% of sex trafficking victims reported at least 1 suicide attempt[69] while being trafficked, 59% had reported previous suicidal ideation,[7] and 44% had self-injurious behaviors.[7] Victims report that if they used non-prescribed substances, they most commonly became dependent on tobacco, alcohol, marijuana, cocaine, crack cocaine, heroin, ecstasy, and/or PCP (phencyclidine). These substances may be used by traffickers to control their victims and by victims themselves for physical and psychological symptom management.[4,5,7,12,23,69–71]

Common Red Flags and Screening Questions

Medical professionals have noted that identification of victims is difficult, and this is often because victims do not readily self-identify. Knowing and recognizing clinical presentation indicators can be helpful to better identify potential victims. Such indicators can be in the victim's outward presentation, medical or social history, and/or physical findings. Box 22.3 provides a list of potential trafficking red flag indicators that can assist medical professionals in recognizing possible victims.[23] Medical professionals can use these indicators to help guide medical history taking, including the use of more direct screening questions to further assess risk. While disclosure of trafficking is *not* the goal of the patient interview, the medical professional will need to assess level of risk so appropriate reports and referrals may be made.

BOX 22.3
Potential Red Flag Indicators of Human Trafficking

Medical Presentation

- Accompanied by overbearing and/or unrelated adult ("friend" or "uncle")
- Accompanying adult does not allow the minor to answer medical questions
- Changing or unknown demographic information
- Suicidality
- Acute physical or sexual assault
- Drug intoxication or sleep deprivation causing disorientation or sedation
- Preventable work-related injury, injury caused by employer or employer's staff

Medical and Social History

- Past suicidality
- Sexually transmitted infections
- Pregnancies/abortions
- Runaway/throwaway/homeless
- Significant school truancies or absences
- Child maltreatment including physical or sexual abuse or neglect
- Exposure to intimate partner violence as a child, or teen dating violence
- Involvement with child protective services or the juvenile justice system
- Substance use history
- Significantly older romantic partner
- Self identifies as LGBTQ (lesbian, gay, bisexual, transgender, queer/questioning) and any of the above
- Has a mental health diagnosis and any of the above

Physical Findings

- Dressed in clothes inadequate for location and/or weather
- Evidence of inflicted trauma
- Withdrawn, scared, fearful, and/or timid around accompanying adult
- Tattoos (eg, gang affiliation, names, pimp)
- Expensive items, clothing, nails, shoes that are inconsistent with presentation or demographics
- Large amounts of cash, hotel keys, or condoms
- Signs of substance use or withdrawal
- Stated age is older than appearance and unable to verify with valid ID

(continued)

BOX 22.3 (*continued*)

Other Concerns

- New to country (immigrant, refugee, or undocumented)
- Doesn't speak English
- Concerning work or living conditions
- Little or no pay; long hours; not allowed to leave, sleeps at work
- Threatened or physically injured by employer or employer's staff

Adapted from Greenbaum J, Crawford-Jakubiak JE; American Academy of Pediatrics Committee on Child Abuse and Neglect. Child sex trafficking and commercial sexual exploitation: health care needs of victims. *Pediatrics.* 2015;135(3):566-574.

Medical Management: Acute Versus Non-acute

The general medical assessment principles for victims of human trafficking apply to both sex and labor trafficking because there is significant overlap in their exposures. Additional elements do apply when assessing and managing victims of acute sexual assault (more often seen with sex trafficking).

Typically, trafficked persons have experienced multiple and intense traumatic events, and these may affect their willingness and ability to provide details of their medical history and participate in parts of the physical examination. Because of this, a trauma-informed, patient-centered, culturally sensitive approach to care is critically important.[11,16,23,69] According to the Substance Abuse and Mental Health Services Administration, a program, organization, or system that is trauma informed "realizes the widespread impact of trauma and understands potential paths for recovery; recognizes the signs and symptoms of trauma in clients, families, staff, and others involved with the system; and responds by fully integrating knowledge about trauma into policies, procedures, and practices, and seeks to actively resist re-traumatization."[74] Such a trauma-informed approach in the medical setting can help set the stage for this, and all future, medical visits for this patient. See Chapter 31 for more information about trauma-informed care and treatment.

Building rapport with victims/patients who present to the medical setting is of utmost importance in establishing trust and a sense of safety. This requires time and active listening, with an open and nonjudgmental demeanor. Before beginning to ask sensitive questions, the medical professional needs to explain the limits of confidentiality so that the patient may choose what to disclose. This demonstrates transparency, shows respect for the patient, and helps prevent a sense of betrayal if and when the medical professional needs to make a report and share information with authorities later in the visit. Informed consent is critical, so the medical professional needs to explain the elements of the visit, including the reasons for asking questions, conducting general and anogenital examinations, testing for STIs, etc. The medical professional should also make it clear that the patient may choose to accept or refuse the various components of the evaluation (ie, may choose which questions to answer and may refuse elements of the examination, workup, and treatment). If safe and feasible, the patient's desires should be respected, even if this means a complete evaluation is not obtained.

Because minors are often reluctant to disclose sex or labor trafficking victimization spontaneously, the best details medical professionals have to guide screening tool implementation and further assessment are all too often contextual. In the medical setting, the medical professional should consider further targeted history gathering to assess the level of risk and vulnerability when a minor has a recent history of being homeless, running away, or being kicked out. When this targeted history is obtained, consider closely the contextual scenario of the events described. Using open-ended questions that solicit narrative description of the minor's exposures while homeless, running away, or having been kicked out, a medical professional may get a contextual disclosure that fits a scenario of victimization, without specific victimization history. This non-leading history gathering should account for the limited time frame for evidence collection and prophylaxis. Any gathered history, if concerning for potential trafficking or exploitation, should be immediately discussed with a local child abuse expert, which may include a sexual assault nurse examiner, a sexual assault response team, and/or a forensic nurse examiner. The reason for this consultation is for expert guidance on the response to, and management of, the patient and potential forensic evidence. The scenarios that relate primarily to labor trafficking may still have some overlap with sex trafficking on more detailed history gathering. Even after a targeted history gathering with this specifically vulnerable population, a lack of disclosure of victimization does not rule out trafficking. If the medical professional is worried about potential exploitation in any form during a patient encounter with a minor, this concern can be reported to the appropriate agencies for further investigation. Knowing the local resources and service agencies for such patients can be key in managing their acute and ongoing care.

Medical professionals often wonder what specific questions they should ask patients to screen for human trafficking when they have a concern. Currently, multiple studies are assessing the validity of trafficking and exploitation screening tools with adolescent and youth populations.[6,75–79]

Questions that can direct the conversation toward historical trafficking or exploitation experiences may include

- Did you ever trade sex of any type for money, drugs, clothing, food, a place to stay, or something else you needed or wanted?
- Did a boyfriend, girlfriend, or anyone else ever ask or force you to have sex of any type with another person?
- Did someone ever ask or force you to undress or strip in public, such as at a party, bar, or strip club?
- Did someone ever ask or force you to pose nude (expose a private part, butt, breast) or perform a sexual act of any type for a photo or video that they took of you?
- Were you (or anyone you work with) ever beaten, hit, yelled at, raped, threatened, or made to feel physical pain for working slowly or for trying to leave the place you work?

It is important to use a victim-centered, trauma-informed approach to the patient history, with the medical professional monitoring the patient for verbal and nonverbal indicators of traumatic stress. Questions about exploitation should be asked only after adequate rapport has been established, the medical professional has explained the reason for sensitive questions, and the patient has been counseled that he or she need not answer any or all of the questions. As noted previously, a disclosure of trafficking is not the ultimate goal of the interview; rather, the medical professional needs to ask only those questions needed to assess the level of risk of exploitation, the safety and well-being of the child, and the health needs that require immediate treatment or patient referral. Questions that go beyond the scope of medical diagnosis and treatment are to be avoided because they risk unnecessarily re-traumatizing the patient. Throughout the interview, the medical professional needs to maintain an open, accepting, nonjudgmental manner and avoid any suggestion of blame, disapproval, or other negative attitude.

The general, non-acute medical management of minor victims of trafficking begins with a thorough and complete medical history (Box 22.4). If the minor is a preadolescent or adolescent, the medical professional should gather the pertinent history with that patient alone or with a medical chaperone as needed. Validated (if available) survey tools to assess for human trafficking and exploitation, teen dating violence, suicidality, depression, and substance use may add substantial information to these assessments. Of course, with any survey tool, there should be a plan in place that guides the evaluation, immediate treatment, and referral of potential positive survey responses. Following the history and with the patient's consent, a complete physical examination should be performed, including vital signs and neurological, musculoskeletal, psychological, and anogenital examinations. Ideally, a second licensed medical professional should accompany the professional performing the physical examination when any breast and anogenital examination is performed. This protects the medical professional and the patient alike.

The acute medical management of minor victims of sex trafficking (Box 22.5) also begins with a thorough and complete medical and social history and review of systems. Similar anogenital examination with photo or video documentation, STI and pregnancy testing and prophylaxis, and evidence collection should be offered as recommended per protocols for prepubescent and pubescent victims of acute sexual assault.[72] See Chapter 10, Medical Evaluation of Suspected Sexual Abuse in Prepubertal Children, and Chapter 11, Medical Management of the Adolescent Who Has Experienced Sexual Abuse or Assault.

BOX 22.4
General, Non-acute Medical Management of Minor Victims of Trafficking[73,80]

- Complete medical and social history, review of systems, and physical examination.
- Evaluation of hydration, nutrition, and growth; include head circumference or body mass index as indicated.
- Documentation of old and/or recent injuries.
- Anogenital examination, with photo or video documentation if possible.
- Assessment of development; include screening for motor, cognitive, and speech delays.
- Assessment of vision and hearing.
- Assessment of dental hygiene and oral health.
- Evaluation of immunization records and starting of appropriate catch-up immunizations during the same visit.
- Assessment for anemia, lead, tuberculosis, and other potential exposures (chemical or infectious); consider other testing for vitamin and mineral deficiencies, if indicated; consider testing for infectious diseases that are endemic in patient's home country, if indicated.
- Assessment for mental health concerns, including risk for self-harm.
- Screening for urine and/or serum alcohol and drugs of abuse, as clinically indicated.
- Testing for pregnancy and sexually transmitted infections as indicated; include gonorrhea, chlamydia, trichomonas, HIV, hepatitis B and C, and syphilis (exposure history should guide anatomical site testing for gonorrhea, chlamydia, and trichomonas).

BOX 22.5
Evidence Collection, Laboratory Testing, and Prophylaxis for Acute Sexual Assault[72]

Evidence Kit Collection

Prepubescent: less than 72 h

Pubescent: less than 96–120 h (or consistent with local law enforcement practices)

Laboratory Testing

Gonorrhea/chlamydia NAAT testing: vaginal/penile, anal, urine

Gonorrhea NAAT testing: oropharyngeal

Trichomonas NAAT testing: vaginal/penile, urine

Serology testing: HIV-1/HIV-2, RPR, hepatitis B virus, hepatitis C virus

Urine: pregnancy

Prophylaxis (May Require Ondansetron With Some Medications for Nausea)

Gonorrhea: ceftriaxone IM

Chlamydia: azithromycin PO

Trichomonas: metronidazole PO

HIV: nPEP; includes regimens of tenofovir, emtricitabine, and raltegravir

Pregnancy: ulipristal or levonorgestrel

Consider hepatitis B and human papillomavirus vaccines as indicated by immunization and exposure histories.

Abbreviations: IM, intramuscular; NAAT, nucleic acid amplification test; nPEP, nonoccupational postexposure prophylaxis; PO, per os (by mouth; oral); RPR, rapid plasma reagin.

Mental Health Considerations

Despite a growing interest in understanding the prevalence and presentations of human trafficking in its various forms in the United States and abroad, robust evidence-based research is still needed to determine best practices for mental health professionals dealing with affected children and adolescents. In their study of women and adolescent female survivors of sex trafficking in the United States, Lederer and Wetzel found that 98.1% of survivors they interviewed had at least 1 self-reported mental health concern. Survivors in that study averaged 12.1 self-reported mental health concerns during trafficking and 10.5 concerns after leaving. These concerns most often included depression, anxiety, acute stress, bipolar disorder, PTSD, depersonalization, multiple personalities, and/or borderline personality disorder.[69]

To date, very little empirical research has been conducted to assess the effectiveness of mental health interventions for youth or adults who have been subject to human trafficking. Therapy approaches have been identified, with best practice guidelines, for treatment of PTSD and other mental health issues associated with trauma in populations experiencing sexual abuse, physical abuse, domestic violence, and torture.[81,82] These may be helpful in treating trafficked persons, but the literature has yet to support this. Overall, there is a consensus among mental health professionals that a multidisciplinary, trauma-informed approach embedded within a system of care is absolutely necessary for survivors of trafficking trauma (see Chapter 31, Trauma-Informed Care and Treatment).

A systematic review of the literature addressing the needs of international survivors of sex trafficking summarized 3 key components essential to successful recovery of survivors.[81,82]

1. Multidisciplinary teams, in coordination with their local medical professionals, must conduct a comprehensive needs assessment.
2. Multidisciplinary teams should comprehensively map the breadth of trauma exposure throughout the trafficking period(s) (eg, number of years, various exposures, extent of victimization).
3. Comprehensive case coordination should be established to maintain a survivor-centered approach to services and resiliency. Without such coordination, teams may find that investigation, legislation, and prosecution take a front seat to the survivor's needs for full recovery.

In the absence of evidence-based treatments for youth who have been commercially sexually exploited, treatment should focus on treating the mental health symptoms and needs with current evidence-based modalities.[81] Some evidence-based modalities that could be adapted for trafficked youth include multisystemic therapy and dialectical behavioral therapy. However, for youth with PTSD, the most studied treatment is trauma-focused cognitive behavioral therapy, which focuses on the interconnectedness of trauma with thoughts, feelings, and behaviors.

Additional attention should be given to the unique psychological effects of trauma bonding, as previously described in this chapter. An article by deYoung and Lowry summarized studies on domestic violence, hostage situations, and victims of incest and found that acts of kindness alternated with physical or sexual violence and/or psychological coercion contributed to a form of bonding based in trauma.[83] Such traumatic bonding may make it psychologically challenging for such victims to break free from their abusers even after being physically separated from them. As summarized by Contreras et al, multiple studies have described a similar trauma bonding that occurs between victims of human trafficking and their traffickers.[84] Not all survivors manifest such bonding with their trafficker, but those who do may take weeks, if not years, to disclose personal, identifiable information about their trafficker. As previously mentioned, establishing rapport, using trauma-informed and trauma-focused services, and making the investigation survivor centered are best practices in attempting to assist survivors through this process.

Furthermore, it is important for the medical professional to keep in mind the high incidences of suicidality and of substance addiction within the trafficked population.[4,12,23,31,69] These are not necessarily coexisting conditions, but one or both are frequently reported by victims. Studies report that 42% to 75% of survivors experienced some form of suicidal ideation and 29% to 64% had at least 1 suicide attempt during, or since, their trafficking victimization. Recognizing the signs of possible exploitation, screening for suicidality and offering appropriate crisis intervention may significantly help prevent future suicide attempts in this population. Trafficked persons may use or misuse alcohol and/or drugs as a result of forced consumption at the hands of traffickers or buyers or through a desire to alleviate the toxic stress they experienced during their victimization. It is not uncommon for survivors to present to a medical professional with altered mental status and/or decreased level of consciousness secondary to drug intoxication. This altered condition renders survivors vulnerable to manipulation by their trafficker and/or buyer(s) and increases the risk of drug-facilitated sexual assault. Because of their drug use, victims are often drawn back to their trafficker, who supplies a steady stream of product in exchange for compliance with sexual demands. Successful recovery programs should include services to address acute suicidality and addiction recovery.[4,12,23,31,69]

Sexual Exploitation via Electronic Media

Electronic communication plays an ever more important and prevalent role in the lives of young people today, shaping the way they learn, grow, form friendships, interact with their community at large, perceive cultural norms, and define relationships. National survey data indicate that more than 92% of American adolescents aged 12 to 17 years access the internet daily and that 71% of them are using more than 1 social networking site (SNS) (eg, Facebook, Instagram, Snapchat, Twitter).[85] These sites allow adolescents to communicate online with the world around them and express themselves through written text, photos, videos, links, emoticons, and "likes."

Sexting

As interpersonal communication via electronic media (eg, texts, emails, chats, gaming) becomes the social norm, the potential for sharing sexually explicit material among those who use such communication methods has increased. This practice of sharing sexual information via electronic devices extends to adolescents, and even children, who frequently use these forms of communication. This sexual information sharing comes in many forms and can range from suggestive to explicit. Sexually explicit messages, more commonly labeled as *sexts,* often include a picture and/or video. The more common research definition of a sext is a message with a picture or video of a person's exposed private parts (penis, vagina, butt, or breasts) or a person performing a sexually explicit act.[86–91] Due to variations in research definitions of sexting, estimates of actual prevalence vary. Prevalence of sexting including producing, distributing, or receiving sexually explicit or suggestive images or videos ranges from 1% to 65%, with averages of 10% to 16% in studies focusing solely on American cohorts of adolescents younger than 18 years.[86–91] Mitchell et al conducted a telephone survey of 1,560 adolescents aged 10 to 17 years and found that 9.6% had appeared in, created, or shared sexually suggestive images or videos.[88] Fleschler Peskin et al conducted a laptop-based survey of 1,034 black and Hispanic urban 10th graders in Texas and found that 21% had sent nude or seminude pictures or videos and 31% had received such media.[89] Strassberg et al used a paper-based survey with 606 southwest US high school students and found that 9% to 27% had sent a sexually explicit cell phone picture and 25% to 65% had received such a picture.[90] A few studies considered adolescent age as a factor and found age to be positively predictive of a higher prevalence of sexting behaviors.[86–88] Sexts may begin on smartphones, but they can quickly be shared with others and even end up online via a myriad of direct links to SNS applications.[89] Once shared electronically, these messages can quickly become widespread and may remain on the internet indefinitely, with some messages potentially meeting legal definitions of child sexual abuse materials (child pornography).[92]

Online Sexual Solicitation and Meeting Offline

Staksrud et al, in their survey of 25,000 European adolescents aged 9 to 16 years, found that adolescents who used SNS encountered significantly more risks online than those who did not. These risks included an increased likelihood to have received sexual messages (46% more likely), to have seen sexual images online (55% more likely), and to have met people offline whom they had first met online (163% more likely).[93]

A minority (3%–4%) of adolescents surveyed in 2000 and 2005 by the Youth Internet Safety Survey experienced online sexual solicitations. These sexual solicitations were defined as solicitors who attempted to establish offline contact, called adolescents on personal phones, or sent adolescents personal mail, money, or gifts.[94] Factors associated with an increased risk for receiving online sexual solicitations include being female, using chat rooms, talking via phone with persons first met online, talking about sex with persons first met online, and concurrent or historical offline physical or sexual abuse.[94–96] Adolescents with a history of offline sexual victimization are at increased risk for online sexual solicitations.[94] Mitchell et al theorized that many of the characteristics of victimized adolescents (eg, isolation, misunderstanding, depression, anxiety, lack of support) influence their capacity to resist or deter victimization. These characteristics are often sought out by "virtual" predators, making these adolescents more vulnerable to online, and subsequently offline, solicitations and revictimization.[94] Noll et al, in their 2013 survey of American female adolescents, concluded that sexual victimization poses a unique risk for online behaviors that may set the stage for provocative social networking and subsequent offline encounters.[97]

Online Grooming and Exploitation

According to the 2016 American Academy of Pediatrics (AAP) technical report, "Children and Adolescents and Digital Media," the internet has many benefits for child education and development but has also created opportunities for the exploitation of children.[98] Online predators can gain access to minors through any and all forms of electronic media communication. Such communication may occur through online gaming, SNSs and applications, instant messaging, special interest or fan sites, chat rooms, and even private and public email accounts. Incidences of child sex trafficking, cyber grooming, and online sexual abuse for private and commercial purposes have increased because of the anonymity of cyberspace.[97,98]

Cyber grooming, for example, often begins with a benign contact online, followed by the building of what may appear to be a trusting, understanding, or even loving relationship. This cyber relationship is, in large part, a virtual reality built around whatever the groomer perceives the child or teen is looking for in a relationship, often misrepresenting the truth. This online relationship may eventually, or even precipitously, lead to the request for personal sexual information, pictures, and/or videos from the child or adolescent. Once shared over the internet or via cellular communication, these files can be nearly impossible to retract or erase completely. Further grooming may include gifts such as jewelry, concert tickets, clothes, and even money sent electronically via gift certificates or through the mail. When the perpetrator feels that the virtual relationship has grown to a point where the child or adolescent may be willing to meet in person offline, he or she may suggest doing so. All too often, this offline meeting, set up by the perpetrator, is to engage in sexual acts with the child or adolescent. Also, children or adolescents may be deceived, tricked, coerced, and even threatened online to meet offline, potentially not even realizing that the person they are meeting or the event they are attending is, in reality, a lure to get the child or adolescent alone. It is not uncommon for these online predators to engage in a sexual act offline with a minor and to video record the encounter. Such sexual material that involves a minor qualifies under most, if not all, legal statutes as online-mediated child sexual abuse (child pornography).[98]

Such online child sexual exploitation, in combination with offline meetings, may lead to the forced recruitment and advertisement of children for commercial sexual acts and other forms of exploitation. The internet may be used to share, sell, trade, and distribute child sexual abuse media, including pictures and videos. It may also be used by human traffickers to facilitate the trafficking of victims, from recruitment and advertisement to sales and transportation. Internet-initiated sex crimes involving offenders who meet and groom children online tend to involve adolescents rather than very young children; 99% of victims in one study were 13 to 17 years old and 48% were 13 to 14 years old. Many of these crimes involve face-to-face sexual contact, which the victim often perceives as "consensual."[98]

Research shows that caregivers generally underestimate the likelihood that their child might engage in online conversation with people they have never met in person, even with adult strangers. Therefore, it is critical that caregivers promote online safety with the children and adolescents they care for, preferably from an early age. It is also advisable that they monitor children's internet use and have an open-door policy with all electronic devices in the home. Parents may choose to use tools such as parental control software to maintain awareness of their children's online activities. Medical professionals, teachers, and caregivers alike should consider asking appropriate questions to their adolescent and preadolescent population to explore social media and internet use and to educate youth about protecting themselves from grooming, exploitation, cyberbullying, and "sextortion." All medical professionals should report any suspicions of online or offline sexual abuse or exploitation according to their local laws on mandatory reporting of child maltreatment.[98]

Sextortion

Persons looking to manipulate others into supplying them with money, information, or sexually explicit pictures or videos, or meeting them offline in person, may do so through various methods of extortion. A newly recognized form of online exploitation that uses sexually sensitive material about a person (eg, conversations, pictures, videos) to extort that individual has been coined "sextortion." Wolak et al describe sextortion as the situation in which a perpetrator threatens to expose sexual material to coerce a victim into providing additional sexual material, engage in offline sexual activity, or agree to some other demand.[99] This emerging online threat to adolescents and even children is being reported to law enforcement and federal agencies with growing frequency. The prevalence in the minor population has yet to be adequately defined. An online report by the US Department of Justice in 2016 describes the sextortion of minors online as significantly increasing as a form of online child exploitation based on more than 1,000 reports by law enforcement investigations.[100]

Various studies have looked at teen dating violence in this era of media-based relationships and have found a co-occurrence of cyber dating violence and sextortion. A 2013 study of 3,745 dating teens at US schools found that 15% of girls and 7% of boys experienced what they labeled "sexual cyber dating abuse."[101] This abuse included being pressured by a partner to send sexual photos or videos, being threatened with exposure or violence if they did not, and/or receiving unwanted sexual photos or videos from their partner. A 2018 survey study of 1,631 youth victims of sextortion aged 18 to 25 years by Wolak et al showed that 572 of the victims were minors when they first experienced this form of sexual exploitation. A staggering 41% were only acquainted with their perpetrator online. The other 59% of minor victims were victimized by someone they knew in person, most often a current or former romantic partner. Of the 572 who experienced sextortion as minors, 75% knowingly provided sexual images to their perpetrators, although 66% of those who provided images stated they did so because of feeling pressured, tricked, threatened, or forced to do so. Only a small percentage (4%) had images stolen via hacking. Fewer than half (49%) of those minor victims came forward while they were minors about their sextortion, and of those, only 33% told a caregiver.[99]

Media-Related Child Sexual Abuse (Child Pornography) and Hands-on Offending

In 2009, Bourke and Hernandez conducted a first-of-its-kind comprehensive comparative study looking into the hands-on offending rates of male prisoners currently serving time in federal prison for possession of child sexual abuse materials (child pornography). These 155 male sex offenders also attended a mandatory sex offender-specific treatment program at this federal prison. They were divided into 2 groups based on their convictions, hands-on (40) versus child sexual abuse materials only (115) and were interviewed multiple times over the course of this 18-month treatment program. By the termination of the treatment program, only 24 of the men denied hands-on offense, an increase of 59% in known hands-on offenders (40 to 131). The total number of disclosed child victims at the end of the treatment program was 1,777, an average of 13.56 victims per hands-on offender. Interviews with these 131 hands-on sex offenders revealed that 65% admitted abusing prepubescent and postpubescent children. Forty percent admitted abusing male and female victims. It was concluded that offending with child sexual abuse materials (child pornography) is a strong diagnostic indicator of hands-on child sexual abuse offense.[102]

Role of Medical Professionals in Media-Related Victim Identification

Medical professionals are, at times, called on to collaborate with local law enforcement, including Internet Crimes Against Children Task Forces, to help medically determine the potential age of an individual based on media evidence (photos or videos) of their genitalia or breasts. Medical professionals trained in pediatric development can, at times, give pubertal development insight to investigative partners on these cases. Such collaboration and medical expertise should be entered into with foresight as to personal exposure and an understanding of diagnostic limitations to avoid outcome bias. In other words, personal exposure to recorded child sexual abuse can potentially have significant vicarious trauma effects on the investigative viewer. Mental preparation and foresight can help prepare the medical professional for this but may not completely mitigate these effects. In addition, the medical professional's opinion is requested in an ongoing investigation, of which the medical professional is overtly aware. Therefore, there exists the potential for outcome bias in determining the pubertal age of an individual depicted in the sexually explicit media.[103,104]

The medical professional should keep in mind the ambiguity in differentiating, for example, between a fully pubertal 15-year-old minor and an 18-year-old adult based solely on depicted genitals or breasts. An individual's face may not be present in the depicted media and, if depicted, may in itself be misleading in determining age. Some research suggests sexual maturation determination based on the child's dentition if depicted in the media, such as in oral fellatio, is the next best option if no determination can be made from the genital or breast development. The presence of deciduous and permanent teeth together is seen in most children younger than 12 years.[103] This, of course, requires that the medical professional feel comfortable in the differentiation between deciduous and permanent dentition. If not, this may require the expertise of a forensic odontologist, who may be more comfortable with this determination. Other variables, such as shaving of the pubic hair, genital tattoos and piercings, depicted clothing styles, and even skin color, can mislead a medical professional to think the individual depicted is older or younger than he or she actually was when the photo or video was taken. Best practice in giving expert opinion in these cases dictates determining whether an individual depicted is prepubertal or postpubertal (age 12 years) and allowing the investigators to more thoroughly evaluate the postpubertal individuals for potential victimization as postpubertal minors. Clear reference of photos of sexual maturity stages are essential, as described in the AAP publication, *Assessment of Sexual Maturity Stages in Girls and Boys.*[103,105]

Prevention

Medical professionals who work with adolescents and children should be aware that these minors are, or will be, very active online. Children and adolescents today are intimately familiar with the navigation of memes, tweets, posts, GIFs, vines, pictures, and videos online. They are also a generation heavily targeted by online predators who may be looking to lure them offline to meet in person, to have them exchange nude pictures or videos, or to exploit them in other forms of sex or even labor trafficking. Prevention of such online abuse as seen with child sexual abuse materials, cyberbullying, and sextortion can best be accomplished through education and training. Parents, caregivers, teachers, coaches, religious leaders, and community leaders, along with these adolescents and children themselves, all need education and training on the potential dangers of social media, media-based relationships, and the sharing of sexually suggestive and explicit material online.[98]

Labor Trafficking

While child labor trafficking is touched on in all sections of this chapter, this dedicated section is provided to highlight this under-recognized form of exploitation. Child labor is permitted in the United States, and federal as well as state laws address the conditions and limitations of child employment.[106,107] In some cases of child labor, there is exploitation, and the exploitation becomes child trafficking when the employer or manager uses force, fraud, or coercion to control the child and convince the victim he or she must continue working.[1,108] The published research on child labor trafficking is relatively sparse, especially on cases identified in the United States. However, like labor trafficking of adults[67,109] and of children around the globe, it is likely fueled by economic need, making children from poor families and communities at high risk.[49] Unaccompanied minors coming to the United States are at risk, especially if undocumented, given their limited resources, cultural barriers, potential immigration issues, and lack of familiarity with US laws and child rights. Children involved in other mass migrations are at risk, as well, whether or not they remain with their family or travel across borders.[48] Homeless and runaway youth and young adults are vulnerable to labor trafficking,[41] especially involving forced drug dealing. As with sex trafficking, increased risk for labor exploitation is associated with persons coming from dysfunctional homes (eg, familial substance abuse, sexual violence, physical violence).[110]

Child labor trafficking in the United States involves a range of settings,[41,49,111] including domestic servitude, factory work, construction, the illicit drug trade, janitorial/cleaning services, traveling sales,[111] agriculture, health and beauty services, begging/peddling, and hotel and restaurant businesses.[49,51,112] Globally, forced labor involves children working in various hazardous settings, including brickkilns,[51] construction,[113] mines and quarries,[114] fisheries,[115] and farms.[109] Children and adolescents may serve as soldiers in armed conflict[48,51] or as forced participants in drug trafficking.[51] Domestic servitude is common, especially among girls.[116] Some children subjected to labor trafficking are also sexually exploited through sexual assault or sex trafficking.[108]

The prevalence of child labor trafficking in the United States is not known, and case tracking is hindered by lack of recognition by authorities, lack of a centralized database, misidentification of trafficked persons, lack of screening, and lack of victim disclosure. Similarly, there is a lack of data to document the frequency with which labor-trafficked children contact medical professionals. However, such contact may occur under a number of conditions, including an injured or ill victim, a child who is the daughter or son of trafficked parents, or a neonate born to a trafficked woman or girl. Potential indicators of labor trafficking include the presence of a domineering companion who speaks for the patient or parent and who is reluctant to leave the patient or parent alone with a medical professional, a parent or child who is apparently afraid of or intimidated by the person accompanying him or her, a patient or parent not in control of his or her own identification documents, or a patient or parent who provides information about exploitative working conditions. As with sex trafficking, forced labor exploitation is associated with major health consequences.

Mandatory Reporting, Referrals, and Resources

Although all US states, districts, and territories have mandatory reporting statutes for suspected child maltreatment, not all of these jurisdictions of the United States have legally included child sex and labor trafficking within their legal definition of child maltreatment and, therefore, mandatory reporting statutes. All medical professionals should understand how sex and labor trafficking of minors is defined in local legal statute with regard to mandatory reporting.[117] Information about laws related to child trafficking may be obtained from the National Human Trafficking Hotline (888/373-7888; https://humantraffickinghotline.org) or Shared Hope International (https://sharedhope.org).

Appropriate law enforcement involvement may occur at the local, state, or federal level, depending on the circumstances of the case. In some areas, small local law enforcement agencies may have little experience with human trafficking cases and may request assistance from specialized state or other task forces. Child protective services may play a critical role in providing services to survivors of sex and labor trafficking. Trafficked persons typically have extensive needs, ranging from immediate (eg, health care, emergency psychiatric assessment/treatment, housing, crisis intervention, food, clothing, interpreter services) to longer term (eg, mental health assessment and therapy, long-term housing, education/job skills training, medical home, immigration assistance, English classes). Depending on location, there may or may not be victim service organizations to fulfill some of these needs. The medical professional may receive assistance in locating resources by contacting the National Human Trafficking Hotline; this hotline has a database of community resources located throughout the United States, although it does not include all organizations and it behooves the medical professional to become aware of agencies and organizations in his or her own area. The hotline also is available to provide guidance and advice to clinicians who have questions about human trafficking, as well as to speak with patients and families. Additional help for the medical professional may be obtained from local child advocacy centers. Typically, these centers provide formal forensic interviews of maltreated and exploited youth, and many also provide medical evaluations and behavioral health services.

Mandatory reporting laws may require the medical professional to contact authorities, even without patient consent. However, referrals to hotlines and community agencies should be made only with the patient's permission (an exception to this may be if the medical professional refers only to a hypothetical case during a discussion with an outside party and does not disclose any protected health information). Ideally, the youth is actively involved in the discussion of referral options and possible resources and helps the medical professional create an appropriate safety plan for follow-up. Furthermore, a "warm handoff" to referral agencies is preferred, with the medical professional or a delegate contacting the organization directly to arrange a referral or helping the trafficked youth to do so. Common health-related referrals for youth who are confirmed survivors of child trafficking, or those felt to be at high risk, are listed in Table 22.2.

Foreign-born trafficking survivors likely will need legal and immigration assistance as well as interpreter services. When a clinician encounters an unaccompanied foreign-born minor suspected of being

TABLE 22.2
Common Health-Related Referrals for Trafficked Persons

Referral	Details
Behavioral health assessment and trauma-focused therapy, if indicated	If acute psychiatric emergency is present, the youth should be referred for immediate assessment
Substance misuse assessment and treatment, if indicated	
Easily accessible, affordable, and acceptable medical home	• Periodic STI and HIV testing • HIV PEP monitoring, HIV PrEP, as indicated • Primary care and anticipatory guidance/harm reduction counseling • Family planning • Immunizations, including HPV vaccine
Second-opinion anogenital examination, if indicated	Sexual assault nurse examiner, sexual assault response team, or child advocacy physician
Child advocacy center	Follow-up examination, HIV PEP monitoring, forensic interview, behavioral health services
Obstetrician/gynecologist, if indicated	
Specialist treatment, if indicated	
LGBTQ resources	Counseling, support, medical treatment, etc

Abbreviations: HPV, human papillomavirus; LGBTQ, lesbian, gay, bisexual, transgender, queer/questioning; PEP, postexposure prophylaxis; PrEP, pre-exposure prophylaxis; STI, sexually transmitted infection.

exploited, it is important for a local, state, or federal official to promptly contact the US Department of Health and Human Services Administration for Children and Families Office of Refugee Resettlement to request assistance for child victims of human trafficking.[118] The Office of Refugee Resettlement will evaluate the case to determine if the child is eligible for federal benefits and services, as well as for the Unaccompanied Refugee Minors Program, a form of federal foster care. The child is not obligated to cooperate with law enforcement to be eligible for assistance.

Foreign-born victims of trafficking may also be eligible to apply for T or U visas, which allow them to remain in the United States for 4 years, receive federally funded benefits and services, and work on obtaining permanent residency status.[119,120] They may also be able to bring family members into the United States. The T visa is specific for victims of human trafficking, while the U visa applies to victims of a variety of crimes, including trafficking and sexual exploitation.

In many cases, the medical professional may have significant concerns about child trafficking but may not have definitive evidence of exploitation. This may occur with survivors who do not feel comfortable disclosing their status, survivors who do not understand that they are being exploited, and youth who are not being trafficked but who are at high risk. In such cases, the medical professional can offer resources to address key vulnerability factors, and counseling on harm reduction techniques. This is demonstrated in the following example:

JT is a 15-year-old cisgender bisexual female who frequently runs away from home and lives on the streets or with various "friends" she meets on the streets. She reports using marijuana, cocaine, and, occasionally, methamphetamines. She has a history of gonorrhea and presents with a vaginal discharge and pelvic pain. She denies exchanging sex for anything of value while living on the streets and reports "getting what she needs" from friends. As her medical professional, you do not have definitive evidence of trafficking, but the youth is at high risk. After assessing and treating her chief concerns, appropriate referrals to consider and discuss with JT include LGBTQ resources; a medical home at a local teen clinic for family planning, periodic STI/HIV testing, possible HIV preexposure prophylaxis, and the human papillomavirus vaccine; possible substance use assessment and treatment (depending on additional information you obtain while taking history); and an accessible behavioral health counseling resource. You might also discuss harm reduction practices, including condom use, the need for regular STI testing and long-acting reversible contraception, interactions of drugs and alcohol and their effects on judgment and risk-taking behavior, common recruitment techniques for sex trafficking, and hotlines such as the National Network for Youth (information for homeless/runaway youth; https://www.nn4youth.org or 202/783-7949) or the National Human Trafficking Hotline (https://humantraffickinghotline.org or 888/373-7888). You might also refer her to a local homeless shelter that serves adolescents and a local food bank.

Central to the process of making referrals and identifying resources is the need for a community-based, multidisciplinary approach. The health sector cannot provide for all the needs of trafficked youth, and building relationships with community service providers who serve these youths can vastly increase the likelihood that a survivor will receive the services he or she needs. Such collaboration requires an initial effort to build relationships with key stakeholders and ongoing work to maintain those relationships and build new ones as the workforce turns over. It is helpful for medical professionals to have an established written protocol for responding to suspected sex and labor trafficking and to youth at risk for such exploitation. Such a protocol not only outlines definitions, risk factors, potential indicators, and trauma-informed strategies for care but also includes a list of reporting and referral agencies, with detailed information about hours of service, eligibility, and type of service offered. This protocol may need to be updated periodically as new victim-serving organizations appear and others disappear. Given the labor-intensive nature of serving trafficked youth, a medical team may delegate various tasks to specific staff members, which will help facilitate the flow of patients through the clinic/hospital. These responsibilities may be clearly outlined in the protocol.

Conclusion

Child trafficking is a complex public health issue in the United States that affects American-born and foreign-born children alike. The health effects may be profound, and medical professionals need to be aware of potential indicators of exploitation so that they are able to respond appropriately and offer services. Reluctance on the part of trafficked persons to disclose their status, their potential inability to recognize their exploitation, and the lack of definitive signs of human trafficking make the process of identification and intervention difficult for medical professionals. However, victims have many needs, and the medical professional may be one of the few professionals with the opportunity to connect the child to service providers. While re-trafficking is common and the medical professional should not expect to permanently "rescue" a child from exploitation, they do have a critical role to play. Medical professionals need to make every effort to build trust and communicate to youth that services are available, that there are adults who are eager to offer assistance, and that the medical professional's health setting is a safe place to seek help. A victim-centered, trauma-informed approach to patient care is an effective way to build this trust and identify the extensive needs of trafficked youth. A community-based, multidisciplinary approach to filling the needs of survivors allows for more comprehensive services to be delivered.

References

1. Pub L No. 106–386, Div A 103(8)
2. United Nations Office of the High Commissioner for Human Rights. *Protocol to Prevent, Suppress and Punish Trafficking in Persons Especially Women and Children, Supplementing the United Nations Convention Against Transnational Organized Crime*. United Nations; 2000. https://www.ohchr.org/EN/ProfessionalInterest/Pages/ProtocolTraffickingInPersons.aspx. Accessed June 7, 2019.
3. Oram S, Stöckl H, Busza J, Howard LM, Zimmerman C. Prevalence and risk of violence and the physical, mental, and sexual health problems associated with human trafficking: systematic review. *PLoS Med*. 2012;9(5):e1001224 PMID: 22666182 https://doi.org/10.1371/journal.pmed.1001224
4. Ottisova L, Hemmings S, Howard LM, Zimmerman C, Oram S. Prevalence and risk of violence and the mental, physical and sexual health problems associated with human trafficking: an updated systematic review. *Epidemiol Psychiatr Sci*. 2016;25(4):317–341 PMID: 27066701 10.1017/S2045796016000135
5. Varma S, Gillespie S, McCracken C, Greenbaum VJ. Characteristics of child commercial sexual exploitation and sex trafficking victims presenting for medical care in the United States. *Child Abuse Negl*. 2015;44:98–105 PMID: 25896617 https://doi.org/10.1016/j.chiabu.2015.04.004
6. Greenbaum VJ, Dodd M, McCracken C. A short screening tool to identify victims of child sex trafficking in the health care setting. *Pediatr Emerg Care*. 2018;34(1):33–37 PMID: 26599463
7. Goldberg AP, Moore JL, Houck C, Kaplan DM, Barron CE. Domestic minor sex trafficking patients: a retrospective analysis of medical presentation. *J Pediatr Adolesc Gynecol*. 2017;30(1):109–115 PMID: 27575407 https://doi.org/10.1016/j.jpag.2016.08.010
8. Edinburgh L, Pape-Blabolil J, Harpin SB, Saewyc E. Assessing exploitation experiences of girls and boys seen at a child advocacy center. *Child Abuse Negl*. 2015;46:47–59 PMID: 25982287 https://doi.org/10.1016/j.chiabu.2015.04.016
9. Kiss L, Pocock NS, Naisanguansri V, et al. Health of men, women, and children in post-trafficking services in Cambodia, Thailand, and Vietnam: an observational cross-sectional study. *Lancet Glob Health*. 2015;3(3):e154–e161 PMID: 25701993 https://doi.org/10.1016/S2214-109X(15)70016-1
10. Willis BM, Levy BS. Child prostitution: global health burden, research needs, and interventions. *Lancet*. 2002;359(9315):1417–1422 PMID: 11978356 https://doi.org/10.1016/S0140-6736(02)08355-1
11. Zimmerman C, Hossain M, Yun K, Roche B, Morison L, Watts C. *Stolen Smiles: A Summary Report on the Physical and Psychological Health Consequences of Women and Adolescents Trafficked in Europe*. London, United Kingdom: London School of Hygiene and Tropical Medicine; 2006
12. Stanley N, Oram S, Jakobowitz S, et al. The health needs and healthcare experiences of young people trafficked into the UK. *Child Abuse Negl*. 2016;59:100–110 PMID: 27552002 https://doi.org/10.1016/j.chiabu.2016.08.001

13. Macias Konstantopoulos W, Ahn R, Alpert EJ, et al. An international comparative public health analysis of sex trafficking of women and girls in eight cities: achieving a more effective health sector response. *J Urban Health*. 2013;90(6):1194–1204 PMID: 24151086 https://doi.org/10.1007/s11524-013-9837-4
14. Deb S, Mukherjee A, Mathews B. Aggression in sexually abused trafficked girls and efficacy of intervention. *J Interpers Violence*. 2011;26(4):745–768 PMID: 20587459 https://doi.org/10.1177/0886260510365875
15. Surtees R. *Re/integraton of Trafficked Persons: Handling "Difficult" Cases 2008. Issues Paper #2: Trafficking Victims Re/integration Programme in Southeast Europe (TVRP)*. Brussels, Belgium: King Baudouin Foundation; 2008. https://www.kbs-frb.be/en/Virtual-Library/2008/295023. Accessed April 9, 2019
16. Greenbaum J. Introduction to human trafficking: who is affected? In: Chisolm-Straker M, Stoklosa H, eds. *Human Trafficking Is a Public Health Issue: A Paradigm Expansion in the United States*. Cham, Switzerland: Springer International; 2017:1–14 https://doi.org/10.1007/978-3-319-47824-1_1
17. Pub L No. 114-22, 129 Stat 227
18. Greijer S, Doek J. *Terminology Guidelines for the Protection of Children from Sexual Exploitation and Sexual Abuse*. Luxembourg: Interagency Working Group on Sexual Exploitation of Children; 2016. http://cf.cdn.unwto.org/sites/all/files/docpdf/terminologyguidelines.pdf. Accessed April 9, 2019
19. US Immigration and Customs Enforcement. Human trafficking and smuggling. https://www.ice.gov/factsheets/human-trafficking. Published January 16, 2013. Accessed April 9, 2019
20. Stransky M, Finkelhor D. How many juveniles are involved in prostitution in the U.S.? Crimes Against Children Research Center website. http://www.unh.edu/ccrc/prostitution/Juvenile_Prostitution_factsheet.pdf. Published 2008. Accessed April 9, 2019
21. UN Office on Drugs and Crime. *Global Report on Trafficking in Persons 2014*. https://www.unodc.org/unodc/en/data-and-analysis/glotip_2014.html. Accessed April 9, 2019
22. Institute of Medicine and National Research Council. *Confronting Commercial Sexual Exploitation and Sex Trafficking of Minors in the United States*. Washington, D.C.: The National Academies Press; 2013
23. Greenbaum J, Crawford-Jakubiak JE; American Academy of Pediatrics Committee on Child Abuse and Neglect. Child sex trafficking and commercial sexual exploitation: health care needs of victims. *Pediatrics*. 2015;135(3):566–574 PMID: 25713283 https://doi.org/10.1542/peds.2014-4138
24. Alliance 8.7. *Global Estimates of Modern Slavery: Forced Labour and Forced Marriage*. Geneva, Switzerland: International Labour Organization; 2017. https://www.ilo.org/wcmsp5/groups/public/---dgreports/---dcomm/documents/publication/wcms_575479.pdf. Accessed June 7, 2019
25. Walls NE, Bell S. Correlates of engaging in survival sex among homeless youth and young adults. *J Sex Res*. 2011;48(5):423–436 PMID: 20799134 https://doi.org/10.1080/00224499.2010.501916
26. Greene JM, Ennett ST, Ringwalt CL. Prevalence and correlates of survival sex among runaway and homeless youth. *Am J Public Health*. 1999;89(9):1406–1409 PMID: 10474560 https://doi.org/10.2105/AJPH.89.9.1406
27. Chettiar J, Shannon K, Wood E, Zhang R, Kerr T. Survival sex work involvement among street-involved youth who use drugs in a Canadian setting. *J Public Health (Oxf)*. 2010;32(3):322–327 PMID: 20061578 https://doi.org/10.1093/pubmed/fdp126

28. Dank M, Yahner J, Madden K, et al. *Surviving the Streets of New York: Experiences of LGBTQ Youth, YMSM, YWSW Engaged in Survival Sex*. Washington, DC: Urban Institute; 2015
29. Davis J, Miles G. "They didn't help me; they shamed me." A baseline study on the vulnerabilities of street-involved boys to sexual exploitation in Manila, Philippines. Love146. https://1at4ct3uffpw1uzzmu191368-wpengine.netdna-ssl.com/wp-content/uploads/2016/01/They-Shamed-Me-.pdf. Published September 2015. Accessed April 9, 2019
30. Curtis R, Terry K, Dank M, Dombrowski K, Khan B. *The Commercial Sexual Exploitation of Children in New York City. Volume 1. The CSEC Population in New York City: Size, Characteristics and Needs*. New York, NY: The City University of New York John Jay College of Criminal Justice; 2008
31. Whitbeck LB, Chen X, Hoyt DR, Tyler KA, Johnson KD. Mental disorder, subsistence strategies, and victimization among gay, lesbian, and bisexual homeless and runaway adolescents. *J Sex Res*. 2004;41(4):329–342 PMID: 15765273 https://doi.org/10.1080/00224490409552240
32. Dennis J. Women are victims, men make choices: the invisibility of men and boys in the global sex trade. *Gend Issues*. 2008;25(1):11–25 https://doi.org/10.1007/s12147-008-9051-y
33. ECPAT-USA. *And Boys Too: An ECPAT-USA Discussion Paper About the Lack of Recognition of the Commercial Sexual Exploitation of Boys in the United States*. Brooklyn, NY: ECPAT-USA; 2013. https://d1qkyo3pi1c9bx.cloudfront.net/00028B1B-B0DB-4FCD-A991-219527535DAB/1b1293ef-1524-4f2c-b148-91db11379d11.pdf. Accessed April 9, 2019
34. Hounmenou C. An initial exploration of prostitution of boys in the West African region. *Child Abuse Negl*. 2017;69:188–200 PMID: 28482251 https://doi.org/10.1016/j.chiabu.2017.04.027
35. Lillywhite R, Skidmore P. Boys are not sexually exploited? A challenge to practitioners. *Child Abuse Rev*. 2006;15(5):351–361 https://doi.org/10.1002/car.952
36. Goździak EM, Bump MN. *Data and Research on Human Trafficking: Bibliography of Research-Based Literature*. Washington, DC: Institute for the Study of International Migration, Walsh School of Foreign Service, Georgetown University; 2008
37. Greenbaum VJ. Commercial sexual exploitation and sex trafficking of children in the United States. *Curr Probl Pediatr Adolesc Health Care*. 2014;44(9):245–269 PMID: 25131563 https://doi.org/10.1016/j.cppeds.2014.07.001
38. Centers for Disease Control and Prevention. Violence prevention. The social-ecological model: a framework for prevention. https://www.cdc.gov/violenceprevention/overview/social-ecologicalmodel.html;. Reviewed January 16, 2019. Accessed April 9, 2019
39. Reid JA. Risk and resiliency factors influencing onset and adolescence-limited commercial sexual exploitation of disadvantaged girls. *Crim Behav Ment Health*. 2014;24(5):332–344 PMID: 24619596 https://doi.org/10.1002/cbm.1903
40. Reid JA, Baglivio MT, Piquero AR, Greenwald MA, Epps N. Human trafficking of minors and childhood adversity in Florida. *Am J Public Health*. 2017;107(2):306–311 PMID: 27997232 https://doi.org/10.2105/AJPH.2016.303564
41. Covenant House; Field Center for Children's Policy, Practice and Research; Loyola University New Orleans Modern Slavery Research Project. Labor and sex trafficking among homeless youth. https://www.covenanthouse.org/homeless-issues/human-trafficking-study. Accessed April 9, 2019
42. Banks D, Kyckelhahn T. *Characteristics of Suspected Human Trafficking Incidents, 2008–2010*. Washington, DC: US Department of Justice, Office of Justice Programs, Bureau of Justice Statistics; 2011. https://www.bjs.gov/content/pub/pdf/cshti0810.pdf. Accessed April 9, 2019

43. US Department of State. *Trafficking in Persons Report. June 2016*. Washington, DC: US Department of State; 2016. http://www.state.gov/documents/organization/258876.pdf. Accessed April 9, 2019
44. UN High Commissioner for Refugees. *Children on the Run: Unaccompanied Children Leaving Central America and Mexico and the Need for International Protection*. Washington, DC: UN High Commissioner for Refugees Regional Office for the United States and the Caribbean; 2014. http://www.unhcr.org/en-us/about-us/background/56fc266f4/children-on-the-run-full-report.html. Accessed April 9, 2019
45. Silverman JG, Decker MR, Gupta J, et al. Experiences of sex trafficking victims in Mumbai, India. *Int J Gynaecol Obstet*. 2007;97(3):221–226 PMID: 17320087
46. Smith LA, Vardaman SH, Snow MA. *The National Report on Domestic Minor Sex Trafficking: America's Prostituted Children*. Vancouver, WA: Shared Hope International; 2009 http://sharedhope.org/wp-content/uploads/2012/09/SHI_National_Report_on_DMST_2009.pdf. Accessed April 9, 2019
47. International Labour Office. *Making Progress Against Child Labour: Global Estimates and Trends 2000–2012. International Programme on the Elimination of Child Labour (IPEC)*. Geneva, Switzerland: International Labour Office; 2013
48. International Centre for Migration Policy Development. *Targeting Vulnerabilities: The Impact of the Syrian War and Refugee Situation on Trafficking in Persons. A Study of Syria, Turkey, Lebanon, Jordan and Iraq*. Vienna, Austria: International Centre for Migration Policy Development; 2015. https://www.icmpd.org/fileadmin/ICMPD-Website/Anti-Trafficking/Targeting_Vulnerabilities_EN__SOFT_.pdf. Accessed April 9, 2019
49. National Human Trafficking Resource Center. Child labor trafficking in the United States. https://traffickingresourcecenter.org/sites/default/files/Child%20Labor%20Trafficking.pdf. Accessed April 9, 2019
50. Free the Slaves. Sex trafficking in Kathmandu's entertainment sector: summary of literature review—December 2015. https://www.freetheslaves.net/wp-content/uploads/2016/02/Kathmandu-Entertainment-Lit-Review-Dec-2015-PUBLIC.pdf. Accessed April 9, 2019
51. Hepburn S, Simon RJ. *Human Trafficking Around the World: Hidden in Plain Sight*. New York, NY: Columbia University Press; 2013
52. Klain E. *Prostitution of Children and Child-Sex Tourism: An Analysis of Domestic and International Responses*. Alexandria, VA: National Center for Missing and Exploited Children; 1999
53. ECPAT International. *The Use of Information and Communication Technologies in Connection With Cases of Child Sex Tourism in East and Southeast Asia*. Bangkok, Thailand: ECPAT International; 2010. https://www.ilo.org/wcmsp5/groups/public/---dgreports/---dcomm/documents/publication/wcms_575479.pdf. Accessed June 7, 2019
54. McIntyre S. *Under the Radar: The Sexual Exploitation of Young Men—Western Canadian Edition*.http://humanservices.alberta.ca/documents/child-sexual-exploitation-under-the-radar-western-canada.pdf. Published 2009. Accessed April 9, 2019
55. Polaris. *More Than Drinks for Sale: Exposing Sex Trafficking in Cantinas and Bars in the U.S.* Washington, DC: Polaris; 2016. https://polarisproject.org/sites/default/files/Cantinas-SexTrafficking-EN.pdf. Accessed April 9, 2019
56. Reid JA. Entrapment and enmeshment schemes used by sex traffickers. *Sex Abuse*. 2016;28(6):491–511 PMID: 25079777 https://doi.org/10.1177/1079063214544334
57. Cole J, Sprang G. Sex trafficking of minors in metropolitan, micropolitan, and rural communities. *Child Abuse Negl*. 2015;40:113–123 PMID: 25151302 https://doi.org/10.1016/j.chiabu.2014.07.015

58. Silverman JG, Raj A, Cheng DM, et al. Sex trafficking and initiation-related violence, alcohol use, and HIV risk among HIV-infected female sex workers in Mumbai, India. *J Infect Dis.* 2011;204(suppl 5):S1229–S1234 PMID: 22043037 https://doi.org/10.1093/infdis/jir540
59. Harris KD. *The State of Human Trafficking in California 2012*. Sacramento, CA: California Department of Justice; 2012. http://oag.ca.gov/sites/all/files/agweb/pdfs/ht/human-trafficking-2012.pdf. Accessed April 9, 2019
60. Carpenter A, Gates J. *The Nature and Extent of Gang Involvement in Sex Trafficking in San Diego County*. San Diego, CA: University of San Diego, Pt. Loma Nazarene University; 2016. https://www.ncjrs.gov/pdffiles1/nij/grants/249857.pdf. Accessed April 9, 2019
61. Goldenberg SM, Silverman JG, Engstrom D, et al. Exploring the context of trafficking and adolescent sex industry involvement in Tijuana, Mexico: consequences for HIV risk and prevention. *Violence Against Women*. 2015;21(4):478–499 PMID: 25648946 https://doi.org/10.1177/1077801215569079
62. Raphael J, Reichert J, Powers M. Pimp control and violence: domestic sex trafficking of Chicago women and girls. *Women Crim Justice*. 2010;20(1-2):89–104 https://doi.org/10.1080/08974451003641065
63. Kiss L, Yun K, Pocock N, Zimmerman C. Exploitation, violence, and suicide risk among child and adolescent survivors of human trafficking in the Greater Mekong Subregion. *JAMA Pediatr.* 2015;169(9):e152278 PMID: 26348864 https://doi.org/10.1001/jamapediatrics.2015.2278
64. Wilson B, Butler LD. Running a gauntlet: a review of victimization and violence in the pre-entry, post-entry, and peri-/post-exit periods of commercial sexual exploitation. *Psychol Trauma*. 2014;6(5):494–504 https://doi.org/10.1037/a0032977
65. McCauley HL, Decker MR, Silverman JG. Trafficking experiences and violence victimization of sex-trafficked young women in Cambodia. *Int J Gynaecol Obstet.* 2010;110(3):266–267 PMID: 20553789 https://doi.org/10.1016/j.ijgo.2010.04.016
66. Turner-Moss E, Zimmerman C, Howard LM, Oram S. Labour exploitation and health: a case series of men and women seeking post-trafficking services. *J Immigr Minor Health*. 2014;16(3):473–480 PMID: 23649665 https://doi.org/10.1007/s10903-013-9832-6
67. Owens C, Dank M, Breaux J, et al. *Understanding the Organization, Operation and Victimization Process of Labor Trafficking in the United States*. Washington, DC: Urban Institute; 2014
68. Dutton DG, Painter S. Emotional attachments in abusive relationships: a test of traumatic bonding theory. *Violence Vict*. 1993;8(2):105–120 PMID: 8193053 https://doi.org/10.1891/0886-6708.8.2.105
69. Lederer LJ, Wetzel CA. The health consequences of sex trafficking and their implications for identifying victims in healthcare facilities. Ann Health Law. 2014;23(1):61–91
70. Chisolm-Straker M, Baldwin S, Gaïgbé-Togbé B, Ndukwe N, Johnson PN, Richardson LD. Health care and human trafficking: we are seeing the unseen. *J Health Care Poor Underserved*. 2016;27(3):1220–1233 PMID: 27524764 https://doi.org/10.1353/hpu.2016.0131
71. Greenbaum J, Bodrick N; American Academy of Pediatrics Committee on Child Abuse and Neglect and Section on International Child Health. Global human trafficking and child victimization. *Pediatrics*. 2017;140(6):e20173138 PMID: 29180462 https://doi.org/10.1542/peds.2017-3138
72. American Academy of Pediatrics. Summaries of infectious diseases. In: Kimberlin DW, Brady MT, Jackson MA, Long SS, eds. *Red Book: 2015 Report of the Committee on Infectious Diseases*. 30th ed. Elk Grove Village, IL: American Academy of Pediatrics; 2015:288–800

73. US Preventive Services Task Force. Published recommendations. https://www.uspreventiveservicestaskforce.org/BrowseRec/Index/browse-recommendations. Updated April 2019. Accessed April 9, 2019
74. Substance Abuse and Mental Health Services Administration. *SAMHSA's Concept of Trauma and Guidance for a Trauma-Informed Approach*. Rockville, MD: Substance Abuse and Mental Health Services Administration; 2014. HHS Publication No. (SMA) 14-4884
75. WestCoast Children's Clinic. Commercial Sexual Exploitation Identification Tool (CSE-IT)—Pilot Version. http://www.westcoastcc.org/wp-content/uploads/2015/04/WCC-CSE_IT-Pilot-14Apr2015.pdf. Published 2014. Accessed April 9, 2019
76. Shared Hope International. *Intervene Practitioner Guide and Intake Tool*. Vancouver, WA: Shared Hope International; 2013
77. Chang KS, Lee K, Park T, et al. Using a clinic-based screening tool for primary care providers to identify commercially sexually exploited children. *J Appl Res Child.* 2015;6:15
78. San Luis Obispo County CSEC Collaborative Response Team. Commercially Sexually Exploited Children (CSEC) Screening Tool. 2014. https://www.cwda.org/sites/main/files/file-attachments/slo-csec-screening-tool.pdf. Accessed June 7, 2019
79. Mays A, Harvill Z, Mejia J. *Sexually Exploited Children Screening Protocol: A Multidisciplinary Model Designed for the Clinical and School Health Setting*. Oakland, CA: The Native American Health Center; 2013
80. American Academy of Pediatrics Committee on Practice and Ambulatory Medicine and Bright Futures Periodicity Schedule Workgroup. 2019 recommendations for preventive pediatric health care. *Pediatrics.* 2019;143(3):e20183971 PMID: 30804073
81. Ijadi-Maghsoodi R, Cook M, Barnert ES, Gaboian S, Bath E. Understanding and responding to the needs of commercially sexually exploited youth: recommendations for the mental health provider. *Child Adolesc Psychiatr Clin N Am.* 2016;25(1):107–122 PMID: 26593123 https://doi.org/10.1016/j.chc.2015.08.007
82. Pascual-Leone A, Kim J, Morrison O-P. Working with victims of human trafficking. *J Contemp Psychother.* 2017;47(1):51–59 https://doi.org/10.1007/s10879-016-9338-3
83. deYoung M, Lowry JA. Traumatic bonding: clinical implications in incest. *Child Welfare.* 1992;71(2):165–175 PMID: 1638904
84. Contreras PM, Kallivayalil D, Herman JL. Psychotherapy in the aftermath of human trafficking: working through the consequences of psychological coercion. *Women Ther.* 2016;40(1–2):31–54
85. Lenhart A, Duggan M, Perrin A, Stepler R, Rainie L, Parker K. *Teens, Social Media & Technology Overview 2015: Smartphones facilitate shifts in communication landscape for teens*. Washington, DC: Pew Research Center's Teens Social Media Technology Project; 2015
86. Klettke B, Hallford DJ, Mellor DJ. Sexting prevalence and correlates: a systematic literature review. *Clin Psychol Rev.* 2014;34(1):44–53 PMID: 24370714 https://doi.org/10.1016/j.cpr.2013.10.007
87. Lenhart A. Teens and Sexting: How and Why Minor Teens Are Sending Sexually Suggestive Nude or Nearly Nude Images via Text Messaging. Washington, DC: Pew Internet & American Life Project, Pew Research Center; 2009. https://www.pewinternet.org/2009/12/15/teens-and-sexting. Accessed April 9, 2019
88. Mitchell KJ, Finkelhor D, Jones LM, Wolak J. Prevalence and characteristics of youth sexting: a national study. *Pediatrics.* 2012;129(1):13–20 PMID: 22144706 https://doi.org/10.1542/peds.2011-1730

89. Fleschler Peskin M, Markham CM, Addy RC, Shegog R, Thiel M, Tortolero SR. Prevalence and patterns of sexting among ethnic minority urban high school students. *Cyberpsychol Behav Soc Netw*. 2013;16(6):454–459 PMID: 23438265 https://doi.org/10.1089/cyber.2012.0452
90. Strassberg DS, McKinnon RK, Sustaíta MA, Rullo J. Sexting by high school students: an exploratory and descriptive study. *Arch Sex Behav*. 2013;42(1):15–21 PMID: 22674035 https://doi.org/10.1007/s10508-012-9969-8
91. Drouin M, Vogel KN, Surbey A, Stills JR. Let's talk about sexting, baby: computer-mediated sexual behaviors among young adults. *Comput Hum Behav*. 2013;29:A25–A30
92. Wolak J, Finkelhor D, Mitchell KJ. How often are teens arrested for sexting? Data from a national sample of police cases. *Pediatrics*. 2012;129(1):4–12 PMID: 22144707 https://doi.org/10.1542/peds.2011-2242
93. Staksrud E, Olafsson K, Livingstone S. Does the use of social networking sites increase children's risk of harm? *Comput Human Behav*. 2013;29(1):40–50 https://doi.org/10.1016/j.chb.2012.05.026
94. Mitchell KJ, Finkelhor D, Wolak J. Youth Internet users at risk for the most serious online sexual solicitations. *Am J Prev Med*. 2007;32(6):532–537 PMID: 17533070 https://doi.org/10.1016/j.amepre.2007.02.001
95. Jones LM, Mitchell KJ, Finkelhor D. Trends in youth internet victimization: findings from three youth internet safety surveys 2000-2010. *J Adolesc Health*. 2012;50(2):179–186 PMID: 22265114 https://doi.org/10.1016/j.jadohealth.2011.09.015
96. Mitchell KJ, Wolak J, Finkelhor D. Trends in youth reports of sexual solicitations, harassment and unwanted exposure to pornography on the Internet. *J Adolesc Health*. 2007;40(2):116–126 PMID: 17259051 https://doi.org/10.1016/j.jadohealth.2006.05.021
97. Noll JG, Shenk CE, Barnes JE, Haralson KJ. Association of maltreatment with high-risk internet behaviors and offline encounters. *Pediatrics*. 2013;131(2):e510–e517 PMID: 23319522 https://doi.org/10.1542/peds.2012-1281
98. Reid Chassiakos YL, Radesky J, Christakis D, Moreno MA, Cross C; American Academy of Pediatrics Council on Communications and Media. Children and adolescents and digital media. *Pediatrics*. 2016;138(5):e20162593 PMID: 27940795
99. Wolak J, Finkelhor D, Walsh W, Treitman L. Sextortion of minors: characteristics and dynamics. *J Adolesc Health*. 2018;62(1):72–79 PMID: 29055647 https://doi.org/10.1016/j.jadohealth.2017.08.014
100. US Department of Justice. *The National Strategy for Child Exploitation Prevention and Interdiction: A Report to Congress*. Washington, DC; US Department of Justice: 2016
101. Zweig JM, Dank M, Yahner J, Lachman P. The rate of cyber dating abuse among teens and how it relates to other forms of teen dating violence. *J Youth Adolesc*. 2013;42(7):1063–1077 PMID: 23412689 https://doi.org/10.1007/s10964-013-9922-8
102. Bourke ML, Hernandez AE. The "Butner study" redux: a report of the incidence of hands-on child victimization by child pornography offenders. *J Fam Violence*. 2009;24(3):183–191 https://doi.org/10.1007/s10896-008-9219-y
103. Cooper SW. The medical analysis of child sexual abuse images. *J Child Sex Abuse*. 2011;20(6):631–642 PMID: 22126107 https://doi.org/10.1080/10538712.2011.627829
104. Wells M, Finkelhor D, Wolak J, Mitchell KJ. Defining child pornography: law enforcement dilemmas in investigations of internet child pornography possession. *Police Pract Res*. 2007;8(3):269–282 https://doi.org/10.1080/15614260701450765
105. Herman-Giddens ME, Bourdony CJ, Dowshen SA, Reiter EO. *Assessment of Sexual Maturity Stages in Girls and Boys*. Elk Grove Village, IL: American Academy of Pediatrics; 2011

106. US Department of Labor. Youth and labor. https://www.dol.gov/general/topic/youthlabor. Accessed April 9, 2019
107. US Department of Labor. State labor laws. https://www.dol.gov/general/topic/youthlabor/statelaborlaws. Accessed April 9, 2019
108. Freedom Network USA. Child trafficking for labor in the United States. Updated April 2015. https://freedomnetworkusa.org/app/uploads/2016/12/HT-and-Child-Labor.pdf. Accessed April 9, 2019
109. Papantoniou-Frangouli M, Dourida V, Diamantopoulou A, Barla E, Kapsalis A. Trafficking for Labour in Greece. Report Prepared in the Frame of the Project: Combating Trafficking in Human Beings—Going Beyond. https://ec.europa.eu/anti-trafficking/sites/antitrafficking/files/2011-03-greek_report_going_beyond_1.pdf. Published February 2011. Accessed April 9, 2019
110. Surtees R. *Labour Trafficking in South-eastern Europe: Developing Prevention and Assistance Programmes*. Vienna, Austria: NEXUS Institute to Combat Human Trafficking; 2007. https://nexushumantrafficking.files.wordpress.com/2015/03/trafficking-for-labour-nexus-paper-2007-final.pdf. Accessed April 9, 2019
111. Polaris. *Knocking at Your Door: Labor Trafficking on Traveling Sales Crews*. Washington, DC: Polaris; 2015. https://polarisproject.org/sites/default/files/Knocking-on-Your-Door-Sales-Crews.pdf. Accessed April 9, 2019
112. Zhang SX. *Looking for a Hidden Population: Trafficking of Migrant Laborers in San Diego County*. Washington, DC: US Department of Justice, National Institute of Justice; 2012
113. Van de Glind H, Coenjaerts C. *Combating Trafficking in Children for Labour Exploitation in the Mekong Sub-region: A Proposed Framework for ILO-IPEC Action and Proceedings of a Mekong Sub-Regional Consultation*. International Labour Organization; 1998. https://www.ilo.org/asia/publications/WCMS_BK_PB_3_EN/lang--en/index.htm. Accessed June 7, 2019
114. International Labour Organization. Child labour in Africa. https://www.ilo.org/ipec/Regionsandcountries/Africa/WCMS_618949/lang--en/index.htm. Accessed June 7, 2019
115. Thomas M. Child traficking in Ghana: an examination of the cultural impact. *Prospect: Journal of International Affairs at UCSD*. 2011. https://prospectjournal.org/2011/09/13/child-traficking-in-ghana/. Accessed June 7, 2019
116. Koseleci N, Kovrova I. Child labour in Bangladesh and India: a preliminary gender-based analysis. Understanding Children's Work Programme Working Paper Series, April 2009. http://www.ucw-project.org/attachment/standard_gender_bangladeshindia_6april20110517_144747.pdf; . Accessed April 9, 2019
117. Atkinson HG, Curnin KJ, Hanson NCUS. state laws addressing human trafficking: education of and mandatory reporting by health care providers and other professionals. *J Human Trafficking*. 2016;2(2):111–138 https://doi.org/10.1080/23322705.2016.1175885
118. US Department of Health and Human Services, Office on Trafficking in Persons. Request for assistance form. https://www.acf.hhs.gov/otip/resource/rfa-0. Accessed June 7, 2019
119. US Citizenship and Immigration Services. Victims of human trafficking: T nonimmigrant status. https://www.uscis.gov/humanitarian/victims-human-trafficking-other-crimes/victims-human-trafficking-t-nonimmigrant-status. Updated May 10, 2018. Accessed April 9, 2019
120. US Citizenship and Immigration Services. Victims of criminal activity: U nonimmigrant status. https://www.uscis.gov/humanitarian/victims-human-trafficking-other-crimes/victims-criminal-activity-u-nonimmigrant-status/victims-criminal-activity-u-nonimmigrant-status. Updated June 12, 2018. Accessed April 9, 2019

PART 5

Pathology of Child Maltreatment

CHAPTER 23

Pathology of Fatal Abuse

Mary Case, MD
Professor
Department of Pathology
St Louis University Health Sciences Center
St Louis, MO

Introduction

Forensic pathologists are a small group of physicians, 400 to 500 in the United States, who have completed 4 to 5 years of residency training in anatomical pathology and usually clinical pathology, as well as a 1-year fellowship in forensic pathology. Forensic pathologists most often work as medical examiners in city, county, or state systems of death investigation. Coroner systems, rather than medical examiner systems, exist in some jurisdictions; usually coroners are lay individuals with no particular educational requirement (in some states, coroners are physicians but not necessarily forensic pathologists). In coroner systems, the coroner acts as the administrator for the office and usually engages the services of a forensic pathologist to carry out autopsies. Medical examiner and coroner systems of death investigation have jurisdiction over deaths that occur suddenly, unexpectedly, and possibly unnaturally, such as homicides, suicides, and accidental deaths. They also have jurisdiction over deaths of concern to public health and welfare, such as possible but unidentified infectious diseases. Medical examiner/coroner systems also investigate certain categories of deaths of concern to the public welfare, including child deaths, unless explained by natural causes at an expected time. Medical examiners and coroners are responsible for certifying deaths in individuals who do not have a treating medical professional who has seen the individual within a reasonably short time before death and who has treated that person for a disease from which he or she might be dying.

Death Investigations

The purpose of the death investigation is to determine cause and manner of death. *Cause of death* refers to the causative injury or event, such as a gunshot wound to the head or a myocardial infarction. *Manner of death* refers to how the cause of death came about and includes natural, accidental, suicidal, homicidal, and undetermined. A *natural manner* is a death brought about by a disease state. An *accidental manner* is a death caused by an unintentional circumstance, such a vehicular collision. *Homicide* means that one individual has caused the death of another individual; this term does not consider intent and is not the same as the legal term *murder,* which does consider intent. A *suicide* is a death that was caused at the hands of the deceased individual. In some deaths, after all information is considered, the medical examiner does not know what the manner of death is and terms it *undetermined. Mechanism of death* refers to the actual pathophysiological derangement that causes death. The mechanism of death in a gunshot wound of the chest is exsanguination. A mechanism of death (eg, exsanguination, cardiac arrest, respiratory arrest) is not an adequate "cause" of death for death certification without stating the initiating factor.

Most state statutes that address the medical examiner/coroner duties provide the medical examiner/coroner the right to carry out forensic autopsies without family permission. When involved with a death that may be a case for the medical examiner or coroner, it is prudent for the attending physician not to ask the family for permission for an autopsy because if the family declines and the medical examiner or coroner needs to carry out an autopsy, it may create a problem with the family. The medical examiner or coroner will consider religious objections to autopsy and endeavor to avoid having to do more than necessary in these cases.

The role of the forensic pathologist/medical examiner in assessing why an individual has died differs from the roles of the various medical professionals who attend the living person and also differs from the role of a hospital pathologist. An autopsy done by a hospital pathologist primarily endeavors to determine why the patient has died, to evaluate the effects of treatment, and to evaluate the accuracy of diagnostic procedures that were performed. Forensic pathologists are charged with determining the cause and manner of death and need to have access to a great deal of material to consider in conjunction with the findings at autopsy. In a medical examiner/coroner case, the investigation begins with the death scene, which is the place where the individual was found dead or injured, although the person may be subsequently transported to medical care and die there. Forensic pathologists do not want to perform autopsies without learning as much as possible about how the death occurred. Other information may become available later, but from the beginning, the information surrounding where the death or injury occurred is needed.

Medicolegal death investigators are the individuals who work in the medical examiner's/coroner's office who receive the calls notifying the office of a death, go to the death scene, and obtain the necessary information from all sources for the forensic pathologists. These investigators interview witnesses, law enforcement, family members, and others, including medical personnel who have information about the deceased. State statute gives the medical examiner or coroner access to whatever information or material (eg, hospital blood or urine specimens) medical personnel have without the need for a subpoena or consideration of the Health Insurance Portability and Accountability Act of 1996.

In a child's death, the investigator will obtain medical records from the entire life of the child, all reports from police and social service agencies, and all information concerning the circumstances of the death, which obviously includes the historical report of how an injury occurred. The US Administration for Children and Families estimates that 1,750 children died from abuse or neglect in fiscal year 2016 (October 2015–September 2016). This number indicates that more than 2 out of every 100,000 children die per year from abuse or neglect in the United States. Of these child fatalities, 70% involved children younger than 3 years, and infants younger than 1 year accounted for nearly 50% of the fatalities.[1] All these child deaths are examined by forensic pathologists to determine their cause and the manner of death as well as other possible forensic issues, such as how long an injury takes to cause death, the mechanism of death, the nature of the injury, whether there was conscious pain and suffering, and how long the injury took to cause loss of consciousness. In child deaths, the investigator comes to the facility where the child died to observe the body as soon as possible and to document photographically such details as injuries, temperature, lividity, and rigor. The body should be handled as little as possible once the child is deceased, and the family or others should not be allowed unsupervised access to the body. Until an examination can be performed, it is not possible to know if evidence such as touch DNA on the body might be a consideration. In most child deaths, the investigator will also carry out a scene investigation. In young infants, most deaths require a scene re-creation to ascertain the position in which the infant was placed to sleep and the position in which the infant was found deceased. There are also cases such as positional asphyxia deaths that require scene visits to document the site of entrapment or the position where found.

Forensic Autopsy

Forensic autopsies are quite different from hospital autopsies. Depending on the nature of the case, the autopsy may include a lengthy external examination of the body to document every mark, injury, and scar and to obtain any forensic evidence on the body. Forensic autopsies may include special dissections not usually performed in hospital autopsies. Such special dissections include incisions to expose the soft tissue of the back, buttocks, extremities, and face to look for injuries and take samples of tissue for microscopic examination. Microscopic examination of this tissue may disclose the nature of injury (eg, blunt, sharp, gunshot wound) and may provide information about the age of an injury. Other special dissections include removal of the eyes, removal of portions of bone or entire bones, removal of the jaws or portions of the jaw, removal of portions of the spinal column, and excarnating ("defleshing") the face.

Evidence obtained from the body could include specimens for toxicology (testing for alcohol, drugs, medications, poison, carbon monoxide), microbiology (cultures for bacterial and viral disease), postmortem chemistry (using the vitreous fluid from the eyes for testing for electrolytes, glucose, urea, creatinine), DNA, or other laboratory testing. During the autopsy, microscopic sections are taken from each organ for determination of disease or lack of disease and injuries are sampled for aging analyses using knowledge of the inflammatory process to evaluate the stage of reaction and healing (Table 23.1).

Sexual assault examinations are performed as needed by forensic pathologists who are trained to do this on dead individuals. Postmortem changes occur to the rectal mucosa, which may be mistaken by treating physicians for lacerations but are easily recognizable to the forensic pathologist. Similarly, dilation of the rectum after death may be misinterpreted by a treating physician as evidence of a sexual assault but is recognized as simply artifact by the forensic pathologist. The forensic pathologist takes appropriate evidence from the orifices as well as swabs from bite marks or other areas of possible bodily fluid deposits or deposition of touch DNA.

TABLE 23.1
Age Estimation of Human Skin Wounds by Histologic Examination

Histologic Parameter	Earliest Appearance	Time of Regular Appearance
Neutrophils	20–30 min	>15 h
Macrophages	3 h	>15 h
Macrophage/gran ratio[a]	20 h	>11 d
Siderophages/hemosiderin	3 d	>7 d
Hematoidin	8 d	Many never positive
Increased fibroblasts	25 h	≥6 d

[a] Ratio of macrophages to granulocytes within inflammatory infiltrate.

Adapted by permission from Springer Nature: Betz P. Histological and enzyme histochemical parameters for the age estimation of human skin wounds. *Int J Legal Med.* 1994;107(2):60–68, copyright 1994.

Forensic pathologists frequently consult with other specialists. These consultants include neuropathologists, odontologists (forensic dentists), forensic anthropologists, radiologists, and toxicologists. These consultants may do their own examinations of the body or body parts. Neuropathologists examine the brain following the autopsy and fixation for the brain. Odontologists examine the teeth and compare them with premortem films and records for age determination and identification. Anthropologists examine the bones for identification, age of the individual, sex determination, racial origin, disease states, and injury analyses. Radiologists may assist with interpretation of imaging issues and in identification of unknown persons using radiological comparisons with premortem images, although generally forensic pathologists interpret their own images and are capable of making identifications from images using premortem and postmortem images. Forensic toxicologists, PhD-level scientists with special expertise in the testing methods, assist with interpreting toxicology results and advise on specimens suitable for different types of analyses. Determination of cause of death from drugs, alcohol, and other substances is the role of the forensic pathologist using the autopsy findings in conjunction with the toxicology results.

Patterns of Abusive Injury

Head Injury

The Centers for Disease Control and Prevention definition of *pediatric abusive head trauma* is an injury to the skull or intracranial contents of an infant or young child (<5 years of age) due to inflicted blunt impact and/or violent shaking. Excluded from the defined cases are unintentional injuries resulting from neglectful supervision and gunshot wounds, stab wounds, and penetrating trauma.[2] The major cause of serious traumatic head injury in infants and young children is inflicted injury; these injuries result in significant morbidity and mortality.[3] The most common cause of death among all inflicted injuries is head injury.[4] A population-based study of abusive head injury in North Carolina found a case rate of 29.7 per 100,000 person-years in infants younger than 1 year and 3.8 per 100,000 person-years in the second year after birth.[3] Inflicted trauma is the third leading cause of all head injuries after falls and motor vehicle crashes.[5] Most who experience inflicted head trauma are younger than 2 years, with a peak incidence from age 2 to 3 months, although the same head injuries may be seen in children as old as 5 years.[6–8] Head injuries account for 75% to 80% of fatal cases of child abuse.[9–11] Most head injuries in young children are accidental from falls or vehicular crashes. Falls are very frequent in young children, but these are overwhelmingly benign when they occur in the home, and even when falls occur from much higher distances they may be nonlethal.[12] Falls are frequently provided as an explanation for injuries caused by abuse, so it is helpful to understand what injuries do occur in falls in young children.[13]

To fully understand traumatic head injuries in young children requires a knowledge of anatomical and developmental differences that exist in the young human that affect how the nervous system is injured. Humans have a longer period of developmental maturation of the nervous system than other species, and there are also marked developmental changes that occur in the skull and neck of the young child, which influence how trauma affects the head. The skull of the young child is very thin and pliable, which serves to make passage through the birth canal easier because the bones can deform under pressure but also renders the skull less protective against impact. Thinner bone fractures more readily and allows the force of impact to pass through more readily. During the first 2 postnatal years, the skull bones become thicker and the diploe develop, which add protection. The fontanelles are particular sites at which force can easily enter the cranial interior. As the fontanelles ossify, the skull becomes more protective of the contents. The human brain is very large at birth and grows rapidly during early life. By age 2 years, the brain will weigh up to 75% of its adult weight, although it is still immature (maturation continues even through the teenage years). The head in early life is very large in proportion to the rest of the body, representing up to 20% of the total body weight compared with only 2% to 3% in the adult. The growth of the calvarium is driven by the growth of the brain. The face of the child develops at a slower rate, driven by the development of the maxillae and mandible, which grow in relationship to development of the secondary dentition. This tooth development takes place around 5 or 6 years of age. During this time, developmental changes occur to the basilar skull regions as well.[14]

The brain is much softer in the infant due to very high water content and has far fewer glial cells than will later develop and which support the brain tissue. The myelin at birth is mainly present in the spinal cord and brain stem and will subsequently begin to develop in the cerebrum during the first year after birth. Myelin is protective against traumatic forces, as demonstrated from evidence that axonal injury occurs at the node of Ranvier where myelin is normally discontinuous.[15] The axons early in life are much smaller than they will be later, and their small size is more vulnerable to damage. The subarachnoid space is shallow in young children so that it offers less buttressing capacity than it will later in life as it becomes deeper.[16] The muscles of the neck of the young child are undeveloped and weak. Obviously, infants early on do not even have the ability to support their own head. One of the principles of head injury in general is that neck strength is of great importance in preventing acceleration/deceleration motion of the head and to keep the head stationary.[17] These unique anatomical and developmental features of the young child's head and brain render young children more vulnerable to the effects of acceleration/deceleration movement of the head and inertial brain motion and more vulnerable to skull fracture.

Mechanisms of traumatic brain injury include static and dynamic injuries depending on the rate at which force is loaded to the head. Static injuries take place over a longer period, greater than 200 milliseconds, and occur primarily to a stationary head when it is crushed by a heavy weight. These injuries result in crushing head injuries with fractures of the calvarium, skull base, and facial skeleton; fragments of bone may penetrate portions of the brain, causing fracture contusions and fracture lacerations. These are not common injuries at any age, but they do occur occasionally in childhood. Because there is no acceleration of the head and thus no inertial brain movement, there may be no loss of consciousness until the brain is totally macerated by the damage. Interestingly, there are children who survive these seemingly extensive injuries.[18,19] Crushing head injuries result from trauma such as a tire running over the head or a heavy object like a TV or piece of furniture falling over onto the head.

The most common mechanism of head injury at all ages is dynamic loading. Dynamic injuries occur when force is loaded quickly to the head in less than 200 milliseconds and the head is caused to move either by direct impact or by a motion to the body that moves both the body and the head abruptly. In the latter circumstance, when the unsupported head moves, it rotates at a point where it attaches to the cervical spine. If this type of impulsive loading is forceful enough, it will cause inertial brain motion inside the cranial cavity, in which there is a separation of the rate at which the skull and the brain move due to their different rigidities and consistency. The dura is firmly attached to the inner table of the skull and will move with it. The bridging veins that arise from the cortical surface of the brain travel from the cortex through the subarachnoid space and arachnoid membrane to the dural sinuses of the dura. Differential movement of the skull/dura and the brain may result in tearing of the bridging veins, which causes subdural bleeding as well as small patches of subarachnoid bleeding where the vein tears. The inertial movement of the brain itself may also cause damage to axonal processes, resulting in traumatic axonal injury.[20–23]

Another aspect of head injury is whether it is a focal injury, diffuse injury, or a combination. *Focal injures* are caused by a direct impact to the head and can be seen by a pathologist with the naked eye. Focal injuries include scalp laceration and contusion, skull fracture, epidural hemorrhage, focal subdural hemorrhage, and certain brain contusions. *Diffuse injuries* are the result of inertial motion of the brain and include interhemispheric diffuse subdural hemorrhage and traumatic diffuse axonal injury. Of clinical interest in distinguishing these injuries is that focal head injuries cause loss of consciousness through the mechanism of increasing intracranial pressure leading to herniation. This type of unconsciousness takes place over some period, so it has a lucid interval. This is in distinction to diffuse injuries, which cause an immediate decrease in the level of conscious as a result of axonal injury at the mesencephalic level of the brain.[23]

Scalp Injury

The scalp is a markedly different type of tissue than other portions of the skin surface of the body at all ages. Skin elsewhere on the body has 2 layers, the epidermis and the dermis, and varies from 0.5 to 3 mm in thickness. The scalp has 5 layers, of which the outmost layer is the skin; then a thick layer of connective tissue consisting of fat and fibrous tissue; then the *galea,* which is a tough layer of dense fibrous tissue; then a layer of loose areolar connective tissue; and finally the *pericranium,* which is the periosteum of the skull bone. These layers have a thickness of about 8 mm. Impact by blunt trauma to the scalp region of the head frequently does not appear as a bruise or contusion at the external skin surface. When there is impact to the head, the impact is frequently visible when the pathologist reflects the scalp and exposes hemorrhage in the underlying tissues of the scalp (Figure 23.1). Imaging by computed tomography (CT) will also demonstrate these areas of soft tissue hemorrhage within the scalp. Some individuals confuse lack of external marks on the scalp as evidence that no internal injury is present, but this is obviously not true.

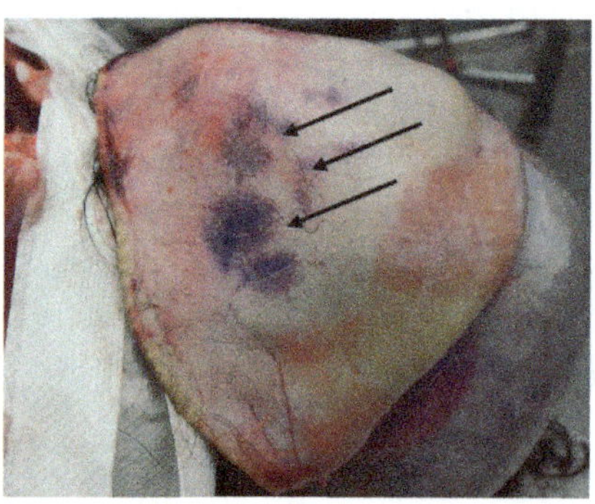

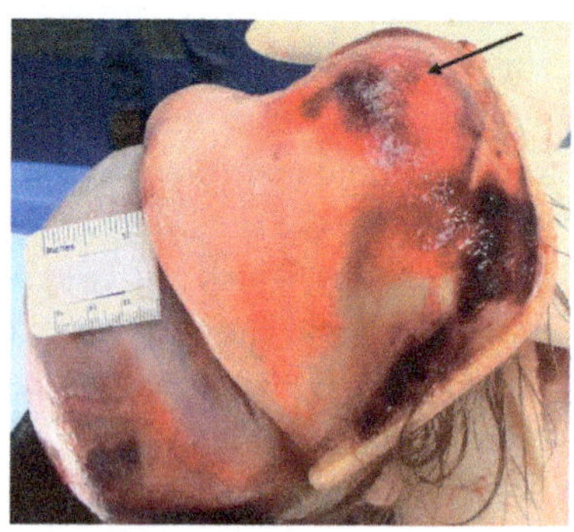

FIGURE 23.1
Reflection of scalp at autopsy to demonstrate multiple subgaleal hemorrhages.

Skull Fracture

The presence of a skull fracture indicates that there has been an impact to the head. Depending on the amount of force delivered by the impact, there may or may not be intracranial injury. Fractures of the skull may be linear, depressed, diastatic, comminuted, or basilar (Figure 23.2). The most common are linear fractures, which may be seen in accidental circumstances without intracranial injury. Diastatic fractures require significant force to separate the cranial sutures. Before the cranial sutures are fused and ossified, the sutures may be separated by brain swelling from any cause; these separations should not be considered fractures, although when seen at autopsy they look quite traumatic and hemorrhagic (Figure 23.3). Comminuted fractures where the skull is fragmented into pieces require very significant force and would not be expected in simple short falls. Decisions about mechanisms of injury require consideration of any bony injury present in conjunction with the presence of any internal injury.

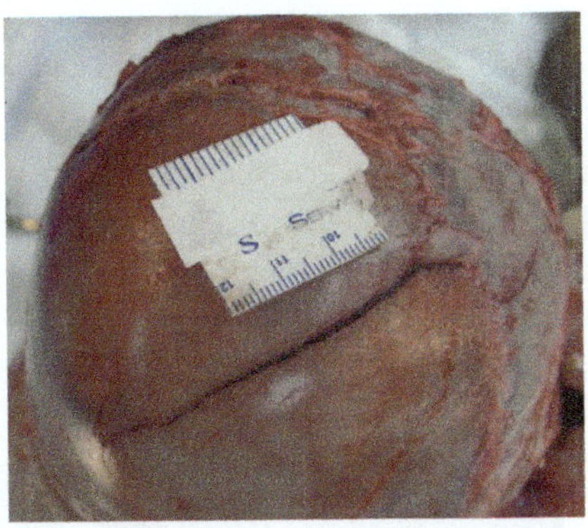

FIGURE 23.2
Linear fracture of the skull.

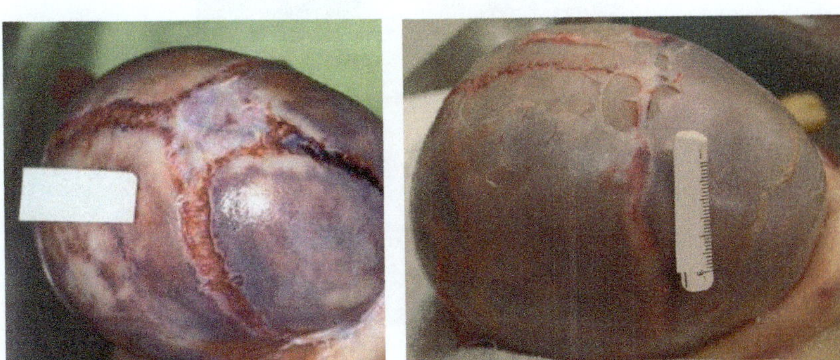

FIGURE 23.3
Separation of the sutures of infants with extreme brain swelling.

Epidural Hemorrhage

Epidural hemorrhages are hemorrhages where the blood is located beneath the bone and over the outer surface of the dura. Most epidural hemorrhages are from accidental mechanisms in young children but, on rare occasions, can be inflicted (Figure 23.4). Epidural hemorrhages are highly associated with skull fracture and are found in association with fracture in 85% of cases, although in young children deformation of the skull can cause epidural bleeding.[24] The bleeding in most epidural hemorrhages arises from damage to a branch of the middle meningeal artery resulting when the dura is separated from the overlying skull when fractured or deformed. Epidural bleeding may also result from tears of a dural sinus or diploic vein. Epidural hemorrhage is a focal contact injury and, in most cases in children, results from a fall with a skull fracture. If the epidural blood becomes a mass lesion resulting in increased intracranial pressure, a child may die from this injury. Not all epidural hemorrhages bleed enough to become space-occupying masses, but some do. It is also possible for a homicidal blow to a stationary head to cause a skull fracture and resulting epidural hemorrhage, which constitutes an inflicted head injury, but these cases are even more rare than deaths from accidental epidural hemorrhages in children.[13]

Epidural hemorrhages occur over the cerebral hemispheres, usually adjacent to the site of the skull fracture that has caused the bleeding, and are usually in the temporal and parietal regions. Epidural bleeding may also occur in the cranial fossae from venous sources of bleeding, and it

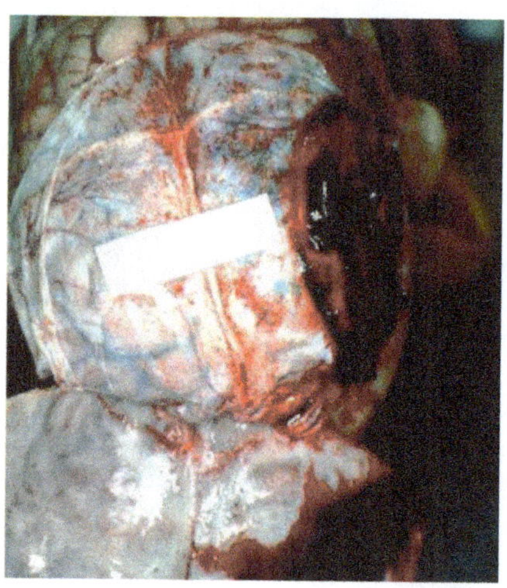

FIGURE 23.4

Epidural hemorrhage in a 7-month-old who was struck on the head to "release devils," fracturing the temporal bone and causing a large epidural hemorrhage.

may take little bleeding in that location to create mass lesions. Epidural hemorrhage flattens out the cerebral convexities; the cortical surface typically has cerebral contusions, which are caused by the adjacent fracture and are thus called *fracture contusions.*

Subdural Hemorrhage

In cases of inflicted neurotrauma, the injuries seen at autopsy are rather uniform and the most common finding is the presence of subdural blood over the cerebral convexities[25] (Figure 23.5). This subdural blood may be a relatively thin layer or film, although in some cases it is present in larger amounts. Subdural hemorrhage is seen in up to 95% of cases of

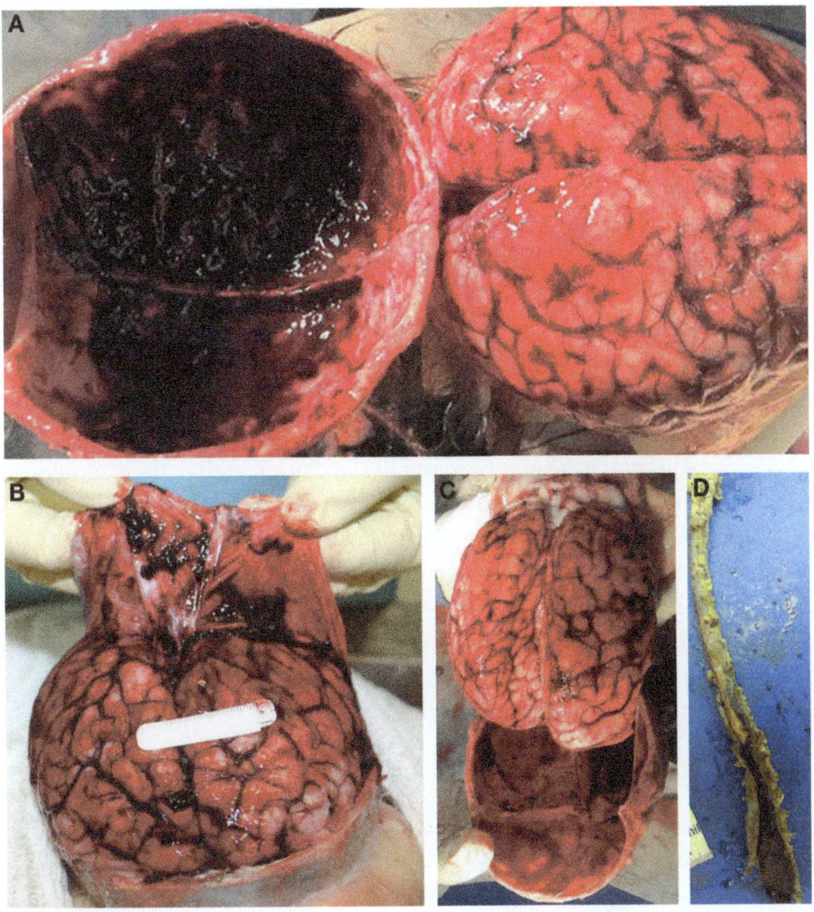

FIGURE 23.5

A–C, Acute subdural hemorrhages at autopsy in young children with inflicted trauma. D, Acute subdural hemorrhage over spinal cord dura.

fatal inflicted head trauma.[11] The number seen at autopsy is considerably different than the number seen by clinicians based on CT scans, which typically find 40% to 55% of cases with subdural hemorrhage. Subdural hemorrhages may be so thin and scant that they do not show up on CT but are visible at autopsy.[8,11,26] Magnetic resonance imaging should be able to visualize thin film subdural blood when CT is not able to do so.[16] The amount of subdural blood may only be a few milliliters. The subdural blood is generally over both cerebral convexities but may be heaviest on one side and, in a few cases, may be unilateral. The subdural bleeding starts in the posterior interhemispheric fissure and then spreads anteriorly and over the convexities.[27] Subdural blood is also frequently found in 1 or more of the cranial fossae in conjunction with the subdural blood seen over the convexities. Subdural blood is also frequently found surrounding the spinal cord and is believed to descend by gravity from the posterior fossa. When subdural hemorrhage is found with skull fracture, the fracture does not need to occur adjacent to the bleeding.

The mechanism causing subdural bleeding in these cases of inflicted trauma is torn bridging veins caused by the inertial motion of the brain's cortical surface away from the overlying skull and attached dura.[28–30] Certain types of subdural hemorrhage would be unlikely in inflicted trauma in a young child, such as a focal area of subdural bleeding on the ventral surface of the brain.[31,32] When a bridging vein tears, it is sometimes possible to visualize that torn vessel on CT images, and sometimes it is detectible at autopsy. These torn bridging veins are found within patches of subarachnoid hemorrhage over the parasagittal regions of the cerebral convexities.[33,34]

Subdural hemorrhage may be found in association with many disorders or conditions, including inflicted trauma in young children, accidental trauma, prenatal and perinatal conditions, surgical manipulation, birth trauma, tumors, metabolic disorders, genetic conditions, autoimmune disorders, coagulopathies, infections, and long-term shunting for hydrocephalus. All these disorders must be considered when evaluating a child with head injury. The detailed workup performed by child abuse pediatricians is designed to include testing and examination for these problems.

Chronic Subdural Hemorrhage

Subdural blood typically resolves into a liquefied clot in 4 to 6 weeks, and then the fluid will be absorbed.[35] In the past, there was some thought that subdural blood aged into chronic subdural hematomas. Newer information shows that few cases of subdural hemorrhage evolve into chronic subdural hematomas.[36–38] Experimental models fail to produce a chronic subdural hematoma from acute subdural blood.[39] When a chronic subdural hematoma does develop, it does so from a subdural hygroma.[40] The space thought of as the subdural space actually does not exist anatomically.[41,42] The dura consists of fibroblasts and extracellular collagen. The most inner layer is the dural border cell layer, which is continuous with the arachnoid outer barrier cell layer. A space may be created within this dura-arachnoid junction by blood entering into the dural border cell layer. Cleaving open this layer by trauma or removal of the calvarium at autopsy thus creates the subdural "space." It is actually an intradural space, but generally it is referred to as a "subdural" space. If the dural border cell layer has been cleaved by trauma and bleeding, when the blood leaves, spinal fluid may in certain circumstances fill the cleaved dural space, resulting in a subdural hygroma.[43,44] Circumstances that would promote persistence of a cleaved intradural space include any cause of lowered intracranial pressure such as foci of brain atrophy or prolonged drainage of cerebrospinal fluid or use of osmotic agents.[45,46] The cleavage of the dural border cell layer can induce proliferation of the border cells to produce a pseudomembrane, which will be associated with the hygroma. Whether the hygroma persists or resolves depends on whether the lowered intracranial pressure persists, in which case the hygroma will remain and may expand. If the intracranial pressure returns to normal, the hygroma will resolve. In those cases in which the hygroma persists, further proliferation of dural border cells may occur with further development of pseudomembranes. The pseudomembranes contain ingrowth of new vessels, which are fragile and may tear, resulting in microhemorrhages with little or no trauma. These repeated microhemorrhages can lead to an enlarging subdural hygroma.[40,47] In infants and young children, it is difficult to distinguish between a subdural hygroma and a chronic subdural hematoma. Before the sutures fuse, if there is post-traumatic brain atrophy, a chronic subdural collection may be tolerated until the sutures fuse and the collection causes a mass effect. The microhemorrhages of the pseudomembrane are not at risk to produce subdural bleeding or to produce neurologic deterioration. These bleeds are microscopic within the membrane.[48]

Exceptional Circumstances of Subdural Hemorrhage

Contact injuries may, rarely, cause a focal area of subdural hemorrhage, which may become problematic if it leads to markedly increased intracranial pressure. These cases are rare but can be fatal. In about 1% to 3% of short falls, a skull fracture occurs.[49–52] A contact focal subdural hemorrhage may result from a skull fracture.[53]

There are also a few rare accidental types of inertial brain motion that have been observed in children and that may cause subdural hemorrhage.

A playground rocking toy was reported to have caused a fatal head injury with subdural bleeding in a 2-year-old.[54] This rocking device was mounted on a heavy spring and could be rocked violently. The 12-year-old brother rocked his 2-year-old sibling on the device; after 4 to 5 minutes of rocking, the child lost his grip and fell forward and struck his head on the handlebars. He became symptomatic after he returned home, was taken for medical care, and died while a subdural hemorrhage was being evacuated. At autopsy, he had bilateral subdural blood, subarachnoid hemorrhage, brain swelling, and bilateral multiple retinal hemorrhages extending out to the ora serrata. There are also a small number of cases of rocking chair injuries in which an inertial mechanism is believed to have possibly occurred. These events occur when toddler-aged children are standing up on a rocking chair facing toward the back of the chair and rocking the chair. If the child loses his/her grip and catapults backward from the chair to strike the floor, these injuries look very much like the injuries found in inflicted head trauma.[13] In these cases, there are thin layers of subdural blood over the cerebral convexities and a few retinal hemorrhages. These are rare cases; in most, only the caregiver and the child are present at time of injury and the history may not even be truthful, but because the mechanism appears feasible, these tend to be attributed to an undetermined manner of death. In these exceptional cases of subdural hemorrhage, it is imperative that a thorough investigation be performed with comprehensive witness interviews and consideration of medical findings before deciding on the manner of death.

Subarachnoid Hemorrhage

Subarachnoid hemorrhage is caused by tearing of bridging veins. The cortical bridging veins are the veins within the subarachnoid space, which empty into the dural sinuses.[30,55] The bridging veins are wrapped with a layer of arachnoid membrane where they emerge from the arachnoid. When the vein is torn, some blood can spill into the subarachnoid space. The subarachnoid bleeding is patchy and may be quite sparse (Figure 23.6). Subarachnoid hemorrhage is present in about 95% of cases of fatal inflicted head trauma.[56] Subarachnoid hemorrhage lies beneath areas of subdural bleeding or is contiguous to the subdural bleeding. Small patches of subarachnoid hemorrhage in association with subdural hemorrhage in cases of inflicted neurotrauma are often seen in the parasagittal regions of the cerebral convexities in locations where bridging veins have torn to produce the subdural bleeding as well as bleeding within the adjacent subarachnoid space (Figure 23.7). In some of these cases, it is possible to detect thromboses of the torn bridging veins and microscopically demonstrate the torn veins with an inflammatory response[34] (Figure 23.8).

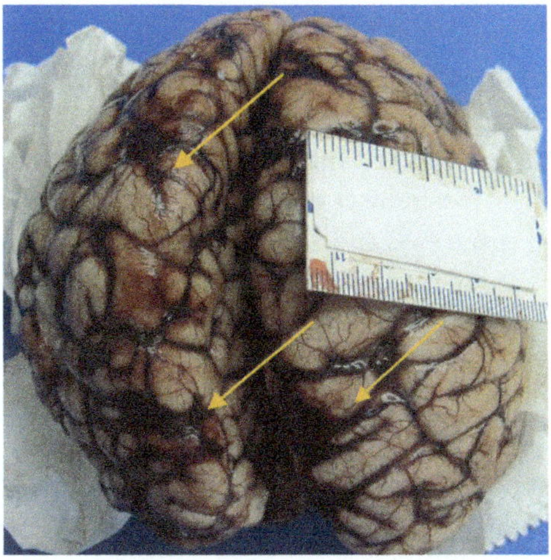

FIGURE 23.6
Subarachnoid hemorrhage in the parasagittal areas over the cerebral convexities.

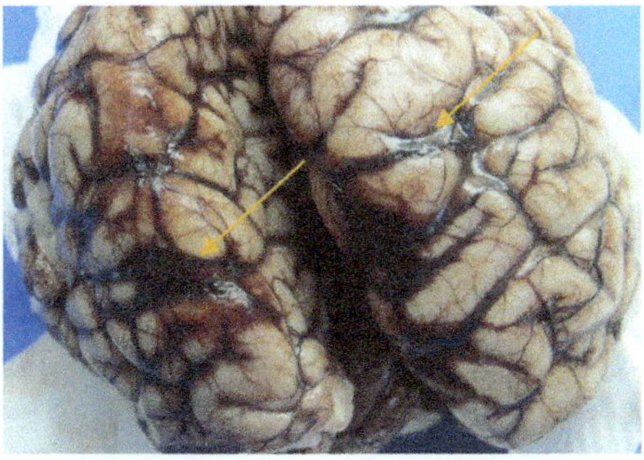

FIGURE 23.7
Subarachnoid hemorrhage at sites of torn bridging veins.

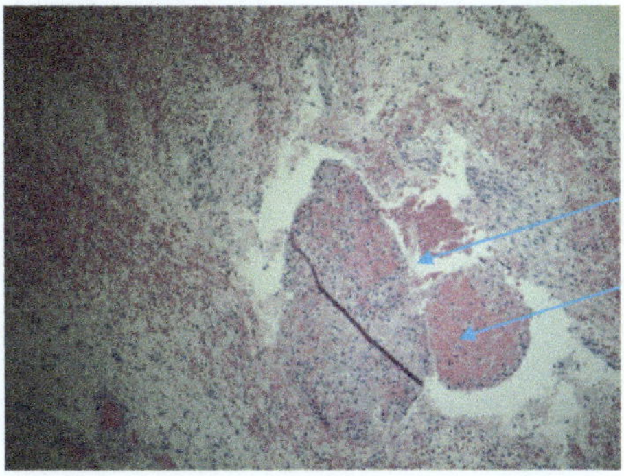

FIGURE 23.8
Medium-power microscopic section of torn bridging veins show inflammatory response to the torn veins.

Retinal Hemorrhage

Forensic pathologists remove the eyes of children in a variety of causes of death, including head injury suspicious for abuse. Forensic pathologists are trained to examine eyes and interpret the findings, although many forensic pathologists feel more comfortable having an ophthalmic pathologist examine the eyes and provide a detailed description.

Retinal hemorrhages are common findings in inflicted head trauma[57] and are described in more detail in Chapter 7, Abusive Head Trauma, and Chapter 8, Ocular Manifestations of Child Abuse. Fatal cases of abusive head trauma have a higher incidence of retinal hemorrhages than are found in living victims, and various studies have found that from 85% to almost 100% of fatal cases have such eye findings.[58–62] The pattern of retinal hemorrhages in child abuse head injuries is usually described as numerous and often found to be too numerous to count, involving all or multiple layers of the retina, and extending far into the periphery of the eye to the ora serrata[63–68] (Figure 23.9). Retinal hemorrhages are more often bilateral than unilateral; unilateral hemorrhages do not correspond to the side of subdural blood, fracture, or evidence of impact.

Another common finding in the retina in abusive head trauma is *retinoschisis,* which is a splitting apart of the retinal layers with blood within the retinoschisis cavity[69] (Figure 23.10). Retinoschisis is thought to result from the traction of the vitreous on the retina when acted on by acceleration/deceleration forces.[29,70] Retinoschisis is highly specific for the acceleration/deceleration forces associated with abusive head trauma and has been reported in only a few other exceptional situations, such as crushing head injury,[71,72] fatal motor vehicle crashes,[73] and an 11-m fall.[74]

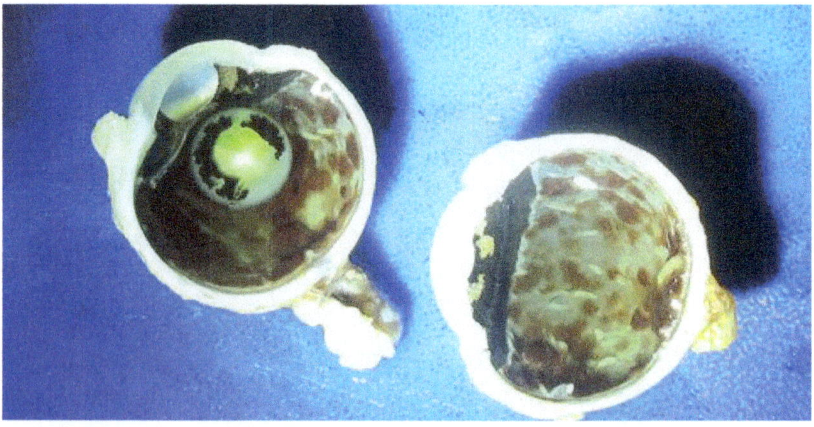

FIGURE 23.9
Bisected eye at autopsy with numerous retinal hemorrhages out to the ora serrata.

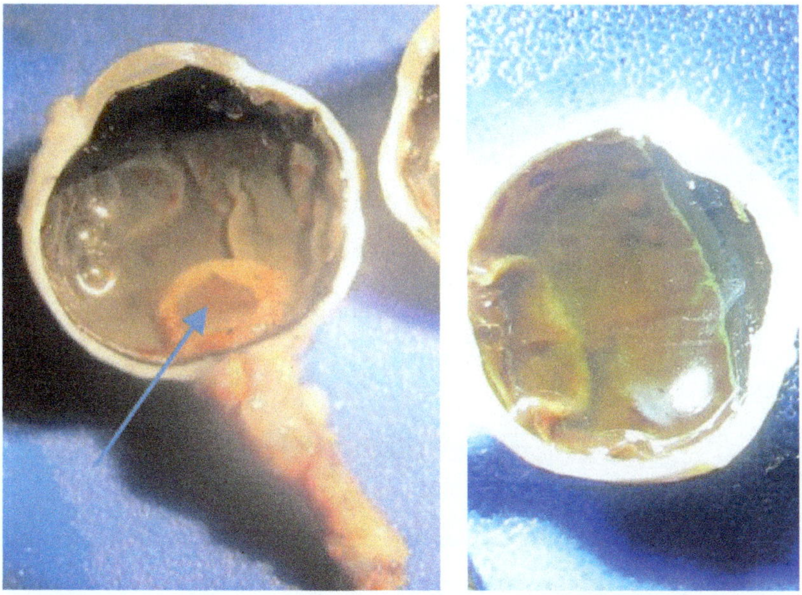

FIGURE 23.10
Bisected eyes at autopsy with retinoschisis.

A number of other diseases and conditions can be associated with retinal hemorrhages. Retinal hemorrhages may be seen in severe accidental trauma, particularly vehicular collisions.[75,76] They are not seen in cases of mild accidental trauma, such as short falls in young children.

Retinal hemorrhages may also be seen in bleeding disorders and coagulopathies, sepsis, meningitis, some newborns, certain genetic conditions, vasculopathies, vascular malformations, megaloblastic anemia, type I osteogenesis imperfecta, infections, intracranial tumors, and some other conditions.[63,77–83] Only in rare cases of resuscitation are retinal hemorrhages found.[84–86] In conditions unrelated to abusive head trauma, the retinal hemorrhages found tend to be few in number and primarily at the posterior pole of the retina. The question of whether retinal hemorrhages are caused by increased intracranial pressure is also sometimes a consideration. Increased intracranial pressure is frequent in head trauma from any cause. In cases of increased intracranial pressure in children without trauma, a few were found to have retinal hemorrhages, but these hemorrhages were different from those seen in abusive head injuries—they were superficial peripapillary hemorrhages or splinter hemorrhages, which were on or adjacent to a swollen optic disk.[87] There is no evidence to support that retinal hemorrhages are caused by resuscitation followed by reperfusion of damaged leaky vessels.[88–91]

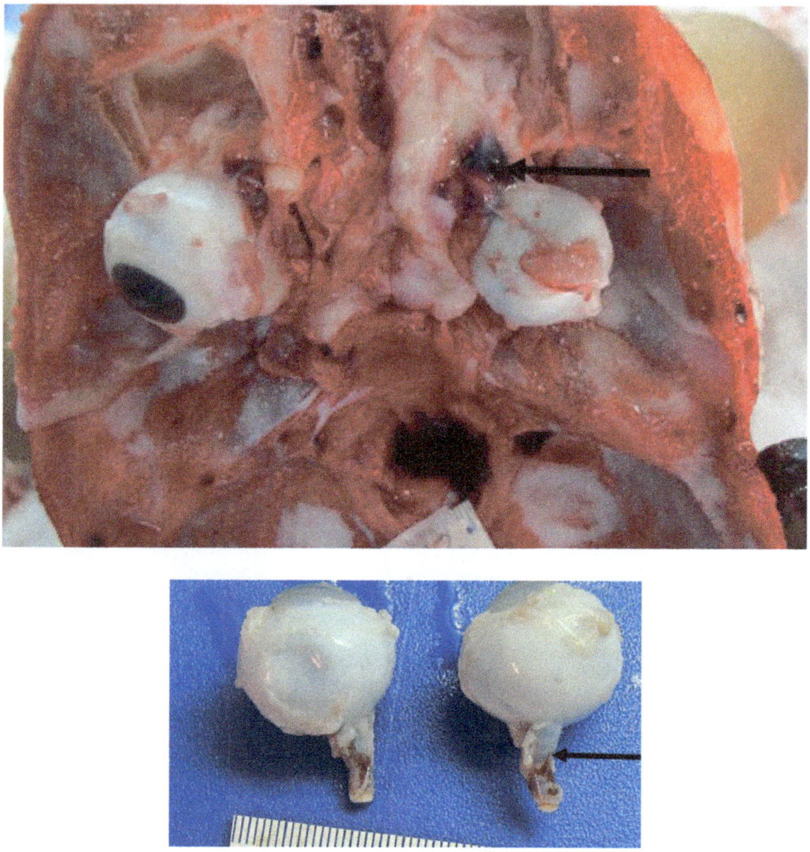

FIGURE 23.11

A, Demonstration of eyes being removed from anterior cranial fossae with hemorrhage in optic nerve sheaths; B, the eyes after removal with optic nerve sheath hemorrhage.

Optic nerve sheath hemorrhage is hemorrhage within the perineural tissue of the optic nerve and is seen in many cases of abusive head trauma, often in association with retinal hemorrhages[70,92,93] (Figure 23.11). Optic nerve sheath hemorrhage without other markers of injury can also be seen in other non-head trauma conditions, such as occasional child asphyxiations, although not with the frequency seen with the retinal hemorrhages of inflicted child head trauma.

Diffuse Axonal Injury

In cases of inflicted head trauma with inertial brain injury, severe rotational acceleration/deceleration forces of the head may result in widespread brain injury called *traumatic axonal injury,* which consists of damage to axons and small blood vessels and, rarely, actual tissue tears.[94–96] The inertial motion of the brain is greatest at the periphery of the brain at the outer cortical surface and extends deeper into the brain in proportion to the severity of the applied force. As the brain distorts and moves from inertia, damage is done to axons and small blood vessels at points where there are changes of structure and anatomy. These areas of damage tend to occur in the subcortical white matter, deep white matter, deep gray matter, and brain stem. In some adults, damage at these sites to the small blood vessels appears as streak or punctate hemorrhages (Figure 23.12). These hemorrhages are not seen in young children and infants with traumatic axonal injury, but there is some evidence that the vessels are damaged, go into spasm, and produce hypoxia but do not bleed. This evidence comes from studies of blast traumatic head injuries in war casualties.[97,98]

Damage to axons may be visible after 18 to 24 hours of survival on routine hematoxylin-eosin staining of brain sections. This axonal damage is very difficult to see in young children because of the small size of the axons. The damaged axons appear as retraction bulbs, which are pink bulbs where axoplasm has accumulated at points of damage to the axon. Beta-amyloid precursor protein (BAPP) immunohistochemical staining allows demonstration of damaged axons as early as 2 hour following injury and makes even very small damaged axons visible on microscopic examination.[99] BAPP is, thus, a useful adjunct for evaluation of damaged axons in young children. Evaluation of BAPP staining requires interpretation of the pattern in which the stain is expressed. Any process that damages an axon can produce a positive expression of the stain. In cases of abusive head injury, the 2 major patterns of BAPP staining

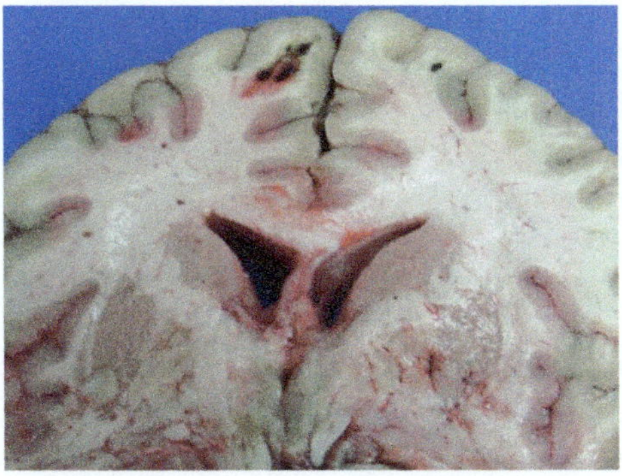

FIGURE 23.12

Adult brain in coronal section showing streak hemorrhages of diffuse axonal injury in left superior frontal gyrus subcortical white matter.

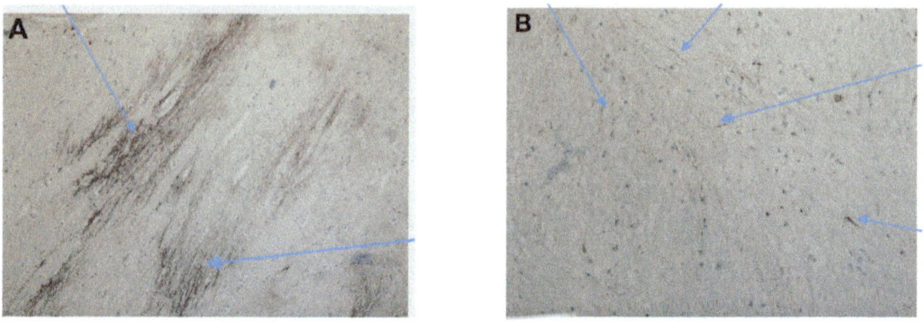

FIGURE 23.13

A, High-power microscopic section with beta-amyloid precursor protein (BAPP) expression in hypoxic pattern with broad areas of axonal damage. B, BAPP expression in traumatic axonal pattern with individual fibers damaged.

of interest are the patterns for traumatic axonal injury and for hypoxic/ischemic axonal injury. The 2 patterns differ in that traumatic axonal injury shows individual damaged axons scattered within fiber tracts, while the hypoxic pattern has broad areas of expression often associated with a vessel and sometimes described as zigzag patterns (Figure 23.13). To evaluate these patterns requires that many sections of brain be taken from above and below the tentorium, including the subcortical and deep white matter, corpus callosum (multiple levels), corpus striatum, midbrain, pons, medulla, and cerebellum. For axonal injury to be considered diffuse it must be found in multiple sites above and below the tentorium. Many cases of abusive head trauma have a mixed pattern of traumatic and hypoxic axonal injury. If the individual dies less than 2 hours after injury, the staining process will usually not be effective. Beta-amyloid precursor protein expression may also be absent in cases in which cerebral perfusion was halted rapidly. In cases of inflicted head injuries, some authors report that few cases demonstrate traumatic axonal injury and that most show evidence of hypoxia.[100,101] As many as 73% of cases of inflicted head trauma have positive expression for BAPP in a traumatic axonal pattern.[56] This latter group of children with inflicted head trauma also demonstrated subgaleal contusions in 76%, skull fractures in 20%, subdural hemorrhage in 91%, and retinal hemorrhages in 80%.

Brain Contusions

The softer consistency of the young brain renders it somewhat less prone to contusion on injury and more prone to tear than the brain at older ages. When there is a fracture of the skull, however, contusions are frequently seen on the adjacent cortical surfaces, and these should be labeled *fracture contusions.* Coup contusions from a direct contact injury without skull fracture are rare in adults and do not often occur in the young brain. When

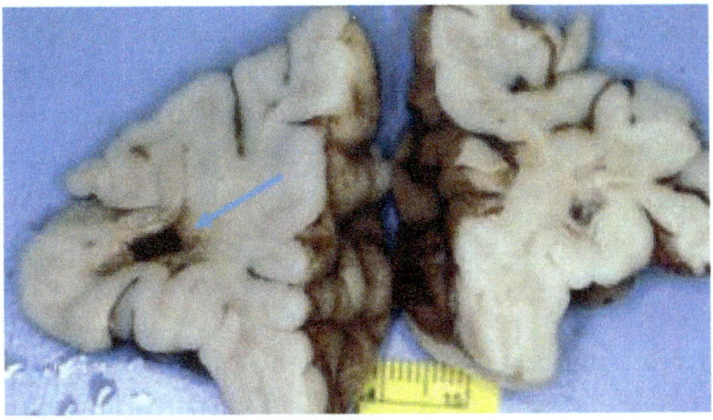

FIGURE 23.14
Infant with contusion tear of subcortical white matter of left frontal lobe.

it does occur, it appears as simply a faint blush on the cortical surface but does not have the hemorrhages typically found within the cortical tissue. Contrecoup contusions caused by a falling head injury, as commonly found in the adult, are not seen before the age of 4 years. There are several reasons for this, including the fact that young children are already close to the surface on which they are falling. They do not fall as a rigid object about a turning torque, so they do not develop the acceleration to the head necessary for contrecoup injury.[102]

A distinct lesion seen in very young infants, usually younger than 5 months, is the contusion tear.[103] *Contusion tears* are slits at the cortex and white matter junction or within the lamina of the cortex (Figure 23.14). These tears of the brain tissue are thought to be caused by the same inertial deformation of the brain, which causes diffuse axonal injury.[104]

Brain Swelling

Brain swelling is nonspecific as to etiology and is seen in many individuals of all ages at autopsy, even when there is only a brief survival. In children with inflicted head injury, most cases show some brain swelling as noted at autopsy by flattening of the cerebral convexities and narrowing of the gyri. This premorbid finding is discussed in Chapter 7, Abusive Head Trauma.

Distraction Injury of the Cervical Spine

A very rare injury to the lower brain stem/upper cervical spinal cord is the distraction injury that occurs when a child's head is grasped by the abuser, the child is suspended by the head with the weight of the body distracting the cervical spine, and the body is shaken violently.[56,105,106] These injuries have been seen in young infants who demonstrated showers of petechial hemorrhages on the neck, face, or chest; bruises on the ears and face; sometimes petechial hemorrhages of the conjunctivae; and sometimes gripping marks on the extremities. In one case, there was a single retinal hemorrhage. These children had contusions of the upper cervical spinal cord and lower medulla. These lesions tend to be hemorrhagic and have been described as hematomyelia (Figure 23.15).

These injuries should be distinguished from an artifact found in patients who are brain dead and have survived a period so that the brain becomes necrotic and softened. The portion of the brain that becomes most softened is the cerebellar tonsils, which can virtually disintegrate,

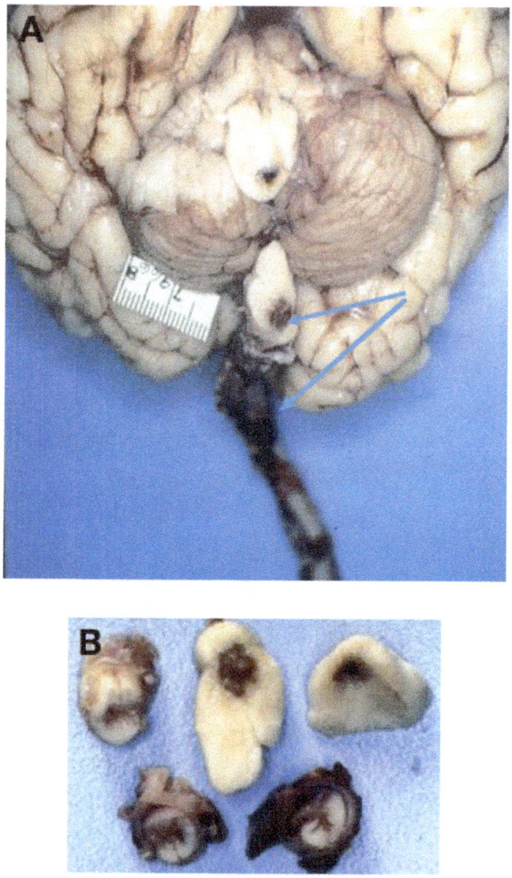

FIGURE 23.15

A, Brain from 4-month-old boy with distraction of cervical spine showing hemorrhage within the lower medulla/upper cervical cord; B, sections with hematomyelia in these regions.

with fragments of cerebellum falling into the subarachnoid space of the cervical spinal cord. These fragments may compress the small vessels, leading to ischemia of the adjacent cervical cord. This ischemia becomes hemorrhagic so that, grossly, these lesions look like the hematomyelia of the distraction injury described previously. Identical lesions can be produced in experimental animal models of brain death.[107]

Remote Severe Abusive Head Trauma

It is estimated that 30% to 50% of young children with severe inflicted head injuries survive some period after sustaining their injuries and do so in significantly debilitated states, with many being in vegetative states.[108] When these children later die from various complications of their devastated neurological state, they should come into the jurisdiction of the medical examiner's/coroner's office. The autosopy for these types of deaths are most appropriately performed by forensic pathologists. The autopsy findings include evidence of the various complicating problems suffered by these children, including chronic and often repeated pulmonary and urinary tract infections, complications related to muscular contractures and therapeutic manipulations performed for those problems, and complications related to their long-term bedridden status. The findings in the head do not allow for establishment of a diagnosis of what initiated the head injury if death occurs many months or years later. However, the proper procedure in medical examiner cases is for the forensic pathologist to consider all the past medical records back to the time of birth along with circumstantial evidence of how and when the injuries occurred. The death, even years later, will be properly certified as due to the initiating head trauma and will be certified as a homicide. The appearance at autopsy is a small cranium containing a small atrophic brain (Figure 23.16).

The growth of the calvarium is driven by the growth of the brain. When a child's brain is injured early in life, it remains as a damaged atrophic brain that does not grow further. The calvarium, therefore, does not grow further after injury. The growth of the face, however, continues at normal rate because its growth is driven by that of the mandible and maxilla, whose growth depends on the development of the secondary dentition. Children with early life brain damage have the appearance of microcephaly with a normal size face, so hair appears abundant on the small head. The brain itself often weighs only 400 g or so and has a "walnut" appearance with collapsed gyri, loss of white matter, foci of cystic encephalomalacia, and enlarged ventricles.

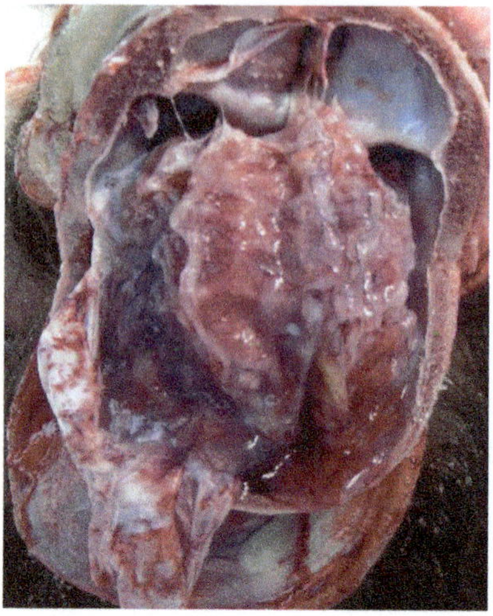

FIGURE 23.16

Thirteen-year-old who sustained abusive head trauma at age 4 months shows very atrophic brain at autopsy within the cranial cavity.

Abusive Chest Trauma

Injuries to the chest include those caused by blunt trauma and those caused by penetrating trauma. *Blunt trauma* is associated with rapid deceleration and is commonly caused by vehicular crashes and by direct blows to the thorax, which can occur from athletic activities or from child abuse. Gunshot wounds, stab wounds, or piercing of the chest from other objects cause *penetrating* injuries; these are less common in children than in adults. The chest of the young child has anatomical features that should be noted. The thorax is very compliant because the bony and cartilaginous structures are extremely flexible.[109] The chest of the small child can be compressed to cause major internal injury without necessarily causing rib fractures. Another difference is that the mediastinum of the child is more moveable than in adults and can shift widely with compression. The more fixed mediastinum of the adult renders the heart and great vessels at risk of deceleration injury, causing laceration of those structures. Young children are at less risk from deceleration injuries unless great force is involved. However, if there is injury to the child's chest resulting in lacerations of the heart or great vessels, the resulting blood loss is critical due to the child's relatively small blood volume, which is 7% to 8% of the body weight.[109] The blood volume of a term neonate is about 80 to 90 mL/kg and about 70 to 75 mL/kg for infants younger than 3 months. An adult's blood volume is 8% to 10% of the body weight; a 5- or 6-year-old reaches that blood volume for

TABLE 23.2
Approximate Blood Volume by Age

Age	Total Blood Volume (mL/kg)
Preterm neonates	90–105
Term newborns	78–86
1-12 mo	73–78
1-3 y	74–82
4–6 y	80–86
7–18 y	83–90
Adults	68–88

Adapted from Costa K. Hematology. In: Hughes HK, Kahl LK, eds. *The Harriet Lane Handbook*. 21st ed. Philadelphia, PA: Elsevier; 2018:364–394. Data from Nathan D, Oski FA. *Hematology of Infancy and Childhood*. Philadelphia, PA: WB Saunders; 1998.

body weight. Many children who sustain thoracic trauma concomitantly have also sustained abdominal or head trauma. Table 23.2 shows approximate blood volume by age.

Laceration of the Heart

Although chest trauma is common in child abuse, it is seldom the direct cause of death. Inflicted trauma may cause rib fractures, lung injury, cardiac injury, hemothorax, pneumothorax, and mediastinal injury. Inflicted blunt chest trauma has been known to cause a laceration of the heart from which the child exsanguinated. Cohle et al reported 6 cases of abusive chest trauma with cardiac lacerations.[110] These children ranged from 9 weeks to 2.5 years of age. Five of the 6 cases had lacerations of the right atrium, and 1 had a laceration of the left ventricle. The confessed mechanisms of injury were striking with a fist, stomping on the child, and drop-kicking the child. Lacerations of the heart in infants and young children are the result of severe blunt trauma caused by vehicular crashes or violent assaults. These are not injuries that can occur in the home from short falls. Of 14 children younger than 15 years reported in studies in the literature on heart lacerations, 3 cases were from vehicular crashes,[111–113] 3 were struck or stomped on the abdomen,[114] 1 was jumped on while on a sled,[115] 1 was a pedestrian struck by a car,[116] 1 was a bicyclist who struck his precordial area on the handlebar during a fall,[117] 1 was a child who fell 2.5 m onto a hard surface,[118] 1 was kicked in the chest by an adult,[119] 1 was thrown off a fast-moving sled and landed with a great impact,[120] 1 was struck by a falling tree limb,[121] 1 was struck in the chest by a 23-kg barbell that fell 1 m,[122] and 1 fell from the first floor of a building.[123] Cardiac trauma is seen only in the most severe trauma and does not occur from cardiopulmonary resuscitation (CPR) or minor trauma.

Rib Fractures

Rib fractures are the most common abusive chest injury. They are fatal in only a few cases, and most rib fractures are found with other lethal injuries.[124] Kleinman noted that rib fractures accounted for 5% to 51% of all fractures in children who had experienced abuse.[125] Rib fractures have a strong association with inflicted child injuries. Barsness et al found that the positive predictive value of a rib fracture as an indicator of nonaccidental trauma was 95%; when historical and clinical circumstances excluded other causes for the rib fractures, the positive predictive value increased to 100%.[126] In that study, rib fractures were the only skeletal injury found in 29% of children who had rib fractures. Bulloch et al noted that rib fractures are uncommon in infancy and, when diagnosed, often raise the suspicion of child abuse.[127] They studied a group of 39 infants younger than 12 months with rib fractures and found these were due to child abuse (82%), accidental injuries (7.7%), birth trauma (2.6%), and bone fragility (7.7%). The accidental mechanisms were a vehicular crash, direct forceful blow, and fall from a height. The children with bone fragility had osteogenesis imperfecta,[1] rickets,[1] and one 23-weeks' gestation neonate with fragile bones due to preterm birth. They concluded that most rib fractures in infants are caused by child abuse.

At autopsy, it is a common finding that children with rib fractures who have experienced abuse have more fractures than do children who have not experienced abuse. Medical professionals have also noted this increased incidence of rib fractures in children who have experienced abuse.[128] In young children, radiographs may not demonstrate acute rib fractures. Because of the recognized difficulty in imaging acute rib fractures, the common forensic practice at autopsy is to strip off the periosteum overlying the ribs to view them directly so that even subtle fractures can be seen. One good technique is to remove the entire rib cage (Figure 23.17). Photographs can be taken showing each fractured rib in situ; then each rib can be dissected out, transected to show grossly any fracture; and then microscopic sections can be taken for determination of the age of the fracture. When the pathologist looks at rib fractures microscopically, the earliest appearance of fracture is a disruption of the bony cortex and adjacent bony trabeculae. Acute hemorrhage is present, and this hemorrhage may persist for several weeks in the living child. As the fracture heals, the microscopic appearance is an inflammatory response with an influx of neutrophils into the fracture site and hematoma. In a few days, mononuclear cells begin to also arrive at the injury site. In 5 to 7 days,

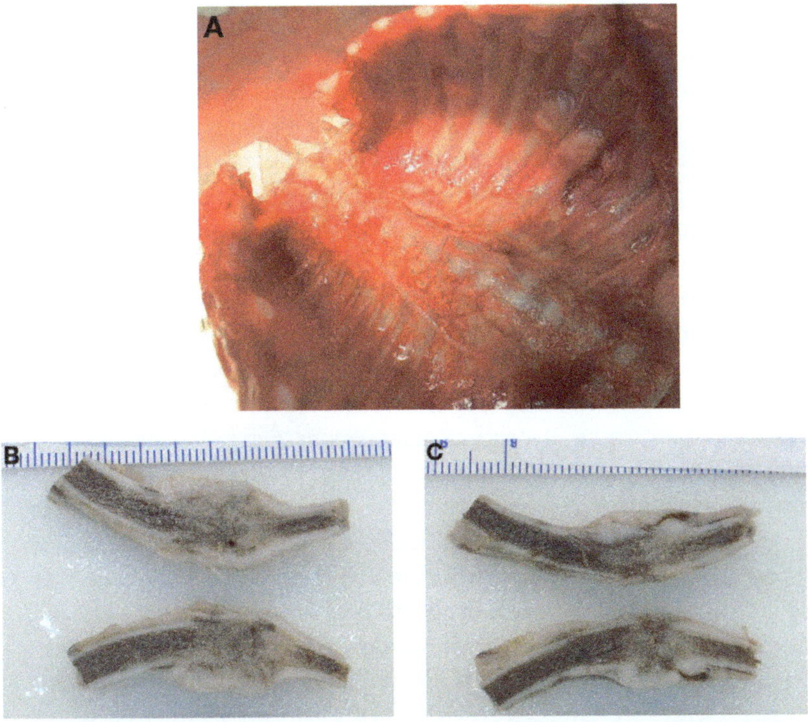

FIGURE 23.17

A, Young infant's rib cage removed at autopsy shows multiple healing rib fractures. B and C, Individual ribs removed and sectioned show healing callus.

the earliest fibroblastic infiltration and granulation formation is seen. This process has now created a soft callus of woven bone, which binds the fracture site. At this time, the gross appearance is a white bulging knob on the bone. The soft callus is gradually remodeled into the hard callus, which is firmer and which further remodels into trabecular bone. This process takes several weeks to months to complete.[129]

Rib fractures may be caused by CPR, although this occurs less commonly in young children than in adults.[130] Fractures associated with CPR tend to be located mainly anterior, while those from abusive injury may be at any point on the rib but most often are posterior. With the institution of the latest method of infant CPR (with the 2 adult hands encircling the infant's chest), more resuscitation-associated rib fractures have been noted at autopsy.[131,132] When these CPR rib fractures are found, they are minimal fractures of the inner surface of the bony cortex and accompanied often by very little hemorrhage.

This chapter's author has seen 3 cases of young infants, 2 to 4 months of age, who were killed by an adult squeezing on the chest. All the perpetrators were the fathers. They performed this squeezing action on multiple occasions, and one father stated that his daughter "liked to be held like that" because when she was crying and the father would squeeze her, she would stop crying. The father did note that on occasion he could hear popping sounds as the ribs broke. The autopsies on these infants demonstrated 27 to 36 rib fractures whose ages varied from very acute to older and very old. The exact mechanism of death in these cases could be either from compression asphyxia, by keeping the chest stationary and not allowing chest excursions for breathing to occur, or that the effect of so many fractured ribs caused a flail chest and instability of the chest and altered breathing. Recently, 2 cases of constrictive asphyxia were reported in the literature. In one case, the father admitted to periodically sitting on his infant daughter to stop her from crying. She was found to have 14 rib fractures but survived. In the other case, a 2-month-old died unexpectedly and was found to have lateral rib fractures bilaterally with callus formation on the postmortem skeletal survey. At autopsy, she was found to have thickening of all the costochondral junctions and lateral rib fractures with callus on the right second through fifth ribs and left third rib with a fresh refracture through the callus. The father ultimately admitted to wrapping the baby tightly in a blanket and holding her to his chest with his arms encircling her until she stopped crying. On the night of her fatal event, he reported squeezing her more tightly than usual until she was quiet.[133]

Abdominal Trauma

Significant blunt trauma injury to the abdomen is a rare type of child abuse but is the second most common cause of death from abuse after head trauma. Of patients hospitalized for abuse in a 2005 study of patients admitted to a large urban pediatric trauma center over a 10-year period, only 1% had abdominal injury.[134] The mortality of this group, however, was 45% to 50%. In a series of 160 child deaths from 1975 to 1985 in a large metropolitan area, 70 were homicides. In a similar series of 72 child deaths from 1986 to 1999 in an adjacent suburban area, 32 were homicides. In the 1975 to 1985 group, 40% died from abdominal injury; in the 1986 to 1999 group, 9% died from abdominal injury. These series of child deaths also collected accidental deaths in children but omitted deaths due to vehicular crashes, drownings outside the home, and gunshot wounds. In those series, there were no accidental deaths from abdominal trauma in children.[124] The literature reflects that about 12% of child abuse deaths are caused by abdominal injuries.[135,136] Abdominal trauma from abuse has a high mortality. To a great extent in fatal cases of abdominal trauma, the high mortality is due to the failure of the perpetrator to seek timely medical care for the injured child. The perpetrator knows he or she has injured the child but hopes to avoid having that fact recognized and hopes for improvement in the child's condition, which fails to happen.

There are unique features of the abdomen of a young child that play a role in the injuries that occur to the abdomen. The abdominal wall in the young child has very little muscle to protect against a blow; also, the young child does not have a reflex to tense the muscle in a protective stance against a blow. Force can pass right through the abdominal wall, and the organs may or may not move away as that force is directed toward the spinal column. The rib cage is widely flared and flexible; thus, the ribs offer little protection to the contents of the abdomen. The abdomen itself is relatively small, so a single blow may injure more than 1 organ.[137] The blood supply of the abdominal contents has some features that reflect on the injuries sustained by blunt trauma. The major blood supply consists of the large arteries coming off the anterior aspect of the aorta, which are the celiac trunk and the superior mesenteric artery. A central blow to the abdomen can cause transection of those arteries or their branches. The celiac trunk and tributaries supply the area around the stomach, pancreas, and proximal small bowel. The superior mesenteric artery is the main blood supply of the small and large bowel. When there is abdominal blunt trauma in small children, a frequent finding at autopsy is a large amount of free blood in the peritoneal cavity and blood within the mesentery along with contusion and tears of the mesentery. Undoubtedly there are tears of branches of the superior mesenteric vessels within the damaged mesentery that had shed this blood. Mesenteric tears are common findings in isolation or in conjunction with other abdominal injury (Figure 23.18). The small blood volume of the young child adversely affects the outcome in abusive blunt abdominal trauma, adding to the significant mortality in these cases.

Fatal abusive abdominal injuries are inflicted by punching with a fist, kicking, or throwing the child to strike a surface and causing deceleration injury to internal structures. Of children dying of abdominal trauma, many do not demonstrate external evidence of impact on the abdomen. Impact to the thin abdominal wall of a small child can pass through the abdominal wall, which contains only a small amount of fat and muscle, and not produce bruising to the abdomen. Therefore, lack of visible bruising to the child's abdomen should not be taken as evidence that trauma has not occurred or that even fatal internal abdominal injury had not been caused. When bruising does occur to the abdomen, it tends to appear as individual knuckle marks

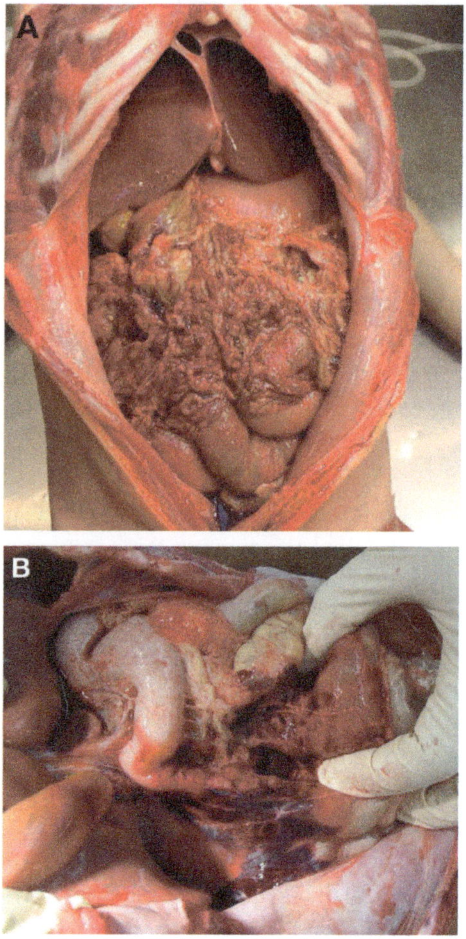

FIGURE 23.18

A, Abdomen of toddler-aged child with massive tears of mesentery. B, Large tear of mesentery.

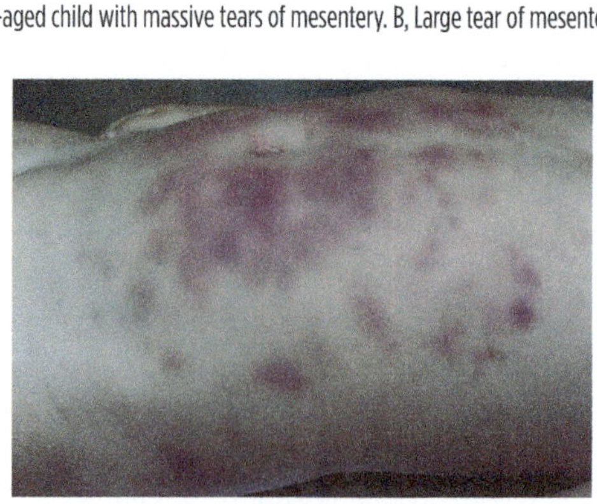

FIGURE 23.19

Child with fatal blunt abdominal trauma with extensive bruising on chest and abdomen.

rather than large areas of contusion (Figure 23.19). This latter type of bruising is frequently scattered over the abdomen and chest.

Lethal inflicted abdominal trauma may damage the liver, kidneys, adrenals, pancreas, mesentery, and portions of the gastrointestinal tract. Most commonly encountered are inflicted injury to the liver, pancreas, mesentery, and proximal small bowel. Accidental abdominal injury is more common to the liver, kidney, and spleen.

Hollow Viscus Injuries

Hollow viscus injury is more common in inflicted trauma than in accidental injury. Obviously, in some cases of accidental or inflicted injury, any of the solid or hollow organs may be damaged. If the liver, mesentery, or other solid organs are damaged, bleeding is the problem that will terminate in hemorrhagic shock, and symptoms leading to the demise will be those of shock. If hollow vicus organs are damaged, the peritoneal cavity will be contaminated with bowel or gastric contents, which will lead to peritonitis, and the child may demonstrate abdominal tenderness, abdominal distention, nausea, vomiting, fever, absent or diminished bowel sounds, peritoneal signs, and inability to eat. The leading abdominal injuries from abuse are liver laceration and laceration of the small bowel.[138–143] The small bowel injuries tend to be in the proximal small bowel near the ligament of Treitz, where the bowel is relatively fixed. Injuries at that point may be a complete or a partial laceration of the bowel wall, and the surrounding mesentery tends to be contused or lacerated as well (Figure 23.20). This portion of the bowel has a rich blood supply, so significant amounts of blood may be lost from

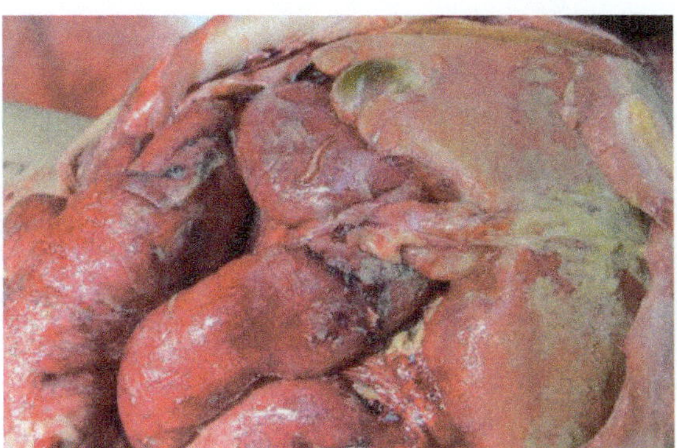

FIGURE 23.20

Child with laceration of the proximal duodenum that was surgically repaired; the child survived 2 days with purulent peritonitis seen at autopsy.

damage in that area. The duodenum is retroperitoneal and deep within the abdominal cavity, so it is protected from minor injury; however, with significant force, it can be damaged by being crushed between the spinal column and the striking force. Injuries to the duodenum from abuse are second in frequency to those from vehicular accidents. At autopsy, the damaged bowel appears dark red or black with the laceration evident by the torn edges, the peritoneal cavity contains purulent fluid, and the peritoneal surfaces are covered with purulent exudate. Microscopic sections of the bowel may help age the inflammatory process and provide a timeline for how long the injury has been present. Younger children seem to die faster from peritonitis and may die within a few hours, whereas older children may survive longer than 24 hours without medical care. If these children with inflicted abdominal injuries were brought to timely medical attention, most would not die. Sometimes the bowel wall itself has hemorrhage within the serosa, which may be present in small focal areas or in widespread areas (Figure 23.21). These serosal hemorrhagic injuries may be found in association with other forms of abuse and are not the cause of death. Lacerations of the stomach may occur from abuse but are relatively rare injuries. Gastric lacerations tend to occur when the stomach is filled with food because, similar to a balloon, an empty viscus will not easily tear, while a filled one will rupture on impact. In 2 documented cases, the children had eaten just before the injury and at autopsy the peritoneal cavity contained the undigested food and evidence of peritonitis.[144] These cases are rare as a result of abusive trauma but occur in older children from accidental trauma, such as a vehicular crash or having a bicycle handlebar forcefully impact the abdomen.

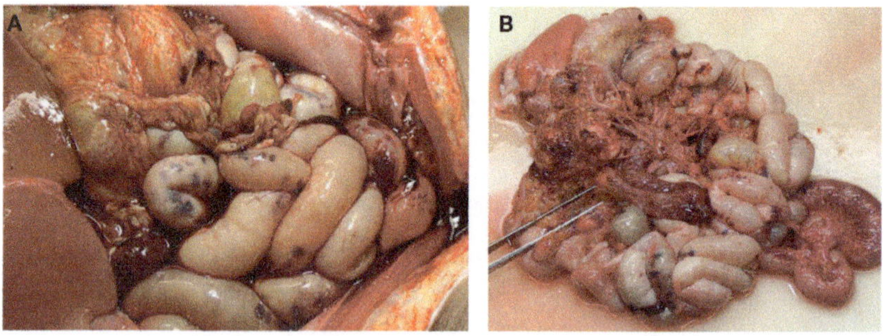

FIGURE 23.21

A, Child with lacerations of mesentery and duodenum with serosal hemorrhages of small bowel. B, Lacerations of mesentery and duodenum.

Liver Lacerations

Liver lacerations are frequently found abusive injuries. Liver trauma varies from small subcapsular hematomas to massive lacerations of the liver, which may transect a portion of the liver or macerate the liver parenchyma (Figure 23.22). The size of the laceration obviously determines the amount and rapidity of the bleeding. Some large liver lacerations can cause death in 15 to 30 minutes. At autopsy, the pathologist usually will measure the amount of blood in the abdominal cavity. The amount of blood in the abdomen can then be used to calculate what portion of the blood volume has been lost, knowing that the total blood volume of a child is around 75 to 80 mL/kg (see Table 23.2).[145] Studies have found that the likelihood of CPR-related abdominal trauma in children is low. A study that gathered data from multiple large Florida medical examiner offices of children dying from inflicted abdominal trauma and control groups of pediatric natural deaths and of non-vehicular accidental blunt abdominal trauma found that of the 320 cases of natural pediatric deaths, all the patients of which had CPR, none had abdominal trauma.[146] In the period from 1981 to 1997, the study found no non-vehicular accidental blunt abdominal traumas. In the 33 child homicides with fatal abdominal injuries, 73% had CPR, and their abdominal trauma did not differ from that seen in the children without CPR. The results of this study are similar to what others have found: CPR does not cause significant liver damage.[130]

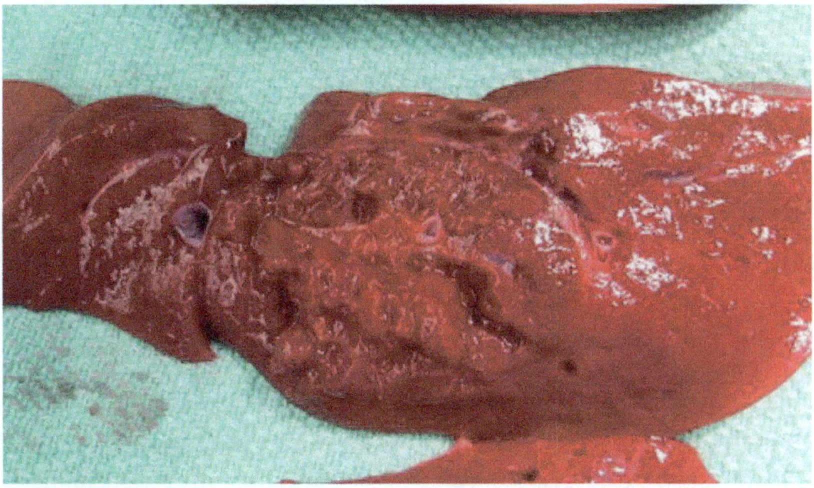

FIGURE 23.22

Liver sliced postmortem into sections showing extensive lacerations and maceration of parenchyma.

Other Solid Abdominal Organ Injury

Injuries to the kidney and spleen are much more frequent in accidental injuries in children than from abuse. Vehicular and bicycle crashes account for most of these injuries. Injuries to these organs can occur in child abuse but are fairly rare. The pancreas is often injured in abusive abdominal trauma and often in conjunction with other injuries such as those to the duodenum, which is nearby anatomically. Lacerations of the pancreas may be partial or total transections.

It is not unusual at autopsy of children dying of abusive injuries, and especially from abdominal injuries, to find evidence of older abdominal injury. This sometimes takes the form of a collection of yellow-stained fluid in the peritoneal cavity, which contains remnants of old blood. It also may be scarring in the mesentery, which appears grossly as fibrotic scars or sometimes is evident only by microscopic evidence of old fibrosis. Dye and colleagues described 4 cases of fatal abdominal inflicted trauma, all of which had older healing abdominal injury evident on microscopic examination.[147]

Blunt Soft Tissue Trauma

Blunt soft tissue trauma is a rare form of abusive injury with extensive external marks of blunt trauma and extensive soft tissue bleeding without injury to internal organs. These children tend to be toddler age or older but, occasionally, may be infants. The external marks of blunt trauma consist of abrasions and bruises on the extremities, chest, back, and buttocks and may have multiple patterned injuries, which indicate a variety of objects having struck the body. The soft tissues of these children are examined postmortem by dissecting into the back, buttocks, and extremities and peeling away the skin surface to demonstrate any areas of bleeding. It is not clear what mechanism causes death in these cases. After death, blood volume cannot be measured because the red blood cell walls begin to disintegrate and the blood undergoes hemolysis. Measurements of hemoglobin and hematocrit cannot be made. In cases of blunt soft tissue trauma, the soft tissues contain large volumes of blood, but it is impossible to judge what portion of the child's blood volume has been lost. Blood loss would be one potential mechanism of death. Another mechanism of death could be stress cardiomyopathy, which has been found in some adults dying exclusively of blunt soft tissue trauma without internal injury.[148] Stress cardiomyopathy may be related to catecholamine release during stress that results in damage to the heart. In the heart, microscopic changes of myofibrillar degeneration and contraction band necrosis are sometimes seen. Pavin and colleagues described 2 such cases of left ventricular dysfunction caused by acute emotional stress.[149] Another possible mechanism is fat embolism, which was reported by Nichols et al as the cause of death in their case of blunt soft tissue trauma in a 2-year-old. The child had extensive blunt traumatic injuries without internal thoracic, abdominal, or cranial injury and without skeletal trauma.[150]

Burns

Burns are discussed in detail in Chapter 3; therefore, this chapter's discussion focuses on fatal cases seen by the medical examiner/coroner. Burns can be caused by scalding, contact, chemical, and flame injury. The most common lethal burns are scalding burns, which are often found in relation to toilet or soiling issues even at a very young age when toilet training would not be a realistic expectation. Knowledge about water temperature is essential in evaluating scalding injuries. At 52.2°C (126°F), it takes 120 seconds to cause full-thickness burning. As the temperature approaches 60°C to 65.6°C (140°F–150°F), the time to full-thickness burns falls to 2 to 3 seconds.[151] Scalding burns are caused by holding a child in hot water, including in tubs, sinks, pans, or showers.

Patterns of scalding burns are helpful in distinguishing whether a burn is inflicted or accidental. When accidental burns from hot water or other liquids or foods occur, these materials generally strike a portion of the body and then move quickly away from the starting area. As the material moves away it loses temperature so that the degree of burning decreases quickly. This is different from inflicted scalds, in which a child is held in hot water, creating large solid areas of burns separated from unburned skin by a sharp line or tidemark.[152] Children placed into hot water will try to remove themselves by moving away or flexing their limbs, which can result in sparing of the inguinal, popliteal, or antecubital areas. Inflicted scalds may have a more symmetrical pattern with stocking or glove distributions. If the burning injury occurs in a bathtub, portions of the body held down may make contact with the tub bottom, and those areas may be spared because the tub surface is cooler than the water.

Because accidental fatal scalds in the home are unlikely, when a fatal scalding injury occurs (Figure 23.23), it must be investigated thoroughly. Scene reenactments must be done in these cases where a trained death investigator goes to the scene and attempts to recreate the circumstances that were purported to have caused the burns. In the course of the reenactment, it may become apparent that such a scenario could not have happened or could not explain the burn pattern sustained. It should be evident to anyone placing a child into hot water that if the child

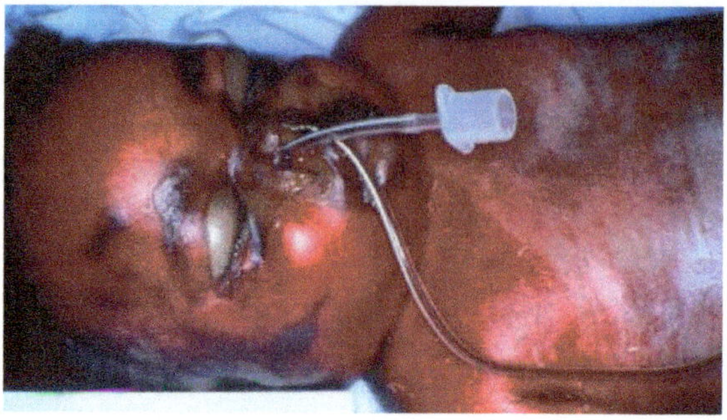

FIGURE 23.23
Ten-month-old held face down in hot water. The child survived overnight in the hospital.

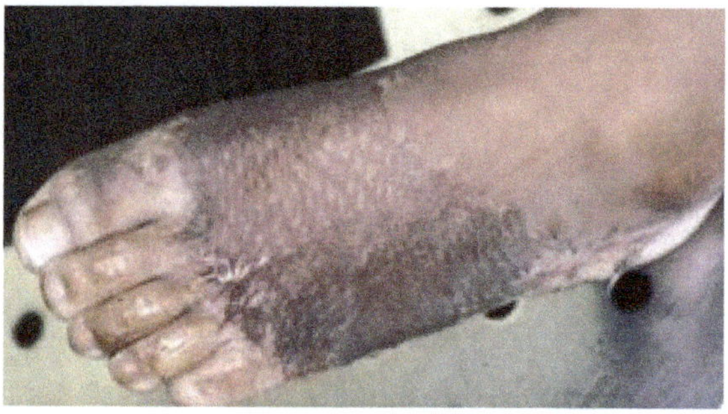

FIGURE 23.24
Child was said to have drowned in a tub, but autopsy showed inflicted abdominal trauma with incidental finding of old burn scar on left foot, which shows grafting. Pattern is suggestive of dipping injury.

demonstrates pain on entering the water, the water is too hot. Even very young infants will register pain and cry when they contact hot water. Water of the temperature necessary to cause full-thickness burns will radiate heat to anyone near the surface of the water, so it would be difficult to place a child into hot water without becoming aware that the water is too hot.

The incidental finding of a contact burn or a contact burn scar is occasionally seen by the medical examiner when doing an autopsy on a child who died from an inflicted injury (Figure 23.24). Such burns are not seen in other child deaths. Contact burns that are full thickness require having the hot object in contact with the skin for several seconds and do not occur from having an object fall onto the child and then fall or bounce off. A number of patterns can be seen in the contact burns noted, such as curling irons, clothing irons, or space heaters or other heating apparatuses. Fatal scald injuries may cause death rapidly due to shock from fluid loss. With delay in care for scald burns, both dehydration leading to shock and secondary infection leading to sepsis can result in a fatality.

Subtle Lethal Abusive Injury

Child abuse deaths can occur in very subtle forms, which include drownings, poisoning, asphyxiation, and various forms of neglect of medical care, nutrition, and safety.[153] These can be difficult cases to interpret, and it is often necessary to establish first the fatal pathophysiological mechanism of death and then, in conjunction with the circumstances from scene investigations along with police and social service and other agency reports, it may become clear how the death was caused.

Drowning

The diagnosis of drowning is always established by exclusion of other causes of death when an individual is seen to become submerged or is found dead in the water. There are no findings at autopsy that conclusively diagnose drowning. When a homicidal drowning occurs in a child, it may be impossible to distinguish that death from an accidental drowning. If a body is removed from the water, a homicidal drowning death may not be recognized as a drowning. These are not common cases but are probably underreported and account for some portion of those deaths called sudden infant death syndrome or other forms of sudden unexpected infant death. Gillenwater et al reported on 205 submersions between 1983 and 1991 in King County, WA, of children younger than 19 years and found that 8% were inflicted drownings.[154] Those who experienced homicidal drownings and near drownings were young, with a median age of 2.1 years; the most common incident site was the bathtub. Griest and Zumwalt described 6 homicidal drownings in young children from newborn to 3 years of age.[155] They noted that accidental drownings were more likely to occur in toddlers and older children in public areas like swimming pools, drainage ditches, lakes, and rivers. Homicidal drownings occurred in the toilet (1 newborn), bathtub (3 cases), living room, and hot springs. Mothers were the perpetrators in 4 cases and fathers in 2 cases.

The manner of death in drowning due to neglectful acts on the part of the caregiver may be considered homicide, accidental, or undetermined, depending on the circumstances. Usually, if the caregiver is impaired by drugs or alcohol, such deaths are considered homicides. If a child is left unattended and drowns, it is also often considered a homicide.

Abuse Deaths by Poisoning

Intentional poisoning deaths from substances such as alcohol, medication, illicit substances, or materials such as water or salt occur but are rare. Zumwalt and Hirsch described a child forced to ingest a large quantity of salt who died as a result.[153] Children have also died from water intoxication as a result of ingesting watered-down formula in large amounts or from being provided large amounts of additional water for other reasons.

Common scenarios of such deaths involve illicit drugs or medication provided to children with the intention of sedating them to stop them from crying or keeping them from "bothering" the caregiver. These deaths are considered homicides, although the intent was not necessarily to kill the child. Another common scenario is when medication that belongs to the caregiver is left in a location that can be obtained and ingested by the child. These deaths are sometimes considered homicides if the medication is negligently left where a child could obtain and ingest it. The opioid epidemic has been accompanied by more deaths in children from homicidal or accidental intoxications. Toxicology screening should be performed on all child deaths. The National Association of Medical Examiners maintains a pediatric toxicology registry, PedTox, as a resource for forensic pathologists to use for evaluation of their cases. For many drugs and medications, lethal levels for young children have not been established, and the PedTox registry contains information on what levels of a variety of substances have been found in children that may be related to their death.

Asphyxiation

Asphyxiation is a category of deaths that result from a failure of oxygen reaching or being used by the cells of the body. Asphyxial mechanisms include suffocation, strangulation, and chemical asphyxia. Suffocation includes entrapment (eg, trapped in a refrigerator), smothering, choking, mechanical asphyxia (eg, heavy weight on the chest to preclude breathing), and gases. In smothering deaths, the nose and mouth are occluded and air cannot reach the lungs. Smothering may be very subtle in young children and may be impossible to detect in some cases. Sometimes, but not always, smothering leaves abrasions and contusions around the face—particularly the nose, lips, gums, or cheeks—so it may be difficult to detect. Sometimes, but not always, smothering will produce petechial hemorrhages of the facial skin, orbital skin, or conjunctivae.[156]

Meadow[156] described 27 young children who were suffocated by their mothers. Suffocation was detected by covert video surveillance or witness, confession, or conviction at trial. In 14 of the cases, there were no marks or any external evidence that suffocation had occurred. Of these 27 children,

90% had had previous apneic episodes, 44% had had previous unexplained disorders, 55% were older than 6 months, and 48% had a dead sibling. DiMaio described 133 homicidal asphyxial deaths, of which 26 were suffocation, and of these, 20 of the victims were children younger than 2 years.[157] Only 1 child had petechial and/or scleral hemorrhage. Infants younger than 12 months are especially likely not to have any injuries resulting from smothering. These deaths may be impossible to distinguish from sudden infant death syndrome or sudden unexpected infant death.

In all child deaths, the autopsy findings must be considered in conjunction with scene investigation, including reenactment, and all aspects of the history, circumstances, and past medical records. Video surveillance has shown that even very young infants can struggle and react vigorously to attempts at smothering.[158]

Investigation of a child death should always include death scene investigation with doll reenactment as well as special attention to items at the scene that might be related to the death. Interviews should be conducted with everyone who was present around the time of death. Finally, while many of these cases may initially be certified as undetermined cause and manner of death, forensic pathologists need to keep an open mind to reconsider additional new information that becomes available even years later.

Older children tend to have more injuries when smothered, and the injuries depend somewhat on what objects are used for the smothering, such as hands, pillows, or blankets. Hands applied to the face may cause fingernail scratches, bruises, and abrasions. Pillows and cloth materials like blankets can cause abrasions and bruises. Injuries may be found to the facial areas of the nose, mouth, lips, cheeks, ears, and chin. Petechiae can occur and, when present, are likely to be on the skin of the face, behind the ears, on the neck or eyelids, and sometimes on the conjunctivae.[159]

Brown et al described in detail 20 cases of homicidal childhood asphyxia deaths.[160] These authors, forensic pathologists who had conducted the autopsies and eventually certified the causes and manners of death, described the autopsy findings and their approaches to deaths of newborns to children 5 years of age. They note that it is common that autopsy alone does not identify the cause of death in an asphyxial death. In 16 of their 20 cases, a ruling of homicide could only be established by a confession by the perpetrator. Three homicidal rulings were made from corroborating witness statements. In only one case, the ruling of homicide was made without either a perpetrator confession or a witness statement. Autopsy findings that these authors considered suggestive of intentional smothering or suffocation included oral and buccal mucosal and facial injuries, frenulum lacerations, and facial or conjunctival petechiae. Petechiae of scleral, conjunctival, or intrathoracic areas were found in 10 of 20 cases. They noted that cases of suspicious deaths in children should have a reexamination for injuries on 1 or more days following the initial autopsy examination, and these should include looking at the intraoral surfaces for trauma as well as injuries seen initially that may display better following autopsy.

Asphyxiation may be carried out by unusual methods and be impossible to detect. Often these deaths are precipitated by a caregiver trying to quiet a crying infant. One such case involved a 6-month-old who was found dead and at autopsy was found to have a baby wipe in the upper airway occluding the epiglottis. When asked, the father who was caring for the child said the infant "grabbed the baby wipe from his hand and swallowed it." Other such cases have been reported in the literature.[161]

In 2 cases of multiple rib fractures that varied from acute to old and very old, the fathers held the infants so tightly around the chest that the chest could not move, and this would stop the infant from crying. During this squeezing on the chest, the ribs would fracture. It is likely that because the rib fractures would be painful, there would be more crying and more squeezing. This squeezing was done over several months. Another father killed 2 of his children by piling folded-up blankets on top of the infants, aged 3 months and 4 months, to muffle their crying. The weight of the blankets and lack of fresh oxygenated air caused the infants to die. These deaths were only recognized as homicidal asphyxiations after the father admitted to what he had done. Another father stated that he found his 9-month-old tightly wrapped in a heavy comforter as though in a cocoon and face down in his crib. In none of these cases did the autopsy provide a cause of death, and the circumstances became known only through scene reenactments with dolls and death scene investigation. The information that came from the reenactment was that the infant had to have been wrapped in the comforter by someone else, and once wrapped in this manner, he could not extricate himself. A series by Brown et al of homicidal asphyxiation describes a similar case, which they describe as "bamboo wrapped."[160]

On rare occasions, infants and young children present to medical care with hypoxic-ischemic encephalopathy (HIE), and despite extensive workup, no etiology of the hypoxia can be found. At autopsy these children demonstrated changes of HIE, but still no cause could be found to explain why the child became hypoxic. A 7-month-old was hospitalized at 4 months of age with seizures and on workup was thought to have herpes encephalitis. When the infant died at 7 months, autopsy showed only HIE with a laminar distribution. The father of this infant later killed a second child by head injury, and in his confession to that death, described that he would hold the first infant with his head over the crib railing, putting pressure on the child's neck, and the child would have seizures. McIntosh et al described a similar child's death.[162] It is imperative that cases of children with HIE without an underlying etiology be investigated thoroughly for the possibility of asphyxial events.

Strangulation in children may also be impossible to detect clinically or at autopsy. This is particularly likely if the hands are used to cause pressure on the child's neck. Ligatures are more likely to cause abrasions on the neck. When a child is manually strangled, the effect may be to close off the airway by collapsing the cartilaginous trachea. In adults and older children, neck pressure is primarily a vascular event with pressure on the jugular veins causing venous return to be precluded and pressure on the carotid arteries causing ischemia. The resulting petechial hemorrhages in the bulbar and palpebral conjunctivae are usually evident, along with bruising and abrasion externally on the neck. Internally, there are usually hemorrhages of neck muscles, and sometimes there are fractures of the laryngeal cartilages or the hyoid bone. Because the airway of the young child is so soft and compliant, it can be totally compressed without leaving an external or internal finding and without petechial hemorrhages. A 911 call was made for a 4-month-old boy who became unresponsive in the care of the mother's boyfriend. Emergency medical services (EMS) responded, performed CPR, and transported the infant to the hospital. The infant survived 2 days in a hypoxic state and came to the medical examiner with the history of having sustained an abusive head injury. At autopsy, the infant had a fractured radius, contusion of the spleen, and massive brain swelling with markedly split sutures but no skull fracture, as had been diagnosed radiologically. No clear cause of death could be established until several months later when additional information came to light. When EMS initially came to the home, a 4-year-old sibling told EMS that he was being sexually abused by the boyfriend, and the boyfriend was arrested. He was put in jail, where he subsequently told a cellmate that he had "strangled" the infant. The cause of death was then certified as strangulation and manner as a homicide.

Medical Child Abuse (Munchausen Syndrome by Proxy/Factitious Illness by Proxy)

Medical child abuse occurs when a parent, usually the mother, fabricates signs and symptoms of illness in a child, who is then taken to medical care and undergoes a workup for a nonexistent illness, resulting in harmful and unnecessary medical procedures and evaluations. These cases have a significant morbidity, and mortality may be as high as 10%.[163] Illness may be created in the child by such harmful practices as giving the child adult blood pressure medication or injecting fecal material into the child.[164–166] The induced or feigned illness is then extensively medically investigated, and the ensuing testing and diagnostic procedures may have devastating effects on the child. The perpetrator of this falsehood receives some type of positive gain by the medical attention directed toward the child. The types of problems created or fictitiously implied in cases of medical child abuse include infections from contaminated materials; poisoning by medications or other substances; use of foreign blood to suggest loss by the child in diapers, urine, or feces; and a myriad of possible problems.

For the forensic pathologist, by far the most common and deadly factitious illness encountered is the apneic episode in which the caregiver states that the child stopped breathing and then was resuscitated by the caregiver. These types of cases illustrate the need for very close examination of the medical records of children with puzzling illnesses and those subjected to multiple hospitalizations for unusual and strange disorders. This review should be performed by child abuse pediatricians who are knowledgeable about factitious illness disorders. Child fatality review panels are appropriate venues for this type of postmortem multidisciplinary investigation as well as other agencies that may collaborate in further interviews with the caregivers or family, such as police, social services, schools, and primary care medical professionals. Sanders and Bursch discuss suggested guidelines for the forensic evaluation of factitious disorders and point out the importance of a thorough medical records review of not just the index child but all the siblings and caregivers involved.[165] This topic is also discussed in detail in Chapter 20, Medical Child Abuse.

Lethal Neglect

Child abuse by neglect may include failure to provide food, water, a safe environment, medical care, education, and emotional support. Young children are dependent on their parents or caregivers to provide all their needs; failure to do so constitutes neglect. Child abuse from neglect is the most common form of child abuse in living children, but those who die from intentional neglect account for a small number.

When death results from failure to provide these essentials, a death may be ruled a homicide. Depending on the jurisdiction and preference of the local medical examiner or coroner, some of these deaths may or may not be considered homicides. These cases can be a challenge to successfully prosecute. In one case, a 9-month-old boy was left unattended in a small room in a house trailer with a temperature above 32.2°C (90°F) due to the use of a space heater. The parents had left the child for up to 2 days while they did drugs. When found, the child was inside a crib on his back with his legs extending through the crib railings. He was in decomposition and showed changes of early mummification from the heat. He did not have vitreous fluid available due to severe dehydration, so his electrolytes could not be evaluated. His death was attributed to "hyperthermia" with another significant condition of severe malnutrition with all growth parameters less than the fifth percentile. The manner of death was homicide. A case of medical neglect involved a 2-year-old who was born very preterm and required endotracheal intubation for a prolonged period, resulting in tracheal stenosis. He was hospitalized for many months and then went to a rehabilitation hospital for several months. He required continuous medical care for his tracheal stenosis involving dilatation, and he remained dependent on a tracheostomy. When he was found dead at home, his tracheostomy tube was out and could not be reinserted because his tracheal opening was 1 to 2 mm. When all his medical records were reviewed, it was evident he had not been taken for medical care for longer than 1 year despite many medical professionals calling the mother to bring him in to be seen. The circumstances were so concerning to the medical professionals that they involved social services, who were concerned enough that they asked the juvenile court to remove the child from the home; that request was denied. His death was considered a homicide.

Neglect of medical care for religious beliefs occasionally causes a child to die. These cases may be handled differently in various medical examiner jurisdictions. They may be certified as homicides when a healthy child develops a treatable condition, such as new-onset diabetes with ketoacidosis and coma, during which the parents would be able to recognize a medical emergency but did not take the child for medical care. Many medical examiners certify these deaths as "natural" in manner and, therefore, many of these cases are never successfully prosecuted.

Starvation is a rare cause of child death from intentional withholding of food. In infants and young children, growth is an ongoing process, and it is possible to discern from a child's height and weight in comparison with standard growth charts how much or how long a child has been deprived of nutrition. Kellogg and Lukefahr described 12 cases of infants and children whose caregivers were prosecuted for starvation, not all of which were fatal.[167] Their subjects ranged from 2.25 months to 13 years old; half of the children died shortly after they came to medical or law enforcement attention, meaning that they were kept hidden from authorities until they were extremely moribund. Access to food was either totally denied or severely restricted. Ten children were considered severely wasted and 2 mildly to moderately wasted. The older children were more likely to survive than were the infants. All the children showed adverse effects of starvation on multiple organs.

Autopsy of a child dying from starvation will demonstrate a child who lacks subcutaneous fat in the abdominal wall, whose bones are very prominent, and whose extremities lack muscle and appear atrophic. The opinion of whether such deaths are from starvation or inanition is based on all the autopsy findings that do not show an alternative process in the body that would conclusively cause death. Many young children who actually die of starvation have other findings at autopsy, such as foci of bronchopneumonia, skin infections or scars from old infections, and atrophy of the thymus, heart, liver, spleen, and kidneys, and may have mucosal erosions of the stomach or ulcerations of the colon.[168,169] A recent case of starvation was a 7-month-old whose 5-year-old sibling was in charge of feeding her. Her meals consisted of small amounts of adult food found in the home, such as pizza. At autopsy she had a total lack of subcutaneous fat. Usually in starvation cases, the bowel is completely empty. This infant had very firm fibrous fecal material in the distal colon (Figure 23.25).

Findings in fatal starvation are summarized in Box 23.1.

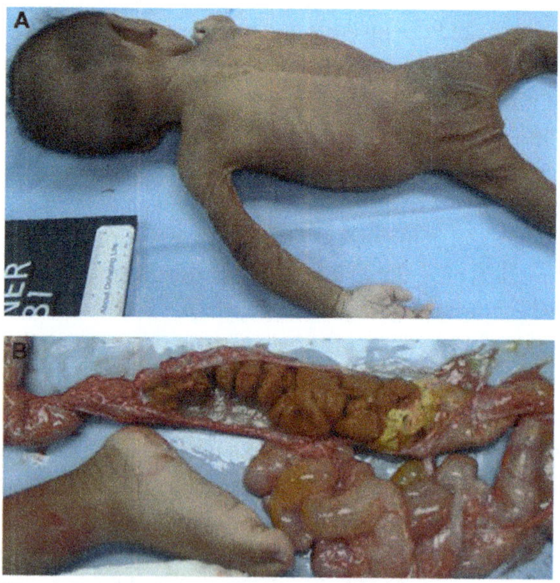

FIGURE 23.25

A, 7-month-old who died from starvation showing lack of fat and muscle; B, distal colon containing firm fibrous fecal material.

BOX 23.1
Gross, Radiographic, and Microscopic Findings in Fatal Starvation

Gross

General emaciation
Prominent joints, facial bones, and ribs
Generalized loss of subcutaneous fat
Muscle atrophy
Temporal wasting
Loss of orbital fat (sunken eyes)
Loss of Bichat fat pad (sunken cheeks)
Redundant skin (especially on thighs, buttocks)
Skin hyperpigmentation or hypopigmentation
Loose, dull, coarse scalp hair
Scalp hair reddish brown, blond, or gray
Edema of limbs, face
Edema of internal organs
Abdominal distention
Empty stomach/small bowel
Small and hard versus mucoid stools
Duodenal stress ulcers
Bowel wall thinning
Decreased organ weights

Radiographic

Delayed bone age
Osteopenia
Nutritional rickets

Microscopic

Fatty infiltration of liver
Atrophic lymph nodes/thymus
Atrophy of brown fat
Decreased size and mass of skeletal muscle fibers
Cardiac myofibrillar degeneration
Atrophy of small bowel mucosa
Decreased white pulp in spleen
Stress involution of adrenals
Hyperkeratosis; epidermal atrophy of skin

Conclusion

Child abuse deaths are relatively common deaths in the medical examiner caseload but are probably the most difficult deaths in terms of certifying the cause and manner of death. All child deaths require extensive investigation of the scene and circumstances, review of the entire medical and family history, and review of all information about the child and family gathered by pediatric consultants and social services. The autopsy contributes valuable information, but the findings can only have meaning when taken in conjunction with all the other historical and investigational information. State statutes often provide medical examiners or coroners access to all information needed to carry out their investigations, including medical records. The need for cooperation among the various agencies that will be involved in the case, including law enforcement, social services, and the juvenile court, as well as those medical professionals who attended or consulted on the child, is paramount. It is not wise for medical professionals to speculate about cause and manner of death in cases that fall under the jurisdiction of the medical examiner or coroner.

If a child death falls under the jurisdiction of the medical examiner or coroner, no further testing or manipulation of the body should occur. Procedures for how to handle the dead are usually part of the hospital's policies and should be familiar to treating medical professionals. It is not advisable to allow the family access to the body for long periods unless supervised by a death investigator or law enforcement representative. While this can be a challenge and risks further trauma to a grieving family, interagency and hospital collaboration on proper policy can be helpful.

Most medical examiners and some coroners are very amenable to postmortem organ and tissue procurement, including in those deaths that are suspected to be from inflicted injury. If the family has given permission to donate, the organ procurement agencies directly contact the medical examiner or coroner. Usually these requests will be allowed by the medical examiner, but this varies by jurisdiction. Organ and tissue procurement should not be considered an impediment in determining the cause and manner of death or in the prosecution of cases of inflicted injury.

References

1. US Department of Health and Human Services; Administration for Children and Families; Administration on Children, Youth and Families; Children's Bureau. *Child Maltreatment 2016*. Washington, DC: US Dept of Health and Human Services; 2018. https://www.acf.hhs.gov/cb/resource/child-maltreatment-2016. Accessed April 9, 2019
2. Parks SE, Annest JL, Hill HA, Karch DL. *Pediatric Abusive Head Trauma: Recommended Definitions for Public Health Surveillance and Research*. Atlanta, GA: Centers for Disease Control and Prevention; 2012

3. Keenan HT, Runyan DK, Marshall SW, Nocera MA, Merten DF, Sinal SH. A population-based study of inflicted traumatic brain injury in young children. *JAMA*. 2003;290(5):621–626 PMID: 12902365 https://doi.org/10.1001/jama.290.5.621
4. Alexander RC, Levitt CJ, Smith W. Abusive head trauma. In: Reece RM, Ludwig S, eds. *Child Abuse: Medical Management and Diagnosis*. 2nd ed. Philadelphia, PA: Lippincott Williams & Wilkins; 2001:47–80
5. Bishop NB. Traumatic brain injury: a primer for primary care physicians. *Curr Probl Pediatr Adolesc Health Care*. 2006;36(9):318–331 PMID: 16996420 https://doi.org/10.1016/j.cppeds.2006.05.004
6. Bruce DA, Zimmerman RA. Shaken impact syndrome. *Pediatr Ann*. 1989;18(8):482–484, 486–489, 492–494 PMID: 2671890 https://doi.org/10.3928/0090-4481-19890801-07
7. Salehi-Had H, Brandt JD, Rosas AJ, Rogers KK. Findings in older children with abusive head injury: does shaken-child syndrome exist? *Pediatrics*. 2006;117(5):e1039–e1044 PMID: 16651283 https://doi.org/10.1542/peds.2005-0811
8. Duhaime AC, Christian CW, Rorke LB, Zimmerman RA. Nonaccidental head injury in infants—the "shaken-baby syndrome." *N Engl J Med*. 1998;338(25):1822–1829 PMID:9632450 https://doi.org/10.1056/NEJM199806183382507
9. Di Maio DJ, Di Maio VS. Neonaticide, infanticide, and child homicide. In: *Forensic Pathology*. 2nd ed. Boca Raton, FL: CRC; 1993
10. Overpeck MD, Brenner RA, Trumble AC, Trifiletti LB, Berendes HW. Risk factors for infant homicide in the United States. *N Engl J Med*. 1998;339(17):1211–1216 PMID: 9780342 https://doi.org/10.1056/NEJM199810223391706
11. Case ME, Graham MA, Handy TC, Jentzen JM, Monteleone JA; National Association of Medical Examiners Ad Hoc Committee on Shaken Baby Syndrome. Position paper on fatal abusive head injuries in infants and young children. *Am J Forensic Med Pathol*. 2001;22(2):112–122 PMID: 11394743 https://doi.org/10.1097/00000433-200106000-00002
12. Case M. Falls from height, physical findings/falls from heights—pediatric. In: Payne-James J, Byard R, eds. *Encyclopedia of Forensic and Legal Medicine*. Oxford: Elsevier; 2015
13. Case ME. Accidental traumatic head injury in infants and young children. *Brain Pathol*. 2008;18(4):583–589 PMID: 18782170 https://doi.org/10.1111/j.1750-3639.2008.00203.x
14. Williams P. Cranial characteristics at different ages. In: William P, ed. *Gray's Anatomy*. 38th ed. New York, NY: Churchill; 1995:607–609
15. Gennarelli TA, Tipperman R, Maxwell WL, Graham DI, Adams JH, Irvine A. Traumatic damage to the nodal axolemma: an early, secondary injury. *Acta Neurochir Suppl (Wien)*. 1993;57:49–52 PMID: 8421954 https://doi.org/10.1007/978-3-7091-9266-5_7
16. Gean AD. *Imaging of Head Trauma*. New York, NY: Raven Press; 1994
17. Cantu RC. Biomechanics of head trauma. In: Cantu RC, ed. *Athletic Head and Spine Injuries*. Philadelphia, PA: WB Saunders; 2000:2–5
18. Duhaime AC, Eppley M, Margulies S, Heher KL, Bartlett SP. Crush injuries to the head in children. *Neurosurgery*. 1995;37(3):401–407 PMID: 7501102 https://doi.org/10.1227/00006123-199509000-00005
19. Prasad MR, Ewing-Cobbs L, Baumgartner J. Crush head injuries in infants and young children: neurologic and neuropsychiatric sequelae. 1999;14(8):496–501 PMID: 10456758
20. Graham DI, McIntosh TK, Maxwell WL, Nicoll JA. Recent advances in neurotrauma. *J Neuropathol Exp Neurol*. 2000;59(8):641–651 PMID: 10952055 https://doi.org/10.1093/jnen/59.8.641
21. Margulies SS, Thibault LE. An analytical model of traumatic diffuse brain injury. *J Biomech Eng*. 1989;111(3):241–249 PMID: 2779190 https://doi.org/10.1115/1.3168373

22. Ommaya AK. Biomechanics of head injury: experimental aspects. In: Ommaya AK, ed. *The Biomechanics of Trauma*. Norwal, CT: Appleton-Century-Crofts; 1985:245–269
23. Ommaya AK, Gennarelli TA. Cerebral concussion and traumatic unconsciousness. Correlation of experimental and clinical observations of blunt head injuries. *Brain*. 1974;97(4):633–654 PMID: 4215541 https://doi.org/10.1093/brain/97.1.633
24. Rivas JJ, Lobato RD, Sarabia R, Cordobés F, Cabrera A, Gomez P. Extradural hematoma: analysis of factors influencing the courses of 161 patients. *Neurosurgery*. 1988;23(1):44–51 PMID: 3173664 https://doi.org/10.1227/00006123-198807000-00010
25. Feldman KW, Bethel R, Shugerman RP, Grossman DC, Grady MS, Ellenbogen RG. The cause of infant and toddler subdural hemorrhage: a prospective study. *Pediatrics*. 2001;108(3):636–646 PMID: 11533330 https://doi.org/10.1542/peds.108.3.636
26. Hymel KP, Rumack CM, Hay TC, Strain JD, Jenny C. Comparison of intracranial computed tomographic (CT) findings in pediatric abusive and accidental head trauma. *Pediatr Radiol*. 1997;27(9):743–747 PMID: 9285736 https://doi.org/10.1007/s002470050215
27. Gennarelli TA, Spielman GM, Langfitt TW, et al. Influence of the type of intracranial lesion on outcome from severe head injury. *J Neurosurg*. 1982;56(1):26–32 PMID: 7054419 https://doi.org/10.3171/jns.1982.56.1.0026
28. Gennarelli TA. Animate models of human head injury. *J Neurotrauma*. 1994;11(4):357–368 PMID: 7837277 https://doi.org/10.1089/neu.1994.11.357
29. Yamashima T, Friede RL. Why do bridging veins rupture into the virtual subdural space? *J Neurol Neurosurg Psychiatry*. 1984;47(2):121–127 PMID: 6707651 https://doi.org/10.1136/jnnp.47.2.121
30. Cheshire EC, Malcomson RDG, Sun P, Mirkes EM, Amoroso JM, Rutty GN. A systematic autopsy survey of human infant bridging veins. *Int J Legal Med*. 2018;132(2):449–461 PMID: 29075919 https://doi.org/10.1007/s00414-017-1714-3
31. Prahlow JA, Rushing EJ, Barnard JJ. Death due to a ruptured berry aneurysm in a 3.5-year-old child. *Am J Forensic Med Pathol*. 1998;19(4):391–394 PMID: 9885938 https://doi.org/10.1097/00000433-199812000-00019
32. Weissgold DJ, Budenz DL, Hood I, Rorke LB. Ruptured vascular malformation masquerading as battered/shaken baby syndrome: a nearly tragic mistake. *Surv Ophthalmol*. 1995;39(6):509–512 PMID: 7660304 https://doi.org/10.1016/S0039-6257(05)80058-X
33. Rambaud C. Bridging veins and autopsy findings in abusive head trauma. *Pediatr Radiol*. 2015;45(8):1126–1131 PMID: 25698365 https://doi.org/10.1007/s00247-015-3285-0
34. Adamsbaum C, Rambaud C. Abusive head trauma: don't overlook bridging vein thrombosis. *Pediatr Radiol*. 2012;42(11):1298–1300 PMID: 22885602 https://doi.org/10.1007/s00247-012-2434-y
35. Cuatico W, Yamamoto R, Howeiler B, Smith R. Spontaneous resolution of subdural hematomas. *J Neurosurg Sci*. 1991;35(3):139–145 PMID: 1774593
36. Dolinskas CA, Zimmerman RA, Bilaniuk LT, Gennarelli TA. Computed tomography of post-traumatic extracerebral hematomas: comparison to pathophysiology and responses to therapy. *J Trauma*. 1979;19(3):163–169 PMID: 458881 https://doi.org/10.1097/00005373-197903000-00006
37. Lee KS, Doh JW, Bae HG, Yun IG. Relations among traumatic subdural lesions. *J Korean Med Sci*. 1996;11(1):55–63 PMID: 8703371 https://doi.org/10.3346/jkms.1996.11.1.55
38. Parent AD. Pediatric chronic subdural hematoma: a retrospective comparative analysis. *Pediatr Neurosurg*. 1992;18(5-6):266–271 PMID: 1476935 https://doi.org/10.1159/000120674
39. Goodell CL, Mealey J Jr. Pathogenesis of chronic subdural hematoma. Experimental studies. *Arch Neurol*. 1963;8(4):429–437 PMID: 13949068 https://doi.org/10.1001/archneur.1963.00460040099009

40. Lee KS, Bae WK, Doh JW, Bae HG, Yun IG. Origin of chronic subdural haematoma and relation to traumatic subdural lesions. *Brain Inj*. 1998;12(11):901–910 PMID: 9839025 https://doi.org/10.1080/026990598121972
41. Haines DE. On the question of a subdural space. *Anat Rec*. 1991;230(1):3–21 PMID: 2064027 https://doi.org/10.1002/ar.1092300103
42. Haines DE, Harkey HL, al-Mefty O. The "subdural" space: a new look at an outdated concept. *Neurosurgery*. 1993;32(1):111–120 PMID: 8421539 https://doi.org/10.1227/00006123-199301000-00017
43. Borzone M, Capuzzo T, Perria C, Rivano C, Tercero E. Traumatic subdural hygromas: a report of 70 surgically treated cases. *J Neurosurg Sci*. 1983;27(3):161–165 PMID: 6663347
44. Murata K. Chronic subdural hematoma may be preceded by persistent traumatic subdural effusion. *Neurol Med Chir (Tokyo)*. 1993;33(10):691–696 PMID: 7505896 https://doi.org/10.2176/nmc.33.691
45. Dierckx RA, Bruyland M, Nuyens Z, Stadnik T, Solheid C, Ebinger G. Non-traumatic subdural hygroma. *Acta Neurol Belg*. 1989;89(5):352–357 PMID: 2517182
46. Mayfrank L, Laborde G, Lippitz B, Reul J. Bilateral chronic subdural haematomas following traumatic cerebrospinal fluid leakage into the thoracic epidural space. *Acta Neurochir (Wien)*. 1993;120(1-2):92–94 PMID: 8434524 https://doi.org/10.1007/BF02001476
47. Kleinman PK, Barnes PD. Head trauma. In: Kleinman PK, ed. *Diagnostic Imaging of Child Abuse*. 2nd ed. St. Louis, MO: Mosby, Inc; 1998
48. Hymel KP, Jenny C, Block RW. Intracranial hemorrhage and rebleeding in suspected victims of abusive head trauma: addressing the forensic controversies. *Child Maltreat*. 2002;7(4):329–348 PMID: 12408245 https://doi.org/10.1177/107755902237263
49. Helfer RE, Slovis TL, Black M. Injuries resulting when small children fall out of bed. *Pediatrics*. 1977;60(4):533–535 PMID: 905018
50. Kravitz H, Driessen G, Gomberg R, Korach A. Accidental falls from elevated surfaces in infants from birth to one year of age. *Pediatrics*. 1969;44(5)(suppl):869–876 PMID: 5375003
51. Lyons TJ, Oates RK. Falling out of bed: a relatively benign occurrence. *Pediatrics*. 1993;92(1):125–127 PMID: 8516057
52. Nimityongskul P, Anderson LD. The likelihood of injuries when children fall out of bed. *J Pediatr Orthop*. 1987;7(2):184–186 PMID: 3558802 https://doi.org/10.1097/01241398-198703000-00014
53. Denton S, Mileusnic D. Delayed sudden death in an infant following an accidental fall: a case report with review of the literature. *Am J Forensic Med Pathol*. 2003;24(4):371–376 PMID: 14634479 https://doi.org/10.1097/01.paf.0000097851.18478.16
54. Sauvageau A, Bourgault A, Racette S. Cerebral traumatism with a playground rocking toy mimicking shaken baby syndrome. *J Forensic Sci*. 2008;53(2):479–482 https://doi.org/10.1111/j.1556-4029.2008.00664.x PMID: 18366585
55. Mortazavi MM, Denning M, Yalcin B, Shoja MM, Loukas M, Tubbs RS. The intracranial bridging veins: a comprehensive review of their history, anatomy, histology, pathology, and neurosurgical implications. *Childs Nerv Syst*. 2013;29(7):1073–1078 PMID: 23456236 https://doi.org/10.1007/s00381-013-2054-3
56. Case ME. Inflicted traumatic brain injury in infants and young children. *Brain Pathol*. 2008;18(4):571–582 PMID: 18782169 https://doi.org/10.1111/j.1750-3639.2008.00204.x
57. Bhardwaj G, Chowdhury V, Jacobs MB, Moran KT, Martin FJ, Coroneo MT. A systematic review of the diagnostic accuracy of ocular signs in pediatric abusive head trauma. *Ophthalmology*. 2010;117(5):983–992.e17 PMID: 20347153 https://doi.org/10.1016/j.ophtha.2009.09.040

58. Kivlin JD. A 12-year ophthalmologic experience with the shaken baby syndrome at a regional children's hospital. *Trans Am Ophthalmol Soc*. 1999;97:545–581 PMID: 10703141
59. Levin A. The ocular findings in child abuse. *American Academy of Ophthalmology Focal Points: Clinical Modules for Ophthalmologists*. 1998;16:1–8,13
60. Levin AV. Ocular manifestations of child abuse. *Pediatr Ophthalmol*. 1990;3:249–265
61. Levin AV. Retinal hemorrhages and child abuse. In: David TJ, ed. *Recent Advances in Paediatrics*. 18th ed. London, England: Churchill Livingston; 2000:151–219
62. Tzioumi D, Oates RK. Subdural hematomas in children under 2 years. Accidental or inflicted? A 10-year experience. *Child Abuse Negl*. 1998;22(11):1105–1112 PMID: 9827315 https://doi.org/10.1016/S0145-2134(98)00093-3
63. Levin AV. Retinal hemorrhage in abusive head trauma. *Pediatrics*. 2010;126(5):961–970 PMID: 20921069 https://doi.org/10.1542/peds.2010-1220
64. Binenbaum G, Mirza-George N, Christian CW, Forbes BJ. Odds of abuse associated with retinal hemorrhages in children suspected of child abuse. *J AAPOS*. 2009;13(3): 268–272 PMID: 19541267 https://doi.org/10.1016/j.jaapos.2009.03.005
65. Maguire SA, Watts PO, Shaw AD, et al. Retinal haemorrhages and related findings in abusive and non-abusive head trauma: a systematic review. *Eye (Lond)*. 2013;27(1):28–36 PMID: 23079748 https://doi.org/10.1038/eye.2012.213
66. Togioka BM, Arnold MA, Bathurst MA, et al. Retinal hemorrhages and shaken baby syndrome: an evidence-based review. *J Emerg Med*. 2009;37(1):98–106 PMID: 19081701 https://doi.org/10.1016/j.jemermed.2008.06.022
67. Christian CW, Taylor AA, Hertle RW, Duhaime AC. Retinal hemorrhages caused by accidental household trauma. *J Pediatr*. 1999;135(1):125–127 PMID: 10393620 https://doi.org/10.1016/S0022-3476(99)70343-4
68. Levin AV. Ophthalmology of shaken baby syndrome. *Neurosurg Clin N Am*. 2002;13(2):201–211, vi PMID: 12391704 https://doi.org/10.1016/S1042-3680(02)00004-9
69. Munger CE, Peiffer RL, Bouldin TW, Kylstra JA, Thompson RL. Ocular and associated neuropathologic observations in suspected whiplash shaken infant syndrome. A retrospective study of 12 cases. *Am J Forensic Med Pathol*. 1993;14(3):193–200 PMID: 8311049 https://doi.org/10.1097/00000433-199309000-00004
70. Greenwald MJ, Weiss A, Oesterle CS, Friendly DS. Traumatic retinoschisis in battered babies. *Ophthalmology*. 1986;93(5):618–625 PMID: 3725321 https://doi.org/10.1016/S0161-6420(86)33688-1
71. Lueder GT, Turner JW, Paschall R. Perimacular retinal folds simulating nonaccidental injury in an infant. *Arch Ophthalmol*. 2006;124(12):1782–1783 PMID: 17159043 https://doi.org/10.1001/archopht.124.12.1782
72. Lantz PE, Sinal SH, Stanton CA, Weaver RG Jr. Perimacular retinal folds from childhood head trauma. *BMJ*. 2004;328(7442):754–756 PMID: 15044292 https://doi.org/10.1136/bmj.328.7442.754
73. Kivlin JD, Currie ML, Greenbaum VJ, Simons KB, Jentzen J. Retinal hemorrhages in children following fatal motor vehicle crashes: a case series. *Arch Ophthalmol*. 2008;126(6):800–804 PMID: 18541842 https://doi.org/10.1001/archopht.126.6.800
74. Moran K, Reddie I, Jacobs M. Severe hemorrhagic retinopathy and traumatic retinoschisis in a 2 year old infant after an 11 meter fall onto concrete. *Acta Paediatr*. 2008;97(suppl 459):149
75. Duhaime AC, Alario AJ, Lewander WJ, et al. Head injury in very young children: mechanisms, injury types, and ophthalmological findings in 100 hospitalized patients younger than 2 years of age. *Pediatrics*. 1992;90(2 Pt 1):179–185 PMID: 1641278
76. Johnson DL, Braun D, Friendly D. Accidental head trauma and retinal hemorrhage. *Neurosurgery*. 1993;33(2):231–235 PMID: 8367044 https://doi.org/10.1227/00006123-199308000-00008

77. Doherty WB, Trubeck M. Significant hemorrhagic retinal lesions in bacterial endocarditis (Roth's spots). *JAMA*. 1931;97(5):308–313 https://doi.org/10.1001/jama.1931.02730050016007
78. Emerson MV, Pieramici DJ, Stoessel KM, Berreen JP, Gariano RF. Incidence and rate of disappearance of retinal hemorrhage in newborns. *Ophthalmology*. 2001;108(1):36–39 PMID: 11150261 https://doi.org/10.1016/S0161-6420(00)00474-7
79. Fraser SG, Horgan SE, Bardavio J. Retinal haemorrhage in meningitis. *Eye (Lond)*. 1995;9(Pt 5):659–660 PMID: 8543098 https://doi.org/10.1038/eye.1995.165
80. Clark RSB, Orr RA, Atkinson CS, Towbin RB, Pang D. Retinal hemorrhages associated with spinal cord arteriovenous malformation. *Clin Pediatr (Phila)*. 1995;34(5):281–283 PMID: 7628174 https://doi.org/10.1177/000992289503400512
81. Lam S, Lam BL. Bilateral retinal hemorrhages from megaloblastic anemia: case report and review of literature. *Ann Ophthalmol*. 1992;24(3):86–90 PMID: 1570927
82. Gayle MO, Kissoon N, Hered RW, Harwood-Nuss A. Retinal hemorrhage in the young child: a review of etiology, predisposed conditions, and clinical implications. *J Emerg Med*. 1995;13(2):233–239 PMID: 7775796 https://doi.org/10.1016/0736-4679(94)00145-6
83. Ganesh A, Jenny C, Geyer J, Shouldice M, Levin AV. Retinal hemorrhages in type I osteogenesis imperfecta after minor trauma. *Ophthalmology*. 2004;111(7):1428–1431 PMID: 15234150 https://doi.org/10.1016/j.ophtha.2003.10.028
84. Kanter RK. Retinal hemorrhage after cardiopulmonary resuscitation or child abuse. *J Pediatr*. 1986;108(3):430–432 PMID: 3950824 https://doi.org/10.1016/S0022-3476(86)80890-3
85. Kramer K, Goldstein B. Retinal hemorrhages following cardiopulmonary resuscitation. *Clin Pediatr (Phila)*. 1993;32(6):366–368 PMID: 8393755 https://doi.org/10.1177/000992289303200610
86. Gilliland MGF, Luckenbach MW. Are retinal hemorrhages found after resuscitation attempts? A study of the eyes of 169 children. *Am J Forensic Med Pathol*. 1993;14(3):187–192 PMID: 8311048 https://doi.org/10.1097/00000433-199309000-00003
87. Binenbaum G, Rogers DL, Forbes BJ, et al. Patterns of retinal hemorrhage associated with increased intracranial pressure in children. *Pediatrics*. 2013;132(2):e430–e434 PMID: 23878052 https://doi.org/10.1542/peds.2013-0262
88. Nonaka A, Kiryu J, Tsujikawa A, et al. Inhibitory effect of ischemic preconditioning on leukocyte participation in retinal ischemia-reperfusion injury. *Invest Ophthalmol Vis Sci*. 2001;42(10):2380–2385 PMID: 11527953
89. Ozbay D, Ozden S, Müftüoğlu S, et al. Protective effect of ischemic preconditioning on retinal ischemia-reperfusion injury in rats. *Can J Ophthalmol*. 2004;39(7):727–732 PMID: 15696762 https://doi.org/10.1016/S0008-4182(04)80066-8
90. Powner MB, Sim DA, Zhu M, et al. Evaluation of nonperfused retinal vessels in ischemic retinopathy. *Invest Ophthalmol Vis Sci*. 2016;57(11):5031–5037 PMID: 27661854 https://doi.org/10.1167/iovs.16-20007
91. Zheng L, Gong B, Hatala DA, Kern TS. Retinal ischemia and reperfusion causes capillary degeneration: similarities to diabetes. *Invest Ophthalmol Vis Sci*. 2007;48(1):361–367 PMID: 17197555 https://doi.org/10.1167/iovs.06-0510
92. Gilliland MG, Luckenbach MW, Chenier TC. Systemic and ocular findings in 169 prospectively studied child deaths: retinal hemorrhages usually mean child abuse. *Forensic Sci Int*. 1994;68(2):117–132 PMID: 7988965 https://doi.org/10.1016/0379-0738(94)90309-3
93. Marshall DH, Brownstein S, Dorey MW, Addison DJ, Carpenter B. The spectrum of postmortem ocular findings in victims of shaken baby syndrome. *Can J Ophthalmol*. 2001;36(7):377–384 PMID: 11794386 https://doi.org/10.1016/S0008-4182(01)80081-8

94. Adams JH, Graham DI, Scott G, Parker LS, Doyle D. Brain damage in fatal non-missile head injury. *J Clin Pathol*. 1980;33(12):1132–1145 PMID: 7451661 https://doi.org/10.1136/jcp.33.12.1132
95. Adams JH, Graham DI, Murray LS, Scott G. Diffuse axonal injury due to nonmissile head injury in humans: an analysis of 45 cases. *Ann Neurol*. 1982;12(6):557–563 PMID: 7159059 https://doi.org/10.1002/ana.410120610
96. Adams JH, Doyle D, Ford I, Gennarelli TA, Graham DI, McLellan DR. Diffuse axonal injury in head injury: definition, diagnosis and grading. *Histopathology*. 1989;15(1):49–59 PMID: 2767623 https://doi.org/10.1111/j.1365-2559.1989.tb03040.x
97. Humphrey JD, Baek S, Niklason LE. Biochemomechanics of cerebral vasospasm and its resolution: I. A new hypothesis and theoretical framework. *Ann Biomed Eng*. 2007;35(9):1485–1497 PMID: 17487586 https://doi.org/10.1007/s10439-007-9321-y
98. Armonda RA, Bell RS, Vo AH, et al. Wartime traumatic cerebral vasospasm: recent review of combat casualties. *Neurosurgery*. 2006;59(6):1215–1225 PMID: 17277684 https://doi.org/10.1227/01.NEU.0000249190.46033.94
99. Sherriff FE, Bridges LR, Sivaloganathan S. Early detection of axonal injury after human head trauma using immunocytochemistry for beta-amyloid precursor protein. *Acta Neuropathol*. 1994;87(1):55–62 PMID: 8140894 https://doi.org/10.1007/BF00386254
100. Geddes JF, Hackshaw AK, Vowles GH, Nickols CD, Whitwell HL. Neuropathology of inflicted head injury in children. I. Patterns of brain damage. *Brain*. 2001;124(Pt 7):1290–1298 PMID: 11408324 https://doi.org/10.1093/brain/124.7.1290
101. Geddes JF, Vowles GH, Hackshaw AK, Nickols CD, Scott IS, Whitwell HL. Neuropathology of inflicted head injury in children. II. Microscopic brain injury in infants. *Brain*. 2001;124(Pt 7):1299–1306 PMID: 11408325 https://doi.org/10.1093/brain/124.7.1299
102. Dawson SL, Hirsch CS, Lucas FV, Sebek BA. The contrecoup phenomenon. Reappraisal of a classic problem. *Hum Pathol*. 1980;11(2):155–166 PMID: 6995266 https://doi.org/10.1016/S0046-8177(80)80136-5
103. Lindenberg R, Freytag E. Morphology of brain lesions from blunt trauma in early infancy. *Arch Pathol*. 1969;87(3):298–305 PMID: 5766255
104. Dias MS, Backstrom J, Falk M, Li V. Serial radiography in the infant shaken impact syndrome. *Pediatr Neurosurg*. 1998;29(2):77–85 PMID: 9792961 https://doi.org/10.1159/000028694
105. Piatt JH Jr, Steinberg M. Isolated spinal cord injury as a presentation of child abuse. *Pediatrics*. 1995;96(4 Pt 1):780–782 PMID: 7567347
106. Parrish R. Isolated cord injury in child abuse [letter]. *Ped Trauma Forensic Newsletter*. 1996
107. Matakas F, Cervos-Navarro J, Schneider H. Experimental brain death. I. Morphology and fine structure of the brain. *J Neurol Neurosurg Psychiatry*. 1973;36(4):497–508 PMID: 4199913 https://doi.org/10.1136/jnnp.36.4.497
108. Barlow K, Thompson E, Johnson D, Minns RA. The neurological outcome of non-accidental head injury. *Pediatr Rehabil*. 2004;7(3):195–203 PMID: 15204571 https://doi.org/10.1080/13638490410001715331
109. Eichelberger MR, Randolph JG. Thoracic trauma in children. *Surg Clin North Am*. 1981;61(5):1181–1197 PMID: 7031929 https://doi.org/10.1016/S0039-6109(16)42540-5
110. Cohle SD, Hawley DA, Berg KK, Kiesel EL, Pless JE. Homicidal cardiac lacerations in children. *J Forensic Sci*. 1995;40(2):212–218 PMID: 7602280 https://doi.org/10.1520/JFS15344J
111. Mozzetti MD, Devin JB, Susselman MS, Lammert GR, Olshaker JS. A pediatric survivor of left ventricular rupture after blunt chest trauma. *Ann Emerg Med*. 1990;19(4):386–389 PMID: 2321824 https://doi.org/10.1016/S0196-0644(05)82341-8

112. Dieter RA III, Anderson AE. Ventricular septal defect caused by nonpenetrating trauma in a 3-year-old child: use of extracorporeal membrane oxygenation in preoperative stabilization. *J Tenn Med Assoc*. 1991;84(10):492–493 PMID: 1758177
113. Merzel DI, Stirling MC, Custer JR. Massive fatal ventricular septal defect due to nonpenetrating chest trauma in a six-year-old boy: the role of early invasive monitoring in an evolving lesion. *Pediatr Emerg Care*. 1985;1(3):138–142 PMID: 3842884 https://doi.org/10.1097/00006565-198509000-00007
114. Cumberland GD, Riddick L, McConnell CF. Intimal tears of the right atrium of the heart due to blunt force injuries to the abdomen. Its mechanism and implications. *Am J Forensic Med Pathol*. 1991;12(2):102–104 PMID: 1882772 https://doi.org/10.1097/00000433-199106000-00003
115. Stein W, Revitch E. Traumatic rupture of the right ventricle—an unusual case. *Am Heart J*. 1942;24(5):703–705 https://doi.org/10.1016/S0002-8703(42)91074-3
116. Smith D, Walker D, Sturridge M. Traumatic left ventricular aneurysm in an 8-year-old child. *Br Heart J*. 1981;45(2):222–224 PMID: 7459180 https://doi.org/10.1136/hrt.45.2.222
117. O'Reilly RJ, Kazenelson G, Spellberg RD. Traumatic pseudoaneurysm of the left ventricle. *Am J Dis Child*. 1970;120(3):252–254 PMID: 5458563
118. Pollak S, Stellwag-Carion C. Delayed cardiac rupture due to blunt chest trauma. *Am J Forensic Med Pathol*. 1991;12(2):153–156 PMID: 1882780 https://doi.org/10.1097/00000433-199106000-00012
119. Rees A, Symons J, Joseph M, Lincoln C. Ventricular septal defect in a battered child. *BMJ*. 1975;1(5948):20–21 PMID: 1120221 https://doi.org/10.1136/bmj.1.5948.20
120. Rosenthal A, Parisi LF, Nadas AS. Isolated interventricular septal defect due to nonpenetrating trauma. *N Engl J Med*. 1970;283(7):338–341 PMID: 4246768 https://doi.org/10.1056/NEJM197008132830704
121. Knapp JF, Sharma V, Wasserman G, Hoover CJ, Walsh I. Ventricular septal defect following blunt chest trauma in childhood: a case report. *Pediatr Emerg Care*. 1986;2(4):242–243 PMID: 3797270 https://doi.org/10.1097/00006565-198612000-00009
122. George DH, Stakiw K, Wright CJ. Fatal accident with weight-lifting equipment: implications for safety standards. *CMAJ*. 1989;140(8):925–926 PMID: 2702529
123. Jebara VA, Acar C, Dervanian P, et al. Traumatic ventricular septal defects. Report of 3 cases with tricuspid valve rupture in 2 cases. *J Cardiovasc Surg (Torino)*. 1992;33(2): 253–255 PMID: 1572889
124. Case ME. Role of the medical examiner in fatal cases of child maltreatment. In: Chadwick DL, Alexander R, Giardino AP, Esernio-Jenssen D, Thackeray JD, eds. *Child Maltreatment*. 4th ed. St. Louis, MO: STM Learning; 2014:299–351
125. Kleinman PK. Bony thoracic. In: Kleinman PK, ed. *Diagnostic Imaging of Child Abuse*. Chicago, IL: Mosby; 1998:110–148
126. Barsness KA, Cha ES, Bensard DD, et al. The positive predictive value of rib fractures as an indicator of nonaccidental trauma in children. *J Trauma*. 2003;54(6):1107–1110 PMID: 12813330 https://doi.org/10.1097/01.TA.0000068992.01030.A8
127. Bulloch B, Schubert CJ, Brophy PD, Johnson N, Reed MH, Shapiro RA. Cause and clinical characteristics of rib fractures in infants. *Pediatrics*. 2000;105(4):E48 PMID: 10742369 https://doi.org/10.1542/peds.105.4.e48
128. Kemp AM, Dunstan F, Harrison S, et al. Patterns of skeletal fractures in child abuse: systematic review. *BMJ*. 2008;337:a1518 PMID: 18832412 https://doi.org/10.1136/bmj.a1518
129. Zumwalt RE, Fanizza-Orphanos AM. Dating of healing rib fractures in fatal child abuse. In: Fenoglio-Presier C, ed. *Advances in Pathology*. St. Louis, MO: Mosby; 1990:193–205

130. Bush CM, Jones JS, Cohle SD, Johnson H. Pediatric injuries from cardiopulmonary resuscitation. *Ann Emerg Med*. 1996;28(1):40–44 PMID: 8669737 https://doi.org/10.1016/S0196-0644(96)70137-3
131. Dolinak D. Rib fractures in infants due to cardiopulmonary resuscitation efforts. *Am J Forensic Med Pathol*. 2007;28(2):107–110 PMID: 17525558 https://doi.org/10.1097/01.paf.0000257392.36528.b8
132. Reyes JA, Somers GR, Taylor GP, Chiasson DA. Increased incidence of CPR-related rib fractures in infants—is it related to changes in CPR technique? *Resuscitation*. 2011;82(5):545–548 PMID: 21353734 https://doi.org/10.1016/j.resuscitation.2010.12.024
133. Vester MEM, Bilo RAC, Nijs HGT, van Rijn RR. Pediatric constrictive asphyxia a rare form of child abuse: a report of two cases. *Forensic Sci Int*. 2018;285:e17–e20 PMID: 29370956 https://doi.org/10.1016/j.forsciint.2018.01.003
134. Wood J, Rubin DM, Nance ML, Christian CW. Distinguishing inflicted versus accidental abdominal injuries in young children. *J Trauma*. 2005;59(5):1203–1208 PMID: 16385300 https://doi.org/10.1097/01.ta.0000196437.07011.b1
135. Kirks DR. Radiological evaluation of visceral injuries in the battered child syndrome. *Pediatr Ann*. 1983;12(12):888–893 PMID: 6657317 https://doi.org/10.3928/0090-4481-19831201-07
136. Ng CS, Hall CM, Shaw DG. The range of visceral manifestations of non-accidental injury. *Arch Dis Child*. 1997;77(2):167–174 PMID: 9301362 https://doi.org/10.1136/adc.77.2.167
137. Huyer D. Abdominal injuries in child abuse. *APSAC Advisor*. 1994;7(3):5–7
138. Kleinman PK, Brill PW, Winchester P. Resolving duodenal-jejunal hematoma in abused children. *Radiology*. 1986;160(3):747–750 PMID: 3488562 https://doi.org/10.1148/radiology.160.3.3488562
139. Cooper A, Floyd T, Barlow B, et al. Major blunt abdominal trauma due to child abuse. *J Trauma*. 1988;28(10):1483–1487 PMID: 3172310 https://doi.org/10.1097/00005373-198810000-00015
140. Kakos GS, Grosfeld JL, Morse TS. Small bowel injuries in children after blunt abdominal trauma. *Ann Surg*. 1971;174(2):238–241 PMID: 5560847 https://doi.org/10.1097/00000658-197108000-00010
141. Ogata M, Tsuganezawa O. An isolated perforation of the jejunum caused by child abuse. A case report. *Am J Forensic Med Pathol*. 1995;16(1):17–20 PMID: 7771376 https://doi.org/10.1097/00000433-199503000-00003
142. Schenk WG III, Lonchyna V, Moylan JA. Perforation of the jejunum from blunt abdominal trauma. *J Trauma*. 1983;23(1):54–56 PMID: 6823001 https://doi.org/10.1097/00005373-198301000-00011
143. Gaines BA, Shultz BS, Morrison K, Ford HR. Duodenal injuries in children: beware of child abuse. *J Pediatr Surg*. 2004;39(4):600–602 PMID: 15065036 https://doi.org/10.1016/j.jpedsurg.2003.12.010
144. Case ME, Nanduri R. Laceration of the stomach by blunt trauma in a child: a case of child abuse. *J Forensic Sci*. 1983;28(2):496–501 PMID: 6864189 https://doi.org/10.1520/JFS11534J
145. Howie SRC. Blood sample volumes in child health research: review of safe limits. *Bull World Health Organ*. 2011;89(1):46–53 PMID: 21346890 https://doi.org/10.2471/BLT.10.080010
146. Price EA, Rush LR, Perper JA, Bell MD. Cardiopulmonary resuscitation-related injuries and homicidal blunt abdominal trauma in children. *Am J Forensic Med Pathol*. 2000;21(4):307–310 PMID: 11111786 https://doi.org/10.1097/00000433-200012000-00001

147. Dye DW, Peretti FJ, Kokes CP. Histologic evidence of repetitive blunt force abdominal trauma in four pediatric fatalities. *J Forensic Sci*. 2008;53(6):1430–1433 PMID: 18808370 https://doi.org/10.1111/j.1556-4029.2008.00883.x
148. Cebelin MS, Hirsch CS. Human stress cardiomyopathy. Myocardial lesions in victims of homicidal assaults without internal injuries. *Hum Pathol*. 1980;11(2):123–132 PMID: 7399504 https://doi.org/10.1016/S0046-8177(80)80129-8
149. Pavin D, Le Breton H, Daubert C. Human stress cardiomyopathy mimicking acute myocardial syndrome. *Heart*. 1997;78(5):509–511 PMID: 9415014 https://doi.org/10.1136/hrt.78.5.509
150. Nichols GR II, Corey TS, Davis GJ. Nonfracture-associated fatal fat embolism in a case of child abuse. *J Forensic Sci*. 1990;35(2):493–499 PMID: 2329342 https://doi.org/10.1520/JFS12853J
151. Moritz AR, Henriques FC. Studies of thermal injury: II. The relative importance of time and surface temperature in the causation of cutaneous burns. *Am J Pathol*. 1947;23(5):695–720 PMID: 19970955
152. King BR. Scald burns should raise the clinician's suspicion for abuse. *Emerg Med News*. 2004;26(11):15–16 https://doi.org/10.1097/00132981-200411000-00012
153. Zumwalt RE, Hirsch CS. Subtle fatal child abuse. *Hum Pathol*. 1980;11(2):167–174 PMID: 7399506 https://doi.org/10.1016/S0046-8177(80)80137-7
154. Gillenwater JM, Quan L, Feldman KW. Inflicted submersion in childhood. *Arch Pediatr Adolesc Med*. 1996;150(3):298–303 PMID: 8603225 https://doi.org/10.1001/archpedi.1996.02170280068013
155. Griest KJ, Zumwalt RE. Child abuse by drowning. *Pediatrics*. 1989;83(1):41–46 PMID: 2909975
156. Meadow R. Suffocation, recurrent apnea, and sudden infant death. *J Pediatr*. 1990;117(3):351–357 PMID: 2391589 https://doi.org/10.1016/S0022-3476(05)81072-8
157. DiMaio VJM. Homicidal asphyxia. *Am J Forensic Med Pathol*. 2000;21(1):1–4 PMID: 10739219 https://doi.org/10.1097/00000433-200003000-00001
158. Southall DP, Stebbens VA, Rees SV, Lang MH, Warner JO, Shinebourne EA. Apnoeic episodes induced by smothering: two cases identified by covert video surveillance. *Br Med J (Clin Res Ed)*. 1987;294(6588):1637–1641 PMID: 3113565 https://doi.org/10.1136/bmj.294.6588.1637
159. Banaschak S, Schmidt P, Madea B. Smothering of children older than 1 year of age-diagnostic significance of morphological findings. *Forensic Sci Int*. 2003;134(2-3):163–168 PMID: 12850412 https://doi.org/10.1016/S0379-0738(03)00135-X
160. Brown TT, Batalis NI, McClain JL, et al. A retrospective study of the investigation of homicidal childhood asphyxia deaths. *J Forensic Sci*. 2018;63(4):1160–1167 PMID: 29044506 https://doi.org/10.1111/1556-4029.13666
161. Krugman SD, Lantz PE, Sinal S, De Jong AR, Coffman K. Forced suffocation of infants with baby wipes: a previously undescribed form of child abuse. *Child Abuse Negl*. 2007;31(6):615–621 PMID: 17617455 https://doi.org/10.1016/j.chiabu.2006.12.012
162. McIntosh BJ, Shanks DE, Whitworth JM. Child abuse by suffocation presenting as hypoxic-ischemic encephalopathy. Report of a patient. *Clin Pediatr (Phila)*. 1994;33(9):561–563 PMID: 8001326 https://doi.org/10.1177/000992289403300909
163. Meadow R. Munchausen syndrome by proxy. *Arch Dis Child*. 1982;57(2):92–98 PMID: 7065720 https://doi.org/10.1136/adc.57.2.92
164. Fish E, Bromfield L, Higgins D. A new name for Munchausen by proxy: defining fabricated or induced illness by carers. *Child Abuse Prev Issues*. 2005;23:2–12

165. Sanders MJ, Bursch B. Forensic assessment of illness falsification, Munchausen by proxy, and factitious disorder, NOS. *Child Maltreat.* 2002;7(2):112–124 PMID: 12020067 https://doi.org/10.1177/1077559502007002003
166. Roesler TA, Jenny C. *Medical Child Abuse: Beyond Munchausen Syndrome by Proxy.* Elk Grove Village, IL: American Academy of Pediatrics; 2008
167. Kellogg ND, Lukefahr JL. Criminally prosecuted cases of child starvation. *Pediatrics.* 2005;116(6):1309–1316 PMID: 16322152 https://doi.org/10.1542/peds.2004-2616
168. Zumwalt RE, Hirsch CS. Pathology of fatal child abuse and neglect. In: Helfer RE, Kempe RS, eds. *The Battered Child.* 4th ed. Chicago, IL: University of Chicago Press; 1987:247–260
169. Winick M, ed. *Hunger Disease: Studies by the Jewish Physicians in the Warsaw Ghetto.* New York, NY: John Wiley & Sons; 1979

CHAPTER 24

SIDS, SUID, and the Child Fatality Review Team Approach to Unexpected Infant Death

Vincent J. Palusci, MD, MS, FAAP
Professor of Pediatrics
New York University School of Medicine
New York, NY

Theresa M. Covington, MPH
Director, Within Our Reach
Alliance for Strong Families and Communities
Washington, DC

Patricia G. Schnitzer, MS, PhD
National Center for Fatality Review and Prevention
Washington, DC

Introduction

Sudden unexpected infant death (SUID) was first described in biblical times, yet there is still confusion about terminology, causation, investigation, and prevention. This chapter summarizes the rapidly changing evidence on unexpected infant deaths to help reduce this ambiguity, defines terminology commonly used to describe the sudden unexpected death of an infant during sleep and the evidence for a diagnostic shift away from the term *sudden infant death syndrome* (SIDS), reviews the epidemiology and current evidence on causes of unexpected infant death and their risk and protective factors, and provides the medical professional with information to help families to provide safe sleep environments and, for those who have experienced the sudden, unexpected loss of a baby, to support the family in the healing process. Information is provided about our current understanding to enhance the likelihood that SUIDs are properly distinguished from maltreatment deaths and review best practices for the multidisciplinary team approach to investigating, understanding, and classifying unexpected infant deaths.

Background

The term *SIDS* was defined in 1969 as "the sudden death of any infant or young child, which is unexpected by history, and in which a thorough postmortem examination fails to demonstrate an adequate cause for death."[1] Twenty years later, the definition was changed by an expert panel convened by the National Institute of Child Health and Human Development (NICHD) to "the sudden death of an infant under one year of age which remains unexplained after a thorough case investigation, including performance of a complete autopsy, examination of the death scene, and review of the clinical history."[2] In the intervening years, thousands of publications have appeared in the medical literature. Biologic mechanisms have been hypothesized and potential risk factors identified in the effort to understand and eliminate SIDS. Confounding the science were numerous stories of multiple SIDS deaths in families that were believed to be the result of apnea but were later found to be homicides.[3] Studies in New Zealand, Australia, and the United Kingdom suggested that non-prone or *supine* sleep could be protective against SIDS. This resulted in prevention initiatives such as the Back to Sleep campaign in the United States in 1992, after which SIDS rates in the United States dramatically declined. This decline stabilized but, since 2000, rates of sudden and unexpected infant deaths have not declined, and it is now thought that the drop in SIDS rate is mostly due to changes in the way deaths are being classified.[4] Improved infant death scene investigations and multidisciplinary case reviews resulted in a diagnostic shift from SIDS to other causes, especially to suffocation and "cause undetermined."[5] Concomitantly, additional research and death scene investigations identified other risk factors in the sleep environment in addition to sleep position. Regardless of the final diagnosis, today as many as 1 in 7 infant deaths and 1 in 3 postneonatal deaths are first attributed to SUID. New strategies are being devised to prevent further deaths by applying what has been learned from basic science, autopsy, scene investigation, and multidisciplinary case reviews.[6]

Definitions

Terminology in the field of SUID has historically been ambiguous, and some terms may overlap or conflict with others. The following definitions are intended to clarify what is meant when each individual term is used;

however, no single, unified system of nomenclature has yet been developed across medical, epidemiological, and forensic systems:

- **Sudden unexpected infant death (SUID):** A sudden and unexpected death, whether later explained or unexplained (including SIDS), occurring before age 1 year and usually occurring in a sleep environment. Sudden unexpected infant death is used to describe a death without obvious cause *but before full investigation.* After investigation, most will be determined to result from 1 of the 3 most frequent types of SUIDs: SIDS, undetermined cause, or accidental suffocation or strangulation in bed.
- **Sudden infant death syndrome (SIDS):** A sudden death of an infant younger than 1 year that remains unexplained *after thorough case investigation,* including performance of a complete autopsy, reenactment of the death scene, and review of the clinical history. Differentiating between SIDS and other SUIDs, such as suffocation, particularly those that occur during an unobserved sleep period, is challenging. The cause of SIDS deaths cannot be determined by autopsy alone and may not be completely resolved after a full case investigation. Specialized techniques, including molecular testing, may be needed to identify previously undiagnosed metabolic and neurologic disorders and cardiac channelopathies.
- **Sudden unexplained death in infancy (SUDI):** A further refinement of SUID to describe a sudden death of an infant younger than 1 year in which investigation, autopsy, medical history review, and appropriate laboratory testing *fail to identify a specific cause* of death. SIDS is one subcategory of an SUDI. Other designations include "undetermined cause." The term *SUDI* has been used interchangeably with SUID in the United Kingdom, but these should not be confused in this chapter.
- **Undetermined infant deaths:** Deaths in which no explanation is found after thorough investigation but for which scene investigation of 10 critical infant sleep environment components[7] does not rule out the possibility that there may be other causes of death, such as asphyxia from hazards in the sleep environment or intentional suffocation.
- **Accidental strangulation or suffocation in bed:** Suffocation, asphyxia, or strangulation when an infant's airway is blocked while in a sleeping environment (eg, from soft bedding, overlay, wedging or entrapment, strangulation).

- **Sleep-related infant death:** Death that occurs during an observed or unobserved sleep period and/or in a sleep environment before cause of death is identified.
- **Child abuse fatality:** The death of an infant or child that is found to be caused by non-accidental trauma and/or that results from one or more forms of neglect, such as malnutrition, dehydration, exposure to the elements, or supervisional or medical care neglect. A more inclusive term is *child maltreatment fatality.* This term may be applied for public health, child death review, or prevention purposes when it is determined that abuse or neglect contributed to a death, but this contribution does not necessarily meet the standard for a medicolegal determination of homicide or for verification of maltreatment by child protective services (CPS).

Epidemiology

Sudden unexpected infant death is the leading cause of postneonatal infant mortality in the United States.[8] One in 3 postneonatal deaths are first attributed to SUID, and sleep-related deaths occur most frequently between 2 and 4 months of age.[9] Fewer than 5% occur during the first month after birth, and after 4 months, the rate decreases progressively such that 90% occur by the age of 6 months. Sudden unexpected infant death initially includes cases of SIDS and SUDI, as well as other causes such as suffocation and strangulation in bed and occult medical causes. In 2013, SIDS and SUID accounted for 39.7 and 87.0 deaths per 100,000 live births, respectively. Since 2000, SIDS rates have remained relatively stable in vital statistics (93.4 per 100,000 live births), but there has been a concomitant increase in suffocation and undetermined causes of death.

SIDS and SUID rates for African American infants (73.3 and 172.5, respectively) and American Indian/Alaskan Native infants (78.3 and 169.6, respectively) remain more than twice those of white infants.[9–12] Deaths have occurred more frequently during the fall and winter months in the northern and southern hemispheres, suggesting that temperature alone is not a causative factor. SIDS rates in Native Americans residing in the northern United States are higher than those in the southwestern part of the country, possibly because of the high prevalence of smoking among the former. The higher prevalence of other SIDS risk factors, such as smoking and bed sharing (ie, an infant sleeping in the same bed or on the same surface with another person or an animal) may account for the higher SIDS rates in Native Americans compared with whites. This differs from *co-sleeping,* which refers to an infant sleeping in the same room as the caregiver(s). Co-sleeping has been associated with decreased SIDS rates. Others have suggested that genetic differences in alcohol metabolism and alcohol abuse may contribute to higher apparent SIDS rates, and that SIDS rates and socioeconomic status are inversely related, with socioeconomic status acting as a confounder, effect modifier, or intermediate variable.[11] More recently, Parks et al[12] suggested that variations in SIDS rates based on race and ethnicity over the past 2 decades are likely driven by changes in known risk factors. As evidence, they note that when significant decreases in soft bedding use occurred across all races in 1993 through 2000, SIDS rates declined for all races. When there were further improvements in safe sleep practices during 2001 through 2010 for white and Hispanic infants, their SIDS rates continued to decline. However, SIDS rates did not decline among black infants, whose safe sleep practices did not improve.

The Diagnostic Shift

As mentioned previously, SIDS rates have remained relatively stable in vital statistics since 2000 (93.4 per 100,000 live births), but there has been a concomitant increase in suffocation and undetermined causes (Figure 24.1). Between 1984 and 2004, infant mortality rates attributed to accidental suffocation and strangulation in bed increased from 2.8 to 12.5 deaths per 100,000 live births. These rates had remained relatively stagnant between 1984 and 1992, and then increased between 1992 and 2004; the most dramatic increase occurred between 1996 and 2004. In contrast, total SUID rates remained stagnant between 1996 and 2004, whereas the proportion of deaths attributed to SIDS declined and that attributed to unknown cause increased.[4] It is widely believed that there has not been an actual increase in SUID but that forensic professionals moved away from SIDS as a diagnostic category—a *diagnostic shift,* with increasing acceptance of findings of SUDI, suffocation, and undetermined causes of death. It is believed that this shift resulted from improved death investigations, a better understanding of sleep environment risk factors, and multidisciplinary case review teams.[5,13] In some jurisdictions, the use of the term *SIDS* has been abandoned altogether in favor of *undetermined* and/or *suffocation.*[14] This shift has made it difficult to understand the true epidemiology of SUID because standards vary so much across jurisdictions. In more recent research, some investigators still study only the diagnosis of SIDS, while others study sleep-related deaths or SUIDs. Risk factors may overlap, and it can be hard to discern relationships of these factors to the different types of SUIDs without carefully looking at the details of the study population included.

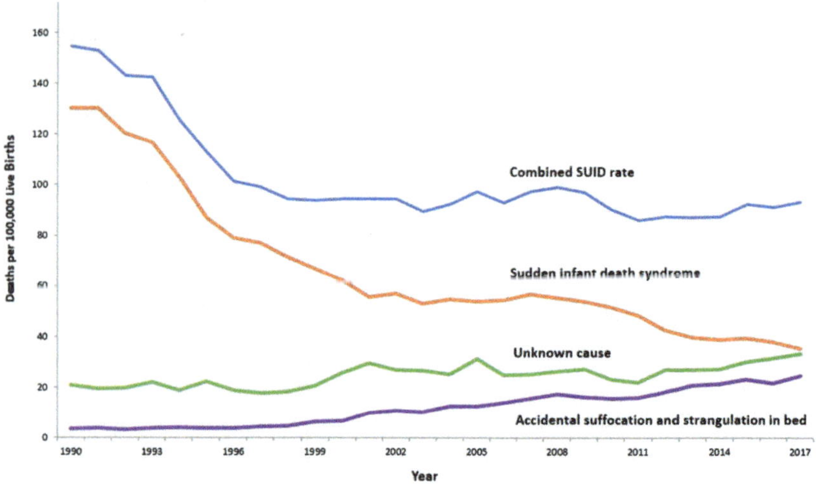

FIGURE 24.1
Trends in sudden unexpected infant death by cause, 1990–2017.
From Centers for Disease Control and Prevention. Sudden unexpected infant death and sudden infant death syndrome: data and statistics. https://www.cdc.gov/sids/data.htm. Reviewed April 10, 2019. Accessed August 7, 2019.

The diagnostic shift has also had an effect on families affected by SUID and on professionals who care for them, including pediatricians who provide services to these family members. Traditionally, families who had experienced SIDS were told that, although the cause was unknown, the syndrome of SIDS likely had a biological cause and the death was not preventable. Today, while better identifying the actual cause of death for vital statistics and prevention, a diagnosis of undetermined or suffocation offers little solace and does not convey either of these possibilities. Crandall et al[15] found that families who were provided a diagnosis other than SIDS reported more detrimental effects, including mental health, negative perceptions of the health field, and increased frustration. Conversely, parents who were given a SIDS diagnosis reported less confusion and higher positive effects.

Case Presentation, Pathology, and Investigation

Thorough death investigations are necessary to identify the causes of SUID. In the absence of postmortem examination, investigation of the circumstances of death, and case review, child maltreatment may be missed, familial genetic diseases may go unrecognized, public health threats are overlooked, inadequate medical care goes undetected, product-safety issues remain unidentified, and progress in understanding the causes and mechanisms of SIDS/SUDI and other causes of unexpected infant death is delayed.

Presentation

The typical presentation of an infant who has died suddenly and unexpectedly is the discovery of an infant who had been fed, put down to sleep, and found later to not be breathing. No outcry indicating distress is typically heard from the infant, and the death is unwitnessed. Infants are reported to be either in the same position as when placed, to have shifted within their sleep space, or to have flipped over. When first discovered unresponsive, some infants show clenching of the fists, occasionally with clutched blanket fibers. Pink, frothy, and/or mucoid oronasal secretions are often reported, but the description of frank blood is very uncommon. Lividity and rigor mortis are not uncommon. Emergency personnel are usually contacted and often initiate cardiopulmonary resuscitation (CPR) in the home and continue these measures until reaching the hospital, where the infant is pronounced dead.

Pathology

An autopsy supplemented by review of the clinical history and circumstances of death is essential in determining the cause and manner of SUID and in making a diagnosis of SIDS.[16] Kumar and colleagues[17] found that a new diagnosis was made at autopsy in 34% of 107 postneonatal infant deaths when these cases were reviewed, with complete concordance seen in only 66%. To address these inconsistencies in SUIDs, autopsy reporting protocols have evolved over time. A standardized protocol for SUID classification[18] was endorsed by the Society for Pediatric Pathology, the National Association of Medical Examiners, and the SIDS Global Strategy Task Force. This protocol, commonly known as the San Diego guidelines, prompts a checklist-guided recording of positive and negative observations required to reach a diagnosis in SUIDs. It also encourages narrative descriptions of abnormalities, supplemented by microscopic, microbiological, and toxicological analyses, and the use of radiographic and photographic imaging. In 2003, an international meeting in Oslo of forensic and pediatric pathologists led to consensus on the diagnostic criteria for SUID and for findings that would exclude the diagnosis of SIDS through cardiac and lung pathology and in genetic and metabolic disorder findings.[19]

To establish a diagnosis of SIDS, autopsy findings should be negative even though some nonspecific findings will be observed. Minor abnormalities that should not be considered lethal are common in SIDS and should not alter the diagnosis. Reddish-blue mottling of the skin indicative of postmortem lividity may occur in dependent portions of the body. The blood in the heart is liquid and often oozes from venipuncture sites. The bladder and rectum are empty. A variety of reported subtle but nonlethal anomalies are neither diagnostic nor specific.[20] Oronasal secretions are observed frequently in SIDS, but oronasal blood is uncommonly reported. In the San Diego SIDS/Sudden Unexplained Death in Childhood (SUDC) Research Project database, some type of oronasal secretion was described in 155 (38%) of 406 cases of sudden infant death.[21] Oronasal blood was described in only 28 (7%) of 406 cases of sudden infant death and could not be attributed to CPR in 14 cases, including 10 (3%) of 300 SIDS cases, 2 (14%) of 14 accidental suffocation cases, and 2 (15%) of 13 undetermined cases.

Intrathoracic petechiae are the most common abnormality seen macroscopically and are identified in more than 80% of SIDS cases.[22] Observations in human postmortem examinations suggest that petechiae limited to the thorax can result from attempting to breathe against an obstructed upper airway in the moments preceding death.[23] However, facial and conjunctival petechiae are exceedingly rare in SIDS cases, and their presence should provoke a search for another cause of death. The relationship between intrathoracic petechiae and a facedown position has also been studied. In the San Diego SIDS/SUDC Research Project database, 36.7% of infants were found with their faces straight down.[21] The severity of intrathoracic petechiae, whether measured by the number of involved intrathoracic organs or by the extent of thymic involvement, was also similar between facedown and other positions.

The lungs in infants who had died of SIDS are congested and variably edematous but not consolidated. Pneumonia evidenced by pulmonary consolidation is not seen with the naked eye, and microscopic interstitial lymphocytic infiltration of the lungs is common but is mild and not to be considered lethal.[24] Occasionally there are mild interstitial lymphocytic infiltrates within the epicardium and/or myocardium, but a diagnosis of myocarditis is precluded by the absence of myocardial necrosis as defined by the Dallas criteria.[25] Molecular autopsy procedures, however, are identifying increasingly more cardiac causes of death, such as channelopathies.[26]

Investigation

Thorough investigation is critical to determining the cause of SUID. For an expanded discussion on improving investigation, the National Center for Fatality Review and Prevention has a publicly available program manual for child death review.[27]

Scene Where the Death Incident Occurred

To address inaccuracies in identifying the cause of death, a comprehensive scene investigation is an essential part of a complete and thorough infant death investigation.[28] There have been major improvements in the quality of SUID scene investigations over the past 20 years, in part because of highly publicized cases in which SIDS deaths were later found to be homicides.[4,29] In addition, in 1996, the US Centers for Disease Control and Prevention (CDC) issued national guidelines for death scene investigation of SUIDs.[30] The CDC followed this release with a national training academy on infant death scene investigation. Many states have adopted the guidelines in full or to their existing investigation protocols. A major change in practice promoted by these guidelines is the performance of a doll reenactment in the sleep environment to help death certifiers determine if suffocation was a possibility.

Health Records of Infant

A review of the infant's health history and status at the time of death should be conducted. It is typical that infants in SUID cases had a minor upper respiratory infection, gastroesophageal symptoms, or fever but not of such a serious nature to have suggested that sudden death was imminent. Historically, upper respiratory infections have been thought to occur at rates similar to those of controls, but gastrointestinal symptoms are slightly more common. Many studies have shown that the risk of SIDS is not increased after diphtheria, tetanus, and pertussis immunization and that any association is coincidental rather than causal.[31,32]

Family Health History

When repetitive, sudden, and unexpected infant deaths occur within a sibship, there should be a thorough evaluation to exclude or confirm conditions that can reoccur in families, such as inborn errors of metabolism, cardiac channelopathies, environmental toxins, unsafe sleep practices, and homicide. While the others are being considered, an analysis of blood and bile may facilitate diagnosis of a fatal inborn error of metabolism. Blood tests for evaluation of many metabolic disorders are now available at low cost. Many medical examiners routinely screen all infants who have experienced SUID for inborn errors of metabolism at autopsy. If an inborn error of metabolism is suspected by autopsy findings (eg, hepatic steatosis) or history (eg, previous unexpected deaths in childhood in the family), the forensic pathologist may elect to retain additional tissues for further analysis, pending the results of the postmortem metabolic screening. Identification of a possible index case warrants referral of the family for comprehensive genetic counseling and additional testing. Whenever the medical examiner is unable to demonstrate an adequate reason for death, a blood sample should be retained for potential future analysis, especially to determine potential genetic disorders.

Team Approach

Current best practices suggest multidisciplinary investigations that bring together law enforcement, emergency medical services, medical examiners/coroners, CPS, prosecutors, and others to ensure a comprehensive investigation.[28] Personnel on first-response teams should be trained to make observations at the scene, including position of the infant, marks on the body, pattern and distribution of livor mortis, body temperature and rigor, type of bed or crib and any defects, amount and position of clothing and bedding, room temperature, type of ventilation and heating, the presence of drugs or alcohol, and reaction of the caregivers. Medics and emergency department personnel should be trained to distinguish normal findings, such as postmortem anal dilation and lividity, from trauma attributable to abuse.

There are, however, continuing challenges to the quality of investigations. Hanzlick[33] listed several, including regional variations in death investigation requirements, lack of peer review, lack of specified standards, credentialing inconsistencies, variations in coroner and/or medical examiner systems, inadequate funding, personnel shortages, lack of government interest, legal influences on medical decisions, and operation of medical examiner/coroner offices outside health care delivery systems. Despite the development of best practices, there is still wide variability in investigation practices across the United States. A recent study analyzed autopsy and death scene investigation data, including key information about the infant sleep environment from 770 SUIDs.[7] The authors found that most deaths (98%) had a death scene investigation that included a narrative description of the circumstances (90%) and witness interviews (88%). Critical information about 10 infant sleep environment components was available for 85% of all SUIDs for all states combined. All 770 deaths had an autopsy performed, which typically included histology, microbiology, other pathology (98%), and toxicology (97%).

These variations extend to case determination as well. In a nationally representative survey in 2014, US medical examiners and coroners were asked to classify SUIDs based on hypothetical scenarios and to describe the evidence considered and investigative procedures used for cause-of-death determination.[34] Among 377 surveys, medical examiners' and coroners' classification of infant deaths varied by scenario. Reliance on investigative procedures to determine cause varied, but 94% indicated using death scene investigations, 88% full autopsy, 85% toxicology analyses, and 82% medical history review. The authors concluded that US medical examiners and coroners apply variable practices to classify and investigate SUID and, thus, they may certify the same deaths differently. This variability influences surveillance and research, affects true understanding of infant mortality causes, and inhibits the ability to accurately monitor and ultimately prevent future deaths.

Causes and Risk Factors for Sudden Infant Death

Almost all of the research on sudden infant deaths has focused specifically on deaths categorized as SIDS. Despite many years of research in the United States and in other countries, the underlying cause of SIDS remains unknown. The *triple risk model* is widely accepted as a way to interpret the 3 factors that appear to interact simultaneously to lead to a SIDS event. These are (1) an underlying physiological vulnerability; (2) an exogenous or environmental stressor (eg, prone sleep position, bed sharing, smoking); and (3) a critical developmental period (the first 6 postnatal months).[35] However, the major differences in investigative and diagnostic reporting practices in the United States among states, jurisdictions, and sometimes even within the same office continue to make it difficult to discern true differences in classification of death as SIDS, undetermined, suffocation, and other SUID causes. It is also difficult to understand the risk factors in each type of SUID and to measure whether efforts to reduce risk factors are successful for specific types of SUID, as most of the research to date has focused only on deaths classified as SIDS.

Much of the research on key underlying physiological vulnerabilities has focused on brain stem abnormalities. Numerous mechanisms have been suggested, but it is generally believed that alterations in the brain stem of vulnerable infants affect arousal mechanisms when an infant is in a hypoxic environment. It has been reported that immature cardiorespiratory autonomic control and failure of arousal responsiveness from sleep are important factors.[36] One study found that more than 40% of infants in a group who died of SIDS had an abnormality in serotonin in brain stem regions critical for homeostatic regulation.[37] Gene polymorphisms relating to serotonin transport and autonomic nervous system development might make affected infants more vulnerable to SIDS.[38] It has also been suggested that genetic mutations associated with cardiac rhythm disturbances such as prolonged QT syndrome, catecholaminergic ventricular paroxysmal tachycardia, and others are responsible for up to 10% of SUIDs.[39,40] Based on these and other studies, it is likely that at least 2% of SUID cases have an identifiable channel defect that may lead to a fatal arrhythmia. The American Academy of Pediatrics (AAP) Task Force on SIDS[41] describes additional research showing other possible physiological associations to SIDS, such as polymorphisms or mutations in genes pertinent to the embryologic origin of the autonomic nervous system or in genes regulating inflammation, energy production, and hypoglycemia.

Exogenous or environmental risk factors for SIDS, suffocation, and undetermined deaths have been identified through epidemiological studies, with most being found to be related to the infant sleep environment. A number of risk and protective factors have been identified (Box 24.1).

A number of meta-analyses have been conducted by the Physiology and Epidemiology working groups of the International Society for the Study and Prevention of Perinatal and Infant Death,[42] and the AAP[41] has developed an evidence base for its updated 2016 guidelines that describe a wide array of risk and protective factors. Numerous studies have found that the risk of SIDS increases as the number of risk factors increases. For example, bed sharing is more hazardous if the caregiver is a smoker and drinks before sleep.[43]

Many studies of SIDS from New Zealand, Australia, Western Europe, Hong Kong, and the United States have found that being placed prone to sleep significantly increases an infant's risk for SIDS.[44,45] Other sleep environment risk factors for SIDS were first identified in the United States through the Chicago Infant Mortality study between 1993 and 1996.[46]

BOX 24.1
Risk and Protective Factors for Sudden Infant Death Syndrome

Risk Factors

- Prone and side positions for infant sleep
- Soft bedding (eg, blankets, pillows, comforters, crib bumpers) and sleep surfaces and objects in a sleep environment
- Non-crib sleep surfaces (eg, couches, adult beds, car seats)
- Bed sharing
- Overheating
- Prenatal and postnatal smoke exposure

Protective Factors

- Pacifier use at sleep time
- Room sharing without bed sharing

Since then, a few studies have tried to expand those risks to all SUID. For example, Schnitzer et al[47] found that only 25% of infants who experienced SUID were sleeping in a crib or on their back when found and 70% were on a surface not intended for infant sleep (eg, adult bed). Importantly, 64% of infants were sharing a sleep surface, and almost half of these infants were sleeping with an adult. Infants whose deaths were classified as suffocation or with undetermined cause were significantly more likely than infants whose deaths were classified as SIDS to be found on a surface not intended for infant sleep and to be sharing that sleep surface.

Bed sharing (sharing a sleep surface with another person or an animal) has emerged as significant risk factor for SIDS and SUID, and a meta-analysis of 11 studies of only SIDS found bed sharing to significantly increase the risk for SIDS.[48] Bed sharing continues to generate controversy, however, between breastfeeding advocates (who believe that bed sharing promotes maternal-infant bonding) and epidemiologists and forensic pathologists (whose concerns center on risk factors that increase the risk for SIDS).[49] However, the AAP, which strongly supports breastfeeding, has recommended that infants are safest when sleeping separately.[9] These recommendations for safe infant sleep environments include evidence that room sharing, as opposed to bed sharing, is protective against SIDS through the first postnatal year.[45]

Cigarette smoking has emerged as an even more important risk factor for SIDS as the supine sleep position has replaced the prone position, and maternal smoking before and/or during gestation and after delivery all increase the risk of SIDS.[43,50] At postmortem examination, pericardial levels of cotinine, a nicotine metabolite, are higher in SIDS cases than in controls.[51]

Descriptions of infants being overdressed, overwrapped, hot, and sweaty when discovered dead have prompted the suggestion that overheating and hyperthermia may be important risk factors of SIDS.[52,53] Elevated ambient temperatures have been associated with apnea in preterm babies, suggesting that apnea might occur in older infants with increased body temperatures. Observations from these studies suggest that thermal stress may be important in SIDS as a result of its adverse effect on arousal, gasping, and laryngeal chemoreflex.

An increasing body of literature suggests that pacifier use can reduce the risk of SIDS. A meta-analysis of 7 published case-control studies calculated summary odds ratios for "usual" and "last sleep" pacifier use and SIDS risk.[54] The odds ratios for pacifier use with "usual" and during "last sleep" were 0.71 and 0.39, respectively.

Differentiating Unexplained Infant Deaths From Child Abuse

When an infant dies unexpectedly, a fundamental goal of investigation is to determine if the death was natural or nonnatural and, if the latter, whether inflicted or noninflicted.[55] The AAP and the National Association of Medical Examiners endorse the universal performance of autopsies on infants who die suddenly and unexpectedly by forensic pathologists experienced in the evaluation of infant death. When Emery et al[56] reviewed the autopsy findings of 60 infant deaths registered as SIDS between 1974 and 1985 in Madison, WI, they found that 10 of those infants had medical diagnoses suggestive of abuse sufficient to explain their deaths. This high rate (17%) had not been seen in other such analyses and called into question the criteria for the SIDS diagnosis. It is difficult, if not impossible, to distinguish among SIDS and accidental or deliberate suffocation because internal injuries cannot be discerned by an external examination.[57,58] There is no anatomic or microscopic feature that is pathognomonic for asphyxial death. Instead, pathologists rely on the investigation, including confessions and witness statements, doll reenactments, and other evidence from the scene. In most cases, the final cause and manner of death rulings of accidental or intentional injuries are dependent on statements or confession by the perpetrator. However, the roles of histology and scene reconstruction cannot be overemphasized.[59] The failure to differentiate fatal child abuse or other causes of death from SIDS/SUDI is costly, and inaccurate vital statistics can lead to inappropriate allocation of limited health care resources. When a cause is not found, a diagnosis of SIDS or undetermined reflects the clear admission that an infant's death remains unexplained.

Epidemiology of Fatal Child Abuse

The US Commission to Eliminate Child Abuse and Neglect Fatalities[60] highlighted the continuing under-ascertainment of child abuse fatalities. Christoffel et al[61] examined 43 unexpected deaths in children brought to Children's Memorial Hospital in Chicago, IL, from 1980 to 1981. Nine of those deaths were the result of child abuse, and in 3 cases the correct diagnosis was established only by postmortem examination. The 2 factors having the highest predictive value for child abuse were the patient being dead on arrival and being younger than 1 year. An interesting observation, however, was that this study included 6 infants who were dead on arrival and who were in the appropriate age group (1–7 months of age) and yet, when subjected to postmortem examination, the results in every instance were consistent with SIDS. In the same journal issue, Kirschner and Stein[62] described 10 cases in which the diagnosis of child abuse was assigned on the basis of incomplete or erroneous medical observation and interpretations (eg, lividity, postmortem anal sphincter dilation, Mongolian blue spots being confused with traumatic lesions). Five of these cases were subsequently diagnosed as SIDS. Both of these articles underscore the need for appropriate evaluation of premortem and postmortem variables for all unwitnessed fatalities.

After studying the problem of infant deaths in Sheffield, England, for more than 25 years, Emery[63] concluded, "Filicide is the probable mechanism of death in approximately 1 in 10 of the unexplained unexpected deaths." Adelson[64] reported details of 46 child homicides in Cuyahoga County, OH, from 1944 to 1960. Ten of the infants were younger than 1 year. Of those, 5 drowned and 3 died of starvation. The cause of death of the other 2 was unknown. Adelson concluded, "Failure to perform autopsies on infants found dead (or said to have been found dead) because they are 'crib deaths'...will inevitably result in the missing of many cases of this type of homicide." Emery and Taylor[65] described a 24-year period in Sheffield, England, during which postperinatal deaths (birth–2 years) were investigated by gathering information about the death scene, obstetric and pediatric care, and autopsy findings and by conducting home visits. Accidental suffocation was thought to be the cause of death in 10% of these cases, and the possibility of active intervention on the part of 1 or both parents was raised in another 10%, a rate consistently double that of overt child abuse in this age group.

It has been suggested that a significant proportion of SUID cases are intentional,[66–68] but the actual percentage of undiagnosed infanticides within the SIDS group is unknown and will probably remain so for the foreseeable future. Asch[69] hypothesized that many cases of sudden infant death were "infanticides, perpetrated by the mother as a specific manifestation of a postpartum depression."

Characteristics of Fatal Child Abuse Cases

It is important to summarize characteristics of these infant fatalities for comparison with SIDS and other forms of SUID. Sidebotham[70] has characterized these deaths among infants as "covert filicide" or "deaths related to, but not directly caused by maltreatment" when maltreatment cannot be determined to be the cause of death. Differentiating child maltreatment in such cases can be challenging.[71] Historically, most overt child abuse fatalities have been associated with certain injuries found on autopsy. Caffey[72] published his seminal article on multiple fractures and subdural hematomas, and Silverman[73] postulated that such injuries were the result of unrecognized trauma. Adelson[64] added factual information about fatal child abuse. Kempe et al[74] coined the phrase *battered child syndrome* and further raised the consciousness of the medical community about the unpleasant truth that infants and children were being physically abused and killed by their parents. Postmortem findings in cases of fatal child abuse included intracranial injuries (diffuse axonal injury, subdural hematoma), abdominal trauma (eg, liver laceration, hollow viscous perforation, intramural hematoma), burns, or drowning.[75–77] It is also critical to distinguish signs of resuscitation and postmortem changes in SIDS/SUID from non-accidental trauma.[58,71,78] Recently, the US Commission to Eliminate Child Abuse and Neglect Fatalities[60] made a number of recommendations to improve child fatality identification and prevention from a number of causes.

Intentional Suffocation

Intentional suffocation is difficult to distinguish from accidental suffocation, SIDS, and other causes. Only a thorough forensic autopsy and testing, a scene investigation, and caregiver interviews will help distinguish between all possible causes of death. The medical community, which had historically repressed the concept of caregivers harming their children, was being educated by new information describing child abuse when Waneta Hoyt in upstate New York was charged with suffocating 5 of her children, all of whom had their deaths initially attributed to SIDS. Two of these children were among 5 cases included in a report by Steinschneider,[79] who postulated that SIDS was the result of prolonged apnea using these 2 deaths from SIDS as examples of this disorder. Firstman and Talan[3,29] skillfully analyzed this case, the implications it had for the SIDS research community, and the effect that it had on medical professionals and many of their patient families. For those parents who had lost babies to SIDS, and for many medical professionals, even the suggestion that some SIDS deaths were actually child murders was painful and unacceptable.

When Meadow[80] reviewed cases of young children suffocated by their mothers, he found 24 of 27 children had histories of previous episodes of apnea, cyanosis, or seizure, and 11 had experienced 10 or more episodes either invented or caused by their mothers. Eighteen of the children were alive, and 9 were dead. In the families of these 27 children, there were 15 older living siblings and 18 who had died suddenly and unexpectedly, 13 of whom had histories of recurrent apnea, cyanosis, or seizures, and most had been certified as SIDS. Meadow drew the distinction between the features seen in this group of suffocated infants and in infants dying of SIDS (Table 24.1).

TABLE 24.1
Features Present in Infants Who Were Intentionally Suffocated and Infants Who Experienced Sudden Infant Death Syndrome

Features	Suffocation (%)	SIDS (%)
Previous apnea	90	<10
Previous unexplained disorder	44	<5
>6 mo	55	<15
Dead sibling	48	2

Abbreviation: SIDS, sudden infant death syndrome.
Reprinted from Meadow R. Suffocation, recurrent apnea, and sudden infant death. *J Pediatr.* 1990;117(3):351–357, copyright 1990, with permission from Elsevier.

Medical Child Abuse (Munchausen Syndrome by Proxy)

Some intentional suffocation deaths and/or descriptions of infants with multiple apneic episodes have been associated with what was first described by Meadow[81] as Munchausen syndrome by proxy, a form of child abuse in which parents induce or report illness in their child with bizarre symptoms and signs without medical explanation. Because parent-induced apnea may be a lethal manifestation, it is now in the differential diagnosis when brief resolved unexplained events (BRUEs) are being evaluated.[82] Berger[83] reported 2 cases of child abuse simulating "near-miss" SIDS. The first case involved a 5-month-old girl who had a history of apnea and cyanotic spells and was extensively evaluated in the hospital for 5 weeks. During unwitnessed bathing of the infant by the mother, the mother ran out of the bathroom calling for help, and the infant was found cyanotic and limp, with bleeding gums and fresh pinch marks on her nose. The second case was a 6-week-old girl with apnea and cyanosis, also hospitalized for several weeks, who had "spells" only when her mother visited. On one of those visits, the mother was discovered holding her hand over the infant's nose and mouth.

Rosen et al[84] reported 2 siblings with recurrent cardiorespiratory arrest who, when removed from the care of the mother, stopped having the episodes. In a later study, Rosen et al[85] described 6 infants referred for evaluation of recurrent infant apnea requiring multiple resuscitation efforts. In 2 cases, the mothers were proven by means of video surveillance to be the perpetrators of the apneic episodes. In a third, the mother had an overt psychiatric disorder. For these 3 infants, the apneic episodes stopped when they were placed with other caregivers. The 3 other infants died within 1 month of leaving the hospital.

Southall et al[86] were able to document what was occurring when they first reported 2 cases of apneic episodes induced by smothering that were detected by covert video surveillance. In 1997, Southall et al reported experience with 39 children referred for evaluation.[87] While in the hospital, the children, ranging in age from 2 to 44 months, were studied by means of covert video surveillance. Thirty-six had been referred for apparent life-threatening events (ALTEs [now known as BRUEs]), 1 for suspected seizure disorder, 1 for failure to thrive, and 1 for suspected strangulation.[82] The number of BRUEs reported by the parents ranged from 2 to more than 50. Forty-six children constituted a control group and were being investigated for BRUEs due to proven medical conditions. Covert video surveillance was accomplished by placing a video camera in each corner of the patients' rooms with a microphone in the ceiling. The infants and children underwent continuous monitoring of transcutaneous oxygen saturation with pulse oximetry and monitoring of breathing movements and electrocardiography. The median time of surveillance was 29 hours. In 30 cases, covert video surveillance revealed attempts at intentional suffocation of the infant. Frank oronasal hemorrhage was reported in 11 of 38 patients with BRUEs but none of the 46 control children. Twelve of the 41 siblings of the children undergoing covert video surveillance had died suddenly and unexpectedly, with 11 being classified as SIDS. After video surveillance, 4 parents admitted to suffocating 8 children, and 1 child died of deliberate poisoning.

Using Autopsy and Radiology to Diagnose Intentional Suffocation

There have been numerous attempts to identify a postmortem marker that could reliably distinguish intentional suffocation from other SUIDs. Oronasal blood, for example, was observed in 60% of previous BRUEs experienced by children and unrelated infants with attempted suffocation.[87] Oronasal blood, however, may also be a postmortem sign of accidental suffocation and in infants who had died of SIDS and were found supine in a safe sleep environment.[21] The presence of intra-alveolar siderophages has also been proposed as evidence of past attempts at inflicted suffocation. The earlier suggestion was that pulmonary interstitial hemosiderin may represent a histologic marker of previous "near-miss" SIDS events.[88] Based on the presence of intra-alveolar siderophages in 2 pairs of siblings who had been repeatedly hospitalized for evaluation of BRUEs before their sudden deaths at home, Becroft and Lockett[89] proposed they may have been victims of imposed suffocation. In the NICHD Cooperative Epidemiological Study, pulmonary intra-alveolar hemorrhage was observed in 66% of more than 700 SIDS cases, but comparisons with infants who died from other causes were not made.[90]

Yukawa et al[91] suggested that pulmonary intra-alveolar hemorrhage of at least moderate severity may be a postmortem marker of overlaying or smothering and that SIDS may be an inappropriate diagnosis. However, infants without a clinical history that suggested either accidental or inflicted suffocation revealed similar severe pulmonary intra-alveolar hemorrhage, as did cases with those histories. Using a similar grading system in 115 SIDS cases, Becroft et al[92] suggested that pulmonary intra-alveolar hemorrhage might be more frequent in infant deaths caused by accidental or inflicted suffocation than in SIDS, even though their study included no control cases and lacked standardized histologic sections of the lungs. Hanzlick[33] found that pulmonary intra-alveolar hemorrhage was common and was possibly enhanced by attempts at CPR and longer postmortem intervals. However, imprecise reporting of results and a complex system of quantifying intra-alveolar siderophages make it difficult to draw comparisons or conclusions. After review of the literature, Forbes and Acland[93] concluded that previous episodes of asphyxiation are not proven by the presence of intra-alveolar siderophages.

The use of radiography in the form of a skeletal survey has been found to be helpful in postmortem examinations for differentiating abuse from other causes of sudden infant death. Radiographic skeletal surveys performed before autopsy may reveal evidence of traumatic skeletal injury or skeletal abnormalities indicative of a naturally occurring illness. Such imaging should only be performed at the direction of the medical examiner/coroner. The presence of both old and new traumatic injuries identified on skeletal survey may suggest inflicted injuries and may lend focus to the postmortem examination, investigation of the circumstances of death, and police investigation. Historically, if obtained at all, imaging of deceased infants included only 1 or 2 images of the entire infant in what came to be called a "babygram." However, a full survey with dedicated images of the entire skeleton should be completed. See Chapter 4, Skeletal Manifestations of Child Abuse, for more information on appropriate studies.

Sleep-Related Neglect Deaths

With the growing trend to diagnose SUIDs as accidental (unintentional) suffocations or undetermined but with known unsafe sleep factors, the role of caregivers in neglecting to provide safe sleep environments is gaining attention from medical professionals and the public.[94] Unfortunately, research in this area has not kept pace with this attention. A number of factors are influencing this increasing awareness of neglect in these deaths among child welfare, public health, and criminal justice professionals, including public education on safe sleep; expanded understanding on the role of substance abuse, especially opiates and medically prescribed or legal recreational use of marijuana,[95] in infant care practices; and the role of child death review teams to document the circumstances in these deaths as a means to improve child welfare and judicial systems' practices. Schnitzer et al[96] conducted an assessment of caregiver responsibility in child deaths, as determined by child death review team members. The study provided vignettes and asked respondents to assign responsibility to the caregiver. In the vignettes describing a sleep-related death, child death review team members assigned more caregiver responsibility when the caregiver had received safe sleep education and a free crib but chose to bed share, compared with the same scenario in which no safe sleep education had been provided. Many state child welfare agencies have responded to the growing number of SUIDs being identified as due to unsafe sleep practices by encouraging investigations of all SUIDs, confirming neglect in cases in which substance use or prior SUID events are known, removing children in families experiencing more than 1 death resulting from unsafe sleep practices, and delivering safe sleep education and/or cribs for families in need. One example is in Illinois, where Department of Children and Family Services policy requires that all sleep-related infant deaths called into its hotline be investigated. It reported that a little more than 6% of these deaths led to findings of neglect in 2016.[97]

Finally, there have been several instances in which prosecutors have obtained criminal convictions in cases in which there were egregious unsafe sleep practices, such as when the caregiver was intoxicated while sleeping with the infant, there were prior deaths in similar circumstances to the caregiver, and/or evidence was provided that caregivers had been given education on safe sleep practices. While there is variability in how these cases are being handled, both criminally and legislatively, there is a trend toward more consistent prosecution of these types of deaths as more is learned about their preventability.

Other Causes of Sudden Unexpected Infant Deaths

Accidents, especially suffocation or strangulation, are a major cause of SUID, and accurate recognition rests not only on the autopsy but on careful scene examination and reconstruction. Accidental causes of death that have been recognized include hangings, wedgings, and foreign body aspiration. Byard et al[98] reported 30 unexpected deaths from asphyxia caused by unsafe sleeping conditions, including suffocation in bedding, from another person's body, hanging from clothing or curtain cords, positional asphyxia, and from plastic bedcovers. Infant deaths while breastfeeding have also been described and are presumably caused by oronasal obstruction. It is important to note that accidental suffocation deaths probably have many of the same sleep environmental risk factors as do SIDS and most undetermined SUIDs.

Hyperthermia has been associated with infant and early childhood death, and careful scene investigation is critical in establishing this diagnosis. Krous et al[21] reported the circumstances of 10 children ranging in age from 53 days to 9 years who died of hyperthermia. Compared with other SUID deaths, these children were older, were exposed more quickly to higher temperatures, and often had more severe skin damage. Those who died in bed were primarily infants exposed to lower environmental temperatures. The presence of intrathoracic petechiae, which were present in nearly all the deaths, suggested terminal gasping had occurred.

Defects in fatty acid metabolism account for a small percentage of sudden infant deaths that have been diagnosed as SIDS.[99] Mild hepatic steatosis is common in SIDS, but severe lipid accumulation in the liver, renal tubular epithelium, and muscle tissues increases the likelihood that a defect in fatty acid metabolism is present. Medium-chain acyl coenzyme A (CoA) dehydrogenase deficiency with autosomal-recessive inheritance is the most common and usually presents with recurrent episodes of hypoglycemia and lethargy or with features clinically indistinguishable from SIDS.[100] There are also defects in short-chain acyl CoA dehydrogenase, long-chain acyl CoA dehydrogenase, and very-long-chain acyl CoA dehydrogenase that can cause SUID. Postmortem or newborn blood specimens can be used to formulate the diagnosis after death.[101]

A variety of benign and malignant neoplasms have been associated with sudden infant and childhood death. These include tumors of the heart and brain, undiagnosed neoplasms such as acute lymphoblastic leukemia and lymphoblastic lymphoma, medulloblastoma complicated by intraventricular hemorrhage, and intraperitoneal rupture of bilateral Wilms tumor.[102,103]

Preventing Sudden Unexpected Infant Death

Pediatricians and others caring for infants should understand the history and efficacy of programs targeting sudden infant death prevention. Since 1992, the AAP has addressed factors that are thought to increase the risk of SIDS by periodically issuing and updating infant safe sleep recommendations.[9] The initial AAP recommendations were a response to compelling evidence associating SIDS with prone sleeping. Following guidance disseminated in 1988 in the Netherlands and adopted by New Zealand, Australia, and the United Kingdom, the AAP guidelines focused primarily on sleep position, specifying that infants should be placed supine for all sleep, including naps. The NICHD adopted this message in 1994 as the cornerstone of its Back to Sleep campaign, a comprehensive public awareness effort that is credited with reducing the incidence of SIDS in the United States. These initiatives were initially followed by dramatic declines in the overall incidence of SIDS.[104,105] By 1995, the annual number of SIDS deaths in the United States declined to approximately 3,000, yielding a rate of approximately 0.5 deaths per 1,000 live births.[106] Revised AAP guidelines released in 2005, 2011, and 2016 attempted to address additional risk factors (eg, smoke exposure, bed sharing, soft or loose bedding, overheating, alcohol or drug use) and protective factors (eg, approved sleep surface, breastfeeding, pacifiers, room sharing, prenatal care, immunizations, supervised tummy time when awake).[10] Unfortunately, SUID remains a significant cause of postneonatal infant death in part because these public health initiatives have not equally reached all segments of the population.[107]

The 2016 AAP guidelines on safe sleep included expanded recommendations for infant safe sleep location, skin-to-skin care for newborns, bedside and in-bed sleepers, and the use of soft bedding after 4 months of age.[9] There are different levels of recommendations based on the quality of evidence available (Box 24.2). The AAP urges that medical professionals, staff in newborn nurseries and neonatal intensive care units, and child care providers should endorse the SIDS risk-reduction recommendations from birth and support the Safe to Sleep campaign. Beyond risk reduction, a "harm reduction" theory has also been suggested as a useful framework for understanding parental motivations for bed sharing and how parents use professional advice on infant sleep and safety, and promoting safe sleep behaviors.[10]

Pediatrician attitudes and anticipatory guidance are important. For example, in the National Infant Sleep Position study, Colson et al[108] found that 36% of the participants reported talking to a doctor about bed sharing. Compared with those who did not talk to a doctor, those who reported their doctors had a negative attitude were less likely to bed share, whereas a neutral attitude was associated with increased bed sharing. Effective harm reduction interventions can target multiple levels, including individual, community, and societal, using tools such as community outreach and education, family and community support, and legal and policy actions.

BOX 24.2
American Academy of Pediatrics Recommendation for Safe Sleep Environments

Level A Recommendations

- Back to sleep for every sleep.
- Use a firm sleep surface.
- Breastfeeding is recommended.
- Room sharing with the infant on a separate sleep surface is recommended.
- Keep soft objects and loose bedding away from the infant's sleep area.
- Consider offering a pacifier at naptime and bedtime.
- Avoid smoke exposure during pregnancy and after birth.
- Avoid alcohol and illicit drug use during pregnancy and after birth.
- Avoid overheating.
- Pregnant women should seek and obtain regular prenatal care.
- Infants should be immunized in accordance with AAP and CDC recommendations.
- Do not use home cardiorespiratory monitors as a strategy to reduce the risk of SIDS.
- Medical professionals, staff in newborn nurseries and NICUs, and child care providers should endorse and model the SIDS risk-reduction recommendations from birth.
- Media and manufacturers should follow safe sleep guidelines in their messaging and advertising.
- Continue the Safe to Sleep campaign, focusing on ways to reduce the risk of all sleep-related infant deaths, including SIDS, suffocation, and other unintentional deaths. Pediatricians and other medical professionals should actively participate in this campaign.

(continued)

BOX 24.2 (continued)

Level B Recommendations

- Avoid the use of commercial devices that are inconsistent with safe sleep recommendations.
- Supervised, awake tummy time is recommended to facilitate development and to minimize development of positional plagiocephaly.

Level C Recommendations

- Continue research and surveillance on the risk factors, causes, and pathophysiologic mechanisms of SIDS and other sleep-related infant deaths, with the ultimate goal of eliminating these deaths entirely.
- There is no evidence to recommend swaddling as a strategy to reduce the risk of SIDS.

Abbreviations: AAP, American Academy of Pediatrics; CDC, Centers for Disease Control and Prevention; NICU, neonatal intensive care unit; SIDS, sudden infant death syndrome.

The following levels are based on the strength of recommendation taxonomy for the assignment of letter grades to each of its recommendations (A, B, or C):

Level A: There is good-quality patient-oriented evidence.

Level B: There is inconsistent or limited-quality patient-oriented evidence.

Level C: The recommendation is based on consensus, disease-oriented evidence, usual practice, expert opinion, or case series for studies of diagnosis, treatment, prevention, or screening.

Note: *Patient-oriented evidence* measures outcomes that matter to patients: morbidity, mortality, symptom improvement, cost reduction, and quality of life; *disease-oriented evidence* measures immediate, physiologic, or surrogate end points that may or may not reflect improvements in patient outcomes (eg, blood pressure, blood chemistry, physiologic function, pathologic findings).

From American Academy of Pediatrics Task Force on Sudden Infant Death Syndrome. SIDS and other sleep-related infant deaths: updated 2016 recommendations for a safe infant sleeping environment. *Pediatrics*. 2016;138(5):e20162938.

Child Death Review

Pediatricians can assist communities in developing additional strategies to prevent SUID. One such activity is child fatality review.[109] Child fatality review teams provide a multidisciplinary, multiagency review of all or most child fatalities that can improve case identification, particularly for sleep-related infant deaths.[110] Teams have identified abuse cases that have been misclassified or misdiagnosed as due to SIDS, natural causes, or unintentional injury.[111] These reviews have a variety of applications. In Milwaukee, WI, they identified many infant deaths with risk factors for unintentional suffocation and SIDS.[112] Herman-Giddens et al[113] reviewed all child homicides in North Carolina from 1985 to 1994 and found that only 68 of 220 homicide cases were properly coded. This under-ascertainment of child maltreatment deaths by almost 60% indicated significant problems in accurately recording the cause and manner of death in children. In Arizona, the state child fatality review team was able to identify and correct an incorrect cause of death in 13% of death certificates and suggested that 38% of all child deaths after the first postnatal month could be prevented.[114] In a report from Georgia, team members reviewed 255 SUID cases and disagreed with the death certificate in 21 cases; 5 cases were reclassified as child abuse based on the team's recommendations.[115]

Multidisciplinary teams have now been established in all US states to review child fatalities, and such reviews offer improved identification of the cause of death and evidence for prevention strategies.[111,116,117] Several types of teams have been created, ranging from those focusing on infant or child deaths with accidental or homicidal manner, to those that review all deaths from all causes. Many routinely review infant deaths attributable to SIDS, SUID, or SUDI and can assist in improved classification of cause of death and services for families. The composition varies, but teams usually consist of representatives from the medical examiner/coroner's office and the district attorney's office, a representative from CPS, and a pediatrician familiar with pediatric diseases and childhood injury. Including a pediatric pathologist and child abuse pediatrician, as well as personnel from the police/sheriff's office and public health nursing, can significantly enhance the expertise of these teams.[109]

Some believe that child fatality review teams can make significant contributions to the protection of children and the prevention of child deaths.[118] One review identified 11 categories with more than 300 recommendations resulting from child fatality review teams in the United States.[119] In Philadelphia, PA, the review process was thought to provide a source of comprehensive data to allow policy makers to formulate solutions.[120] A number of problem areas in Michigan's child welfare system were identified by reviewing child maltreatment fatalities, and most were addressed by the state CPS agency with changes in law, policy, or practice. There was then a reduction in the number of findings and in the number of deaths associated with those findings over time.[117]

Supporting Families and Reducing Trauma

Pediatricians have important roles in providing clinical care, support for the family and investigation, and prevention after the sudden, unexpected death of an infant. Those working in acute care settings have a number of important tasks once an infant is pronounced dead.[121] Most sudden infant deaths occur at home. Parents are shocked, bewildered, and distressed. Historically, coroners were reluctant to burden families at this difficult time with an investigation, and many infant deaths have historically been labeled as SIDS so as not to upset the family.[57,122] Parents who are innocent of blame in their child's death often feel responsible nonetheless and imagine ways in which they might have contributed to or prevented the tragedy. Additional steps are now recommended to address family needs in addition to conducting a thorough investigation.[123,124] The appropriate medical professional response to every child death must be compassionate, empathic, supportive, and non-accusatory. Inadvertent comments and unnecessary questioning by medical personnel and investigators are likely to cause additional stress.[125] Grief and long-term effects of such stress are significant, especially for remaining children in the home, and can be lifelong with significant effects on the parents in addition to any siblings of the deceased infant.[126] It is important for those in contact with parents during this time to remain non-accusatory and to allow them to begin the process of grieving while a thorough death investigation is conducted. This is true even when there are concerns of fatal child maltreatment.[71]

The pediatrician, family physician, and pathologist must know which course to follow in relating to the family after the death of an infant. If child abuse is suspected, the pediatrician or family physician must fulfill mandated legal obligations to report the death and suspected abuse to the appropriate authorities. Sympathy and support for the family are still required. Complicating this evaluation is the potential polarization between those who believe that a sympathetic approach to parents losing their infant is the highest priority, and those whose training and experience have convinced them that fatal child abuse is distressingly common, especially because sudden infant death cases can often not be distinguished from intentional suffocation in the absence of a confession by the perpetrator.[127]

When a previously healthy infant has died unexpectedly in the absence of external evidence of injury or with initial history or scene findings suggestive of another cause or manner of death, parents may be informed that initial findings are suggestive of SIDS or SUDI and that other causes and mechanisms of death will be excluded only by thorough investigation of the circumstances of death, complete postmortem examination, and review of case records.[121] Parents should be given a clearly stated, honest, and forthright conclusion even if that conclusion lacks the solidity of a specific diagnosis such as pneumonia or congenital heart disease.[15] Good communication with parents should ensure an adequate explanation that undetermined does not necessarily imply that the death is "suspicious." Furthermore, designating the cause of death as undetermined should not diminish the parents' access to appropriate grief counseling. It should be explained to parents that the investigation might enable them and their physician to understand why their infant died and how other children in the family, including children born later, might be affected.

Depending on local protocols and statutes, and if permitted by the medical examiner, the family may be given an opportunity to see and hold the infant once death has been pronounced.[128] It is suggested that an unrelated observer remain with the family throughout this period to serve as a witness should questions arise about whether there were alterations to the body after death, possibly to hide or remove evidence. Professionals need to be able to address the many issues that require attention, including baptism, grief counseling, funeral arrangements, religious support, termination of breastfeeding, and the reactions of surviving siblings.[124,129] All parents should be provided with information about SUID and how to contact the medical examiner/coroner office and the local SIDS support group.[130,131]

Counseling Families After a Death

A decedent's primary care medical professional has important information to share about the infant and family history and the possibility of medical causes for the infant's death. The medical professional's prior relationship with a family can serve as the basis for additional support and referrals to be provided in the community. Pediatricians do not replace the medical examiner/coroner's role in investigation and communication with the family, but they can serve to interpret findings for the family and help them determine if medical follow-up or testing is needed for surviving children or adults. Although repetitive sudden and unexpected infant deaths occurring within the same family should compel investigators to consider the possibility of serial homicide, it is important to remember that serial infant deaths within a sibship can also be explained by a heritable disorder undefined and unrecognized at the time of investigation, 2 separate and unrelated natural disease processes, or an unrecognized environmental hazard. When an infant's sudden and unexpected death has been thoroughly evaluated and alternate genetic, environmental, accidental, or inflicted causes of death have been carefully excluded, parents should be informed that the risk in subsequent children is not likely increased.

Recurrence of SIDS within a family is an important counseling issue for future pregnancies, given that many parents of infants who die of SIDS may wish to have subsequent children. The possibility of genetically transmitted inborn errors of metabolism or other conditions must be considered, and questions of a forensic nature should also be raised. In a 14-year study of subsequent siblings of infants who had died of SIDS in Norway[132] and in a Washington study over 16 years,[133] the SIDS risk in siblings was almost 4 times the risk among the general population. A comparison of SIDS occurrences between siblings of infants who died of SIDS and infants from matched control families revealed no statistically significant differences in SIDS rates or in total infant mortality rates. With the exclusion from the SIDS statistics of some of the deaths now thought to be due to inborn errors of metabolism, the chances for recurrent SIDS in families seem even less likely. It should be noted that many of these studies were reported before implementation of initiatives promoting supine sleep position and avoidance of smoke exposure. There is a growing impression among pediatric and forensic pathologists that an increasingly higher proportion of SIDS cases have more complex risk factor interactions than was found before the implementation of the Back to Sleep campaign.[134] In a setting of socioeconomic deprivation, unsafe sleep environments, and persistence of the prone sleeping position and continued exposure to tobacco smoke, the recurrence risk may be increased. Additional studies are needed to address this issue.

Looking Ahead

A number of initiatives are now being implemented to improve the diagnosis, understanding, and prevention of these deaths. In March 2015, the NICHD held a workshop, "Sudden Unexpected Death in Fetal Life Through Early Childhood: New Opportunities,"[135] which recommended the application of new technologies and "omics" approaches to accelerate research. The major advances in delineating the intrinsic vulnerabilities to sudden death in early life continue to come from epidemiologic, neural, cardiac, metabolic, genetic, and physiologic research, with some commonalities among cases of unexplained stillbirth, SIDS, and sudden unexplained death in childhood observed.

To standardize classification of SUID in the United States and to improve our ability to understand the different risk and protective factors across the wide array of possible causes, the CDC created a national SUID Case Registry[6] to collect "accurate and consistent population-based data about the circumstances and events surrounding SUID cases, to improve the completeness and quality of SUID case investigations, to categorize SUID cases by the use of a decision-making algorithm with standardized definitions...and to assist program planners and policy makers with identifying targeted strategies to reduce potentially preventable infant deaths."[6] The National Institutes of Health is also funding 3 research centers to study the case review report findings, medical data, and DNA findings. As of this writing, 17 states were conducting statewide SUID surveillance and 5 states were participating in the CDC registry in limited jurisdictions.

Matshes and Lew[55] have worked to improve classifications used in SUID cases. They recommend that infants found dead in a safe sleep environment with no historical elements of concern and who had normal autopsy and laboratory work results should be classified as undetermined cause of death. When there are markers of an unsafe sleep environment in absence of admitted overlay, wedging, or accidental strangulation or suffocation, and an autopsy that finds a natural disease process that negatively affected cardiac or respiratory function, the case should be classified as accidental manner with probable asphyxia or natural disease as a cause. Negative autopsy findings in this category would indicate an undetermined or probable mechanical asphyxia cause of death. The finding of bed sharing or other concerns of overlay or wedging would move the findings to accidental manner with variable asphyxia as a cause.

The Global Action and Prioritization of Sudden Infant Death Project is an international consensus process that aimed to define and direct future research by investigating the priorities of expert and lay members of the SUID community across countries.[136] Researchers, clinicians, counselors, educators, and affected parents from 25 countries identified 3 main themes for future research: (1) a better understanding of mechanisms underlying SUID; (2) ensuring best practice in data collection, management, and sharing; and (3) a better understanding of target populations and more effective communication of risk.

In the United States, SUID prevention activities are occurring with public education, media campaigns, improvements in agency policies requiring assessments of sleep environments during home visits and provision of cribs, requirements for hospitals to provide safe sleep education and modeling, and numerous other ways. There is now a national certification program available for hospitals to obtain designation as "safe infant sleep" hospitals. Continuing professional education is available to train nurses and physicians in safe sleep practices. Many communities not only distribute cribs to families but provide cardboard boxes as temporary safe sleep places for infants. The federal government continues to support prevention efforts through the Safe to Sleep campaign and its safe sleep curricula for American Indians, "Healthy Native Babies."[130]

Conclusion

To improve case identification, investigation, diagnosis, and reporting, SUID should be classified as SIDS or SUDI only when all of the critical elements of investigation are completed. Pediatricians should offer their expertise to investigators to ensure that child abuse is accurately identified as a cause of death when appropriate. They should participate on local or state child death review teams. They should continue to provide safe sleep education to all families with young children using the AAP recommendations as a standard of practice. Finally, they should provide support to bereaved families and counseling on the possible inheritable cause of SUID.

References

1. Beckwith JB. Discussion of terminology and definition of the sudden infant death syndrome. In: Bergman AB, Beckwith JB, Ray CG, eds. Proceedings of the Second International Conference on the Causes of Sudden Death in Infants. Seattle, WA: University of Washington Press; 1970:14–22
2. Willinger M, James LS, Catz C. Defining the sudden infant death syndrome (SIDS): deliberations of an expert panel convened by the National Institute of Child Health and Human Development. *Pediatr Pathol*. 1991;11(5):677–684 PMID: 1745639 https://doi.org/10.3109/15513819109065465
3. Firstman R, Talan J. *The Death of Innocents: A True Story of Murder, Medicine, and High-Stakes Science*. New York, NY: Bantam Books; 1997
4. Shapiro-Mendoza CK, Tomashek KM, Anderson RN, Wingo J. Recent national trends in sudden, unexpected infant deaths: more evidence supporting a change in classification or reporting. *Am J Epidemiol*. 2006;163(8):762–769 PMID: 16582034 https://doi.org/10.1093/aje/kwj117
5. Bowman L, Hargrove T, Hoffman L. *Saving Babies: Exposing Sudden Infant Death*. Scripps Howard New Services; 2007. https://www.nwsids.org/Exposing%20SIDS.pdf. Accessed June 10, 2019
6. Shapiro-Mendoza CK, Camperlengo L, Ludvigsen R, et al. Classification system for the Sudden Unexpected Infant Death Case Registry and its application. *Pediatrics*. 2014;134(1):e210–e219 PMID: 24913798 https://doi.org/10.1542/peds.2014-0180
7. Erck Lambert AB, Parks SE, Camperlengo L, et al. Death scene investigation and autopsy practices in sudden unexpected infant deaths. *J Pediatr*. 2016;174:84–90.e1 PMID: 27113380 https://doi.org/10.1016/j.jpeds.2016.03.057
8. Shapiro-Mendoza CK, Colson ER, Willinger M, Rybin DV, Camperlengo L, Corwin MJ. Trends in infant bedding use: National Infant Sleep Position study, 1993-2010. *Pediatrics*. 2015;135(1):10–17 PMID: 25452654 https://doi.org/10.1542/peds.2014-1793
9. American Academy of Pediatrics Task Force on Sudden Infant Death Syndrome. SIDS and other sleep-related infant deaths: updated 2016 recommendations for a safe infant sleeping environment. *Pediatrics*. 2016;138(5):e20162938 PMID: 27940804 https://doi.org/10.1542/peds.2016-2938
10. Altfeld S, Peacock N, Rowe HL, et al. Moving beyond "abstinence-only" messaging to reduce sleep-related infant deaths. *J Pediatr*. 2017;189:207–212 PMID: 28838726 https://doi.org/10.1016/j.jpeds.2017.06.069
11. Kinney HC, Randall LL, Sleeper LA, et al. Serotonergic brainstem abnormalities in Northern Plains Indians with the sudden infant death syndrome. *J Neuropathol Exp Neurol*. 2003;62(11):1178–1191 PMID: 14656075 https://doi.org/10.1093/jnen/62.11.1178
12. Parks SE, Erck Lambert AB, Shapiro-Mendoza CK. Racial and ethnic trends in sudden unexpected infant deaths: United States, 1995–2013. *Pediatrics*. 2017;139(6):e20163844 PMID: 28562272 https://doi.org/10.1542/peds.2016-3844
13. Cutz E. The disappearance of sudden infant death syndrome: has the clock turned back? *JAMA Pediatr*. 2016;170(4):315–316 PMID: 26833064 https://doi.org/10.1001/jamapediatrics.2015.4172

14. Nashelsky M, Pinckard KJ. The death of SIDS. *Acad Forensic Pathol.* 2011;1(1):92–99 https://doi.org/10.23907/2011.010
15. Crandall LG, Reno L, Himes B, Robinson D. The diagnostic shift of SIDS to undetermined: are there unintended consequences? *Acad Forensic Pathol.* 2017;7(2):212–220 https://doi.org/10.23907/2017.022
16. Mitchell E, Krous HF, Donald T, Byard RW. An analysis of the usefulness of specific stages in the pathologic investigation of sudden infant death. *Am J Forensic Med Pathol.* 2000;21(4):395–400 PMID: 11111805 https://doi.org/10.1097/00000433-200012000-00020
17. Kumar P, Taxy J, Angst DB, Mangurten HH. Autopsies in children: are they still useful? *Arch Pediatr Adolesc Med.* 1998;152(6):558–563 PMID: 9641709 https://doi.org/10.1001/archpedi.152.6.558
18. Krous HF. Instruction and reference manual for the International Standardized Autopsy Protocol for Sudden Unexpected Infant Death. *J SIDS Infant Mortal.* 1996;1:203–246
19. Rognum TO, Arenstad M, Bajanowski T, et al. State of the art conference on the stratification of SUID: consensus on diagnostic criteria for the exclusion of SIDS. *Nordisk Rettsmedisin NR.* 2003:49–88. https://www.ispid.org/fileadmin/user_upload/textfiles/Exclusion_of_SIDS_2003.pdf. Accessed April 10, 2019
20. Vawter GF, Kozakewich PHW. Aspects of morphologic variation amongst SIDS victims. In: Tildon JT, Roeder RL, Steinschneider A, eds. *Sudden Infant Death Syndrome.* New York, NY: Academic Press; 1983:163–170
21. Krous HF, Nadeau JM, Byard RW, Blackbourne BD. Oronasal blood in sudden infant death. *Am J Forensic Med Pathol.* 2001;22(4):346–351 PMID: 11764900 https://doi.org/10.1097/00000433-200112000-00003
22. Krous HF. The microscopic distribution of intrathoracic petechiae in sudden infant death syndrome. *Arch Pathol Lab Med.* 1984;108(1):77–79 PMID: 6546345
23. Beckwith JB. Observations on the pathologic anatomy of SIDS. In: Bergman AB, Beckwith JB, Ray CG, eds. *Proceedings of the Second International Conference on the Causes of Sudden Death in Infants.* Seattle, WA: University of Washington Press; 1970:83–107
24. Krous HF, Nadeau JM, Silva PD, Blackbourne BD. A comparison of respiratory symptoms and inflammation in sudden infant death syndrome and in accidental or inflicted infant death. *Am J Forensic Med Pathol.* 2003;24(1):1–8 PMID: 12604990 https://doi.org/10.1097/01.PAF.0000051520.92087.C3
25. Aretz HT. Myocarditis: the Dallas criteria. *Hum Pathol.* 1987;18(6):619–624 PMID: 3297992 https://doi.org/10.1016/S0046-8177(87)80363-5
26. Ackerman MJ, Siu BL, Sturner WQ, et al. Postmortem molecular analysis of SCN5A defects in sudden infant death syndrome. *JAMA.* 2001;286(18):2264–2269 PMID: 11710892 https://doi.org/10.1001/jama.286.18.2264
27. Covington TM, Foster V, Rich SK, eds. *A Program Manual for Child Death Review.* Okemos, MI: The National Center for Child Death Review; 2005, https://www.ncfrp.org/wp-content/uploads/NCRPCD-Docs/ProgramManual.pdf. Accessed June 5, 2019
28. Diebold Hargrave KL. Best practices: infant death scene recreation and investigation. *Acad Forensic Pathol.* 2011;1(4):356–361 https://doi.org/10.23907/2011.049
29. Firstman R, Talan J. SIDS and infanticide. In: Byard RW, Krous HF, eds. *Sudden Infant Death Syndrome: Problems, Progress & Possibilities.* London, United Kingdom: Arnold; 2001:291–300
30. Centers for Disease Control and Prevention. *Sudden, Unexplained Infant Death Investigation: Guidelines for the Scene Investigator.* Atlanta, GA: Centers for Disease Control and Prevention; 2007

31. Bouvier-Colle MH, Flahaut A, Messiah A, Jougla E, Hatton F. Sudden infant death and immunization: an extensive epidemiological approach to the problem in France—winter 1986. *Int J Epidemiol*. 1989;18(1):121–126 PMID: 2722354 https://doi.org/10.1093/ije/18.1.121
32. Silvers LE, Ellenberg SS, Wise RP, Varricchio FE, Mootrey GT, Salive ME. The epidemiology of fatalities reported to the vaccine adverse event reporting system 1990-1997. *Pharmacoepidemiol Drug Saf*. 2001;10(4):279–285 PMID: 11760487 https://doi.org/10.1002/pds.619
33. Hanzlick R. Pulmonary hemorrhage in deceased infants: baseline data for further study of infant mortality. *Am J Forensic Med Pathol*. 2001;22(2):188–192 PMID: 11394757 https://doi.org/10.1097/00000433-200106000-00016
34. Shapiro-Mendoza CK, Parks SE, Brustrom J, et al. Variations in cause-of-death determination for sudden unexpected infant deaths. *Pediatrics*. 2017;140(1):e20170087 PMID: 28759406 https://doi.org/10.1542/peds.2017-0087
35. Filiano JJ, Kinney HC. A perspective on neuropathologic findings in victims of the sudden infant death syndrome: the triple-risk model. *Biol Neonate*. 1994;65(3-4):194–197 PMID: 8038282 https://doi.org/10.1159/000244052
36. Paterson DS, Trachtenberg FL, Thompson EG, et al. Multiple serotonergic brainstem abnormalities in sudden infant death syndrome. *JAMA*. 2006;296(17):2124–2132 PMID: 17077377 https://doi.org/10.1001/jama.296.17.2124
37. Haynes RL, Frelinger AL III, Giles EK, et al. High serum serotonin in sudden infant death syndrome. *Proc Natl Acad Sci U S A*. 2017;114(29):7695–7700 PMID: 28674018 https://doi.org/10.1073/pnas.1617374114
38. Moon RY, Horne RS, Hauck FR. Sudden infant death syndrome. *Lancet*. 2007;370 (9598):1578–1587 PMID: 17980736 https://doi.org/10.1016/S0140-6736(07)61662-6
39. Ackerman MJ. State of postmortem genetic testing known as the cardiac channel molecular autopsy in the forensic evaluation of unexplained sudden cardiac death in the young. *Pacing Clin Electrophysiol*. 2009;32(suppl 2):S86–S89 PMID: 19602172 https://doi.org/10.1111/j.1540-8159.2009.02393.x
40. Cunningham KS, Pollanen M. Evolution of a molecular autopsy program from within a death investigation system. *Acad Forensic Pathol*. 2015;5(2):211–220 https://doi.org/10.23907/2015.024
41. Moon RY; American Academy of Pediatrics Task Force on Sudden Infant Death Syndrome. SIDS and other sleep-related infant deaths: evidence base for 2016 updated recommendations for a safe infant sleeping environment. *Pediatrics*. 2016;138(5):e20162940 PMID: 27940805 https://doi.org/10.1542/peds.2016-2940
42. Hauck FR, Thompson JM, Tanabe KO, Moon RY, Vennemann MM. Breastfeeding and reduced risk of sudden infant death syndrome: a meta-analysis. *Pediatrics*. 2011;128(1):103–110 PMID: 21669892 https://doi.org/10.1542/peds.2010-3000
43. Blair PS, Sidebotham P, Pease A, Fleming PJ. Bed-sharing in the absence of hazardous circumstances: is there a risk of sudden infant death syndrome? An analysis from two case-control studies conducted in the UK. *PLoS One*. 2014;9(9):e107799 PMID: 25238618 https://doi.org/10.1371/journal.pone.0107799
44. Taylor JA, Krieger JW, Reay DT, Davis RL, Harruff R, Cheney LK. Prone sleep position and the sudden infant death syndrome in King County, Washington: a case-control study. *J Pediatr*. 1996;128(5 Pt 1):626–630 PMID: 8627433 https://doi.org/10.1016/S0022-3476(96)80126-0
45. Mitchell EA, Brunt JM, Everard C. Reduction in mortality from sudden infant death syndrome in New Zealand: 1986-92. *Arch Dis Child*. 1994;70(4):291–294 PMID: 8185361 https://doi.org/10.1136/adc.70.4.291

46. Hauck FR, Herman SM, Donovan M, et al. Sleep environment and the risk of sudden infant death syndrome in an urban population: the Chicago Infant Mortality Study. *Pediatrics*. 2003;111(5 Pt 2):1207–1214 PMID: 12728140
47. Schnitzer PG, Covington TM, Dykstra HK. Sudden unexpected infant deaths: sleep environment and circumstances. *Am J Public Health*. 2012;102(6):1204–1212 PMID: 22515860 https://doi.org/10.2105/AJPH.2011.300613
48. Tappin D, Ecob R, Brooke H. Bedsharing, roomsharing, and sudden infant death syndrome in Scotland: a case-control study. *J Pediatr*. 2005;147(1):32–37 PMID: 16027691 https://doi.org/10.1016/j.jpeds.2005.01.035
49. Vennemann MM, Hense HW, Bajanowski T, et al. Bed sharing and the risk of sudden infant death syndrome: can we resolve the debate? *J Pediatr*. 2012;160(1):44–48.e2 PMID: 21868032 https://doi.org/10.1016/j.jpeds.2011.06.052
50. MacDorman MF, Cnattingius S, Hoffman HJ, Kramer MS, Haglund B. Sudden infant death syndrome and smoking in the United States and Sweden. *Am J Epidemiol*. 1997;146(3):249–257 PMID: 9247009 https://doi.org/10.1093/oxfordjournals.aje.a009260
51. Milerad J, Rajs J, Gidlund E. Nicotine and cotinine levels in pericardial fluid in victims of SIDS. *Acta Paediatr*. 1994;83(1):59–62 PMID: 8193474 https://doi.org/10.1111/j.1651-2227.1994.tb12953.x
52. Bass M, Kravath RE, Glass L. Death-scene investigation in sudden infant death. *N Engl J Med*. 1986;315(2):100–105 PMID: 3724796 https://doi.org/10.1056/NEJM198607103150206
53. Stanton AN. Sudden infant death. Overheating and cot death. *Lancet*. 1984;2(8413):1199–1201 PMID: 6150244 https://doi.org/10.1016/S0140-6736(84)92753-3
54. Li DK, Willinger M, Petitti DB, Odouli R, Liu L, Hoffman HJ. Use of a dummy (pacifier) during sleep and risk of sudden infant death syndrome (SIDS): population based case-control study. *BMJ*. 2006;332(7532):18–22 PMID: 16339767 https://doi.org/10.1136/bmj.38671.640475.55
55. Matshes EW, Lew EO. An approach to the classification of apparent asphyxial infant deaths. *Acad Forensic Pathol*. 2017;7(2):200–211 https://doi.org/10.23907/2017.021
56. Emery JL, Chandra S, Gilbert-Barness EF. Findings in child deaths registered as sudden infant death syndrome (SIDS) in Madison, Wisconsin. *Pediatr Pathol*. 1988;8(2):171–178 PMID: 3045783 https://doi.org/10.3109/15513818809022294
57. Coe JI, Hartman EE. Sudden unexpected death in infancy. *J Pediatr*. 1960;56(6):786–794 PMID: 13810850 https://doi.org/10.1016/S0022-3476(60)80316-2
58. Case ME. Distinguishing accidental from inflicted head trauma at autopsy. *Pediatr Radiol*. 2014;44(suppl 4):S632–S640 PMID: 25501735 https://doi.org/10.1007/s00247-014-3061-6
59. Brown TT, Batalis NI, McClain JL, et al. A retrospective study of the investigation of homicidal childhood asphyxial deaths. *J Forensic Sci*. 2018;63(4):1160–1167 PMID: 29044506 10.1111/1556-4029.13666
60. US Commission to Eliminate Child Abuse and Neglect Fatalities. Within Our Reach: A National Strategy to Eliminate Child Abuse and Neglect Fatalities. Washington, DC: Government Printing Office; 2016. https://www.acf.hhs.gov/sites/default/files/cb/cecanf_final_report.pdf. Accessed April 10, 2019
61. Christoffel KK, Zieserl EJ, Chiaramonte J. Should child abuse and neglect be considered when a child dies unexpectedly? *Am J Dis Child*. 1985;139(9):876–880 PMID: 4036919 https://doi.org/10.1001/archpedi.1985.02140110030023
62. Kirschner RH, Stein RJ. The mistaken diagnosis of child abuse. A form of medical abuse? *Am J Dis Child*. 1985;139(9):873–875 PMID: 4036918 https://doi.org/10.1001/archpedi.1985.02140110027022

63. Emery JL. Infanticide, filicide, and cot death. *Arch Dis Child*. 1985;60(6):505–507 PMID: 4015166 https://doi.org/10.1136/adc.60.6.505
64. Adelson L. Slaughter of the innocents. A study of forty-six homicides in which the victims were children. *N Engl J Med*. 1961;264(26):1345–1349 PMID: 13681464 https://doi.org/10.1056/NEJM196106292642606
65. Emery JL, Taylor EM. Investigation of SIDS [Letter]. *N Engl J Med*. 1986;315(26):1675–1677 PMID: 3785340 https://doi.org/10.1056/NEJM198612253152611
66. Cashell AW. Homicide as a cause of the sudden infant death syndrome. *Am J Forensic Med Pathol*. 1987;8(3):256–258 PMID: 3673987 https://doi.org/10.1097/00000433-198708030-00012
67. Bajanowski T, Vennemann M, Bohnert M, Rauch E, Brinkmann B, Mitchell EA; GeSID Group. Unnatural causes of sudden unexpected deaths initially thought to be sudden infant death syndrome. *Int J Legal Med*. 2005;119(4):213–216 PMID: 15830244 https://doi.org/10.1007/s00414-005-0538-8
68. Milroy CM, Kepron C. Ten percent of SIDS cases are murder—or are they? *Acad Forensic Pathol*. 2017;7(2):163–170 https://doi.org/10.23907/2017.018
69. Asch SS. Crib deaths: their possible relationship to post-partum depression and infanticide. *J Mt Sinai Hosp N Y*. 1968;35(3):214–220 PMID: 5239550
70. Sidebotham P. Fatal child maltreatment. In: Dixon L, Perkins DF, Hamilton-Giachritsis C, Craig LA. The Wiley Handbook of What Works in Child Maltreatment: An Evidence-Based Approach to Assessment and Intervention in Child Protection. Hoboken, NJ: John Wiley and Sons; 2017:48–70
71. Palusci VJ, Kay AJ, Moon RY, et al; American Academy of Pediatrics Council on Child Abuse and Neglect, Section on Child Death Review and Prevention, and Task Force on Sudden Infant Death Syndrome; National Association of Medical Examiners. Identifying child abuse fatalities during infancy. *Pediatrics*. In press
72. Caffey J. Multiple fractures in the long bones of infants suffering from chronic subdural hematoma. *Am J Roentgenol Radium Ther*. 1946;56(2):163–173 PMID: 20995763
73. Silverman FN. The roentgen manifestations of unrecognized skeletal trauma in infants. *Am J Roentgenol Radium Ther Nucl Med*. 1953;69(3):413–427 PMID: 13016844
74. Kempe CH, Silverman FN, Steele BF, Droegemueller W, Silver HK. The battered-child syndrome. *JAMA*. 1962;181(1):17–24 PMID: 14455086 https://doi.org/10.1001/jama.1962.03050270019004
75. Brown RH. The battered child syndrome. *J Forensic Sci*. 1976;21(1):65–70 PMID: 1249557 https://doi.org/10.1520/JFS10338J
76. Christian CW, Block R; American Academy of Pediatrics Committee on Child Abuse and Neglect. Abusive head trauma in infants and children. *Pediatrics*. 2009;123(5):1409–1411 PMID: 19403508 https://doi.org/10.1542/peds.2009-0408
77. Lauer B, ten Broeck E, Grossman M. Battered child syndrome: review of 130 patients with controls. *Pediatrics*. 1974;54(1):67–70 PMID: 4834303
78. Reece RM. Fatal child abuse and sudden infant death syndrome: a critical diagnostic decision. *Pediatrics*. 1993;91(2):423–429 PMID: 8424022
79. Steinschneider A. Prolonged apnea and the sudden infant death syndrome: clinical and laboratory observations. *Pediatrics*. 1972;50(4):646–654 PMID: 4342142
80. Meadow R. Suffocation, recurrent apnea, and sudden infant death. *J Pediatr*. 1990; 117(3):351–357 PMID: 2391589 https://doi.org/10.1016/S0022-3476(05)81072-8
81. Meadow R. Munchausen syndrome by proxy. The hinterland of child abuse. *Lancet*. 1977;2(8033):343–345 PMID: 69945 https://doi.org/10.1016/S0140-6736(77)91497-0
82. Tieder JS, Bonkowsky JL, Etzel RA, et al; American Academy of Pediatrics Subcommittee on Apparent Life Threatening Events. Brief resolved unexplained events (formerly

apparent life-threatening events) and evaluation of lower-risk infants. *Pediatrics*. 2016;137(5):e20160590 PMID: 27244835

83. Berger D. Child abuse simulating "near-miss" sudden infant death syndrome. *J Pediatr*. 1979;95(4):554–556 PMID: 480032 https://doi.org/10.1016/S0022-3476(79)80763-5
84. Rosen CL, Frost JD Jr, Bricker T, Tarnow JD, Gillette PC, Dunlavy S. Two siblings with recurrent cardiorespiratory arrest: Munchausen syndrome by proxy or child abuse? *Pediatrics*. 1983;71(5):715–720 PMID: 6835753
85. Rosen CL, Frost JD Jr, Glaze DG. Child abuse and recurrent infant apnea. *J Pediatr*. 1986;109(6):1065–1067 PMID: 3783332 https://doi.org/10.1016/S0022-3476(86)80301-8
86. Southall DP, Stebbens VA, Rees SV, Lang MH, Warner JO, Shinebourne EA. Apnoeic episodes induced by smothering: two cases identified by covert video surveillance. *Br Med J (Clin Res Ed)*. 1987;294(6588):1637–1641 PMID: 3113565 https://doi.org/10.1136/bmj.294.6588.1637
87. Southall DP, Plunkett MC, Banks MW, Falkov AF, Samuels MP. Covert video recordings of life-threatening child abuse: lessons for child protection. *Pediatrics*. 1997;100(5):735–760 PMID: 9346973 https://doi.org/10.1542/peds.100.5.735
88. Stewart S, Fawcett J, Jacobson W. Interstitial haemosiderin in the lungs of sudden infant death syndrome: a histological hallmark of 'near-miss' episodes? *J Pathol*. 1985;145(1):53–58 PMID: 3968606 https://doi.org/10.1002/path.1711450105
89. Becroft DM, Lockett BK. Intra-alveolar pulmonary siderophages in sudden infant death: a marker for previous imposed suffocation. *Pathology*. 1997;29(1):60–63 PMID: 9094180 https://doi.org/10.1080/00313029700169554
90. Valdes-Dapena M, McFeeley PA, Hoffmanh HJ, et al. *"Classic" or Typical Histologic Findings in SIDS*. Washington, DC: Armed Forces Institute of Pathology; 1993
91. Yukawa N, Carter N, Rutty G, Green MA. Intra-alveolar haemorrhage in sudden infant death syndrome: a cause for concern? *J Clin Pathol*. 1999;52(8):581–587 PMID: 10645227 https://doi.org/10.1136/jcp.52.8.581
92. Becroft DM, Thompson JM, Mitchell EA. Nasal and intrapulmonary haemorrhage in sudden infant death syndrome. *Arch Dis Child*. 2001;85(2):116–120 PMID: 11466185 https://doi.org/10.1136/adc.85.2.116
93. Forbes A, Acland P. What is the significance of haemosiderin in the lungs of deceased infants? *Med Sci Law*. 2004;44(4):348–352 PMID: 15573974 https://doi.org/10.1258/rsmmsl.44.4.348
94. Brandon M, Bailey S, Belderson P, Larsson B. The role of neglect in child fatality and serious injury. *Child Abuse Rev*. 2014;23(4):235–245 https://doi.org/10.1002/car.2320
95. Nappe TM, Hoyte CO. Pediatric death due to myocarditis after exposure to cannabis. *Clin Pract Cases Emerg Med*. 2017;1(3):166–170 PMID: 29849306 https://doi.org/10.5811/cpcem.2017.1.33240
96. Schnitzer PG, Covington TM, Kruse RL. Assessment of caregiver responsibility in unintentional child injury deaths: challenges for injury prevention. *Inj Prev*. 2011;17 (suppl 1):i45–i54 PMID: 21278098 https://doi.org/10.1136/ip.2010.027094
97. Chicago Tribune Editorial Board. Editorial: infant death and DCFS: is unsafe sleep abusive? https://www.chicagotribune.com/news/opinion/editorials/ct-edit-cosleep-dcfs-child-abuse-20171116-story.html. Published November 22, 2017. Accessed April 10, 2019
98. Byard RW, Beal S, Bourne AJ. Potentially dangerous sleeping environments and accidental asphyxia in infancy and early childhood. *Arch Dis Child*. 1994;71(6):497–500 PMID: 7726607 https://doi.org/10.1136/adc.71.6.497
99. Bennett MJ, Powell S. Metabolic disease and sudden, unexpected death in infancy. *Hum Pathol*. 1994;25(8):742–746 PMID: 8056419 https://doi.org/10.1016/0046-8177(94)90241-0

100. Harpey JP, Charpentier C, Paturneau-Jouas M. Sudden infant death syndrome and inherited disorders of fatty acid beta-oxidation. *Biol Neonate*. 1990;58(suppl 1):70–80 PMID: 2265221 https://doi.org/10.1159/000243301
101. Bennett MJ, Rinaldo P. The metabolic autopsy comes of age. *Clin Chem*. 2001;47(7): 1145–1146 PMID: 11427443
102. Krous HF, Chadwick AE, Isaacs H Jr. Tumors associated with sudden infant and childhood death. *Pediatr Dev Pathol*. 2005;8(1):20–25 PMID: 15803214 https://doi.org/10.1007/s10024-004-7077-z
103. Somers GR, Smith CR, Perrin DG, Wilson GJ, Taylor GP. Sudden unexpected death in infancy and childhood due to undiagnosed neoplasia: an autopsy study. *Am J Forensic Med Pathol*. 2006;27(1):64–69 PMID: 16501353 https://doi.org/10.1097/01.paf.0000203267.91806.ed
104. Fleming PJ, Blair PS, Bacon C, et al; Confidential Enquiry into Stillbirths and Deaths Regional Coordinators and Researchers. Environment of infants during sleep and risk of the sudden infant death syndrome: results of 1993-5 case-control study for confidential inquiry into stillbirths and deaths in infancy. *BMJ*. 1996;313(7051):191–195 PMID: 8696193 https://doi.org/10.1136/bmj.313.7051.191
105. Mitchell EA, Thompson JMD. Co-sleeping increases the risk of SIDS, but sleeping in the parents' bedroom lowers it. In: Rognum TO, ed. *Sudden Infant Death Syndrome: New Trends in the Nineties*. Oslo, Norway: Scandinavian University Press; 1995:266–269
106. Anderson RN, Kochanek KD, Murphy SL. Report of final mortality statistics, 1995. *Mon Vital Stat Rep*. 1997;45(suppl 2):66–69
107. Willinger M, Hoffman HJ, Wu KT, et al. Factors associated with the transition to nonprone sleep positions of infants in the United States: the National Infant Sleep Position Study. *JAMA*. 1998;280(4):329–335 PMID: 9686549 https://doi.org/10.1001/jama.280.4.329
108. Colson ER, Willinger M, Rybin D, et al. Trends and factors associated with infant bed sharing, 1993–2010: the National Infant Sleep Position Study. *JAMA Pediatr*. 2013;167(11):1032–1037 PMID: 24080961 https://doi.org/10.1001/jamapediatrics.2013.2560
109. American Academy of Pediatrics Committee on Child Abuse and Neglect; Committee on Injury, Violence, and Poison Prevention; and Council on Community Pediatrics. Child fatality review. *Pediatrics*. 2010;126(3):592–596 PMID: 20805149
110. Covington TM. The US National Child Death review case reporting system. *Inj Prev*. 2011;17(suppl 1):i34–i37 PMID: 21278095 https://doi.org/10.1136/ip.2010.031203
111. Schnitzer PG, Covington TM, Wirtz SJ, Verhoek-Oftedahl W, Palusci VJ. Public health surveillance of fatal child maltreatment: analysis of 3 state programs. *Am J Public Health*. 2008;98(2):296–303 PMID: 17538060 https://doi.org/10.2105/AJPH.2006.087783
112. Brixey SN, Kopp BC, Schlotthauer AE, Collier A, Corden TE. Use of child death review to inform sudden unexplained infant deaths occurring in a large urban setting. *Inj Prev*. 2011;17(suppl 1):i23–i27 PMID: 21278093 https://doi.org/10.1136/ip.2010.027037
113. Herman-Giddens ME, Brown G, Verbiest S, et al. Underascertainment of child abuse mortality in the United States. *JAMA*. 1999;282(5):463–467 PMID: 10442662 https://doi.org/10.1001/jama.282.5.463
114. Rimsza ME, Schackner RA, Bowen KA, Marshall W. Can child deaths be prevented? The Arizona Child Fatality Review Program experience. *Pediatrics*. 2002;110(1 Pt 1):e11 PMID: 12093992 https://doi.org/10.1542/peds.110.1.e11
115. Luallen JJ, Rochat RW, Smith SM, O'Neil J, Rogers MY, Bolen JC. Child fatality review in Georgia: a young system demonstrates its potential for identifying preventable childhood deaths. *South Med J*. 1998;91(5):414–419 PMID: 9598846 https://doi.org/10.1097/00007611-199805000-00001

116. Palusci VJ, Covington TM. Child maltreatment deaths in the U.S. National Child Death Review Case Reporting System. *Child Abuse Negl*. 2014;38(1):25–36 PMID: 24094272 https://doi.org/10.1016/j.chiabu.2013.08.014
117. Palusci VJ, Yager S, Covington TM. Effects of a Citizens Review Panel in preventing child maltreatment fatalities. *Child Abuse Negl*. 2010;34(5):324–331 PMID: 20347145 https://doi.org/10.1016/j.chiabu.2009.09.018
118. Hochstadt NJ. Child death review teams: a vital component of child protection. *Child Welfare*. 2006;85(4):653–670 PMID: 17039823
119. Douglas EM, Cunningham JM. Recommendations from child fatality review teams: results of a US nationwide exploratory study concerning maltreatment fatalities and social service delivery. *Child Abuse Rev*. 2008;17(5):331–351 https://doi.org/10.1002/car.1044
120. Onwuachi-Saunders C, Forjuoh SN, West P, Brooks C. Child death reviews: a gold mine for injury prevention and control. *Inj Prev*. 1999;5(4):276–279 PMID: 10628916 https://doi.org/10.1136/ip.5.4.276
121. American Academy of Pediatrics Committee on Pediatric Emergency Medicine; American College of Emergency Physicians Pediatric Emergency Medicine Committee; Emergency Nurses Association Pediatric Committee. Death of a child in the emergency department. *Pediatrics*. 2014;134(1):198–201 PMID: 24958579 https://doi.org/10.1542/peds.2014-1245
122. Cowgill BM. *Rest Uneasy: Sudden Infant Death Syndrome in twentieth-century America* [thesis or dissertation]. Cincinnati, OH: University of Cincinnati; 2015. http://rave.ohiolink.edu/etdc/view?acc_num=ucin1439282125. Accessed April 10, 2019
123. American Academy of Pediatrics Committee on Child Abuse and Neglect and Committee on Community Health Services. Investigation and review of unexpected infant and child deaths. *Pediatrics*. 1999;104(5):1158–1160 PMID: 10545567 https://doi.org/10.1542/peds.104.5.1158
124. American Academy of Pediatrics Committee on Psychosocial Aspects of Child and Family Health. The pediatrician and childhood bereavement. *Pediatrics*. 2000;105(2):445–447 PMID: 10654974 https://doi.org/10.1542/peds.105.2.445
125. Levetown M; American Academy of Pediatrics Committee on Bioethics. Communicating with children and families: from everyday interactions to skill in conveying distressing information. *Pediatrics*. 2008;121(5):e1441–e1460 PMID: 18450887 https://doi.org/10.1542/peds.2008-0565
126. Garner AS, Shonkoff JP, Siegel BS, et al; American Academy of Pediatrics Committee on Psychosocial Aspects of Child and Family Health; Committee on Early Childhood, Adoption, and Dependent Care; Section on Developmental and Behavioral Pediatrics. Early childhood adversity, toxic stress, and the role of the pediatrician: translating developmental science into lifelong health. *Pediatrics*. 2012;129(1):e224–e231 PMID: 22201148 https://doi.org/10.1542/peds.2011-2662
127. Rudd RA, Marain LC, Crandall L. To hold or not to hold: medicolegal death investigation practices during unexpected child death investigations and the experiences of next of kin. *Am J Forensic Med Pathol*. 2014;35(2):132–139 PMID: 24781400 https://doi.org/10.1097/PAF.0000000000000089
128. Wender E; CAmerican Academy of Pediatrics Committee on Psychosocial Aspects of Child and Family Health. Supporting the family after the death of a child. *Pediatrics*. 2012;130(6):1164–1169 PMID: 23184104 https://doi.org/10.1542/peds.2012-2772
129. National Sudden Infant Death Syndrome/Infant Death Resource Center. Responding to a sudden, unexpected infant death: the professional's role. https://www.ncemch.org/suid-sids/documents/SIDRC/ProfessionalRole.pdf. Revised 2004. Accessed April 10, 2019

130. McClain M, Arnold J, Longchamp E, Shaefer J. *Bereavement Counseling for Sudden Infant Death Syndrome (SIDS) and Infant Mortality: Core Competencies for the Health Care Professional.* McLean, VA: Association of SIDS and Infant Mortality Programs; 2004. https://www.nwsids.org/documents/BereavementCounselingforInfantMortality.pdf. Accessed June 10, 2019
131. First Candle. Who We Are and What We Do. https://firstcandle.org/about-us. Accessed June 10, 2019
132. Irgens LM, Oyen N, Skjaerven R. Recurrence of sudden infant death syndrome among siblings. *Acta Paediatr Suppl.* 1993;82(suppl 389):23–25 PMID: 8374185 https://doi.org/10.1111/j.1651-2227.1993.tb12869.x
133. Peterson DR, Sabotta EE, Daling JR. Infant mortality among subsequent siblings of infants who died of sudden infant death syndrome. *J Pediatr.* 1986;108(6):911–914 PMID: 3712156 https://doi.org/10.1016/S0022-3476(86)80926-X
134. Blair PS, Sidebotham P, Berry PJ, Evans M, Fleming PJ. Major epidemiological changes in sudden infant death syndrome: a 20-year population-based study in the UK. *Lancet.* 2006;367(9507):314–319 PMID: 16443038 https://doi.org/10.1016/S0140-6736(06)67968-3
135. Goldstein RD, Kinney HC, Willinger M. Sudden unexpected death in fetal life through early childhood. *Pediatrics.* 2016;137(6):e20154661 PMID: 27230764 https://doi.org/10.1542/peds.2015-4661
136. Hauck FR, McEntire BL, Raven LK, et al. Research priorities in sudden unexpected infant death: an international consensus. *Pediatrics.* 2017;140(2):e20163514 PMID: 28751613 https://doi.org/10.1542/peds.2016-3514

PART 6

Professional Issues in Child Maltreatment

CHAPTER 25

Photodocumentation

John D. Melville, MD, MS, FAAP
Associate Professor of Pediatrics
Medical University of South Carolina
Charleston, SC

In contrast with traditional medical services, when a medical professional provides diagnostic services to children alleged to have experienced abuse, the medical professional's documentation directly benefits the patient. Clinical documentation is often read and considered by child protection authorities, attorneys, judges, and other professionals charged to protect children.

The medical professional's documentation is the definitive evidence of the injuries of a child who has experienced abuse. Modalities for documenting physical findings may include written description, drawing, and photodocumentation. Written and photographic documentation play complementary roles.[1]

Although a written description of physical findings remains an important aspect of documentation, it is incumbent on the medical professional to obtain adequate photographic documentation of visible lesions. Photodocumentation, whether still or video, provides the clearest demonstration that the findings the examiner reports as present are, indeed, present. Some states[2] permit or require medical professionals with concern for child abuse "to take or cause to be taken" color photographs of any areas of visible trauma.

High-quality photodocumentation benefits the patient as follows:

- Photographs allow the medical professional to obtain a second opinion of unclear findings. Absent a high-quality photograph or video, the ability to provide such an opinion is severely compromised.
- Imaging during a first visit can be compared with findings during a repeat visit should the child have healing of acute lesions or should new allegations arise.
- In cases that go to litigation, photographic imaging can provide a record for an opposing expert to review. This may prevent the need for the child to be reexamined by an opposing expert.
- Magnification is often needed to appreciate subtle genital findings.

While the only adequate justification for genital photography would be a benefit to the child, additional benefits accrue to the medical and legal systems.

- Peer review is increasingly important in the field of child abuse diagnosis[3,4] as a mechanism of education and accountability. Peer review is limited, if not impossible, without high-quality still or video documentation.
- Medical professionals can review photos and video in preparation for trial testimony. Because trials may occur several years following the examination, photodocumentation is necessary to recall specific details related to the diagnosis.
- Still photographs and videos are useful in court to demonstrate significant findings to the judge and jury. However, images of sexual abuse, given their subtlety to a lay observer, are probably less useful than images of physical abuse.

Photodocumentation of injuries thought to be the result of abuse is emerging as a standard of care,[5] especially in cases of sexual abuse. Although some authors suggest that written documentation may be acceptable for physical abuse injuries,[6] photographs are strongly preferred.

Equipment

The traditional format for documentation of visible lesions was 35-mm still photography. Early camera systems recommended for photographing a child who had experienced sexual abuse ranged from 35-mm close-up systems[7,8] to colposcope-based still and video cameras.[9–13]

More recently, digital still and video imaging[14] have replaced 35-mm slide and print photography. Digital still cameras include

- *Cell phone cameras.* Despite the ubiquity and convenience of these devices, the quality of cell phone photographs is frequently suboptimal. Because of limited photographic capabilities, as well as privacy concerns, the routine use of cell phones to document abusive injuries is not advised.
- *Point-and-shoot cameras* are inexpensive and frequently provide sufficient-quality photos to examiners with minimal training or experience.
- *Digital single-lens reflex (DSLR) cameras* are more expensive and have the potential to take the best clinical photographs. Training and experience are needed to realize the additional benefits

provided by these devices. When used properly, however, a DSLR camera with an appropriate lens and flash provides magnification and clarity that cannot be accomplished with simpler cameras.

Historically, the colposcope has been the instrument of choice for photographically documenting anogenital injuries. While the colposcope provides unsurpassed magnification, the price is prohibitive for many medical professionals. Digital single-lens reflex and video cameras can also provide quality genital photodocumentation. Regardless of the device used, a tripod or colposcope stand provides a significant benefit.

More recently, video has been used to document genital examinations. Video provides a number of benefits over still photography.

- Certain genital findings,[14] particularly the mature hymen, are easier to appreciate when observing them in motion, such as when the examiner runs the edge with a cotton swab or uses the balloon of a Foley catheter.
- Viewing the findings on a television or computer monitor, rather than through an eyepiece on the scope, allows the examiner to maintain visual contact with the child and quickly respond to changes in demeanor.
- Some children would like to view the examination on the screen along with the examiner. This can decrease anxiety and improve cooperation. It can also help the child learn about his or her body and feel a sense of participation and control throughout the examination.
- The examination can be recorded in its entirety for future reference.
- In children with limited ability to cooperate with the examination, review of the video frequently reveals brief glimpses of diagnostic findings that were missed on live examination.

Image Storage

Digital still cameras typically save images in JPEG format. Most digital cameras can be configured to save images at a variety of resolution and compression settings. Similarly, most digital video cameras contain a variety of compression options. While image compression is acceptable[15] for forensic images, larger file sizes are recommended. Files captured in a compressed format, such as JPEG, should not be recompressed. When selecting image or video storage formats, it is vital to review the stored photos and ensure that they maintain adequate image quality.

A disadvantage of digital technologies relative to film is the ease with which digital data can be modified, stolen, or lost. To reassure the court of the photographs' validity, medical professionals must be able to explain specific policies for handling and security of digital images. Images stored on write-once media, such as writable CDs or DVDs, are protected from accidental modifications but are more vulnerable to loss. Many practices store digital images in an electronic health record or network file managed by a hospital information technology department.

Photographs taken during a child abuse evaluation are sensitive medical records. Each center must have policies and procedures addressing the appropriate access and release of clinical photographs. Requirements to release photos in response to various legal documents, such as subpoenas, court orders, or parental requests, vary widely by jurisdiction within the United States. Local legal advice is essential in formulating these policies.

Photographing Children

Obtaining quality photographs is dependent on the patient's cooperation. An expert photographer gains this cooperation with a combination of compassion and firmness. Like any pediatric examination, when photographing a child, it is important to explain what is going to happen in language that the child will understand.[16,17]

When explained well, most children tolerate photography by a confident examiner without apparent distress.[17–19] Expressed fears[18,20] that genital photography will trigger traumatic memories of sexual abuse or production of pornography are rarely encountered in clinical practice. Many examiners directly explain to the child that genital examinations and photography are appropriate only in medical settings. This may be more important if the examiner is using cameras that do not look like "medical instruments."

Some school-aged children or adolescents may refuse photographic documentation or genital examination, despite the examiner's best efforts. This refusal should be respected.[21] Forced examinations are uniformly poor quality and reinforce the child's inability to prevent others from touching the child's body. Examinations under sedation or anesthesia should be reserved for urgent medical indications.

Photography begins during the general medical examination. Begin by photographing the patient label and the patient's face. A comprehensive skin examination includes photographing any rashes, sores, or lesions. Photographing all skin lesions, including those unrelated to abuse, allows the examiner to answer "negative" questions that may arise after the examination.

If a purported finding was not photographed, the examiner can confidently state that the finding was not present at the time of the examination.

For each injury, take a minimum of 3 still photographs. An orienting photograph demonstrates the position of the injury on the body, including whether the lesion is on the right or left side of the body. The lesion of interest should nearly fill the frame of a detail photograph. Lastly, a photograph with a ruler allows accurate measurement. A dedicated forensic scale, such as the American Board of Forensic Odontology No. 2[22] is preferred in these photos. Some examiners include patient identification on the ruler used in measurement photographs.

In some cases, particularly with a moving child with a lot of skin injuries, video can be used, or the still camera may be set to sports mode, in which photos are shot 3 to 5 times per second. Usually, this means the flash is off, but with high-end cameras and good room lighting (particularly if full-spectrum fluorescent lights are used in the room), color rendition can be quite good and motion blur eliminated. Video frames, however, have significantly lower resolution than still shots. When possible, still photography is the preferred method for documenting nongenital injuries.

As mentioned earlier, genital photography typically includes magnified photographs or videos from a mounted camera. Orienting and measurement shots are frequently unnecessary for genital injuries. Current National Children's Alliance accreditation guidelines recommend photodocumentation of normal and abnormal anogenital examinations.[5]

In general, no photograph or video from a child abuse examination should be discarded. This action could be viewed as destruction of evidence.[23] Some examiners have suggested that a very poor image, such as one completely out of focus or blurred because of movement, can be deleted in the camera before it is downloaded. This practice, however, remains controversial, and its acceptability differs by jurisdiction within the United States. Local legal advice is essential prior to deleting examination images or video.

Photodocumentation supplements, rather than replaces, written documentation of the examiner's findings. Following the examination, review the photographs and document the associated findings. Findings can be documented on a body diagram or other standardized form. Occasionally, findings, especially bruises, are more apparent on live examination than in photographs. Shadows or lighting irregularities can create artifacts in photos that are not actually present. Documenting these variances soon after the examination preserves the examiner's live impressions and prevents them from being impeached by comparison with the photographs.

Problems in Photodocumentation

A forensic photograph can be evaluated for 4 independent attributes: focus, sharpness, exposure, and color rendition.

Focus

A focused photograph shows sharp details without distortion caused by the camera lens. For a certain lens setting, objects a set distance from the lens will be in focus, and with close-up photography the distance between in and out of focus may be a few centimeters. Thus, it makes less sense to ask, "Is this photo in focus?" than to ask, "What in this photo is in focus?" Consider Figure 25.1. In Figure 25.1A, the hair is in focus at the expense of the ear bruising, which is the injury of interest. Figure 25.1B is properly focused. A fundamental skill for new photographers is the ability to look through the viewfinder or at the monitor and quickly identify the elements that are properly focused.

When an autofocus camera is used, the camera has to "guess" where the focus should be. Most cameras will select objects that are close to the camera, are near the center of the image, and have high contrast. When photographing the female genitalia, this often results in a fine photograph of the examiner's gloves, at the expense of the genital structures that were the intended subject (Figure 25.2). Some cameras have settings to restrict the autofocus to the center point of the frame.

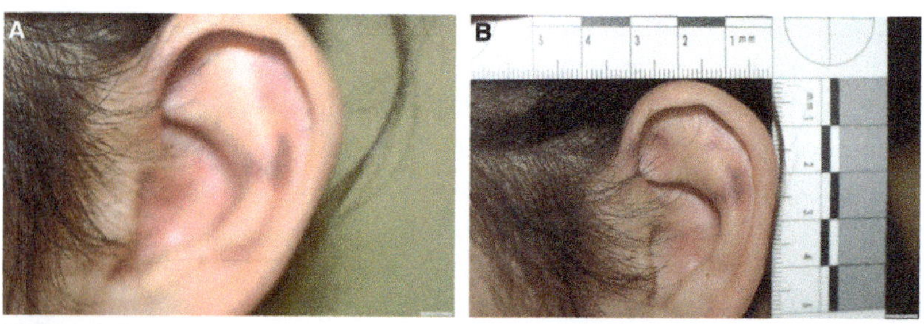

FIGURE 25.1

For a certain focus setting, objects a specific distance from the lens will be in focus. Thus, it is less correct to call a photo "in focus" or "out of focus" than to ask, "What is in focus?" In A, the hair in front of the ear is in focus, and the bruises on the ear are out of focus. This is because most cameras will autofocus on the nearest object. In B, the ear bruises are in proper focus.

From Melville J. Digital photography in child protection. In: Anderst JD, ed. *Visual Diagnosis of Child Abuse*. 4th ed. Elk Grove Village, IL: American Academy of Pediatrics; 2017.

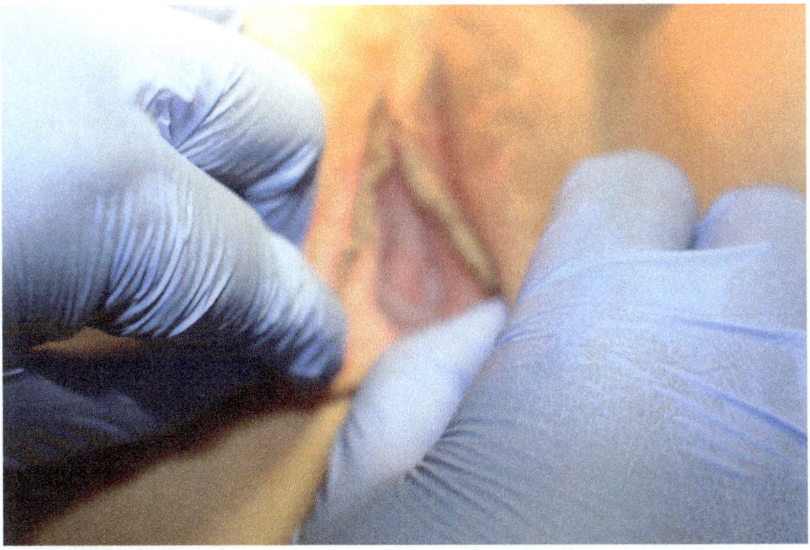

FIGURE 25.2
Use of an autofocus camera results in a photograph focused on the examiner's gloves rather than the patient's genitals.

Sharpness

Blur, or the opposite of sharpness, also creates images with a "smudged" appearance, but due to a completely different reason. Examine Figure 25.3. Figure 25.3A is actually well focused, but motion during the photograph has caused blur. Motion of the camera or the subject will cause blur. Taking blur-free photos of an active toddler can be a challenge. Use of additional light and a flash can increase a camera's shutter speed and reduce blur. Young children may need assistance holding still for accurate photography.

Exposure

The camera must compute a proper shutter speed to allow precisely the right amount of light to fall on the image sensor. When the camera computes incorrectly, overexposure (Figure 25.4) or underexposure (Figure 25.5) may result. Clinical examiners should photograph using automatic exposure settings. If a photograph is poorly exposed, often simply retaking the photo will result in a better exposure. If poor exposures persist, increasing or decreasing ambient lights or the camera's flash may help the camera do a better job.

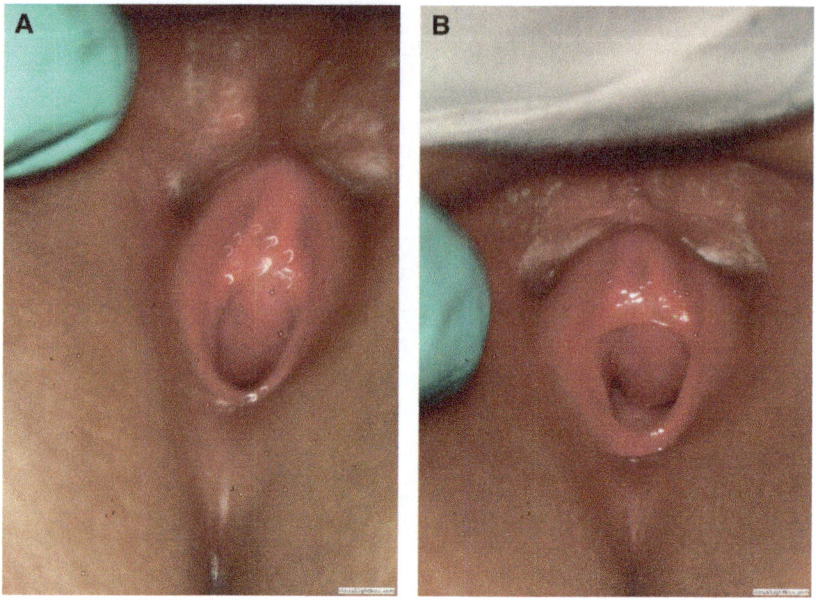

FIGURE 25.3

A, This image is fairly well focused. The photo looks blurry because the colposcope was bumped while taking the photograph. Motion blur can occur when the camera or patient is moving. Increasing the available light will decrease shutter time and make motion blur less of a problem. B, Same photograph as A but without the motion blur.
From Melville J. Digital photography in child protection. In: Anderst JD, ed. *Visual Diagnosis of Child Abuse.* 4th ed. Elk Grove Village, IL: American Academy of Pediatrics; 2017. Copyright Nancy Kellogg, MD.

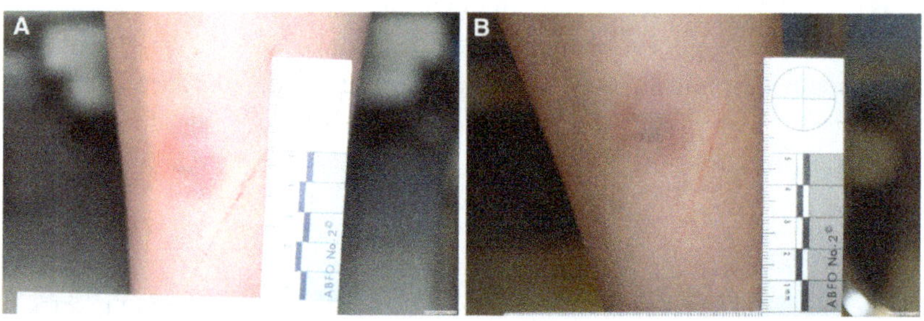

FIGURE 25.4

A, This image is overexposed, meaning the camera let in too much light. Many of the details are obscured in the overly bright areas of the image. B, A properly exposed photograph is showing the same injury. Most clinically used cameras manage exposure automatically. Often simply taking another photo, or a photo from a different angle, will allow the camera to expose the photograph correctly. Sometimes turning off the flash will allow inexpensive cameras to expose close-up photographs correctly.
From Melville J. Digital photography in child protection. In: Anderst JD, ed. *Visual Diagnosis of Child Abuse.* 4th ed. Elk Grove Village, IL: American Academy of Pediatrics; 2017. Copyright Nancy Kellogg, MD.

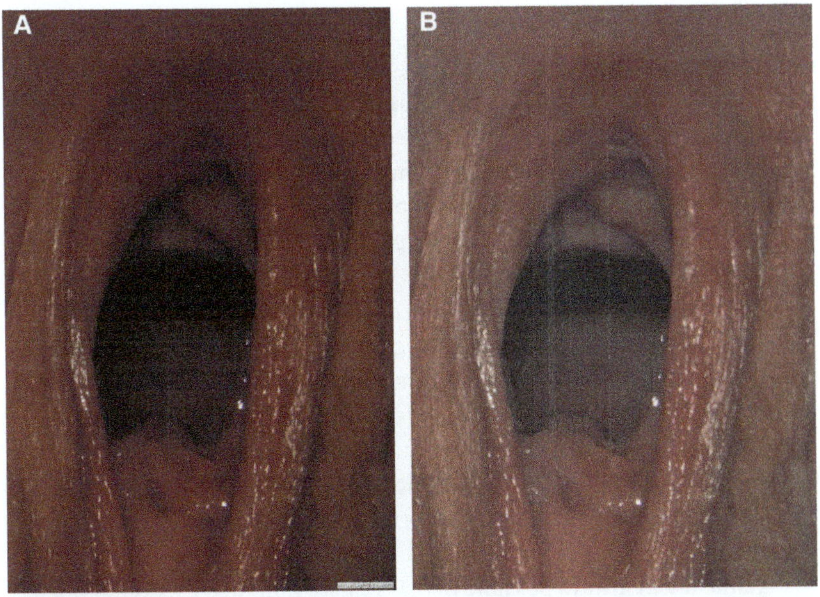

FIGURE 25.5

A, This image is underexposed—the camera did not let enough light in and the details are obscured in darkness. Just like overexposure, the best way to fix an underexposure is usually to take another photo and let the camera try again. If this does not work, using additional light or a flash can be helpful. B, An attempt to correct the exposure of image A using an image editing program.

From Melville J. Digital photography in child protection. In: Anderst JD, ed. *Visual Diagnosis of Child Abuse*. 4th ed. Elk Grove Village, IL: American Academy of Pediatrics; 2017. Copyright Nancy Kellogg, MD.

Color Rendition

Extremely accurate color rendition using digital photography is a difficult problem and beyond the skills of most medical professionals. A few simple techniques, such as properly setting the white balance on the camera, will provide adequate color fidelity for virtually all clinical encounters. If the exact color of a specific finding is important, examiners are advised to note the finding in written documentation.

Legal Issues

Consent

Although many child abuse laws state[24] that permission is not needed if photographs are obtained as a part of a child abuse evaluation,[2] going through the process of obtaining consent can establish an alliance with the family. A variety of consent forms are available.

Accuracy

When printing stills and video for legal purposes it is important to create as exact a copy as possible. This means that the image should not be modified or cropped and, if printed, that print should be on high-quality photographic paper using a high-quality color printer. Black-and-white copies on plain inkjet or laser paper are almost worthless. Many courtrooms now embrace digital display technologies, making printing unnecessary.

Concerns that digital photographs might not be accepted in court have not happened in practice. In 2019, digital images are routinely admitted to courts in the United States, and there have been few, if any, reports of images being excluded simply because they were recorded digitally. In the United States, the Federal Bureau of Investigation Scientific Working Group on Imaging Technologies endorses the use of digital imaging, image compression, and digital image enhancement in the criminal justice system.[15]

While it was always possible to manipulate film images, digital image alteration is easier and does not require a darkroom. This presents both opportunity and danger: computer image analysis can enlighten or distort our evaluation of photographs. Unfortunately, the line between enhancing and editing a digital image is often very thin. The solution, though, is simple: preserve original images for courtroom use. If copies are electronically enhanced or analyzed, clearly state the procedures used and present the original and enhanced photographs. Some examiners will use digital enhancement to clarify or understand findings but do not make a diagnosis based on findings that are not visible in the unenhanced image.

Admissibility

To be used in court, photographs must be properly verified and relevant.[25] Each jurisdiction has specific rules of evidence that govern what kinds of evidence are allowed in court. This chapter will discuss the US Federal Rules of Evidence.[26] The rules in most US states are similar.

The attorney is responsible for seeing that a photograph is verified prior to it being admitted in court. Verification[26] is typically accomplished when the photographer testifies that the photograph fairly and accurately represents what the photographer saw at the time the photograph was taken. Reviewing photographs shortly after taking them, and documenting the same, allows the photographer to confidently testify to the photo's accuracy.

Relevance[26] is a judicial decision. To be admitted in court, a photograph must help the judge or jury decide some contested fact. Photographs may have evidentiary value and still be excluded as excessively prejudicial to the defendant. Photos with excessive amounts of blood or that otherwise appeal to the jury's emotions are more likely to be excluded as prejudicial.[26] The trial judge decides if the probative value outweighs the prejudicial danger.

In some cases, a child is severely injured, and the initial appearance may be very inflammatory. An excellent technique is to take photos before and after wounds are cleaned and then additional photos after the wounds are dressed. Photos are admitted or excluded individually, so the examiner need not worry about how prejudicial the initial photos may be because the later photos will be clearly admissible.

Conclusion

Visualization and documentation technology and equipment have evolved alongside our understanding of the pathophysiology of child abuse. Early magnification tools, such as otoscopes and eye loupes, have given way to colposcopes and close-up video cameras attached to high-resolution monitors. The earliest documentation techniques included words and drawings. Fortunately, the ready availability of still and video documentation formats affords clinicians the opportunity to use visual documentation to obtain a second opinion, participate in peer review, and facilitate teaching.

Currently accepted documentation techniques include still and video photography, which should be augmented with thorough written descriptions of findings.[1] The colposcope has been a valuable tool for enhancing visualization through magnification and offers the ability to obtain digital video and still images effortlessly. Less expensive alternatives to a colposcope are now available. For many, a decision whether to use a colposcope or another form of imaging equipment is based on a number of issues, including cost, ease of use, compatibility with existing systems, and availability of technical assistance. Regardless of the method of obtaining images, photodocumentation of significant findings must be considered a standard of care for any medical professional providing diagnostic and treatment services to children alleged to have experienced sexual abuse.

Acknowledgment

The author expresses gratitude to Dr Larry Ricci, who wrote an earlier edition of this text.

References

1. Melville JD, Lukefahr JL, Cornell J, Kellogg ND, Lancaster JL. The effect of image quality on the assessment of child abuse photographs. *Pediatr Emerg Care*. 2013;29(5):607–611 PMID: 23603650 https://doi.org/10.1097/PEC.0b013e31828e848e
2. Child Welfare Information Gateway. *Immunity for Reporters of Child Abuse and Neglect*. Washington, DC: US Dept of Health and Human Services, Children's Bureau; 2019. https://www.childwelfare.gov/pubPDFs/immunity.pdf. Accessed April 4, 2019
3. Starling SP, Frasier LD, Jarvis K, McDonald A. Inter-rater reliability in child sexual abuse diagnosis among expert reviewers. *Child Abuse Negl*. 2013;37(7):456–464 PMID: 23398966 https://doi.org/10.1016/j.chiabu.2013.01.002
4. Frasier LD, Thraen I, Kaplan R, Goede P. Development of standardized clinical training cases for diagnosis of sexual abuse using a secure telehealth application. *Child Abuse Negl*. 2012;36(2):149–155 PMID: 22405479 https://doi.org/10.1016/j.chiabu.2011.06.006
5. National Children's Alliance. *Standards for Accredited Members*: 2017 Edition. http://www.nationalchildrensalliance.org/wp-content/uploads/2015/06/NCA-Standards-for-Accredited-Members-2017.pdf. Accessed April 4, 2019
6. Christian CW; American Academy of Pediatrics Committee on Child Abuse and Neglect. The evaluation of suspected child physical abuse. *Pediatrics*. 2015;135(5):e1337–e1354 PMID: 25917988 https://doi.org/10.1542/peds.2015-0356
7. Cordell W, Zollman W, Karlson H. A photographic system for the emergency department. *Ann Emerg Med*. 1980;9(4):210–214 PMID: 7369566 https://doi.org/10.1016/S0196-0644(80)80009-6
8. Ricci LR. Medical forensic photography of the sexually abused child. *Child Abuse Negl*. 1988;12(3):305–310 PMID: 3167620 https://doi.org/10.1016/0145-2134(88)90043-9
9. McCann J. Use of the colposcope in childhood sexual abuse examinations. *Pediatr Clin North Am*. 1990;37(4):863–880 PMID: 2199919 https://doi.org/10.1016/S0031-3955(16)36940-1
10. Soderstrom RM. Colposcopic documentation. An objective approach to assessing sexual abuse of girls. *J Reprod Med*. 1994;39(1):6–8 PMID: 8169919
11. Teixeira WR. Hymenal colposcopic examination in sexual offenses. *Am J Forensic Med Pathol*. 1981;2(3):209–215 PMID: 7325130 https://doi.org/10.1097/00000433-198109000-00004
12. Woodling BA, Heger A. The use of the colposcope in the diagnosis of sexual abuse in the pediatric age group. *Child Abuse Negl*. 1986;10(1):111–114 PMID: 3955420 https://doi.org/10.1016/0145-2134(86)90039-6
13. Woodling BA, Kossoris PD. Sexual misuse: rape, molestation, and incest. *Pediatr Clin North Am*. 1981;28(2):481–499 PMID: 7243374 https://doi.org/10.1016/S0031-3955(16)34010-X
14. Killough E, Spector L, Moffatt M, Wiebe J, Nielsen-Parker M, Anderst J. Diagnostic agreement when comparing still and video imaging for the medical evaluation of child sexual abuse. *Child Abuse Negl*. 2016;52:102–109 PMID: 26746111 https://doi.org/10.1016/j.chiabu.2015.12.007
15. Scientific Working Group on Imaging Technologies. Guidelines for image processing. In: *Scientific Working Group on Imaging Technologies Guidelines for the Forensic Imaging Practitioner*. Version 2.1. Scientific Working Group on Imaging Technologies; 2010
16. Ricci LR. Photographing the physically abused child. Principles and practice. *Am J Dis Child*. 1991;145(3):275–281 PMID: 2003475 https://doi.org/10.1001/archpedi.1991.02160030043018

17. Steward MS, Schmitz M, Steward DS, Joye NR, Reinhart M. Children's anticipation of and response to colposcopic examination. *Child Abuse Negl*. 1995;19(8):997–1005 PMID: 7583758 https://doi.org/10.1016/0145-2134(95)00061-C
18. Mears CJ, Heflin AH, Finkel MA, Deblinger E, Steer RA. Adolescents' responses to sexual abuse evaluation including the use of video colposcopy. *J Adolesc Health*. 2003;33(1):18–24 PMID: 12834993 https://doi.org/10.1016/S1054-139X(03)00043-0
19. Scribano PV, Hornor G, Rhoda D, Curran S, Stevens J. Multi-informant assessment of anxiety regarding ano-genital examinations for suspected child sexual abuse (CSA). *Child Abuse Negl*. 2010;34(8):602–609 PMID: 20605630 https://doi.org/10.1016/j.chiabu.2010.01.006
20. Muram D, Aiken MM, Strong C. Children's refusal of gynecologic examinations for suspected sexual abuse. *J Clin Ethics*. 1997;8(2):158–164 PMID: 9302633
21. Issac R. The physical examination when child abuse is suspected. In: Jenny C, ed. *Child Abuse and Neglect: Diagnosis, Treatment, and Evidence*. St Louis, MO: Saunders; 2011:64 https://doi.org/10.1016/B978-1-4160-6393-3.00009-9
22. Hyzer WG, Krauss TC. The bite mark standard reference scale—ABFO No. 2. *J Forensic Sci*. 1988;33(2):498–506 PMID: 3373166 https://doi.org/10.1520/JFS11963J
23. Spring GE. Evidence photography: an overview. *J Biol Photogr*. 1987;55(4):129–132 PMID: 3436918
24. Narang SK, Melville JD. Legal issues in child maltreatment. *Pediatr Clin North Am*. 2014;61(5):1049–1058 PMID: 25242715 https://doi.org/10.1016/j.pcl.2014.06.016
25. Flower MS. Photographs in the courtroom. Getting it straight between you and your professional photographer. *North Ky State Law Forum*. 1974;2:184
26. Supreme Court of the United States. *Federal Rules of Evidence: 2019 Edition*. https://www.rulesofevidence.org. Accessed April 4, 2019

CHAPTER 26

Reporting Abuse, Managing Uncertainty, and Other Legal Issues

Sandeep K. Narang, MD, JD, FAAP
Associate Professor of Pediatrics
Northwestern University Feinberg School of Medicine
Division Head, Child Abuse Pediatrics
Ann and Robert H. Lurie Children's Hospital of Chicago
Chicago, IL

Kristine Campbell, MD, MSc, FAAP
Associate Professor
Division of Child Protection and Family Health
Department of Pediatrics
University of Utah School of Medicine
Primary Children's Hospital Center for Safe and Healthy Families
Salt Lake City, UT

Kirsten Simonton, MD, FAAP
Assistant Professor of Pediatrics
Northwestern University Feinberg School of Medicine
Attending Physician
Division of Child Abuse Pediatrics
Ann and Robert H. Lurie Children's Hospital of Chicago
Chicago, IL

There are few circumstances in medicine that have greater intersection with law than a suspected case of child abuse. In fact, medical professionals engaged in the clinical care of child maltreatment are becoming increasingly knowledgeable of various medicolegal issues pertaining to child maltreatment, as well as the legal process that ensues. This chapter focuses on the effect of law on medical practice related to child abuse and neglect. It provides an overview of legal principles, without focusing on the law of individual states, with regard to reporting abuse. It examines the difficulties uncertainty brings in the clinical evaluation of suspected abuse. Additionally, it reviews general legal concepts and principles related to confidentiality, documentation, evidence, and testimony in child abuse. For more case or locale-specific information, it is wise to consult a local attorney about the laws of your state.

The Medical Professional's Role in the Legal System

The medical professional's role in the legal system has expanded considerably over the last 2 decades. In addition to the traditional roles of examining children, reporting cases of child abuse, and testifying as an expert witness, medical professionals increasingly participate in the review of cases outside the traditional medical setting, such as participation in hospital- and community-based multidisciplinary teams, child death review teams, and, more recently, telemedicine. *Telemedicine* is defined as the delivery of clinical services via electronic and telecommunication technologies (see https://www.hrsa.gov/rural-health/telehealth/index.html). Child abuse pediatrics has explored the use of telemedicine in cases of suspected child sexual abuse and found positive results in delivery of high-quality clinical care and patient satisfaction.[1]

The medical professional's judgment about whether a child's injury or death results from abuse is central to the investigative process in physical abuse and child homicide cases. Coordination between the medical professional and investigating agencies is essential to ensure that conclusions are accurate.

Medical professionals recognize the value of actively participating in training efforts to improve other professionals' knowledge of medical issues. Many medical professionals serve as "medical mentors," sharing medical literature and training materials with attorneys and other professionals, conducting meetings to discuss current developments, and giving lectures and seminars.

Mental health professionals have also witnessed an expansion of their role in the legal system. Psychologists and psychiatrists are now increasingly involved with forensic aspects of sexual abuse cases, providing insights into the behaviors and motivations of sex offenders, as well as into the risk for recidivism. Mental health professionals have also become increasingly important in the sentencing process, informing the courts about issues involving risk management in the community, recommending appropriate probation conditions or levels of community supervision or registration, and conducting assessments that can be used to determine rehabilitative potential and needs. Finally, laws in many states mandate mental health treatment of offenders, in addition to services afforded to victims.

As practice in this area continues to expand, medical and mental health professionals can anticipate that their roles in the legal system will continue to develop.

Reporting Child Abuse

Mandated Reporting

Professionals who work with children are required to report suspected abuse and neglect to designated authorities. Passage of the Child Abuse Prevention and Treatment Act in 1973 set standards for mandated reporting as a condition for federal funding and expanded the state reporting requirements nationwide. Currently, state laws differ in their mandated reporter specifications. Some states require all people to report concerns for child abuse and neglect, while others identify specific professionals, such as medical and mental health professionals, social workers, teachers, and child care providers. Physicians are considered mandated reporters in all states. When not included in state law as a mandated reporter, any individual is permitted to report concerns for abuse or neglect, referred to as *permissive reporting*. When making a report while working at an institution such as a hospital or clinic, internal institutional policies may be in place that address the process of reporting. These policies do not relieve a mandated reporter of the responsibility to report but should be reviewed and followed.[2]

Specific state statutes including mandated reporter qualifications, procedures for making referrals to child protective services (CPS), and reporter confidentiality can be found though the Child Welfare Information Gateway, a service of the Administration for Children and Families division of the US Department of Health and Human Services (https://www.childwelfare.gov/topics/systemwide/laws-policies/state).

Expanded Mandated Reporting

The consequences of child maltreatment can include ongoing mental, physical, and behavioral health problems with substantial economic and societal costs. The introduction of mandated reporting laws in the United States resulted in significant increases in the number of total and confirmed maltreatment reports.[3] Due to the success in encouraging the identification of abuse and neglect, and the interest in mitigating long-term consequences of maltreatment, many states have expanded or considered expanding mandated reporting laws in recent years. In some cases, consideration is made for universal mandatory reporting (UMR), under which all citizens are legally required to initiate a report when they have reason to suspect child maltreatment. As of 2016, 18 states and Puerto Rico have instituted UMR laws.[2] Some work has shown an increase in overall reporting rates under UMR laws, as well as improved detection of child neglect and identification of families at risk for maltreatment (eg, experiencing domestic violence or substance use).[4–6] However, an increase in the reporting rate of confirmed physical or sexual abuse has not yet been demonstrated.[6] There have been no studies to date that examine the effect of UMR on the outcomes of individual children who experienced abuse or neglect. Possible unintended negative consequences of UMR can include instances of unnecessary resources used by CPS and a diffusion of responsibility whereby individuals may assume that a report will be generated elsewhere. Additionally, low-income and minority families are likely to be disproportionately affected by expanded reporting laws.[7] The goal to improve identification of children experiencing maltreatment remains critical to effectively protect and treat children. The strategy to achieve that goal has yet to be clearly defined and may ultimately involve a variety of efforts, including the purposeful expansion of mandated reporters in conjunction with public health education and training on the identification of child abuse and neglect.

Standard to Report

Barriers to reporting have been identified among medical professionals working with children and include uncertainty in the diagnosis of abuse or neglect, fear of relationship disruption with the child or caregiver, time limitations, and lack of confidence in the system's effectiveness to respond appropriately to reports.[8] It is important to note that reporters do not have the burden of providing proof that abuse or neglect has occurred. Rather, reporters are required only to report the facts and circumstances that led to a suspicion of abuse or neglect. Postponing a report until all doubt is eliminated risks violating reporting laws and potentially placing the child in danger. While many states require reporters to provide their name and contact information, all states have statutes to maintain the confidentiality of abuse and neglect reports, with strict regulations on circumstances necessitating the release of that information. The reporting laws override the ethical duty to protect confidential client information. Additionally, the reporting requirement overrides privileges for confidential communications between professionals and patients. States provide immunity from civil liability for individuals who report suspected maltreatment. However, civil and criminal penalties may result if a medical professional fails to report suspected abuse.

The reporting requirement is triggered when a medical professional possesses a prescribed level of suspicion that a child is experiencing abuse or neglect. The terms used to describe the triggering level of suspicion vary slightly from state to state and include *cause to believe, reasonable cause to believe, known or suspected abuse,* and *observation or examination which discloses evidence of abuse.*[2] Despite differences, the intended basic meaning of the reporting laws is the same across the country. Reporting is required when a professional has information that would lead a reasonable person to believe abuse or neglect is likely. At face value, this is a simple mandate. In practice, however, uncertainty about legal and medical definitions of "reasonable cause" or "suspected abuse" is common.

Medical Uncertainty in Child Abuse

Medicine is the science of uncertainty and the art of probability.[9]

An uncomfortable challenge in the medical evaluation of and response to suspected child abuse is the use of legal notions of certainty—*reasonable certainty, preponderance of the evidence,* and *beyond a reasonable doubt*—to describe medical experiences of uncertainty—*rule out, empiric therapy,* or *differential diagnosis.* While uncertainty influences clinical decision-making in the evaluation and reporting of suspected child abuse,[10,11] it is hardly unique to such cases. Medical uncertainty exists in the outpatient clinic with a toddler responding with hand-flapping and echolalia, in the delivery room with a neonate delivered at the cusp of viability, and in the emergency department with a 3-month-old with unexplained bruising. Recognized and acknowledged, uncertainty supports the art of medical practice, encouraging medical professionals to elicit family preferences in treatment decisions, invite hope to coexist alongside grim prognoses, and introduce creativity and innovation in the setting of ambiguity.[12–15] When ignored or denied, uncertainty inhibits effective communication with colleagues and patients, supports stubborn reliance on implicit biases and heuristic experience, and contributes to medical professional stress and burnout.[16,17] In 2011, Srivastava proposed 3 critical steps in dealing with medical uncertainty: acknowledging our own feelings about uncertainty, harnessing available scientific evidence to reduce uncertainty, and learning to communicate uncertainty.[18] While decision-making in cases of suspected child abuse has unique characteristics that may amplify the experience of uncertainty, reliance on these core medical competencies can reduce uncertainty where possible and manage uncertainty when it remains unresolved.[19,20]

Acknowledging Medical Uncertainty

Despite rising attention to the topic of medical uncertainty, a strong expectation for certainty continues to influence the teaching and practice of medicine. This expectation is reinforced with advances in scientific evidence that provide ever-increasing specificity and certainty in the diagnosis of and prognosis for disease. This focus on certainty is not unreasonable; it is a necessary prerequisite for the provisional diagnosis of autism spectrum disorder in a toddler, the intubation and resuscitation of a neonate with apnea who is bradycardic, or the recognition of physical abuse in an infant with bruises. For each of these cases, however, the point at which uncertainty tilts toward the certainty required to support medical interventions varies by diagnosis, prognosis, treatment, patient, and clinician. Medical professionals have traditionally been asked by legal colleagues to pronounce that a diagnosis of child maltreatment has achieved a level of *reasonable medical certainty,* a concept that has no established definition within medicine. It may be appropriate to suggest that reasonable medical certainty is best defined as a tipping point between watchful waiting and clinical intervention for a likely diagnosis. This threshold reflects a complex interplay of scientific evidence, personal preferences, and reasoned inferences and deductions rather than a constant with an accepted predictive probability.[21–23]

Diagnostic Uncertainty

The tradition of the differential diagnosis is an explicit reflection of medical uncertainty. Presented with a patient who has an unknown illness, the differential diagnosis first reflects all possible explanations for the presenting signs and symptoms. This list of possibilities is narrowed, expanded, and reordered as new information is gathered through iterative medical evaluation. In an idealized world, this diagnostic process proceeds until a single etiology surfaces as the best explanation for a patient's condition. In reality, however, medical professionals frequently manage multiple working diagnoses before a single diagnosis rises to the top of the differential. It is important to recognize that diagnostic certainty may not be reached in a time frame relevant to medical decision-making. In these cases, empiric treatments may be initiated if the benefit of early intervention outweighs the risk of unnecessary treatment. The febrile neonate is rapidly started on antibiotics while awaiting culture results; chemotherapy is held until a bone marrow biopsy confirms the diagnosis of leukemia.

In the medical evaluation of suspected child maltreatment, the differential diagnosis may include accidental and inflicted injury, normal variants and unrecognized medical conditions, and misunderstanding or misinterpretations of legal requirements, social expectations, or child behaviors (Figure 26.1). While the specifics of these possibilities differ across physical abuse, sexual abuse, and neglect, each case should be approached with a systematic evaluation of a robust differential diagnosis

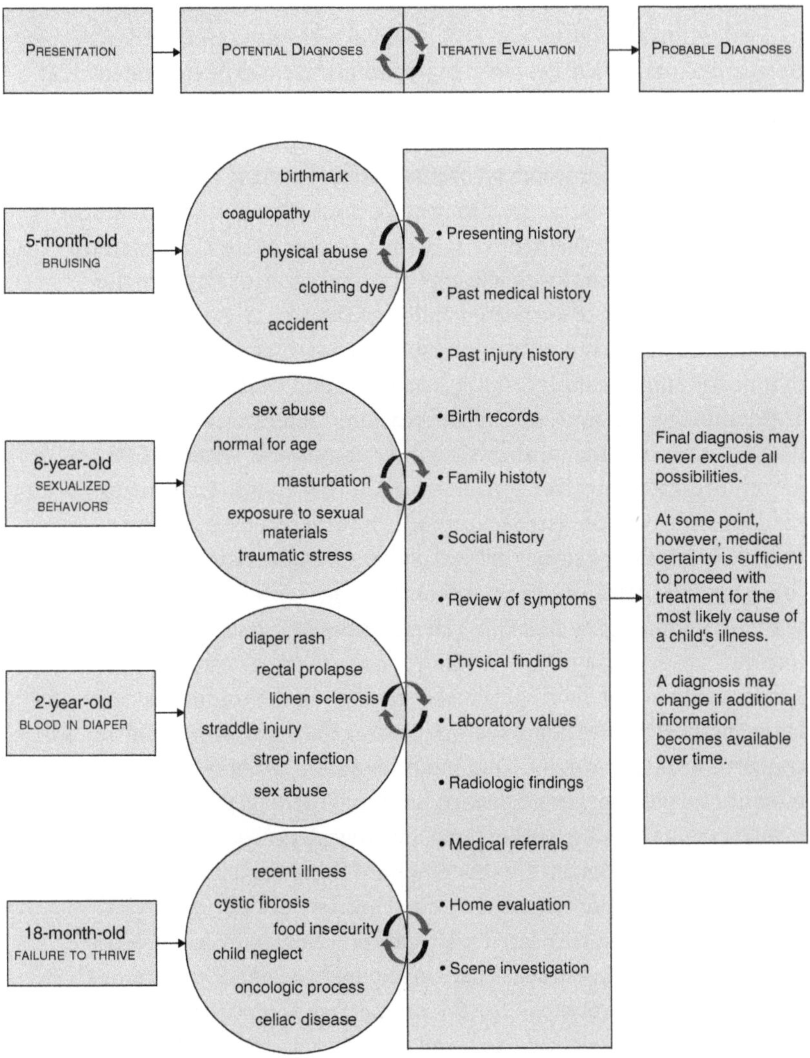

FIGURE 26.1
Medical evaluation of suspected child maltreatment.

before arriving at a diagnosis of maltreatment. When possible, parents should be made aware of this diagnostic process to provide assurance that all reasonable alternatives to a diagnosis of abuse are being fairly evaluated. A medical professional may initiate a referral to CPS at any point in this diagnostic process. In some cases, a referral to CPS reflects an end point—a moment in which all other possible explanations for a child's presenting symptoms have been excluded and the professional has achieved diagnostic certainty. In many other cases, however, a referral to CPS is one step in the iterative process of diagnostic evaluation.

Prior efforts to define a level of medical certainty associated with the decision to make a CPS referral in hypothetical cases of suspected child maltreatment have failed to identify a clear reporting threshold.[24,25] While this has been interpreted by some as a lack of consistency in the meaningful interpretation of mandated reporting requirements of suspected maltreatment, it may more honestly reflect the dual role of child welfare involvement in arriving at a diagnosis. Child welfare and law enforcement investigations often play a critical role in the medical evaluation of suspected child maltreatment. A multidisciplinary investigation after the sudden unexpected death of an infant is a critical diagnostic step in differentiating sudden infant death syndrome, accidental overlay, and abusive suffocation.[26] A definitive medical diagnosis of child sexual abuse is almost impossible without CPS and law enforcement involvement. In addition to serving as a primary medical intervention with safety planning and resource referrals, these investigations supply critical collateral information required for diagnostic certainty and not otherwise accessible to the medical team. Acknowledging that CPS referral more often reflects diagnostic uncertainty than diagnostic certainty in the medical evaluation of suspected maltreatment is critical to reshaping the traditional relationship between these professional sectors. Rather than simply passing along concerns of maltreatment from medical system to child welfare agency, meaningful collaboration between referring medical professionals and investigating CPS caseworkers may improve diagnostic certainty, reduce error, and ensure optimal management of these difficult cases.

Even with comprehensive, multidisciplinary evaluation, diagnostic uncertainty around suspected maltreatment may persist. Unresolved uncertainty may encourage reliance on perceived child, parent, or household risk factors to judge the probability of maltreatment.[27] At these moments, it is critical to recall that there is no causal link between well-described population risk factors—child disability, young parents, household poverty—and child maltreatment. In cases with persistent diagnostic uncertainty but high social risk, medical uncertainty should be shared honestly with child welfare and law enforcement colleagues even if this reduces the likelihood that such cases will be fully investigated, substantiated or prosecuted. For these reasons, it is critical that medical professionals "lean in" to cases with diagnostic uncertainty and learn to work with children and families to identify resources and supports that may reduce maltreatment risk moving forward.

Prognostic Uncertainty

There is a strong expectation that medical professionals have the ability to precisely and unambiguously predict the outcome of a treatment, the probability of 5-year survival, or the moment when aggressive treatments should be set aside in favor of palliative care.[14,15] In cases of suspected child maltreatment, pressure from external agencies to provide evaluations of the effect of abuse on patients may encourage medical professionals to make pronouncements about future risk despite uncertain supporting evidence. Prognostic information—regarding clinical outcomes and future risk—should be provided with acknowledgment of uncertainty when appropriate and with clear understanding of the statistical limitations of such predictions.[28]

Prognostic uncertainty should arise in statements estimating the probability of post-traumatic stress disorder (PTSD) among children who experience sexual abuse, developmental disability for children who experience abusive head trauma, or behavioral problems for children identified as having experienced neglect. While each experience of maltreatment increases a risk for lifetime health consequences, prognostic data estimating the effect of each of these experiences is limited by available research. More importantly, perhaps, the long-term outcomes associated with each of these experiences are shaped by genetic risk, biological response, cumulative exposures to toxic stress, and the quality of environmental supports available in the weeks and years following maltreatment.[29–31] This message of uncertainty, while less useful to those seeking to demonstrate harms, may offer hope to children and families who have experienced maltreatment.

Reducing Medical Uncertainty

Medical uncertainty arises from multiple sources within an encounter with a patient. Individual medical professionals may experience insecurity in eliciting a history for possible sexual abuse, planning a complete laboratory evaluation in a child with multiple fractures, or deciding whether a particular bruise is concerning for abuse. Classifying uncertainties into distinct "bins" is a constructive approach to reducing uncertainty in some cases and acknowledging unresolved uncertainty in others[20,32–34] (Figure 26.2).

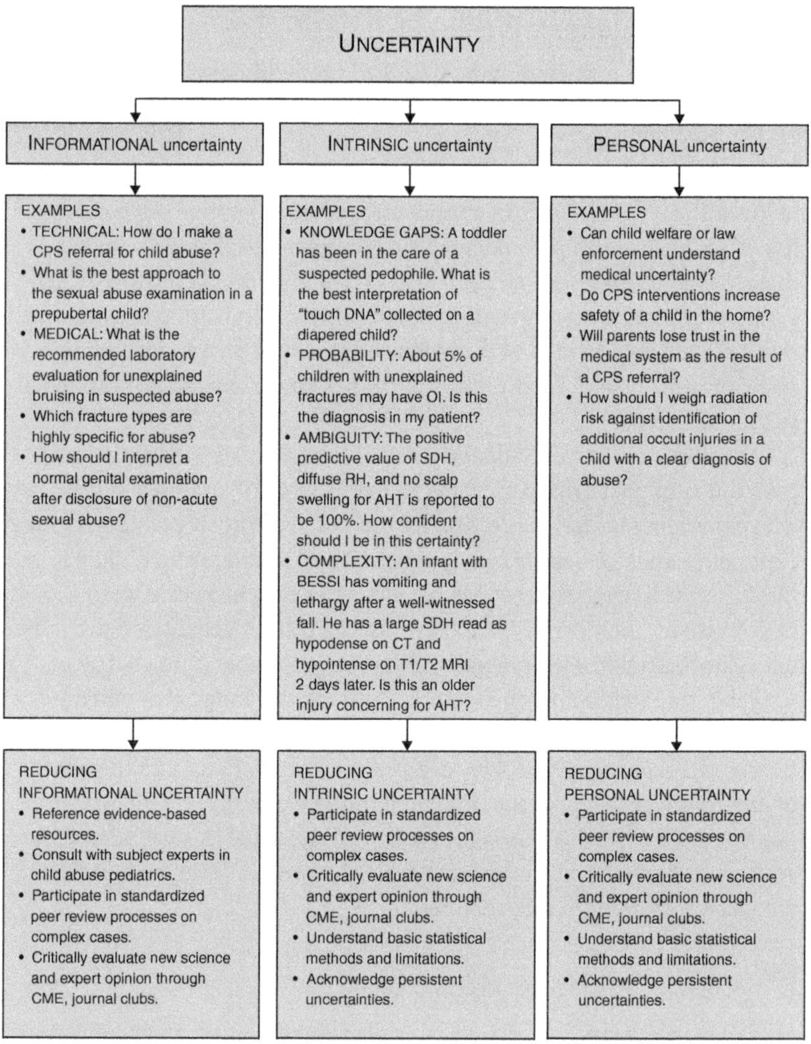

FIGURE 26.2

Classifying, acknowledging, and reducing uncertainty.

Abbreviations: AHT, abusive head trauma; BESSI, benign expansion of the subdural spaces of infancy; CME, continuing medical education; CPS, child protective services; CT, computed tomography; MRI, magnetic resonance imaging; OI, osteogenesis imperfecta; RH, retinal hemorrhage; SDH, subdural hematoma.

Informational Uncertainty

Informational uncertainty arises routinely in medical practice, often in the form of straightforward technical questions. How does one make a referral for suspected child maltreatment—and what will happen after that? What is the probability of hemophilia as a cause of unexplained bruising in an infant, and what is the recommended evaluation? What is the differential diagnosis for vaginal bleeding in a 4-year-old, and what are the best approaches to the physical examination? These challenges may arise in the context of diagnosis, prognosis, or treatment decisions but have the shared characteristic of being answerable to a reasonable level of certainty. Within the context of a complex case, however, these informational uncertainties may become entangled with multifaceted ambiguities rather than being systematically recognized and addressed. Data resources widely available in many medical settings provide up-to-date expert opinion and evidence that can resolve many of these informational uncertainties. Subspecialty consultants, medical educators, and peer reviewers are well positioned as both objective outsiders and content experts to identify and clarify informational uncertainty when a difficult case is presented. In suspected child maltreatment, nonmedical sources such as CPS caseworkers and law enforcement investigators may also help to reduce medical uncertainty by clarifying critical information not available through medical evaluation alone (eg, the bathwater temperature in a scald burn, the height of a kitchen counter).

Intrinsic Uncertainty

Intrinsic uncertainty is more likely than informational uncertainty to persist even with complete medical evaluation and response, and typically it reflects limits to certainty based on scientific knowledge. In some cases, intrinsic uncertainty reflects true gaps in medical evidence. Recognition of this form of intrinsic uncertainty can be challenging, however, because it requires acknowledgment of known and potential unknown unknowns. Historical examples of intrinsic uncertainty may be seen with the evolution of understanding of normal variants in prepubertal genital findings, which at one time were interpreted as indicators of healed genital trauma.[35,36] Current examples may lie in uncertainty related to subdural hemorrhage in association with enlargement of the subarachnoid space in infants, the precision of dating subdural collections on neuroimaging, and the role of biological mechanisms in development of PTSD in children after sexual abuse.[37–39] Research in the coming years and decades will increase understanding of each of these issues, but uncertainty must be acknowledged until then. Intrinsic uncertainty also reflects inherent ambiguities arising from application of population-based scientific evidence to the individual patient. Probabilities, confidence intervals, and clinical complexities make the expectation of absolute certainty in any individual case almost impossible.[33]

Personal Uncertainty

Personal uncertainty further complicates the medical evaluation of suspected child maltreatment by introducing patient-centered questions that may be in conflict with the legal mandate to report suspicion of child maltreatment. Fundamental principles of medical ethics including nonmaleficence (do no harm) and beneficence (provide benefit) may contribute to personal uncertainty of medical professionals who doubt the effect of social and legal interventions on the holistic health and well-being of an individual patient.[10,11,40–42] In traditional medical decision-making, personal uncertainty is best addressed through conversations exploring patient priorities and goals. In cases of child maltreatment, however, assessment of patient goals may be challenged by the patient's age, potential conflicting priorities for patients and parents, and legal requirements that may supersede patient, family, or medical professional preferences in the management of suspected child maltreatment. Medical professionals may more effectively manage personal uncertainties by working collaboratively with families and child welfare caseworkers to optimize child well-being and respond to family needs within the legal structure of the state.

Communicating Medical Uncertainty

Personal histories of experience with uncertainty around a rare diagnosis or an uncertain prognosis suggest that families recognize and resent obfuscation and appreciate clarity around the sources and meaning of medical uncertainty.[14,43] Unfortunately, there is little, if any, research to guide how medical professionals should communicate medical uncertainty in any clinical context.[44] This lack of guidance is magnified when faced with communicating uncertainty of a diagnosis of child maltreatment to patients, parents, or community agencies. Common sense suggests that medical professionals may underestimate certainty when communicating with parents to avoid uncomfortable conversations; for example, explaining that a CPS referral is simply a matter of routine or providing assurances that alternate explanations are just as likely "in cases like these." Conversely, medical professionals may overestimate certainty when presenting to a CPS intake line to ensure that a case receives a thorough and rapid response despite persistent uncertainty in the medical evaluation. Reflecting medical uncertainty to nonmedical communities can be challenging and may result in misunderstanding. Waiting for the final results of a factor XIII assay may introduce several days of uncertainty for nonmedical partners even while medical professionals have already reached a point of reasonable medical certainty and are relying on the working diagnosis of child maltreatment to make treatment recommendations. It is critical to recognize that each audience may achieve a threshold for certainty in a different time frame—or may never share the same level of certainty around a diagnosis of child maltreatment.

In the absence of research to guide communication in these cases, medical professionals involved in the evaluation of and response to suspected child maltreatment should develop personal scripts to clarify the sources and effects of uncertainty to parents and community colleagues. Families and community partners should be allowed to understand that uncertainty about a case does not mean that maltreatment has not occurred, just as a failure to substantiate a CPS investigation does not indicate that a child is not at risk for traumatic stress or for future maltreatment.[45,46] Moreover, if the primary goal of a diagnosis of child maltreatment is the future safety of the patient and other children in the household, absolute certainty of the diagnosis may not be a requirement. Safety planning, parent training, social supports, mental health therapy, and other interventions may be appropriate options to recommend even in a context where uncertainty precludes a strong legal response.

Importance of Documentation

Medical professionals are in an excellent position to document medicolegally important information in suspected child abuse cases. Careful, thorough, and objective documentation provides relevant clinical context, with minimization of facts that can bias or skew an evaluation and impression. Additionally, without careful and objective documentation, medical professionals run the risk of not remembering important clinical details about a particular case months or years later when the professional is called as a witness and asked to recall specific facts about a case.

Confidential Records and Privileged Communications

Children who have experienced abuse and neglect interact with many professionals. Each professional who comes in contact with the child documents the interaction. Much of this information is confidential and must be protected from inappropriate disclosure. Confidentiality arises from 3 sources: the broad ethical duty to protect confidential information, laws that make certain records confidential, and privileges that apply in legal proceedings.

Ethical Duty to Safeguard Confidential Information

The ethical principles of medicine, nursing, and other professions require professionals to safeguard confidential information revealed by patients. The principles of medical ethics of the American Medical Association require physicians to "safeguard patient confidences within the constraints of the law."[47] The Hippocratic oath states, "Whatsoever I shall see or hear in the course of my profession...if it be what should not be published abroad, I will never divulge, holding such things to be holy secrets." The Code of Ethics for Nurses of the American Nurses Association states that nurses safeguard the patient's right to privacy by carefully protecting information of a confidential nature.[48]

Laws That Make Patient Records Confidential

Every state has laws that make certain records confidential. Some of the laws pertain to records compiled by government agencies such as CPS, public hospitals, and the juvenile court. Other laws govern records created by professionals and institutions in the private sector such as physicians, psychotherapists, and private hospitals. The federal Health Insurance Portability and Accountability Act (HIPAA) also controls the confidentiality of some of these records.

Despite legal protections, confidential records may be ordered to be produced in child abuse proceedings through a variety of means. Records may be subpoenaed by a grand jury or an attorney. A judge may order release of records. In appropriate cases, the judge considering release of records conducts a private or "in camera" inspection of the records to determine their appropriateness for release.

Privileged Communications

The ethical duty to protect confidential information applies in all settings. In legal proceedings, however, certain professionals have an additional duty to protect confidential information. The law prohibits disclosure during legal proceedings of confidential communications between certain professionals and their patients. These laws are called *privileges.*

Unlike the across-the-board ethical obligation to protect confidential patient information, privileges apply only in legal proceedings. Privileges clearly apply when professionals testify in court and are asked to reveal privileged information. Privileges also apply during legal proceedings outside the courtroom. For example, in most civil cases, and in some criminal cases, attorneys take pretrial depositions of potential witnesses. During a deposition, questions may be asked that call for disclosure of privileged information. If this occurs, the professional or one of the attorneys should raise the privilege issue.

Communication between a patient and a professional is privileged when 3 requirements are fulfilled. First, the communication (oral or written) must be between a patient and a professional with whom privileged communication is possible. All states have some form of physician-patient and psychotherapist-patient privilege. Not all professionals are covered by privilege statutes, however. For example, if a patient communicates with a psychotherapist who is not covered by privilege law, no privilege applies. (A privilege may apply if the therapist not covered by a privilege is working under the supervision of a therapist who is covered by a privilege.) Of course, the fact that a privilege does not apply does nothing to undermine the therapist's ethical duty to protect confidential information.

In legal proceedings, the presence or absence of a privilege is important. In court, a professional may have to answer questions that require disclosure of information the professional is ethically bound to protect. By contrast, the professional generally does not have to answer questions that require disclosure of privileged information. Thus, in legal proceedings a privilege gives protection to confidentiality that is not available under the ethical duty to protect confidential information.

The second requirement for a privilege to apply is that the patient must seek professional services. The patient must consult the professional to obtain advice or therapy. If the patient enters therapy, the privilege applies to confidential communications leading up to and during therapy. If the patient does not formally enter therapy, the privilege may nevertheless apply to confidential communications between the patient and the professional. For example, a patient may consult a physician who refers the patient to a second professional. Communication between the patient and the referring physician is privileged even though the patient does not receive treatment from the referring physician.

The third requirement of privilege law is that only communications that the patient intends to be confidential are privileged. The privilege covers confidential statements from the patient to the professional. The privilege also covers statements by the professional to the patient. Thus, privilege is a 2-way street. Privilege generally does not attach to communications that the patient intends to be released to other people.

The presence of a third person when a patient discloses information may or may not eliminate the confidentiality required for privilege. The deciding factor usually is whether the third person is needed to assist the professional. For example, suppose a physician is conducting a physical examination and interview of a child. The presence of a nurse during the examination does not undermine the confidentiality of information revealed to the doctor. Furthermore, the presence of a child's parents need not defeat privilege. Again, the important factor is whether the third person is needed to assist the professional. A privilege is not destroyed when colleagues consult about cases.

Privileged communications remain privileged when the relationship with the patient ends. In most situations, the patient's death does not end the privilege.

The privilege belongs to the patient, not the professional. In legal parlance, the patient is the *holder* of the privilege. As the privilege holder, the patient can prevent the professional from disclosing privileged information in legal proceedings. For example, suppose a treating physician is subpoenaed to testify about a patient. While the physician is on the witness stand, an attorney asks a question that calls for privileged information. At that point, the patient's attorney should object. The patient's attorney asserts the privilege on behalf of the privilege holder—the patient. The judge then decides whether a privilege applies. If the patient's attorney fails to object to a question calling for privileged information, or if the patient is not represented by an attorney, the professional may assert the privilege on behalf of the patient. Indeed, the professional has an ethical duty to assert the privilege if no one else does. The professional might turn to the judge and say, "Your Honor, I would rather not answer that question because answering would require disclosure of information I believe is privileged." When the judge learns that a privilege may exist, the judge decides whether the question should be answered.

Disclosure of Confidential and Privileged Information

Patient Consent

Patient consent plays the central role in release of confidential or privileged information. As Gutheil and Appelbaum observed, "With rare exceptions, identifiable data can be transmitted to third parties only with the patient's explicit consent."[49] A competent adult may consent to release of privileged information to attorneys, courts, or anyone else. The patient's consent should be informed and voluntary. The professional should explain any disadvantages of disclosing confidential information.

For example, the patient may be told that release to third persons may waive privileges that would otherwise apply.

A professional who discloses confidential information without patient consent can be sued. With an eye toward such lawsuits, Gutheil and Appelbaum wrote, "It is probably wise for therapists always to require the written consent of their patients before releasing information to third parties. Written consent is advisable for at least 2 reasons: (1) it makes clear to both parties involved that consent has, in fact, been given and (2) if the fact, nature, or timing of the consent should ever be challenged, a documentary record exists. The consent should be made a part of the patient's [medical record]."[49]

When the patient is a child, parents normally have authority to make decisions about confidential and privileged information. When a parent is accused of abusing or neglecting a child, however, it may not be appropriate for the parent to make decisions about the child's confidential information. In the event of a conflict between the interests of the child and a parent, a judge may appoint someone else, such as a guardian ad litem, to make decisions about confidential and privileged information. Unfortunately, appointment of a guardian ad litem cannot always be accomplished in a timely fashion. Two examples among many possible scenarios illustrate the problem.

The first involves the request for authorization to donate organs when a child sustains fatal injuries as a result of abuse. This situation occurs particularly in abusive head trauma cases. The child may be declared brain dead and remain on life support to prolong opportunities to harvest organs. In this situation, the parent may be a suspect in the investigation while at the same time asked to authorize medical procedures that may affect the evidence uncovered in a subsequent autopsy. The necessity of harvesting the organs at a particular time may not permit the time necessary to appoint a guardian ad litem to authorize the procedure. In some jurisdictions, laws authorizing the harvesting of organs from donors may override even the ability of the medical examiner to intercede.

The second example involves situations in which a child has been removed from a parent's care as a result of allegations of abuse or neglect. Despite removal, the parent retains certain parental rights and, therefore, may have authority to authorize release of confidential records to the parent himself or herself or the parent's attorney. Parents may desire to obtain therapeutic records of the child or other confidential records to discredit the child as a witness or to support the parent's defense. In many instances, the child's attorney or the prosecutor are not aware that such records are being sought and are not in a position to object. Moreover, the custodian of the records may be unaware that a criminal or juvenile court proceeding is underway against the parent, suggesting the need for caution in the release of records.

Limitations of the Physician-Patient Privilege

Privileges are not absolute. In many states, for example, the physician-patient privilege applies only in civil cases and is not applicable in criminal trials. Thus, in a criminal trial, confidential communications between patient and doctor that would normally be privileged may have to be revealed. In most states, the psychotherapist-patient privilege applies in civil and criminal cases, making the psychotherapist-patient privilege broader than the physician-patient privilege.

Evidentiary Issues and Testimony

There are numerous evidentiary and procedural legal rules that are relevant to a child maltreatment scenario. A comprehensive coverage of those rules is beyond the scope of this chapter. However, certain concepts, such as hearsay, qualification as an expert, and providing testimony in court are more commonplace for the child maltreatment clinician and, thus, warrant some exposition. For a more detailed examination of legal issues arising in child maltreatment, refer to Myers.[50,51]

Hearsay

Hearsay is a statement (a) made outside of the courtroom, (b) recounted by the person to whom the statement was made, and (c) offered as evidence of the truth of the statement's contents.[51] The rule in all states is that hearsay statements are inadmissible unless the statements meet the requirements of an exception to the rule against hearsay. Many children disclose abuse to medical professionals. Less commonly, some caregivers also admit harmful acts against children to medical professionals. Caregiver's and children's statements made during the clinical evaluation process have clinical and forensic value. Caregiver's and children's statements describing abuse are hearsay but can be admitted in court as evidence when certain conditions are satisfied. (On occasion, a child's statement to a medical professional can be used in court as non-hearsay. The intricacies of non-hearsay uses of children's statements are beyond the scope of this chapter.)

For example, while 4-year-old Beth is being examined by a physician, she points to her genital area and says, "Daddy put his pee-pee in me down there. Then he took it out and shook it up and down and white stuff came out." Beth's words are compelling evidence of abuse. In subsequent criminal proceedings against Beth's father, the prosecutor would call the examining physician as a witness and ask the physician to repeat Beth's words and to describe her gesture. Before the doctor could speak, however, the defense attorney would most likely raise the objection that Beth's words and gesture are hearsay.

To determine whether Beth's description of abuse is hearsay, the judge analyzes Beth's words in terms of the following definition: a child's words are hearsay when (a) the child's words were intended by the child to describe something that happened, (b) the child's words were spoken before the court proceeding at which the words are repeated by someone who heard the child speak, and (c) the child's words are offered in court to prove that what the child said actually happened.

Analysis of Beth's words reveals that they are hearsay. First, Beth intended to describe something that happened. Second, Beth made her statement before a court proceeding at which the prosecutor asks the physician to repeat Beth's words. Finally, the prosecutor is offering Beth's words to prove that what Beth said actually happened. Beth's gesture is also hearsay. The gesture was nonverbal communication intended by Beth to describe abuse. The judge would sustain a hearsay objection unless an attorney can persuade the judge that Beth's words and gesture meet the requirements of an exception to the rule against hearsay. In Beth's case, as in many other child abuse cases, the prosecutor's ability to convince the judge that Beth's hearsay statement meets the requirements of an exception to the hearsay rule depends as much on the documentation of the physician as on the legal acumen of the prosecutor.

Exceptions to the Hearsay Rule

Although the rule against hearsay has at least 30 exceptions, only a few play a day-to-day role in child abuse and neglect litigation. For extensive analysis of children's hearsay statements see Myers.[51]

Excited Utterance Exception

An *excited utterance* is a hearsay statement that relates to or describes a startling event. The statement must be made while the child is under the emotional stress caused by the startling event. The theory behind the excited utterance exception is that statements made under significant stress are generally reliable. All states have a version of the excited utterance exception. There are numerous factors a judge considers in determining whether a hearsay statement is an excited utterance.

- **Nature of the event.** Some events are more startling than others, and judges consider the likely effect a particular event would have on a child of similar age and experience. In most cases, sexual or physical abuse is sufficiently startling to satisfy the excited utterance exception.

- **Amount of time elapsed between the startling event and the child's statement relating to the event.** The more time that passes between a startling event and a child's statement describing the event, the less likely a judge is to conclude that the statement is an excited utterance. Although passage of time is important, elapsed time is not dispositive. Appellate courts and trial judges have approved delays ranging from a few minutes to many hours. The medical professional can assist the court in this determination, when feasible, by documenting as precisely as possible how much time passed between the abuse and the child's statement.
- **Indications the child was emotionally upset when the child spoke.** Judges consider whether the child was crying, frightened, or otherwise upset when the statement was made. If the child was injured or in pain, the judge is more likely to find an excited utterance.
- **Child's speech pattern.** In some cases, the way a child speaks, such as pressured or hurried speech, can indicate excitement. Such observations documented by the medical professional can be helpful.
- **Extent to which the child's statement was spontaneous.** Spontaneity is a critical factor in the excited utterance exception. The more spontaneous a statement, the more likely it meets the requirements of the exception.
- **Questions used to elicit the child's statement.** Asking questions does not necessarily destroy the spontaneity required for the excited utterance exception. As questions become suggestive, however, spontaneity may dissipate, undermining applicability of the exception.
- **First safe opportunity.** In many cases, children who have experienced abuse remain under the control of the abuser for hours or days after an abusive incident. When the child is finally released to a trusted adult the child has the first safe opportunity to disclose what happened. A child's statement at the first safe opportunity may qualify as an excited utterance even though considerable time has elapsed since the abuse occurred. It is important to document threats communicated to the child, experiences of physical abuse or corporal punishment, and the child's expressions of fear.
- **Rekindled excitement.** A startling event such as abuse may be followed by a period of calm during which excitement abates.

> If the child is subsequently exposed to a stimulus that reminds the child of the startling event, the child's excitement may be rekindled. Rekindled excitement sometimes satisfies the excited utterance exception to the rule against hearsay.

Although not of paramount importance, medical professionals should understand that thorough documentation of spontaneous statements made under stress, with descriptions of the stressful events, child's behavioral response to those events, and other relevant factors, can assist courts in gaining a clear picture of events surrounding a child's (or caregiver's) statements.

Medical Diagnosis or Treatment Exception

Nearly all states have a *diagnosis or treatment* exception to the hearsay rule for certain statements to professionals providing diagnostic or treatment services. The professional to whom the individual speaks may be a physician, psychiatrist, psychologist, nurse, social worker, paramedic, emergency medical technician, or other technician. The exception includes statements describing medical history and present symptoms (eg, pain, other complaints) and statements about the cause of the illness or injury.

In some cases, the child is the one who provides the information that is admissible under the diagnosis or treatment exception. Sometimes, however, an adult caregiver describes the child's history and symptoms to the professional. Courts have held that as long as the adult caregiver's motive is to obtain treatment for the child, the adult caregiver's statements are admissible under the exception.

The primary rationale for the diagnosis or treatment exception is that hearsay statements to professionals providing diagnostic or treatment services are reliable because the patient has an incentive to be truthful with the professional. This rationale is generally applicable for most medical scenarios. However, the child abuse scenario, in which a caregiver (who may be a perpetrator) is providing the medical information, presents challenges to this rationale. There could be variable motivations (eg, custody battle, self-preservation) that dilute the inherent reliability of this rationale. Thus far, however, courts have held that a parent's statements to a medical professional in the child maltreatment scenario may still be admissible under this hearsay exception, but an "exacting inquiry" must be made by the court about the purpose of the statements being for medical diagnosis or treatment.[52]

Another consideration for the applicability of this hearsay exception is the understanding of the declarant about the value or benefit of being truthful to medical professionals. For many older children and adolescents, this is known. Some young children, however, may not understand the need for accuracy and candor with medical professionals. When a child does not understand that personal well-being may be affected by the accuracy of what is said, the rationale for the diagnosis or treatment exception evaporates, and the judge may rule that the child's hearsay statement does not satisfy the exception.

Courts have held that the diagnosis or treatment exception has its clearest application with children receiving care in a traditional medical, setting such as a hospital, clinic, or physician's office, where most children have at least some understanding of doctors and nurses and the importance of telling the doctor "what really happened." Courts are less certain about the applicability of the diagnosis or treatment exception with psychotherapy, where the child may not understand the importance of accuracy. Yet, when there is evidence that the child understood the need for accuracy with a mental health professional, judges generally conclude that the diagnosis or treatment exception extends to psychotherapy.

In summary, important points with regard to the diagnosis or treatment hearsay exception are

- When clinically applicable, discussing with the child the health-related importance of candid medical information.
- Providing detailed documentation of the medical encounter, including verbal statements as well as nonverbal communication/behavior that is pertinent to diagnosis or treatment. Because a principal component of diagnostic information is the child's or caregiver's history, it is prudent for the medical professional to include a specific statement in his or her documentation that the medical history is pertinent to diagnosis and/or treatment.
- If the child identifies the perpetrator, the medical professional should document the particulars of how that disclosure came to be. Establishing the rationale of why the identity of the perpetrator is pertinent to diagnosis or treatment (eg, testing for sexually transmitted infection, safety planning, mental health treatment) will augment the applicability of this hearsay exception for those statements.

Residual Hearsay Exceptions

Most states have a hearsay exception known as a *residual* or *catchall* exception that allows use in court of reliable hearsay statements that do not meet the requirements of one of the traditional exceptions (ie, excited utterance, medical diagnosis or treatment). In addition to the general residual exception, most states have a special residual exception for statements by children in child abuse cases.

When a child's hearsay statement is offered under a residual or child hearsay exception, the most important question is whether the statement is reliable. Professionals who interview, examine, and treat children play an indispensable role in documenting the information courts may consider in assessing the applicability of this exception. Accordingly, it will be helpful to the court if the following information is documented:

- **Spontaneity.** The more spontaneous a child's statement, the more likely a judge will find it reliable.
- **Statements elicited by questioning.** The reliability of a child's statement may be influenced by the type of questions asked. When questions are suggestive or leading, the possibility increases that the questioner influenced the child's statement. Medical professionals should ask open-ended, non-leading questions (eg, who, what, when, how) when gathering history from children. The smaller the number of suggestive and leading questions, the more likely a judge is to conclude that a child's statement is reliable.
- **Consistent statements**. Reliability may be enhanced if the child's description of abuse is consistent over time.
- **Child's affect and emotion when hearsay statement was made.** When a child's emotions are consistent with the child's statement, the reliability of the statement may be enhanced.
- **Play or gestures that corroborate the child's hearsay statement.** The play or gestures of a young child may strengthen confidence in the child's statement. For example, the child's use of dolls may support the reliability of the child's statement.
- **Developmentally unusual sexual knowledge.** A young child's developmentally unusual knowledge of sexual acts or anatomy supports the reliability of the child's statement.
- **Idiosyncratic detail.** Presence in a child's statement of idiosyncratic details points to reliability. An example includes children who describe age-appropriate visual details, smells, and tastes associated with rectal, vaginal, or oral sex.[53]
- **Child's or adult's motive to fabricate.** Evidence that the child or an adult had or lacked a motive to fabricate affects reliability.

- **Medical evidence of abuse.** The child's statement may be corroborated by medical evidence.
- **Changes in child's behavior.** When a child's behavior alters in a way that corroborates the child's description of abuse, it may be appropriate to place increased confidence in the child's statement.

None of the foregoing factors is a litmus test for reliability. Judges consider the totality of circumstances to evaluate reliability, and professionals can assist the legal system by thoroughly documenting information and observations involved in the child maltreatment evaluation.

Effect of the Constitution on Hearsay

The Sixth Amendment of the US Constitution, with its Confrontation Clause, dictates that certain hearsay statements are inadmissible against defendants in criminal cases. Two decisions of the US Supreme Court, *Crawford v Washington*[54] and *Davis v Washington*,[55] define the effect of the Confrontation Clause on the admission of hearsay in criminal cases. Before discussing *Crawford* and *Davis*, however, it is important to mention 2 subsidiary conditions. First, if the child who made a hearsay statement is able to testify in court and be cross-examined by the defense attorney about the hearsay, the Confrontation Clause is satisfied and the child's hearsay can be admitted without affronting the Confrontation Clause. (Of course, the hearsay still has to meet the requirements of an exception to the rule against hearsay.) Second, the limits on hearsay imposed by the Confrontation Clause apply only in criminal cases. Thus, in child protection proceedings in juvenile or family court—which are civil, not criminal—the Confrontation Clause is inapplicable; *Crawford* and *Davis* do not apply.

In a criminal prosecution, when the prosecutor offers a child's hearsay statement against the defendant, *Crawford* and *Davis* come into play. As stated previously, if the child can testify and be cross-examined about the hearsay, the Confrontation Clause is satisfied. However, when the child is unable to testify in court, the question under *Crawford* and *Davis* is whether the child's hearsay statement was *testimonial* when it was made. If the child's hearsay was testimonial, it cannot be admitted against the defendant. On the other hand, if the child's statement was non-testimonial, the Confrontation Clause places no limit on use of the statement against the defendant.

The word *testimonial* is somewhat of a term of art. Under *Crawford* and *Davis*, a hearsay statement can be testimonial even though it bears no resemblance to testimony in court. Hearsay is testimonial when a reasonable person in the position of the speaker would appreciate that the statement could be used in later criminal proceedings. For example, a person's answers to questions during formal police interrogation at a police station are testimonial because a reasonable person in that situation could reasonably appreciate that the police are asking questions to conduct an investigation and gathering evidence for possible use in court. Children's hearsay statements to parents, relatives, teachers, friends, foster parents, babysitters, and other non–law enforcement individuals are typically non-testimonial.

Statements to child protection social workers are sometimes testimonial and sometimes not. A statement to a social worker is testimonial if the social worker's primary purpose in questioning a child is to gather evidence. Judges generally rule that children's statements during formal forensic interviews at child advocacy centers are testimonial, although the Minnesota Supreme Court held to the contrary in *State v Bobadilla*.[56]

Hearsay statements to physicians, nurses, and other medical professionals are generally considered non-testimonial when the professional's primary motive for questioning the child is clinical.[57–59] The fact that the professional is aware of the forensic implications of communicating with children about maltreatment does not alter this conclusion. In *State v Moses*,[60] the Washington Court of Appeals concluded that a domestic violence victim's statements to a doctor were non-testimonial. The court wrote, "Courts that have addressed *Crawford's*[54] impact on statements admitted under the medical diagnosis or treatment exception focus on the purpose of the [victim's] encounter with the health care provider....In cases where courts have found such statements to health care providers are testimonial, the prosecutorial purpose of the medical examination has been clear."[60] Thus, factors establishing a primary medical purpose for an examination will bolster the conclusion that statements made in the course of that evaluation are non-testimonial.

Providing Testimony in Court

Medical professionals may be called to testify in a variety of legal proceedings related to child maltreatment—criminal trials, juvenile dependency hearings, child support or custody cases in family court, malpractice actions, pretrial expert testimony hearings (ie, *Frye* or *Daubert* hearings), and governmental administrative hearings (eg, licensure or revocation of licensure). Burdens of proof vary in the various legal proceedings. In criminal trials, the state will seek to prove the guilt of a defendant "beyond a reasonable doubt." Judges often provide juries with instructions for clarification as to what that standard means. There is no standard judicial instruction on "beyond a reasonable doubt." One sample instruction put forth by the US Judicial Center states[61]

> "[T]he government has the burden of proving the defendant guilty beyond a reasonable doubt. Some of you may have served as jurors in civil cases, where you were told that it is only necessary to prove that a fact is more likely true than not true. In criminal cases, the government's proof must be more powerful than that. It must be beyond a reasonable doubt.
>
> Proof beyond a reasonable doubt is proof that leaves you firmly convinced of the defendant's guilt. There are very few things in this world that we know with absolute certainty, and in criminal cases the law does not require proof that overcomes every possible doubt. If, based on your consideration of the evidence, you are firmly convinced that the defendant is guilty of the crime charged, you must find him guilty. If on the other hand, you think there is a real possibility that he is not guilty, you must give him the benefit of the doubt and find him not guilty."

In civil proceedings, litigants, including government officials (eg, CPS), will typically attempt to establish findings by "a preponderance of the evidence" so they can obtain orders about child custody, visitation, or support or establish negligent action. In jury instructions, *preponderance of the evidence* is typically clarified as evidence that makes the conclusion or determination "more likely than not." Stated another way, a preponderance of the evidence means the greater weight of the evidence.[62] Occasionally, when termination of parental rights is at stake, the burden of proof may be slightly raised to "by clear and convincing evidence."

In any event, it is important for medical professionals to realize that their diagnostic or expert opinion thresholds are not to be conflated with the level of burden of proof required by a particular legal forum. Medical professionals may be required to couch their in-court expert opinions to a "reasonable degree of medical certainty." But this expression is not meant to require medical professionals to maintain the same level of diagnostic certainty as that required by a particular court (ie, diagnostic certainty is not required to be beyond a reasonable doubt for a criminal trial, or just by a preponderance of the evidence for juvenile dependency hearing); the 2 are unrelated. Medical professionals should understand that the pro forma legal expression of "to a reasonable degree of medical certainty" is more a surety to the courts that the medical professional has exercised due diligence in the attainment of the correct diagnosis, as that would be exercised in any other similar medical scenario.

Diagnostic certainty in an opinion should be tethered to the clinical requirements of the medical scenario. Thus, if clinical exigency exists to treat or save a patient, diagnostic certainty is secondary. For example, in a newborn presenting with sepsis, knowing the exact organism that is causing the sepsis does not take precedence over starting broad-spectrum antibiotics. The same principle holds for the child maltreatment scenario. If clinical exigency permits, achieving the greatest degree of diagnostic certainty is preferable (irrespective of the legal forum in which the diagnostic impression will be expressed).

Unfortunately, child maltreatment cases have long been affected by physicians who give irresponsible testimony.[63] Irresponsible testimony includes, but is not limited to, testimony for which the expert is insufficiently qualified, testimony based on theories that have not been substantiated by well-conducted medical studies, and testimony on theories that have not gained wide acceptance in the medical community. Given the gravitas of the child maltreatment case, medical professionals should strive to provide objective medical information to the court, adherent to the highest ethical principles. Some of the American Academy of Pediatrics ethical guidelines for the provision of expert testimony are listed in Box 26.1.

BOX 26.1
American Academy of Pediatrics Recommendations for Physician Expert Witness Testimony

1. Should be actively and meaningfully engaged in clinical practice in the medical specialty or area of medicine about which they testify, including knowledge of or experience in performing the skills and practices at issue to the lawsuit.
2. Should render an opinion only after reviewing sufficient medical records and documents to enable the formation of unbiased and accurate conclusions.
3. Should present testimony that reflects the generally accepted standard within the specialty or area of practice, including those held by a significant minority.
4. Should provide objective, valid opinions that are well supported by their clinical experience and the best evidence-based medical literature, regardless of whether it is to be used by the plaintiff/prosecutor or defendant.
5. Should testify to matters only within their expertise. If asked about matters outside of their expertise, physicians should refrain from testifying on those matters.
6. Should testify in cases of abuse and neglect, especially if they have special knowledge and/or extensive experience in the field. General pediatricians testifying in these cases may wish to consult with subspecialists in child abuse pediatrics.
7. Must not enter into agreements in which compensation for expert witness work is contingent on the outcome of the case.

Adapted from Paul SR, Narang SK; American Academy of Pediatrics Committee on Medical Liability and Risk Management. Expert witness participation in civil and criminal proceedings. *Pediatrics*. 2017;139(3):e20163862.

Subpoenas

A medical professional's first formalized contact with the testimonial process will come in the form of a subpoena. A subpoena, issued by a court, typically at the request of an attorney, is a court order and cannot be ignored. Refusal to obey a subpoena can be punished as contempt of court. A subpoena notifies a witness that he or she is needed to present evidence in court. The 2 types of subpoenas a medical professional may encounter are a subpoena requiring an individual to appear at a designated time and place to provide testimony, sometimes called a *subpoena ad testificandum,* and a subpoena requiring a person to produce records or documents, sometimes called a *subpoena duces tecum.*

Because a subpoena suspends typical rules for medical confidentiality, it is important to read carefully what disclosures are commanded (and therefore allowed) by the subpoena. A subpoena, however, does not override privileges such as physician-patient and psychotherapist-patient. The subpoena for testimony requires the professional to appear, but the subpoena does not mean the professional has to disclose privileged information. A judge decides whether a privilege applies and whether a professional has to answer questions or release records.

When a medical professional receives any subpoena, an initial prudent action is to call the attorney who issued the subpoena to determine what the attorney actually seeks. Often, the attorney will inform the medical professional exactly what testimony or documents are required and what facts or opinions to which the attorney hopes the medical professional will testify. Care should be taken during such conversations to avoid disclosing privileged information. If a medical professional receives a subpoena for a medical record that he or she did not create, the professional should notify the attorney issuing the subpoena of the appropriate custodian of the medical record instead of disclosing the record. If doubts exist concerning how to respond to a subpoena, it is prudent for the medical professional to consult with hospital legal counsel or risk management or an attorney knowledgeable about such matters.

Preparation for Expert Testimony

In preparation for court testimony, the medical professional should make it a priority to be thoroughly familiar with the medical facts of the case. Although many courts will permit a witness to refer to notes during testimony, demonstrating a thorough command of the medical facts of the case (ie, the patient's name, age, and dates seen; high points of the history; and injuries found) will enhance the medical professional's credibility as an expert. Additionally, the medical professional should be familiar with the patient's entire medical record, because questions are sometimes asked about conditions unrelated to abuse or neglect.

When a medical professional prepares to testify, it is important to meet with the attorney for whom the expert will testify. Nothing about pretrial conferences is ethically or legally improper. The law allows experts to base their testimony on all sources of data that are relied on by experts in the field. The materials do not have to be independently admissible in court. Thus, hearsay that would be inadmissible in court may be relied on by an expert in formulating testimony. The expert should review relevant literature and anticipate that the opposing attorney will be at least partially familiar with the literature and may use it to try to impeach testimony during cross-examination.

In preparing to testify, the medical professional should ask the attorney whether he or she will testify primarily as a *fact* witness or as an *expert* witness. A fact witness may testify only to the specific facts that the witness has seen, heard, felt, etc. He or she is not accorded the latitude by the rules of evidence to express opinions; those are reserved for expert witnesses.

If being called as an expert witness, it is important to know whether there will be an opposing expert witness(es) and what his or her likely medical theories will be. It may also be helpful to learn of the style, demeanor, and level of sophistication of opposing counsel and whether the case will be tried before a judge or a jury. Finally, it is important to review with the attorney requesting the testimony what questions will be asked during direct examination and what are the anticipated lines of cross-examination.

The expert witness should be prepared to discuss similarities and differences between the expert's opinion and the opinions of other experts and whether differences between opinions can be reconciled. In some instances, the opposing expert has written articles that can be reviewed. Further preparation includes creating and discussing any exhibits, charts, or demonstrative aids that will be used during testimony. Exhibits may have to be shared with opposing counsel prior to trial.

Judge as Gatekeeper for Admissibility of "Reliable" Scientific Evidence

The American judicial system (an *adversarial* judicial system) is systemically engineered to permit a "battle of the experts."[64] American judges have long lamented being placed in the position of having to discern "reliable" scientific or expert testimony in the battlefield of experts.[65] Additionally, judges have understood that, with rare exceptions, jurors are not scientists and are not in a good position to critically evaluate the scientific foundation for expert testimony. Historically, American jurisprudence has vacillated between 2 legal tests for assisting judiciary in the determination of reliable scientific or medical expert testimony: the *Frye* standard (*general acceptance* test) or the *Daubert* standard (general acceptance plus other factors).

In *Frye v United States*,[66] the Court of Appeals for the District of Columbia examined the issue of evaluating the reliability of novel scientific principles underlying expert testimony when it was confronted with a precursor of the modern polygraph or lie detector. The court ruled that expert testimony based on novel scientific principles cannot be admitted in court until the principles are "generally accepted" as reliable by the relevant scientific community.

For most of the 20th century, *Frye* was the dominant test in the United States for evaluating the admissibility of novel scientific evidence. Over the years, however, particularly in the 1980s, *Frye* was subjected to a steady drumbeat of criticism from judges and scholars. The basic criticism was that the *Frye* requirement of general acceptance had the undesirable effect of excluding scientific evidence that had yet to achieve general acceptance but that was nevertheless sufficiently reliable for use in court. Criticism of *Frye* culminated in the US Supreme Court 1993 decision in *Daubert v Merrell Dow Pharmaceuticals, Inc.*[67] In *Daubert*, the Supreme Court rejected *Frye* and replaced it with a new test for scientific evidence.

Under *Daubert*, the Supreme Court made the trial judge the gatekeeper for *all* scientific evidence, not just novel scientific evidence. As was the case with *Frye*, under *Daubert* an attorney could object that expert testimony is based on unreliable scientific principles and request a hearing, now called a *Daubert* hearing. Unlike *Frye*, however, where the only issue at the hearing was general acceptance by the scientific community, the judge conducting a *Daubert* hearing considers all evidence that sheds light on reliability.

In *Daubert*, the Supreme Court wrote that judges conducting *Daubert* hearings should consider the following factors:

- *Falsifiability.* Has the scientific principle underlying the proposed expert testimony been subjected to testing under the scientific method?
- *Peer review.* Has the principle been subjected to peer review and publication?
- *Error rate.* Is there an established error rate when using the principle?
- Borrowing from *Frye*, *general acceptance.* Is the principle generally accepted as reliable in the scientific community?

The *Daubert* court stated that these factors were not a litmus test for reliability but just factors for consideration in the judge's overall assessment of the *methodology* the expert used in arriving at his or her opinion.

Following *Daubert*, there was uncertainty as to whether *Daubert* applied to expert testimony that combines science and professional judgment and interpretation. Thus, does *Daubert* apply to expert testimony from engineers as well as physicians and mental health professionals (who combine scientific knowledge with professional or clinical judgment)? In 1999, the Supreme Court answered in the affirmative with its decision in *Kumho Tire Company, Ltd v Carmichael*.[68] In *Kumho* the Supreme Court ruled, *"Daubert's* general holding—setting forth the trial judge's 'gatekeeping' obligation—applies not only to testimony based on 'scientific' knowledge, but also to testimony based on 'technical' and 'other specialized' knowledge." In *Kumho*, the court reiterated that the trial judge should consider all evidence shedding light on the reliability of expert testimony. The Supreme Court rulings in *Daubert* and *Kumho* are only binding on federal courts and do not compel individual states to abandon *Frye*. As of 2017, a slight majority of states had jettisoned *Frye* in favor of *Daubert*. Interestingly, surveys of state judges have confirmed judicial misunderstanding of the *Daubert* criteria and its consequent difficulty and variability in application.[69]

In many child maltreatment cases involving expert testimony, there is no request for a hearing under *Frye* or *Daubert*. The expert gets on the witness stand, is qualified, testifies, is cross-examined, and that is the end of it. *Frye* and *Daubert* do not come up. Indeed, a few states (eg, California, Florida) have a rule that *Frye* and *Daubert* generally do not apply to opinion testimony. *Frye* or *Daubert* only arises when an attorney believes expert testimony offered by the opponent is based on demonstrably unreliable scientific principles. In such cases, the attorney requests a *Frye* or *Daubert* hearing in an effort to exclude the expert testimony.

Qualification as an Expert

While medical professionals may feel uncomfortable testifying as an expert in child maltreatment, it is important to remember that the definition of *expert* in this context is actually quite broad, and the level of expertise required to qualify as an expert witness is relatively low. The Federal Rules of Evidence define an *expert* as anyone with "scientific, technical, or other specialized knowledge" that would assist the judge or jury in deciding the case.[70] Courts have repeatedly held that one need not be the foremost authority on child maltreatment or understand every nuance of the subject to qualify as an expert.[51] With this minimal threshold in mind, physicians qualify to testify on many matters within their specialty, and sometimes on matters outside of their specialty. Although a physician who does not specialize in child abuse will pass the relatively low threshold required to provide some forms of expert testimony, professionals who lack advanced training and experience in child maltreatment should be careful to avoid exceeding their level of expertise. Medical professionals who are unsure about proper testimony in a child maltreatment case should consult with a child abuse pediatrician for further guidance.

Before a medical professional may testify as an expert witness, a judge must be convinced that the medical professional possesses sufficient knowledge, skill, experience, training, and education to qualify as an expert. In a guided process by the calling attorney, the professional takes the witness stand and answers questions about his or her education, specialized training, publications, prior court qualifications, and relevant experience. Occasionally, the judge asks some additional questions. After establishing the medical professional's qualifications to be rendered an expert, the calling attorney will ask the judge to recognize the witness as an expert in a particular subject matter. The opposing attorney has the right to question the medical professional in an effort to persuade the judge that the professional should not be allowed to testify as an expert. Such questioning by the opposing attorney is called *voir dire*. When the professional's qualifications are obvious, there usually is no voir dire. Being qualified as an expert entitles the medical professional to offer opinions in court, a privilege not inured to other witnesses.[71]

Forms of Expert Testimony

Expert testimony may take several forms, including

- A factual recitation of what the expert observed, tested for, or documented
- An opinion
- Answers to hypothetical questions
- A brief educational exposition providing technical or clinical information for the judge or jury
- Testimony rebutting another witness or expert's theories

Often more than one of these forms is used during testimony.

Opinion Testimony

Expert witnesses in child maltreatment are permitted to offer opinions that touch on the ultimate factual issue in the case. For example, in a physical abuse case, one ultimate factual issue for the jury (or judge) is whether a child's injuries were accidental or inflicted. When a defendant is on trial for rape, penetration is an issue of ultimate fact. It is here, in the use of overlapping medical and legal terminology (ie, abuse), that some courts have limited the vernacular that medical professionals can use. Some courts have required medical professionals to use other, similar terms, such as *non-accidental,* to connote the same medical definition as *abuse.*[72] Medical professionals in child maltreatment should understand that courts exercise this function in efforts to avoid confusing juries and to satisfy the rules of evidence, such as 704(b), where an expert should not opine an ultimate issue for the jury, and 403, where the probative value of evidence should not be substantially outweighed by its prejudicial effect.

It is for this reason that medical professionals should *not* use terminology, either in testimony or in medical documentation, that comments on the mental state (or, in legal terms, mens rea) of a perpetrator. Not only is this arguably an improper role for medical professionals, but this is yet another ultimate issue for the jury or judge. Words such as "intentional," "reckless," or "negligent" should be avoided, because they are common mens rea elements of criminal offenses that lawyers must prove.

Medical professionals can testify about the nature of a child's injuries, the likely mechanism or cause of injury, the degree of force required to produce injury, whether injuries are consistent with a caregiver's explanation, whether injuries are consistent with child abuse, and whether a child's injuries were inflicted or accidental. In some circumstances, experts may opine or be asked to opine whether certain injuries were caused by someone of adult strength, or whether the child's symptomology would have been immediate or possibly delayed. In neglect cases, experts commonly offer an opinion that a child's failure to thrive was caused by parental behavior and not by some medical condition or physical abnormality. In sexual abuse cases, medical experts offer opinions about whether findings of physical examination are consistent with penetrative acts or sexually transmitted infection. When rendering such opinions, the medical professional should recognize (and communicate to the court) that such opinions may be exclusively based on personal experience or have limited evidence base in the medical literature.

Brief Expositions to Educate the Jury

Experts may testify in the form of a brief exposition that provides the jury with information on technical, clinical, or scientific issues. For example, in sexual abuse cases, the defense often asserts that a child's delayed reporting, inconsistent disclosures, or recantation means the child cannot be believed. An expert witness can inform the jury of the reasons for delayed disclosure, delayed reporting, partial or piecemeal disclosures, and recantations. Similarly, in physical abuse cases, experts inform the jury about pertinent aspects of anatomy and physiology, how the body responds to injury, symptoms associated with injuries, the timing and dating of injuries, the role that the history plays in diagnosis, and other matters. The expert witness may also be asked to summarize relevant literature.

This form of expert testimony plays an important role in maltreatment litigation. It not only amplifies the medical professional's persona of an educator but bolsters credibility of the expert witness. However, these expositions must be brief, because "narratives" are frowned on by courts and impermissible by the rules of evidence. Therefore, it is important for the calling attorney and the medical professional to review direct examination questions prior to trial to minimize long narrations. It is in this process that demonstrative tools (eg, photographs, anatomical drawings) can facilitate the educational process of the jury and/or judge.

The Hypothetical Question

In some instances, expert testimony is elicited in response to a hypothetical question. A hypothetical question generally directs the witness to assume that certain facts have been established. The judge will sometimes inform the jurors that they are only to consider the answer to the hypothetical question if all the facts assumed to be true by the expert are established by other evidence. For example, in a physical abuse case in which the testifying expert witness is not a treating physician, an attorney seeks to ascertain an expert's opinion on the likelihood of immediate symptoms versus delayed symptomology. The attorney offering the doctor's testimony says, "Now Doctor, let me ask you to assume that the following facts are true: that the child's eating, feeding, and sleeping patterns were all normal before the 911 call was placed, and the child was described as acting 'normal' by the caregiver for days prior to the onset of symptoms. Based on these facts, Doctor, would it be reasonable for a child with this extent of brain injury to have been acting in such a manner for days prior to presentation for medical care?"

Attorneys cross-examining expert witnesses will often ask hypothetical questions. The cross-examiner may try to undermine the expert's opinion by presenting a hypothetical set of facts that differs from the facts described by the expert. Chadwick and Krous[73] observe that it is "common to encounter hypothetical questions based on hypotheses that are extremely unlikely, and the witness may need to point out the unlikelihood." When asked about a hypothetical set of facts, listen to the premised facts carefully. If there are sufficient gaps in the hypothetical that do not permit an opinion to be rendered, the expert may so state and ask for additional information or facts before being able to render opinion on the hypothetical. In some circumstances, a hypothetical question may be proffered to induce a *possible* scenario. In such circumstances, it would be reasonable for an expert to opine that "anything is possible," but his or her medical expert opinion is confined to reasonable probabilities, not any possibilities.

Cross-examination and Impeachment of Expert Witnesses

Testifying begins with direct examination. During direct examination, the expert witness answers questions from the attorney who asked the expert to testify. After direct examination, the opposing attorney has the right to cross-examine the expert witness. Cross-examination is sometimes followed by redirect examination. Some common forms and themes of cross-examination are discussed in the following sections.

Positive and Negative Cross-examination

Cross-examination can be broken down into 2 types: positive and negative. With *positive* cross-examination, the cross-examining attorney does not attack the expert. Rather, the attorney questions the expert in a positive—even friendly—way, seeking agreement from the expert on certain facts or inferences that may be helpful to the attorney's client. With *negative* cross-examination, by contrast, the attorney seeks to undermine (impeach) the expert's testimony. A cross-examining attorney who plans to employ both types of cross-examination typically begins with positive questioning in the hopes of eliciting favorable testimony from the expert.

Asking Only Leading Questions on Cross-examination

The key to a successful cross-examination is controlling what the witness says in response to the questions. This is best accomplished by asking only questions that require short, specific answers, preferably limited to "yes" or "no." These are known as *leading* questions and are only permissible by courtroom procedure on cross-examination. If done on direct examination (outside of the circumstance of laying foundation), an attorney will be confronted with an "objection, leading." In fact, experienced cross-examiners almost never ask non-leading questions during cross-examination. The cross-examiner keeps the witness hemmed in with such leading questions and seldom asks "why" or "how" something happened. "Why" and "how" questions relinquish control to the expert.

When an expert attempts to explain an answer to a leading question, the cross-examiner may interrupt and say, "Please just answer 'yes' or 'no.'" If the expert persists, the cross-examiner may ask the judge to admonish the expert to limit answers to the questions asked. Medical professionals should understand that such methods are not attempts to frustrate but merely well-established courtroom procedure. While it may be frustrating, medical professionals should listen carefully to questions asked and answer them if answerable. If answering requires conjecture, assumptions, or premises not stated in the question, experts are advised to respond in a manner that indicates the inability to answer the question as stated. One example might be, "Sir/ma'am, it is not possible for me to answer the question with a simple 'yes' or 'no.' May I explain myself?" Another tactic may be to appeal to the judge that the question is not answerable as asked. Judges sometimes may permit witnesses to amplify their opinion during cross-examination, but most often will advise the witness to answer the question asked, if possible, and that opportunity for amplification or clarification will be afforded on redirect examination.

Impeaching an Expert Witness: Bias and Undermining the Expert's Facts, Inferences, or Conclusions

One of the most common cross-examination techniques with expert witnesses is to portray the expert as biased. This may be personal, professional, philosophical, financial, or some other form of bias. One of the more common methods for demonstrating a professional bias is to portray the medical expert as preferential to, or an *advocate* for, one side. An attorney may attempt to infer this by inquiring of the medical professional's determinations of abuse versus non-abuse in clinical care. Another manner is to infer a preference for testifying for one particular legal side or another (ie, testifying almost exclusively for the prosecution or defense). Medical professionals can insulate themselves from these inferences by, first, having ready their general clinical statistics on diagnostic impressions (ie, relative percentages of abuse determinations versus non-abuse/indeterminate determinations) and, second, by making themselves available to consult or testify for both sides. It is not lost on judges or juries that treating clinicians have no say in the side that calls them to testify. However, expert consultations or testimony exclusively for one side or another can bolster the inference of partiality.

Another practical consideration for minimizing claims of bias is willingness to talk with both legal sides prior to trial when the medical professional is a treating clinician (and not exclusively a consulting expert for the purposes of trial). When engaging in this practice, the medical professional should establish some boundaries and exercise some caution. First and foremost, he or she should ensure that the attorney with whom he or she is about to speak has appropriate HIPAA release or authorization for discussing protected health information. Second, it is a wise practice to inform the attorney that no *informal* audio or video recording (ie, not a deposition or without a court-appointed stenographer for recording purposes) will be permitted of the discussion. This is to prevent any potential impeachment at trial with unofficial transcripts of recordings.

Additionally, bias can be suggested by demonstrating an expert who is unwilling to change an opinion when confronted with data that conflict with the opinion. It is good medicolegal practice to acknowledge, especially in documentation, that you are willing to look at additional data that could alter your medical impression.

Aside from portraying bias, another common cross-examination theme is to attack the facts, inferences, or conclusions that comprise the basis of the expert's opinion. This is a typical scenario in which a cross-examining attorney may ask the professional a hypothetical question on the stand with changed facts. Rather than attack the doctor's facts, inferences, and conclusions during cross-examination, the attorney may limit cross-examination to pinning the doctor down to a limited set of facts, inferences, and conclusions and then, when the doctor has left the witness stand, offer another expert to contradict the data supporting the doctor's testimony.

Finally, a cross-examining attorney may seek to undermine the expert's testimony by confronting the expert with books or articles (called *learned treatises* or *evidence-based literature*) that seem to contradict the expert's opinion or basis for his or her opinion. Because attorneys are not scientists and their aptitude and proclivity for reviewing and understanding scientific literature varies, this is an uncommon practice fraught with danger for the attorney. The rules on impeachment with learned treatises vary from state to state. However, there is agreement on one thing: when an expert is confronted with a select sentence or a paragraph from a larger article or chapter, the expert has the right to put the selected passage in context by reading surrounding material. If confronted with this scenario on the stand, the expert should state something to the effect of, "Counsel, I cannot comment on the sentence you have selected unless I first read the entire article. If you will permit me to read the article, I'll be happy to answer your question about a particular sentence or paragraph out of that article."

Courtroom Testimony Pearls: Maintain Professional Demeanor, Listen to Questions Carefully, and Ask for Clarification When Applicable

The experienced expert witness refuses to be cajoled, dragged, or tricked into verbal sparring with the cross-examiner. The medical professional is at all times just that—professional. Given the aggression of some cross-examiners—aggression that is sometimes laced with error, misinterpretation, and even personal attack—it is a challenge to maintain a calm, professional demeanor on the witness stand. Yet, the professional must do just that. Fact finders (ie, judges, juries) are people. They have unstated norms and expectations of respect, courtesy, and humility. In the professional sparring of cross-examination, the one who loses calm or demonstrates aggression or arrogance in tone, words, or behavior is the one who has lost the argument. Judges and juries want, and expect, the medical professional to be data driven, objective, open-minded, and, most of all, humble and courteous. This does not mean the expert witness should be submissive or easily suggestible. It means that respected medical professionals will express confidence when challenged, not vacillate or equivocate in the face of attack, but concede weak points and acknowledge conflicting evidence or data gaps.

Achieving the end goal of being an expert for the court is a skill. Much like skills of physical examination, it requires actual experience and repetition. Ten basic pearls of good testimony to be practiced include

1. Sit attentively and with good posture in the witness stand.
2. Listen to each question carefully.
3. When answering more than a "yes" or "no" question, turn to the fact finder (ie, judge, jury) and speak to him, her, or them.
4. When questioning becomes heated or aggressive, briefly pause and breathe before answering and be mindful to maintain a nonaggressive tone in response.
5. Do not be arrogant, flippant, or petty.
6. Try to answer each question with a data focus; when feasible, state that "The data indicate...."
7. When providing medical information, use plain English; if using medical terms, make conscious efforts to explain them in plain English.
8. Know the medical facts of the case well.
9. Be ready to concede limitations of facts or gaps in medical literature.
10. Do not speculate or exaggerate.

Liability

A medical professional's liability risk in child maltreatment cases stems from 3 general areas: reporting maltreatment, diagnosing maltreatment (eg, malpractice actions and civil actions related to deprivation of constitutional rights), and providing expert testimony. Although a medical professional may encounter other adverse actions (eg, civil suits for defamation or battery, administrative complaints to state licensing boards), these are less common and, therefore, beyond the scope of this chapter. As a general rule, to minimize liability risk, it is prudent for a medical professional to closely review his or her employment malpractice insurance policy and to have a discussion with his or her institution's risk management and/or legal counsel to understand well its coverage and limitations with regard to child maltreatment practice.

However, equally as important as protecting oneself from potential financial liability, a professional should be cognizant of the emotional liability the legal process can exact when a medical professional is sued. The negative feelings of having one's professional reputation besmirched, of losing decision-making control when in the legal forum, and of being judged by a process that may not seem very fair, all factor into emotional trauma that can affect a medical professional. Medical professionals should be aware that the American Academy of Pediatrics, as well as other professional medical societies, have support resources for medical professionals who have been or are being sued.

Liability Associated With Reporting Maltreatment

All US jurisdictions provide reporters of abuse some form of immunity from liability when reports of suspected abuse are made in good faith. *Good faith* means that a reporter must genuinely suspect that a child has been abused or neglected.[74] Some states afford reporters a *presumption of good faith,* meaning that the good faith of the reporter is assumed until it is disproved. Conversely, many jurisdictions will revoke a reporter's immunity when reports are deemed false or are maliciously made. More than half of jurisdictions specify civil or criminal penalties for false reporting.[2]

The statutory immunity for reporting abuse often does not extend to other aspects of child protection cases (eg, performing case reviews, taking photographs, providing testimony in a judicial proceeding).[75] For example, approximately 36 jurisdictions provide immunity to reporters who participate in any judicial proceedings that may arise from a child abuse report, but only 26 jurisdictions provide immunity to reporters who "assist with" or "participate in" a child maltreatment investigation.[75] Thus, it is prudent for medical professionals to be familiar with the governing statute in their jurisdiction.

If immunity represents one side of the reporting coin, *liability* represents the other. Almost all states list penalties for mandatory reporters who *fail to report* suspected abuse or neglect.[2] Penalties can include fines and/or imprisonment. In most states, failure to report is a misdemeanor, but in a few states, repeat failures to report or failure to report serious abusive injuries are regarded as potential felony offenses. Despite known underreporting of suspected abuse, charges against medical professionals for failure to report have been infrequent.[76] When charges have been brought, court records reveal that most cases were thrown out.

Liability Associated With Diagnosing Maltreatment

The diagnosis of maltreatment, like any medical diagnosis, is subject to malpractice liability. Medical professionals can be found negligent in their medical duty in either not having recognized or diagnosed abuse or in diagnosing abuse when another medical diagnosis explains the findings. Prevalence of malpractice liability related to a diagnosis of child maltreatment is unknown but believed to be low. Factors that affect malpractice suit prevalence include the breadth of the immunity language in individual state reporting laws and the presence or absence of malpractice liability caps in the particular state.

In addition to malpractice risk, medical professionals involved in child maltreatment cases are also susceptible to civil suits known as *1983 actions*—suits brought by parents under 42 USC §1983, a federal statute that affords US citizens civil redress against the state for violations of constitutional rights. Typically, parents allege that medical professionals who assist CPS in the process of removing children from their custody violate their constitutional rights to be free from "unlawful seizures" under the Fourth Amendment and their right to "familial relations" under the Fourteenth Amendment of the US Constitution.[77] As with malpractice liability, the prevalence of these suits is unknown but believed to be uncommon. For the most part, these actions have been unsuccessful in the courts.[78] However, even the successful defeat of these actions is not without costs to medical professionals, such as loss of time, higher malpractice costs, and significant emotional anguish. Thus, it is prudent for medical professionals to review their malpractice insurance coverage policies to ensure that those policies contain sufficiently broad language to provide coverage for expert testimony and other involvement in the child abuse evaluation and treatment process.

Liability Associated With Providing Expert Testimony in Maltreatment Cases

The determination of whether a medical professional's expert testimony constitutes the practice of medicine (and, therefore, is subject to malpractice liability) is variable from jurisdiction to jurisdiction.

Some professional medical organizations and courts have deemed the provision of expert testimony as the practice of medicine; others have not.[79] Florida, for example, requires a medical professional to attain an "expert witness certificate" prior to providing testimony the state.[80] In essence, Florida requires out-of-state medical professionals to first attain a limited measure of Florida licensure prior to providing testimony in that state or be subject to liability for the unlawful practice of medicine. Arizona courts, however, have held differently.[81] Thus, medical expert witnesses should be cognizant of potential licensure requirements in other states where they provide expert testimony.

In addition to potential malpractice liability, physician expert witnesses are also subject to civil and criminal liability for the provision of false testimony (ie, perjury). Although the prosecution of perjury related to the provision of expert testimony is an extremely uncommon occurrence, medical professionals should always strive to provide expert testimony that is reliable, honest, unbiased, and based on evidence-based scientific principles. Failure to do so opens the medical professional to potential embarrassment on cross-examination, potential grievance with professional societies or state medical boards, and, more rarely, other civil or criminal legal action. Some professional medical societies (eg, American Association of Neurological Surgeons, American Academy of Orthopaedic Surgeons) have taken the vanguard position of being more active in the regulation of unethical or unreliable expert testimony with a variety of disciplinary measures (ie, censure, probation, suspension, or expulsion).[82] Others have sought to combat inappropriate expert testimony by publishing examples of unethical expert testimony or by requiring members to sign an affirmation statement promising to provide ethical expert testimony. Thus, medical professionals should be aware of the mandates of their professional society.

In summary, medical professional liability in child maltreatment cases can arise from a variety of circumstances. Medical professionals should be well acquainted with the governing laws of reporting and testimony in their jurisdiction, of the specific mandates of their professional society and state medical board, and of the provisions of coverage of their malpractice insurance. If medical professionals have additional or more case-specific questions, it may be prudent to consult with their local child abuse pediatrician or hospital counsel.

Conclusion

The professions of medicine and law sometimes seem like ships passing in the night. Yet, if children are to be protected, medical professionals and attorneys must put aside their differences and work together.

Only genuine interdisciplinary cooperation holds realistic hope of reducing the tragic number of children who experience abuse and neglect.

Acknowledgment

The authors wish to acknowledge the contributions of John E.B. Myers, JD, in writing the original version of this chapter.

References

1. Miyamoto S, Dharmar M, Boyle C, et al. Impact of telemedicine on the quality of forensic sexual abuse examinations in rural communities. *Child Abuse Negl.* 2014;38(9):1533–1539 PMID: 24841062 https://doi.org/10.1016/j.chiabu.2014.04.015
2. Child Welfare Information Gateway. US Department of Health and Human Services, Children's Bureau Washington, DC. Mandatory reporters of child abuse and neglect 2016. https://www.childwelfare.gov/topics/systemwide/laws-policies/statutes/manda. Accessed June 6, 2019
3. Zellman G, Fair C. Preventing and reporting abuse. In: Myers JEB, Berliner L, Briere JN, Hendrix CT, eds. *The APSAC Handbook of Child Maltreatment.* Thousand Oaks, CA: Sage; 2002:449–475
4. Krase KS, DeLong-Hamilton TA. Comparing reports of suspected child maltreatment in states with and without universal mandated reporting. *Child Youth Serv Rev.* 2015;50:96–100 https://doi.org/10.1016/j.childyouth.2015.01.015
5. Palusci VJ, Vandervort FE, Lewis JM. Does changing mandated reporting laws improve child maltreatment reporting in large U.S. counties? *Child Youth Serv Rev.* 2016;66: 170–179 https://doi.org/10.1016/j.childyouth.2016.05.002
6. Ho GW, Gross DA, Bettencourt A. Universal mandatory reporting policies and the odds of identifying child physical abuse. *Am J Public Health.* 2017;107(5):709–716 PMID: 28323475 https://doi.org/10.2105/AJPH.2017.303667
7. Raz M. Unintended consequences of expanded mandatory reporting laws. *Pediatrics.* 2017;139(4):e20163511 PMID: 28292874 https://doi.org/10.1542/peds.2016-3511
8. Jones R, Flaherty EG, Binns HJ, et al; Child Abuse Reporting Experience Study Research Group. Clinicians' description of factors influencing their reporting of suspected child abuse: report of the Child Abuse Reporting Experience Study Research Group. *Pediatrics.* 2008;122(2):259–266 PMID: 18676541 https://doi.org/10.1542/peds.2007-2312
9. Bean RB. *Osler Aphorisms, From His Bedside Teachings and Writings.* New York, NY: Henry Schuman, Inc; 1950
10. Talsma M, Bengtsson Boström K, Östberg AL. Facing suspected child abuse—what keeps Swedish general practitioners from reporting to child protective services? *Scand J Prim Health Care.* 2015;33(1):21–26 PMID: 25676563 https://doi.org/10.3109/02813432.2015.1001941
11. Flaherty EG, Sege RD, Griffith J, et al; PROS Network; NMAPedsNet. From suspicion of physical child abuse to reporting: primary care clinician decision-making. *Pediatrics.* 2008;122(3):611–619 PMID: 18676507 https://doi.org/10.1542/peds.2007-2311
12. Wellbery C. The value of medical uncertainty? *Lancet.* 2010;375(9727):1686–1687 PMID: 20480942 https://doi.org/10.1016/S0140-6736(10)60725-8
13. Simpkin AL, Schwartzstein RM. Tolerating uncertainty—the next medical revolution? *N Engl J Med.* 2016;375(18):1713–1715 PMID: 27806221 https://doi.org/10.1056/NEJMp1606402

14. Han PK. The need for uncertainty: a case for prognostic silence. *Perspect Biol Med.* 2016;59(4):567–575 PMID: 28690246 https://doi.org/10.1353/pbm.2016.0049
15. Smith AK, White DB, Arnold RM. Uncertainty—the other side of prognosis. *N Engl J Med.* 2013;368(26):2448–2450 PMID: 23802514 https://doi.org/10.1056/NEJMp1303295
16. Luther VP, Crandall SJ. Commentary: ambiguity and uncertainty: neglected elements of medical education curricula? *Acad Med.* 2011;86(7):799–800 PMID: 21715991 https://doi.org/10.1097/ACM.0b013e31821da915
17. Katz J. Why doctors don't disclose uncertainty. *Hastings Cent Rep.* 1984;14(1):35–44 PMID: 6715153 https://doi.org/10.2307/3560848
18. Srivastava R. Dealing with uncertainty in a time of plenty. *N Engl J Med.* 2011;365(24):2252–2253 PMID: 22168641 https://doi.org/10.1056/NEJMp1109456
19. Deutsch SA. A struggle for certainty—protecting the vulnerable. *N Engl J Med.* 2015;372(6):506–507 PMID: 25651244 https://doi.org/10.1056/NEJMp1409627
20. Wray CM, Loo LK. The diagnosis, prognosis, and treatment of medical uncertainty. *J Grad Med Educ.* 2015;7(4):523–527 PMID: 26692960 https://doi.org/10.4300/JGME-D-14-00638.1
21. Dias MS, Boehmer S, Johnston-Walsh L, Levi BH. Defining "reasonable medical certainty" in court: what does it mean to medical experts in child abuse cases? *Child Abuse Negl.* 2015;50:218–227 PMID: 26589362 https://doi.org/10.1016/j.chiabu.2015.10.027
22. Myers JE. What is the meaning of "reasonable medical certainty"? Your guess is as good as mine. *Child Abuse Negl.* 2015;50:228–231 PMID: 26686005 https://doi.org/10.1016/j.chiabu.2015.11.008
23. Narang SK. The unreasonableness of "reasonable medical certainty." *Child Abuse Negl.* 2015;50:232–233 PMID: 26686006 https://doi.org/10.1016/j.chiabu.2015.11.009
24. Levi BH, Brown G. Reasonable suspicion: a study of Pennsylvania pediatricians regarding child abuse. *Pediatrics.* 2005;116(1):e5–e12 PMID: 15995018 https://doi.org/10.1542/peds.2004-2649
25. Levi BH, Crowell K. Child abuse experts disagree about the threshold for mandated reporting. *Clin Pediatr (Phila).* 2011;50(4):321–329 PMID: 21138854 https://doi.org/10.1177/0009922810389170
26. American Academy of Pediatrics Task Force on Sudden Infant Death Syndrome. SIDS and other sleep-related infant deaths: updated 2016 recommendations for a safe infant sleeping environment. *Pediatrics.* 2016;138(5):e20162938 PMID: 27940804 https://doi.org/10.1542/peds.2016-2938
27. Keenan HT, Cook LJ, Olson LM, Bardsley T, Campbell KA. Social intuition and social information in physical child abuse evaluation and diagnosis. *Pediatrics.* 2017;140(5):e20171188 PMID: 29074609 https://doi.org/10.1542/peds.2017-1188
28. Dyer C. Professor Roy Meadow struck off. *BMJ.* 2005;331(7510):177 PMID: 16037430 https://doi.org/10.1136/bmj.331.7510.177
29. Binder EB, Bradley RG, Liu W, et al. Association of FKBP5 polymorphisms and childhood abuse with risk of posttraumatic stress disorder symptoms in adults. *JAMA.* 2008;299(11):1291–1305 PMID: 18349090 https://doi.org/10.1001/jama.299.11.1291
30. Dubowitz H, Papas MA, Black MM, Starr RH Jr. Child neglect: outcomes in high-risk urban preschoolers. *Pediatrics.* 2002;109(6):1100–1107 PMID: 12042549 https://doi.org/10.1542/peds.109.6.1100
31. Keenan HT, Hooper SR, Wetherington CE, Nocera M, Runyan DK. Neurodevelopmental consequences of early traumatic brain injury in 3-year-old children. *Pediatrics.* 2007;119(3):e616–e623 PMID: 17332181 https://doi.org/10.1542/peds.2006-2313
32. Beresford EB. Uncertainty and the shaping of medical decisions. *Hastings Cent Rep.* 1991;21(4):6–11 PMID: 1938352 https://doi.org/10.2307/3562993

33. Han PK, Klein WM, Arora NK. Varieties of uncertainty in health care: a conceptual taxonomy. *Med Decis Making*. 2011;31(6):828–838 PMID: 22067431 https://doi.org/10.1177/0272989X10393976
34. Moles RL, Asnes AG. Has this child been abused? Exploring uncertainty in the diagnosis of maltreatment. *Pediatr Clin North Am*. 2014;61(5):1023–1036 PMID: 25242713 https://doi.org/10.1016/j.pcl.2014.06.009
35. Krugman RD. The more we learn, the less we know "with reasonable medical certainty"? *Child Abuse Negl*. 1989;13(2):165–166 PMID: 2743176 https://doi.org/10.1016/0145-2134(89)90001-X
36. McCann J, Wells R, Simon M, Voris J. Genital findings in prepubertal girls selected for nonabuse: a descriptive study. *Pediatrics*. 1990;86(3):428–439 PMID: 2388791
37. Oh DL, Jerman P, Silvério Marques S, et al. Systematic review of pediatric health outcomes associated with childhood adversity. *BMC Pediatr*. 2018;18(1):83 PMID: 29475430 https://doi.org/10.1186/s12887-018-1037-7
38. McCrory E, De Brito SA, Viding E. The link between child abuse and psychopathology: a review of neurobiological and genetic research. *J R Soc Med*. 2012;105(4):151–156 PMID: 22532655 https://doi.org/10.1258/jrsm.2011.110222
39. Notterman DA, Mitchell C. Epigenetics and understanding the impact of social determinants of health. *Pediatr Clin North Am*. 2015;62(5):1227–1240 PMID: 26318949 https://doi.org/10.1016/j.pcl.2015.05.012
40. Campbell KA, Cook LJ, LaFleur BJ, Keenan HT. Household, family, and child risk factors after an investigation for suspected child maltreatment: a missed opportunity for prevention. *Arch Pediatr Adolesc Med*. 2010;164(10):943–949 PMID: 20921352 https://doi.org/10.1001/archpediatrics.2010.166
41. Campbell KA, Thomas AM, Cook LJ, Keenan HT. Longitudinal experiences of children remaining at home after a first-time investigation for suspected maltreatment. *J Pediatr*. 2012;161(2):340–347 PMID: 22480699 https://doi.org/10.1016/j.jpeds.2012.02.039
42. Flaherty EG, Jones R, Sege R; Child Abuse Recognition Experience Study Research Group. Telling their stories: primary care practitioners' experience evaluating and reporting injuries caused by child abuse. *Child Abuse Negl*. 2004;28(9):939–945 PMID: 15450760 https://doi.org/10.1016/j.chiabu.2004.03.013
43. Aquino J. The significance of unknown significance. *Acad Pediatr*. 2017;17(8):799–800 PMID: 28919573 https://doi.org/10.1016/j.acap.2017.09.007
44. Politi MC, Han PK, Col NF. Communicating the uncertainty of harms and benefits of medical interventions. *Med Decis Making*. 2007;27(5):681–695 PMID: 17873256 https://doi.org/10.1177/0272989X07307270
45. Hussey JM, Marshall JM, English DJ, et al. Defining maltreatment according to substantiation: distinction without a difference? *Child Abuse Negl*. 2005;29(5):479–492 PMID: 15970321 https://doi.org/10.1016/j.chiabu.2003.12.005
46. Kohl PL, Jonson-Reid M, Drake B. Time to leave substantiation behind: findings from a national probability study. *Child Maltreat*. 2009;14(1):17–26 PMID: 18971346 https://doi.org/10.1177/1077559508326030
47. American Medical Association. Code of Medical Ethics: Overview. https://www.ama-assn.org/delivering-care/ethics/code-medical-ethics-overview. Accessed June 10, 2019
48. American Nurses Association. *Code of Ethics for Nurses With Interpretive Statements*. Silver Spring, MD: American Nurses Association; 2015. https://www.nursingworld.org/coe-view-only. Accessed June 10, 2019
49. Gutheil TG, Appelbaum PS. *Clinical Handbook of Psychiatry and the Law*. New York, NY: McGraw-Hill; 1982

50. Myers JEB. *Legal Issues in Child Abuse and Neglect Practice*. 2nd ed. Thousand Oaks, CA: SAGE Publications; 1998
51. Myers JEB. *Myers on Evidence of Interpersonal Violence: Child Maltreatment, Intimate Partner Violence, Rape, Stalking, and Elder Abuses*. 5th ed. New York, NY: Aspen Law & Business; 2011
52. *United States v Yazzie,* CA9, 59 F3d 807 (1995)
53. Jones DPH. *Interviewing the Sexually Abused Child: Investigation of Suspected Abuse*. Gaskell, United Kingdom: Royal College of Psychiatrists; 1992
54. *Crawford v Washington,* 541 US 36 (2004)
55. *Davis v Washington,* 126 US 2266 (2006)
56. *State v Bobadilla,* 709 NW2d 243 (MN 2006)
57. *State v Blue,* 717 NW2d 558 (ND 2006)
58. *Commonwealth v DeOliveria,* 849 NE2d 243 (MA 2006)
59. *Hobgood v State,* 926 So2d 847 (MS 2006)
60. *State v Moses,* 119 P3d 906 (Wash Ct App 2005)
61. Weinstein JB, Dewsbury I. Comment on the meaning of 'proof beyond a reasonable doubt.' *Law Probab Risk*. 2006;5(2):167–173 https://doi.org/10.1093/lpr/mgl016
62. Judicial Council of California. Civil jury instructions. https://www.justia.com/trials-litigation/docs/caci/200/200/. Published 2017. Accessed June 3, 2019
63. Leventhal JM, Edwards GA. Flawed theories to explain child physical abuse: what are the medical-legal consequences? *JAMA*. 2017;318(14):1317–1318 PMID: 28975235 https://doi.org/10.1001/jama.2017.11703
64. World Bank Group. Comparative study on expert witnesses in court proceedings. https://openknowledge.worldbank.org/handle/10986/2991. Published June 30, 2010. Accessed June 3, 2019
65. Hand L. Historical and practical considerations regarding expert testimony. *Harv Law Rev*. 1901;15(1):40–58 https://doi.org/10.2307/1322532
66. *Frye v United States,* 293 F 1013 (DC Cir 1923)
67. *Daubert v Merrell Dow Pharmaceuticals, Inc,* 509 US 579 (1993)
68. *Kumho Tire Company, Ltd v Carmichael,* 526 US 137 (1999)
69. Gatowski SI, Dobbin SA, Richardson JT, Ginsburg GP, Merlino ML, Dahir V. Asking the gatekeepers: a national survey of judges on judging expert evidence in a post-Daubert world. *Law Hum Behav*. 2001;25(5):433–458 PMID: 11688367 https://doi.org/10.1023/A:1012899030937
70. Federal Rules of Evidence. Rule 702. Testimony by expert witnesses. Legal Information Institute website. https://www.law.cornell.edu/rules/fre/rule_702. Accessed June 3, 2019
71. Federal Rules of Evidence. Rule 703. Bases of an expert. Legal Information Institute website. https://www.law.cornell.edu/rules/fre/rule_703. Accessed June 3, 2019
72. *State v Holzknecht,* 157 Wash App 754, 238 P3d 1233 (2010)
73. Chadwick DL, Krous HF. Irresponsible testimony by medical experts in cases involving the physical abuse and neglect of children. *Child Maltreat*. 1997;2(4):313–321 https://doi.org/10.1177/1077559597002004004
74. US Department of Health and Human Services; Administration for Children and Families; Administration on Children, Youth, and Families; Children's Bureau. Report to Congress on immunity from prosecution for professional consultation in suspected and known instances of child abuse and neglect. https://www.acf.hhs.gov/sites/default/files/cb/capta_immunity_rptcongress.pdf. Published June 2013. Accessed June 3, 2019
75. Child Welfare Information Gateway. Immunity for reporters of child abuse and neglect. https://www.childwelfare.gov/pubPDFs/immunity.pdf. Accessed June 3, 2019

76. Heath B. Few penalties for keeping child abuse secret. *USA Today*. http://usatoday30.usatoday.com/news/nation/story/2012-01-02/unreported-child-abuse/51981108/1. Updated December 16, 2011. Accessed June 3, 2019
77. Hoult J. The evidentiary admissibility of parental alienation syndrome: science, law, and policy. *Child Leg Rights J*. 2006;26:1–61
78. Myers JEB. *A Mother's Nightmare—Incest: A Practical Legal Guide for Parents and Professionals*. Thousand Oaks, CA: Sage; 1997
79. American Academy of Psychiatry and the Law. Report 18 of the Board of Trustees of the American Medical Association (1-98). Expert witness testimony (reference committee B). https://www.aapl.org/AMA_expert_witness.htm. Accessed June 3, 2019
80. Florida Board of Medicine. Expert witness certificate. http://www.flboardofmedicine.gov/licensing/expert-witness-certificate. Accessed June 3, 2019
81. *Seisinger v Siebel*, 220 AZ 85; 203 P3d 483
82. Kesselheim AS, Studdert DM. Professional oversight of physician expert witnesses: an analysis of complaints to the Professional Conduct Committee of the American Association of Neurological Surgeons, 1992–2006. *Ann Surg*. 2009;249(1):168–172. PMID: 19106694. https://doi.org/10.1097/SLA.0b013e31818a14ef

CHAPTER 27

Caring for Those Who Care: Vicarious Trauma and Burnout

Antonia Chiesa, MD
University of Colorado School of Medicine
Kempe Center for the Prevention and Treatment of Child Abuse and Neglect
Children's Hospital Colorado
Aurora, CO

Sasha Svendsen, MD, FAAP
UMass Memorial Children's Medical Center
Westborough, MA
University of Massachusetts Medical School
Worcester, MA

"The capacity for compassion and empathy seems to be at the core of our ability to do the work and at the core of our ability to be wounded by the work." Charles Figley

Introduction

Health care is considered the helping science. Medical professionals are attracted to medical practice out of an altruistic concern for others. This characteristic also makes medical professionals vulnerable to emotional stress when exposed to the suffering of others. The stress is understandable; however, if negative emotions go unchecked, there can be serious consequences for the medical professional. Ironically, the degree to which one is committed to the work may increase susceptibility to stressors. While some may cope better than others, no one is entirely immune. All medical professionals are at risk, and work within the field of child maltreatment carries unique challenges.

Scope of the Problem

Since the first extensive, national study in 2011 of physician burnout, which documented a 45% rate of at least one burnout symptom and higher rates of burnout compared with other professionals,[1] a multitude of other studies have confirmed the phenomenon.[2–4] Burnout is not unique to one subspecialty or dependent on length of practice. The phenomenon crosses all specialty domains and types of professional. Due to workforce shortages in the field of child maltreatment and the inherently challenging patient care, professionals in this field may be at particular risk.[5] Trainees may be more vulnerable, with reported burnout rates of up to 75%.[6–8] Besides the emotional burden, physician burnout can lead to decreased productivity, as gauged by sick leave and the ability to work and remain in the same job.[9]

Research in this area is growing and informing intervention. Current knowledge is based on a limited number of available tools and challenges with study design (mostly small cross-sectional studies dependent on self-report and subject to recall bias).[10] Furthermore, many of the studies do not examine the same outcome or obtain data from a single site or specialty, making generalizability more difficult. Despite these issues in research, lack of recognition is no longer an issue. Burnout and its consequences indicate a crisis in the health care field, necessitating a call to action among medical professionals and systems.

As part of recognition of the importance of establishing healthy stress responses early in one's career, there has been focus on professionalism standards within medical education. The Accreditation Council for Graduate Medical Education (ACGME) has prioritized curriculum development aimed to promote resilience and prevent burnout. These efforts are often embedded within the domain of professional development. The American Board of Pediatrics, in collaboration with the ACGME, created relevant pediatric milestones regarding professionalism. Milestones focus on how stress can affect professional behavior, emphasizing the importance of self-awareness, help-seeking behaviors, conduct, conflict management, and adaptability.[11] Similarly, 1 of the 4 Entrustable Professional Activities created for the child abuse pediatrics subspecialty includes the development of behaviors and strategies to cope with the stresses of caring for patients who have experienced maltreatment.[12] Relevant work in this area crosses specialties, and user-friendly tools are available that can assist educators in the dialogue around managing difficult emotions and creating individual wellness plans.[13]

Definitions

Varying language has been used to describe the emotional stress associated with the workplace and, more specifically, working with others who have experienced trauma. Definitions are often used interchangeably, but when examined there are subtle, important differences among concepts. Establishing a framework is essential to identify, measure, and assess intervention strategies.

Terms used to describe the negative emotional effect of work within the caring professions include *vicarious trauma, compassion fatigue, posttraumatic stress disorder* (*PTSD*), *toxic stress, secondary trauma,* and *burnout.* Conceptually, these states exist on a continuum and may fluctuate over time depending on an individual's experiences. The following definitions help to differentiate similar constructs:

- **Secondary trauma:** A relatively immediate response whereby, following an indirect exposure to a traumatic event or series of events, the service provider internalizes the experience of his or her client and may begin to feel or exhibit post-traumatic symptoms similar to those expressed by the client.[14] Secondary trauma can occur following a single episode, whereas vicarious trauma results from the accumulation of experiences over time.[15]
- **Vicarious trauma:** The cumulative effect on the service provider of being repeatedly exposed to the trauma experienced by clients through empathetic engagement that affects the provider's worldview.[16] Vicarious trauma may exhibit similar symptoms to burnout and compassion fatigue, such as emotional exhaustion. Responses may be apparent in multiple facets of life.[17]
- **Compassion fatigue:** Succinctly put, "the stress resulting from helping or wanting to help a traumatized or suffering person."[15] This term also has general applicability to anyone in a caregiving role and describes the result of the repetitive and stressful nature of caregiving that has a negative effect on the empathic ability of the caregiver.[18] This reduced capacity can manifest suddenly, often resulting in a disinterest or inability of the caregiver to bear the suffering of another.[15] The individual may also experience unexplained emotions, such as fear or sadness, in the absence of a triggering event.[16]
- **Burnout:** "A syndrome of emotional exhaustion, depersonalization, and reduced personal accomplishment that can occur among individuals who do 'people work' of some kind."[19] Burnout is a work-related cumulative process occurring over time in response to repetitive job stress.[20] It can lead to feeling overextended, depleted, and cynical, resulting in decreased efficacy at work.[21,22] Reaching burnout is a prolonged process and is typically associated with the work environment itself.

Warning Signs

Regardless of the label, the signs and symptoms of emotional stress are varied and can affect many domains of functioning. Stress is an inevitable part of life. The physiologic response to stress is helpful in certain situations, prompting the release of cortisol and priming the individual for action. How an individual responds to stress is likely multifactorial, a complex interplay of genetics, environment, and developmental factors; however, prolonged and overwhelming stress can lead to adverse and exaggerated behavioral and physiologic symptoms.[23]

Physical and cognitive symptoms can include fatigue, somatic complaints, sleep dysfunction, inability to concentrate or make decisions, disillusionment, poor memory, emotional lability, and apathy.[24] Behavioral and emotional reactions can include hyperarousal, withdrawal, loss of humor, guilt, and feelings of helplessness. Depression, anxiety, and even suicide are among the most severe outcomes. All these factors can increase risk of medical error and lapses in patient safety protocols.[25]

Assessment Tools

Challenges with terminology have complicated the development of a universal tool for measuring the signs and symptoms of workplace stress within health care. Burnout was first described decades ago through the clinical observations of Freudenberger, a psychiatrist, who observed many different physical and mental symptoms among clinical staff.[26] Attempts to measure burnout included structured interviews and projected drawings, although many were rejected by the research community. These early efforts raised issues of inter-rater reliability and the need for self-report tools.

The Maslach Burnout Inventory (MBI) was first published in 1981 and is intended for use for those in the human services or "people professions." It is a 22-item self-assessment tool that measures the 3 domains of burnout: emotional exhaustion, depersonalization, and personal achievement.[27] The MBI is the most popular and widely used measurement of burnout and has emerged as the gold standard assessment tool.[28]

The Copenhagen Burnout Inventory (CBI) was subsequently developed in the Netherlands. This tool recognizes exhaustion as the primary component of burnout and measures personal, work-related, and client-related realms.[29] The CBI has been shown to be useful in measuring burnout in those working in the human service sector, including caseworkers and child welfare professionals.

Another commonly used tool is the Professional Quality of Life (ProQOL) measure.[30] This tool has been in use since 1995 and examines the positive and negative effects experienced by individuals who help those who have experienced trauma.[31] The ProQOL measures these effects in the domains of compassion satisfaction and compassion fatigue and classifies burnout and secondary trauma as subscales of compassion fatigue.

While not a comprehensive list, other measurement tools include the Satisfaction with Life Scale, used to measure an individual's global life satisfaction[32]; the Compassion Satisfaction/Fatigue Self-Test for Helpers, which measures the 3 subscales of compassion fatigue, burnout, and compassion satisfaction[33,34]; and the Mayo Clinic Well-Being Index, developed by physicians, which measures multiple dimensions of well-being and may identify those whose distress may negatively affect their medical practice.[35] Depending on institution-specific issues and desired outcomes for evaluation, tools should be examined closely for relevance.

Risk Factors

There is no doubt that medical professionals across all specialties are at risk of developing burnout. Those on the front line of care may be at higher risk (eg, emergency medicine, family medicine, internal medicine).[1] Similarly, those specialists who are consistently confronted with high acuity and life-or-death situations (eg, emergency medicine, critical care, hematology/oncology) may also be at increased risk for burnout.

Child maltreatment professionals are no exception and face unique challenges. In a small survey of 56 physicians specializing in child abuse, 77% reported having negative experiences from their work, including verbal and physical threats, formal complaints made to the employment institution, adverse media attention, and lawsuits.[36] Participation in the legal process is an expected part of the job, but court appearances have been identified as a major stressor of child abuse pediatrics and emergency medicine specialists.[37] Additionally, family interactions can be challenging for child maltreatment professionals, especially during the early stages of patient evaluation as families struggle to accept a diagnosis of abuse. A shortage of medical professionals working in the field may exacerbate other stressors, which can lead to increased feelings of isolation and emotional burden.

Burnout is not only an issue for the medical professional; others involved in the child welfare system are equally at risk. Training and experience for law enforcement and social workers can vary. Busy caseloads, high turnover rates, and level of experience may limit the longevity and function of individuals in these roles and may also contribute to burnout.[34]

Well-being and Resilience

Being affected by this work and the stories of trauma is inevitable. Therefore, it is imperative to acknowledge the effect these experiences have on a medical professional. The ability to intellectually and psychologically process information in a healthy manner is integral to sustaining compassionate care. Just as there are many terms used to describe the emotional toll of this work, there are also multiple terms to describe medical professional resilience. These include *fulfillment, satisfaction, engagement,* and *well-being,* all of which can be applied to the personal and professional realms. From a broad perspective, *resilience* may be conceptualized as one's ability to adapt to adversity.[38] The literature on resilience and resilience theory is extensive and ranges from studies on the inherent characteristics of an individual's personality to organizational structuring and strategies to promote engagement.[39,40]

Compassion satisfaction, or one's sense of fulfillment in the professional interaction with others, is believed to play a critical role in mitigating the effects of burnout.[41] The concept of *well-being* focuses on a sense of being fully engaged in all aspects of one's life, or a sense of "life satisfaction."[10] It has been suggested that well-being is attained when the 3 psychological needs of autonomy, competence, and relatedness are fulfilled.[10,42] Job satisfaction, self-awareness, mindfulness, and self-reflection have been shown to have a positive effect on individuals' perceptions of well-being,[34,43] along with restful sleep and exercise.[44]

Resilience in the face of adversity is most achievable when other factors of health and functioning are optimal. The concept of wellness or well-being is a helpful construct to consider when discussing individual resources, which may deplete or improve one's ability to cope with stress. Wellness includes physical and mental health as well as connectedness within society. Eight dimensions of wellness have been described (Figure 27.1).[45] Strengths or weaknesses in each domain can affect the others. It is important to note that wellness does not imply a lack of stress. Rather, this framework can be used to help focus efforts, which affect an individual's ability to cope with stresses. For each dimension, there are specific interventions to improve functioning and promote wellness.

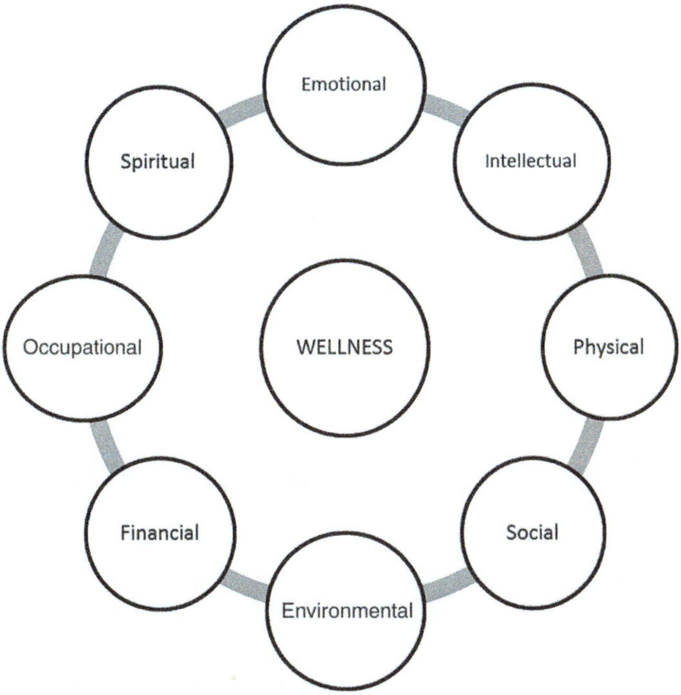

FIGURE 27.1
Eight dimensions of wellness.
1. *Spiritual* wellness does not necessarily equate to religion. This concept refers to the core values and morals for an individual. For some, it is related to understanding one's existence and meaning in life.
2. *Emotional* wellness refers to managing emotions and coping with the challenges of life.
3. *Intellectual* well-being means that one is satisfied with cognitive pursuits, not just at work but also in one's personal life, such as hobbies. It is important to keep an active, curious, and engaged mind and to maintain opportunities for learning.
4. *Physical* wellness includes health, exercise, nutrition, and sleep. Preventive care and access to treatment are key.
5. *Social* wellness is about finding connection and community, at work and in one's personal life. Finding time for joy with others is vital. Strong and positive relationships can be basis of support in times of stress.
6. *Environmental* wellness implies that an individual has a safe, clean, healthy environment. One should have a sense of comfort within personal surroundings.
7. *Financial* wellness includes living within a budget, planning for a secure future, and being able to meet one's needs.
8. *Occupational* wellness refers to feeling successful and productive at work, as well as finding meaning in and connecting work to personal values.
Adapted from Substance Abuse and Mental Health Services Administration. Wellness Initiative. The Eight Dimensions of Wellness. https://www.samhsa.gov/wellness-initiative/eight-dimensions-wellness. Accessed January 18, 2017.

Workplace Issues

The promotion of well-being and resilience in the workplace has become a primary focus of many organizations and institutions. Efforts should be integrated into multiple domains: on a personal level, within operational teams, and on a broader systems level. The profound effect of burnout on the individual has been shown to increase morbidity and mortality, including cardiovascular disease, substance use, depression, and suicide.[7,46–50] With regard to team function, patient care and satisfaction can be significantly affected. Perceived isolation and lack of social support in the professional setting contribute to frustration and decrease job satisfaction.[51,52] Promoting professionalism, consistent communication, and a supportive work environment are imperative. From a broader systems perspective, there are significant implications to the organization when the economic burdens and costs associated with burnout, such as high turnover and decreased productivity, are minimized.

The structure of the work environment can profoundly influence burnout. Flexibility and control over daily schedule are recognized as important to a sense of balance in the workplace. When the institution places value on recognizing the individual's needs and then creates opportunities for reflection and protected time to explore other professional interests and provides some flexibility within the day-to-day schedule, the entire system can benefit.

The US health care system is increasingly complex, and navigating the work environment can be exhausting and overwhelming. Professionals must keep current with a vast knowledge base for diagnosis and treatment. Changes in payment and incentive systems can add to financial stressors. Organizational models where physicians are employees rather than independent practitioners can lead to a sense of reduced autonomy. New regulatory and Maintenance of Certification requirements are time-consuming and not necessarily perceived as relevant. Quality and safety efforts are a worthy focus but require additional attention from already busy medical professionals. Commonly, medical professionals report feeling increasingly burdened by the bureaucratic tasks of their jobs, such as charting within the electronic medical record. Advances in technology designed to improve the workplace may decrease time for more meaningful human interactions.

Rates of burnout are reportedly increasing, with a particular effect noted on younger physicians in training. For medical students and residents, stressors appear to be different when compared with early career physicians. For trainees, issues around autonomy and academic performance are common. Depression and fatigue appear to be contributing factors despite work hour restrictions. For the early career physician, scores for quality of life and accomplishment improve but pressures related to adjusting to new work responsibilities are reported.[53,54] Recognizing and addressing burnout with colleagues and coworkers is important, and the effect of burnout on trainees cannot be underestimated. It has been demonstrated that residents perceive autonomy, competence building, social connection, sleep, and time away from work as the factors that most contribute to their sense of well-being.[10] Training institutions are tasked with addressing burnout and resilience training in the educational curriculum. The strategies and resources used vary widely. The limited data available on the utility and efficacy of these interventions make standardization difficult. However, duty work hour restrictions in residency have consistently been shown to be associated with lower rates of emotional exhaustion and burnout.[55] While some improvements have been made, the data suggest that burnout is multifactorial and must be addressed with attention to changes that affect systemic and individual factors.

Risk of burnout is not just related to the individual personality traits of the professional. In fact, system issues such as workplace conditions, lack of control in decision-making, time and productivity requirements, and mismatch between medical professional and organizational priorities have been identified as major factors related to burnout.[56] Medical professionals are increasingly taxed by these issues, which can affect autonomy and work-life balance.[25] The increasing demands of the workplace are exacerbated by a lack of resources. System-level factors highlight the importance of shared responsibility between the individual medical professional, work units, institutions, and national organizations. See Box 27.1 for a suggested approach to organizational intervention.[57]

As mentioned earlier, medical professional burnout can lead to high turnover rates and lower productivity, creating financial incentives for institutions to address resilience; however, effectiveness and affordably of interventions remain a concern for institutions. Economic costs of burnout can be calculated for organizations.[22] Experts argue that interventions are often justified in light of overall cost and safety considerations.[22]

Some larger organizations have created specific offices to address personnel support on a system-wide scale. Specifically, efforts geared toward peer-to-peer support and coordinated through a centralized office have proven successful.[58] Other studies have identified specific workplace cultural considerations that are most closely associated with medical professional satisfaction.[59] A chaotic work environment, poor communication, distrust in the organization, and misalignment of values between medical professionals and leaders predict poor satisfaction.[59] When interventions are tailored to improve these areas, a significant effect can be made.

BOX 27.1
Components of System-Level Efforts to Address Resilience in the Workplace

Organizational Awareness That Medical Professional Resilience Is a Priority

Recognition of key drivers of medical professional engagement

- Workload
- Efficiency and resources
- Meaning in work
- Culture and values
- Control/flexibility in practice
- Social support and community at work
- Work-life integration

Engaged Leadership

Effective interventions

- Based on data and need
- Specific to individual unit dynamics

Community Within the Workplace

Incentive structure

Rewards beyond financial incentives

Culture of Care That Is Congruent With Values

Work-life integration

- Consider flexible work schedules
- Examine benefits system

Resources for Individuals

Research in the Area of Medical Professional Resilience

Adapted from Shanafelt TD, Noseworthy JH. Executive leadership and physician well-being: nine organizational strategies to promote engagement and reduce burnout. *Mayo Clinic Proc.* 2017;92(1):129–146.

Prevention: Self-awareness, Social Connections, and Self-care

Given the increase in recognition and effect of burnout within all fields of medicine, there has been growing attention to prevention efforts and strategies. In the process, a notable shift has occurred from a negative construct of combating burnout to a more positive approach of promoting resilience and well-being. The discussion that follows focuses on resilience strategies from this perspective. These efforts are multidimensional, with options to affect the individual, the team, and the system at large.

Opportunities to debrief and discuss experiences in real time have been recognized as an essential component to promote resilience. Debriefing sessions are not therapy sessions. Rather, they provide an opportunity for the care team to discuss emotions regarding challenging or difficult cases. Debriefings are facilitated by someone who has no experience with the case who helps to ensure a confidential and supportive environment. The facilitator can also help to identify and refer individual team members to more intensive support services if needed.

In a systematic review evaluating well-being in residency, the 3 main factors associated with resident well-being were autonomy, competence building, and strong social connection.[10] Furthermore, when asked to identify aspects of the ideal learning environment, residents expressed a desire for increased opportunities for personal interaction and discussion with faculty.[60] While there are some advantages to online education modules, such as flexibility and ease of distribution, the same study emphasized the need to focus on in-person and individualized interactions.[60] These interactions not only provide space for trainees to develop supportive relationships with colleagues but also create opportunities for mentors to model professionalism through their own behavior and practice. Role modeling by faculty and co-fellows in addition to informal discussions with attendings were overwhelmingly perceived to be a helpful strategy in graduate medical education efforts to promote skill development in the areas of professionalism and humanism.[61]

The multidisciplinary nature of addressing child maltreatment can help combat some of the inherent pressures of work in the field. A team approach in child abuse cases has become a common standard of practice. Organization of the team may differ, but regardless of the team's primary function, decision-making is shared among the group. This multidisciplinary approach addresses the complex nature of cases, which require expertise in medical, legal, mental health, and social service domains. A multidisciplinary practice can offer relief from the emotional burden, intellectual challenges, and risk management questions involved with individual cases. At their best, multidisciplinary teams will make assessments easier and members will learn from and feel supported by colleagues.

Self-awareness is a vital component to burnout prevention. Medical professionals must be able to accept that some stress is to be expected, and efforts should be made to preemptively adhere to boundaries between work and personal functioning. This includes prioritizing personal well-being and striving to achieve balance between work and personal life. Additionally, professionals must acknowledge when experiencing the physical, cognitive, emotional or behavioral side effects of secondary trauma. It is important not to over-pathologize, acknowledging that without recognition of the problem there can be no response. Ideally, this recognition comes before serious individual consequences. When self-care is routinely incorporated into practice, symptoms are prevented. Nedrow and colleagues offer the following 4 questions as a tool for self-reflection.[62] Implicit within them is validation of the internal struggles medical professionals often feel.

1. How can I take care of myself so that I can be of service to others?
2. How can I strive for excellence and at the same time have compassion for myself when I don't have all the answers or I make a mistake?
3. How can I offer my expertise to cure illness and at the same time stay open to what my patients have to teach me about their own healing?
4. How can I maintain an empathetic connection with my patients and at the same time protect myself?

Research consistently demonstrates that supportive personal relationships have an effect on health and well-being.[63,64] While the exact mechanism is unknown, healthy relationships and participation within a larger social network may reduce the consequences of stress and improve emotional health. This, in turn, may positively influence attitudes and health-related behaviors.[64] Supports include relatives, friends, and work peers who are trusted and available to listen in times of stress or to help identify unhealthy behaviors. Informal relationships are important; however, more formal professional peer group activities, such as Finding Meaning in Medicine, Balint groups, and Caritas Coaches have proven beneficial.[65–67] These peer groups meet on a regular basis and give professionals the opportunity to share stories and dialogue about the socioemotional aspects of care.

The term *self-care* is often used in discussions about resilience. It can refer to individual practices outside of the workplace or more specific evidence-based stress management strategies. Too often, the discussion is centered around basic health care practices such as exercise, leisure activities, nutrition, and sleep. Other approaches that more intentionally focus on personal connections and support, reflection, and confronting the emotional burden of working in health care have proven to be important adjuncts to traditional self-care strategies.

Some of the most effective and well-studied interventions involve individual practices such as stress management training, mindfulness, and creating habits that promote a positive psychological perspective.[40,62,68,69] These interventions help, in part, by guiding an individual on how to focus attention and efforts. Some borrow from elements of cognitive behavioral therapy.[23] For example, cognitive reframing or reappraisal techniques emphasize the recognition of negative, often inaccurate, cognitive and behavioral attitudes. Once these attitudes are identified, the individual seeks to reexamine, or reframe, the situation from a more positive perspective.[23] This skill may be particularly helpful for the medical professional with perfectionist tendencies and for those who feel overwhelmed or inadequate.[62] Identification with spiritual beliefs and practices has also been demonstrated as a protective factor for burnout.[70]

Positive psychology is a conceptual framework focused on an individual's strengths to achieve optimal functioning with regard to purpose, meaning, and fulfillment in life.[71] Negative emotions and experiences are not ignored, but positive emotions are cultivated so that an individual can thrive and flourish. "Three good things" is a practice derived from this framework that may promote resilience. In this practice, positive experiences are considered throughout the day. At the end of the day, the individual reflects on 3 things that went well and his or her role in the success.[69]

One of the most commonly researched practices in health care is *mindfulness*,[72–74] a contemplative practice that can include meditation and emphasizes a nonjudgmental, reflective mental state anchored in the present moment. The goal is to promote clarity of mind, compassion, and self-awareness. Mindfulness practices can include activities that can be done in any environment, including during clinical work.[73] Some mindfulness interventions have combined training with other exercises intended to improve self-reflection, such as narrative writing or active listening.[72] Studies have shown improvement in medical professional well-being and positive emotional outcomes.[74]

There are many strategies for the promotion of resilience for the medical professional.[62,68,75] While not comprehensive, Box 27.2 presents 5 domains of interpersonal functioning that can have a positive effect on resilience and suggested strategies within each domain. Therapy or counseling with a mental health professional is an important option, especially if symptoms are serious or functioning is impaired. Starting with achievable goals is advisable. Fortunately, available resources are likely to increase with time, given the increased awareness of these issues among medical professionals.

BOX 27.2
Five Domains of Interpersonal Functioning That Can Have a Positive Effect on Resilience and Suggested Strategies for Improvements Within Each Domain

Self-awareness

Mindfulness
Self-reflection
Journaling
Healthy boundaries
Acknowledgment of strengths and weakness

Purpose

Spiritual practice
Connecting with mission
Meaningful patient interactions
Values appraisal

Connection

Community
Relationships
Peer groups
Debriefing
Mentorship

Self-care

Exercise
Good nutrition
Therapy
Practicing self-compassion
Hobbies and leisure activities
Meditation

Cultivating a Positive Mindset

Positive psychology
Practicing appreciation and gratitude ("3 good things")
Reframing
Active and generous listening
Keeping a record of successes/kudos as a reminder of positive experiences

References

1. Shanafelt TD, Boone S, Tan L, et al. Burnout and satisfaction with work-life balance among US physicians relative to the general US population. *Arch Intern Med.* 2012;172(18):1377–1385 PMID: 22911330 https://doi.org/10.1001/archinternmed.2012.3199
2. Lee RT, Seo B, Hladkyj S, Lovell BL, Schwartzmann L. Correlates of physician burnout across regions and specialties: a meta-analysis. *Hum Resour Health.* 2013;11(1):48 PMID: 24074053 https://doi.org/10.1186/1478-4491-11-48
3. Keswani RN, Taft TH, Coté GA, Keefer L. Increased levels of stress and burnout are related to decreased physician experience and to interventional gastroenterology career choice: findings from a US survey of endoscopists. *Am J Gastroenterol.* 2011;106(10):1734–1740 PMID: 21979198 https://doi.org/10.1038/ajg.2011.148
4. Ariely D, Lanier WL. Disturbing trends in physician burnout and satisfaction with work-life balance: dealing with malady among the nation's healers. *Mayo Clin Proc.* 2015;90(12):1593–1596 PMID: 26653295 https://doi.org/10.1016/j.mayocp.2015.10.004
5. Bennett S, Plint A, Clifford TJ. Burnout, psychological morbidity, job satisfaction, and stress: a survey of Canadian hospital based child protection professionals. *Arch Dis Child.* 2005;90(11):1112–1116 PMID: 16243862 https://doi.org/10.1136/adc.2003.048462
6. Ishak WW, Lederer S, Mandili C, et al. Burnout during residency training: a literature review. *J Grad Med Educ.* 2009;1(2):236–242 PMID: 21975985 https://doi.org/10.4300/JGME-D-09-00054.1
7. Dyrbye LN, Thomas MR, Massie FS, et al. Burnout and suicidal ideation among U.S. medical students. *Ann Intern Med.* 2008;149(5):334–341 PMID: 18765703 https://doi.org/10.7326/0003-4819-149-5-200809020-00008
8. Shanafelt TD, Bradley KA, Wipf JE, Back AL. Burnout and self-reported patient care in an internal medicine residency program. *Ann Intern Med.* 2002;136(5):358–367 PMID: 11874308 https://doi.org/10.7326/0003-4819-136-5-200203050-00008
9. Dewa CS, Loong D, Bonato S, Thanh NX, Jacobs P. How does burnout affect physician productivity? A systematic literature review. *BMC Health Serv Res.* 2014;14(1):325 PMID: 25066375 https://doi.org/10.1186/1472-6963-14-325
10. Raj KS. Well-being in residency: a systematic review. *J Grad Med Educ.* 2016;8(5):674–684 PMID: 28018531 https://doi.org/10.4300/JGME-D-15-00764.1
11. Spector ND, Trimm RF, eds. *Teaching, Promoting and Assessing Professionalism Across the Continuum: A Medical Educator's Guide.* https://www.abp.org/professionalism-guide. Accessed April 4, 2019
12. American Board of Pediatrics. Entrustable Professional Activities for subspecialties. https://www.abp.org/subspecialty-epas. Accessed April 4, 2019
13. American Academy of Pediatrics. Resilience curriculum: resilience in the face of grief and loss. https://www.aap.org/en-us/advocacy-and-policy/aap-health-initiatives/hospice-palliative-care/Pages/Resilience-Curriculum.aspx. Accessed April 4, 2019
14. Baird K, Kracen AC. Vicarious traumatization and secondary traumatic stress: a research synthesis. *Couns Psychol* Q. 2006;19(2):181–188 https://doi.org/10.1080/09515070600811899
15. Figley CR. Compassion fatigue as secondary traumatic stress disorder: an overview. In: Figley CR, ed. *Compassion Fatigue: Coping With Secondary Traumatic Stress Disorder In Those Who Treat The Traumatized.* New York: Brunner Mazel; 1995:1–20

16. Pearlman LA, Saakvitne KW. Treating therapists with vicarious traumatization and secondary traumatic stress disorder. In: Figley CR, ed. *Compassion Fatigue: Coping With Secondary Traumatic Stress Disorder In Those Who Treat The Traumatized*. New York, NY: Brunner Mazel; 1995:150–177
17. Best Start Meilleur Départ. *When Compassion Hurts: Burnout, Vicarious Trauma and Secondary Trauma in Prenatal and Early Childhood Service Providers*. https://resources.beststart.org/product/j13e-when-compassion-hurts-manual. Published 2012. Accessed April 4, 2019
18. van Mol MM, Kompanje EJ, Benoit DD, Bakker J, Nijkamp MD. The prevalence of compassion fatigue and burnout among healthcare professionals in intensive care units: a systematic review. *PLoS One*. 2015;10(8):e0136955 PMID: 26322644 https://doi.org/10.1371/journal.pone.0136955
19. Maslach C. *Burnout–the Cost of Caring*. Englewood Cliffs, NJ: Prentice-Hall; 1982
20. Cherniss C. Staff Burnout: Job Stress in the Human Services. Beverly Hills, CA: Sage Publications; 1980
21. Maslach C, Leiter MP. Early predictors of job burnout and engagement. *J Appl Psychol*. 2008;93(3):498–512 PMID: 18457483 https://doi.org/10.1037/0021-9010.93.3.498
22. Shanafelt T, Goh J, Sinsky C. The business case for investing in physician well-being. *JAMA Intern Med*. 2017;177(12):1826–1832 PMID: 28973070 https://doi.org/10.1001/jamainternmed.2017.4340
23. Southwick SM, Charney DS. The science of resilience: implications for the prevention and treatment of depression. *Science*. 2012;338(6103):79–82 PMID: 23042887 https://doi.org/10.1126/science.1222942
24. Salvagioni DAJ, Melanda FN, Mesas AE, González AD, Gabani FL, Andrade SM. Physical, psychological and occupational consequences of job burnout: a systematic review of prospective studies. *PLoS One*. 2017;12(10):e0185781 PMID: 28977041 https://doi.org/10.1371/journal.pone.0185781
25. Rothenberger DA. Physician burnout and well-being: a systematic review and framework for action. *Dis Colon Rectum*. 2017;60(6):567–576 PMID: 28481850 https://doi.org/10.1097/DCR.0000000000000844
26. Schaufeli WB, Enzmann D, Girault N. Measurement of burnout: a review. In: Schaufeli WB, Maslach C, Marek T, eds. *Professional Burnout: Recent Developments in Theory and Research*. Philadelphia, PA: Taylor & Francis; 1993:199–215
27. Maslach CJ, Jackson SE, Leiter MP. *Maslach Burnout Inventory Manual*. 3rd ed. Palo Alto, CA: Consulting Psychologists Press; 1996
28. Schaufeli WB, Bakker AB, Hoogduin K, Schaap C, Kladler A. On the clinical validity of the Maslach burnout inventory and the burnout measure. *Psychol Health*. 2001;16(5):565–582 PMID: 22804499 https://doi.org/10.1080/08870440108405527
29. Kristensen TS, Borritz M, Villadsen E, Christensen KB. The Copenhagen Burnout Inventory: A new tool for the assessment of burnout. *Work Stress*. 2005;19(3):192–207
30. Hudnall Stamm B. *Professional Quality of Life: Compassion Satisfaction and Fatigue Version 5 (ProQOL)*. http://www.proqol.org/uploads/ProQOL_5_English.pdf. Published 2009. Accessed April 4, 2019
31. Jacobs LM, Nawaz MK, Hood JL, Bae S. Burnout among workers in a pediatric health care system. *Workplace Health Saf*. 2012;60(8):335–344 PMID: 22850134 https://doi.org/10.1177/216507991206000803
32. Diener E, Emmons RA, Larsen RJ, Griffin S. The Satisfaction With Life Scale. *J Pers Assess*. 1985;49(1):71–75 PMID: 16367493 https://doi.org/10.1207/s15327752jpa4901_13
33. Figley CR, Stamm BH. *Psychometric Review of Compassion Fatigue Self Test. Measurement of Stress, Trauma, and Adaptation*. Lutherville, MD: Sirdran Press; 1996:127–130

34. Conrad D, Kellar-Guenther Y. Compassion fatigue, burnout, and compassion satisfaction among Colorado child protection workers. *Child Abuse Negl.* 2006;30(10):1071–1080 PMID: 17014908 https://doi.org/10.1016/j.chiabu.2006.03.009
35. Dyrbye LN, Varkey P, Boone SL, Satele DV, Sloan JA, Shanafelt TD. Physician satisfaction and burnout at different career stages. *Mayo Clin Proc.* 2013;88(12):1358–1367 PMID: 24290109 https://doi.org/10.1016/j.mayocp.2013.07.016
36. Flaherty EG, Sege RD. Are the protectors protected? Paper presented at: Pediatric Academic Society Annual Meeting; 2007; Toronto, Ontario, Canada
37. Johnson CF. Child abuse as a stressor of pediatricians. *Pediatr Emerg Care.* 1999;15(2): 84–89 PMID: 10220074 https://doi.org/10.1097/00006565-199904000-00002
38. McFadden PCA, Taylor B. Resilience and burnout in child protection social work: individual and organisational themes from a systematic literature review. *Br J Soc Work.* 2014;45(11):1546–1563
39. Bonanno GA, Galea S, Bucciarelli A, Vlahov D. What predicts psychological resilience after disaster? The role of demographics, resources, and life stress. *J Consult Clin Psychol.* 2007;75(5):671–682 PMID: 17907849 https://doi.org/10.1037/0022-006X.75.5.671
40. West CP, Dyrbye LN, Erwin PJ, Shanafelt TD. Interventions to prevent and reduce physician burnout: a systematic review and meta-analysis. *Lancet.* 2016;388(10057): 2272–2281 PMID: 27692469 https://doi.org/10.1016/S0140-6736(16)31279-X
41. Stamm BH. Measuring compassion satisfaction as well as fatigue: developmental history of the compassion satisfaction and fatigue test. In: Figley CR, ed. *Treating Compassion Fatigue (Psychosocial Stress Series).* New York, NY: Brunner-Routledge; 2013:107–119
42. Ryan RM, Deci EL. Self-regulation and the problem of human autonomy: does psychology need choice, self-determination, and will? *J Pers.* 2006;74(6):1557–1585 PMID: 17083658 https://doi.org/10.1111/j.1467-6494.2006.00420.x
43. Epstein RM. Mindful practice. *JAMA.* 1999;282(9):833–839 PMID: 10478689 https://doi.org/10.1001/jama.282.9.833
44. Lebensohn P, Dodds S, Benn R, et al. Resident wellness behaviors: relationship to stress, depression, and burnout. *Fam Med.* 2013;45(8):541–549 PMID: 24129866
45. Substance Abuse and Mental Health Services Administration. Wellness Initiative. The Eight Dimensions of Wellness. https://www.samhsa.gov/wellness-initiative/eight-dimensions-wellness. Accessed January 18, 2017
46. Ahola K, Väänänen A, Koskinen A, Kouvonen A, Shirom A. Burnout as a predictor of all-cause mortality among industrial employees: a 10-year prospective register-linkage study. *J Psychosom Res.* 2010;69(1):51–57 PMID: 20630263 https://doi.org/10.1016/j.jpsychores.2010.01.002
47. Oreskovich MR, Shanafelt T, Dyrbye LN, et al. The prevalence of substance use disorders in American physicians. Am J Addict. 2015;24(1):30–38 PMID: 25823633 https://doi.org/10.1111/ajad.12173
48. Oreskovich MR, Kaups KL, Balch CM, et al. Prevalence of alcohol use disorders among American surgeons. Arch Surg. 2012;147(2):168–174 PMID: 22351913
49. Shanafelt TD, Balch CM, Dyrbye L, et al. Special report: suicidal ideation among American surgeons. Arch Surg. 2011;146(1):54–62 PMID: 21242446
50. Pompili M, Innamorati M, Narciso V, et al. Burnout, hopelessness and suicide risk in medical doctors. *Clin Ter.* 2010;161(6):511–514 PMID: 21181078
51. Koeske GKR, Koeske RD. A preliminary test of a stress-strain-outcome model for reconceptualization of the burnout phenomenon. *J Soc Serv Res.* 1993;17(3–4):107–135 https://doi.org/10.1300/J079v17n03_06

52. Lewandowski CA. Organizational factors contributing to worker frustration: the precursor to burnout. *J Sociol Soc Welf.* 2003;30(4):175–185
53. Dyrbye LN, West CP, Satele D, et al. Burnout among U.S. medical students, residents, and early career physicians relative to the general U.S. population. *Acad Med.* 2014;89(3):443–451 PMID: 24448053 https://doi.org/10.1097/ACM.0000000000000134
54. McClafferty H, Brown OW; American Academy of Pediatrics Section on Integrative Medicine, Committee on Practice and Ambulatory Medicine. Physician health and wellness. *Pediatrics.* 2014;134(4):830–835 PMID: 25266440 https://doi.org/10.1542/peds.2014-2278
55. Busireddy KR, Miller JA, Ellison K, Ren V, Qayyum R, Panda M. Efficacy of interventions to reduce resident physician burnout: a systematic review. *J Grad Med Educ.* 2017;9(3):294–301 PMID: 28638506 https://doi.org/10.4300/JGME-D-16-00372.1
56. Linzer M, Konrad TR, Douglas J, et al. Managed care, time pressure, and physician job satisfaction: results from the physician worklife study. *J Gen Intern Med.* 2000;15(7): 441–450 PMID: 10940129 https://doi.org/10.1046/j.1525-1497.2000.05239.x
57. Shanafelt TD, Noseworthy JH. Executive leadership and physician well-being: nine organizational strategies to promote engagement and reduce burnout. *Mayo Clin Proc.* 2017;92(1):129–146 PMID: 27871627 https://doi.org/10.1016/j.mayocp.2016.10.004
58. Shanafelt TD, Lightner DJ, Conley CR, et al. An organization model to assist individual physicians, scientists, and senior health care administrators with personal and professional needs. *Mayo Clin Proc.* 2017;92(11):1688–1696 PMID: 29101937 https://doi.org/10.1016/j.mayocp.2017.08.020
59. Linzer M, Sinsky CA, Poplau S, Brown R, Williams E; Healthy Work Place Investigators. Joy in medical practice: clinician satisfaction in the healthy work place trial. *Health Aff (Millwood).* 2017;36(10):1808–1814 PMID: 28971927 https://doi.org/10.1377/hlthaff.2017.0790
60. Daskivich TJ, Jardine DA, Tseng J, et al. Promotion of wellness and mental health awareness among physicians in training: perspective of a national, multispecialty panel of residents and fellows. *J Grad Med Educ.* 2015;7(1):143–147 PMID: 26217450 https://doi.org/10.4300/JGME-07-01-42
61. Garvey KC, Kesselheim JC, Herrick DB, Woolf AD, Leichtner AM. Graduate medical education in humanism and professionalism: a needs assessment survey of pediatric gastroenterology fellows. *J Pediatr Gastroenterol Nutr.* 2014;58(1):34–37 PMID: 23863327 https://doi.org/10.1097/MPG.0b013e3182a4e5c9
62. Nedrow A, Steckler NA, Hardman J. Physician resilience and burnout: can you make the switch? *Fam Pract Manag.* 2013;20(1):25–30 PMID: 23418835
63. Thoits PA. Mechanisms linking social ties and support to physical and mental health. *J Health Soc Behav.* 2011;52(2):145–161 PMID: 21673143 https://doi.org/10.1177/0022146510395592
64. Umberson D, Montez JK. Social relationships and health: a flashpoint for health policy. *J Health Soc Behav.* 2010;51(suppl):S54–S66 PMID: 20943583 https://doi.org/10.1177/0022146510383501
65. Remen Institute for the Study of Health and Illness at Wright State University Boonshoft School of Medicine. Finding meaning discussion groups. http://www.rishiprograms.org/finding-meaning-discussion-groups. Accessed April 4, 2019
66. Watson J, Brewer BB. Caring science research: criteria, evidence, and measurement. *J Nurs Adm.* 2015;45(5):235–236 PMID: 25906128 https://doi.org/10.1097/NNA.0000000000000190
67. Scheingold L. Balint work in England: lessons for American family medicine. *J Fam Pract.* 1988;26(3):315–320 PMID: 3279157

68. Zwack J, Schweitzer J. If every fifth physician is affected by burnout, what about the other four? Resilience strategies of experienced physicians. *Acad Med*. 2013;88(3): 382–389 PMID: 23348093 https://doi.org/10.1097/ACM.0b013e318281696b
69. Rippstein-Leuenberger K, Mauthner O, Bryan Sexton J, Schwendimann R. A qualitative analysis of the Three Good Things intervention in healthcare workers. *BMJ Open*. 2017;7(5):e015826 PMID: 28611090 https://doi.org/10.1136/bmjopen-2017-015826
70. Wachholtz A, Rogoff M. The relationship between spirituality and burnout among medical students. *J Contemp Med Educ*. 2013;1(2):83–91 PMID: 25485165 https://doi.org/10.5455/jcme.20130104060612
71. Seligman ME, Csikszentmihalyi M. Positive psychology. An introduction. *Am Psychol*. 2000;55(1):5–14 PMID: 11392865 https://doi.org/10.1037/0003-066X.55.1.5
72. Krasner MS, Epstein RM, Beckman H, et al. Association of an educational program in mindful communication with burnout, empathy, and attitudes among primary care physicians. *JAMA*. 2009;302(12):1284–1293 PMID: 19773563 https://doi.org/10.1001/jama.2009.1384
73. Fortney L, Luchterhand C, Zakletskaia L, Zgierska A, Rakel D. Abbreviated mindfulness intervention for job satisfaction, quality of life, and compassion in primary care clinicians: a pilot study. *Ann Fam Med*. 2013;11(5):412–420 PMID: 24019272 https://doi.org/10.1370/afm.1511
74. Shapiro SL, Schwartz GE, Bonner G. Effects of mindfulness-based stress reduction on medical and premedical students. *J Behav Med*. 1998;21(6):581–599 PMID: 9891256 https://doi.org/10.1023/A:1018700829825
75. Epstein RM, Krasner MS. Physician resilience: what it means, why it matters, and how to promote it. *Acad Med*. 2013;88(3):301–303 PMID: 23442430 https://doi.org/10.1097/ACM.0b013e318280cff0

PART 7

Outcomes

CHAPTER 28

Caring for Children in Out-of-Home Care

Heather Forkey, MD, FAAP
Associate Professor
Department of Pediatrics
University of Massachusetts Medical School
Worcester, MA

Wynne Morgan, MD
Assistant Professor
Department of Psychiatry
University of Massachusetts Medical School
Worcester, MA

Introduction

Removal of children from their family of origin and admission to foster care is and should be reserved for situations in which the children's health and safety are deemed to be at imminent risk. Foster care is intended to be a temporary setting to provide for the safety, health, and well-being of children until they can be reunified with their family or an alternative permanent setting (adoptive, guardianship, or emancipation) can be identified. Due to the exposures and stressors that precipitate removal; the uncertainty, upheaval, and losses associated with placement and seeking permanency; and the physiologic responses to these traumas, children in foster care often have a significant health burden. Familiarity with the medical needs common to children in foster care, attention to cross-agency communication, and incorporation of the emerging science of toxic stress and trauma into care for these children allow the medical professional to have a positive effect on the health trajectory for this most vulnerable group.

Epidemiology

At the end of fiscal year (FY) 2016 there were an estimated 437,465 children in foster care in the United States.[1] That year, 273,539 children entered care, and of the 250,248 children who exited foster care during FY 2016, 51% reunited with their parent or primary caregiver, 23% were adopted, 8% were emancipated, 10% went to live with a guardian, 7% went to live with another relative, and 2% had other outcomes.[1–3] These numbers reflect several trends. The number of children in care on any given day hit a high of 523,616 in 2002. Legislative and child welfare efforts to preserve families by diverting them to in-home support services and engaging extended families as resources for children who could not safely remain at home, and attention to shortening the time to permanency through reunification, kinship care, guardianship, or adoption, resulted in a decline in the number of children in foster care to a low of 399,546 in 2012.[2,4] Interestingly, these declines occurred despite an increase in child abuse reports and the numbers of children in foster care who had experienced multiple forms of maltreatment and were diagnosed as emotionally disturbed.[5]

The number of children in care has increased each year since 2012, and reports associate the opioid epidemic with increases in the number of children in foster care. In 2005, parental drug abuse was noted as at least a partial reason for placement for 22% of children entering foster care. In 2016 that number was up to 34%.[1] Additionally, the surge of unaccompanied refugee minors in 2014 through 2016 affected the number of children in foster care.[6]

Minorities and children living in poverty are overrepresented in foster care, although there has been a reduction of black children in child welfare placement since 1999.[4] In 2016, 23% of children in placement were black/non-Hispanic, 21% were Hispanic, and 7% were multiracial. As with other aspects of child welfare, concerns exist regarding conscious and unconscious bias affecting rates of removal of minority and poor children from their family of origin.[7]

Legislation Overview

The primary responsibility for child welfare services rests with the states; however, states must comply with federal legislation to receive funding for the care and keeping of children in child welfare. Each state has its own set of regulations and programs to serve its children and families, but most financial support comes from the federal government. The bulk of federal support for child welfare, foster care, and adoption comes through titles IV-B and IV-E of the Social Security Act. These programs are administered by the US Department of Health and Human Services and include

- Title IV-B Child Welfare Service and Promoting Safe and Stable Families (formerly known as Family Preservation) programs: Provides funds to support families in their own home when the child is at risk of out-of-home placement due to abuse or neglect.
- Title IV-E Foster Care Program: Provides funding for children in out-of-home care.

- Title IV-E Adoption Assistance Program: Provides financial support to promote adoption when it is determined that a child cannot be returned to the parent's home.
- Title IV-E Chafee Foster Care Independence Program: Assists youth aging out of foster care with job training and independent living support to help attain self-sufficiency and permits states to extend Medicaid coverage to youth who are aging out of foster care. Medicaid was extended further (to age 26 years) by the Patient Protection and Affordable Care Act.[8]

The Indian Child Welfare Act was enacted in 1978 to prevent the breakup of American Indian and Alaskan Native families. The Indian Child Welfare Act set federal requirements that apply to state child custody proceedings involving an American Indian/Alaska Native child who is a member of or eligible for membership in a federally recognized tribe. It requires child welfare to specifically work to prevent the need for removal and to take measures to keep American Indian/Alaska Native children in relative care and within their tribal community and culture whenever safe and possible.[8]

Entry and Exit From Care

Almost all children entering foster care are placed involuntarily by court order, most for reasons of maltreatment (70%) in the form of neglect, physical abuse, sexual abuse, emotional abuse, or abandonment. Neglect of basic nutritional, educational, or medical needs, or lack of supervision, is the most commonly cited reason for placement, as findings of child physical abuse and sexual abuse have declined.[9,10] Many children experience multiple types of abuse, and more than 80% have been exposed to violence, including community and domestic violence.[1] Even before placement, it is not uncommon for children from these chaotic households to have had multiple caregivers, with varying levels of experience with or commitment to the child, thus further affecting their risk of experiencing abuse and ability to form healthy attachments.[11,12] Removal may occur urgently after a first-time report to child protective services or, at the other extreme, after prolonged involvement with child welfare during which preventive strategies have been exhausted. In either case, removal itself is yet another trauma for these children, even when it provides a new sense of safety and stability.[11,13]

When concerns of abuse or neglect are raised, an investigation is undertaken by child welfare. If allegations of maltreatment are felt to be credible (or *founded*), a determination of whether it is safe for the child to remain at home is made. Most often, it is determined that a child can stay at home and services to support the family are offered. When child welfare determines that a child is at imminent risk if he or she remains at home, a child is removed. A court hearing must occur within 72 hours to authorize that removal.

The remaining 30% of admissions are predominantly teens placed by the courts because of their own behaviors or because parents are seeking mental health services, cannot manage their behaviors, or abandon them. Less commonly, children are placed because caregivers' health, incarceration, or mental health issues preclude their ability to care for children at home. In many of these cases, the children involved have experienced the same adversities as the children placed involuntarily, including abuse, domestic violence exposure, parental substance abuse, and mental health concerns.[14]

Approximately 50% of children and teens will experience more than 1 foster care placement, and 25% will have 3 or more placements. Placement stability can affect a child's ability to later achieve permanency. Placements can be disrupted for many reasons, including reasons related to the child, the foster placement, or the biological family. While a child's behavioral issues extant prior to a stay in foster care may lead to placement instability, behavior problems can increase due to placement instability itself.[15,16] Children who enter care with a sibling are more likely to experience placement disruption compared with those without siblings.[17] Unfortunately, systems issues, such as policy mandates, often lead to placement changes, although the child welfare system may also move children for reasons that are more child-centric, such as keeping sibling groups together or moving to a relative placement.[18]

Although many children (approximately 50%) cycle through foster care in weeks to months, approximately 10% to 20% remain in the system for years. The largest determinant of length of stay is the biological family's level of cooperation with the individualized case plan for the family, although minority children, older children, children with severe behavioral and developmental disabilities, and children who are part of large sibling groups are almost twice as likely to remain in care longer.[1,3,5]

Regardless of the reason for placement, foster care is intended to be a temporary situation to allow caregivers to obtain the support and services they need to reunify with their children. Family service plans are created for each child, which delineate what services will be provided and what caregivers are expected to do to regain their children. These cases are reviewed by child welfare and the courts at regular intervals for the cooperation and compliance of the birth family with meeting the safety and other needs of the child. While the principle of "best interest of the child" guides decisions, reunification with the parent is usually the goal of foster care.

Understanding that some families will not have the capacity to safely care for the children, most child welfare agencies engage in *concurrent planning,* which means that child welfare works to find alternate sources of permanency for a child should reunification not be possible.[19] If a child has been in care for 18 months or 15 of the previous 22 months, the state must begin termination of parental rights. Once parental rights are terminated, a child is freed for adoption.[8]

Types of Placement, Permanency, and Aging Out

Removal of any length is traumatic and adds to the adversities that lead to placement. Foster placements can be an opportunity for healing and support and are most effective when they are stable,[15] nurturing, and supportive.[11] Improved health status, mental health, school attendance, and school success have all been linked to stable healthy foster placements,[20,21] and the value of a quality and invested foster home can be life changing for a child. However, placements are challenged by factors related to the child, administrative decisions, court judgements, and the foster family. A child's needs can be complex, and both in-home and congregate settings can be challenging and even inappropriate if the setting cannot provide the skills, attention, patience, and support to meet a child's needs.[19] Medical professionals should understand the setting a child is in, advocate for the most supportive setting, and be attentive to signs that a child is not thriving or is experiencing further abuse in a foster placement.

The placement of a child in foster care should be determined by the needs of the child and is supposed to be in the least restrictive environment. Nonrelative family, kinship, specialized, and therapeutic foster care are in-home settings. Congregate care in a group home or other highly structured setting is designed for children with behavioral or health issues that make in-home placement difficult; 13% of children in foster care will spend some time in congregate care.[1] Four percent of children reside in pre-adoptive homes.[1] Table 28.1 reviews the types of placements and some of the benefits and challenges of each.

While in placement, visits with biological parents are mandated. These are regularly scheduled, are usually supervised by child welfare staff, and offer an opportunity for birth parents and children to interact. Additionally, they allow child welfare to observe the quality of parent-child interactions and, at best, to have the parent and child participate in evidence-based attunement or trauma therapies together.[35,36] Unfortunately, visitation is also a challenge for everyone involved, and foster families are often frustrated that anticipation of and response to

TABLE 28.1
Foster Placement Settings[12,13,22-33]

Foster Placement Setting	% of Those in Care	Description	Benefits	Challenges
Nonrelative foster homes	45%	Placement in a home of an unrelated caregiver. Stipends provided by the state. Training by the state (often minimal) with certification of the home as meeting safety standards. State (with age-related guideline) determines number of children who can be fostered in a home, usually 4–6.	Training and home certification by state agency. Reimbursement for clothing, stipend to cover child costs.	Reimbursement often does not fully cover costs; foster parents usually have to cover about $\frac{1}{3}$ of costs. Foster parents often feel inadequately supported by child welfare, especially with medical and mental health needs of children. Training is often minimal.
Kinship homes	30% of formal foster care 4–8x as many in informal kinship arrangements	Caregivers who have an established relationship with the child, such as relatives, godparents, or family friends. Formal kinship is care provided by relatives as foster care under auspices of the state. Informal kinship arrangements are all other caregiving provided by relative in the absence of a parent.	More likely to be a setting the child is familiar with, less disruptive. May be in same neighborhood/ school. Fewer developmental and behavioral health concerns. More stable placements.	Caregivers more likely to be less resourced, older, have health concerns.[34] May have more unsupervised contact with birth parent. Less likely to get needed health care. Less support from child welfare (none if informal kinship).
Treatment or therapeutic foster care	Subset of unrelated foster care	Out-of-home care by foster parents who typically receive additional supports and services and, sometimes, specialized training to care for children with a wide variety of needs, including emotional, behavioral, or medical.	More training, support, and subsidy to care for children with specialized needs. Lower child to parent ratios than in routine foster care. Studies of those following treatment protocols with fidelity can demonstrate good results.	In some instances, training and support are minimal. Outcomes for children in these settings need more study.

(continued)

TABLE 28.1 (*continued*)

Foster Placement Setting	% of Those in Care	Description	Benefits	Challenges
Group homes (residential treatment)	6%	Congregate care facilities that care for children with behavioral health issues that make placement in a home difficult. Usually used for older children and adolescents.	Continuous supervision by trained staff improves safety and oversight of children in need of more intensive services.	No federal laws or regulations regarding training of staff, quality, or standards; thus, standard of care varies. The shortage of foster homes has led to use of this setting for children without behavioral needs.
Institutional care	8%	Children with significant medical or mental health needs are cared for in long-term care or inpatient settings.	Provides most intensive services for children at most need.	Expensive. Most restrictive setting.
Independent living	1%	Youth preparing to emancipate from foster care live in supervised independent settings.	Allows older teen to "try out" living on their own, with some supervision and support. Designed to prepare youth for independence. Youth may prefer this to foster home.	Degree of supervision and support varies widely by program. Does not appear to protect young adults from some common negative outcomes (eg, homelessness, unemployment).

visits can be disruptive to a child. Biological parents may bring to the visits their frustration with child welfare or may demonstrate the mental health or substance use concerns that led to placement. Biological parents may make unrealistic promises about reunification or may trigger trauma reactions in children. The visits can place emotional strain on children by reminding them of the separation and can generate a conflict of loyalties between biological and foster parents.[37] It is helpful for medical professionals to provide anticipatory guidance to foster parents regarding visits (see the Anticipatory Guidance section later in this chapter). Preparing a child for the visit with discussion of what to expect, including expected return to foster parent home, and building routines around visit days (return to foster home with a consistent and well-delineated routine of certain foods, games, books or bedtime ritual) can help to ease the disruptive nature of these visits.

While foster placement is intended to be a short-term arrangement, when reunification cannot be achieved, relative placement, adoption, or legal guardianship is investigated. In 2016, 51% of children exited foster care for reunification with parents or relatives, while 23% were adopted. The 9% who emancipate annually usually do so on their 18th birthday, although legislation, including the Chaffee Independence Act of 1999 and Fostering Connections to Success and Increasing Adoptions Act of 2008, have expanded funding to states to allow teens who are in school or job training to remain in foster care up to age 21 years.[38] *Other planned permanent living arrangement* and *another planned permanent living arrangement* are terms created by the Adoption and Safe Families Act of 1997 to replace the term *long-term foster care*. With other planned permanent living arrangements, child welfare maintains care and custody of the youth and arranges a living situation in which the youth is expected to remain until adulthood.[39]

Outcomes Data

Outcomes for alumni from foster care reflect the many challenges facing these youth. Foster care alumni are likely to be underemployed, undereducated, and overrepresented among the homeless and are likely to experience significant mental health problems even after controlling for economic status.[40–44] Young women who were in foster care are more likely than peers to have given birth by age 21 years, and young men who were in foster care are more likely to have fathered a child by age 21 years.[45,46]

The outcomes for children who reunify or are adopted are less clear. There is some literature indicating that children who are adopted or remain in long-term stable foster or kinship care fare better than children who return to parents. About 30% of children who are returned to their families reenter care within 1 year.[47] Reunified youth have a greater likelihood of substance abuse, arrest, poor mental health outcomes, more school failure, and dropping out of school.[48] Approximately 9% to 24% of adoptions disrupt (before finalization) or dissolve (after finalization).[49] Failed adoptions are more common for adolescents, with the youth's behavior being the most frequently cited reason.[50]

Physical Health

Nature of Physical Health Problems

The adversities that lead to foster placement can have significant health consequences for children. Poor health outcomes for children in foster care, both in the short term and into adulthood, have been linked to exposure to drugs in utero, insufficient prenatal care, preterm birth, exposure to environmental toxins, poor nutrition, and exposure to HIV, hepatitis, tuberculosis, and other communicable disease.[51,52] Poor health outcomes have also been linked to exposure to adverse childhood experiences, including chronic neglect, community and household violence, and physical, sexual, and emotional abuse.[22,53–58] In addition to the direct effects of toxins and infection, we now understand that the pathophysiology of the stress response and consequent behavioral adaptations affects health not just in childhood but over the life course, and that these toxic stressors have a multiplicative effect on health and amplify the effect of environmental stressors.[53–58]

Descriptive studies documenting the health of children in foster care over the past 30 years have had consistent findings, demonstrating that physical, mental, and developmental health issues plague most children in care—30% to 80% have at least 1 health concern, 30% have a chronic health concern, and 10% are medically complex.[55,59–62] These morbidity findings suggest that after decades of descriptive studies, we have yet to significantly lessen the health burden for these children. Additionally, children in foster care are the "canary in the coal mine"—often the first and most severely affected by epidemics that plague the nation's youth. Although early studies documented higher rates of failure to thrive in foster youth than the general population,[63,64] now obesity rates for children in foster care are higher than for matched peers who are not in foster care.[65,66] Pregnancy rates are higher among teen women in care,[23,45] and dental decay affects many children in foster care.[61,67]

Developmental and mental health consequences for these children are similarly concerning.[12,62,68,69] Sixty percent of children in care who are younger than 5 years have a developmental concern,[69] and 40% of school-aged children in care have educational delay or learning disabilities.[59] Up to 80% have significant mental health needs.[13,70] Common issues include language, social adaptive, and fine motor skill delays in young children and educational delays related to learning disabilities and cognitive issues in older children.[19] Increasing evidence indicates that early childhood insults, neglect, maltreatment, and environmental toxins affect the active and vulnerable growing brain, increasing the chance of developmental delay.[12,71] *Complex trauma,* or the repeated and severe insults children in foster care have been exposed to, can limit neurocognitive development and lead to lower IQ.[72] In particular, executive function, memory, impulse control, and problem-solving are negatively affected by these traumas.[14,73] Once a child is in foster care, placement instability, school disruption, behavioral health issues, and truancy magnify these issues and often result in poor educational outcomes and lower graduation rates among children in foster care.[42]

Medical Management

Despite the health issues noted previously, prior to placement in foster care, few of the children have received routine pediatric health care.[74] Much of the health care these children do receive prior to and during foster care is delivered in emergency departments.[75,76] The circumstances of abuse and neglect that often lead to placement further compromise child health.[51,75,77] Therefore, standards to guide the health evaluations and health care of children in foster care have been developed to address the unmet needs of this underserved population. The American Academy of Pediatrics (AAP) District II New York State Task Force on Health Care for Children in Foster Care[78] and Child Welfare League of America[79] have guidelines for the health care of children in foster care developed by expert consensus in the mid-2000s and late 1980s, respectively. Subsequently, evidence-based studies have further informed medical management and increased attention to the effect of adversity and trauma on the health of this population. Guidance presented here includes these standards supplemented with recent literature and consensus to address current health epidemics and recent advances in understanding of the effect of adversities on the health of children in foster placement.[14,80–82]

Yet, even when the standards and literature are scrupulously followed, it is also important for medical professionals to be "foster care friendly," attending to the needs of a group of children who have been profoundly affected by traumas of multiple types. Features of this readiness include[14,19,83]

- Longer appointments for initial screening and comprehensive and ongoing care
- Developing health summaries or health documents to share pertinent information with foster parents and child welfare
- Clear lines of communication with child welfare agencies and point people in the medical office and the child welfare agency to facilitate information transfer
- Open access or easily scheduled appointments to meet the needs of children who may abruptly face removal from home or placement disruptions
- Familiarity with terminology referring to court proceedings, biological parents, foster parents, and child welfare practices
- Sensitivity of all office staff and clinicians to the emotions associated with being in foster care and coming for medical care
- Understanding of the effect of trauma on a child's reactions and responses and strategies to reduce triggers and reexperiencing, which can occur with medical care

Initial Screening

At the time of placement, children are often removed from unhealthy and dangerous situations, may have experienced acute or chronic abuse, have untreated chronic illness, and/or have had exposure to infection and infestations. These traumas, as well as the trauma of removal, has an effect on the immune system and inflammatory mediators, further affecting the health of children at the time of placement.[58] To address this acute need, the AAP recommends that children entering foster care have a screening health evaluation within 72 hours of placement,[19] although infants and those with acute or chronic illness or injury should be seen more urgently. Regional standards and regulations for the timing of initial evaluations vary, although most suggest a medical evaluation within 7 days of entering foster care. Table 28.2 summarizes the timing, goals, and components of this evaluation.

Goals of the initial screening are to identify urgent health issues requiring treatment or further evaluation, including infection, infestation, pregnancy, injury, and acute or chronic illness; identify findings consistent with abuse or neglect; identify and address urgent mental health issues; provide urgent medications or treatments to maintain health; and provide information to child welfare and foster caregivers to inform placement.[19,78] In particular, child welfare and foster parents often benefit from anticipatory guidance on how trauma may affect health and behavior.[14]

Every effort should be made to obtain and review medical, developmental, and mental health history. Medications and durable medical equipment to treat physical and behavioral health conditions should be made available in the new home. Brief developmental and mental health screening should be conducted using standardized screening tools for significant developmental delay, major depression, suicidal thoughts, and violent behavior. A targeted examination should focus on vital signs, growth parameters, skin, joints, and genitalia to make sure injury, infection, and infestations are not missed.[19,83] Any necessary workup should be undertaken and/or subspecialist referrals made for children who require further evaluation or who have been lost to follow-up for previously identified physical or mental health issues.

Providing the caregiver and child welfare with all available health information will help ease the transition for the child and family. This includes providing the caregiver with necessary prescriptions or medical equipment. Foster parents identify the lack of health information and difficulty obtaining that information as one of their most significant frustrations.[24] The medical professional should discuss specific care instructions directly with the foster caregivers and caseworker.

TABLE 28.2
Initial Screening of Children Entering Foster Care

Timing		Goals	Components
Standard AAP guideline	Within 72 h	1. Identify acute health care issues requiring immediate attention or further evaluation and referral. 2. Provide health information to child welfare and foster families to appropriately care for child. a. Guidance on effect of trauma on health and behavior b. Specific health guidance on patient health issues (eg, asthma, epilepsy, obesity) c. Specific health guidance on medications including psychotropic medication	1. Review medical records including medications. 2. Review trauma history. 3. Mental health screening for acute issues. 4. Adolescent health screening: pregnancy and STIs. 5. Physical examination targeting a. Measurement of vital signs, height, weight, and head circumference b. Examination of skin for bruises, burns, scars, or other trauma c. Examination of joints for range of motion, deformities, or limitations in function d. Genital and anal examination e. Examination of hair and skin for infestations such as lice or scabies f. Pregnancy and STI testing as appropriate
Regional regulations	Up to 7 d		
Acute needs • Child younger than 3 y • Child with chronic health or mental health issues or significant developmental delay • Child with acute illness • Child with acute mental health concern • Child suspected of having experienced abuse or neglect	Within 24 h		

Abbreviations: AAP, American Academy of Pediatrics; STI, sexually transmitted infection.

Comprehensive Evaluation

A comprehensive health assessment should be performed 30 days into placement.[19,78] It can take time to amass a child's full medical, mental health, immunization, and trauma history. Children often change placements from a "hotline" or urgent setting to a more stable foster or kin setting in the first weeks of placement and may also change child care or school settings. Child welfare personnel supervising the child's case may change in the first weeks of placement as the initial investigation staff transitions the child to ongoing or pre-adoptive units and staff. As children transition into foster care, the adjustment to a new living situation, the losses associated with removal, and the behaviors that may have allowed them to adapt and survive previously can all emerge and present challenges to the caregivers and staff working with the child. Often it is not until 30 days into care that the health information, caregiving team, placement setting, child care and school assignment, and emotional challenges are identified.

The goals of the comprehensive evaluation are to review all the available health information; identify and treat physical and mental health conditions; complete or refer for more complete assessment of developmental, mental health, educational, and dental needs; identify and address trauma-related behavior and the child's adaptation to foster care; and provide anticipatory guidance related to emotional effects of trauma and loss, visitation with parents, court schedules, and safety.[19,78] See Table 28.3 for a summary of the comprehensive evaluation.

TABLE 28.3
Comprehensive Evaluation

Aspect	Goals	Component
Health information review	Obtain health, developmental, mental health history.	1. Child welfare to facilitate obtaining records. 2. Consider alternative sources to obtain information: child care, school, immunization registry, child welfare records. 3. Medical, behavioral, developmental, and social history information sharing among pediatrician, foster family, and child welfare will facilitate care.
Confidentiality	Know rules for own state.	Caregivers (foster parents, medical professionals) have right to information to care for child.
Consent	Know rules for own state.	1. Foster parent cannot consent or refuse routine care. 2. Consent through child welfare.
History and physical examination	1. Identify and address health concerns of child, foster caregiver, and child welfare. 2. Identify health issues that may have been overlooked or undertreated or that are newly developed.	1. Speak to child alone. 2. Speak to caregiver separately from child about sleep, eating, toileting, and behavior. 3. Complete unclothed examination as tolerated and with attention to trauma triggers. 4. Physical examination with attention to abuse, inflammation, allergy, metabolism. 5. Dental examination.

(continued)

TABLE 28.3 (*continued*)

Aspect	Goals	Component
Screening	1. Evaluate for hearing and vision loss. 2. Evaluate for infectious disease. 3. Evaluate for effect of nutritional concerns. 4. Evaluate for toxin exposure (lead). 5. Evaluate for reproductive health issues. 6. Evaluate developmental and mental health with trauma focus.	1. Hearing and vision screen. 2. CBC. 3. Lead if <6 y or developmentally delayed. 4. HIV, hepatitis B and C, RPR (and maybe *Neisseria gonorrhoeae, Chlamydia, Trichomonas)* if concern for vertical transmission, sexual abuse, or sexually active. 5. Consider tuberculin screen if high risk exposure. 6. Developmental screen. 7. Mental health screen. 8. Trauma screen.
Immunization	Confirm/update immunization status.	1. Give vaccines if needed. 2. Update vaccine records.
Anticipatory guidance	Address issues for foster families, child welfare, and youth that help to explain behaviors, normalize experiences, address issues unique to foster care, and trauma.	Review • Adjustment to home • How biological or other children in home are adapting to new child in foster placement • Visits with biological parents • Sexual health issues with adolescents • Extracurricular activities, hobbies, faith-based groups

Abbreviations: CBC, complete blood cell count; RPR, rapid plasma reagin.

Health Information Review

It is the responsibility of the child welfare agency to facilitate health information transfer to the medical professional, although this process can be difficult to achieve. Birth parents may be unavailable, unwilling, or unable to provide information about a child's prior health care, and caseworkers and medical office staff may need to contact former medical professionals, schools, child care providers, and immunization registries to access health information. Child welfare agencies or their designees have the authority to consent for the sharing of health information when a parent's consent cannot be obtained, unless the child has been placed in foster care voluntarily (and then parents retain that right). Many localities and child welfare agencies have had "medical passports," which are designed to collect, maintain, and facilitate the transfer of up-to-date health information between medical professionals and child welfare. Unfortunately, the paper versions of these documents have had limited success, although electronic records hold promise. Some medical homes and foster care medical clinics have created standardized formats for collecting and reporting information in the electronic medical record, thus streamlining some of the information transfer process.[19] The information that should be obtained, and the possible sources of that information, are listed in Table 28.4.

Consent and Confidentiality

Confusion often arises regarding who can consent for medical care of a child in foster care and with whom health information can be shared. Consent and confidentiality laws vary by state and locality, so medical professionals need to become familiar with their own state's regulations. Medical professionals are often called on to provide a spectrum of care and interpret and explain health information to a variety of people working with a child, so understanding these issues is essential. In general, caregivers for the child (including caseworkers, foster parents, and medical professionals) have access to all health information about children in their care. Exceptions include reproductive health and sometimes HIV-related issues. In most states, birth parents or legal guardians retain the right to consent for treatment, but general medical consent is usually obtained from the parent or guardian by child welfare at the time of placement to cover routine care. This usually includes physical examinations, immunizations, and noninvasive treatments. Mental health evaluations, surgery, and sedation usually require separate informed consent from a parent or guardian. Once a child has had parental rights terminated and is free for adoption, the child welfare agency is usually the consenting party. Consent for psychotropic medications differ from state to state and may involve approval from the court. *Adolescents,* defined as "minor[s] with the capacity to consent," have the right to make their own reproductive health care decisions. Emergency care can be provided if no consenting party is available. Foster parents, although they do have physical care of the child, do not have rights to consent to (or deny) medical care.[19]

History and Physical Examination

During the comprehensive assessment, the medical professional should speak with the foster and birth parents (when it is safe and appropriate for them to participate), child welfare representative, and child (if verbal). Starting a visit

TABLE 28.4
Health Information Sources

Source	Information
Birth record	Neonatal exposures Birth history Newborn screening results
Medical record	Growth charts Allergies Medications Prior diagnoses Hospitalizations Surgeries Immunizations Vision and hearing screenings/evaluations Family history Durable medical equipment Sexual health/family planning record
Immunization registry	Immunization records
Child care records	Immunizations Prior medical professional information
School records	Immunizations Prior medical professional information Educational evaluations, IEP Developmental testing
Early Intervention	Developmental evaluations
Child welfare	Child welfare evaluations Court investigations Trauma history Demographic information Health insurance information
Mental health records	Mental health history Mental health evaluations Trauma history

Abbreviation: IEP, Individual Education Plan.

with attention specifically to the child or youth, including time alone to identify the history of placement and address his or her feelings about the separation and current placement, visitation, and functioning at school, as well as his or her understanding of the family plan, helps to frame the child's care and begin with the child's needs.[13,14,19] It is often helpful to gather the caregiver's and child welfare's health concerns both with and without the child. Caregivers may express frustration or confusion at child behaviors, which are often related to the histories of trauma and loss. Caregiver negativity can further traumatize the child and reinforce his or her sense of unworthiness, so these important discussions should be held privately while the child is occupied by other staff.

The physical examination should be as complete as the child can tolerate. Physical touch can be associated with abusive trauma for children in foster care, so the medical professional should attend to a child's anxiety about the examination. Children may need to keep their clothes on for the examination or return for multiple visits if anxiety is too high. It can be helpful, as age appropriate, to explain the examination before and during the visit (eg, "I'm going to check inside your ears now to make sure they are healthy") to reduce the risk that palpation and orifice examination will trigger a fight-or-flight response.

During the physical examination, specific issues to attend to include

- Child abuse and neglect screening should be conducted. Children in foster care have often been exposed to multiple types of maltreatment prior to placement and have some risk in placement, and disclosure or findings may bring up issues not previously identified. A complete unclothed physical examination, including genital examination, is indicated, as tolerated by the patient.
- It is important to assess growth parameters, because failure to thrive and, more commonly, obesity are not uncommon issues for children in foster care.[62,65]
- Dental caries is common to children in foster care due to exposures and poor access to dental care.[84,85] Oral examinations and referral for further dental care are indicated.
- Neuroendocrine changes can affect the immune and inflammatory response. In part, increased risk of infection, increased rates of asthma and allergy, and increased risk of metabolic syndrome can all be linked to trauma and should be specifically considered and addressed in this population.[58,86]

Immunization Status

Every effort to determine immunization status should be employed (eg, obtaining child care or school records, reviewing immunization registries [see Table 28.4]), because children entering foster care may be incompletely immunized, although visits to various medical professionals with poor record management may also lead to over-vaccination.[19,87] If records are unavailable, children should be considered at risk and be immunized.

Screening

The comprehensive evaluation affords the opportunity to screen for many of the health issues more common to children in foster care than their peers.

- Screening for hearing and vision is critical for children in foster care, who are 3 times more likely than peers to have hearing and vision problems.[77,88]
- Because poor nutrition puts children at risk for anemia, a complete blood cell count should be measured.
- A lead level is indicated for children 6 months to 6 years of age.[89]
- Children entering foster care are often at risk of tuberculosis from exposure to high-risk populations, sexually transmitted infections (STIs) from vertical transmission, and/or sexual abuse. Therefore, tuberculosis, HIV, syphilis, and hepatitis B and C testing should be considered. Low yield has been noted on some of these studies in regional reviews; thus, targeted screening may be considered. Child-specific risk factors and health conditions may increase the risk to any individual child.[90,91]
- Pregnancy and STI testing should be considered for all sexually active adolescents. History of sexual abuse can decrease the age at which children become sexually active, increase number of lifetime partners, and increase risk of STI; thus, this should be considered for all children who are pubertal.[92–94]
- Developmental and mental health screens should be administered with follow-up referral for comprehensive evaluations as needed. Screening should be performed according to the AAP "Recommendations for Preventive Pediatric Health Care."[95] Young children (<36 months) who are in foster care due to maltreatment are automatically eligible for Early Intervention services and should be referred for these in-home services.[8]

- Educational evaluations can be helpful, because school failure and learning issues are common to children in foster care.[59] Placement issues including absenteeism, changing schools, and missing classes due to court can have a negative effect on educational success,[20] but learning disabilities, cognitive and processing delays, and attention and behavior concerns that limit school functioning often go unaddressed for children in foster care. Questioning child welfare staff or schools directly about a child's needs and supports and, if concerns are raised, advocating for a multidisciplinary team educational evaluation to create an Individual Education Plan or Section 504 plan through the school district should be part of the comprehensive evaluation.[13]
- The medical professional can probe for information about trauma by asking simple open-ended questions to the foster caregiver, such as, "Do you know of any really scary or upsetting things that happened to (child's name) before (he/she) came to live with you?"[96] Alternatively, a formal screening tool, such as the Trauma Symptom Checklist, may be used to provide the medical professional with more objective data.[80,97,98] A variety of screening tools can be found through AAP resources[82,99] and the National Child Traumatic Stress Network (www.nctsn.org).

Anticipatory Guidance

Education and counseling are critical components of preventive health care encounters, especially for children in foster care. Because of traumatic histories, sleep problems (eg, difficulty falling asleep, staying asleep, early waking, nightmares), eating issues (eg, hoarding, overeating, picky eating), and toileting issues (eg, enuresis, encopresis, constipation) are common effects of trauma from increased sympathetic tone and alterations of the reticular activating system and satiety center.[82] Discussing adjustment to the home (for the child and the foster family, including the foster parents' biological children), grief and separation, visits with biological parents, and behavior issues, all with a trauma lens, can help to put these expected responses into a framework for the foster family and child.

The medical professional should affirm that these responses and behaviors are to be expected and represent a normal reaction to unhealthy threats that have resulted in healthy and unhealthy coping strategies. Caregivers who listen calmly, validate the child's emotions without reinforcing them, and reassure the child of the caregivers' support and affection will help the child's brain and body to learn new, more adaptive ways to respond to a new, safer environment.

Because usual parenting practices may not be effective with children who have experienced trauma, it is important to give foster caregivers alternative, trauma-specific ways to respond. Children who have experienced harsh parenting in the family of origin may be triggered by discipline that is restrictive in nature, and all forms of physical discipline should be avoided. Even before symptoms occur, in a high-risk population such as children in foster care, it can be helpful to provide trauma-specific anticipatory guidance.[82,100]

Specific attention should be paid to visits with the biological family. Biological parents may be unreliable in following through with plans for these visits or may be limited in their emotional self-control associated with the child's removal in the presence of the child. Even when biological parents are present for their children at visits, the opportunity to interact with biological parents can reopen the pain of the separation or create confusion for the child about foster parent/biological parent roles and allegiance. Preparing foster parents for this by identifying the visit as a stressor, recommending specific routines before and after visits (eg, pizza and the same favorite movie every time the child returns from a visit), and identifying concrete ways to reassure the child during the transitions (eg, making cards for mommy, looking at pictures of the biological and foster family) can significantly ease this process.

For adolescents in foster care, the comprehensive examination may be one of the only settings that provides an opportunity to discuss the issues of safety, sexuality, and teen risks.[101] For foster youth, the adults who usually assume responsibility for discussing these topics are absent, and child welfare and foster parents do not see this as their role. Therefore, there is a need for the medical professional to provide anticipatory guidance around these issues. Frank and open discussion of family planning and sexual safety, with attention to the trauma issues that may have affected the teen, has the potential to have a significant effect on an adolescent in foster care. Adolescent girls with a history of foster care placement have reported earlier age at first intercourse and a greater number of lifetime partners compared with those in the general population.[93] Foster care is also associated with higher risk of STIs.[92]

Ongoing Health Care

Different models for provision of ongoing health care have been successful, including continuity of care with the pre-foster placement medical professional, evaluation in a specialized foster care clinic followed by ongoing care with the prior medical professional or a new medical home, or becoming established in a new medical home for the initial evaluation and ongoing care. Once a child enters foster care, the medical professional ideally should remain the same, despite changes in foster placement or insurance coverage, to maximize access and continuity of care.[102] Multidisciplinary teams, which can combine health, developmental, and mental health resources, can be an efficient and comprehensive option,[63,103] but most children will receive their care in community-based settings. Regardless, coordination of care with child welfare, continuity, and regular access can have a positive effect on the health of children in foster settings.[19]

Consensus recommendations suggest preventive pediatric visits should be conducted on a more frequent schedule for the child in foster care. This augmented schedule is necessary because of the history of trauma, health burden at placement, and multiple environmental and social issues that can adversely affect health and development. This includes visits monthly for the first 6 months after birth, every 2 months for ages 6 to 12 months, every 3 months for ages 1 to 2 years, and every 6 months thereafter.[19,78] In fact, additional visits may be indicated depending on the stability of placement and changes in the child's physical health or severity of chronic conditions, emotional health, or living situation. Recent studies indicate that after children leave foster care, they are far less likely to receive routine health care.

Health Care Financing

Medicaid funds health care for children in foster care. Beginning in 2014, through a mandate in the Affordable Care Act, youth who age out of foster care remain eligible for Medicaid coverage until age 26 years.[8] However, although Medicaid is responsible for the full spectrum of services these children require, Medicaid payments usually do not adequately cover the time required to address the complex needs of these children and extent of care coordination that is often necessary to address those needs.[104] There have been some successes from Medicaid managed care plans designed with the needs of these children in mind,[105] although concerns about these plans include the rationing of services and disruptions to care when children are moved outside the coverage area for the managed care plan.[19,104] Some medical home models rely on supplemental funding besides Medicaid payments to provide the range of services necessary, through external grant funding, contracts with child welfare agencies, or local public health resources.[19]

Meanwhile, when children in foster care do not receive the coordinated services of a medical professional attuned to their needs, costs rise and preventive services are missed. A number of studies have demonstrated that children in foster care use a high proportion of Medicaid dollars but remain in poor health, accessing expensive inpatient medical, psychiatric, and emergency department services rather than primary and preventive continuity care.[74,76,106]

Mental Health Care

Youth in the child welfare system have specialized mental health needs. These specialized needs stem from stressors related to events that brought the youth into care, often including chronic traumas, separation from their family of origin, and placement into a complex system of care that, at times, struggles to meet the individual need of each child.[107] Youth in foster care have often had multiple traumatic experiences within the context of a chaotic family environment and poverty, without the psychosocial or parenting supports needed to buffer the negative effects of trauma on development.[14] Neurobiological research has demonstrated that the effects of early traumatic experiences on brain development and subsequent changes in psychological and physiological responses can be profound, leading to significant challenges for many youth involved in the child welfare system.[108] These children in foster care have higher rates of mental health disorders, such as depression and attention-deficit/hyperactivity disorder (ADHD), when compared with age-matched peers, with a poorer recovery and prognosis.[77,109–111] With these higher rates of mental health needs, youth in the child welfare system have increased behavioral health expenditures when compared with youth who are not in foster care.[112,113] Despite these increased rates of mental health disorders and high rates of service utilization, many youth still struggle with inadequate care, with only 19% to 50% of those in need of behavioral health services receiving them.[114–117]

Assessing Psychological Concerns

Assessing mental health concerns for youth in the child welfare system takes a coordinated effort among all members of the youth's care team, including communication with the child welfare agency, therapeutic team, school system, and legal team. Information about in utero exposures, birth and early development, and family history are important pieces to a child mental health evaluation, especially in young children, which means that collateral information and history are essential to accurately diagnose youth in foster care and develop a comprehensive trauma-informed treatment plan.[118,119]

Teasing out trauma-related symptoms from other diagnoses such as ADHD or oppositional defiant disorder can be difficult and may require consultation with a mental health professional with expertise in this vulnerable population. Many trauma-related symptoms overlap with other psychiatric disorders. Along with using specific trauma screens in the office (see Chapter 31, Trauma-Informed Care and Treatment), medical professionals working with traumatized youth should gather information around behavioral concerns in areas including school, child care, and home. It is useful to develop a timeline for when behaviors started in relation to any stressful or new events (eg, trauma, visitation with parent, move from placement). For example, if inattention and hyperactivity symptoms started after a traumatic incident, the inattention is more likely to be related to trauma symptoms of dissociation and hypervigilance than to ADHD. Trauma symptoms are frequently mistaken for behavior problems. Youth in foster care who have experienced multiple traumas are frequently identified as "problem children" when, in reality, the unwanted behaviors result from the expected trauma response of emotional lability and impulsivity after a traumatic event.[25,108] Medical and mental health professionals are in a position to educate the school system, caregivers, and child welfare about the nature of the trauma-reactive behaviors, helping to create more empathy for the youth while also building trauma-informed care across systems.[118,119]

Mental health safety screening is also important for pediatricians to assess when working with youth in the child welfare system. Youth who have been exposed to trauma are more likely to have suicidal ideation and attempts as well as self-injurious behaviors, making it essential that safety questions are asked and reassessed regularly.[109,120] Other concerning behaviors to screen for in a developmentally appropriate manner include fire setting, violence toward animals, urges to run, substance use, harm to others, and concerning sexualized behaviors.

Evidence-based Psychosocial Supports

First-line treatment of youth with mental health concerns is psychosocial interventions. Evidence-based, trauma-informed therapeutic supports are essential for youth in the child welfare system, given the high rates of traumatic experiences and symptoms of trauma seen in this population.[14,80,83,115,121] With the wide variety of treatments available, medical professionals can search the evidence base of a particular intervention through the National Registry of Evidence-based Programs and Practices or the California Evidence-Based Clearinghouse for Child Welfare to ensure their patients are receiving appropriate interventions.[85,122] Table 28.5 lists well-established psychosocial interventions that have a strong evidence base within families involved with child welfare.

TABLE 28.5
Evidence-based Psychosocial Interventions for Youth in Foster Care

Name of Intervention	Target Population	Length of Treatment	Brief Description	Key Concepts
Alternatives for Families: A Cognitive-Behavioral Therapy (AF-CBT)[123]	Age: 5–17 y Mode: individual, family	20 sessions 1–1.5 h each	• Targets family where physical abuse and harsh, excessive punishment have been used. • Methods are designed for use with children who have experienced physical abuse who present with externalizing behavior problems, notably aggressive behavior. • Addresses caregiver-child conflicts.	• Divided into 3 components: child directed, caregiver directed, and family systems directed. • Each component uses CBT framework to provide psychoeducation, process past hostility/physical abuse, assess automatic thoughts around aggression, and train in feeling identification, expression, and management skills. • Aims to help families develop prosocial management principles and problem-solving to serve as alternatives to physical discipline.
Attachment, Self-Regulation, and Competency (ARC) model[124]	Age: 2–21 y Mode: individual, family, group, systems	• Dependent on individual and mode of treatment. • Number of sessions range from 12 to >50.	• Targets youth exposed to complex trauma. • Grounded in attachment theory and early childhood development. • Addresses how a child's entire system of care can become trauma informed to better support trauma-focused therapy and factors promoting resilience.	• Three primary domains: attachment, self-regulation, and competency. • Fourth domain, trauma experience integration, draws from skills addressed in the first 3. • Each domain identifies primary targets called *building blocks* for assessment and intervention. • Develops a framework for work with systems, caregivers, and the child/youth.

(continued)

TABLE 28.5 (*continued*)

Name of Intervention	Target Population	Length of Treatment	Brief Description	Key Concepts
Parent-Child Interaction Therapy (PCIT)[125]	Age: 2–12 y Mode: individual, family, systems	12–20 sessions	• Targets youth exposed to interpersonal complex trauma. • Theoretical bases stem from developmental, social learning and attachment theory. • Uses highly specified, step-by-step, live-coached sessions with both the parent/caregiver and the child. • Emphasis is on changing negative parent/caregiver-child patterns.	• Two-stage approach aimed at relationship enhancement and child behavioral management. • The caregiver is coached in relationship-building skills: praise, reflection, imitation, description, and enthusiasm (PRIDE). • Caregiver and child participate in relationship-enhancement treatment sessions with a live coach. • Coach reinforces positive discipline program, including effective delivery of commands and strategies designed to increase compliance. • Parents are provided immediate feedback about their progress and mastery of skills. The skills are gradually expanded for use in everyday situations.
Trauma-Focused Cognitive Behavioral Therapy (TF-CBT)[126]	Age: 3–21 y Mode: individual and family	12–25 sessions 60- to 90-min session divided between youth and caregiver	• Targets youth with emotional difficulties relating to ≥1 traumatic life event(s), including complex trauma. • Addresses multiple domains of trauma, including, but not limited to, externalizing behavior problems, relationship and attachment problems, school problems, and cognitive problems. • Skills for regulating affect, behavior, thoughts, and relationships; trauma processing; and enhancing safety, trust, parenting skills, and family communication.	• Uses CBT skills taught to both caregiver and child with the framework to create an environment for the youth to retell his or her trauma narrative in a caring way. • Steps to implement therapy outlined in PRACTICE components: *p*sychoeducation to both parent and child, *r*elaxation skills for parent and youth, *a*ffective modulation tailored to youth, *c*ognitive coping, *t*rauma narrative, *i*n vivo mastery of trauma reminders, *c*onjoint youth-parent session, *e*nhancing safety.

Psychotropic Medications and Youth in Foster Care

Youth in foster care are at high risk for the inappropriate use of psychotropic medications. Numerous studies have outlined concern for overprescribing and under-prescribing of psychotropic medications to youth in foster care.[127–130] A variety of factors contribute to inappropriate prescribing, including placement disruptions, lack of communication among medical professionals and across agencies, unknown early mental health history, unknown family psychiatric history, lack of access to care, and lack of trauma-informed practice. Pediatric medical professionals can often feel pressure to prescribe medication to address behavioral health concerns when foster care placement is at risk and/or when mental health services and foster parent training are unavailable. Alternatively, pediatric medical professionals may be asked to renew, stop, or restart medications originally prescribed by other medical professionals, with little health information to support their use or modification.[14] Pressure to prescribe psychotropic medication is also fed by the lack of information about child trauma and misidentification of trauma symptoms as other mental health conditions such as ADHD.[131]

Inappropriate prescribing resulting from frequent placement disruptions is a particular vulnerability for youth in foster care. As a youth moves from one psychotropic prescriber to another, key information about why a medication was started or how a diagnosis was determined is often lost. The consequences of this lack of information are compounded by other information gaps, including family mental health history, early developmental history, abuse history, and prior response to medication, leaving youth at risk for layering of psychotropic medications—medications are added but never removed. When trauma symptoms are misinterpreted as other mental health diagnoses, the risk of further inappropriate medicating increases.

Placement type also predicts the use of psychotropic medications. Youth in kinship or home placements have been found to have lower rates of psychotropic use and behavioral health concerns as compared with youth placed in residential or group settings. Male gender and older age have also been shown to have increased rates of psychotropic use.[132] Nationally, there are geographical differences, and there are concerns of underuse of psychotropic medications in some areas, with 40-fold differences from area to area.[129]

Over the past decade, there has been specific concern about the increased use of antipsychotics in the foster care population. Although the use of second-generation antipsychotics has increased in the general pediatric

Medicaid population,[133] the rate of use among youth in foster care has increased disproportionately.[127,128,133,134] Inappropriate psychotropic prescribing practices came to a head in 2011 following the release of the 2011 US Government Accountability Office report calling for improved psychotropic oversight for youth in state custody.[135] This report looked at Medicaid claims data from 5 different states and compared rates of antipsychotic use in youth in and out of foster care. This analysis showed higher rates of psychotropic prescribing among youth in foster care in all 5 states and higher rates of inappropriate prescribing in all youth. The 2011 report was followed by a 2012 US Government Accountability Office report that shed light on the need for not just psychotropic oversight but clinical oversight, noting that upward of 30% of youth in foster care who received a psychotropic medication didn't receive psychosocial interventions for which they were eligible. The US Administration for Children and Families survey from 2012 outlined the need for state psychotropic oversight programs for youth in state custody to target concerns about psychotropic medication patterns, characterizing prescribing practices as "too many, too much, and too young" as well as highlighting concern around lack of evidence-based psychosocial interventions.[136]

The Child and Family Services Improvement and Innovation Act (PL 112–34) was signed into law in 2011, requiring states to develop an oversight system and coordination of health care services for youth in foster care and specifying that states must set up protocols for appropriate use and monitoring of psychotropic medication. These protocols vary from state to state, but all must balance timely access to appropriate medications while limiting high-risk regimens and provide oversight of medications and appropriate psychosocial services.[137]

The concept of deprescribing psychotropic medications has emerged in response to these concerns. *Deprescribing* is a structured approach to drug discontinuation designed to use the lowest effective dose and least amount of medication to optimize the regimen. Two drugs from the same class should not be used simultaneously. When presented with patients on polypharmacy, a medical professional should review the current medications and doses and consider slowly reducing the pharmacotherapy. This process may be best achieved in coordination with psychiatric medicine colleagues. The general principle is to target medications that have the highest risk profiles and lowest benefits while also taking into account the patient's voice surrounding medication regimen. Efforts led by Christopher Bellonci, MD, are ongoing to develop deprescribing guidelines that provide best practices for prescribers to optimize the most effective medications and reduce ineffective and duplicative medication regimens.[138,139]

Starting Psychotropic Medication

When used judiciously, medications can be helpful and even lifesaving for youth struggling with a mental health condition. Medications should be considered to treat a mental health disorder when therapy alone has not been effective and when there are significant safety concerns. Medications should be used at the lowest effective dose, monitored regularly, and assessed for possible discontinuation following a period of relative stability. Medication should always be used with therapeutic supports in youth in foster care. Close communication with a therapeutic team, including caregivers and the education system, is critical to ensure appropriate psychosocial services are also being provided to the youth. Before starting medication, youth voice and choice around medication should be considered. This is particularly important when a child is involved with child welfare, a setting in which youth often feel they have no control over what happens to them. Along with the youth's perspective on medication, it is also important to consider the family of origin's concerns and questions about medications. To best manage the medication concerns, needs, and management, it may be important to continue to be engaged with both foster parents and the biological family. By affirming parental voice as well as the child voice, the prescriber will promote engagement and motivation with treatment.[118,119,140]

Consultation with a child and adolescent psychiatrist should be considered for complex cases when first-line medications have not been effective or there is a significant safety concern. Pediatricians should seek an emergency mental health evaluation if there are urgent safety concerns with a youth in their care.

Consent for Psychotropic Medications

Consent for psychotropic medications varies by state, and medical professionals should become familiar with the rules of their locality. Consent may reside with parents or guardian if rights have not been terminated, although in some states, consent for psychotropic medication resides within the child welfare agency at the time of removal even if rights have not been terminated. Occasionally, state child welfare agencies elect for consent for a specific class of medication, such as antipsychotics, to be determined by court process rather than child welfare or family of origin.[141]

Special Populations Within Foster Care

There are some populations of youth in foster care who should be recognized as having even more significant challenges than the general population of children in foster care. While all of this chapter's guidance is appropriate for these children and teens as well, it is important to consider the pertinent risk factors and challenges for children and youth in these situations and augment services as appropriate. When children from these subgroups are encountered in practice, the medical professional will need increased vigilance to the standards of care to achieve the best outcome possible.

Unaccompanied Immigrant Children

Unaccompanied children immigrating to the United States from Central America and other regions has increased in recent years, and up to 35% are eventually placed in long-term foster care in the United States. These children may be served by the US Office of Refugee Resettlement as well as child welfare. Many of these children have histories of trauma, loss, mental illness, and unmet medical needs that are like other children in foster care. However, these issues are compounded by issues of acculturation, language barriers, limited connections in the community, and ambiguous legal status.[6,142]

Additional considerations for these children include

- Specific attention to risks of infectious disease, parasitic disease, and immunization status. Medical and immunization records are often difficult to access, and catch-up vaccine schedules, tuberculin testing, and stool testing for ova and parasites should be considered.
- Culturally sensitive trauma and mental health assessments and treatment may not be commonly available in the community. Medical professionals should partner with mental health colleagues to best address the needs of these children, who may have experienced violence, trafficking, separation, and loss. Resources specifically for this population are available from the National Child Traumatic Stress Network.[143]
- Limited formal education, language barriers, and transient placements challenge educational attainment for the unaccompanied immigrant patient. Educational assessments, in partnership with the local school district, should be a part of the evaluation for these children.

Children With Significant Medical, Cognitive, or Mental Health Needs

Children with significant medical, cognitive, or mental health needs can come to foster care with health issues both known and unknown. A small percentage of children with significant needs have profound medical or cognitive impairment and are usually placed in long-term care facilities, especially those who are dependent on technology for activities of daily living. Children with complex cardiac, renal, neurologic, or other systems issues; children with autism spectrum disorder or significant cognitive delay; or children with severe mental illness may come into care with little health information or supports. The role of the medical professional in obtaining, reviewing, and interpreting health records and documentation of previous evaluations; evaluating current health status; and evaluating need for urgent or acute intervention is crucial. Children with needs that surprise and overwhelm caregivers can have multiple placement disruptions or inappropriate placement in congregate care. By partnering with child welfare and foster caregivers, explaining the conditions and supports needed, and facilitating referrals, evaluations, and care planning, best placement and care can be identified.[19,144]

Children With Juvenile Justice Involvement

Youth involved with child welfare who later are served by juvenile justice, or those youth involved with juvenile justice who also spend time in foster care, are called *crossover youth, dual-status youth, dual-jurisdiction youth,* and *dually adjudicated youth.* Pathways to this status include arrest while in foster care or while involved with the child welfare system; identification of maltreatment on arrest, leading to child welfare referral; or referral to child welfare when a youth's time in juvenile justice ends and no safe home can be identified for the youth. In one study, 10% of youth leaving juvenile justice were served by child welfare within 1 year of release.[145] Characteristics of these youth included significant maltreatment history[146,147] and history of witnessing domestic violence; parents with history of criminal justice and substance use problems; being of color (more likely as compared with the general, child welfare, and juvenile justice populations); being male gender (although the difference in number between males and females in the dual-jurisdiction group is smaller than among the general delinquency population); special education issues, problems at school, and mental health and/or substance use problems; and likely living in a group home at the time of arrest.[148,149]

Compared with youth involved only in child welfare or probation, the dually involved youth are more likely to have poor outcomes, including adult criminal justice involvement; more likely to be on public welfare; 2 to 3 times more likely to access health, mental health, and substance use services (and access multiple services) within the first years after emancipation; and less likely to be employed, with lower earnings than peers.[150] Despite this high risk of negative outcomes, there is no coordinated system of identification of crossover youth within child welfare, there is limited engagement of child welfare with the court and legal system, there is poor coordination with the educational and behavioral health systems and, ultimately, and probably most significantly, a failure to recognize the effect of trauma on behavior.[151]

Medical professionals for these youth can help to bridge the information divide and emphasize the need to have access to trauma-informed mental health services for these youth. Medical professionals may need to guide caregivers or child welfare in obtaining educational assessments and substance use services.

Pregnant and Parenting Teens in Foster Care

As with the foster care population as a whole, youth who are pregnant or parenting are not homogeneous. Some youth enter the foster care system when they become pregnant or already have a child or children, while others become pregnant once in foster care. As noted previously, teens in foster care are more likely to become pregnant and to parent a child than peers who are not in foster care.[46,152] As legislation has allowed states to extend the age youth can remain in foster care from 18 to 21 years, more youth who are pregnant or parenting are in custody than in the past.

As previously noted, outcomes for adolescents transitioning out of care are poor. Youth who are pregnant or parenting are even more likely to demonstrate the poor outcomes seen in all foster youth—to drop out of school, be unemployed or underemployed, and be homeless. The children born to youth in foster care have increased challenges as well. Children born to teen parents are more likely to be born preterm, have school difficulties, and have higher rates of incarceration later in life. Children born to youth in foster care are, by some estimates, 5 times more likely to spend time in foster care than children of same-aged mothers who are not in foster care.[43,46,153]

Pregnant and parenting youth can be served in a variety of placements. Options include living with a relative or adult with whom the teen has a strong attachment, a foster home with special training to help youth with parenting skills, or a residential treatment setting where young parents and babies can be together while the parent can get treatment for mental health and trauma issues. The setting should promote attachment of the parent and baby and provide assistance with parenting skills, while allowing the youth to continue schooling, medical care, and mental health services.[154]

Medical professionals can support youth in foster care with comprehensive medical services, prenatal and antenatal care, and connection to supports such as the Special Supplemental Nutrition Program for Women, Infants, and Children and Early Intervention for the infant or toddler. Particular attention to the developmental needs of both the adolescent and young child, with an understanding of how trauma can affect development and parenting, can help to ameliorate the negative outcomes most common to both the teen and her child.[154]

LGBTQ Youth

Children and adolescents who identify as lesbian, gay, bisexual, transgender, and queer/questioning (LGBTQ) face unique developmental challenges, placing them at risk for medical and mental health vulnerabilities.[155,156] When LBGTQ youth are involved with child welfare, another layer of strain is added that requires specialized attention and care. Research has shown that LBGTQ youth are overrepresented in foster care, more likely to experience multiple placement disruptions, and more likely to reside in a group placement, and have increased challenges reaching permanency.[157] These vulnerabilities leave youths at high risk for homelessness as well. Medical professionals working with LGBTQ youth in an out-of-home placement should review the current placement setting to ensure the living environment is safe and affirming.[158]

Significant health and mental health disparities exist for LGBTQ youth. Those LGBTQ youth involved with child welfare are at high risk for exposure to complex trauma related to events that brought them into foster care, such as neglect and abuse, coupled with the high rate of bullying and violence experienced by this population as a sexual minority. Whether or not they are in foster care, LGBTQ youth have higher rates of depression, substance use, and suicide, indicating a need for medical professionals to assess mental health needs, including safety, and ensure appropriate referrals to therapeutic resources are made. Baseline LGBTQ youth are also at risk of unsafe sexual practices, leading to higher rates of unintended pregnancy and STIs including HIV.[155] Medical professionals working with this population should be aware of the added complexities an out-of-home placement can have on the medical and mental health needs of LGBTQ youth.

Conclusion

Children in foster care are at high risk for persistent and chronic physical, emotional, and developmental conditions because of multiple and cumulative adverse events in their lives. Pediatric medical professionals can have a significant effect on the health and wellness of these patients and can best serve them with an understanding of the legal, administrative, and medical issues that affect the lives of these children. Child welfare agencies and pediatricians should work together to implement the standards for health care and mental health care of children in foster care outlined by the AAP, American Academy of Child and Adolescent Psychiatry, and the Child Welfare League of America in the past and informed by the science of today. Pediatricians can help improve the health and well-being of children in foster care by performing timely and thorough medical evaluations, providing continuity of care, playing an active advocacy role, and practicing compassionate, trauma-informed care.

References

1. US Department of Health and Human Services; Administration for Children and Families; Administration on Children, Youth, and Families; Children's Bureau. The AFCARS Report. *No.* 24: Preliminary FY 2016 Estimates as of October 20, 2017. https://www.acf.hhs.gov/sites/default/files/cb/afcarsreport24.pdf. Accessed April 11, 2019
2. Child Welfare Information Gateway. Foster Care Statistics 2016. Washington, DC: US Department of Health and Human Services, Children's Bureau; 2017. https://www.childwelfare.gov/pubs/factsheets/foster. Accessed April 11, 2019
3. US Department of Health and Human Services, Administration for Children and Families, Children's Bureau. Trends in foster care and adoption. https://www.acf.hhs.gov/cb/resource/trends-in-foster-care-and-adoption. Accessed April 11, 2019
4. US Department of Health and Human Services, Administration for Children and Families, Children's Bureau. Data Brief 2013–1: Recent Demographic Trends in Foster Care. https://www.acf.hhs.gov/cb/resource/data-brief-trends-in-foster-care-1. Published September 13, 2013. Accessed April 11, 2019
5. Conn AM, Szilagyi MA, Franke TM, Albertin CS, Blumkin AK, Szilagyi PG. Trends in child protection and out-of-home care. *Pediatrics*. 2013;132(4):712–719 PMID: 24062369 https://doi.org/10.1542/peds.2013-0969
6. Kandel W. *Unaccompanied Alien Children: An Overview*. Washington, DC: Congressional Research Service; January 2017. https://fas.org/sgp/crs/homesec/R43599.pdf. Accessed October 17, 2017.
7. Hill R. *Synthesis of Research on Disproportionality in the Child Welfare System: An Update*. Washington, DC: The Casey CSSP-Family Alliance for Racial Equality; 2006
8. Child Welfare Information Gateway. Major federal legislation concerned with child protection, child welfare, and adoption. Fact Sheet current through March 2015. https://www.childwelfare.gov/pubPDFs/majorfedlegis.pdf. Accessed April 11, 2019
9. Finkelhor D, Turner H, Ormrod R, Hamby SL. Trends in childhood violence and abuse exposure: evidence from 2 national surveys. *Arch Pediatr Adolesc Med*. 2010;164(3):238–242 PMID: 20194256 https://doi.org/10.1001/archpediatrics.2009.283
10. Finkelhor D, Turner HA, Shattuck A, Hamby SL. Violence, crime, and abuse exposure in a national sample of children and youth: an update. *JAMA Pediatr*. 2013;167(7):614–621 PMID: 23700186 https://doi.org/10.1001/jamapediatrics.2013.42
11. Hillen T, Gafson L. Why good placements matter: pre-placement and placement risk factors associated with mental health disorders in pre-school children in foster care. *Clin Child Psychol Psychiatry*. 2015;20(3):486–499 PMID: 24733375 https://doi.org/10.1177/1359104514530733

12. Leslie LK, Gordon JN, Lambros K, Premji K, Peoples J, Gist K. Addressing the developmental and mental health needs of young children in foster care. *J Dev Behav Pediatr*. 2005;26(2):140–151 PMID: 15827467 https://doi.org/10.1097/00004703-200504000-00011
13. Szilagyi M. The pediatric role in the care of children in foster and kinship care. *Pediatr Rev*. 2012;33(11):496–508 PMID: 23118315 https://doi.org/10.1542/pir.33-11-496
14. Forkey H, Szilagyi M. Foster care and healing from complex childhood trauma. *Pediatr Clin North Am*. 2014;61(5):1059–1072 PMID: 25242716 https://doi.org/10.1016/j.pcl.2014.06.015
15. Rubin DM, O'Reilly AL, Luan X, Localio AR. The impact of placement stability on behavioral well-being for children in foster care. *Pediatrics*. 2007;119(2):336–344 PMID: 17272624 https://doi.org/10.1542/peds.2006-1995
16. Chamberlain P, Price JM, Reid JB, Landsverk J, Fisher PA, Stoolmiller M. Who disrupts from placement in foster and kinship care? *Child Abuse Negl*. 2006;30(4):409–424 PMID: 16600372 https://doi.org/10.1016/j.chiabu.2005.11.004
17. Carnochan S, Moore M, Austin MJ. Achieving placement stability. *J Evidence-Based Soc Work*. 2013;10(3):235–253 PMID: 23705653 https://doi.org/10.1080/15433714.2013.788953
18. James S. Why do foster care placements disrupt? An investigation of reasons for placement change in foster care. *Soc Serv Rev*. 2004;78(4):601–627 https://doi.org/10.1086/424546
19. Szilagyi MA, Rosen DS, Rubin D, Zlotnik S; American Academy of Pediatrics Council on Foster Care, Adoption, and Kinship Care, Committee on Adolescence, and Council on Early Childhood. Health care issues for children and adolescents in foster care and kinship care. *Pediatrics*. 2015;136(4):e1142–e1166 PMID: 26416934 https://doi.org/10.1542/peds.2015-2656
20. Zorc CS, O'Reilly AL, Matone M, Long J, Watts CL, Rubin D. The relationship of placement experience to school absenteeism and changing schools in young, school-aged children in foster care. *Child Youth Serv Rev*. 2013;35(5):826–833 PMID: 23645948 https://doi.org/10.1016/j.childyouth.2013.02.006
21. Rubin DM, Alessandrini EA, Feudtner C, Mandell DS, Localio AR, Hadley T. Placement stability and mental health costs for children in foster care. *Pediatrics*. 2004;113(5):1336–1341 PMID: 15121950 https://doi.org/10.1542/peds.113.5.1336
22. Fisher PA, Stoolmiller M, Gunnar MR, Burraston BO. Effects of a therapeutic intervention for foster preschoolers on diurnal cortisol activity. *Psychoneuroendocrinology*. 2007;32(8-10):892–905 PMID: 17656028 https://doi.org/10.1016/j.psyneuen.2007.06.008
23. Sakai C, Lin H, Flores G. Health outcomes and family services in kinship care: analysis of a national sample of children in the child welfare system. *Arch Pediatr Adolesc Med*. 2011;165(2):159–165 PMID: 21300656 https://doi.org/10.1001/archpediatrics.2010.277
24. Greiner MV, Ross J, Brown CM, Beal SJ, Sherman SN. Foster caregivers' perspectives on the medical challenges of children placed in their care: implications for pediatricians caring for children in foster care. *Clin Pediatr (Phila)*. 2015;54(9):853–861 PMID: 25561697 https://doi.org/10.1177/0009922814563925
25. Fisher PA, Gunnar MR, Dozier M, Bruce J, Pears KC. Effects of therapeutic interventions for foster children on behavioral problems, caregiver attachment, and stress regulatory neural systems. *Ann N Y Acad Sci*. 2006;1094(1):215–225 PMID: 17347353 https://doi.org/10.1196/annals.1376.023
26. Stein REK, Hurlburt MS, Heneghan AM, et al. Health status and type of out-of-home placement: informal kinship care in an investigated sample. *Acad Pediatr*. 2014;14(6):559–564 PMID: 25439154 https://doi.org/10.1016/j.acap.2014.04.002

27. Dozier M, Albus K, Fisher PA, Sepulveda S. Interventions for foster parents: implications for developmental theory. *Dev Psychopathol*. 2002;14(4):843–860 PMID: 12549706 https://doi.org/10.1017/S0954579402004091
28. Barnett ER, Jankowski MK, Butcher RL, Meister C, Parton RR, Drake RE. Foster and adoptive parent perspectives on needs and services: a mixed methods study. *J Behav Health Serv Res*. 2018;45(1):74–89 PMID: 28852992 https://doi.org/10.1007/s11414-017-9569-4
29. Macdonald GM, Turner W. Treatment foster care for improving outcomes in children and young people. *Cochrane Database Syst Rev*. 2008;23(1):CD005649 PMID: 18254087 https://doi.org/10.1002/14651858.CD005649.pub2
30. Stacks AM, Partridge T. Infants placed in foster care prior to their first birthday: differences in kin and nonkin placements. *Infant Ment Health J*. 2011;32(5):489–508 PMID: 28520253 https://doi.org/10.1002/imhj.20311
31. Rubin DM, Downes KJ, O'Reilly AL, Mekonnen R, Luan X, Localio R. Impact of kinship care on behavioral well-being for children in out-of-home care. *Arch Pediatr Adolesc Med*. 2008;162(6):550–556 PMID: 18524746 https://doi.org/10.1001/archpedi.162.6.550
32. Fowler PJ, Marcal KE, Zhang J, Day O, Landsverk J. Homelessness and aging out of foster care: a national comparison of child welfare-involved adolescents. *Child Youth Serv Rev*. 2017;77:27–33 PMID: 29056803 https://doi.org/10.1016/j.childyouth.2017.03.017
33. Jones LP. Former foster youth's perspectives on independent living preparation six months after discharge. *Child Welfare*. 2014;93(1):99–126 PMID: 26030989
34. Blustein J, Chan S, Guanais FC. Elevated depressive symptoms among caregiving grandparents. *Health Serv Res*. 2004;39(6 Pt 1):1671–1689 PMID: 15533181 https://doi.org/10.1111/j.1475-6773.2004.00312.x
35. Chinitz S, Guzman H, Amstutz E, Kohchi J, Alkon M. Improving outcomes for babies and toddlers in child welfare: a model for infant mental health intervention and collaboration. *Child Abuse Negl*. 2017;70:190–198 PMID: 28622589 https://doi.org/10.1016/j.chiabu.2017.05.015
36. Taplin S, Bullen T, McArthur M, Humphreys C, Kertesz M, Dobbins T. KContact, an enhanced intervention for contact between children in out-of-home care and their parents: protocol for a cluster randomised controlled trial. *BMC Public Health*. 2015;15(1):1134 PMID: 26573144 https://doi.org/10.1186/s12889-015-2461-3
37. Taplin S, Mattick RP. Supervised contact visits: results from a study of women in drug treatment with children in care. *Child Youth Serv Rev*. 2014;39(suppl C):65–72 https://doi.org/10.1016/j.childyouth.2014.01.023
38. Pergamit M, McDaniel M, Hawkins A. *Housing Assistance for Youth Who Have Aged Out of Foster Care: The Role of the Chaffee Foster Care Independence Program*. Washington, DC: Urban Institute for the US Department of Health and Human Services Office of the Assistant Secretary for Planning and Evaluation; 2012. https://aspe.hhs.gov/basic-report/housing-assistance-youth-who-have-aged-out-foster-care. Accessed April 11, 2019
39. American Bar Association Center on Children and the Law, Juvenile Law Center. *Issue Brief: The Role of the Courts in Implementing the Older Youth Provisions of the Strengthening Families Act.* http://jlc.org/sites/default/files/publication_pdfs/ABAIssueBrief-SFAforCourts-Feb2016_0.pdf. Published February 2016. Accessed April 11, 2019
40. Reilly T. Transition from care: status and outcomes of youth who age out of foster care. *Child Welfare*. 2003;82(6):727–746 PMID: 14736032

41. Ahrens KR, Garrison MM, Courtney ME. Health outcomes in young adults from foster care and economically diverse backgrounds. *Pediatrics*. 2014;134(6):1067–1074 PMID: 25367543 https://doi.org/10.1542/peds.2014-1150
42. Pecora PJ, Kessler RC, O'Brien K, et al. Educational and employment outcomes of adults formerly placed in foster care: results from the Northwest Foster Care Alumni Study. *Child Youth Serv Rev*. 2006;28(12):1459–1481 https://doi.org/10.1016/j.childyouth.2006.04.003
43. Dworsky A, Courtney M. The risk of teenage pregnancy among transitioning foster youth: implications for extending state care beyond age 18. *Child Youth Serv Rev*. 2010;32(10):1351–1356 https://doi.org/10.1016/j.childyouth.2010.06.002
44. Dworsky A, Napolitano L, Courtney M. Homelessness during the transition from foster care to adulthood. *Am J Public Health*. 2013;103(S2)(suppl 2):S318–S323 PMID: 24148065 https://doi.org/10.2105/AJPH.2013.301455
45. Putnam-Hornstein E, Hammond I, Eastman AL, McCroskey J, Webster D. Extended foster care for transition-age youth: an opportunity for pregnancy prevention and parenting support. *J Adolesc Health*. 2016;58(4):485–487 PMID: 26853490 https://doi.org/10.1016/j.jadohealth.2015.11.015
46. Combs KM, Begun S, Rinehart DJ, Taussig H. Pregnancy and childbearing among young adults who experienced foster care. *Child Maltreat*. 2018;23(2):166–174 PMID: 29034732 https://doi.org/10.1177/1077559517733816
47. Wulczyn F. Family reunification. *Future Child*. 2004;14(1):94–113 PMID: 15072020 https://doi.org/10.2307/1602756
48. Taussig HN, Clyman RB, Landsverk J. Children who return home from foster care: a 6-year prospective study of behavioral health outcomes in adolescence. *Pediatrics*. 2001;108(1):E10 PMID: 11433089 https://doi.org/10.1542/peds.108.1.e10
49. Child Welfare Information Gateway. Adoption Disruption and Dissolution. Washington, DC: US Department of Health and Human Services, Children's Bureau; 2012. https://www.childwelfare.gov/pubPDFs/s_disrup.pdf. Accessed April 11, 2019
50. Rushton A, Dance C. The adoption of children from public care: a prospective study of outcome in adolescence. *J Am Acad Child Adolesc Psychiatry*. 2006;45(7):877–883 PMID: 16832325 https://doi.org/10.1097/01.chi.0000220850.86768.e8
51. Jee SH, Barth RP, Szilagyi MA, Szilagyi PG, Aida M, Davis MM. Factors associated with chronic conditions among children in foster care. *J Health Care Poor Underserved*. 2006;17(2):328–341 PMID: 16702718 https://doi.org/10.1353/hpu.2006.0062
52. Tooley UA, Makhoul Z, Fisher PA. Nutritional status of foster children in the U.S.: implications for cognitive and behavioral development. *Child Youth Serv Rev*. 2016;70(suppl C):369–374 PMID: 28626279 https://doi.org/10.1016/j.childyouth.2016.10.027
53. Garner AS, Shonkoff JP, Siegel BS, et al; American Academy of Pediatrics Committee on Psychosocial Aspects of Child and Family Health; Committee on Early Childhood, Adoption, and Dependent Care; and Section on Developmental and Behavioral Pediatrics. Early childhood adversity, toxic stress, and the role of the pediatrician: translating developmental science into lifelong health. *Pediatrics*. 2012;129(1):e224–e231 PMID: 22201148 https://doi.org/10.1542/peds.2011-2662
54. Shonkoff JP, Garner AS, Siegel BS, et al; American Academy of Pediatrics Committee on Psychosocial Aspects of Child and Family Health; Committee on Early Childhood, Adoption, and Dependent Care; and Section on Developmental and Behavioral Pediatrics. The lifelong effects of early childhood adversity and toxic stress. *Pediatrics*. 2012;129(1):e232–e246 PMID: 22201156 https://doi.org/10.1542/peds.2011-2663

55. Leslie LK, Gordon JN, Meneken L, Premji K, Michelmore KL, Ganger W. The physical, developmental, and mental health needs of young children in child welfare by initial placement type. *J Dev Behav Pediatr*. 2005;26(3):177–185 PMID: 15956866 https://doi.org/10.1097/00004703-200506000-00003
56. Clougherty JE, Levy JI, Kubzansky LD, et al. Synergistic effects of traffic-related air pollution and exposure to violence on urban asthma etiology. *Environ Health Perspect*. 2007;115(8):1140–1146 PMID: 17687439 https://doi.org/10.1289/ehp.9863
57. Cameron JL, Eagleson KL, Fox NA, Hensch TK, Levitt P. Social origins of developmental risk for mental and physical illness. *J Neurosci*. 2017;37(45):10783–10791 PMID: 29118206 https://doi.org/10.1523/JNEUROSCI.1822-17.2017
58. Johnson SB, Riley AW, Granger DA, Riis J. The science of early life toxic stress for pediatric practice and advocacy. *Pediatrics*. 2013;131(2):319–327 PMID: 23339224 https://doi.org/10.1542/peds.2012-0469
59. Ringeisen H, Casanueva C, Urato M, Cross T. Special health care needs among children in the child welfare system. *Pediatrics*. 2008;122(1):e232–e241 PMID: 18595968 https://doi.org/10.1542/peds.2007-3778
60. Halfon N, Mendonca A, Berkowitz G. Health status of children in foster care. The experience of the Center for the Vulnerable Child. *Arch Pediatr Adolesc Med*. 1995;149(4):386–392 PMID: 7704166 https://doi.org/10.1001/archpedi.1995.02170160040006
61. Chernoff R, Combs-Orme T, Risley-Curtiss C, Heisler A. Assessing the health status of children entering foster care. *Pediatrics*. 1994;93(4):594–601 PMID: 8134214
62. Steele JS, Buchi KF. Medical and mental health of children entering the Utah foster care system. *Pediatrics*. 2008;122(3):e703–e709 PMID: 18762506 https://doi.org/10.1542/peds.2008-0360
63. Simms MD. The foster care clinic: a community program to identify treatment needs of children in foster care. *J Dev Behav Pediatr*. 1989;10(3):121–128 PMID: 2473095 https://doi.org/10.1097/00004703-198906000-00001
64. Wyatt DT, Simms MD, Horwitz SM. Widespread growth retardation and variable growth recovery in foster children in the first year after initial placement. *Arch Pediatr Adolesc Med*. 1997;151(8):813–816 PMID: 9265884 https://doi.org/10.1001/archpedi.1997.02170450063010
65. Schneiderman JU, Smith C, Arnold-Clark JS, Fuentes J, Duan L, Palinkas LA. Overweight and obesity among Hispanic children entering foster care: a preliminary examination of polyvictimization. *Child Maltreat*. 2013;18(4):264–273 PMID: 24137014 https://doi.org/10.1177/1077559513508236
66. Schneiderman JU, Leslie LK, Arnold-Clark JS, McDaniel D, Xie B. Pediatric health assessments of young children in child welfare by placement type. *Child Abuse Negl*. 2011;35(1):29–39 PMID: 21316106 https://doi.org/10.1016/j.chiabu.2010.06.007
67. Randsalu LS, Laurell L. Children in out-of-home care are at high risk of somatic, dental and mental ill health. *Acta Paediatr*. 2018;107(2):301–306 PMID: 28986993 10.1111/apa.14108
68. American Academy of Pediatrics Committee on Early Childhood, Adoption, and Dependent Care. Developmental issues for young children in foster care. *Pediatrics*. 2000;106(5):1145–1150 PMID: 11061791 https://doi.org/10.1542/peds.106.5.1145
69. Jee SH, Szilagyi M, Ovenshire C, et al. Improved detection of developmental delays among young children in foster care. *Pediatrics*. 2010;125(2):282–289 PMID: 20064864 https://doi.org/10.1542/peds.2009-0229
70. Simms MD, Dubowitz H, Szilagyi MA. Health care needs of children in the foster care system. *Pediatrics*. 2000;106(4)(suppl):909–918 PMID: 11044143

71. Oswald SH, Heil K, Goldbeck L. History of maltreatment and mental health problems in foster children: a review of the literature. *J Pediatr Psychol*. 2010;35(5):462–472 PMID: 20007747 https://doi.org/10.1093/jpepsy/jsp114
72. Greeson JK, Briggs EC, Kisiel CL, et al. Complex trauma and mental health in children and adolescents placed in foster care: findings from the National Child Traumatic Stress Network. *Child Welfare*. 2011;90(6):91–108 PMID: 22533044
73. Cicchetti D, Rogosch FA, Howe ML, Toth SL. The effects of maltreatment and neuroendocrine regulation on memory performance. *Child Dev*. 2010;81(5):1504–1519 PMID: 20840237 https://doi.org/10.1111/j.1467-8624.2010.01488.x
74. Johnson CSP, Wulczyn F. *Raising the Bar for Health and Mental Health Services for Children in Foster Care: Developing a Model of Managed Care*. New York, NY: Council of Family and Child Caring Agencies; 2013
75. Jee SH, Antonucci TC, Aida M, Szilagyi MA, Szilagyi PG. Emergency department utilization by children in foster care. *Ambul Pediatr*. 2005;5(2):102–106 PMID: 15780011 https://doi.org/10.1367/A04-068R.1
76. Rubin DM, Alessandrini EA, Feudtner C, Localio AR, Hadley T. Placement changes and emergency department visits in the first year of foster care. *Pediatrics*. 2004;114(3): e354–e360 PMID: 15342897 https://doi.org/10.1542/peds.2003-0594-F
77. Turney K, Wildeman C. Mental and physical health of children in foster care. *Pediatrics*. 2016;138(5):e20161118 PMID: 27940775 https://doi.org/10.1542/peds.2016-1118
78. American Academy of Pediatrics District II New York State Task Force on Health Care for Children in Foster Care. *Fostering Health: Health Care for Children and Adolescents in Foster Care*. 2nd ed. Elk Grove Village, IL: American Academy of Pediatrics; 2005
79. Child Welfare League of America. *Standards for Health Care Services for Children in Out-of-Home Care*. Washington, DC: Child Welfare League of America, Inc; 1988
80. Forkey H, Morgan W, Schwartz K, Sagor L. Outpatient clinic identification of trauma symptoms in children in foster care. *J Child Fam Stud*. 2016;25(5):1480–1487 https://doi.org/10.1007/s10826-015-0331-3
81. American Academy of Pediatrics. Healthy Foster Care America: health issues and needs. https://www.aap.org/en-us/advocacy-and-policy/aap-health-initiatives/healthy-foster-care-america/Pages/Health-Issues.aspx. Accessed April 11, 2019
82. American Academy of Pediatrics, Dave Thomas Foundation for Adoption. Helping Foster and Adoptive Families Cope With Trauma. Elk Grove Village, IL: American Academy of Pediatrics; 2015. https://www.aap.org/en-us/advocacy-and-policy/aap-health-initiatives/healthy-foster-care-america/Documents/Guide.pdf. Accessed April 11, 2019
83. Schilling S, Fortin K, Forkey H. Medical management and trauma-informed care for children in foster care. *Curr Probl Pediatr Adolesc Health Care*. 2015;45(10):298–305 PMID: 26381646 https://doi.org/10.1016/j.cppeds.2015.08.004
84. Melbye M, Huebner CE, Chi DL, Hinderberger H, Milgrom P. A first look: determinants of dental care for children in foster care. *Spec Care Dentist*. 2013;33(1):13–19 PMID: 23278144 https://doi.org/10.1111/j.1754-4505.2012.00312.x
85. Melbye ML, Chi DL, Milgrom P, Huebner CE, Grembowski D. Washington state foster care: dental utilization and expenditures. *J Public Health Dent*. 2014;74(2):93–101 PMID: 23889590 https://doi.org/10.1111/jphd.12027
86. Dantzer R, O'Connor JC, Freund GG, Johnson RW, Kelley KW. From inflammation to sickness and depression: when the immune system subjugates the brain. *Nat Rev Neurosci*. 2008;9(1):46–56 PMID: 18073775 https://doi.org/10.1038/nrn2297
87. US Government Accountability Office. *Foster Care: Health Needs of Many Young Children Are Unknown and Unmet*. Washington, DC: US Government Accountability Office; 1995

88. Takayama JI, Wolfe E, Coulter KP. Relationship between reason for placement and medical findings among children in foster care. *Pediatrics*. 1998;101(2):201–207 PMID: 9445492 https://doi.org/10.1542/peds.101.2.201
89. Chung EK, Webb D, Clampet-Lundquist S, Campbell C. A comparison of elevated blood lead levels among children living in foster care, their siblings, and the general population. *Pediatrics*. 2001;107(5):E81 PMID: 11331731 https://doi.org/10.1542/peds.107.5.e81
90. Greiner MV, Beal SJ, Nause K, Staat MA, Dexheimer JW, Scribano PV. Laboratory screening for children entering foster care. *Pediatrics*. 2017;140(6):e20163778 PMID: 29141915 https://doi.org/10.1542/peds.2016-3778
91. Szilagyi M, Schulte E. Issues related to laboratory screening for children and adolescents entering foster care. *Pediatrics*. 2017;140(6):e20173075 PMID: 29141917 https://doi.org/10.1542/peds.2017-3075
92. Ahrens KR, Richardson LP, Courtney ME, McCarty C, Simoni J, Katon W. Laboratory-diagnosed sexually transmitted infections in former foster youth compared with peers. *Pediatrics*. 2010;126(1):e97–e103 PMID: 20547646 https://doi.org/10.1542/peds.2009-2424
93. Boyer D, Fine D. Sexual abuse as a factor in adolescent pregnancy and child maltreatment. *Fam Plann Perspect*. 1992;24(1):4–11, 19 PMID: 1601126 https://doi.org/10.2307/2135718
94. Ahrens KR, McCarty C, Simoni J, Dworsky A, Courtney ME. Psychosocial pathways to sexually transmitted infection risk among youth transitioning out of foster care: evidence from a longitudinal cohort study. *J Adolesc Health*. 2013;53(4):478–485 PMID: 23859955 https://doi.org/10.1016/j.jadohealth.2013.05.010
95. American Academy of Pediatrics Committee on Practice and Ambulatory Medicine and Bright Futures Periodicity Schedule Workgroup. 2017 recommendations for preventive pediatric health care. *Pediatrics*. 2017;139(4):e20170254 PMID: 28213605 https://doi.org/10.1542/peds.2017-0254
96. Cohen JA, Kelleher KJ, Mannarino AP. Identifying, treating, and referring traumatized children: the role of pediatric providers. *Arch Pediatr Adolesc Med*. 2008;162(5):447–452 PMID: 18458191 https://doi.org/10.1001/archpedi.162.5.447
97. Briere J. *Trauma Symptom Checklist for Children (TSCC): Professional Manual*. Odessa, FL: Psychological Resources Inc; 1996
98. Briere J. *Trauma Symptom Checklist for Young Children (TSCYC): Professional Manual*. Odessa, FL: Psychological Assessment Resources; 2005
99. American Academy of Pediatrics. Healthy Foster Care America: trauma guide: trauma toolbox for primary care. https://www.aap.org/en-us/advocacy-and-policy/aap-health-initiatives/healthy-foster-care-america/Pages/Trauma-Guide.aspx. Accessed April 11, 2019
100. Vasileva M, Petermann F. Posttraumatic stress symptoms in preschool children in foster care: the influence of placement and foster family environment. *J Trauma Stress*. 2017;30(5):472–481 PMID: 29077996 https://doi.org/10.1002/jts.22217
101. Christian CW, Schwarz DF. Child maltreatment and the transition to adult-based medical and mental health care. *Pediatrics*. 2011;127(1):139–145 PMID: 21149424 https://doi.org/10.1542/peds.2010-2297
102. Jaudes KP, Champagne V, Harden A, Masterson J, Bilaver LA. Expanded medical home model works for children in foster care. *Child Welfare*. 2012;91(1):9–33 PMID: 22894013
103. Greiner MV, Beal SJ. Developing a health care system for children in foster care. *Health Promot Pract*. 2018;19(4):621–628 PMID: 28905635 https://doi.org/10.1177/1524839917730045

104. Leslie LK, Kelleher KJ, Burns BJ, Landsverk J, Rolls JA. Foster care and Medicaid managed care. *Child Welfare*. 2003;82(3):367–392 PMID: 12769396
105. Bright MA, Kleinman L, Vogel B, Shenkman E. Visits to primary care and emergency department reliance for foster youth: impact of Medicaid managed care. *Acad Pediatr.* 2018;18(4):397–404 PMID: 29081362 https://doi.org/10.1016/j.acap.2017.10.005
106. DiGiuseppe DL, Christakis DA. Continuity of care for children in foster care. *Pediatrics.* 2003;111(3):e208–e213 PMID: 12612273 https://doi.org/10.1542/peds.111.3.e208
107. Stirling J Jr, Amaya-Jackson L, Amaya-Jackson L; American Academy of Pediatrics Committee on Child Abuse and Neglect and Section on Adoption and Foster Care; American Academy of Child and Adolescent Psychiatry; National Center for Child Traumatic Stress. Understanding the behavioral and emotional consequences of child abuse. *Pediatrics*. 2008;122(3):667–673 PMID: 18762538 https://doi.org/10.1542/peds.2008-1885
108. Sege RD, Harper Browne C. Responding to ACEs with HOPE: health outcomes from positive experiences. *Acad Pediatr*. 2017;17(7S):S79–S85 PMID: 28865664 https://doi.org/10.1016/j.acap.2017.03.007
109. Heneghan A, Stein RE, Hurlburt MS, et al. Mental health problems in teens investigated by U.S. child welfare agencies. *J Adolesc Health*. 2013;52(5):634–640 PMID: 23375826 https://doi.org/10.1016/j.jadohealth.2012.10.269
110. Heim C, Shugart M, Craighead WE, Nemeroff CB. Neurobiological and psychiatric consequences of child abuse and neglect. *Dev Psychobiol*. 2010;52(7):671–690 PMID: 20882586 https://doi.org/10.1002/dev.20494
111. Heim C, Newport DJ, Mletzko T, Miller AH, Nemeroff CB. The link between childhood trauma and depression: insights from HPA axis studies in humans. *Psychoneuroendocrinology*. 2008;33(6):693–710 PMID: 18602762 https://doi.org/10.1016/j.psyneuen.2008.03.008
112. Harman JS, Childs GE, Kelleher KJ. Mental health care utilization and expenditures by children in foster care. *Arch Pediatr Adolesc Med*. 2000;154(11):1114–1117 PMID: 11074852 https://doi.org/10.1001/archpedi.154.11.1114
113. dosReis S, Zito JM, Safer DJ, Soeken KL. Mental health services for youths in foster care and disabled youths. *Am J Public Health*. 2001;91(7):1094–1099 PMID: 11441737 https://doi.org/10.2105/AJPH.91.7.1094
114. McCue Horwitz S, Hurlburt MS, Heneghan A, et al. Mental health problems in young children investigated by U.S. child welfare agencies. *J Am Acad Child Adolesc Psychiatry*. 2012;51(6):572–581 PMID: 22632617 https://doi.org/10.1016/j.jaac.2012.03.006
115. Hurlburt MS, Leslie LK, Landsverk J, et al. Contextual predictors of mental health service use among children open to child welfare. *Arch Gen Psychiatry*. 2004;61(12):1217–1224 PMID: 15583113 https://doi.org/10.1001/archpsyc.61.12.1217
116. Leslie LK, Hurlburt MS, Landsverk J, Barth R, Slymen DJ. Outpatient mental health services for children in foster care: a national perspective. *Child Abuse Negl*. 2004;28(6):699–714 PMID: 15193856 https://doi.org/10.1016/j.chiabu.2004.01.004
117. Libby AM, Orton HD, Barth RP, et al. Alcohol, drug, and mental health specialty treatment services and race/ethnicity: a national study of children and families involved with child welfare. *Am J Public Health*. 2006;96(4):628–631 PMID: 16507729 https://doi.org/10.2105/AJPH.2004.059436
118. American Academy of Child and Adolescent Psychiatry. *A Guide for Community Child Serving Agencies on Psychotropic Medications for Children and Adolescents*. http://www.aacap.org/app_themes/aacap/docs/press/guide_for_community_child_serving_agencies_

on_psychotropic_medications_for_children_and_adolescents_2012.pdf. Published February 2012. Accessed April 11, 2019

119. Lee T, Fouras G, Brown R; American Academy of Child and Adolescent Psychiatry (AACAP) Committee on Quality Issues (CQI). Practice parameter for the assessment and management of youth involved with the child welfare system. *J Am Acad Child Adolesc Psychiatry*. 2015;54(6):502–517 PMID: 26004666 https://doi.org/10.1016/j.jaac.2015.03.005
120. Heneghan A, Stein RE, Hurlburt MS, et al. Health-risk behaviors in teens investigated by U.S. Child Welfare Agencies. *J Adolesc Health*. 2015;56(5):508–514 PMID: 25744208 https://doi.org/10.1016/j.jadohealth.2015.01.007
121. Sege RD, Amaya-Jackson L; American Academy of Pediatrics Committee on Child Abuse and Neglect and Council on Foster Care, Adoption, and Kinship Care; American Academy of Child and Adolescent Psychiatry Committee on Child Maltreatment and Violence; National Center for Child Traumatic Stress. Clinical considerations related to the behavioral manifestations of child ,altreatment. *Pediatrics*. 2017;139(4):e20170100 PMID: 28320870 https://doi.org/10.1542/peds.2017-0100
122. Pears KC, Fisher PA, Kim HK, Bruce J, Healey CV, Yoerger K. Immediate effects of a school readiness intervention for children in foster care. *Early Educ Dev*. 2013;24(6): 771–791 PMID: 24015056 https://doi.org/10.1080/10409289.2013.736037
123. Kolko DJ, Baumann BL, Herschell AD, Hart JA, Holden EA, Wisniewski SR. Implementation of AF-CBT by community practitioners serving child welfare and mental health: a randomized trial. *Child Maltreat*. 2012;17(1):32–46 PMID: 22278087 https://doi.org/10.1177/1077559511427346
124. Kinniburgh KJ, Blaustein M, Spinazzola J, van der Kolk BA. Attachment, self-regulation, and competency: a comprehensive intervention framework for children with complex trauma. *Psychiatr Ann*. 2005;35(5):424–430 https://doi.org/10.3928/00485713-20050501-08
125. Thomas R, Zimmer-Gembeck MJ. Parent-child interaction therapy: an evidence-based treatment for child maltreatment. *Child Maltreat*. 2012;17(3):253–266 PMID: 22942167 https://doi.org/10.1177/1077559512459555
126. Smith P, Yule W, Perrin S, Tranah T, Dalgleish T, Clark DM. Cognitive-behavioral therapy for PTSD in children and adolescents: a preliminary randomized controlled trial. *J Am Acad Child Adolesc Psychiatry*. 2007;46(8):1051–1061 PMID: 17667483 https://doi.org/10.1097/CHI.0b013e318067e288
127. Zito JM, Safer DJ, de Jong-van den Berg LT, et al. A three-country comparison of psychotropic medication prevalence in youth. *Child Adolesc Psychiatry Ment Health*. 2008;2(1):26 PMID: 18817536 https://doi.org/10.1186/1753-2000-2-26
128. Zito JM, Safer DJ, Sai D, et al. Psychotropic medication patterns among youth in foster care. *Pediatrics*. 2008;121(1):e157–e163 PMID: 18166534 https://doi.org/10.1542/peds.2007-0212
129. Leslie LK, Raghavan R, Hurley M, Zhang J, Landsverk J, Aarons G. Investigating geographic variation in use of psychotropic medications among youth in child welfare. *Child Abuse Negl*. 2011;35(5):333–342 PMID: 21620160 https://doi.org/10.1016/j.chiabu.2011.01.012
130. Raghavan R, McMillen JC. Use of multiple psychotropic medications among adolescents aging out of foster care. *Psychiatr Serv*. 2008;59(9):1052–1055 PMID: 18757601 https://doi.org/10.1176/ps.2008.59.9.1052
131. Webb E. Poverty, maltreatment and attention deficit hyperactivity disorder. *Arch Dis Child*. 2013;98(6):397–400 PMID: 23564836 https://doi.org/10.1136/archdischild-2012-303578

132. Raghavan R, Zima BT, Andersen RM, Leibowitz AA, Schuster MA, Landsverk J. Psychotropic medication use in a national probability sample of children in the child welfare system. *J Child Adolesc Psychopharmacol*. 2005;15(1):97–106 PMID: 15741791 https://doi.org/10.1089/cap.2005.15.97
133. Constantine R, Tandon R. Changing trends in pediatric antipsychotic use in Florida's Medicaid program. *Psychiatr Serv*. 2008;59(10):1162–1168 PMID: 18832502 https://doi.org/10.1176/ps.2008.59.10.1162
134. Rubin D, Matone M, Huang YS, dosReis S, Feudtner C, Localio R. Interstate variation in trends of psychotropic medication use among Medicaid-enrolled children in foster care. *Child Youth Serv Rev*. 2012;34(8):1492–1499 https://doi.org/10.1016/j.childyouth.2012.04.006
135. US Government Accountability Office. Foster Children: HHS Guidance Could Help States Improve Oversight of Psychotropic Prescriptions. Washington, DC: US Government Accountability Office; 2011. https://www.gao.gov/assets/590/586570.pdf. Accessed April 11, 2019
136. US Government Accountability Office. *Children's Mental Health*: Concerns Remain about Appropriate Services for Children in Medicaid and Foster Care. Washington, DC: US Government Accountability Office; 2012. https://www.gao.gov/assets/660/650716.pdf. Accessed April 11, 2019
137. Mackie TI, Hyde J, Palinkas LA, Niemi E, Leslie LK. Fostering psychotropic medication oversight for children in foster care: a national examination of states' monitoring mechanisms. *Adm Policy Ment Health*. 2017;44(2):243–257 PMID: 26860953 https://doi.org/10.1007/s10488-016-0721-x
138. Gupta S, Cahill JD. A prescription for "deprescribing" in psychiatry. *Psychiatr Serv*. 2016;67(8):904–907 PMID: 26975524 https://doi.org/10.1176/appi.ps.201500359
139. Baker M, Bellonci C, Huefner J, Hilt R, Carlson G. Polypharmacy and the pursuit of appropriate prescribing for children and adolescents. *Child Adolesc Psychopharmacol News*. 2017;22(1):1–7 https://doi.org/10.1521/capn.2017.22.1.1
140. American Academy of Child and Adolescent Psychiatry. Recommendations about the use of psychotropic medications for children and adolescents involved in child-serving systems. https://www.aacap.org/App_Themes/AACAP/docs/clinical_practice_center/systems_of_care/AACAP_Psychotropic_Medication_Recommendations_2015_FINAL.pdf. Published 2015. Accessed April 11, 2019
141. Naylor MW, Davidson CV, Ortega-Piron DJ, Bass A, Gutierrez A, Hall A. Psychotropic medication management for youth in state care: consent, oversight, and policy considerations. *Child Welfare*. 2007;86(5):175–192 PMID: 18422054
142. Crea TM, Lopez A, Hasson RG, Evans K, Palleschi C, Underwood D. Unaccompanied immigrant children in long term foster care: identifying needs and best practices from a child welfare perspective. *Child Youth Serv Rev*. 2018;92:56–64 https://doi.org/10.1016/j.childyouth.2017.12.017
143. National Child Traumatic Stress Network. Unaccompanied migrant children. https://www.nctsn.org/resources/unaccompanied-migrant-children. Published 2015. Accessed July 14, 2019
144. Diaz A, Edwards S, Neal WP, et al. Foster children with special needs: the Children's Aid Society experience. *Mt Sinai J Med*. 2004;71(3):166–169 PMID: 15164129
145. Cusick GR, Goerge RM, Bell KC. *From Corrections to Community: The Juvenile Reentry Experience as Characterized by Multiple Systems Involvement*. Chicago, IL: Chapin Hall Center for Children at the University of Chicago; 2009

146. Yampolskaya S, Armstrong MI, McNeish R. Children placed in out-of-home care: risk factors for involvement with the juvenile justice system. *Violence Vict.* 2011;26(2): 231–245 PMID: 21780537 https://doi.org/10.1891/0886-6708.26.2.231
147. Dannerbeck A, Yan J. Missouri's crossover youth: examining the relationship between their maltreatment history and risk of violence. *OJJDP Journal of Juvenile Justice.* 2011;1(1):78–92
148. Jonson-Reid M, Barth RP. From placement to prison: the path to adolescent incarceration from child welfare supervised foster or group care. *Child Youth Serv Rev.* 2000;22(7):493–516 https://doi.org/10.1016/S0190-7409(00)00100-6
149. Jonson-Reid M, Barth RP. From maltreatment report to juvenile incarceration: the role of child welfare services. *Child Abuse Negl.* 2000;24(4):505–520 PMID: 10798840 https://doi.org/10.1016/S0145-2134(00)00107-1
150. Culhane DP, Metraux S, Moreno M. *Young Adult Outcomes of Exiting Dependent or Delinquent Care in Los Angeles County.* Los Angeles: County of Los Angeles; 2011. https://c.ymcdn.com/sites/www.naccchildlaw.org/resource/resmgr/docs/young_adult_outcomes_of_yout.pdf. Accessed July 1, 2019
151. Herz DLP, Lutz L, Stewart M, Tuell J, Wiig J. *Addressing the Needs of Multi-System Youth: Strengthening the Connection between Child Welfare and Juvenile Justice.* Washington, D.C.: The Center for Juvenile Justice Reform and Robert F. Kennedy Children's Action Corps; 2012
152. Dworsky A, DeCoursey J. *Pregnant and Parenting Foster Youth: Their Needs, Their Experiences.* Chicago, IL: Chapin Hall at the Univeristy of Chicago; 2009
153. Center for the Study of Social Policy. *Improving Outcomes for Pregnant and Parenting Youth in Foster Care: Federal Policy Recommendations.* Washington, DC: Center For the Study of Social Policy; 2011. https://www.cssp.org/reform/child-welfare/pregnant-and-parenting-youth/Improving-Outcomes-for-Pregnant-and-Parenting-Youth-in-Foster-Care_Federal-Policy-Recommendations.pdf. Accessed December 5, 2017
154. Center for the Study of Social Policy. *Pregnant and Parenting Youth in Foster Care Part I: A Guide to Service Improvements.* Washington, DC: Center for the Study of Social Policy. https://www.cssp.org/publications/child-welfare/pregnant-and-parenting-youth/Pregnant-and-Parenting-Youth-in-Foster-Care-Service-Recommendations-Guide.pdf. Accessed December 5, 2017
155. Levine DA; American Academy of Pediatrics Committee on Adolescence. Office-based care for lesbian, gay, bisexual, transgender, and questioning youth. *Pediatrics.* 2013;132(1):e297–e313 PMID: 23796737 https://doi.org/10.1542/peds.2013-1283
156. Adelson SL; American Academy of Child and Adolescent Psychiatry (AACAP) Committee on Quality Issues (CQI). Practice parameter on gay, lesbian, or bisexual sexual orientation, gender nonconformity, and gender discordance in children and adolescents. *J Am Acad Child Adolesc Psychiatry.* 2012;51(9):957–974 PMID: 22917211 https://doi.org/10.1016/j.jaac.2012.07.004
157. Annie E. Casey Foundation. *LGBTQ in Child Welfare: A Systemic Review of the Literature.* Baltimore, MD: The Annie E. Casey Foundation; 2016. https://www.aecf.org/resources/lgbtq-in-child-welfare. Accessed April 11, 2019
158. Child Welfare League of America; American Bar Association Center on Children and the Law: Opening Doors for LGBTQ Youth in Foster Care Project; Elze DE; et al. *Recommended Practices to Promote the Safety and Well-Being of Lesbian, Gay, Bisexual, Transgender, and Questioning (LGBTQ) Youth and Youth at Risk of or Living with HIV in Child Welfare Settings.* New York, NY: Lambda Legal; 2012. https://www.lambdalegal.org/publications/recommended-practices-youth. Accessed April 11, 2019

CHAPTER 29

Medical and Psychological Sequelae of Child Abuse and Neglect

Mary E. Moffatt, MD, FAAP
University of Missouri Kansas City School of Medicine
Department of Pediatrics
Children's Mercy Hospital, Kansas City
Kansas City, MO

Introduction

The long-term sequelae of child abuse and neglect may manifest months to years afterward. Long-term effects may result directly from the physical injuries sustained (eg, abusive head trauma, fractures, burn injury, abdominal trauma) or from the physiological stress responses, altered brain development and dysfunction, maladaptive coping strategies, and health-threatening behaviors that develop as a consequence.

This chapter provides a framework for understanding the consequences of child abuse and neglect on a neuroendocrine-immune basis and using an ecobiodevelopmental model, based on the current literature and research on adverse childhood experiences (ACEs) and toxic stress. It is imperative that all medical professionals recognize the potential long-term effects of child maltreatment, which may manifest across the life trajectory, to institute appropriate interventions that reduce or eliminate the associated morbidity and improve outcomes.

Overview of Research

Initial Studies on Adverse Childhood Experiences

Most of the data compiled prior to the work of Dr Vincent Felitti and his research team[1] were amassed from patients' recollections during psychological counseling sessions, medical examinations and assessments, or surveys conducted during clinic visits for patients meeting certain screening criteria. However, a large proportion of the published research prior to the 1990s has significant methodological flaws that limit the reliability and generalizability of the data, including the use of select populations, the absence of control populations, the inconsistent definition of neglect and abuse, the presence of multiple confounding variables, and the presence of significant recall and selection biases.[1]

Development of the Adverse Childhood Experiences (ACE) screening instrument (Box 29.1)[1] helped standardize the way in which clinicians collect information about a patient's lifetime exposure to ACEs, including abuse and neglect. Using the ACE instrument, Felitti et al[1–12] conducted several large-scale surveys within the Kaiser Permanente health system to examine the relationship between ACEs and a variety of health behaviors and outcomes.

The most widely cited of the studies involved a survey of 13,494 adults using the ACE instrument.[1] Each of the respondents also had completed an independent standardized medical evaluation, which allowed researchers to examine the associations between the survey responses and the respondents' health states. More than 50% of the respondents reported at least 1 category of exposure on the ACE instrument; 25% reported 2 or more categories of childhood exposures. The study determined that subjects who had reported multiple items on the ACE instrument had increased health risks for adult disease (ie, ischemic heart disease, cancer, chronic lung disease, skeletal fractures, and liver disease) and negative health behaviors (ie, alcoholism, smoking, substance use, depression, suicide attempts, obesity, inactivity, and sexual promiscuity).[1–12]

Although studies employing the ACE instrument provide the best available data on the long-term consequences of child abuse and neglect,

BOX 29.1
Adverse Childhood Experiences Instrument

The Adverse Childhood Experiences questionnaire queried 7 categories of specific childhood events and quantified the frequency with which such events were experienced.

Psychological Abuse

While you were growing up during your first 18 years, did a parent or other adult in the household

1. Often or very often swear at, insult, or put you down?
2. Often or very often act in a way that made you afraid that you would be physically hurt?

(continued)

BOX 29.1 (*continued*)

Physical Abuse

While you were growing up during your first 18 years, did a parent or other adult in the household

1. Often or very often push, grab, shove, or slap you?
2. Often or very often hit you so hard that you had marks or were injured?

Sexual Abuse

While you were growing up during your first 18 years, did an adult or person at least 5 years older ever

1. Touch or fondle you in a sexual way?
2. Have you touch their body in a sexual way?
3. Attempt oral, anal, or vaginal intercourse with you?
4. Actually have oral, anal, or vaginal intercourse with you?

Substance Use

While you were growing up during your first 18 years, did you

1. Live with anyone who was a problem drinker or alcoholic?
2. Live with anyone who used street drugs?

Mental Illness

While you were growing up during your first 18 years

1. Was a household member depressed or mentally ill?
2. Did a household member attempt suicide?

Mother Treated Violently

While you were growing up during your first 18 years, was your mother (or stepmother)

1. Sometimes, often, or very often pushed, grabbed, slapped, or had something thrown at her?
2. Sometimes, often, or very often kicked, bitten, hit with a fist, or hit with something hard?
3. Ever repeatedly hit over at least a few minutes?
4. Ever threatened with, or hurt by, a knife or gun?

Criminal Behavior in Household

While you were growing up in the first 18 years

1. Did a household member go to prison?

Adapted from Felitti VJ, Anda RF, Nordenberg D, et al. Relationship of childhood abuse and household dysfunction to many of the leading causes of death in adults. The Adverse Childhood Experiences (ACE) Study. *Am J Prev Med*. 1998;14(4):245-258, copyright 1998, with permission from Elsevier.

the data are subject to certain limitations.[1] Most importantly, the ACE studies suffer from potential recall bias. For example, adults with poor medical and/or psychological health may be more inclined to link their problems to and lay blame on ACEs. Similarly, adults with good health but who were also abused as children may fail to report having experienced ACEs. In both of these cases, the sample population may not be representative of the actual population. Additionally, the associations made between ACE status and long-term health effects are correlations and do not prove causality, although Felitti et al[1–12] demonstrated dose-dependent relationships between the number of ACE categories endorsed and the risk for adult disease and negative health behaviors.

These limitations notwithstanding, the ACE studies, as well as subsequent similarly conducted studies, have provided much evidence for what is currently known about child abuse and neglect and its long-term effect on health. Since the original ACE studies, there has been significant work focused on ACEs in correlation with health status as a developing child. Conceptually, our understanding of how pervasive, persistent adversity in childhood affects brain development and function has grown and causal pathways related to the effect of toxic stress[13–15] have been proposed.

Toxic Stress and the Neuroendocrine-Immune Network

Toxic stress is defined as extreme, frequent, or extended activation of the physiological stress response in a developing child, without the buffering presence of a supportive adult.[13–15] Early adversity, including the trauma of child abuse and neglect, lack of nurturance and social support, and poverty, is linked to biological adaptation through the neuroendocrine-immune network.[16] Through hormones, signaling molecules, receptors, and neurotransmitters, adversity affects brain development and function, especially during sensitive and critical periods in early life, as well as physical health across the life trajectory.[15] Central to the systemic response is the hypothalamic-pituitary-adrenal (HPA) axis, which manages the response of other body systems to a stressor. Unfortunately, toxic stress in young children dysregulates the HPA axis and has negative effects on the brain and body. There is also evidence for the deleterious effects of prenatal maternal stress on the developing child.[16] A suboptimal caregiving environment before and after birth can result in epigenetic changes altering gene expression and, thus, protein synthesis.[15,16] Inadequate early caregiving and nurturance can also negatively affect a child's immunocompetence.[16] The ecobiodevelopmental model of disease and wellness, endorsed by the American Academy of Pediatrics in 2012,[14,15] views health as an interaction between ecology such as the early developmental environment (physical, nutritional, psychosocial) and biology, at the molecular and cellular level in a dynamic yet cumulative manner over time.[17] Using this ecobiodevelopmental framework helps us to understand how toxic stress and its effect on the developing brain leads to maladaptive coping patterns and fragmented social networks, increasing the risk for health-threatening behaviors, disease states (physical and mental), academic underachievement, and economic disadvantage later in life.[13–15] Individual resilience factors, such as intelligence, capacity and willingness to learn, high self-esteem, optimism, ability to regulate emotion and behavior, and genetic predisposition to diminished stress reactivity, can effectively modulate the negative effects of toxic stress for some children.[15,16,18] The important role of evidence-based cognitive behavioral therapy to help mitigate effects of toxic stress and trauma must also be emphasized.[19,20] A secure attachment to, and a stable relationship with, a nurturing adult who understands how to best respond to a child's maladaptive responses is also essential to optimizing well-being and outcomes.[19] Medical professionals caring for children and adolescents who are demonstrating maladaptive or dysregulated behaviors, as sequelae of child maltreatment or other adversity experienced, should advocate for the child to have a safe, stable, nurturing environment and to receive evidence-based, trauma-focused therapy and/or other therapeutic services so as to give the child the best chance for positive physical, psychological, and social outcomes.

Adverse Childhood Experiences and Child/Youth Health

A small collection of studies has evaluated the effect of ACEs on childhood health.[21–24] Four prospective studies[21–24] from the Consortium of Longitudinal Studies of Child Abuse and Neglect found that children who were at risk for, or who had experienced, child maltreatment experienced significant ACEs and that ACEs predicted health outcomes in early childhood, middle childhood, and early adolescence. ACEs were assessed as 4 categories of maltreatment—psychological maltreatment, physical abuse, sexual abuse, and neglect—and as 4 categories of household dysfunction—caregiver's substance or alcohol abuse, caregiver's depressive symptoms, caregiver being treated violently, and criminal behavior in the household, per the ACEs used in the Centers for Disease Control and Prevention and Kaiser ACE studies.[1] Child protective services data were used to classify the type of maltreatment reported for each child. Caregivers completed surveys about substance use, depressive symptoms, intimate partner violence, and imprisonment of anyone in the child's household at different time points during the child's first 16 years after birth. Youth health was assessed by caregiver completion of the Child Health Assessment, Child Life Events, and the Child Behavior Checklist and by asking caregivers if the child had an illness that required medical attention. Children and youth completed the Child Health and Development survey and the Youth Self-Report and were asked if they had an illness that required medical attention.

In the 2009 study by Flaherty et al,[22] 37% of the children at age 12 years had a health complaint: poor health rated by the child and/or caregiver, illness requiring a doctor, or somatic complaints reported by the child and/or caregiver. For children with ACE score 5 or higher, somatic complaints and any health problem were significant associations. Any complaint of poor health and illness requiring a doctor was strongly associated with increased ACEs during years 7 to 12 after the child's birth. The results suggested that dosage effects of ACEs on child health may emerge over time.

The next study[23] evaluated whether a dose-response relationship for ACEs and health problems at age 14 years could be demonstrated. Timing of exposure to ACEs was also evaluated as occurring in the first 6 years after birth, the second 6 years after birth, or recently from 12 to 14 years of age. A graded relationship between ACE exposure and any health problem was found. An adversity index score of 2 or more (ACE score ≥ 2) was associated with an odds ratio (OR) of 8.91 or higher for somatic concerns (number of ACEs ever ≥ 2, somatic concerns OR = 8.91, 95% CI, 1.15–68.83). As well, 2 or more concurrent ACEs during age 13 to 14 years was associated with increased ORs for poor health classification by caregiver, somatic concerns, and any health problem. The authors concluded that ACEs, including child maltreatment, influence health, illness, and somatic complaints beginning in childhood and continuing into adolescence.

A 2015 study[24] that is similar in design to the previously discussed work included additional data on child health. This study included earlier self-reported health at 6, 12, 14, and 16 years of age by each youth and by his or her caregiver when the child was 6, 12, and 14 years old. Caregivers also completed the Child Behavior Checklist when the child was 6, 12, 14, and 16 years and were asked if the child had an illness that required medical attention. At 16 years of age, youth were asked if they had an illness that required medical attention. Finally, at 18 years of age, each study participant was asked about his or her degree of health worry in the past month, use of medical care for a serious or ongoing health problem, or needing medical care for a serious health problem but not seeking it, and to rank his or her health compared with others of the same age. Child protective services data were analyzed more in depth than in previous studies.[22,23] Similar to the findings of Flaherty et al,[21] exposure to ACEs was found to be highest in early childhood (0–6 years) and decreased through late childhood (12–16 years). The chronic ACE group, who had ACE score 2 or more over all 3 periods in childhood (early, 0–6 years; late, 6–12 years; teen, 12–16 years), had significantly higher likelihood of ever experiencing caregiver substance use, depression, victimization, and household criminal behavior. This group had more health worries and more medical care than the low ACE group, who consistently had low ACE scores across all years. Chronic exposure to ACEs over childhood was found in this study to predict health worries and self-reported use of medical care at age 18 years.

With regard to the effect of early exposure to multiple stressors, Kerker et al[25] examined the prevalence of ACEs among young children, aged 18 months through 5 years, who underwent investigation by child protective services but remained in their homes, to evaluate if any proximal consequences of adversity could be noted in young children. Their results suggest that the effects of adverse experiences may occur almost immediately in terms of mental health, chronic medical conditions, and social development. In multivariable logistic regression analyses, the number of ACEs predicted the Child Behavior Checklist score for children 36 to 71 months, such that for each additional ACE a child had a 32% increase in the odds of having a problem score on the Child Behavior Checklist (OR 1.32, 95% CI, 1.14–1.53). As well, each additional ACE for a child aged 36 to 71 months was associated with 21% increased odds of having a chronic medical condition (OR 1.21, 95% CI, 1.05–1.40). Children aged 36 to 71 months were found to have increased odds of having a socialization problem (OR 1.32 for low Vineland Adaptive Behavior Scales socialization score, 95% CI, 1.12–2.78). In vulnerable populations, early ACEs may lead to early mental health, chronic medical, and social development problems.

Beyond physical health effects, ACEs in early childhood have been found to affect kindergarten outcomes in terms of teacher-reported academic and behavioral problems.[26] Experiencing 3 or more ACEs in early childhood was found to be associated with below-average performance or problems in each outcome this study examined: language and literacy skills (adjusted odds ratio [AOR] 1.8, 95% CI, 1.1–2.9) and math skills (AOR 1.8, 95% CI, 1.1–2.9), attention problems (AOR 3.5, 95% CI, 1.8–6.5), social problems (AOR 2.7, 95% Ci, 1.4–5.0), and aggression (AOR 2.3, 95% CI, 1.2–4.6). The findings indicate a predisposition for affected children to low educational attainment and adult literacy, which are both, in turn, related to poor health. Similarly, analysis of data from the 2011–2012 National Survey of Children's Health demonstrated that children with 2 or more ACEs were 2.67 times more likely to repeat a grade in school, compared with children with no such adverse experiences.[27]

Deprivation Dwarfism

Those who do not suffer the direct consequences of physical abuse may still experience failure to thrive (FTT) or growth impairment.[28] There are reports of those who experienced child abuse and neglect who have deprivation (psychosocial) dwarfism, defined as residual infant-like appearance, wasting, and stunting of growth.[29] With appropriate recognition and intervention, most notably through establishing a nurturing caregiver relationship and living environment, FTT or growth impairment may be reversed.[30] While data suggest that children with abuse-related FTT may catch up in physical growth, children may not make a similar recovery in terms of neurodevelopment.[31,32] See Chapter 17, Failure to Thrive, for an in-depth discussion of growth impairment related to child maltreatment.

Physical Abuse Outcomes

As one might expect, abusive head trauma has severe and life-altering consequences for a high number of those who experience it. Although abdominal trauma is the second most lethal form of physical abuse, those who experience it do well in the long term. Burn injury, as expected, leaves children with permanent scarring affecting function and appearance. Children with inflicted fractures are at low risk for poor outcome in terms of skeletal function.

Abusive Head Trauma

Abusive head trauma, involving inertial and/or impact injury to the child's brain, can result in severe, permanent sequelae for children who experience it.[31,33–35] Neurodevelopmental sequelae may involve a number of domains, including neurological, cognitive, visual, developmental, and behavioral. Abusive head trauma can also be lethal. Death from inflicted head trauma is reported to occur in approximately 13% to 36% of cases and exceeds the 6% to 12% mortality rate for non-inflicted head injuries.[31] Neuropathologic changes occurring after traumatic brain injury have been reported.[36] Directly after brain injury, there is often cortical and subcortical injury, including contusion, hemorrhage, hypoxic-ischemic damage, axonal damage, and cerebral edema. As acute lesions resolve, permanent damage becomes evident, including the development of encephalopathies, such as multicystic encephalomalacia, porencephaly, generalized white matter attenuation, diffuse cortical atrophy, microgyria, ulegyria, or hydrocephalus ex vacuo. Non-injured areas may also undergo reorganization, leading to progressive cortical dysplasia with cytoarchitectural disorganization, laminar obliteration, or morphological and functional synaptic reorganization of neurons.[36–40] The changes occurring in the damaged and undamaged portions of the brain may influence the child's subsequent neurologic and psychological maturation.[36,40]

Lack of Consensus for Assessing Neurodevelopmental Outcomes

There is not consensus on the outcome measure to apply in assessing long-term neurodevelopmental outcomes after abusive head trauma. Many measures, at different points in time, can be and have been applied, including neurological examination, caregiver report, outcome scales such as the Glasgow Outcome Scale (GOS), as well as medical and cognitive assessments of the affected child. Regardless of the lack of consensus on how to assess outcomes, studies reporting outcomes 5 or more years post-injury show high rates of impairments in several domains, including neurological, cognitive, visual, developmental, and behavioral.[41]

Neurodevelopmental Deficits

Neurological deficits include cortical-subcortical atrophy, microcephaly, delayed psychomotor development and motor deficits, gross and fine motor function impairment, hydrocephalus, posttraumatic epilepsy that is often intractable, sensory deficits such as sensorineural deafness, visual impairment and dysfunction, and blindness.[41] Cognitive deficits such as speech and language difficulties involving production and impaired comprehension, intellectual disability of various degrees, memory deficits, disrupted executive functioning, and challenges with social skills have all been described.[41] Deficits tend to emerge over time as developmental demands increase and cognitive processes are expected to be more developed, such that children who appear normal or fully recovered soon after the injury quite often are noticed and labeled as disabled 6 months to 5 years later.[42] Thus, prolonged, close monitoring of cognitive development, including executive skills, is warranted, particularly given the normal course of frontal lobe maturation continuing into early adulthood. Behavior and sleep disorders have not been studied as much as long-term outcomes, but when studied, they have been noted in more than half of children who have experienced abusive head trauma.[41] Disordered sleep and behavior can become particularly noticeable as the affected infant becomes a toddler at 2 to 3 years of age. Features such as frontal lobe injury, speech and language challenges, and environmental factors likely all contribute to and compound behavior and sleep disorders.[41] Adaptive behaviors such as communication, daily living skills, and socialization are also challenges for the child as he or she matures from infant to toddler and beyond. From a cognitive standpoint, academic underachievement and need for special education are common, including multidisciplinary team support, adaptive housing, and vocational training.[41]

Pre- and Post-injury Features Affect Outcomes

Pre- and post-injury features affect long-term outcomes. Pre-injury environmental and demographic features, as well as pre-injury medical or developmental abnormalities and unrecognized trauma, are associated with worse outcomes and mortality.[41] Infant age younger than 6 months at time of injury is not consistently associated with poor prognosis in the literature. Post-injury environmental features including adverse caregiving environments with emotional abuse, neglect, repeat injury, unaddressed or uncontrolled seizures, and medical complications are also contributory to outcomes.[41] Not only is abusive head trauma associated with increased costs to society early in the trajectory due to more severe injury, higher morbidity and mortality, and longer hospital stay than accidental head injury, but also with increased costs after discharge from the hospital for the lifetime of care involving high use of ancillary medical resources, lost parental wages due to caring for affected children, need for special education, and reduced productivity and earning potential of those who reach adulthood.[41]

Comprehensive, systematic long-term care, including timely formal cognitive testing, is required to monitor development, detect challenges or deficits, and implement adequate interventions to reduce impairment, enhance quality of life and independence, and minimize family burden of caregiving. In-depth study of children who experienced abusive head trauma from infancy or early toddlerhood into early adulthood, describing and assessing interventions, is also much needed despite the obvious challenge of high attrition rates for affected children and their families. Future research should focus on more systematic, prospective, very long-term outcome studies, given that outcome and autonomy in adulthood are largely unknown.[41]

Association of Acute Injury Clinical Variables and Outcomes

Glasgow Outcome Scale

There have been attempts to identify early on which children are more likely to have poor prognosis based on acute injury variables that are associated with functional outcome.[43] This type of information is desirable so medical professionals can counsel caregivers appropriately and implement systems of care to follow affected children closely over the long term. The study by Rhine et al[43] used the primary outcome GOS at the initial follow-up visit after injury to describe outcomes. The GOS was initially described in 1975 by Jennet and Bond and is a standard outcome descriptor for adult traumatic brain injury.[44] In addition to GOS, the study by Rhine et al[43] incorporated secondary outcome measures regarding functional deficits based on the need for interventional services and/or medication from 2 separate follow-up visits and included neurobehavior problems, motor deficits, need for tracheostomy, and meeting age-appropriate milestones. Similar to the findings from previous studies, bivariate analyses while controlling for age at and time of injury demonstrated that low Glasgow Coma Scale (GCS) component scores, need for neurosurgical intervention, seizures in first week, initial hyperglycemia, need for mechanical ventilation more than 10 days, duration of stay in the intensive care unit (ICU) longer than 10 days, and neuroimaging reflecting cerebral edema or loss of gray-white differentiation were significantly related to poor outcome. The presence of retinal hemorrhage in this study was not found to be a significant predictor of functional outcome, perhaps due to the small sample size. However, the literature to date on the presence of retinal hemorrhages and outcome after abusive head trauma is conflicting.[43] Children in the study demonstrated functional deficits within multiple developmental domains, including newly identified functional deficits for some children who attended a second follow-up visit (mean of 12.7 months post-injury). Consistent with previously published studies, age at injury was not a significant predictor of GOS.

The findings in this study underscore the necessity of long-term follow-up, including neuropsychological testing of school-aged children who experienced abusive head trauma, even for affected children who initially seem to be doing fairly well. Complicated social situations, as well as legal and custody issues, were found to contribute to the ability to follow children who experienced abusive head trauma long term and were noted to confound the prognosis. Pediatric-specific functional outcome scales and other acute injury variables, along with hypoxia and hypotension, are likely important considerations for future prospective work examining clinical predictors of outcome for children who experienced abusive head trauma.[43]

Evaluation of Seizures, Pediatric Intensive Care Unit Admission, Mechanical Ventilation, and Outcomes

The most useful study to date correlating the development outcome of children who experienced abusive head trauma to clinical features appears to be that by Greiner et al.[45] This study evaluated the presence or absence of seizures, the presence or absence of intubation, and the presence or absence of admission to the pediatric ICU with developmental testing of children having a diagnosis of abusive head trauma and seen for follow up in the post-injury growth and development clinic. The developmental testing involved use of the Capute Scales, which consist of testing of 2 domains to determine the presence of atypical development in 2 areas of cognitive development: visual-motor functioning and expressive and receptive language. The Cognitive Adaptive Test is used as a test for visual-motor development, and the Clinical Linguistic and Auditory Milestone Scale is used as a test for language development. Children previously diagnosed with abusive head trauma underwent follow-up testing 2 to 35 months from the time of injury. The average follow-up time for children in the study was 12 months, and if a child attended more than 1 follow-up visit, the last obtained developmental scores were used for analysis. A total of 71 patients diagnosed with abusive head trauma were identified. Thirty-four patients had early onset seizures, 21 were intubated, and 35 were admitted to the pediatric ICU. When evaluating the presence of seizures at time of injury, 34 patients were noted to have seizure activity and 18 of those children were later tested. Twelve children with seizures were diagnosed with cognitive adaptive delay, 11 were diagnosed with language delay, and 12 were diagnosed with global developmental delay. Twenty-one patients were intubated at time of injury and were followed up in the post-injury growth and development clinic; 12 had cognitive adaptive delay, 11 had language delay, and 12 had global developmental delay. Pediatric ICU admission in and of itself was found to be associated with worse developmental outcomes, in terms of the 35 patients with diagnosed abusive head trauma who were admitted to the pediatric ICU. However, when the intubated patients were removed from the pediatric ICU admission group, the association between pediatric ICU admission and developmental delay was not found to be significant. The use of presence or absence of seizures and presence or absence of intubation as a means of early clinical assessment after abusive head trauma is better than the use of GCS given its poor interobserver agreement and limited utility due to lack of scores noted or recorded in the first 24 hours post-injury. The findings in the study by Greiner et al[45] indicate that the presence of seizures and the need for intubation at the time of abusive head trauma are significantly correlated with poor developmental outcome.

The use of the Capute Scales for assessment of neurodevelopmental outcome after abusive head trauma is both unique and beneficial; also, the scales are not difficult to administer and are not subject to inter-rater reliability, which are features making other outcome scales less desirable.[45] While admission to the pediatric ICU did not significantly correlate with poor developmental outcome, of the 8 patients *not* admitted to the pediatric ICU, 7 were found to be borderline for delay and 1 was diagnosed with global developmental delay. Thus, the need for close developmental follow-up for all patients diagnosed with abusive head trauma is evident, regardless of where they are admitted. A group discussed as having special risk for development of later sequelae is children who are borderline for delay because learning problems may not be as apparent and functional deficits may not prompt screening. Longitudinal, systematic developmental testing in this group could reveal needs to be addressed to optimize outcomes.[45] Prospective study of early clinical features and neuroradiology features correlated with meaningful developmental testing, such as the Capute Scales, may also be a fruitful area for future research focus.[45]

Evaluation of Neuroimaging Features, Clinical Features, and Outcomes

Both early and late neuroradiology studies performed on young children who have experienced abusive head trauma have assessed for correlations among imaging findings, clinical features, and neurological sequelae. The results of a few studies with some overlapping findings are discussed in this section. Additional study appears necessary to fully appreciate the significance of imaging findings and outcomes for affected children.

The study by Ilves et al[46] aimed to evaluate the value of early radiology studies and clinical features for predicting long-term neurodevelopmental outcomes and find correlations between long-term neurological and radiological sequelae in infants with abusive head trauma. This small study involved 24 infants who were divided into 2 groups: those with GCS of 3 to 8 for at least 6 hours or impairment in consciousness for more than 24 hours, and those with GCS of 9 to 15 and with consciousness impairment for less than 24 hours. All 24 infants had clinical assessments and initial computed tomography (CT) or magnetic resonance imaging (MRI) within 3 days of admission to the hospital. Acute radiological outcome was noted as imaging finding 1 to 3 days after admission on CT head and/or MRI brain imaging; early radiological outcome was noted as imaging finding 4 days to 3 months after admission; and late radiological outcome was noted as imaging finding at least 9 months post-injury. The mean age at injury was 4 months (range, 4 days–12 months); 2 children died, 3 had severe disability, and 2 had good recovery. Twenty-two infants had follow-up visits for more than 9 months post-injury (range, 28 months–9 years). Only low initial GCS (≤8) on the first day correlated with poor neurodevelopmental outcome (severe disability or death). In this study, retinal hemorrhages, seizures on admission, fractures including skull fracture, and need for neurosurgical procedure did not correlate with poor neurodevelopmental outcome. In terms of acute imaging findings, cerebral edema and focal changes in the basal ganglia were found to be significantly correlated with poor neurodevelopmental outcome. New focal intracerebral findings, decrease in white matter, and severe atrophy noted on early neuroimaging were also found to be significantly correlated with poor outcome.

Attempts to use findings on early neuroimaging to predict long-term neurodevelopmental outcomes for children diagnosed with abusive head trauma have also been studied by others. Tanoue and colleagues[47] published in this regard after assessing CT head and/or MRI brain imaging performed up to 3 days after admission to the hospital, and neuroimaging performed 4 days to 1 month later, in relation to GOS. In this small study of 28 children with mean age of 7.2 months (range, 5 days–18 months), 4 children died, 5 were found to be severely disabled, and 12 had good recovery. The mean time of neurological follow-up was 4 years and 7 months (range, 2 years 3 months–9 years). Neuroimaging findings noted during the first 3 days after admission that were significantly associated with poor long-term outcome included changes in the basal ganglia or brain stem, diffuse edema, transtentorial herniation, subarachnoid hemorrhage, and parenchymal injury. Skull fracture was not found to be associated with poor outcome in this study. Neuroimaging findings, noted 4 days to 1 month after injury for 14 survivors, that were significantly associated with poor long-term outcomes were changes in the basal ganglia or brain stem and parenchymal injury, as well as severe atrophy. Given the small number of patients in this study,[47] evaluation of a large series of patients with abusive head trauma having neuroradiology findings and with detailed long-term neuropsychological assessments would be helpful to determine if neuroimaging is useful and reliable for predicting prognosis.

Tanoue et al[48] also evaluated the utility of apparent diffusion coefficient (ADC) values from early and follow-up MRI brain imaging to predict outcomes after abusive head trauma. In a population of 18 children with abusive head trauma aged 1 to 18 months, ADC maps were available for review for 14 children; 11 had early MRI of the head within 4 days of admission to the hospital, and 5 had imaging 8 days to 1 month after admission. Again, GOS was used to assess the neurodevelopmental outcome at the last follow-up visit (mean, 3 years; range, 4 months–5 years). In the study population, 1 child died, 2 had severe disability, and 6 had good recovery. Apparent diffusion coefficient values on early MRI in all brain regions described in this study were significantly associated with poor neurodevelopmental outcomes (ie, severe disability). However, only ADC values in the basal ganglia, thalamus, brain stem, and corpus callosum were significantly associated with poor outcomes when imaging 5 days to 1 month post-admission to the hospital was evaluated. Further study of the utility of ADC maps in predicting long-term neurodevelopmental outcomes is warranted using a large population of children with abusive head trauma and prospective neuropsychological testing before ADC can be reliably used to predict outcome in a meaningful manner.[48]

Fractures and Skeletal Injury

Complications from non-accidental fractures in children are not well described in child abuse literature or in pediatric orthopedic literature, but they seem to be rare. However, all fractures in children have possibility for complications.

More immediate complications include vascular and nerve injury, although they may be underrecognized. Arterial laceration, hemorrhage, and intimal injury are possible sequelae when fractures affect nearby arterial structures.[49] Findings of concern for vascular injury on examination can be evaluated further by imaging. Sensory and motor deficits due to nerve injury are not particularly common sequelae of fractures in children, but upper extremity nerve injury, particularly ulnar nerve injury, is more common than lower extremity nerve injury.[49] Some neurovascular injuries will require surgical attention. For children who are comatose, including children with abusive head trauma, secondary nerve injury developing as a result of limb positioning is important to be aware of, and prevention is essential. The ulnar, radial, and peroneal nerves are particularly susceptible.[49] Compartment syndrome can accompany pediatric extremity fractures, crush injuries, and burns. Although fat embolism as a sequelae of long bone fracture in children occurs, children are not commonly symptomatic.[49]

Longer-term complications of fractures include malunion when bony fragments of a fracture are not initially satisfactorily reduced or aligned or there is loss of fracture reduction. Clearly, failure to seek medical care after a fracture also places a child at risk for malunion. Malunion can result in cosmetic and functional deficits, which can require orthopedic surgery for improvement. Late angulation of proximal tibia metaphyseal fractures in young children is reported as a common complication.[49,50] Observation of the progressive valgus deformity is advisable because many improve spontaneously. Limb length discrepancies are well known sequelae of extremity fractures in children.[50] Overgrowth of the femur after fracture, and sometimes of the ipsilateral tibia, is common,[50] but overgrowth in the upper extremity after fracture is not common.[51] Discrepancy less than 2 cm does not tend to affect knee mechanics or stride.[52] Physeal injury of bones with large physes can result in growth arrest or slowing due to formation of a bony bridge, called a bony bar, across some or all of the cartilage,[52] such that the affected limb is shortened and/or has angular deformity.[50] Younger children with physeal injury have poorer prognosis. Normal growth of the physis can also be affected by epiphyseal injury. Nonunion in children is rare, tending to occur mostly in the tibial diaphysis and fractures about the elbow, particularly the lateral humeral condyle.[50,51] Nonunion is associated with high energy traumatic mechanisms and open fractures with extensive soft tissue injury and infection. Refracture can occur, even up to 12 months after original injury, as a result of stress to the fragile union at the site of the original fracture incurred during physical activity or repeat trauma to the area.[50,51]

Myositis ossificans, ectopic bone formation in muscle, tends to occur after soft tissue injury, causing a hematoma, which then calcifies, in association with fractures of the pelvis, or after burn injury.[49] Reflex sympathetic dystrophy, thought to be related to autonomic instability, can occur after a trivial injury to an extremity.[49] Although this is more common in adolescent girls, children of all ages may exhibit symptoms. The laboratory workup result is often negative, and this helps to exclude differential diagnoses. Radiography may show generalized osteoporosis in the affected area of the limb. In addition to addressing psychological features, weight-bearing, vigorous active exercises, and direct skin stimulation are usually beneficial.

Burn Injury

In general, most US children who suffer burn injury affecting less than 90% of the total body surface area (BSA) are now expected to survive due to improved and more effective critical and burn care than has been available in previous eras.[53] Ensuring quality of life for these patients is also receiving equal focus in initial resuscitative and therapeutic efforts.[53] Physical complications and sequelae from accidental and abusive burn injury are similar. Burn injuries to the limbs may impair an individual's ability to write, ambulate, or perform activities of daily living. Facial burns may affect an individual's self-esteem as well as others' perception of the individual (eg, as manifest through the inability to obtain employment). With appropriate rehabilitation and therapy, however, burn victims with significant injury (up to 40% of the total BSA) may enjoy a typical quality of life.[54] Prevention of hypertrophic scarring, a frequent complication of burn injury in children, may be an important aspect to ensuring quality of life given that hypertrophic scarring can cause functional and cosmetic problems.[55] Burn size (total BSA), epithelialization delayed beyond 10 to 14 days, and multiple surgical procedures were each shown in logistic regression analysis to be associated with increased risk for hypertrophic scar formation.

Where accidental and abusive burn sequelae likely differ most in terms of outcomes is the severity of adverse behavioral and mental health outcomes. Children of all ages frequently experience traumatic stress after burn injury, including classical symptoms of hyperarousal, avoidance, and reexperiencing of the event. Two phases of trauma, the burn trauma and the recovery trauma, were identified as central to the burn experience in a qualitative research study of 12 children, aged 8 to 15 years, who sustained accidental burn injury ranging from 1% to 20% of their total BSA.[56] The knowledge or realization that one's burn trauma was the intentional act of a caregiver likely compounds the posttraumatic stress and psychological sequalae, although this does not appear to have been explicitly studied to date.

Abdominal Trauma

Abusive abdominal trauma is the second most lethal form of child physical abuse,[57] and infants with abusive abdominal injury require admission to the hospital more often than toddlers. Children admitted to the hospital with inflicted abdominal trauma undergo more procedures than children admitted for accidental abdominal trauma and have greater length of stay,[57] as one might expect for the more severe injuries seen in children who have experienced abuse. Absent or lack of accurate history for children presenting with abdominal trauma may contribute to misdiagnosis, increased testing to formulate a diagnosis, and delay in appropriate treatment. Children with abusive abdominal trauma more commonly have pancreatic and hollow viscus injury than children with accidental abdominal trauma.[57–60] As such, delayed presentation as peritonitis or pancreatitis develops may result in the child being more severely ill at the time he or she is brought for medical care and requiring longer hospitalization. Long-term consequences of inflicted abdominal trauma are not well documented in the literature, although it seems that if children survive, their abdominal injuries heal well. One study has found an association with reported nausea and vomiting for children aged 12 years who had a history of physical abuse.[61] This study did not explore abdominal trauma as an isolated feature of physical abuse.

Sexual Abuse Outcomes

Sequelae from sexual abuse endured during childhood can involve physical and mental health. Although the precise cause for most of the nongynecologic sequelae is not clear, the role of the neuroendocrine system appears paramount given the number of somatic disorders associated with a history of child sexual abuse, particularly those involving the gastrointestinal (GI) system. Child sexual abuse is also linked to a number of gynecologic and sexual health issues. This section reports on physical health outcomes related to sexual abuse. A more in-depth discussion can be found in Chapter 10, Medical Evaluation of Suspected Sexual Abuse in Prepubertal Children, and Chapter 11, Medical Management of the Adolescent Who Has Experienced Sexual Abuse or Assault.

Sexual Abuse and Somatic Disorders

Significant association between a history of sexual abuse and a lifetime diagnosis of functional GI disorders, nonspecific chronic pain, psychogenic seizures, and chronic pelvic pain has been found by a systematic review and meta-analysis that set out to assess the association between sexual abuse and lifetime diagnosis of somatic disorders,[62] given the strong evidence that exists to support a link between child sexual abuse and mental health sequelae. No statistically significant association was found between a history of sexual abuse and a lifetime diagnosis of fibromyalgia, obesity, or headache. When history of sexual abuse specifically including rape was analyzed, though, significant association with a lifetime diagnosis of fibromyalgia, functional GI disorders, and chronic pelvic pain was found. Neuroendocrine maladaptation, including HPA axis dysregulation, is speculated to mediate the noted associations.

Gastrointestinal Disorders

Multiple reports link GI disturbances (eg, functional abdominal pain, irritable bowel syndrome [IBS], non-ulcer dyspepsia) and diseases (eg, liver disease) to a history of prior sexual abuse.[1,7,63–66] One study reported that the overall prevalence of sexual abuse in GI clinic patients approached 44%.[64] The explanations for this association are myriad. For example, the alteration in patterns of gastric secretion after the delivery of bad news was first reported in 1929[67]; subsequent research has confirmed the effects of psychological stress on GI secretion and GI motility.[68] The physiological basis for these symptoms is believed to be a result of disturbances to neurotransmitter signaling in the GI nervous system.[68] Research in the field of IBS and inflammatory bowel disease (IBD) has demonstrated the effects of severe, sustained life stressors on the modulation of GI symptoms.[69,70]

While the precise etiology of GI symptoms in those with a history of childhood sexual abuse is unknown, current research indicates a higher than normal incidence of GI disturbances in this population.[71] Felitti[71] noted this association when examining the prevalence of GI complaints among survey respondents who had reported multiple categories on the ACE instrument. Sixty-four percent of those respondents with a history of ACEs had GI symptoms or complaints, compared with 39% without a history of ACEs.[71] In a similarly designed study that used a mailed questionnaire in patients with GI symptoms or complaints, 41% of women and 11% of men reported some type of prior abuse.[63]

In particular, functional abdominal disturbances such as IBS have been noted to occur more frequently among patients with a history of childhood sexual abuse.[63] Irritable bowel syndrome is typically characterized by a history of 3 or more months of recurrent abdominal pain, usually relieved by a bowel movement; changes in the frequency or consistency of stool; disturbed defecation at least 25% of the time (ie, altered stool frequency, form, or passage); and an association with bloating or the sensation of abdominal distention.[68] Other symptoms reported by patients include nausea, early satiety, dysphagia, lethargy, back pain, thigh pain, urinary frequency, urinary urgency, dyspareunia, and/or symptoms of fibromyalgia.[68]

Initial studies correlating IBS with a history of sexual abuse were based on questionnaires that queried female GI clinic patients about their history of prior sexual abuse, their GI symptoms, and their use of health services. Fifty-three percent of those with functional GI disturbances (ie, IBS) reported a history of sexual abuse, while only 37% of those with organic GI disease (ie, IBD) reported a history of sexual abuse.[64] In a similar study comparing patients with IBS to patients with IBD, 54% versus 5%, respectively, had a history of severe abuse during childhood or sexual assault as an adult.[72] Finally, in a study evaluating 105 subjects with IBS, IBD, or other GI disorders, investigators reported that patients with IBS had a much higher frequency of sexual abuse as a child when compared with the patients with IBD or other GI disorders.[66]

Other GI diseases have been linked to a history of adverse childhood events, including liver disease.[1,7] In one survey using the ACE instrument, those who reported at least 1 ACE category demonstrated a 1.2- to 1.6-fold increase in the risk of self-reported liver disease; a 2.6-fold increase was observed for respondents who endorsed 6 or more ACE categories.[7] Investigators postulated that this link between liver disease and ACEs is mediated, in part, by the development of adverse health behaviors (eg, alcoholism, substance use, sexual promiscuity) that may increase the risk of viral and/or alcohol-induced liver disease.[7] Lending weight to such theory, after adjusting for such adverse health behaviors, the association between ACEs and the development of liver disease was significantly reduced.[7]

Gynecologic Conditions and Sexual Health

The association between gynecologic conditions, sexual health, and a history of ACEs has been widely cited in the literature.[1,73–75] Women who report a history of sexual abuse during childhood are at greater risk for acquiring sexually transmitted infections (STIs), experiencing teen pregnancy, having multiple sexual partners, or experiencing repeat episodes of abuse when compared with individuals without a history of childhood abuse.[74,76–80] The long-term conditions associated with a history of ACEs range from problems with adult sexual adjustment (eg, dissatisfaction with adult sexual relationships, problems with intimacy), to the practice of risky sexual behaviors (eg, sexual promiscuity, drug and alcohol use), to the development of actual physical complaints (eg, chronic pelvic pain, fibromyalgia).[11,81]

Sexual Promiscuity and Sexually Transmitted Infections

Felitti et al[1] investigated the relationship between the presence of ACEs and risky sexual behaviors such as sexual promiscuity, which may increase the risk of developing subsequent medical diseases (eg, STIs, pelvic inflammatory disease, HIV infection) and their complications (eg, pain and discomfort, infertility). In one large survey study, investigators estimated the prevalence of having 50 or more sexual intercourse partners to be 6.8% among respondents reporting 4 or more ACE categories, compared with 3.0% among those reporting no ACE categories.[1] They demonstrated that subjects who reported 1 ACE category had an adjusted OR of 1.7 (95% CI 1.3, 2.3) for having 50 or more sexual intercourse partners. When compared with those subjects reporting no ACE categories, the OR increased to 3.2 (95% CI 2.1, 5.1) for subjects reporting 4 or more ACE categories.[1] Likewise, individuals who report ACEs seem to be at higher risk for contracting STIs.[1,75] In one study, the prevalence of ever having an STI was 16.7% among those respondents reporting 4 or more ACE categories, compared with 5.6% among those reporting no ACE categories.[1] Those subjects reporting a single ACE category have an adjusted OR of 1.4 (95% CI 1.1, 1.7) for ever having had an STI, when compared with those subjects reporting no ACE categories.[1] The OR increased to 2.5 (95% CI 1.9, 3.2) for those subjects reporting 4 or more ACE categories.[1] When examined in detail, the ACE categories most associated with ever having had an STI were (from most to least) criminal behavior in household, sexual abuse, emotional abuse, and physical abuse.[1]

Disorders of Sexual Adjustment

Those who experience sexual abuse during childhood may be at risk for developing disorders of sexual adjustment in adult life.[82,83] In a randomized, community-based study that queried participants about the effect of childhood sexual abuse on their adult sexual relationships, 50% of the respondents reported that a history of incestuous sexual abuse during childhood had affected their sexual adjustment as adults.[74] In particular, females who had a history of abuse including sexual intercourse were more likely to experience dissatisfaction with their adult sexual relationships.[74] Those who experienced childhood sexual abuse have described having problems with intimacy, specifically by experiencing a sense of insecurity or having disorganized attachments,[84,85] which is manifest by an increased incidence of separation and divorce among those who experienced abuse.[86,87]

Chronic Pelvic Pain

Certain gynecologic conditions have been associated with a history of ACEs. Although the data are conflicting, there are reports that chronic pelvic pain occurs at an increased frequency among patients who report having had some type of ACE.[88,89] In one often-cited study, when participants who had chronic pelvic pain, headache, or no pain complaints were questioned about a history of childhood sexual abuse, individuals with chronic pelvic pain had a significantly higher lifetime prevalence of major sexual abuse (ie, genital-genital contact, penetration) than individuals in the comparison groups.[88] Another similar study demonstrated a significant relationship between experiencing major sexual abuse before the age of 15 years and developing chronic pelvic pain later in life, although there was no significant difference in the lifetime prevalence of sexual abuse between the chronic pelvic pain and comparison groups.[89]

Behavioral and Mental Health Conditions

Behavioral and mental health conditions are common outcomes for children who have experienced child maltreatment. The sequelae may manifest as posttraumatic stress disorder (PTSD), internalizing or externalizing behaviors, risk-taking behaviors, formal diagnosis of depression or anxiety, suicidality, and other problematic behaviors. Knowledge gained during work focused on the effect of early life adversity on the developing brain and physiological response to such stressors leading to maladaptive coping skills and behaviors provides a framework for understanding these outcomes and developing therapeutic measures aimed to mitigate them.[13–15,32] As well, there is hope that by recognizing and addressing these effects there can be prevention of the adult diseases (physical and mental) rooted in childhood adversity on a population-health basis.

Posttraumatic stress disorder is a traumatic-specific psychiatric diagnosis described in the *Diagnostic and Statistical Manual of Mental Disorders,* 5th Edition.[90] Children who have experienced or witnessed violence, including child abuse or neglect, can experience PTSD. Key symptoms diagnostic of the disorder include 1) persistent reexperience of the traumatic event through intrusive thoughts, dreams, and feelings (ie, flashbacks); 2) avoidance of stimuli that remind the child of the event(s) or trigger thoughts or feelings; 3) negative alterations in cognitions and mood disrupting the emotional status and belief system of the child; and 4) altered arousal and reactivity that affect the child's behavior (ie, hyperarousal).[19,20,90]

In addition, those who experience child maltreatment are known to suffer internalizing problems such as depression and anxiety.[19,20] Suicidal ideation, self-harming behavior, and suicide are well known as sequelae of abuse and neglect, particularly for adolescents. Some children demonstrate externalizing problems such as oppositional defiant disorder and conduct disorder.[19,20] Anger and aggression are not uncommon. Problems with substance use may develop during preadolescence and adolescence as a means of coping with the adversity endured. Many children receive a diagnosis of attention-deficit/hyperactivity disorder based on difficulty paying attention and other behaviors they exhibit.[19,20] Elucidating a trauma history may lead to better understanding on the part of the medical professional and caregivers as to the basis for the child's emotions and behaviors, as well as lead to a more appropriate diagnosis and approach to treatment. Behavior problems are understandable in the context of adversity and toxic stress and neuroendocrine-immune network and biological adaptation/maladaptation (discussed at the beginning of this chapter). Dramatic emotional reactions, seeming out of proportion or inappropriate to the eliciting stimuli; emotional dysregulation paralleling the flight-or-fight response; challenging behaviors; and difficulty with daily routines can be common experiences for caregivers of children who have experienced trauma.[20] In turn, caregivers in the home and school environments who lack understanding or empathy may respond negatively or in an escalating fashion and even punish the child for the undesirable behavior, which can compound the problem and act as positive reinforcement of the child's maladaptive emotional response system and ensuing behaviors.[19,20]

Mitigating the situation involves establishment of a secure attachment for the child, who has previously experienced a disordered attachment, with a nurturing adult who can consistently and appropriately respond to the child's needs,[91,92] which, in turn, helps the child develop trust and learn social communication skills.[93] Additionally, the child can learn how to recognize and regulate his or her emotions, similar to the way infants with an attentive mother or caregiver and non-frightening environment do. As a result, the parent-child interaction is not impaired, and the child can reap the benefits and grow or develop on a social-emotional basis.

Adolescents, in particular, are at risk for significant behavior and mental health conditions. The trauma history may be more complex given the duration of exposure, multiple experiences of trauma and abuse, and chaotic relationships experienced on a cumulative basis by the teen. Impaired self-efficacy and self-perception[94] and cognitive and emotion dysregulation may manifest as risk-taking behaviors involving smoking, alcohol, and drugs, as well as sexual reactivity.[19,20] The intersection of mental health conditions and physical health problems can become more evident during adolescence. This is consistent with the basis of the original ACE studies,[1–12] which exposed the link among adult diseases, health-threatening behaviors, and ACEs.

Exploration of a child's psychosocial history, comprehensive mental assessment, and referral to therapeutic services are critical steps to helping children and adolescents with mental health and behavioral conditions resulting from ACEs and other trauma. Caregivers in each of a child's environments need education and assistance on how to best help the child. Education on how the emotional responses and behaviors of traumatized children differ from those who have not experienced trauma[19,20] and the use of positive parenting strategies is often necessary.[95–97] Parent-child interaction therapy for children aged 2 to 7 years and their parents is a therapeutic modality with demonstrated benefit.[20] Evidence-based, trauma-focused psychotherapy can also aid in the rehabilitation of the child's misperceptions, traumatic stress responses, and maladaptive coping.[20] In particular, cognitive behavioral therapy has proven efficacy in the treatment of pediatric PTSD.[19,20] Examples include trauma-focused cognitive behavioral therapy, which was originally developed for children who experienced child sexual abuse, and other cognitive behavioral therapy focused on children who have experienced abuse.[98] Those now responsible for the care of the child may also benefit from mental health therapy, especially if they, too, have unaddressed symptoms or are having difficulties handling the effect of the child's issues on the family's functioning. Pharmacotherapy prescribed by a psychiatrist who specializes in children and adolescents may be necessary as adjunctive treatment of a traumatized child's hyperarousal symptoms.[19,20]

Adult Mental Health Conditions

The risk of behavior and mental health conditions clearly extends into adulthood; those who experienced childhood abuse and neglect have repeatedly been shown to have an increased risk for developing PTSD, depression, anxiety, dissociative disorder, and suicidality during adulthood.[6,87,99,100] Complementary theories have been reported in the psychology literature, citing that adult psychopathology in those who experienced childhood abuse occurs as a consequence of a chronic form of PTSD rooted in chronic neurophysiological changes.[101–104] Depression is one of the most frequent mental health concerns among adults who experienced child abuse.[1,6,9] Individuals with a history of ACEs are also at an increased risk for attempting suicide.[10] Posttraumatic stress disorder and other anxiety-related disorders are also observed at increased frequency.[105–107] Emotional distress can manifest as adult behaviors and unhealthy lifestyles, which can result in related medical conditions and diseases.

Behavior-Related Medical Conditions

The effect of a history of ACEs on the development of psychosomatic and behavioral conditions, which can result in physical medical conditions whose etiology is thought to be, in large part, due to underlying psychological stressors, has been well described.[1] Behaviors and conditions may include eating disorders[108]; tobacco, alcohol, and illicit drug use; and medical conditions such as obesity[1,8,71,108,109] and its related disorders, such as chronic obstructive pulmonary disease, liver disease, and chronic pain syndromes.[1,88,110] The etiology of such behaviors is thought to be multifactorial, including the notion of disordered eating as an adaptive coping mechanism[1] and/or having a distorted body image or misperception of weight.[71] Individuals with obesity and overeating disorders are at increased risk for developing serious long-term health consequences, such as ischemic heart disease or diabetes. Similarly, it has been suggested that anorexia nervosa and bulimia are associated with a history of ACEs.[111–113] Alcohol, tobacco, and illicit drug use occur at an increased frequency among adults who experienced child abuse, perhaps as a coping mechanism; each has deleterious long-term health consequences, such as heart and liver disease, STIs (eg, HIV, hepatitis), psychiatric illness, and multiple psychosocial problems.[1,9,12,114,115] Chronic pain disorders, specifically fibromyalgia, have been linked to abuse occurring during childhood or adulthood.[116,117] The severity of the abuse has been significantly correlated with the self-reported measures of physical disability and pain, psychiatric distress, sleep quality, and ability to cope with stress.[116]

Conclusion

Using the neuroendocrine-immune pathway and ecobiodevelopmental framework, we have deepened our understanding of the lifelong risk for poor health and disease states associated with ACEs and toxic stress. It is hoped with more widespread distribution of this knowledge throughout society, especially in the early childhood, health care, and education sectors, that recognition and mitigation as well as prevention efforts will change the trajectory for children, decreasing their exposure to ACEs in general and ameliorating outcomes for those who are exposed. It will be interesting to see if increased provision of trauma-focused therapy and trauma-informed, secure, stable, nurturing relationships for children who have experienced child maltreatment can improve population health.

References

1. Felitti VJ, Anda RF, Nordenberg D, et al. Relationship of childhood abuse and household dysfunction to many of the leading causes of death in adults. The Adverse Childhood Experiences (ACE) Study. *Am J Prev Med*. 1998;14(4):245–258 PMID: 9635069 https://doi.org/10.1016/S0749-3797(98)00017-8
2. Dube SR, Miller JW, Brown DW, et al. Adverse childhood experiences and the association with ever using alcohol and initiating alcohol use during adolescence. *J Adolesc Health*. 2006;38(4):444.e1–444.e10 PMID: 16549308 https://doi.org/10.1016/j.jadohealth.2005.06.006
3. Anda RF, Felitti VJ, Bremner JD, et al. The enduring effects of abuse and related adverse experiences in childhood. A convergence of evidence from neurobiology and epidemiology. *Eur Arch Psychiatry Clin Neurosci*. 2006;256(3):174–186 PMID: 16311898 https://doi.org/10.1007/s00406-005-0624-4
4. Dong M, Anda RF, Felitti VJ, et al. Childhood residential mobility and multiple health risks during adolescence and adulthood: the hidden role of adverse childhood experiences. *Arch Pediatr Adolesc Med*. 2005;159(12):1104–1110 PMID: 16330731 https://doi.org/10.1001/archpedi.159.12.1104
5. Dong M, Giles WH, Felitti VJ, et al. Insights into causal pathways for ischemic heart disease: adverse childhood experiences study. *Circulation*. 2004;110(13):1761–1766 PMID: 15381652 https://doi.org/10.1161/01.CIR.0000143074.54995.7F

6. Chapman DP, Whitfield CL, Felitti VJ, Dube SR, Edwards VJ, Anda RF. Adverse childhood experiences and the risk of depressive disorders in adulthood. *J Affect Disord*. 2004;82(2):217–225 PMID: 15488250 https://doi.org/10.1016/j.jad.2003.12.013
7. Dong M, Dube SR, Felitti VJ, Giles WH, Anda RF. Adverse childhood experiences and self-reported liver disease: new insights into the causal pathway. *Arch Intern Med*. 2003;163(16):1949–1956 PMID: 12963569 https://doi.org/10.1001/archinte.163.16.1949
8. Williamson DF, Thompson TJ, Anda RF, Dietz WH, Felitti V. Body weight and obesity in adults and self-reported abuse in childhood. *Int J Obes Relat Metab Disord*. 2002;26(8):1075–1082 PMID: 12119573 https://doi.org/10.1038/sj.ijo.0802038
9. Anda RF, Whitfield CL, Felitti VJ, et al. Adverse childhood experiences, alcoholic parents, and later risk of alcoholism and depression. *Psychiatr Serv*. 2002;53(8):1001–1009 PMID: 12161676 https://doi.org/10.1176/appi.ps.53.8.1001
10. Dube SR, Anda RF, Felitti VJ, Chapman DP, Williamson DF, Giles WH. Childhood abuse, household dysfunction, and the risk of attempted suicide throughout the life span: findings from the Adverse Childhood Experiences Study. *JAMA*. 2001;286(24):3089–3096 PMID: 11754674 https://doi.org/10.1001/jama.286.24.3089
11. Hillis SD, Anda RF, Felitti VJ, Nordenberg D, Marchbanks PA. Adverse childhood experiences and sexually transmitted diseases in men and women: a retrospective study. *Pediatrics*. 2000;106(1):E11 PMID: 10878180 https://doi.org/10.1542/peds.106.1.e11
12. Anda RF, Croft JB, Felitti VJ, et al. Adverse childhood experiences and smoking during adolescence and adulthood. *JAMA*. 1999;282(17):1652–1658 PMID: 10553792 https://doi.org/10.1001/jama.282.17.1652
13. Shonkoff JP. Building a new biodevelopmental framework to guide the future of early childhood policy. *Child Dev*. 2010;81(1):357–367 PMID: 20331672 https://doi.org/10.1111/j.1467-8624.2009.01399.x
14. Garner AS, Shonkoff JP, Siegel BS, et al; American Academy of Pediatrics Committee on Psychosocial Aspects of Child and Family Health; Committee on Early Childhood, Adoption, and Dependent Care; Section on Developmental and Behavioral Pediatrics. Early childhood adversity, toxic stress, and the role of the pediatrician: translating developmental science into lifelong health. *Pediatrics*. 2012;129(1):e224–e231 PMID: 22201148 https://doi.org/10.1542/peds.2011-2662
15. Shonkoff JP, Garner AS, Siegel BS, et al; American Academy of Pediatrics Committee on Psychosocial Aspects of Child and Family Health; Committee on Early Childhood, Adoption, and Dependent Care; Section on Developmental and Behavioral Pediatrics. The lifelong effects of early childhood adversity and toxic stress. *Pediatrics*. 2012;129(1):e232–e246 PMID: 22201156 https://doi.org/10.1542/peds.2011-2663
16. Johnson SB, Riley AW, Granger DA, Riis J. The science of early life toxic stress for pediatric practice and advocacy. *Pediatrics*. 2013;131(2):319–327 PMID: 23339224 https://doi.org/10.1542/peds.2012-0469
17. Garner AS. Thinking developmentally: the next evolution in models of health. *J Dev Behav Pediatr*. 2016;37(7):579–584
18. Traub F, Boynton-Jarrett R. Modifiable resilience factors to childhood adversity for clinical pediatric practice. *Pediatrics*. 2017;139(5):e20162569 PMID: 28557726 https://doi.org/10.1542/peds.2016-2569
19. Stirling J Jr, Amaya-Jackson L, Amaya-Jackson L; American Academy of Pediatrics Committee on Child Abuse and Neglect and Section on Adoption and Foster Care; American Academy of Child and Adolescent Psychiatry; National Center for Child Traumatic Stress. Understanding the behavioral and emotional consequences of child abuse. *Pediatrics*. 2008;122(3):667–673 PMID: 18762538 https://doi.org/10.1542/peds.2008-1885

20. Sege RD, Amaya-Jackson L; American Academy of Pediatrics Committee on Child Abuse and Neglect and Council on Foster Care, Adoption, and Kinship Care; American Academy of Child and Adolescent Psychiatry Committee on Child Maltreatment and Violence; National Center for Child Traumatic Stress. Clinical considerations related to the behavioral manifestations of child maltreatment. 2017;139(4):e20170100 PMID: 28320870 https://doi.org/10.1542/peds.2017-0100
21. Flaherty EG, Thompson R, Litrownik AJ, et al. Effect of early childhood adversity on child health. *Arch Pediatr Adolesc Med*. 2006;160(12):1232–1238 PMID: 17146020 https://doi.org/10.1001/archpedi.160.12.1232
22. Flaherty EG, Thompson R, Litrownik AJ, et al. Adverse childhood exposures and reported child health at age 12. *Acad Pediatr*. 2009;9(3):150–156 PMID: 19450774 https://doi.org/10.1016/j.acap.2008.11.003
23. Flaherty EG, Thompson R, Dubowitz H, et al. Adverse childhood experiences and child health in early adolescence. *JAMA Pediatr*. 2013;167(7):622–629 PMID: 23645114 https://doi.org/10.1001/jamapediatrics.2013.22
24. Thompson R, Flaherty EG, English DJ, et al. Trajectories of adverse childhood experiences and self-reported health at age 18. *Acad Pediatr*. 2015;15(5):503–509 PMID: 25441654 https://doi.org/10.1016/j.acap.2014.09.010
25. Kerker BD, Zhang J, Nadeem E, et al. Adverse childhood experiences and mental health, chronic medical conditions, and development in young children. *Acad Pediatr*. 2015;15(5):510–517 PMID: 26183001 https://doi.org/10.1016/j.acap.2015.05.005
26. Jimenez ME, Wade R Jr, Lin Y, Morrow LM, Reichman NE. Adverse experiences in early childhood and kindergarten outcomes. *Pediatrics*. 2016;137(2):e20151839 PMID: 26768347 https://doi.org/10.1542/peds.2015-1839
27. Bethell CD, Newacheck P, Hawes E, Halfon N. Adverse childhood experiences: assessing the impact on health and school engagement and the mitigating role of resilience. *Health Aff (Millwood)*. 2014;33(12):2106–2115 PMID: 25489028 https://doi.org/10.1377/hlthaff.2014.0914
28. Block RW, Krebs NF; American Academy of Pediatrics Committee on Child Abuse and Neglect, Committee on Nutrition. Failure to thrive as a manifestation of child neglect. *Pediatrics*. 2005;116(5):1234–1237 PMID: 16264015 https://doi.org/10.1542/peds.2005-2032
29. Oates RK. Similarities and differences between nonorganic failure to thrive and deprivation dwarfism. *Child Abuse Negl*. 1984;8(4):439–445 PMID: 6542816 https://doi.org/10.1016/0145-2134(84)90025-5
30. Black MM, Dubowitz H, Hutcheson J, Berenson-Howard J, Starr RH Jr. A randomized clinical trial of home intervention for children with failure to thrive. *Pediatrics*. 1995;95(6):807–814 PMID: 7539121
31. Barlow KM, Thomson E, Johnson D, Minns RA. Late neurologic and cognitive sequelae of inflicted traumatic brain injury in infancy. *Pediatrics*. 2005;116(2):e174–e185 PMID: 16061571 https://doi.org/10.1542/peds.2004-2739
32. Teicher MH, Andersen SL, Polcari A, Anderson CM, Navalta CP. Developmental neurobiology of childhood stress and trauma. *Psychiatr Clin North Am*. 2002;25(2): 397–426, vii–viii PMID: 12136507 https://doi.org/10.1016/S0193-953X(01)00003-X
33. Makaroff KL, Putnam FW. Outcomes of infants and children with inflicted traumatic brain injury. *Dev Med Child Neurol*. 2003;45(7):497–502 PMID: 12828406 https://doi.org/10.1111/j.1469-8749.2003.tb00947.x
34. Keenan HT, Runyan DK, Nocera M. Child outcomes and family characteristics 1 year after severe inflicted or noninflicted traumatic brain injury. *Pediatrics*. 2006;117(2):317–324 PMID: 16452349 https://doi.org/10.1542/peds.2005-0979

35. Barlow K, Thompson E, Johnson D, Minns RA. The neurological outcome of non-accidental head injury. *Pediatr Rehabil.* 2004;7(3):195–203 PMID: 15204571 https://doi.org/10.1080/13638490410001715331
36. Marín-Padilla M, Parisi JE, Armstrong DL, Sargent SK, Kaplan JA. Shaken infant syndrome: developmental neuropathology, progressive cortical dysplasia, and epilepsy. *Acta Neuropathol.* 2002;103(4):321–332 PMID: 11904751 https://doi.org/10.1007/s00401-001-0470-z
37. Marín-Padilla M. Developmental neuropathology and impact of perinatal brain damage. I: hemorrhagic lesions of neocortex. *J Neuropathol Exp Neurol.* 1996;55(7): 758–773 PMID: 8965092 https://doi.org/10.1097/00005072-199607000-00002
38. Marín-Padilla M. Developmental neuropathology and impact of perinatal brain damage. II: white matter lesions of the neocortex. *J Neuropathol Exp Neurol.* 1997;56(3):219–235 PMID: 9056536 https://doi.org/10.1097/00005072-199703000-00001
39. Marín-Padilla M. Developmental neuropathology and impact of perinatal brain damage. III: gray matter lesions of the neocortex. *J Neuropathol Exp Neurol.* 1999;58(5):407–429 PMID: 10331430 https://doi.org/10.1097/00005072-199905000-00001
40. Marín-Padilla M. Perinatal brain damage, cortical reorganization (acquired cortical dysplasias), and epilepsy. *Adv Neurol.* 2000;84:153–172 PMID: 11091865
41. Chevignard MP, Lind K. Long-term outcome of abusive head trauma. *Pediatr Radiol.* 2014;44(S4)(suppl 4):S548–S558 PMID: 25501726 https://doi.org/10.1007/s00247-014-3169-8
42. Bonnier C. [Outcome after non-accidental head injury in children]. *Arch Pediatr.* 2006;13(6):531–533 PMID: 16697574 https://doi.org/10.1016/j.arcped.2006.03.113
43. Rhine T, Wade SL, Makoroff KL, Cassedy A, Michaud LJ. Clinical predictors of outcome following inflicted traumatic brain injury in children. *J Trauma Acute Care Surg.* 2012;73(4)(suppl 3):S248–S253 PMID: 23026962 https://doi.org/10.1097/TA.0b013e31826b0062
44. Jennett B, Bond M. Assessment of outcome after severe brain damage. *Lancet.* 1975;1(7905):480–484 PMID: 46957 https://doi.org/10.1016/S0140-6736(75)92830-5
45. Greiner MV, Lawrence AP, Horn P, Newmeyer AJ, Makoroff KL. Early clinical indicators of developmental outcome in abusive head trauma. *Childs Nerv Syst.* 2012;28(6):889–896 PMID: 22367916 https://doi.org/10.1007/s00381-012-1714-z
46. Ilves P, Lintrop M, Talvik I, Sisko A, Talvik T. Predictive value of clinical and radiological findings in inflicted traumatic brain injury. *Acta Paediatr.* 2010;99(9):1329–1336 PMID: 20377537 https://doi.org/10.1111/j.1651-2227.2010.01820.x
47. Tanoue K, Matsui K, Nozawa K, Aida N. Predictive value of early radiological findings in inflicted traumatic brain injury. *Acta Paediatr.* 2012;101(6):614–617 PMID: 22353249 https://doi.org/10.1111/j.1651-2227.2012.02635.x
48. Tanoue K, Aida N, Matsui K. Apparent diffusion coefficient values predict outcomes of abusive head trauma. *Acta Paediatr.* 2013;102(8):805–808 PMID: 23631484 https://doi.org/10.1111/apa.12281
49. Stans AA. Complications of fractures in children. In: Mencio GA, Swiontkowski MF, eds. *Green's Skeletal Trauma in Children.* 5th ed. Philadelphia, PA: Elsevier Saunders; 2015:105–129 https://doi.org/10.1016/B978-0-323-18773-2.00007-X
50. Riccio AI, Wilson PL, Wimberly RL. Lower extremity injuries. In: Herring JA, ed. *Tachdjian's Pediatric Orthopedics.* 5th ed. Philadephia, PA: Elsevier Saunders; 2014:1353–1516
51. Herring JA, Ho C. Upper extremity injuries. In: Herring JA, ed. *Tachdjian's Pediatric Orthopedics.* 5th ed. Philadephia, PA: Elsevier Saunders; 2014:1245–1352
52. Sarwark JF, LaBella CR. *Pediatric Orthopedics and Sports Injuries: A Quick Reference Guide.* Elk Grove Village, IL: American Academic of Pediatrics; 2010

53. Tompkins RG, Liang MH, Lee AF, Kazis LE; Multi-Center Benchmarking Study Working Group. The American Burn Association/Shriners Hospitals for Children Burn Outcomes Program: a progress report at 15 years. *J Trauma Acute Care Surg*. 2012;73(3 suppl 2): S173–S178 PMID: 22929544 https://doi.org/10.1097/TA.0b013e318265c53e
54. Druery M, Brown TL, Muller M. Long term functional outcomes and quality of life following severe burn injury. *Burns*. 2005;31(6):692–695 PMID: 16129223 https://doi.org/10.1016/j.burns.2005.03.001
55. Wallace HJ, Fear MW, Crowe MM, Martin LJ, Wood FM. Identification of factors predicting scar outcome after burn injury in children: a prospective case-control study. *Burns Trauma*. 2017;5(1):19 PMID: 28680887 https://doi.org/10.1186/s41038-017-0084-x
56. McGarry S, Elliott C, McDonald A, Valentine J, Wood F, Girdler S. Paediatric burns: from the voice of the child. *Burns*. 2014;40(4):606–615 PMID: 24041516 https://doi.org/10.1016/j.burns.2013.08.031
57. Lane WG, Dubowitz H, Langenberg P, Dischinger P. Epidemiology of abusive abdominal trauma hospitalizations in United States children. *Child Abuse Negl*. 2012;36(2):142–148 PMID: 22398302 https://doi.org/10.1016/j.chiabu.2011.09.010
58. Wood J, Rubin DM, Nance ML, Christian CW. Distinguishing inflicted versus accidental abdominal injuries in young children. *J Trauma*. 2005;59(5):1203–1208 PMID: 16385300 https://doi.org/10.1097/01.ta.0000196437.07011.b1
59. Trokel M, DiScala C, Terrin NC, Sege RD. Blunt abdominal injury in the young pediatric patient: child abuse and patient outcomes. *Child Maltreat*. 2004;9(1):111–117 PMID: 14871002 https://doi.org/10.1177/1077559503260310
60. Barnes PM, Norton CM, Dunstan FD, Kemp AM, Yates DW, Sibert JR. Abdominal injury due to child abuse. *Lancet*. 2005;366(9481):234–235 PMID: 16023514 https://doi.org/10.1016/S0140-6736(05)66913-9
61. van Tilburg MA, Runyan DK, Zolotor AJ, et al. Unexplained gastrointestinal symptoms after abuse in a prospective study of children at risk for abuse and neglect. *Ann Fam Med*. 2010;8(2):134–140 PMID: 20212300 https://doi.org/10.1370/afm.1053
62. Paras ML, Murad MH, Chen LP, et al. Sexual abuse and lifetime diagnosis of somatic disorders: a systematic review and meta-analysis. *JAMA*. 2009;302(5):550–561 PMID: 19654389 https://doi.org/10.1001/jama.2009.1091
63. Talley NJ, Fett SL, Zinsmeister AR, Melton LJ III. Gastrointestinal tract symptoms and self-reported abuse: a population-based study. *Gastroenterology*. 1994;107(4):1040–1049 PMID: 7926457 https://doi.org/10.1016/0016-5085(94)90228-3
64. Drossman DA, Leserman J, Nachman G, et al. Sexual and physical abuse in women with functional or organic gastrointestinal disorders. *Ann Intern Med*. 1990;113(11):828–833 PMID: 2240898 https://doi.org/10.7326/0003-4819-113-11-828
65. Drossman DA, Talley NJ, Leserman J, Olden KW, Barreiro MA. Sexual and physical abuse and gastrointestinal illness. Review and recommendations. *Ann Intern Med*. 1995;123(10):782–794 PMID: 7574197 https://doi.org/10.7326/0003-4819-123-10-199511150-00007
66. Ross CA. Childhood sexual abuse and psychosomatic symptoms in irritable bowel syndrome. *J Child Sex Abuse*. 2005;14(1):27–38 PMID: 15914403 https://doi.org/10.1300/J070v14n01_02
67. Cannon WB. *Bodily Changes in Pain, Hunger, Fear and Rage: An Account of Recent Researches Into the Function of Emotional Excitement*. 2nd ed. New York, NY: D. Appleton and Company; 1920
68. Sleisenger MH, Feldman M, Friedman LS, Brandt LJ. *Sleisenger & Fordtran's Gastrointestinal and Liver Disease: Pathophysiology, Diagnosis, Management*. 8th ed. Philadelphia, PA: Saunders; 2006

69. Bradesi S, McRoberts JA, Anton PA, Mayer EA. Inflammatory bowel disease and irritable bowel syndrome: separate or unified? *Curr Opin Gastroenterol*. 2003;19(4):336–342 PMID: 15703574 https://doi.org/10.1097/00001574-200307000-00003
70. Quigley EM. Disturbances of motility and visceral hypersensitivity in irritable bowel syndrome: biological markers or epiphenomenon. *Gastroenterol Clin North Am*. 2005;34(2):221–233, vi PMID: 15862931 https://doi.org/10.1016/j.gtc.2005.02.010
71. Felitti VJ. Long-term medical consequences of incest, rape, and molestation. *South Med J*. 1991;84(3):328–331 PMID: 2000519 https://doi.org/10.1097/00007611-199103000-00008
72. Walker EA, Katon WJ, Roy-Byrne PP, Jemelka RP, Russo J. Histories of sexual victimization in patients with irritable bowel syndrome or inflammatory bowel disease. *Am J Psychiatry*. 1993;150(10):1502–1506 PMID: 8379554 https://doi.org/10.1176/ajp.150.10.1502
73. Fromuth ME. The relationship of childhood sexual abuse with later psychological and sexual adjustment in a sample of college women. *Child Abuse Negl*. 1986;10(1):5–15 PMID: 3955429 https://doi.org/10.1016/0145-2134(86)90026-8
74. Mullen PE, Martin JL, Anderson JC, Romans SE, Herbison GP. The effect of child sexual abuse on social, interpersonal and sexual function in adult life. *Br J Psychiatry*. 1994;165(1):35–47 PMID: 7953055 https://doi.org/10.1192/bjp.165.1.35
75. Senn TE, Carey MP, Vanable PA, Coury-Doniger P, Urban M. Characteristics of sexual abuse in childhood and adolescence influence sexual risk behavior in adulthood. *Arch Sex Behav*. 2007;36(5):637–645 PMID: 17192833 https://doi.org/10.1007/s10508-006-9109-4
76. Gorcey M, Santiago JM, McCall-Perez F. Psychological consequences for women sexually abused in childhood. *Soc Psychiatry*. 1986;21(3):129–133 PMID: 3750024 https://doi.org/10.1007/BF00582682
77. Nagy S, DiClemente R, Adcock AG. Adverse factors associated with forced sex among southern adolescent girls. *Pediatrics*. 1995;96(5 Pt 1):944–946 PMID: 7478840
78. Russell DEH. *The Secret Trauma: Incest in the Lives of Girls and Women*. New York, NY: Basic Books; 1986
79. Springs FE, Friedrich WN. Health risk behaviors and medical sequelae of childhood sexual abuse. *Mayo Clin Proc*. 1992;67(6):527–532 PMID: 1434879 https://doi.org/10.1016/S0025-6196(12)60458-3
80. Fergusson DM, Horwood LJ, Lynskey MT. Childhood sexual abuse, adolescent sexual behaviors and sexual revictimization. *Child Abuse Negl*. 1997;21(8):789–803 PMID: 9280383 https://doi.org/10.1016/S0145-2134(97)00039-2
81. Gunter J. Chronic pelvic pain: an integrated approach to diagnosis and treatment. *Obstet Gynecol Surv*. 2003;58(9):615–623 PMID: 12972837 https://doi.org/10.1097/01.OGX.0000083225.90017.01
82. Herman JL, Hirschman L. *Father-Daughter Incest*. Cambridge, MA: Harvard University Press; 2000
83. Finkelhor D. *Child Sexual Abuse: New Theory and Research*. New York, NY: Free Press; 1984
84. Jehu D, Gazan M, Klassen C. *Beyond Sexual Abuse: Therapy with Women Who Were Childhood Victims*. New York, NY: Wiley; 1988
85. Briere J, Runtz M. Multivariate correlates of childhood psychological and physical maltreatment among university women. *Child Abuse Negl*. 1988;12(3):331–341 PMID: 3167621 https://doi.org/10.1016/0145-2134(88)90046-4
86. Beitchman JH, Zucker KJ, Hood JE, daCosta GA, Akman D. A review of the short-term effects of child sexual abuse. *Child Abuse Negl*. 1991;15(4):537–556 PMID: 1959086 https://doi.org/10.1016/0145-2134(91)90038-F
87. Mullen PE, Romans-Clarkson SE, Walton VA, Herbison GP. Impact of sexual and physical abuse on women's mental health. *Lancet*. 1988;1(8590):841–845 PMID: 2895362 https://doi.org/10.1016/S0140-6736(88)91600-5

88. Walling MK, Reiter RC, O'Hara MW, Milburn AK, Lilly G, Vincent SD. Abuse history and chronic pain in women: I. Prevalences of sexual abuse and physical abuse. *Obstet Gynecol.* 1994;84(2):193–199 PMID: 8041529
89. Lampe A, Sölder E, Ennemoser A, Schubert C, Rumpold G, Söllner W. Chronic pelvic pain and previous sexual abuse. *Obstet Gynecol.* 2000;96(6):929–933 PMID: 11084180
90. American Psychiatric Association, ed. *Diagnostic and Statistical Manual of Mental Disorders.* 5th ed. Washington, DC: American Psychiatric Association Press; 2013
91. Bowlby J. *Attachment and Loss.* 2nd ed. New York, NY: Basic Books; 1982
92. Lieberman AF, Amaya-Jackson L. Reciprocal influences of attachment and trauma: using a dual lens in the assessment and treatment of infants, toddlers, and preschoolers. In: Berlin LJ, Ziv Y, Amaya-Jackson L, Greenberg MT, eds. *Enhancing Early Attachments: Theory, Research, Intervention and Policy.* New York, NY: Guildford Press; 2005:100–124
93. Putnam F. Developmental neurobiology of disrupted attachment: lessons from animal models and child abuse research. In: Berlin LJ, Ziv Y, Amaya-Jackson L, Greenberg MT, eds. *Enhancing Early Attachments: Theory, Research, Intervention and Policy.* New York, NY: Guildford Press; 2005:100–124
94. Amaya-Jackson L, Derosa RR. Treatment considerations for clinicians in applying evidence-based practice to complex presentations in child trauma. *J Trauma Stress.* 2007;20(4):379–390 PMID: 17823959 https://doi.org/10.1002/jts.20266
95. Centers for Disease Control and Prevention, National Center for Injury Prevention and Control, Division of Violence Prevention. *Children Benefit When Parents Have Safe, Stable, Nurturing Relationships.* https://www.cdc.gov/violenceprevention/pdf/SSNRs-for-Parents.pdf. Accessed July 14, 2019
96. American Academy of Pediatrics. Trauma Toolbox for Primary Care. https://www.aap.org/en-us/advocacy-and-policy/aap-health-initiatives/healthy-foster-care-america/Pages/Trauma-Guide.aspx#trauma. Accessed May 29, 2019
97. The National Child Traumatic Stress Network. All NCTSN resources. https://www.nctsn.org/resources/all-nctsn-resources. Accessed May 29, 2019
98. Child Welfare Information Gateway. Cognitive behavioral therapy. https://www.childwelfare.gov/search/?addsearch=cognitive+behavioral+therapy. Accessed May 29, 2019
99. Edwards VJ, Holden GW, Felitti VJ, Anda RF. Relationship between multiple forms of childhood maltreatment and adult mental health in community respondents: results from the adverse childhood experiences study. *Am J Psychiatry.* 2003;160(8):1453–1460 PMID: 12900308 https://doi.org/10.1176/appi.ajp.160.8.1453
100. Mullen PE, Martin JL, Anderson JC, Romans SE, Herbison GP. Childhood sexual abuse and mental health in adult life. *Br J Psychiatry.* 1993;163(06):721–732 PMID: 8306113 https://doi.org/10.1192/bjp.163.6.721
101. Bryer JB, Nelson BA, Miller JB, Krol PA. Childhood sexual and physical abuse as factors in adult psychiatric illness. *Am J Psychiatry.* 1987;144(11):1426–1430 PMID: 3674223 https://doi.org/10.1176/ajp.144.11.1426
102. Craine LS, Henson CE, Colliver JA, MacLean DG. Prevalence of a history of sexual abuse among female psychiatric patients in a state hospital system. *Hosp Community Psychiatry.* 1988;39(3):300–304 PMID: 3356438 https://doi.org/10.1176/ps.39.3.300
103. Lindberg FH, Distad LJ. Post-traumatic stress disorders in women who experienced childhood incest. *Child Abuse Negl.* 1985;9(3):329–334 PMID: 4052838 https://doi.org/10.1016/0145-2134(85)90028-6
104. Finkelhor D. The trauma of child sexual abuse: two models. *J Interpers Violence.* 1987;2(4):348–366 https://doi.org/10.1177/088626058700200402

105. Schumm JA, Briggs-Phillips M, Hobfoll SE. Cumulative interpersonal traumas and social support as risk and resiliency factors in predicting PTSD and depression among inner-city women. *J Trauma Stress*. 2006;19(6):825–836 PMID: 17195981 https://doi.org/10.1002/jts.20159
106. Mulder RT, Beautrais AL, Joyce PR, Fergusson DM. Relationship between dissociation, childhood sexual abuse, childhood physical abuse, and mental illness in a general population sample. *Am J Psychiatry*. 1998;155(6):806–811 PMID: 9619154
107. Fergusson DM, Horwood LJ, Lynskey MT. Childhood sexual abuse and psychiatric disorder in young adulthood: II. Psychiatric outcomes of childhood sexual abuse. *J Am Acad Child Adolesc Psychiatry*. 1996;35(10):1365–1374 PMID: 8885591 https://doi.org/10.1097/00004583-199610000-00024
108. Gustafson TB, Sarwer DB. Childhood sexual abuse and obesity. *Obes Rev*. 2004;5(3):129–135 PMID: 15245381 https://doi.org/10.1111/j.1467-789X.2004.00145.x
109. Felitti VJ. Childhood sexual abuse, depression, and family dysfunction in adult obese patients: a case control study. *South Med J*. 1993;86(7):732–736 PMID: 8322078 https://doi.org/10.1097/00007611-199307000-00002
110. Walling MK, O'Hara MW, Reiter RC, Milburn AK, Lilly G, Vincent SD. Abuse history and chronic pain in women: II. A multivariate analysis of abuse and psychological morbidity. *Obstet Gynecol*. 1994;84(2):200–206 PMID: 8041530
111. Smolak L, Murnen SK. A meta-analytic examination of the relationship between child sexual abuse and eating disorders. *Int J Eat Disord*. 2002;31(2):136–150 PMID: 11920975 https://doi.org/10.1002/eat.10008
112. Léonard S, Steiger H, Kao A. Childhood and adulthood abuse in bulimic and nonbulimic women: prevalences and psychological correlates. *Int J Eat Disord*. 2003;33(4):397–405 PMID: 12658669 https://doi.org/10.1002/eat.10176
113. Romans SE, Gendall KA, Martin JL, Mullen PE. Child sexual abuse and later disordered eating: a New Zealand epidemiological study. *Int J Eat Disord*. 2001;29(4):380–392 PMID: 11285575 https://doi.org/10.1002/eat.1034
114. Dube SR, Felitti VJ, Dong M, Chapman DP, Giles WH, Anda RF. Childhood abuse, neglect, and household dysfunction and the risk of illicit drug use: the adverse childhood experiences study. *Pediatrics*. 2003;111(3):564–572 PMID: 12612237 https://doi.org/10.1542/peds.111.3.564
115. Dube SR, Anda RF, Felitti VJ, Edwards VJ, Croft JB. Adverse childhood experiences and personal alcohol abuse as an adult. *Addict Behav*. 2002;27(5):713–725 PMID: 12201379 https://doi.org/10.1016/S0306-4603(01)00204-0
116. Walker EA, Keegan D, Gardner G, Sullivan M, Bernstein D, Katon WJ. Psychosocial factors in fibromyalgia compared with rheumatoid arthritis: II. Sexual, physical, and emotional abuse and neglect. *Psychosom Med*. 1997;59(6):572–577 PMID: 9407574 https://doi.org/10.1097/00006842-199711000-00003
117. Finestone HM, Stenn P, Davies F, Stalker C, Fry R, Koumanis J. Chronic pain and health care utilization in women with a history of childhood sexual abuse. *Child Abuse Negl*. 2000;24(4):547–556 PMID: 10798843 https://doi.org/10.1016/S0145-2134(00)00112-5

CHAPTER 30

Neurobiological Consequences of Childhood Maltreatment

Emma Jane Rose, PhD
Assistant Research Professor
Associate Director, Program for Translational Research on Adversity and Neurodevelopment
Edna Bennett Pierce Prevention Research Center
The Center for Healthy Children
The Pennsylvania State University
University Park, PA

Diana H. Fishbein, PhD
Director, Program for Translational Research on Adversity and Neurodevelopment
Edna Bennett Pierce Prevention Research Center
Professor, Department of Human Development and Family Studies
The Pennsylvania State University
University Park, PA

Introduction

The effect of childhood maltreatment extends far beyond the immediate trauma endured by children who experience abuse and neglect. Those who experience abuse, neglect, and other forms of maltreatment during their formative years often exhibit cognitive and behavioral deficits and impaired social cognition.[1–5] In addition, a history of childhood maltreatment predicts heightened risk for a range of mental health disorders, such as posttraumatic stress disorder (PTSD) and other anxiety disorders, depression, and substance use disorder (SUD).[1,6–8] The increased risk for these psychiatric conditions does not only occur in concert with episodes of maltreatment; rather, it is pervasive across the life span.

Underlying many mental health diagnoses associated with childhood maltreatment are trauma-related modifications in a system of overlapping networks in the brain.[6–9] This potential for maltreatment to modify neural systems is aided by the protracted trajectory of normal human neurodevelopment—maturation of the human brain lasts well into emerging and early adulthood, providing multiple opportunities to critically affect development—and by the fact that neurodevelopment is strongly influenced by experiential factors.[10,11] Childhood maltreatment engenders neurodevelopmental changes through the promotion of biological processes (physiological, hormonal, and neurochemical) that affect both structure and function in brain regions that are critical for adaptive, optimal functioning.[11,12] Commonly involved networks include those that support affective processes, such as fear, threat, and reward, and those that are critical for cognitive control and flexibility. Maltreatment exerts lasting changes on brain regions and networks via an effect on cortisol and catecholamines, hormonal factors relating to stress and trauma. These hormonal changes, in turn, affect processes underlying the differentiation of brain structures across development.[11,13]

Not all individuals who show these neurodevelopmental changes develop subsequent mental health disorders; for those who do, there is considerable variation in symptoms, diagnoses, severity, and outcomes. Moreover, while many maltreatment-related changes in neurobiology are detrimental and lead to poor mental health, these effects may not all be, at their core, maladaptive. For example, changes in brain structure and function that often characterize risk for later mental health disorders may have, paradoxically, originated as a means of adapting to the trauma, allowing the child to cope with a toxic developmental environment in the short term.[6]

Despite evidence of the neurobiological effects of childhood maltreatment, there is not a clear understanding of the mechanisms by which maltreatment affects neurodevelopmental trajectories in relation to mental health disorders.[14] This impedes the determination of which children may be most at risk[15] and, thus, has limited our ability to prevent adverse mental health outcomes. A more complete understanding of the neurobiological trajectories following childhood maltreatment must include a determination of trauma-related changes that potentially arise as a result of neurobiological *adaptations*.

This chapter summarizes the outcomes of brain imaging studies focusing on individuals who have experienced childhood maltreatment. It considers neuroimaging findings reflective of changes in brain structure and function in maltreated individuals with and without psychiatric histories and the relative differences and similarities between these groups, as well as across studies and developmental stages. It also delineates the mechanisms and pathways that underlie associations between maltreatment and neurodevelopment and outlines potential mediators and moderators of this relationship (eg, abuse type, timing, and chronicity; genetic factors; sex differences).

As such, this chapter aims to describe the most consistent and pertinent neurobiological outcomes in those who experience childhood maltreatment and subsequently develop mental health conditions, compared with those who do not experience negative mental health outcomes; consider potential mechanisms that underlie these neurobiological changes; and elucidate critical mediators and moderators of the relationship between maltreatment and neurobiology. Given the implications of these findings, the chapter also aims to outline the implications for prevention and treatment, including whether or not maltreatment-related changes in the brain are malleable and, if so, if they can be effectively targeted (or even reversed) with appropriate interventions, and discuss experimental limitations that constrain our current understanding of the neurobiological consequences of childhood maltreatment and highlight future directions to address these concerns.

Neurobiological Outcomes in Children Who Experience Maltreatment

Psychopathology

A history of maltreatment predicts around 45% of childhood-onset and 30% of adult-onset psychiatric disorders[16] and is associated with more severe forms of adverse mental health outcomes.[17,18] Those with such a history experience mental health problems with earlier onset, greater severity, and less responsivity to treatment, compared with individuals without a history of maltreatment.[1,6] According to the theory of latent vulnerability, childhood maltreatment leads to changes in multiple levels of cognitive and neurobiological functioning as a means of "recalibrating" in response to adversity or trauma.[14] In the long term, this systems-level change increases the risk for poor mental health. From this postulation, it follows that neurobiological systems affected by maltreatment should be measurable in childhood and serve as biomarkers for the risk of psychiatric diagnosis in adolescence and/or adulthood.

Posttraumatic Stress Disorder

Anxiety disorders (ie, PTSD, obsessive-compulsive disorder, generalized anxiety disorder, social phobia, and panic disorder) are the most common mental health disorders in the United States.[19] While genetic risk plays a role in their prevalence,[20] exposure to psychosocial stressors, such as child abuse or neglect, significantly increases the likelihood of their development. Of these disorders, one of the most common among those who experience maltreatment is PTSD. A history of childhood maltreatment increases the lifetime likelihood of a diagnosis of PTSD by almost 5 times.[21] Moreover, having experienced maltreatment and other types of childhood adversity appears to make individuals more susceptible to developing PTSD following a trauma experienced in adulthood.[22] As with most other psychopathologies, maltreated individuals who develop PTSD have a tendency toward more severe and complex symptoms, are more likely to have a comorbid diagnosis (eg, depression), and, consequently, are also at increased risk of being designated as having "complex PTSD."[23,24]

Posttraumatic stress disorder can be thought of as a disorder of recovery, where an individual continues to reexperience a traumatic event that has already passed. Through the learning process of conditioning, reminders of the trauma help to cause the fear response to persist.[25] Key brain areas involved in the extinction of fear response that are highly sensitive to stress and are involved in learning and memory include the amygdala, hippocampus, anterior cingulate cortex, and ventromedial prefrontal cortex. Morphological studies of the brain in those who have experienced childhood maltreatment and subsequently develop PTSD in adulthood have found smaller volumes in all of these brain regions.[26,27] However, the precise relationship between volume in these regions and PTSD is not yet clear.

With regard to brain function in PTSD secondary to childhood maltreatment, it is interesting to note that a number of studies have found maltreatment-related variability in activity in those same regions that are structurally implicated in the failed extinction of the fear response. A history of childhood trauma in those with PTSD has been shown to correlate with activation in the anterior cingulate cortex during the processing of threat-related stimuli, such as fearful or angry faces.[28,29] For example, patients with complex PTSD *and* a history of childhood sexual or physical abuse show increased activation in brain regions that are involved in cognitive control, including the anterior cingulate cortex, when presented with trauma-related words.[30] Similarly, PTSD following childhood sexual abuse has been linked to reduced hippocampal activity while recalling facts or performing other functions of declarative memory.[31] Moreover, PTSD following childhood maltreatment has been shown to affect the functional connectivity of extinction-related brain areas, such as the amygdala,[32] and may specifically predict altered ventral prefrontal-subcortical connectivity.[33]

Collectively, these outcomes suggest that variability in structural volume, function, and functional connectivity in extinction-related brain regions may be one pathway by which childhood maltreatment leads to

PTSD, either in youth or adulthood. However, further longitudinal work is needed to delineate the pertinent neurobiological mechanisms that underlie risk for or resilience to PTSD following maltreatment.[34]

Major Depressive Disorder

The seminal Adverse Childhood Experiences (ACE) study (see Chapter 29, Medical and Psychological Sequelae of Child Abuse and Neglect) provided some of the strongest evidence to date for the association between childhood maltreatment and major depressive disorder (MDD),[35] with the authors demonstrating that the risk for MDD was not only predicted by maltreatment-related adversity but that risk increased linearly with the number of ACEs and in a dose-dependent manner. This environmental link between maltreatment and MDD is further supported by twin studies that suggest a relatively minor role of heritability in the risk for depression[36] and prospective longitudinal studies that have revealed a 2-fold increase in MDD in those with a history of childhood maltreatment.[16,21] As with many of the other psychopathologies, depression appears earlier in maltreated individuals and is more intractable.[17] Depressed patients with a history of childhood maltreatment also show more severe symptoms, including mood, neurovegetative, and endogenous symptoms, and higher rates of comorbidities, compared with those with depression without this history.[17]

From a neurobiological perspective, one of most relevant outcomes is evidence of maltreatment-related reduction in hippocampal volume in MDD. Across multiple studies, there is strong support for reduced hippocampal volume in those diagnosed with MDD, so much so that it is commonly considered a key biomarker of this disorder. However, a pivotal study by Vythilingam and colleagues in women with MDD found that only those participants who had a history of childhood physical or sexual abuse exhibited MDD-related reductions in hippocampal volume.[37] This finding has not only been replicated in multiple other studies,[38–40] but it has been suggested that the evidence of reduced hippocampal volume is more consistent in adults with a history of childhood maltreatment, regardless of the presence or absence of MDD, than it is for MDD alone.[1,41,42] Accordingly, reduced hippocampal volume may be a consequence of early trauma that serves as a potential risk factor for MDD.[1]

Additional structural deficits in depressed patients with a history of childhood maltreatment may include widespread alterations in white matter, such as reduced white matter volume[43] and altered diffusivity,[44,45] and reduced prefrontal gray matter volume,[39] including orbitofrontal cortex and dorsomedial prefrontal cortex.[38] Deficits in dorsomedial prefrontal cortex in healthy controls and unmedicated patients with affective disorders with a history of emotional maltreatment suggests that reduced volume in this region is a potential marker of childhood maltreatment rather than of affective disorders per se.[46] In contrast, gray matter reductions in orbitofrontal cortex have been noted in patients with MDD *and* a history of childhood maltreatment compared with patients without such experiences,[47] which may signal a combined effect of MDD and maltreatment, although the absence of controls with a history of maltreatment in this study precludes delineating whether structural deficits in orbitofrontal cortex are indicative of childhood maltreatment more generally (ie, in the absence of psychopathology).

Familial risk for MDD is one factor that potentially influences the interplay between childhood maltreatment, MDD, and structural variability in the brain; some studies have considered how these factors may vary according to familial risk for MDD. For example, among healthy individuals with a history of childhood maltreatment, having a first-degree relative with a history of MDD has been associated with reduced volume in the hippocampus, dorsolateral prefrontal cortex (dlPFC), medial prefrontal cortex, and anterior cingulate cortex,[48] as well as in the insula and orbitofrontal cortex, compared with those who do not have a family history of MDD.[49] While further exploration of the relative contributions of familial versus environmental risk is required, especially to reconcile differences between these 2 comparatively small neuroimaging studies, these outcomes suggest a combined genetic and environmental risk underlying structural abnormalities in MDD, perhaps mediated by epigenetic modifications.

Neurobiological effects of childhood maltreatment in those with depression extend to variability in brain function. As with structural findings, it appears that maltreatment contributes substantially to some "classic" neurobiological features in MDD. Compared with healthy individuals, those with MDD reliably show an increased response to negative stimuli in the amygdala, insula, and dorsal anterior cingulate and lower response in the dorsal striatum and dlPFC.[50] Explorations of the functional correlates of MDD in those with and without a history of childhood maltreatment have found diminished reward-dependent activity in the ventral striatum as a function of emotional neglect, which predicts the emergence of depressive symptoms in adolescents[51] and reduced functional connectivity strength in prefrontal-limbic-thalamic-cerebellar circuitry during resting (ie, while not engaged in goal-directed tasks) in depressed patients who experienced childhood maltreatment.[52] Moreover, a history of emotional maltreatment is associated with enhanced activity in the amygdala in response to emotional faces and hypoactivity in the medial prefrontal cortex during the encoding and recognition of emotional words, regardless of patient status (ie, control vs MDD) or illness severity.[53,54] A history of early life trauma has also been associated with failed inhibition in a functional network involving medial prefrontal cortex and the amygdala, which underlies emotional regulation, in those with MDD and a history of maltreatment but not in patients without such history.[55] Collectively, these data suggest that emotional maltreatment in childhood enhances the risk for depression through a dual process of "blunting" higher order cognitive processing and enhancing lower order emotional processes.[53]

Psychosis

The possibility of developing psychotic disorders, such as schizophrenia, is markedly increased in those who experience childhood trauma.[56–60] Moreover, childhood maltreatment influences the trajectory of psychosis, with maltreated cohorts showing more severe symptoms[61,62] and greater stress sensitivity than peers who have not been maltreated.[63] Multiple studies have considered the relationships between childhood maltreatment, psychosis, and brain structure. In one early study, Sheffield and colleagues found that a history of childhood sexual abuse, but not other types of maltreatment, predicted a reduction in total gray matter volume in patients with psychosis and that, within a segment of the prefrontal cortex, volume was negatively correlated with the severity of sexual abuse.[64] Similarly, Cancel et al found that total gray matter volume was negatively correlated with emotional neglect scores in patients with psychosis.[65] These authors also found that as the severity of emotional neglect increased, volume in the dlPFC decreased, which, in turn, predicted the severity of disorganization in patients.

The structural neurobiological effects of childhood maltreatment in those with psychosis include aspects of structural connectivity, such as variation in measurable aspects of the "intactness" of white matter. The integrity of white matter appears to be negatively affected by early childhood stress and trauma,[66] and there is a high degree of similarity in the white matter tracts affected by ACEs and those that show psychosis-related variability.[67–69] Using diffusion tensor imaging (ie, a magnetic resonance imaging technique for mapping white matter tracts in the brain) in a relatively homogenous sample of patients with schizophrenia, Poletti and colleagues found a negative correlation between the severity of adverse experiences and fractional anisotropy (ie, a quantifiable measure that relates to the organization and integrity of white matter fibers) in several white matter tracts (ie, corona radiata, thalamic radiations, corpus callosum, cingulum bundle, superior longitudinal fasciculus, inferior fronto-occipital fasciculus, and uncinate fasciculus).[70] Lower fractional anisotropy values are indicative of reduced fiber coherence and integrity, so these outcomes suggest that more severe trauma leads to greater deficits in white matter connectivity and that, consequently, childhood maltreatment may contribute to an increased risk for psychosis via an effect on the structural connectivity of corticolimbic networks.

Substance Use Disorder

A number of studies point to childhood maltreatment as a potent risk factor for substance use and dependence.[71] An estimated 40% to 50% of individuals who experience maltreatment in childhood develop a substance use problem in their lifetime.[72] Correspondingly, a history of child abuse or neglect is highly prevalent in adults with SUD, and those with such a history begin using illicit substances twice as often as peers who have not been maltreated and are more likely to use substances earlier in adolescence.[72,73] This effect does not appear to be specific to substance use of one type or another; indeed, childhood maltreatment predicts higher rates of use for a range of substances in adulthood, including nicotine,[74] alcohol,[75,76] methamphetamine,[77] heroin,[78] and cocaine.[79] Moreover, the effect of trauma extends beyond an increased risk for substance use; it also contributes to patterns of substance use and long-term outcomes. For example, substance-dependent individuals with a history of maltreatment are more likely than those without such history to experience severe negative consequences of substance use,[80] are at increased risk of dropping out of treatment,[81] and are more likely to relapse after being abstinent.[82] While substance use following childhood maltreatment can be associated with higher rates and greater severity of other psychopathologies, such as PTSD, anxiety, and depression,[83–86] it is important to note that substance use subsequent to maltreatment can occur without a comorbid diagnosis.[87]

Neurobiological changes at the level of brain structure and function are associated with childhood maltreatment and SUD[1,41,88–90] and are often found in overlapping regions and networks. Disentangling the specific contributions of maltreatment per se versus those changes that arise in response to early and sustained use of substances presents an interesting challenge. Research in this domain must aim to understand the contributions of maltreatment and SUD to brain development independently, as well as the interactive neurodevelopmental effects specifically related to being an individual with a history of maltreatment who develops an SUD. A recent review of the neurocognitive evidence of neurobiological pathways underlying the risk for SUD in childhood maltreatment, by Puetz and McCrory, considered evidence of compromise in 3 interconnected systems that may heighten SUD vulnerability. The evidence presented in that review regarding functional and structural changes in the brain that underlie addictive propensities in individuals who have experienced maltreatment is summarized here.[91]

Reward Processing

Perturbations of the mesocorticolimbic and nigrostriatal pathways that constitute the brain's reward system are a primary feature of SUD.[92,93] Functional and structural alterations in the regions that lie along these pathways are ubiquitous for SUD across a range of substances[94,95] and appear to be associated with a reduced sensitivity to natural rewards and a potent increase in the perceived value of drugs and drug-related cues.[96] Behaviorally, children and adolescents who experience maltreatment are less sensitive to monetary rewards than peers who have not been maltreated, in a manner that suggests heightened impulsivity and reduced goal-directed behavior.[97] Functional imaging studies of reward processing indicate that childhood maltreatment makes positive or rewarding cues less compelling and that this is associated with reduced activation in midbrain regions typically linked to reward anticipation.[98,99] Structural deficits along reward pathways have also been found in maltreated groups, including volumetric deficits in the anterior cingulate cortex and striatum[100,101] and reduced white matter integrity in fronto-striatal pathways.[102]

Executive Control Function

Deficits in executive control function, such as cognitive control and response inhibition, are another key feature of SUD.[103] Along with impairments in emotional regulation,[104] SUD-related variability in executive control function underlies the behavioral impulsivity that is stereotypical of individuals who are dependent on substances.[105] Executive control function deficits are found consistently in maltreated people and appear to be driven by prefrontal cortical deficits.[91] Related structural deficits are, for example, seen in key executive control function regions such as dlPFC and medial prefrontal cortex,[46,106] orbitofrontal cortex,[88,107–109] and anterior cingulate cortex.[101] In addition, adolescents with a history of physical and sexual abuse show increased prefrontal activation (including in the dorsal anterior cingulate cortex) during effortful control, compared with peers who have not been maltreated.[110] While not many neuroimaging studies have specifically considered the contributions of childhood maltreatment to brain function in dependent adults, related effects in regions associated with emotion regulation and cognitive control may be a key factor in the increased risk of relapse in individuals with an SUD and a history of maltreatment versus peers.[111]

Threat Processing

Affective processing is often compromised in SUD[112,113] and significantly affected by maltreatment.[114] Individuals in both groups, independently and combined, are more sensitive to threat-related stimuli, such as angry or fearful faces,[115,116] and are more likely to avoid threat-related cues.[15,117] The amygdala is critical for these types of threat-related responses, due in part to its role in detecting salient environmental stimuli.[118] While there is inconsistent evidence of maltreatment-related structural variability in the amygdala,[119,120] the available evidence reliably points to a relationship to variability in amygdala function. For example, multiple studies suggest that children who have been maltreated show heightened amygdala activity in response to angry faces, compared with controls.[121] The amygdala is also an area of interest in SUDs because it appears to be involved in drug craving.[122,123] While relatively few studies have considered the role of the amygdala in SUD specifically in maltreated groups, there is some evidence to support the notion that, in individuals with a history of maltreatment who develop substance use and dependence, the ability of some drugs of abuse (eg, alcohol) to induce anxiolytic effects by attenuating activity in the amygdala may be a driving factor in substance use behaviors.[124]

Nonclinical Cohorts

As noted in the previous section, childhood maltreatment is consistently associated with an increased propensity for a range of mental health diagnoses across the life span. However, not all individuals who experience maltreatment develop symptoms of psychiatric illness.[125] Indeed, some individuals with a history of maltreatment are comparatively resilient to mental health problems, despite potentially showing evidence of neurobiological effects. There is also considerable variation in the presentation of mental health disorders. Determining the similarities and differences in neurobiological outcomes in those who have experienced maltreatment and either do or do not develop subsequent mental health symptoms has great potential to guide the design and refinement of effective interventions. For example, the delineation of putatively adaptive neurobiological modifications in relatively resilient individuals (ie, those changes in brain structure and function that allow the individual to adapt effectively to the stressful experience of abuse or neglect) may provide biomarkers for determining the efficacy of evidence-based intervention strategies, helping to ascertain which approaches work for which individuals and under what circumstances, or even biological targets in the prevention and/or treatment of negative sequelae.

An important caveat is that, even in the absence of mental health symptoms, resilient individuals may still experience negative consequences, such as neurocognitive dysfunction, as a result of changes in underlying neurobiology. Neurobiological alterations may, in effect, interfere with development of adaptations that would otherwise allow the individual to maintain function in other domains. Alternatively, changes that may be adaptive in an earlier developmental phase to meet existing environmental challenges may lead to negative outcomes later in development. Studies are needed to ascertain whether neurobiological changes that appear to be adaptive with regard to mental health do so at the expense of function in other domains. Further delineating these complex pathways will be useful in the design of interventions that address dysfunction while preserving or further strengthening other critical processes.

Differential Pathways: Clinical Versus Nonclinical Cohorts

Clearly, constitutional characteristics and internal psychological processes interact with environmental conditions to affect mental health outcomes.[126] A rapidly growing body of evidence indicates that those who experience childhood maltreatment and do not develop mental health disorders differ from those who do in neurobiological, psychophysiological, and behavioral responses to stress.[127] Thus, while maladaptive stress responses associated with maltreatment may exacerbate poor psychological functioning, stress does not invariably result in a mental health disorder. The lack of a universal relationship between stress and psychiatric disorder suggests that stress triggers a predisposition to such problems in an already vulnerable neurobiological system.[128] Because stress adaptations and mental health disorders are interrelated, have reciprocal influences, and have similar neurobehavioral manifestations, the issue of whether psychiatric disorders are moderators or outcomes cannot be entirely untangled. Literature consistently indicates that susceptibility to a mental health disorder is largely genetic, and expression of that susceptibility may be conferred through experience (eg, stress).[129] Future longitudinal neuroimaging studies are likely to provide more sensitive and specific markers of the neurobehavioral dimensions underlying mental health diagnoses that are differentially associated with different types of maltreatment (eg, abuse vs neglect). A multisystem approach to this issue of who is more at risk versus those who are comparatively resilient has the potential to provide a comprehensive picture of how maltreatment relates to vulnerable neurocognitive networks, thereby increasing risk for mental health disorders.

Moderators of the relationship between childhood maltreatment and subsequent mental health disorders include an increased sensitivity to consequences or an adaptive coping style that may provide insulation from a poor outcome, perhaps preventing development of a mental health disorder.[130] On the other hand, the relationship between maltreatment and mental health disorders may become amplified in the presence of later experiences, such as substance use or domestic violence, via bidirectional interactions with stress adaptations.[131] Furthermore, aspects of parenting style, family structure, and neighborhood characteristics may either exacerbate or inhibit negative psychological outcomes.[132–134] Thus, even when exposures to stressors are similar, individual outcomes can be quite different. To advance scientific understanding of risk and resilience and inform prevention and treatment, it is crucial to explore whether individual differences in effects of stressors on neurobiology and behavior lead to different pathways and outcomes.

The Role of Stress Neurobiology

There are many similarities in the alterations of brain circuits in individuals with mental health disorders and those who experience severe and/or chronic stress and adversity. Furthermore, dysfunctions in the neurocognitive and emotion regulatory functions underpinned by these circuits are often found in individuals with mental illness and those who have experienced trauma or other adversities, including childhood maltreatment[135] (Figure 30.1). This observation is instructive because it suggests that maltreatment may increase risk for mental health disorders via its effects on aspects of brain structure and function that mediate the stress response, irrespective of the specific type of trauma. While the existing literature cannot fully support this mechanistic hypothesis, consistent findings implicating brain networks involved in stress responses to maltreatment and in a range of mental health disorders, as well as the high rate of co-occurrence of maltreatment and various psychopathologies, provides some tantalizing clues about how childhood maltreatment exerts its effects. At a minimum, their comorbidity appears to exacerbate poor outcomes for those who have experienced maltreatment and compromise treatment success.[136–139]

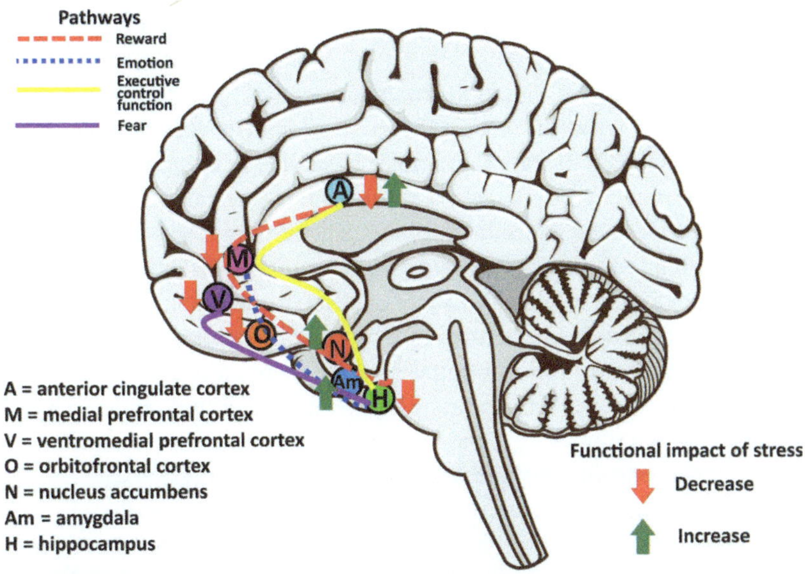

FIGURE 30.1

The functional effect of stress on brain regions and pathways related to childhood maltreatment. Shown here are those brain regions that have been consistently implicated in the neurobiological effects of maltreatment (either functionally or structurally) and which are known to be functionally affected (increased or decreased) by the experience of stress. (For the anterior cingulate cortex, some studies indicate an increase in activity with stress, while others indicate a decrease.) The depiction of individual pathways shown here is not neuroanatomically accurate; rather, the figure depicts simply the links between different, spatially distinct regions that show coordinated activity in the support of particular cognitive and affective processes that are affected by maltreatment and stress and for which disruption may underlie many of the maladaptive outcomes associated with childhood maltreatment.

Stress adaptations have been defined as a process involving perception, interpretation, response, and adjustment to harmful, threatening, or challenging events.[140] This conceptualization involves 4 facets of stress adaptation: nature and severity of the events that cause stress (ie, stressors), cognitive and emotional processes used to evaluate and appraise the events and determine available coping responses, biological responses and adaptations needed to cope, and behavioral and cognitive responses to the events.[141] Cumulative exposure to stressors can exhaust available internal and external resources, leading to maladaptations in response to daily challenges and to future acutely stressful events, thus exerting long-term effects on behavioral pathways. For some, these maladaptations appear to sensitize responses to later acute stressors; for others, they may lead to a desensitization of stress responses. Both orientations may be related to risk for mental health disorders since the neural and behavioral systems responsible for stress adaptations are the same systems implicated in mental health.[142] In effect, both stress and mental health problems are processed by, and may subsequently alter, the same neural network.[143]

More often than not, childhood maltreatment is typified by its chronicity or severity. Chronic or severe stress, in turn, exerts an effect on stress signaling pathways that impair the ability of the prefrontal cortex to exert cognitive control over more reflexive responses. Indeed, maltreatment-related neurodevelopmental deficits or delays in mesocorticolimbic circuits may underlie the compromise of regulatory functions mediated by this network of prefrontal and limbic regions.[144,145] As a result, the experience of maltreatment may compromise social, behavioral, cognitive, and emotional functioning in profound ways. One such consequence is the predominance of reflexive versus reflective reactions, which translates to greater impulsivity and compromised executive decision-making and deliberation. Cumulative stressor exposures can further perturb hormonal systems (eg, cortisol) that modulate these functions[146]; chronically elevated levels of stress hormones can reduce volume of the hippocampus, impairing memory and decision-making.[147,148] Psychophysiological studies also show effects of stress on autonomic responses such as heart rate, which, when perturbed, are associated with poor behavioral and emotional regulation and cognitive and coping skill deficits.[149–151] These physiological and behavioral stress responses activate the same neural systems found altered in many mental health disorders, including the dopaminergic mesocorticolimbic circuitry,[152] the implications being that the response to stress and the severity of mental health disorders may be heightened. The functional consequences of alterations in these neurobehavioral processes are poor stress adaptations manifested as impaired coordination between social, cognitive, psychological, and emotional responses thought to be critical in self-regulation of behavior and emotion.

The model depicted in Figure 30.2 applies a developmental psychopathology approach to delineating the relationships between childhood maltreatment, stress neurobiology, and mental health outcomes by considering the influence of individual and environmental transactions on the development of mental health disorders; the influence of individual differences in stress adaptations on onset, maintenance, worsening, or improvement in mental health symptomatology; multiple pathways (*equifinality*) to mental health disorders via cognitive, emotional, and physiologic dysregulation resulting from exposure to cumulative stress; and the influence of childhood behavioral and emotional problems and other psychosocial variables associated with future adaptation.[153,154] The aim of the model is to illustrate how cumulative exposure to stressors might influence the development and integrity of stress adaptations, as

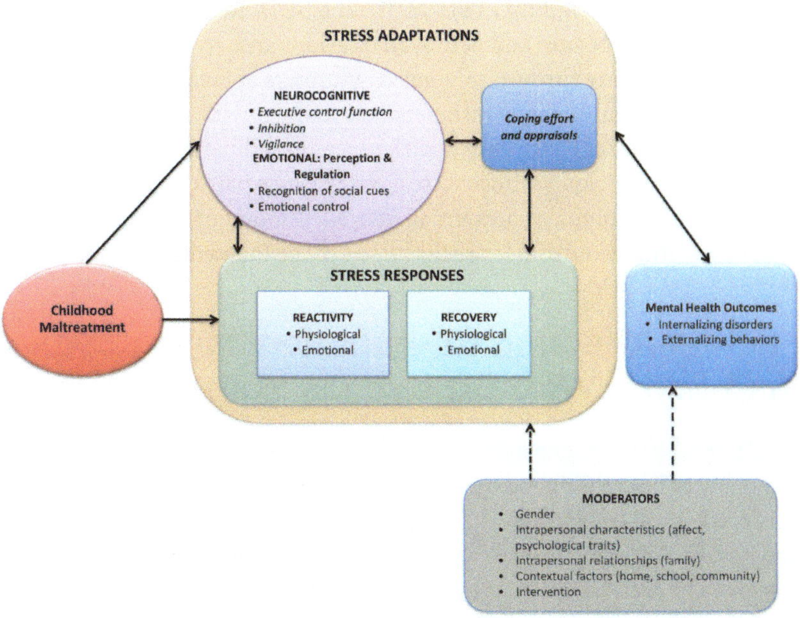

FIGURE 30.2

The relationship between childhood maltreatment, stress adaptations, and transitions to maladaptive mental health outcomes. This diagram shows the stress adaptation pathways by which the experience of maltreatment may lead to poor mental health, including physiological and emotional stress responses, neurocognitive functions, and emotion regulation and perception. In addition to stress-related mechanisms, whether or not the experience of maltreatment ultimately leads to psychopathology is moderated by a number of individual level and contextual factors (shown here in the gray box).

defined by neurocognitive and emotion regulatory functions, physiological reactivity and sensitivity to stress stimuli, and recovery of these functions to baseline. Integrity of these functions, in turn, influences effectiveness of coping efforts. Given the malleability of the prefrontal cortex in the context of environmental inputs, the focus is on executive control function, which is modulated by the prefrontal cortex, including decision-making, inhibition, sensitivity to consequences, and regulation of emotional responses. Responses throughout this system are also altered by stressful experiences over time and implicated in the ability to cope with future stressors. These responses include psychophysiological processes such as hypothalamic-pituitary-adrenal (HPA) axis function (eg, cortisol) and electrophysiological indexes (eg, heart rate, respiratory sinus arrhythmia, pulse transit time).[150,151] Deficits in neurocognition, emotion regulation, and physiological responses are associated with maladaptive coping strategies, which can further impair decision-making and self-regulation.[155] This constellation of alterations in biological and psychological processes is, in turn, related to a variety of mental health disorders, including PTSD, MDD, and SUD. The relationships between stress exposure and neural adaptations and, in turn, mental health disorders are further influenced by a range of factors (eg, gender, interpersonal relationships, intrapersonal characteristics, contextual factors) that further contribute to differences in individual propensity for mental health problems. Those factors that may be particularly pertinent for the influence of maltreatment on neurodevelopmental trajectories leading to adverse outcomes are discussed in the following section.

Factors Affecting Neurobiological Outcomes in Children Who Experience Maltreatment

Maltreatment-Dependent Factors

The study of how childhood maltreatment exerts an influence on neurobiological trajectories is a comparatively young field of study and has tended to focus on those with a history of sexual or physical abuse or children who witnessed domestic violence. In many studies, participants are selected on the basis of existing psychopathology, such as PTSD, and/or may have been exposed to multiple types of trauma and adversity. Furthermore, multiple types of abuse or neglect are often regarded under the single category of maltreatment. In light of studies that suggest differential associations between types of maltreatment (eg, emotional abuse vs physical abuse or neglect) and specific patterns of brain structure and function,[156] it is critical that the field aims to more fully delineate variations and similarities in neurobiological outcomes relative to maltreatment type. Given that the type of trauma experienced is an important factor in clinical outcomes (eg, those who have experienced sexual abuse are at increased risk for self-harm and eating disorders[157,158]), it seems reasonable to assume that the type of maltreatment experienced by any given individual may be a critical factor in the neurodevelopmental effects observed and the risk for specific outcomes later in life.

In addition to the critical issue of how the type of maltreatment might influence neurodevelopmental outcomes, other factors that might be important to consider are the timing and chronicity of abuse. As with type of maltreatment, there is not currently sufficient literature to conclude precisely how timing and chronicity may affect brain development, either alone or in combination with other aspects of trauma and key environmental factors. Nonetheless, neurocognitive studies suggest that children who experience trauma earlier and with greater chronicity may be more likely to show dysregulation in the types of neurocognitive processes that are known to be relevant to psychopathological outcomes, such as executive control function or emotion regulatory deficits.[135] It is possible that earlier trauma or trauma at times of developmental sensitivity (ie, so-called critical periods) may lead to distinctive or particularly detrimental outcomes by disrupting normative development, which may, in turn, be exacerbated by chronic, unrelenting trauma throughout development.

Maltreatment-Independent Factors

Genetic Factors

Genetic vulnerabilities play a significant role in whether an individual will experience maltreatment-related neuroadaptations that lead to mental health disorders, and those genetic vulnerabilities that mediate or moderate how the brain responds to stress may be particularly relevant. Emerging literature points to an association among childhood maltreatment, psychiatric diagnosis, and a common variant of the brain-derived neurotrophic factor (BDNF) gene. Gene BDNF plays an important role in neurodevelopment through the promotion of neuronal survival and supporting neuronal migration and is involved in synaptic sprouting and remodeling.[159–161] Genetic susceptibilities for psychiatric illness have been associated with a single-nucleotide polymorphism (SNP) that results in the substitution of valine (Val) for methionine (Met) at codon 66 of the gene. This SNP is commonly known as *Val66Met* and is linked to a reduction in the levels of biologically available BDNF.[162]

In terms of psychopathology, having a Met allele for *Val66Met* is associated with increased risk for affective disorders, especially those that occur following childhood trauma.[163–165] Being a Met "carrier" also predicts reduced volume in the hippocampus and subcallosal medial prefrontal cortex in adults who experienced childhood maltreatment, regardless of mental health status (ie, healthy adult or adult with depression).[166–170] Conversely, individuals who are homozygous for the Val allele and experience early life stress show increased amygdala volume, which, in turn, is associated with increased anxiety.[168]

Intriguingly, the influence of BDNF on maltreatment-dependent changes in brain structure appears to vary across developmental trajectories. For example, in one study of 4- to 12-year-olds who had been institutionalized between 0 and 5 years of age, institutionalization at this early stage of development was associated with reduced gray matter volume in hippocampus in Val homozygotes and increased amygdala volume in Met carriers,[171] which is the opposite of what has been noted in adults with histories of childhood maltreatment (ie, reduced volumes are more typically noted for Met carriers). Marusak and colleagues considered the association between this *Val66Met* variant and limbic gray matter volume in a sample of youth (7–15 years old) with high sociodemographic risk for trauma.[172] They found that in youth without trauma, being a Met carrier predicted greater volumes in the right subcallosal area and the right hippocampus and that lower hippocampal volume predicted higher levels of anxiety. Collectively, these studies suggest that the *Val66Met* variant may moderate the effect of maltreatment on volume in regions of the limbic system that are critical for affective functioning and, depending on the type and timing of trauma, may be a key factor in the development of anxiety and related mental health disorders.

Other genes that may play a role in the structural effects of childhood maltreatment include the *FKBP5* gene[173] and the oxytocin receptor gene (*OXTR*).[174] The *FKBP5* gene is a critical regulator of HPA-axis sensitivity, and activity and variants of this gene (eg, rs1360780) appear to be associated with PTSD and depression in individuals who experience childhood maltreatment.[175–177] Grabe and colleagues found that, in a large community sample, those who were homozygous for the T allele of rs1360780 and had experienced maltreatment showed reduced volumes in widespread regions of the brain, including insula, superior and middle temporal gyri, hippocampus, amygdala, and anterior cingulate cortex, compared with C carriers with histories of maltreatment. In light of the role of these brain regions in affective processing, the investigators suggest that being homozygous for the T allele of this SNP may increase the likelihood of affective disorders following childhood maltreatment.[173]

Similarly, there is an *OXTR* SNP (rs53576) that appears to moderate the association between maltreatment and structural alterations in regions that are important for affective processing. Individuals who are homozygous for the G allele of this SNP show higher levels of functioning in a number of prosocial domains,[178–180] including reward dependence,[181] while A carriers appear to experience a range of negative socioemotional outcomes.[182–184] Dannlowski and colleagues found that healthy adults who were GG homozygotes but not A-allele carriers (ie, AA or AG individuals) exhibited a significant negative correlation between volume in the ventral striatum and Childhood Trauma Questionnaire scores and a positive correlation between striatal volume and reward dependence. Furthermore, carrying a G allele for this SNP predicted increased responsiveness to emotional facial expressions in the amygdala.[174] These outcomes suggest that an increased sensitivity to social cues, expected to be facilitated by the G allele and which would normally be considered to be advantageous, may be detrimental in the face of early trauma.

Sex Differences

Sex may moderate individual responses to maltreatment that, in turn, contribute to differences in mental health and resilience outcomes.[185,186] Yet, there are discrepancies in the literature as to whether males or females are more susceptible to the adverse neurobehavioral effects of stressors in general and childhood maltreatment specifically and in ways that make them more or less prone to particular mental health problems.[185] For example, a recent review and meta-analysis found that associations between childhood maltreatment and mood disorders (eg, depression, anxiety) were larger for females compared with males. However, the authors concluded that there is currently insufficient evidence to definitively support sex-based differences in affective outcomes.[187] It has been suggested that there is a generally increased vulnerability among females relative to males to mood disorders and other internalizing disorders, while males are more vulnerable to externalizing behaviors.[188] Furthermore, given that females are more susceptible to experiencing certain types of trauma (eg, sexual abuse), while males are at heightened risk of others (eg, physical abuse),[189] it is possible that stressful experiences may produce somewhat different neurobehavioral effects depending on the nature of the experience, sex, or both. In either case, the sexes may be prone to somewhat distinctive neurobiological effects that place them at differential risk for mental illness in response to maltreatment. For example, studies suggest that the incidence of physical and sexual abuse in childhood, as well as dysfunctional families and maltreatment, is more pervasive among females with mental health problems relative to males.[190]

There is some evidence that neurobiological responses to maltreatment may differ between males and females, including in ways that confer greater risk for certain mental health problems. The adrenal cortex is more sensitive to stress in females, producing greater amounts of stress hormones, which can negatively alter mood.[191] Also, while estrogens are neuroprotective in response to stressors, the cyclic fluctuations of estrogens and progesterone serve to amplify the response to stressors, which confers susceptibility to behavioral and mental health disorders.[192] In addition, females may be more prone to negative affect in response to subjective perceptions of stress than males,[193] thereby increasing risk for mental health disorders. On the other hand, sex differences within developing brain structures such as the prefrontal cortex, amygdala, and hippocampus suggest that neurobehavioral responses to stress may offer some protection to females against poor outcomes.[194–196] The behavioral response to stress among females is better characterized as "tend and befriend,"[195] involving the use of social interactions and supports to provide protection against the stressful agent or its detrimental consequences. Females' advanced language and memory skills[197–199] and processing of emotional and social cues[200] may also protect them from neurocognitive damage that would otherwise develop in response to stress. Thus, protective factors may further amplify sex-based differences in sensitivity in their unequal exposure to maltreatment and either buffer or otherwise contribute to somewhat different pathways for the sexes. This is an area ripe for further exploration given the significant implications for the development of sex-specific interventions.

Implications for Intervention

An eventual understanding of the effect of childhood maltreatment on neural circuitry and the cognitive processes it supports is critical for developing effective and timely interventions that serve to prevent the onset of mental health disorders later in life. Although much remains to be further investigated, many researchers and clinicians argue that sufficient evidence has already been amassed to warrant investments in well-targeted preventive interventions. Two avenues for prevention are necessary to disrupt the pathway from maltreatment to mental health disorders. First, children identified as having experienced maltreatment should receive immediate services and programs that have been shown to work. An array of evidence-based practices is appropriate for preventing or attenuating traumatic stress symptoms that lead to mental health disorders. Second, inarguably, public health strategies that reduce exposure in the first place are of the utmost importance. Enhanced knowledge about the effects of maltreatment on the brain promises to provide greater precision in our ability to prevent mental health disorders as well as to direct public educational campaigns and other public health strategies to increase awareness and influence policy.

A growing number of neuroscience studies are focused on elucidating the underlying pathogenesis of preventable mental and behavioral problems, kindling a growing excitement about the potential for neuroscience to inform development of more precision-based preventive intervention approaches. A more comprehensive understanding of the neurobiological moderators and mediators of risk for and resilience to mental health disorders in the context of childhood maltreatment, and the effect of interventions on these neural signatures, has the potential to help delineate more precisely what works for whom, why, and under what circumstances. Neuroimaging is increasing our understanding of variability in treatment response through the identification of biomarkers for psychopathology. Proximal biomarkers in prevention studies are similarly needed to provide targets for preventive intervention, detect which subgroups are more or less receptive, predict intervention response, and broadly improve outcomes. Important advances in research including neuroimaging and other biomarker investigations have revealed activity within neural circuits that is associated with behavioral change in response to intervention, potentially conferring protection from mental health disorders. The application of early neuroimaging to well-established, longitudinal prevention strategies could well reveal malleable neural dimensions of functioning commonly implicated in mental health disorders and related characteristics, such as reduced cognitive control and emotion dysregulation. A better understanding of these functional dimensions and their neural correlates could identify malleable brain-behavior biomarkers as targets for improving the effects of preventive intervention.

Of specific relevance here, neurobiological research to date suggests that the type, chronicity, and timing of maltreatment may exert differential influences on neural substrates of executive control functions that are often associated with mental health disorders. For example, differences in maturational trajectories between limbic and frontal regions likely contribute to variability in the effects on neurobehavioral functioning and, in turn, mental health outcome type and severity.[201] As structures that underpin affect (eg, amygdala) mature prior to full formation and connectivity of the hippocampus and other structures that support executive control function in adolescence, susceptibility of the brain to altered growth patterns and/or damage from adverse psychosocial and environmental influences is heightened. As a result, maltreatment experienced during this period may compromise prefrontal control over affective responses.[202] Furthermore, because the prefrontal cortex takes so long to mature, the cognitive processes that depend on it may remain particularly vulnerable until early adulthood. In younger children, maltreatment may affect the building blocks of executive control function such as attention, working memory, verbal learning, and impulse control. The significance of these developmental differences is an important consideration in the design and targeting of interventions that more precisely focus on strengthening potentially weakened neural functions and connections, thereby mitigating the damage and increasing resilience.

The promise for this line of research is that outcomes will inform future directions in the field by identifying relevant targets within neurobiological and neurobehavioral pathways that are influenced by maltreatment and that should respond to prevention and treatment interventions. In turn, mental health disorders are likely to be significantly affected by preventing their development, attenuating their severity, and/or increasing their responsiveness to intervention. Furthermore, this research aims to illuminate individual differences in those who are resilient to shed light on factors that can be strengthened by more specifically targeted interventions rather than those directed toward a heterogeneous population with varying needs.[203] One such approach is to design interventions around regulatory processes that are potentially malleable.[201,202,204] For example, pharmacological or psychosocial therapies designed to stimulate activity of the amygdala and its connections (eg, akin to deep brain stimulation in depression)[205,206] and to reinforce adaptive prefrontal cortex inhibitory control may normalize cognitive and emotion regulatory deficits. A rapidly expanding body of empirical work also has emerged on the neuroscience of mindfulness effects.[207] Neuroimaging and electrophysiological studies with adults suggest that mindfulness interventions influence the neurobiological mechanisms that target regulatory and affective processes.[208–212]

Another intriguing possibility is the potential preventive effect of educating caregivers, educators, and public health and social welfare policy makers about approaches that address differential developmental pathways in youth who are exposed to abuse and neglect. For example, early enrichment, tactile stimulation, stress reduction, and other environmental enhancements early in life may strengthen prefrontal cortex cognitive control and enlarge the striatum to improve emotion regulation.[213] Current therapies can be inefficient because program components are not mapped to underlying etiologies.[214,215] Targeting components to factors that predict maltreatment-related psychopathology, which may confer differential vulnerability to mental health disorders, is likely to influence intervention responsivity and substantially improve outcomes. Future work to gain a better understanding of influences on varying outcomes for translation will guide more effective and targeted interventions. Perhaps most compelling is the potential for this line of work to reform educational systems and public health policies to understand the harm induced by childhood maltreatment across the life span and reduce exposure in the first place.

Limitations and Future Directions

Despite the wealth of evidence supporting profound neurodevelopmental effects of childhood maltreatment and ensuing psychiatric and other poor health outcomes, there remain significant gaps in our understanding of the mechanistic pathways of the effect of maltreatment in the short and longer term. This is, in part, exacerbated by methodological limitations, including the small sample sizes that often characterize neuroimaging investigations. Although this is usually due to logistical and financial concerns, such studies can be underpowered to detect the more subtle effects on neural biomarkers of maltreatment that likely portend mental health problems and related poor outcomes. In addition, most studies adopt cross-sectional designs that are not capable of providing information regarding neurobiological mechanisms or pathways or, therefore, establishing causal relationships between childhood maltreatment and specific neural markers. Moreover, with a cross-sectional approach there is little or no guarantee that the chosen time point of measurement is optimal for detecting maltreatment-related change in brain structure, function, or connectivity. The timing of assessment relative to maltreatment may be critical, and variability in the type of trauma and other factors may directly influence this association. An additional concern with the current literature on the neurobiological effects of maltreatment is the overreliance on retrospective self-report. As one might expect, a participant's ability to accurately remember and report the trauma that they experienced can be compromised, the longer the time between trauma and report becomes. For example, as time passes, individuals may become more prone to forgetting specific aspects or incidences of trauma that they experienced, especially those that occurred in early childhood, and may not be able to accurately recall the effect these experiences had on them. Finally, current reports of associations between maltreatment and neurobiological factors are sometimes compromised by inadequate matching of maltreated and control samples, especially for factors such as IQ and socioeconomic status that are linked independently to the types of altered brain function and structure that lead to poor mental health outcomes.[6,216]

It is hoped that future studies of the neurobiological sequelae of childhood maltreatment adopt a prospective longitudinal approach, with repeated brain imaging assessments over multiple years and developmental periods in larger samples that are well characterized regarding trauma histories and for other pertinent factors. Moreover, control and experimental samples should be closely matched for key personal and demographic factors. Recruiting participants closely to the time of trauma occurring has the advantage of allowing researchers to accurately assess maltreatment type and severity and to monitor neurodevelopmental pathways that unfold following childhood maltreatment. In larger, well-matched cohorts, this will facilitate a delineation of the mechanisms of neurobiological development specifically related to trauma and a determination of more subtle, smaller effects.

Conclusion

While childhood maltreatment crosses all social boundaries, the distribution of affected families is uneven; the concentration is higher among those who live in resource-poor, stressful environments, which can affect parenting and family contexts and pose a threat to children who are exposed to unstable lifestyles, violence, and crime. These risk factors are likely to act at the neurodevelopmental level, given the brain's dependence on experience, to exacerbate poor outcomes. Additional studies are needed to determine the interactive effect of maltreatment and other psychosocial risks on neurobiology and subsequent functional outcomes.

Although research in this area has overwhelmingly focused on the risks associated with maltreatment, far less is known about protective mechanisms—psychosocial and neurobiological—underlying differential child outcomes. Research shows that psychosocial protective factors can deflect the path toward mental health disorders in the long term, even in the presence of maltreatment but especially when it is detected and stopped.[217] For example, the influence of familial protective factors (eg, parental warmth, involvement, bonding, effective management practices, cohesion) on stress adaptations can potentially attenuate risk for behavioral maladjustments and poor social competency skills that often precede mental health disorders. Determining the effects of protective factors on neurodevelopment is, thus, equally as important to developing approaches to reduce exposure to maltreatment and effectively address the consequences when it does occur. In essence, the effects of risk and protective factors on neurodevelopment in the context of childhood maltreatment have yet to be fully elucidated.

In sum, to break intergenerational patterns of stressors related to childhood maltreatment and its effect on children's risk for mental health problems, there is a critical need to understand the role of neurobiological liability factors in poor outcomes. Additionally, the neurobiological mechanisms need to be identified by which protective factors operate to buffer the subgroup of children who do not develop psychopathology in spite of exposure to these adverse psychosocial conditions. Identification of neurobiological mechanisms that underlie poor versus adaptive outcomes has significant implications for designing interventions that focus on building resilience. Although there are several evidence-based preventive and treatment intervention programs, many children and adults with a history of maltreatment do not respond to these programs and, therefore, likely require more intensive interventions targeted to their individual liabilities. Individual differences in outcome may be a function of the ability of risk and protective factors to influence neurobiological stress adaptations. Thus, to effectively prevent maladaptations, the relationship between environmental, neurobiological, and genetic liabilities must be better understood.

References

1. Teicher MH, Samson JA. Childhood maltreatment and psychopathology: a case for ecophenotypic variants as clinically and neurobiologically distinct subtypes. *Am J Psychiatry*. 2013;170(10):1114–1133 PMID: 23982148 https://doi.org/10.1176/appi.ajp.2013.12070957
2. Gould F, Clarke J, Heim C, Harvey PD, Majer M, Nemeroff CB. The effects of child abuse and neglect on cognitive functioning in adulthood. *J Psychiatr Res*. 2012;46(4):500–506 PMID: 22336639 https://doi.org/10.1016/j.jpsychires.2012.01.005
3. Flynn M, Cicchetti D, Rogosch F. The prospective contribution of childhood maltreatment to low self-worth, low relationship quality, and symptomatology across adolescence: a developmental-organizational perspective. *Dev Psychol*. 2014;50(9):2165–2175 PMID: 25046123 https://doi.org/10.1037/a0037162
4. Puetz VB, Viding E, Palmer A, et al. Altered neural response to rejection-related words in children exposed to maltreatment. *J Child Psychol Psychiatry*. 2016;57(10):1165–1173 PMID: 27457415 https://doi.org/10.1111/jcpp.12595
5. Puetz VB, Zweerings J, Dahmen B, et al. Multidimensional assessment of neuroendocrine and psychopathological profiles in maltreated youth. *J Neural Transm (Vienna)*. 2016;123(9):1095–1106 PMID: 26875183 https://doi.org/10.1007/s00702-016-1509-6
6. Teicher MH, Samson JA. Annual research review: enduring neurobiological effects of childhood abuse and neglect. *J Child Psychol Psychiatry*. 2016;57(3):241–266 PMID: 26831814 https://doi.org/10.1111/jcpp.12507
7. Teicher MH, Samson JA, Anderson CM, Ohashi K. The effects of childhood maltreatment on brain structure, function and connectivity. *Nat Rev Neurosci*. 2016;17(10):652–666 PMID: 27640984 https://doi.org/10.1038/nrn.2016.111
8. De Bellis MD. The psychobiology of neglect. *Child Maltreat*. 2005;10(2):150–172 PMID: 15798010 https://doi.org/10.1177/1077559505275116
9. Bremner JD. Long-term effects of childhood abuse on brain and neurobiology. *Child Adolesc Psychiatr Clin N Am*. 2003;12(2):271–292 PMID: 12725012 https://doi.org/10.1016/S1056-4993(02)00098-6
10. Sánchez MM, Ladd CO, Plotsky PM. Early adverse experience as a developmental risk factor for later psychopathology: evidence from rodent and primate models. *Dev Psychopathol*. 2001;13(3):419–449 PMID: 11523842 https://doi.org/10.1017/S0954579401003029
11. Teicher MH, Andersen SL, Polcari A, Anderson CM, Navalta CP. Developmental neurobiology of childhood stress and trauma. *Psychiatr Clin North Am*. 2002;25(2):397–426, vii–viii PMID: 12136507 https://doi.org/10.1016/S0193-953X(01)00003-X
12. Teicher MH, Tomoda A, Andersen SL. Neurobiological consequences of early stress and childhood maltreatment: are results from human and animal studies comparable? *Ann N Y Acad Sci*. 2006;1071(1):313–323 PMID: 16891580 https://doi.org/10.1196/annals.1364.024

13. Rinne-Albers MA, van der Wee NJ, Lamers-Winkelman F, Vermeiren RR. Neuroimaging in children, adolescents and young adults with psychological trauma. *Eur Child Adolesc Psychiatry*. 2013;22(12):745–755 PMID: 23553572 https://doi.org/10.1007/s00787-013-0410-1
14. McCrory EJ, Viding E. The theory of latent vulnerability: reconceptualizing the link between childhood maltreatment and psychiatric disorder. *Dev Psychopathol*. 2015;27(2):493–505 PMID: 25997767 https://doi.org/10.1017/S0954579415000115
15. McCrory EJ, Gerin MI, Viding E. Annual research review: childhood maltreatment, latent vulnerability and the shift to preventative psychiatry—the contribution of functional brain imaging. *J Child Psychol Psychiatry*. 2017;58(4):338–357 PMID: 28295339 https://doi.org/10.1111/jcpp.12713
16. Green JG, McLaughlin KA, Berglund PA, et al. Childhood adversities and adult psychiatric disorders in the national comorbidity survey replication I: associations with first onset of DSM-IV disorders. *Arch Gen Psychiatry*. 2010;67(2):113–123 PMID: 20124111 https://doi.org/10.1001/archgenpsychiatry.2009.186
17. Nanni V, Uher R, Danese A. Childhood maltreatment predicts unfavorable course of illness and treatment outcome in depression: a meta-analysis. *Am J Psychiatry*. 2012;169(2):141–151 PMID: 22420036 https://doi.org/10.1176/appi.ajp.2011.11020335
18. Cutajar MC, Mullen PE, Ogloff JR, Thomas SD, Wells DL, Spataro J. Schizophrenia and other psychotic disorders in a cohort of sexually abused children. *Arch Gen Psychiatry*. 2010;67(11):1114–1119 PMID: 21041612 https://doi.org/10.1001/archgenpsychiatry.2010.147
19. National Institute of Mental Health. Statistics. https://www.nimh.nih.gov/health/statistics/index.shtml. Updated January 2018. Accessed June 3, 2019
20. Shimada-Sugimoto M, Otowa T, Hettema JM. Genetics of anxiety disorders: genetic epidemiological and molecular studies in humans. *Psychiatry Clin Neurosci*. 2015;69(7):388–401 PMID: 25762210 https://doi.org/10.1111/pcn.12291
21. Scott KM, Smith DR, Ellis PM. Prospectively ascertained child maltreatment and its association with DSM-IV mental disorders in young adults. *Arch Gen Psychiatry*. 2010;67(7):712–719 PMID: 20603452 https://doi.org/10.1001/archgenpsychiatry.2010.71
22. Xie P, Kranzler HR, Poling J, et al. Interactive effect of stressful life events and the serotonin transporter 5-HTTLPR genotype on posttraumatic stress disorder diagnosis in 2 independent populations. *Arch Gen Psychiatry*. 2009;66(11):1201–1209 PMID: 19884608 https://doi.org/10.1001/archgenpsychiatry.2009.153
23. Cloitre M, Stolbach BC, Herman JL, et al. A developmental approach to complex PTSD: childhood and adult cumulative trauma as predictors of symptom complexity. *J Trauma Stress*. 2009;22(5):399–408 PMID: 19795402 https://doi.org/10.1002/jts.20444
24. Sher L. Childhood abuse, suicidal behavior and the concept of post-traumatic mood disorder. *Med Hypotheses*. 2008;71(5):809–810 PMID: 18694629 https://doi.org/10.1016/j.mehy.2008.07.007
25. Yehuda R, LeDoux J. Response variation following trauma: a translational neuroscience approach to understanding PTSD. *Neuron*. 2007;56(1):19–32 PMID: 17920012 https://doi.org/10.1016/j.neuron.2007.09.006
26. Thomaes K, Dorrepaal E, Draijer N, et al. Reduced anterior cingulate and orbitofrontal volumes in child abuse-related complex PTSD. *J Clin Psychiatry*. 2010;71(12):1636–1644 PMID: 20673548 https://doi.org/10.4088/JCP.08m04754blu
27. Kitayama N, Quinn S, Bremner JD. Smaller volume of anterior cingulate cortex in abuse-related posttraumatic stress disorder. *J Affect Disord*. 2006;90(2-3):171–174 PMID: 16375974 https://doi.org/10.1016/j.jad.2005.11.006

28. Herringa RJ, Phillips ML, Fournier JC, Kronhaus DM, Germain A. Childhood and adult trauma both correlate with dorsal anterior cingulate activation to threat in combat veterans. *Psychol Med*. 2013;43(7):1533–1542 PMID: 23171514 https://doi.org/10.1017/S0033291712002310
29. Fonzo GA, Flagan TM, Sullivan S, et al. Neural functional and structural correlates of childhood maltreatment in women with intimate-partner violence-related posttraumatic stress disorder. *Psychiatry Res*. 2013;211(2):93–103 PMID: 23154098 https://doi.org/10.1016/j.pscychresns.2012.08.006
30. Herzog JI, Niedtfeld I, Rausch S, et al. Increased recruitment of cognitive control in the presence of traumatic stimuli in complex PTSD. *Eur Arch Psychiatry Clin Neurosci*. 2019;269(2):147–159 PMID: 28712089 https://doi.org/10.1007/s00406-017-0822-x
31. Bremner JD, Vythilingam M, Vermetten E, et al. MRI and PET study of deficits in hippocampal structure and function in women with childhood sexual abuse and posttraumatic stress disorder. *Am J Psychiatry*. 2003;160(5):924–932 PMID: 12727697 https://doi.org/10.1176/appi.ajp.160.5.924
32. Aghajani M, Veer IM, van Hoof MJ, Rombouts SA, van der Wee NJ, Vermeiren RR. Abnormal functional architecture of amygdala-centered networks in adolescent posttraumatic stress disorder. *Hum Brain Mapp*. 2016;37(3):1120–1135 PMID: 26859310 https://doi.org/10.1002/hbm.23093
33. Birn RM, Patriat R, Phillips ML, Germain A, Herringa RJ. Childhood maltreatment and combat posttraumatic stress differentially predict fear-related fronto-subcortical connectivity. *Depress Anxiety*. 2014;31(10):880–892 PMID: 25132653 https://doi.org/10.1002/da.22291
34. Morey RA, Haswell CC, Hooper SR, De Bellis MD. Amygdala, hippocampus, and ventral medial prefrontal cortex volumes differ in maltreated youth with and without chronic posttraumatic stress disorder. *Neuropsychopharmacology*. 2016;41(3):791–801 PMID: 26171720 https://doi.org/10.1038/npp.2015.205
35. Felitti VJ, Anda RF, Nordenberg D, et al. Relationship of childhood abuse and household dysfunction to many of the leading causes of death in adults. The Adverse Childhood Experiences (ACE) Study. *Am J Prev Med*. 1998;14(4):245–258 PMID: 9635069 https://doi.org/10.1016/S0749-3797(98)00017-8
36. Lyons MJ, Eisen SA, Goldberg J, et al. A registry-based twin study of depression in men. *Arch Gen Psychiatry*. 1998;55(5):468–472 PMID: 9596050 https://doi.org/10.1001/archpsyc.55.5.468
37. Vythilingam M, Heim C, Newport J, et al. Childhood trauma associated with smaller hippocampal volume in women with major depression. *Am J Psychiatry*. 2002;159(12):2072–2080 PMID: 12450959 https://doi.org/10.1176/appi.ajp.159.12.2072
38. Chaney A, Carballedo A, Amico F, et al. Effect of childhood maltreatment on brain structure in adult patients with major depressive disorder and healthy participants. *J Psychiatry Neurosci*. 2014;39(1):50–59 PMID: 23900024 https://doi.org/10.1503/jpn.120208
39. Frodl T, Reinhold E, Koutsouleris N, Reiser M, Meisenzahl EM. Interaction of childhood stress with hippocampus and prefrontal cortex volume reduction in major depression. *J Psychiatr Res*. 2010;44(13):799–807 PMID: 20122698 https://doi.org/10.1016/j.jpsychires.2010.01.006
40. Opel N, Redlich R, Zwanzger P, et al. Hippocampal atrophy in major depression: a function of childhood maltreatment rather than diagnosis? *Neuropsychopharmacology*. 2014;39(12):2723–2731 PMID: 24924799 https://doi.org/10.1038/npp.2014.145

41. Dannlowski U, Stuhrmann A, Beutelmann V, et al. Limbic scars: long-term consequences of childhood maltreatment revealed by functional and structural magnetic resonance imaging. *Biol Psychiatry*. 2012;71(4):286–293 PMID: 22112927 https://doi.org/10.1016/j.biopsych.2011.10.021
42. Teicher MH, Anderson CM, Polcari A. Childhood maltreatment is associated with reduced volume in the hippocampal subfields CA3, dentate gyrus, and subiculum. *Proc Natl Acad Sci USA*. 2012;109(9):E563–E572 PMID: 22331913 https://doi.org/10.1073/pnas.1115396109
43. Peng H, Ning Y, Zhang Y, et al. White-matter density abnormalities in depressive patients with and without childhood neglect: a voxel-based morphometry (VBM) analysis. *Neurosci Lett*. 2013;550:23–28 PMID: 23831354 https://doi.org/10.1016/j.neulet.2013.06.048
44. Frodl T, Carballedo A, Fagan AJ, Lisiecka D, Ferguson Y, Meaney JF. Effects of early-life adversity on white matter diffusivity changes in patients at risk for major depression. *J Psychiatry Neurosci*. 2012;37(1):37–45 PMID: 22008179 https://doi.org/10.1503/jpn.110028
45. Ugwu ID, Amico F, Carballedo A, Fagan AJ, Frodl T. Childhood adversity, depression, age and gender effects on white matter microstructure: a DTI study. *Brain Struct Funct*. 2015;220(4):1997–2009 PMID: 24744150 https://doi.org/10.1007/s00429-014-0769-x
46. van Harmelen AL, van Tol MJ, van der Wee NJ, et al. Reduced medial prefrontal cortex volume in adults reporting childhood emotional maltreatment. *Biol Psychiatry*. 2010;68(9):832–838 PMID: 20692648 https://doi.org/10.1016/j.biopsych.2010.06.011
47. Ahn SJ, Kyeong S, Suh SH, Kim JJ, Chung TS, Seok JH. What is the impact of child abuse on gray matter abnormalities in individuals with major depressive disorder: a case control study. *BMC Psychiatry*. 2016;16(1):397 PMID: 27842522 https://doi.org/10.1186/s12888-016-1116-y
48. Carballedo A, Lisiecka D, Fagan A, et al. Early life adversity is associated with brain changes in subjects at family risk for depression. *World J Biol Psychiatry*. 2012;13(8):569–578 PMID: 22515408 https://doi.org/10.3109/15622975.2012.661079
49. Opel N, Zwanzger P, Redlich R, et al. Differing brain structural correlates of familial and environmental risk for major depressive disorder revealed by a combined VBM/pattern recognition approach. *Psychol Med*. 2016;46(2):277–290 PMID: 26355299 https://doi.org/10.1017/S0033291715001683
50. Hamilton JP, Etkin A, Furman DJ, Lemus MG, Johnson RF, Gotlib IH. Functional neuroimaging of major depressive disorder: a meta-analysis and new integration of base line activation and neural response data. *Am J Psychiatry*. 2012;169(7):693–703 PMID: 22535198 https://doi.org/10.1176/appi.ajp.2012.11071105
51. Hanson JL, Hariri AR, Williamson DE. Blunted ventral striatum development in adolescence reflects emotional neglect and predicts depressive symptoms. *Biol Psychiatry*. 2015;78(9):598–605 PMID: 26092778 https://doi.org/10.1016/j.biopsych.2015.05.010
52. Wang L, Dai Z, Peng H, et al. Overlapping and segregated resting-state functional connectivity in patients with major depressive disorder with and without childhood neglect. *Hum Brain Mapp*. 2014;35(4):1154–1166 PMID: 23408420 https://doi.org/10.1002/hbm.22241
53. van Harmelen AL, van Tol MJ, Dalgleish T, et al. Hypoactive medial prefrontal cortex functioning in adults reporting childhood emotional maltreatment. *Soc Cogn Affect Neurosci*. 2014;9(12):2026–2033 PMID: 24493840 https://doi.org/10.1093/scan/nsu008
54. van Harmelen AL, van Tol MJ, Demenescu LR, et al. Enhanced amygdala reactivity to emotional faces in adults reporting childhood emotional maltreatment. *Soc Cogn Affect Neurosci*. 2013;8(4):362–369 PMID: 22258799 https://doi.org/10.1093/scan/nss007

55. Grant MM, White D, Hadley J, et al. Early life trauma and directional brain connectivity within major depression. *Hum Brain Mapp*. 2014;35(9):4815–4826 PMID: 24737710 https://doi.org/10.1002/hbm.22514
56. Mullen PE, Martin JL, Anderson JC, Romans SE, Herbison GP. Childhood sexual abuse and mental health in adult life. *Br J Psychiatry*. 1993;163(06):721–732 PMID: 8306113 https://doi.org/10.1192/bjp.163.6.721
57. Janssen I, Krabbendam L, Bak M, et al. Childhood abuse as a risk factor for psychotic experiences. *Acta Psychiatr Scand*. 2004;109(1):38–45 PMID: 14674957 https://doi.org/10.1046/j.0001-690X.2003.00217.x
58. Spauwen J, Krabbendam L, Lieb R, Wittchen HU, van Os J. Impact of psychological trauma on the development of psychotic symptoms: relationship with psychosis proneness. *Br J Psychiatry*. 2006;188(06):527–533 PMID: 16738342 https://doi.org/10.1192/bjp.bp.105.011346
59. Morgan C, Kirkbride J, Leff J, et al. Parental separation, loss and psychosis in different ethnic groups: a case-control study. *Psychol Med*. 2007;37(4):495–503 PMID: 17094816 https://doi.org/10.1017/S0033291706009330
60. Bendall S, Jackson HJ, Hulbert CA, McGorry PD. Childhood trauma and psychotic disorders: a systematic, critical review of the evidence. *Schizophr Bull*. 2008;34(3):568–579 PMID: 18003630 https://doi.org/10.1093/schbul/sbm121
61. Heins M, Simons C, Lataster T, et al. Childhood trauma and psychosis: a case-control and case-sibling comparison across different levels of genetic liability, psychopathology, and type of trauma. *Am J Psychiatry*. 2011;168(12):1286–1294 PMID: 21955935 https://doi.org/10.1176/appi.ajp.2011.10101531
62. Rosenberg SD, Lu W, Mueser KT, Jankowski MK, Cournos F. Correlates of adverse childhood events among adults with schizophrenia spectrum disorders. *Psychiatr Serv*. 2007;58(2):245–253 PMID: 17287383 https://doi.org/10.1176/ps.2007.58.2.245
63. Lardinois M, Lataster T, Mengelers R, Van Os J, Myin-Germeys I. Childhood trauma and increased stress sensitivity in psychosis. *Acta Psychiatr Scand*. 2011;123(1):28–35 PMID: 20712824 https://doi.org/10.1111/j.1600-0447.2010.01594.x
64. Sheffield JM, Williams LE, Woodward ND, Heckers S. Reduced gray matter volume in psychotic disorder patients with a history of childhood sexual abuse. *Schizophr Res*. 2013;143(1):185–191 PMID: 23178105 https://doi.org/10.1016/j.schres.2012.10.032
65. Cancel A, Comte M, Truillet R, et al. Childhood neglect predicts disorganization in schizophrenia through grey matter decrease in dorsolateral prefrontal cortex. *Acta Psychiatr Scand*. 2015;132(4):244–256 PMID: 26038817 https://doi.org/10.1111/acps.12455
66. Siehl S, King JA, Burgess N, Flor H, Nees F. Structural white matter changes in adults and children with posttraumatic stress disorder: a systematic review and meta-analysis. *Neuroimage Clin*. 2018;19:581–598 PMID: 29984166 https://doi.org/10.1016/j.nicl.2018.05.013
67. Ellison-Wright I, Nathan PJ, Bullmore ET, et al. Distribution of tract deficits in schizophrenia. *BMC Psychiatry*. 2014;14(1):99 PMID: 24693962 https://doi.org/10.1186/1471-244X-14-99
68. Lee DY, Smith GN, Su W, et al. White matter tract abnormalities in first-episode psychosis. *Schizophr Res*. 2012;141(1):29–34 PMID: 22863549 https://doi.org/10.1016/j.schres.2012.06.042
69. Peters BD, Dingemans PM, Dekker N, et al. White matter connectivity and psychosis in ultra-high-risk subjects: a diffusion tensor fiber tracking study. *Psychiatry Res*. 2010;181(1):44–50 PMID: 19954931 https://doi.org/10.1016/j.pscychresns.2009.10.008

70. Poletti S, Mazza E, Bollettini I, et al. Adverse childhood experiences influence white matter microstructure in patients with schizophrenia. *Psychiatry Res*. 2015;234(1):35–43 PMID: 26341951 https://doi.org/10.1016/j.pscychresns.2015.08.003
71. Edalati H, Krank MD. Childhood maltreatment and development of substance use disorders: a review and a model of cognitive pathways. *Trauma Violence Abuse*. 2016;17(5):454–467 PMID: 25964275 https://doi.org/10.1177/1524838015584370
72. Dube SR, Felitti VJ, Dong M, Chapman DP, Giles WH, Anda RF. Childhood abuse, neglect, and household dysfunction and the risk of illicit drug use: the adverse childhood experiences study. *Pediatrics*. 2003;111(3):564–572 PMID: 12612237 https://doi.org/10.1542/peds.111.3.564
73. Pirard S, Sharon E, Kang SK, Angarita GA, Gastfriend DR. Prevalence of physical and sexual abuse among substance abuse patients and impact on treatment outcomes. *Drug Alcohol Depend*. 2005;78(1):57–64 PMID: 15769558 https://doi.org/10.1016/j.drugalcdep.2004.09.005
74. Mingione CJ, Heffner JL, Blom TJ, Anthenelli RM. Childhood adversity, serotonin transporter (5-HTTLPR) genotype, and risk for cigarette smoking and nicotine dependence in alcohol dependent adults. *Drug Alcohol Depend*. 2012;123(1-3):201–206 PMID: 22172222 https://doi.org/10.1016/j.drugalcdep.2011.11.013
75. Klanecky A, McChargue DE, Bruggeman L. Desire to dissociate: implications for problematic drinking in college students with childhood or adolescent sexual abuse exposure. *Am J Addict*. 2012;21(3):250–256 PMID: 22494227 https://doi.org/10.1111/j.1521-0391.2012.00228.x
76. Fenton MC, Geier T, Keyes K, Skodol AE, Grant BF, Hasin DS. Combined role of childhood maltreatment, family history, and gender in the risk for alcohol dependence. *Psychol Med*. 2013;43(5):1045–1057 PMID: 22883538 https://doi.org/10.1017/S0033291712001729
77. Meade CS, Watt MH, Sikkema KJ, et al. Methamphetamine use is associated with childhood sexual abuse and HIV sexual risk behaviors among patrons of alcohol-serving venues in Cape Town, South Africa. *Drug Alcohol Depend*. 2012;126(1-2):232–239 PMID: 22717338 https://doi.org/10.1016/j.drugalcdep.2012.05.024
78. Wang Z, Du J, Sun H, Wu H, Xiao Z, Zhao M. Patterns of childhood trauma and psychological distress among injecting heroin users in China. *PLoS One*. 2010;5(12):e15882 PMID: 21209959 https://doi.org/10.1371/journal.pone.0015882
79. Afifi TO, Henriksen CA, Asmundson GJ, Sareen J. Childhood maltreatment and substance use disorders among men and women in a nationally representative sample. *Can J Psychiatry*. 2012;57(11):677–686 PMID: 23149283 https://doi.org/10.1177/070674371205701105
80. Asberg K, Renk K. Substance use coping as a mediator of the relationship between trauma symptoms and substance use consequences among incarcerated females with childhood sexual abuse histories. *Subst Use Misuse*. 2012;47(7):799–808 PMID: 22468563 https://doi.org/10.3109/10826084.2012.669446
81. Claus RE, Kindleberger LR. Engaging substance abusers after centralized assessment: predictors of treatment entry and dropout. *J Psychoactive Drugs*. 2002;34(1):25–31 PMID: 12003110 https://doi.org/10.1080/02791072.2002.10399933
82. Heffner JL, Blom TJ, Anthenelli RM. Gender differences in trauma history and symptoms as predictors of relapse to alcohol and drug use. *Am J Addict*. 2011;20(4):307–311 PMID: 21679261 https://doi.org/10.1111/j.1521-0391.2011.00141.x
83. Bernstein DP, Stein JA, Handelsman L. Predicting personality pathology among adult patients with substance use disorders: effects of childhood maltreatment. *Addict Behav*. 1998;23(6):855–868 PMID: 9801721 https://doi.org/10.1016/S0306-4603(98)00072-0

84. Douglas KR, Chan G, Gelernter J, et al. Adverse childhood events as risk factors for substance dependence: partial mediation by mood and anxiety disorders. *Addict Behav*. 2010;35(1):7–13 PMID: 19720467 https://doi.org/10.1016/j.addbeh.2009.07.004
85. Ellason JW, Ross CA, Fuchs DL. Lifetime axis I and II comorbidity and childhood trauma history in dissociative identity disorder. *Psychiatry*. 1996;59(3):255–266 PMID: 8912944 https://doi.org/10.1080/00332747.1996.11024766
86. Ellason JW, Ross CA, Sainton K, Mayran LW. Axis I and II comorbidity and childhood trauma history in chemical dependency. *Bull Menninger Clin*. 1996;60(1):39–51 PMID: 8742671
87. Fetzner MG, McMillan KA, Sareen J, Asmundson GJ. What is the association between traumatic life events and alcohol abuse/dependence in people with and without PTSD? Findings from a nationally representative sample. *Depress Anxiety*. 2011;28(8):632–638 PMID: 21769995 https://doi.org/10.1002/da.20852
88. Hanson JL, Chung MK, Avants BB, et al. Early stress is associated with alterations in the orbitofrontal cortex: a tensor-based morphometry investigation of brain structure and behavioral risk. *J Neurosci*. 2010;30(22):7466–7472 PMID: 20519521 https://doi.org/10.1523/JNEUROSCI.0859-10.2010
89. Ersche KD, Jones PS, Williams GB, Turton AJ, Robbins TW, Bullmore ET. Abnormal brain structure implicated in stimulant drug addiction. *Science*. 2012;335(6068):601–604 PMID: 22301321 https://doi.org/10.1126/science.1214463
90. Robbins TW, Gillan CM, Smith DG, de Wit S, Ersche KD. Neurocognitive endophenotypes of impulsivity and compulsivity: towards dimensional psychiatry. *Trends Cogn Sci*. 2012;16(1):81–91 PMID: 22155014 https://doi.org/10.1016/j.tics.2011.11.009
91. Puetz VB, McCrory E. Exploring the relationship between childhood maltreatment and addiction: a review of the neurocognitive evidence. *Curr Addict Rep*. 2015;2(4):318–325 PMID: 26550550 https://doi.org/10.1007/s40429-015-0073-8
92. Diekhof EK, Falkai P, Gruber O. Functional neuroimaging of reward processing and decision-making: a review of aberrant motivational and affective processing in addiction and mood disorders. *Brain Res Brain Res Rev*. 2008;59(1):164–184 PMID: 18675846 https://doi.org/10.1016/j.brainresrev.2008.07.004
93. Haber SN, Knutson B. The reward circuit: linking primate anatomy and human imaging. *Neuropsychopharmacology*. 2010;35(1):4–26 PMID: 19812543 https://doi.org/10.1038/npp.2009.129
94. Koob GF, Volkow ND. Neurobiology of addiction: a neurocircuitry analysis. *Lancet Psychiatry*. 2016;3(8):760–773 PMID: 27475769 https://doi.org/10.1016/S2215-0366(16)00104-8
95. Volkow ND, Koob GF, McLellan AT. Neurobiologic advances from the brain disease model of addiction. *N Engl J Med*. 2016;374(4):363–371 PMID: 26816013 https://doi.org/10.1056/NEJMra1511480
96. Garavan H, Ross TJ, Murphy K, Roche RA, Stein EA. Dissociable executive functions in the dynamic control of behavior: inhibition, error detection, and correction. *Neuroimage*. 2002;17(4):1820–1829 PMID: 12498755 https://doi.org/10.1006/nimg.2002.1326
97. Guyer AE, Nelson EE, Perez-Edgar K, et al. Striatal functional alteration in adolescents characterized by early childhood behavioral inhibition. *J Neurosci*. 2006;26(24):6399–6405 PMID: 16775126 https://doi.org/10.1523/JNEUROSCI.0666-06.2006
98. Dillon DG, Holmes AJ, Birk JL, Brooks N, Lyons-Ruth K, Pizzagalli DA. Childhood adversity is associated with left basal ganglia dysfunction during reward anticipation in adulthood. *Biol Psychiatry*. 2009;66(3):206–213 PMID: 19358974 https://doi.org/10.1016/j.biopsych.2009.02.019

99. Mehta MA, Gore-Langton E, Golembo N, Colvert E, Williams SC, Sonuga-Barke E. Hyporesponsive reward anticipation in the basal ganglia following severe institutional deprivation early in life. *J Cogn Neurosci*. 2010;22(10):2316–2325 PMID: 19929329 https://doi.org/10.1162/jocn.2009.21394
100. Cohen RA, Grieve S, Hoth KF, et al. Early life stress and morphometry of the adult anterior cingulate cortex and caudate nuclei. *Biol Psychiatry*. 2006;59(10):975–982 PMID: 16616722 https://doi.org/10.1016/j.biopsych.2005.12.016
101. Kelly PA, Viding E, Wallace GL, et al. Cortical thickness, surface area, and gyrification abnormalities in children exposed to maltreatment: neural markers of vulnerability? *Biol Psychiatry*. 2013;74(11):845–852 PMID: 23954109 https://doi.org/10.1016/j.biopsych.2013.06.020
102. Behen ME, Muzik O, Saporta AS, et al. Abnormal fronto-striatal connectivity in children with histories of early deprivation: a diffusion tensor imaging study. *Brain Imaging Behav*. 2009;3(3):292–297 PMID: 19727404 https://doi.org/10.1007/s11682-009-9071-6
103. Clark DB, Chung T, Martin CS, et al. Adolescent executive dysfunction in daily life: relationships to risks, brain structure and substance use. *Front Behav Neurosci*. 2017;11:223 PMID: 29180956 https://doi.org/10.3389/fnbeh.2017.00223
104. Mandavia A, Robinson GG, Bradley B, Ressler KJ, Powers A. Exposure to childhood abuse and later substance use: indirect effects of emotion dysregulation and exposure to trauma. *J Trauma Stress*. 2016;29(5):422–429 PMID: 27622844 https://doi.org/10.1002/jts.22131
105. Ross S, Peselow E. The neurobiology of addictive disorders. *Clin Neuropharmacol*. 2009;32(5):269–276 PMID: 19834992 https://doi.org/10.1097/WNF.0b013e3181a9163c
106. Tomoda A, Polcari A, Anderson CM, Teicher MH. Reduced visual cortex gray matter volume and thickness in young adults who witnessed domestic violence during childhood. *PLoS One*. 2012;7(12):e52528 PMID: 23300699 https://doi.org/10.1371/journal.pone.0052528
107. De Brito SA, Viding E, Sebastian CL, et al. Reduced orbitofrontal and temporal grey matter in a community sample of maltreated children. *J Child Psychol Psychiatry*. 2013;54(1):105–112 PMID: 22880630 https://doi.org/10.1111/j.1469-7610.2012.02597.x
108. Eluvathingal TJ, Chugani HT, Behen ME, et al. Abnormal brain connectivity in children after early severe socioemotional deprivation: a diffusion tensor imaging study. *Pediatrics*. 2006;117(6):2093–2100 PMID: 16740852 https://doi.org/10.1542/peds.2005-1727
109. Govindan RM, Makki MI, Wilson BJ, Behen ME, Chugani HT. Abnormal water diffusivity in corticostriatal projections in children with Tourette syndrome. *Hum Brain Mapp*. 2010;31(11):1665–1674 PMID: 20162597 https://doi.org/10.1002/hbm.20970
110. McLaughlin KA, Peverill M, Gold AL, Alves S, Sheridan MA. Child maltreatment and neural systems underlying emotion regulation. *J Am Acad Child Adolesc Psychiatry*. 2015;54(9):753–762 PMID: 26299297 https://doi.org/10.1016/j.jaac.2015.06.010
111. Elton A, Smitherman S, Young J, Kilts CD. Effects of childhood maltreatment on the neural correlates of stress- and drug cue-induced cocaine craving. *Addict Biol*. 2015;20(4):820–831 PMID: 25214317 https://doi.org/10.1111/adb.12162
112. Spechler PA, Orr CA, Chaarani B, et al; IMAGEN Consortium. Cannabis use in early adolescence: evidence of amygdala hypersensitivity to signals of threat. *Dev Cogn Neurosci*. 2015;16:63–70 PMID: 26347227 https://doi.org/10.1016/j.dcn.2015.08.007
113. Verdejo-García A, Pérez-García M, Bechara A. Emotion, decision-making and substance dependence: a somatic-marker model of addiction. *Curr Neuropharmacol*. 2006;4(1):17–31 PMID: 18615136 https://doi.org/10.2174/157015906775203057

114. Hein TC, Monk CS. Research review: neural response to threat in children, adolescents, and adults after child maltreatment—a quantitative meta-analysis. *J Child Psychol Psychiatry*. 2017;58(3):222–230 PMID: 27778344 https://doi.org/10.1111/jcpp.12651
115. Leist T, Dadds MR. Adolescents' ability to read different emotional faces relates to their history of maltreatment and type of psychopathology. *Clin Child Psychol Psychiatry*. 2009;14(2):237–250 PMID: 19293321 https://doi.org/10.1177/1359104508100887
116. Trick L, Kempton MJ, Williams SC, Duka T. Impaired fear recognition and attentional set-shifting is associated with brain structural changes in alcoholic patients. *Addict Biol*. 2014;19(6):1041–1054 PMID: 25123156 https://doi.org/10.1111/adb.12175
117. Richardson GB, Freedlander JM, Katz EC, Dai CL, Chen CC. Impulsivity links reward and threat sensitivities to substance use: a functional model. *Front Psychol*. 2014;5:1194 PMID: 25386147 https://doi.org/10.3389/fpsyg.2014.01194
118. Schlund MW, Cataldo MF. Amygdala involvement in human avoidance, escape and approach behavior. *Neuroimage*. 2010;53(2):769–776 PMID: 20600966 https://doi.org/10.1016/j.neuroimage.2010.06.058
119. Woon FL, Hedges DW. Hippocampal and amygdala volumes in children and adults with childhood maltreatment-related posttraumatic stress disorder: a meta-analysis. *Hippocampus*. 2008;18(8):729–736 PMID: 18446827 https://doi.org/10.1002/hipo.20437
120. Ahmed-Leitao F, Spies G, van den Heuvel L, Seedat S. Hippocampal and amygdala volumes in adults with posttraumatic stress disorder secondary to childhood abuse or maltreatment: a systematic review. *Psychiatry Res Neuroimaging*. 2016;256:33–43 PMID: 27669407 https://doi.org/10.1016/j.pscychresns.2016.09.008
121. McCrory EJ, De Brito SA, Kelly PA, et al. Amygdala activation in maltreated children during pre-attentive emotional processing. *Br J Psychiatry*. 2013;202(4):269–276 PMID: 23470285 https://doi.org/10.1192/bjp.bp.112.116624
122. Padula CB, McQueeny T, Lisdahl KM, Price JS, Tapert SF. Craving is associated with amygdala volumes in adolescent marijuana users during abstinence. *Am J Drug Alcohol Abuse*. 2015;41(2):127–132 PMID: 25668330 https://doi.org/10.3109/00952990.2014.966198
123. Wrase J, Makris N, Braus DF, et al. Amygdala volume associated with alcohol abuse relapse and craving. *Am J Psychiatry*. 2008;165(9):1179–1184 PMID: 18593776 https://doi.org/10.1176/appi.ajp.2008.07121877
124. Sripada CS, Angstadt M, McNamara P, King AC, Phan KL. Effects of alcohol on brain responses to social signals of threat in humans. *Neuroimage*. 2011;55(1):371–380 PMID: 21122818 https://doi.org/10.1016/j.neuroimage.2010.11.062
125. Collishaw S, Pickles A, Messer J, Rutter M, Shearer C, Maughan B. Resilience to adult psychopathology following childhood maltreatment: evidence from a community sample. *Child Abuse Negl*. 2007;31(3):211–229 PMID: 17399786 https://doi.org/10.1016/j.chiabu.2007.02.004
126. Caspi A, McClay J, Moffitt TE, et al. Role of genotype in the cycle of violence in maltreated children. *Science*. 2002;297(5582):851–854 PMID: 12161658 https://doi.org/10.1126/science.1072290
127. Hassel S, McKinnon MC, Cusi AM, Macqueen GM. An overview of psychological and neurobiological mechanisms by which early negative experiences increase risk of mood disorders. *J Can Acad Child Adolesc Psychiatry*. 2011;20(4):277–288 PMID: 22114609
128. Connor-Smith JK, Compas BE, Wadsworth ME, Thomsen AH, Saltzman H. Responses to stress in adolescence: measurement of coping and involuntary stress responses. *J Consult Clin Psychol*. 2000;68(6):976–992 PMID: 11142550 https://doi.org/10.1037/0022-006X.68.6.976

129. Gutman DA, Nemeroff CB. Persistent central nervous system effects of an adverse early environment: clinical and preclinical studies. *Physiol Behav*. 2003;79(3):471–478 PMID: 12954441 https://doi.org/10.1016/S0031-9384(03)00166-5
130. Wu G, Feder A, Cohen H, et al. Understanding resilience. *Front Behav Neurosci*. 2013;7:10 PMID: 23422934 https://doi.org/10.3389/fnbeh.2013.00010
131. Hussey JM, Chang JJ, Kotch JB. Child maltreatment in the United States: prevalence, risk factors, and adolescent health consequences. *Pediatrics*. 2006;118(3):933–942 PMID: 16950983 https://doi.org/10.1542/peds.2005-2452
132. Schultz D, Jaycox LH, Hickman LJ, et al. The relationship between protective factors and outcomes for children exposed to violence. *Violence Vict*. 2013;28(4):697–714 PMID: 24047048 https://doi.org/10.1891/0886-6708.VV-D-12-00005
133. Afifi TO, Macmillan HL. Resilience following child maltreatment: a review of protective factors. *Can J Psychiatry*. 2011;56(5):266–272 PMID: 21586192 https://doi.org/10.1177/070674371105600505
134. Lansford JE, Malone PS, Stevens KI, Dodge KA, Bates JE, Pettit GS. Developmental trajectories of externalizing and internalizing behaviors: factors underlying resilience in physically abused children. *Dev Psychopathol*. 2006;18(1):35–55 PMID: 16478551 https://doi.org/10.1017/S0954579406060032
135. Cowell RA, Cicchetti D, Rogosch FA, Toth SL. Childhood maltreatment and its effect on neurocognitive functioning: timing and chronicity matter. *Dev Psychopathol*. 2015;27(2):521–533 PMID: 25997769 https://doi.org/10.1017/S0954579415000139
136. Kaplan MJ, Klinetob NA. Childhood emotional trauma and chronic posttraumatic stress disorder in adult outpatients with treatment-resistant depression. *J Nerv Ment Dis*. 2000;188(9):596–601 PMID: 11009333 https://doi.org/10.1097/00005053-200009000-00006
137. Kleindienst N, Limberger MF, Ebner-Priemer UW, et al. Dissociation predicts poor response to dialectial behavioral therapy in female patients with borderline personality disorder. *J Pers Disord*. 2011;25(4):432–447 PMID: 21838560 https://doi.org/10.1521/pedi.2011.25.4.432
138. Wolf EJ, Miller MW, Reardon AF, Ryabchenko KA, Castillo D, Freund R. A latent class analysis of dissociation and posttraumatic stress disorder: evidence for a dissociative subtype. *Arch Gen Psychiatry*. 2012;69(7):698–705 PMID: 22752235 https://doi.org/10.1001/archgenpsychiatry.2011.1574
139. Zanarini MC, Laudate CS, Frankenburg FR, Reich DB, Fitzmaurice G. Predictors of self-mutilation in patients with borderline personality disorder: A 10-year follow-up study. *J Psychiatr Res*. 2011;45(6):823–828 PMID: 21129758 https://doi.org/10.1016/j.jpsychires.2010.10.015
140. Lazarus RS, Folkman S. *Stress, Appraisal, and Coping*. New York, NY: Springer; 1984
141. Sinha R. How does stress increase risk of drug abuse and relapse? *Psychopharmacology (Berl)*. 2001;158(4):343–359 PMID: 11797055 https://doi.org/10.1007/s002130100917
142. McEwen BS. Neurobiological and systemic effects of chronic stress. *Chronic Stress (Thousand Oaks)*. 2017;1:1 PMID: 28856337 https://doi.org/10.1177/2470547017692328
143. Saal D, Dong Y, Bonci A, Malenka RC. Drugs of abuse and stress trigger a common synaptic adaptation in dopamine neurons. *Neuron*. 2003;37(4):577–582 PMID: 12597856 https://doi.org/10.1016/S0896-6273(03)00021-7
144. Davidson RJ, Sutton SK. Affective neuroscience: the emergence of a discipline. *Curr Opin Neurobiol*. 1995;5(2):217–224 PMID: 7620310 https://doi.org/10.1016/0959-4388(95)80029-8

145. Dichter GS, Damiano CA, Allen JA. Reward circuitry dysfunction in psychiatric and neurodevelopmental disorders and genetic syndromes: animal models and clinical findings. *J Neurodev Disord*. 2012;4(1):19 PMID: 22958744 https://doi.org/10.1186/1866-1955-4-19
146. Huether G. Stress and the adaptive self-organization of neuronal connectivity during early childhood. *Int J Dev Neurosci*. 1998;16(3-4):297–306 PMID: 9785126 https://doi.org/10.1016/S0736-5748(98)00023-9
147. Nelson CA, Carver LJ. The effects of stress and trauma on brain and memory: a view from developmental cognitive neuroscience. *Dev Psychopathol*. 1998;10(4):793–809 PMID: 9886227 https://doi.org/10.1017/S0954579498001874
148. Sapolsky RM. Why stress is bad for your brain. *Science*. 1996;273(5276):749–750 PMID: 8701325 https://doi.org/10.1126/science.273.5276.749
149. Gunnar MR, Nelson CA. Event-related potentials in year-old infants: relations with emotionality and cortisol. *Child Dev*. 1994;65(1):80–94 PMID: 8131656 https://doi.org/10.2307/1131367
150. Sinha R, Robinson J, O'Malley S. Stress response dampening: effects of gender and family history of alcoholism and anxiety disorders. *Psychopharmacology (Berl)*. 1998;137(4):311–320 PMID: 9676889 https://doi.org/10.1007/s002130050624
151. Szabo A. The combined effects of orthostatic and mental stress on heart rate, T-wave amplitude, and pulse transit time. *Eur J Appl Physiol Occup Physiol*. 1993;67(6):540–544 PMID: 8149934 https://doi.org/10.1007/BF00241651
152. Belujon P, Grace AA. Regulation of dopamine system responsivity and its adaptive and pathological response to stress. *Proc Biol Sci*. 2015;282(1805):20142516 PMID: 25788601 https://doi.org/10.1098/rspb.2014.2516
153. Glantz MD, Leshner AI. Drug abuse and developmental psychopathology. *Dev Psychopathol*. 2000;12(4):795–814 PMID: 11202044 https://doi.org/10.1017/S0954579400004120
154. Rutter M, Sroufe LA. Developmental psychopathology: concepts and challenges. *Dev Psychopathol*. 2000;12(3):265–296 PMID: 11014739 https://doi.org/10.1017/S0954579400003023
155. Wadsworth ME. Development of maladaptive coping: a functional adaptation to chronic, uncontrollable stress. *Child Dev Perspect*. 2015;9(2):96–100 PMID: 26019717 https://doi.org/10.1111/cdep.12112
156. De Bellis MD, Zisk A. The biological effects of childhood trauma. *Child Adolesc Psychiatr Clin N Am*. 2014;23(2):185–222, vii PMID: 24656576 https://doi.org/10.1016/j.chc.2014.01.002
157. Wonderlich SA, Brewerton TD, Jocic Z, Dansky BS, Abbott DW. Relationship of childhood sexual abuse and eating disorders. *J Am Acad Child Adolesc Psychiatry*. 1997;36(8):1107–1115 PMID: 9256590 https://doi.org/10.1097/00004583-199708000-00018
158. Weierich MR, Nock MK. Posttraumatic stress symptoms mediate the relation between childhood sexual abuse and nonsuicidal self-injury. *J Consult Clin Psychol*. 2008;76(1):39–44 PMID: 18229981 https://doi.org/10.1037/0022-006X.76.1.39
159. Ortiz-López L, Vega-Rivera NM, Babu H, Ramírez-Rodríguez GB. Brain-derived neurotrophic factor induces cell survival and the migration of murine adult hippocampal precursor cells during differentiation in vitro. *Neurotox Res*. 2017;31(1):122–135 PMID: 27663583 https://doi.org/10.1007/s12640-016-9673-x
160. Scharfman HE, MacLusky NJ. Differential regulation of BDNF, synaptic plasticity and sprouting in the hippocampal mossy fiber pathway of male and female rats. *Neuropharmacology*. 2014;76(Pt C):696–708 PMID: 23660230 https://doi.org/10.1016/j.neuropharm.2013.04.029

161. Yang J, Harte-Hargrove LC, Siao CJ, et al. proBDNF negatively regulates neuronal remodeling, synaptic transmission, and synaptic plasticity in hippocampus. *Cell Rep*. 2014;7(3):796–806 PMID: 24746813 https://doi.org/10.1016/j.celrep.2014.03.040
162. Chen ZY, Jing D, Bath KG, et al. Genetic variant BDNF (Val66Met) polymorphism alters anxiety-related behavior. *Science*. 2006;314(5796):140–143 PMID: 17023662 https://doi.org/10.1126/science.1129663
163. Aguilera M, Arias B, Wichers M, et al. Early adversity and 5-HTT/BDNF genes: new evidence of gene-environment interactions on depressive symptoms in a general population. *Psychol Med*. 2009;39(9):1425–1432 PMID: 19215635 https://doi.org/10.1017/S0033291709005248
164. Kaufman J, Yang BZ, Douglas-Palumberi H, et al. Brain-derived neurotrophic factor-5-HTTLPR gene interactions and environmental modifiers of depression in children. *Biol Psychiatry*. 2006;59(8):673–680 PMID: 16458264 https://doi.org/10.1016/j.biopsych.2005.10.026
165. Wichers M, Kenis G, Jacobs N, et al. The BDNF Val(66)Met x 5-HTTLPR x child adversity interaction and depressive symptoms: an attempt at replication. *Am J Med Genet B Neuropsychiatr Genet*. 2008;147B(1):120–123 PMID: 17579366 https://doi.org/10.1002/ajmg.b.30576
166. Frodl T, Skokauskas N, Frey EM, Morris D, Gill M, Carballedo A. BDNF Val66Met genotype interacts with childhood adversity and influences the formation of hippocampal subfields. *Hum Brain Mapp*. 2014;35(12):5776–5783 PMID: 25044977 https://doi.org/10.1002/hbm.22584
167. Carballedo A, Morris D, Zill P, et al. Brain-derived neurotrophic factor Val66Met polymorphism and early life adversity affect hippocampal volume. *Am J Med Genet B Neuropsychiatr Genet*. 2013;162B(2):183–190 PMID: 23341118 https://doi.org/10.1002/ajmg.b.32130
168. Gatt JM, Nemeroff CB, Dobson-Stone C, et al. Interactions between BDNF Val66Met polymorphism and early life stress predict brain and arousal pathways to syndromal depression and anxiety. *Mol Psychiatry*. 2009;14(7):681–695 PMID: 19153574 https://doi.org/10.1038/mp.2008.143
169. Joffe RT, Gatt JM, Kemp AH, et al. Brain derived neurotrophic factor Val66Met polymorphism, the five factor model of personality and hippocampal volume: implications for depressive illness. *Hum Brain Mapp*. 2009;30(4):1246–1256 PMID: 18548532 https://doi.org/10.1002/hbm.20592
170. Gerritsen L, Tendolkar I, Franke B, et al. BDNF Val66Met genotype modulates the effect of childhood adversity on subgenual anterior cingulate cortex volume in healthy subjects. *Mol Psychiatry*. 2012;17(6):597–603 PMID: 21577214 https://doi.org/10.1038/mp.2011.51
171. Casey BJ, Glatt CE, Tottenham N, et al. Brain-derived neurotrophic factor as a model system for examining gene by environment interactions across development. *Neuroscience*. 2009;164(1):108–120 PMID: 19358879 https://doi.org/10.1016/j.neuroscience.2009.03.081
172. Marusak HA, Kuruvadi N, Vila AM, et al. Interactive effects of BDNF Val66Met genotype and trauma on limbic brain anatomy in childhood. *Eur Child Adolesc Psychiatry*. 2016;25(5):509–518 PMID: 26286685 https://doi.org/10.1007/s00787-015-0759-4
173. Grabe HJ, Wittfeld K, Van der Auwera S, et al. Effect of the interaction between childhood abuse and rs1360780 of the FKBP5 gene on gray matter volume in a general population sample. *Hum Brain Mapp*. 2016;37(4):1602–1613 PMID: 26813705 https://doi.org/10.1002/hbm.23123

174. Dannlowski U, Kugel H, Grotegerd D, et al. Disadvantage of social sensitivity: interaction of oxytocin receptor genotype and child maltreatment on brain structure. *Biol Psychiatry*. 2016;80(5):398–405 PMID: 26858213 https://doi.org/10.1016/j.biopsych.2015.12.010
175. Binder EB. The role of FKBP5, a co-chaperone of the glucocorticoid receptor in the pathogenesis and therapy of affective and anxiety disorders. *Psychoneuroendocrinology*. 2009;34(suppl 1):S186–S195 PMID: 19560279 https://doi.org/10.1016/j.psyneuen.2009.05.021
176. Appel K, Schwahn C, Mahler J, et al. Moderation of adult depression by a polymorphism in the FKBP5 gene and childhood physical abuse in the general population. *Neuropsychopharmacology*. 2011;36(10):1982–1991 PMID: 21654733 https://doi.org/10.1038/npp.2011.81
177. Zimmermann P, Brückl T, Nocon A, et al. Interaction of FKBP5 gene variants and adverse life events in predicting depression onset: results from a 10-year prospective community study. *Am J Psychiatry*. 2011;168(10):1107–1116 PMID: 21865530 https://doi.org/10.1176/appi.ajp.2011.10111577
178. Rodrigues SM, Saslow LR, Garcia N, John OP, Keltner D. Oxytocin receptor genetic variation relates to empathy and stress reactivity in humans. *Proc Natl Acad Sci USA*. 2009;106(50):21437–21441 PMID: 19934046 https://doi.org/10.1073/pnas.0909579106
179. Kogan A, Saslow LR, Impett EA, Oveis C, Keltner D, Rodrigues Saturn S. Thin-slicing study of the oxytocin receptor (OXTR) gene and the evaluation and expression of the prosocial disposition. *Proc Natl Acad Sci USA*. 2011;108(48):19189–19192 PMID: 22084107 https://doi.org/10.1073/pnas.1112658108
180. Saphire-Bernstein S, Way BM, Kim HS, Sherman DK, Taylor SE. Oxytocin receptor gene (OXTR) is related to psychological resources. *Proc Natl Acad Sci USA*. 2011;108(37):15118–15122 PMID: 21896752 https://doi.org/10.1073/pnas.1113137108
181. Tost H, Kolachana B, Hakimi S, et al. A common allele in the oxytocin receptor gene (OXTR) impacts prosocial temperament and human hypothalamic-limbic structure and function. *Proc Natl Acad Sci USA*. 2010;107(31):13936–13941 PMID: 20647384 https://doi.org/10.1073/pnas.1003296107
182. Lucht MJ, Barnow S, Sonnenfeld C, et al. Associations between the oxytocin receptor gene (OXTR) and affect, loneliness and intelligence in normal subjects. *Prog Neuropsychopharmacol Biol Psychiatry*. 2009;33(5):860–866 PMID: 19376182 https://doi.org/10.1016/j.pnpbp.2009.04.004
183. van Roekel E, Verhagen M, Engels RC, Goossens L, Scholte RH. Oxytocin receptor gene (OXTR) in relation to loneliness in adolescence: interactions with sex, parental support, and DRD2 and 5-HTTLPR genotypes. *Psychiatr Genet*. 2013;23(5):204–213 PMID: 23838880 https://doi.org/10.1097/YPG.0b013e328363f631
184. Wang J, Qin W, Liu B, et al. Neural mechanisms of oxytocin receptor gene mediating anxiety-related temperament. *Brain Struct Funct*. 2014;219(5):1543–1554 PMID: 23708061 https://doi.org/10.1007/s00429-013-0584-9
185. Samplin E, Ikuta T, Malhotra AK, Szeszko PR, Derosse P. Sex differences in resilience to childhood maltreatment: effects of trauma history on hippocampal volume, general cognition and subclinical psychosis in healthy adults. *J Psychiatr Res*. 2013;47(9):1174–1179 PMID: 23726669 https://doi.org/10.1016/j.jpsychires.2013.05.008
186. Sperry DM, Widom CS. Child abuse and neglect, social support, and psychopathology in adulthood: a prospective investigation. *Child Abuse Negl*. 2013;37(6):415–425 PMID: 23562083 https://doi.org/10.1016/j.chiabu.2013.02.006

187. Gallo EAG, Munhoz TN, Loret de Mola C, Murray J. Gender differences in the effects of childhood maltreatment on adult depression and anxiety: a systematic review and meta-analysis. *Child Abuse Negl*. 2018;79:107–114 PMID: 29428878 https://doi.org/10.1016/j.chiabu.2018.01.003
188. Eaton NR, Keyes KM, Krueger RF, et al. An invariant dimensional liability model of gender differences in mental disorder prevalence: evidence from a national sample. *J Abnorm Psychol*. 2012;121(1):282–288 PMID: 21842958 https://doi.org/10.1037/a0024780
189. Asscher JJ, Van der Put CE, Stams GJ. Gender differences in the impact of abuse and neglect victimization on adolescent offending behavior. *J Fam Violence*. 2015;30(2):215–225 PMID: 25663744 https://doi.org/10.1007/s10896-014-9668-4
190. MacMillan HL, Fleming JE, Streiner DL, et al. Childhood abuse and lifetime psychopathology in a community sample. *Am J Psychiatry*. 2001;158(11):1878–1883 PMID: 11691695 https://doi.org/10.1176/appi.ajp.158.11.1878
191. Kudielka BM, Kirschbaum C. Sex differences in HPA axis responses to stress: a review. *Biol Psychol*. 2005;69(1):113–132 PMID: 15740829 https://doi.org/10.1016/j.biopsycho.2004.11.009
192. Shansky RM, Glavis-Bloom C, Lerman D, et al. Estrogen mediates sex differences in stress-induced prefrontal cortex dysfunction. *Mol Psychiatry*. 2004;9(5):531–538 PMID: 14569273 https://doi.org/10.1038/sj.mp.4001435
193. Myin-Germeys I, Krabbendam L, Delespaul PA, van Os J. Sex differences in emotional reactivity to daily life stress in psychosis. *J Clin Psychiatry*. 2004;65(6):805–809 PMID: 15291657 https://doi.org/10.4088/JCP.v65n0611
194. Rose AB, Merke DP, Clasen LS, et al. Effects of hormones and sex chromosomes on stress-influenced regions of the developing pediatric brain. *Ann N Y Acad Sci*. 2004;1032(1):231–233 PMID: 15677417 https://doi.org/10.1196/annals.1314.027
195. Klein LC, Corwin EJ. Seeing the unexpected: how sex differences in stress responses may provide a new perspective on the manifestation of psychiatric disorders. *Curr Psychiatry Rep*. 2002;4(6):441–448 PMID: 12441024 https://doi.org/10.1007/s11920-002-0072-z
196. Taylor SE, Kemeny ME, Reed GM, Bower JE, Gruenewald TL. Psychological resources, positive illusions, and health. *Am Psychol*. 2000;55(1):99–109 PMID: 11392870 https://doi.org/10.1037/0003-066X.55.1.99
197. Rentz DM, Dekhtyar M, Sherman J, et al. The feasibility of at-home iPad cognitive testing for use in clinical trials. *J Prev Alzheimers Dis*. 2016;3(1):8–12 PMID: 26998469 https://doi.org/10.14283/jpad.2015.78
198. Marrocco J, McEwen BS. Sex in the brain: hormones and sex differences. *Dialogues Clin Neurosci*. 2016;18(4):373–383 PMID: 28179809
199. Burman DD, Bitan T, Booth JR. Sex differences in neural processing of language among children. *Neuropsychologia*. 2008;46(5):1349–1362 PMID: 18262207 https://doi.org/10.1016/j.neuropsychologia.2007.12.021
200. Kret ME, De Gelder B. A review on sex differences in processing emotional signals. *Neuropsychologia*. 2012;50(7):1211–1221 PMID: 22245006 https://doi.org/10.1016/j.neuropsychologia.2011.12.022
201. Maccari S, Krugers HJ, Morley-Fletcher S, Szyf M, Brunton PJ. The consequences of early-life adversity: neurobiological, behavioural and epigenetic adaptations. *J Neuroendocrinol*. 2014;26(10):707–723 PMID: 25039443 https://doi.org/10.1111/jne.12175
202. Stanis JJ, Andersen SL. Reducing substance use during adolescence: a translational framework for prevention. *Psychopharmacology (Berl)*. 2014;231(8):1437–1453 PMID: 24464527 https://doi.org/10.1007/s00213-013-3393-1

203. Diamond A. Biological and social influences on cognitive control processes dependent on prefrontal cortex. *Prog Brain Res*. 2011;189:319–339 PMID: 21489397 https://doi.org/10.1016/B978-0-444-53884-0.00032-4
204. Tottenham N. Human amygdala development in the absence of species-expected caregiving. *Dev Psychobiol*. 2012;54(6):598–611 PMID: 22714586 https://doi.org/10.1002/dev.20531
205. McLaughlin KA, Sheridan MA, Nelson CA. Neglect as a violation of species-expectant experience: neurodevelopmental consequences. *Biol Psychiatry*. 2017;82(7):462–471 PMID: 28392082 https://doi.org/10.1016/j.biopsych.2017.02.1096
206. Thayer JF, Hansen AL, Saus-Rose E, Johnsen BH. Heart rate variability, prefrontal neural function, and cognitive performance: the neurovisceral integration perspective on self-regulation, adaptation, and health. *Ann Behav Med*. 2009;37(2):141–153 PMID: 19424767 https://doi.org/10.1007/s12160-009-9101-z
207. McLaughlin KA, Sheridan MA, Lambert HK. Childhood adversity and neural development: deprivation and threat as distinct dimensions of early experience. *Neurosci Biobehav Rev*. 2014;47:578–591 PMID: 25454359 https://doi.org/10.1016/j.neubiorev.2014.10.012
208. Màsse LC, Tremblay RE. Behavior of boys in kindergarten and the onset of substance use during adolescence. *Arch Gen Psychiatry*. 1997;54(1):62–68 PMID: 9006402 https://doi.org/10.1001/archpsyc.1997.01830130068014
209. Paquola C, Bennett MR, Lagopoulos J. Understanding heterogeneity in grey matter research of adults with childhood maltreatment—a meta-analysis and review. *Neurosci Biobehav Rev*. 2016;69:299–312 PMID: 27531235 https://doi.org/10.1016/j.neubiorev.2016.08.011
210. Paquola C, Bennett MR, Hatton SN, Hermens DF, Groote I, Lagopoulos J. Hippocampal development in youth with a history of childhood maltreatment. *J Psychiatr Res*. 2017;91:149–155 PMID: 28364595 https://doi.org/10.1016/j.jpsychires.2017.03.019
211. Paquola C, Bennett MR, Hatton SN, Hermens DF, Lagopoulos J. Utility of the cumulative stress and mismatch hypotheses in understanding the neurobiological impacts of childhood abuse and recent stress in youth with emerging mental disorder. *Hum Brain Mapp*. 2017;38(5):2709–2721 PMID: 28256777 https://doi.org/10.1002/hbm.23554
212. Sheridan MA, McLaughlin KA. Dimensions of early experience and neural development: deprivation and threat. *Trends Cogn Sci*. 2014;18(11):580–585 PMID: 25305194 https://doi.org/10.1016/j.tics.2014.09.001
213. Costello EJ, Erkanli A, Federman E, Angold A. Development of psychiatric comorbidity with substance abuse in adolescents: effects of timing and sex. *J Clin Child Psychol*. 1999;28(3):298–311 PMID: 10446679 https://doi.org/10.1207/S15374424jccp280302
214. Bonanno GA. Loss, trauma, and human resilience: have we underestimated the human capacity to thrive after extremely aversive events? *Am Psychol*. 2004;59(1):20–28 PMID: 14736317 https://doi.org/10.1037/0003-066X.59.1.20
215. Kaplow JB, Curran PJ, Dodge KA; Conduct Problems Prevention Research Group. Child, parent, and peer predictors of early-onset substance use: a multisite longitudinal study. *J Abnorm Child Psychol*. 2002;30(3):199–216 PMID: 12041707 https://doi.org/10.1023/A:1015183927979
216. Hart H, Rubia K. Neuroimaging of child abuse: a critical review. *Front Hum Neurosci*. 2012;6:52 PMID: 22457645 https://doi.org/10.3389/fnhum.2012.00052
217. Meng X, Fleury MJ, Xiang YT, Li M, D'Arcy C. Resilience and protective factors among people with a history of child maltreatment: a systematic review. *Soc Psychiatry Psychiatr Epidemiol*. 2018;53(5):453–475 PMID: 29349479 https://doi.org/10.1007/s00127-018-1485-2

CHAPTER 31

Trauma-Informed Care and Treatment

Brooks Keeshin, MD, FAAP
Assistant Professor
Department of Pediatrics
University of Utah
Salt Lake City, UT

Lindsay Dianne Shepard, LCSW, MSW, MSC
Program Manager
Department of Pediatrics
University of Utah
Therapist
Center for Safe and Healthy Families
Primary Children's Hospital
Salt Lake City, UT

Kara Byrne, PhD
Assistant Research Professor
College of Social Work
University of Utah
Salt Lake City, UT

Delaney is a 16-year-old with her General Educational Development (GED), driver's permit, first job, and first semester of online college classes, but she almost did not make it to this point. Delaney was sexually abused by her maternal uncle from the time she was about 4 to 7 years old. Delaney describes knowing and feeling like something was not quite right about how her uncle would "help" her with toileting and bathing, but she was 11 or 12 years old before she better understood that he had sexually abused her. Filled with shame, guilt, and a barrage of overwhelming and confusing feelings, Delaney says she spiraled out of control. By the time she was 15 years old, she was failing out of school, drinking and doing drugs, sleeping around, running away from home, self-harming, and planning her suicide. Her parents—dad, stepmom, and mom—had continuously tried to figure out what was wrong with her. They had taken her to her medical professional multiple times. Some of her medical professional appointments were for her sexual health, a couple were about her acting out, and a few addressed chronic abdominal pain, for which she also presented to the emergency department (ED) multiple times a year.

Then one day, when she was 15, after an otherwise unremarkable argument with her stepmom, Delaney summoned all of her courage. With a soft voice and tears in her eyes, Delaney told her stepmom of the abuse by her uncle. It suddenly became clear. The question was never, "What is wrong with you?" It was, "What happened to you?"

The next weeks after telling were a blur of emotions and interviews. Delaney's disclosure resulted in her uncle's arrest and then a series of court dates. When Delaney saw her uncle at the first court date, she was inundated with emotional, mental, and physical responses. She wanted to scream, cry, throw up, and escape all at once. She was sweating. Her heart was racing. Her thoughts flooded with memories, thoughts of worthlessness, disgust, and hate. After court, it felt like she could not shake it. She ended up in the ED and then the inpatient hospital for concerns of suicide. She went home with a safety plan and an outpatient therapy referral, but she never went to therapy. A few months later, she went back to the ED and then the inpatient hospital following a suicide attempt. This time, though, she was discharged with an outpatient therapy appointment at an agency offering trauma-specific evidence-based treatments. Delaney worked with her therapist almost weekly for about 8 months. She received trauma-focused cognitive behavioral therapy (TF-CBT). By the time of her therapy graduation, she had attained her GED and driver's permit, started her job, and begun her online college classes.

Delaney made it to this point, but could her journey have been less traumatic? And what role might her medical professional have played? This chapter presents what medical professionals need to know and do to provide trauma-informed care. The first few sections define trauma-informed care, review its application in primary care, and describe the role of the medical professional. The remainder of the chapter is more directive in what medical professionals need to know and do about trauma, particularly for children and teens who have experienced abuse or maltreatment.

Defining Trauma-Informed Care

Trauma-informed care is a strengths-based, overarching framework emphasizing the effect of trauma in the approach to working with individuals and families and in designing systems of care within organizations.[1] Trauma-informed care is based on assumptions encompassed in the 4 Rs: *realizing, recognizing, responding,* and resisting *re-traumatization*.[2] A trauma-informed program, organization, or system "*realizes* the widespread impact of trauma and understands potential paths for recovery; *recognizes* the signs and symptoms of trauma in clients, families, staff, and others involved with the system; *responds* by fully integrating knowledge about trauma into policies, procedures, and practices; and seeks to actively resist *re-traumatization*."[2] These components point to the critical importance in a health care system of understanding the prevalence of trauma; its effect on individuals, families, and communities; and the best interventions to actively treat and prevent unnecessary distress and re-traumatization among the patients and families served. Given the abundance of literature on trauma-informed care, it is important to be cognizant of the many terms and definitions associated with it, including *trauma-specific services* and *trauma-informed systems.*

Trauma-specific services are promising or evidence-based interventions that specifically treat the effects of trauma, including traumatic stress and other associated disorders such as substance use and mental disorders.[2] A discerning medical professional should be aware of evidence-based trauma-specific interventions and services to ensure appropriate referral and follow-up. Some examples of trauma-specific services, which are also described in greater detail later in the chapter, are TF-CBT, parent-child interaction therapy (PCIT), child-parent psychotherapy (CPP), and child and family traumatic stress intervention (CFTSI).

Whereas trauma-specific services aim to treat the individual and family, trauma-informed systems take a macro approach to treating trauma by ensuring that larger systems of care incorporate trauma-informed care across and between their agencies. This contributes to a "comprehensive continuum of care available and accessible to all traumatized children and their families."[3] Components of a trauma-informed system include "a knowledgeable workforce, committed organizations, and skilled professionals."[3] Clinicians can create a system within their own clinic while collaborating with a larger system of trauma-informed clinics and agencies to ensure effective and consistent patient access to trauma-informed care.

To learn more about trauma-informed care, visit the US Substance Abuse and Mental Health Services Administration (SAMHSA)–Health Resources and Services Administration Center for Integrated Health Solutions (https://www.integration.samhsa.gov/clinical-practice/trauma-informed) and the National Child Traumatic Stress Network (NCTSN) (https://www.nctsn.org).

How Trauma-Informed Care Is Developing in Primary Care Settings

In their 2015 systematic review, Flynn and colleagues identified 5 studies that examined the effect of primary care interventions to treat children at risk for traumatic stress.[4] In general, trauma-informed primary care programs employed universal or targeted screening, focused on younger children, and used outcome measures related to reducing risk of child abuse and other forms of childhood trauma (with secondary measures looking at proxies for childhood trauma as well as internalizing and externalizing behaviors).[4] Although medical professionals are generally accepting of these interventions and families rated trauma-informed programs with a high level of satisfaction, few measurable differences regarding child outcomes have been demonstrated.[4] For example, Safe Environment for Every Kid reduces possible child abuse and neglect and severe physical assault when delivered in a high-risk population but produces no differences in potentially traumatic experiences when delivered in a less at-risk population.[5]

Several conceptual models for trauma-informed care have already been developed that warrant further study. The Pediatric Integrated Care Collaborative has developed a toolkit that introduces trauma-informed care concepts to a primary care practice and encourages the use of Plan-Do-Study-Act cycles to thoughtfully and systematically incorporate concepts of trauma-informed care within the pediatric primary care setting.[6] Researchers from the Children's Hospital of Philadelphia have conceptualized trauma-informed care as a separate but overlapping and complementary framework to family-centered care, which has been adopted in numerous pediatric inpatient and outpatient settings across the country (visit https://www.healthcaretoolbox.org for more information)[7] (Figure 31.1). Additionally, centers around the country are experimenting with the use of standardized screeners and responses to potentially traumatized children and their families. One such approach is the use of a brief trauma exposure and symptom screening tool currently being tested in primary care settings in Utah. This screening and complementary decision-support tool assists the medical team in identifying and responding to 3 main factors in children with known trauma exposures: mandated reporting, potential suicidality, and traumatic stress symptoms that would warrant evidence-based trauma-specific interventions or referrals (see https://utahpips.org).

Of additional note, a growing and robust body of research demonstrates the effectiveness of integrated care. *Integrated care* is a heterogeneous concept but generally refers to the acquisition of behavioral health through primary care settings. A review by Asarnow and colleagues in 2015 demonstrated that integrated care trials for pediatric mental health fared considerably better than care as usual. In general, treatment studies demonstrated a greater effect than prevention-focused interventions, children and adolescents both saw gains in integrated care, and mental health interventions as a group were generally more

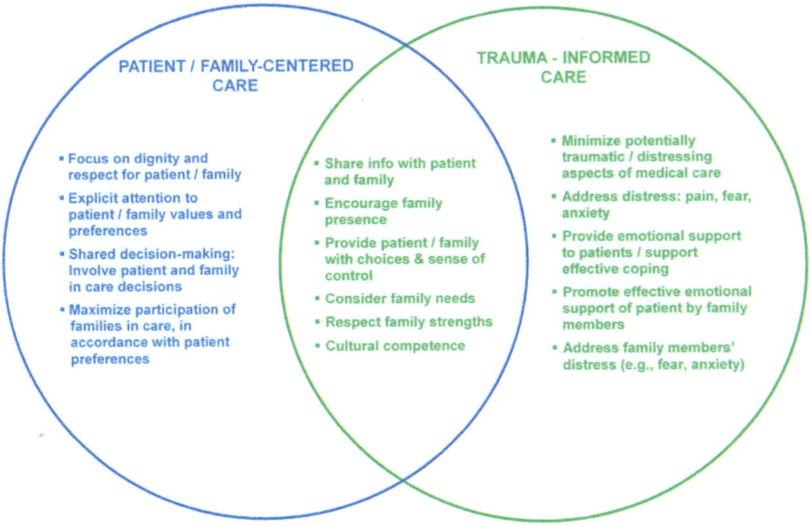

FIGURE 31.1
Family-centered and trauma-informed care.
Reprinted from Center for Pediatric Traumatic Stress. Improving quality of care. *Health Care Toolbox.* https://www.healthcaretoolbox.org/how-providers-make-a-difference/improving-quality-of-care-2.html. Updated October 12, 2015. Accessed August 26, 2019.

successful than substance use integrated care.[8] Although no traumatic stress interventions were included in this meta-analysis, it is likely that the findings are generalizable to children who have experienced trauma who have internalizing and externalizing symptoms.[8]

Role of the Medical Professional in Trauma-Informed Care

About 75% of all children in the United States have seen a medical professional within the past 6 months, most often a primary care professional, regardless of race (69%–81% averages across races) or family income (73%–78% range over income groups).[9] This predictable contact with youth makes frontline medical professionals ideal for identifying past trauma experiences and assessing for traumatic stress. While rates of lifetime exposure to trauma for children vary, one pediatric primary care clinic noted that more than 90% of patients seen identified trauma exposure and 25% of them endorsed full or partial criteria for posttraumatic stress disorder (PTSD).[10] For youth exposed to trauma, their medical professional can be a critical player when it comes to responding to traumatic stress and referring to services and mental health treatment.[11]

Indeed, often schools and health care systems are children's primary points of entry to needed mental health resources.[3] "Seventy-five percent of children under age 12 see a pediatrician at least once per year, whereas 4% see a mental health professional."[12] Medical professionals also typically have a safe and calm rapport with their patients, wherein the patients might feel comfortable disclosing or talking about potentially traumatic events.[11] Because of their frequent contact, trusted relationship, and connections to resources, medical professionals are key to youth safety and healing from the adverse effects of trauma.

However, to be successful, trauma-informed systems require trauma-informed medical professionals. In pediatric health care, this means professionals who *realize* "the widespread impact of trauma and understand potential paths for recovery"; *recognize* "the signs and symptoms of trauma in clients, families, staff, and others involved with the system"; *respond* "by fully integrating knowledge about trauma into policies, procedures, and practices"; and seek to actively resist *re-traumatization*.[2] The next few sections detail what medical professionals need to know (*realize* and *recognize*) about trauma and what they can do about trauma (*respond* and resist *re-traumatization*).

What Medical Professionals Need to Know About Trauma

While trauma is a robust field of theory, research, and practice, there are some definitions, key concepts, and research with which every medical professional should be familiar.

Definitions of Trauma

By way of definitions, Sege, Amaya-Jackson, and the American Academy of Pediatrics (AAP) Committee on Child Abuse and Neglect and Council on Foster Care, Adoption, and Kinship Care; the American Academy of Child and Adolescent Psychiatry (AACAP) Committee on Child Maltreatment and Violence; and the National Center for Child Traumatic Stress distinguish the following commonly used terms: *adverse childhood experiences* (ACEs), *trauma, child traumatic stress, toxic stress,* and *PTSD* (Box 31.1).[16]

Trauma and *traumatic stress* are the most frequently used terms in this chapter, wherein *trauma* is in reference to an intense or harmful event or experience and *traumatic stress* refers to the emotional, mental, and physical responses to trauma exposure.

BOX 31.1
Commonly Used Terms in Trauma-Informed Care

Adverse childhood experiences: Emotional, physical, or sexual abuse; emotional or physical neglect; domestic violence; parental substance use; parental mental illness; parental separation or divorce; or incarceration of a household member.[13]

Trauma: Psychological trauma occurs when a child experiences an intense event that threatens or causes harm to his or her emotional and physical well-being.[14]

Child traumatic stress: The intense fear and stress response occurring when children are exposed to traumatic events that overwhelm their ability to cope with what they have experienced.

Toxic stress: Term introduced by Garner et al and the American Academy of Pediatrics.[15] Defined as excessive or prolonged activation of the physiologic stress response systems in the absence of the buffering protection afforded by stable, responsive relationships.

Posttraumatic stress disorder: Set of psychiatric symptoms meeting *Diagnostic and Statistical Manual of Mental Disorders*, 5th Edition, criteria after a person has experienced, witnessed, or learned of a close family member experiencing an event involving actual or threatened death, serious injury, or sexual violation.

Adapted from Sege RD, Amaya-Jackson L; American Academy of Pediatrics Committee on Child Abuse and Neglect and Council on Foster Care, Adoption, and Kinship Care; American Academy of Child and Adolescent Psychiatry Committee on Child Maltreatment and Violence; National Center for Child Traumatic Stress. Clinical considerations related to the behavioral manifestations of child maltreatment. *Pediatrics*. 2017;139(4):e20170100.

Key Concepts of Trauma

The most important concepts for medical professionals to understand about trauma might be best summarized by the 12 Core Concepts of the NCTSN.[17] These 12 items define the effect of traumatic experiences on children and support the importance of trauma-informed assessment and intervention (Box 31.2).

Prevalence of Trauma

Up to 80% of children report experiencing at least one significant traumatic event in childhood,[18] such as a disaster, automobile crash, accidental injury, life-threating medical diagnosis, child maltreatment, exposure to community violence, or war or terrorism. More specifically, about 1 in 6 American girls and 1 in 25 American boys have experienced sexual assault[19–21]; about 17% of American youth have experienced forms of

BOX 31.2
National Child Traumatic Stress Network 12 Core Concepts for Childhood Traumatic Stress

1. Traumatic experiences are inherently complex.

Every traumatic event is made up of different traumatic moments, each of which includes varying degrees of objective life threat, physical violation, and witnessing of injury or death. Children's thoughts and actions (or inaction) during various moments may lead to feelings of conflict at the time and to feelings of confusion, guilt, regret, and/or anger afterward.

2. Trauma occurs within a broad context that includes children's personal characteristics, life experiences, and current circumstances.

The child's own experience, personality, and environment affect his or her own appraisal of traumatic events and may exacerbate the adverse effects of trauma.

3. Traumatic events often generate secondary adversities, life changes, and distressing reminders in children's daily lives.

Children's exposure to trauma reminders can serve as additional sources of distress. Secondary adversities may significantly affect functioning in trauma survivors.

4. Children can exhibit a wide range of reactions to trauma and loss.

Posttraumatic stress and grief reactions can develop over time into psychiatric disorders (eg, posttraumatic stress disorder, separation anxiety, depression), may disrupt major domains of child development, and may reduce children's level of functioning at home, at school, and in the community.

5. Danger and safety are core concerns in the lives of traumatized children.

Lack of physical and psychological safety can be magnified in a child's mind. Ensuring children's physical safety is foundational to restoring the sense of a protective shield.

6. Traumatic experiences affect the family and broader caregiving systems.

Caregivers' own concerns may impair their ability to support children who have experienced trauma. The ability of caregiver systems to provide support is an important contributor to children's and families' adjustment.

7. Protective and promotive factors can reduce the adverse effect of trauma.

Protective factors buffer the adverse effects of trauma and its stressful aftermath, whereas promotive factors generally enhance children's positive adjustment regardless of whether risk factors are present. The presence of these factors (ie, positive attachment to a caregiver, reliable social support, environment) can enhance children's ability to resist, or to "bounce back" from adversities.

(continued)

BOX 31.2 (*continued*)

8. Trauma and post-trauma adversities can strongly influence development.

Trauma and post-trauma adversities can profoundly influence children's acquisition of developmental competencies and their capacity to reach important developmental milestones. Trauma and its aftermath can lead to developmental disruptions (regressive behavior, reluctance, or inability to participate in developmentally appropriate activities), and developmental accelerations such as leaving home at an early age and engagement in precocious sexual behavior.

9. Developmental neurobiology underlies children's reactions to traumatic experiences.

Children's capacities to appraise and respond to danger are linked to an evolving neurobiology of brain structures, neurophysiological pathways, and neuroendocrine systems. Traumatic experiences evoke strong biological responses that can persist and alter the normal course of neurobiological maturation. Exposure to multiple traumatic experiences carries a greater risk.

10. Culture is closely interwoven with traumatic experiences, response, and recovery.

Culture can profoundly affect the ways in which children and their families respond to traumatic events, including how they express distress and disclose personal information to others.

11. Challenges to the social contract, including legal and ethical issues, affect trauma response and recovery.

Traumatic experiences often constitute a violation of expectations of the child, family, community, and society. The perceived success or failure of these institutional responses may exert a profound influence on the course of children's post-trauma adjustment and on their evolving beliefs regarding family, work, and civic life.

12. Working with trauma-exposed children can evoke distress in providers that makes it more difficult for them to provide good care.

Medical professionals often encounter personal and professional challenges as they confront details of children's traumatic experiences and life adversities. Proper self-care is an important part of providing quality care.

Adapted from National Child Traumatic Stress Network Core Curriculum on Childhood Trauma Task Force. *The 12 Core Concepts: Concepts for Understanding Traumatic Stress Responses in Children and Families. Core Curriculum on Childhood Trauma.* Los Angeles, CA, and Durham, NC: UCLA-Duke University National Center for Child Traumatic Stress; 2012. https://www.nctsn.org/sites/default/files/resources//the_12_core_concepts_for_understanding_traumatic_stress_responses_in_children_and_families.pdf. Accessed July 14, 2019.

physical punishment and abuse that left noticeable marks, bruises, welts, burns, or cuts[21]; up to 70% have witnessed serious community violence[21]; approximately 20% to 25% have experienced a human-made or natural disaster[21]; and anywhere from 20% to 66% of all youth have been exposed to multiple traumatic events.[18,21] The National Survey of Children's Exposure to Violence also shows alarming rates of children exposed to trauma not just in their lifetime but each year.[20] Moreover, children who are minorities, including those who are part of federally recognized tribes, are disproportionately exposed to and affected by trauma.[22,23]

Of concern with trauma associated specifically with child maltreatment is that exposures might go undetected or unreported[16] and can often be multiple and concurrent, such as experiencing sexual abuse over a number of years or experiencing neglect and exposure to substance use.[3,18,21] Furthermore, concerns of child maltreatment can involve children in the welfare system where they are exposed to additional stressors such as home removal, multiple out-of-home placements, and new caregivers, schools, and peers.[3] Trauma from child abuse and maltreatment is of great concern because of its potentially intimate nature, disruption to home and family, and significant risk of poor health and mental health outcomes.[13,24]

Trauma-Protective Factors and Resilience

In spite of the potential negative effects of trauma, there is cause for hope. Studies of certain trauma therapies show efficacy for recovery for children with symptoms.[25–27] Furthermore, resilience studies indicate some children demonstrate minimal distress or are only temporarily affected by trauma before returning to their previous level of functioning.[28,29] Some resilient and protective factors have been identified as helpful to children withstanding or recovering from trauma. These include supportive parents, friends, family, school, and community; a safe environment; personal high self-esteem and self-efficacy; reassuring spiritual and cultural beliefs; personal talents or skills (eg, academics, arts, athletics); coping skills; access to social resources; strong relationships; minimal trauma exposure; and connectedness to school, health, and behavioral health providers.[28,29] Interestingly, some researchers have also started to look into post-traumatic growth, or the possibility of positive outcomes following trauma exposure, for which there is some evidence in children.[30]

Risks and Cost of Trauma

Some traumas can be life altering and have lingering effects on children and their environments. While it is normal to have a response to trauma, some children exposed to trauma will develop symptoms of traumatic stress, "the intense fear and stress response occurring when children are exposed to traumatic events that overwhelm their ability to cope with what they have experienced."[16] About 16% (95% CI, 11.5–21.5) of children exposed to trauma meet the criteria for PTSD, with particularly higher rates among girls exposed to interpersonal trauma (32.9%; 95% CI, 19.8–49.3).[24] Symptoms, such as nightmares, intrusive thoughts, flashbacks, avoidance, hypervigilance, or somatic complaints, may linger or even intensify. Children's functioning may change or regress at school, home, and/or socially. Youth might also present with behaviors of concern, such as self-harm, suicidal intent or attempts, substance use, or other risk-taking behaviors. Furthermore, adverse effects of traumatic stress can extend well into adulthood. The seminal Adverse Childhood Experiences study identified relationships between adverse event exposure in childhood and a number of negative health and mental health outcomes, including suicide, early pregnancy, sexually transmitted infections, mental health comorbidities, substance use, obesity, chronic illness, heart disease, cancer, liver disease, and even early death.[13] Parallel to this significant human cost, the Perryman Group has estimated that each first-time case of child maltreatment in the United States will have lifetime economic costs of $1.8 million per child who experiences maltreatment.[31] At minimum, these risk and cost data warn against the consequences of doing nothing and the importance of trauma-informed care.

Traumatic Stress Symptoms

Traumatic stress is characterized by responses of intense fear and stress to traumatic events.[16] While these responses are normal and healthy for survival and coping at the time of the event and often for a short time after, their persistence can become maladaptive and disruptive. Common symptoms include an onset and/or intensifying of sleep problems, intrusive thoughts, flashbacks, avoidance, hypervigilance, and general mood dysregulation. Some children experience somatic complaints, or unexplained physical complaints, such as headaches, stomachaches, chest pain, or weight change. Substance use and suicidality can also co-occur and are of great concern.

Traumatic stress can be comorbid with other disorders, particularly preexisting conditions. However, traumatic stress can also go undiagnosed or be misdiagnosed as other conditions with similar symptom profiles. As examples, children with prominent trauma symptoms of arousal and hypervigilance might be confused for having attention-deficit/hyperactivity disorder (ADHD) or anxiety; youth with significant trauma symptoms of avoidance, negative affect, mood dysregulation, and suicidal intent might be solely identified for depression; or children who have panic attacks in response to trauma reminders might be misdiagnosed with anxiety or a panic disorder. Of particular note for medical professionals, traumatic stress symptoms can also present as physical health concerns that are actually somatic complaints. A few studies have documented a relationship between trauma exposure and health concerns such as asthma, allergies, gastrointestinal issues, and headaches.[32] However, in relation to trauma, stomachaches or headaches can come from stress, poor sleep, changes to routine, or avoidance. Chest pain or symptoms of asthma, such as shortness of breath, can come from trauma-induced stress, panic attacks, and anxiety. Weight change can come from emotional coping, stress, and body image or connectivity issues post trauma. Because of possible similar symptom profiles with other health and mental health conditions, it is important for medical professionals to be trauma informed. This is not to say that someone with ADHD, depression, anxiety, irritable bowels, asthma, or weight change cannot also have traumatic stress comorbid to these conditions, but the under-detection of trauma exposure and the mis- and underdiagnosis of traumatic stress is concerning. Correctly identifying trauma can help the medical professional understand the etiology of the child's symptoms as well as indicate appropriate trauma-specific evidence-based treatment. A trauma-informed medical professional *realizes* the importance of responding to trauma and *recognizes* its symptoms. A simple application of this knowledge directs trauma-informed medical professionals to screen for trauma or rule it out before making diagnostic, treatment, and referral decisions for health and mental health conditions with similar symptom profiles.

The most important diagnoses with which to be familiar for traumatic stress are acute stress disorder and PTSD. The American Psychiatric Association *Diagnostic and Statistical Manual of Mental Disorders,* 5th Edition (*DSM-5*), provides full criteria for acute stress disorder and PTSD.[32] Generally speaking, acute stress disorder is characterized by a combination of intrusive thoughts or memories, negative mood, dissociative, avoidance, and arousal symptoms for the first month following exposure to a traumatic event.[32] Posttraumatic stress disorder is when traumatic stress symptoms persist for longer than 1 month, including a minimum of 1 intrusive symptom, 1 avoidance symptom, 2 negative cognition or mood symptoms, and 2 symptoms of hyperarousal.[32] In children who meet criteria for PTSD, it is important to consider whether the dissociative modifier is applicable, which indicates if the child experiences *depersonalization* ("persistent or recurrent experiences of feeling detached from, and as if one were an outside observer of, one's mental processes or body"[32]) or *derealization* ("persistent or recurrent experiences of unreality of surroundings"[32]). Of note for children younger than 7 years, the criteria for PTSD are somewhat simplified in that avoidance and many of the symptoms of negative or decreased cognition and mood are joined into one large category. This is in recognition that young children may not understand the connection between trauma reminders and distress and, therefore, may not engage in avoidant activities, or simply that because of their age they lack the ability to control enough of their environment that they can effectively avoid trauma reminders. When considering diagnoses for child traumatic stress, the AAP also has a trauma guide that includes a helpful resource on this topic, "Diagnoses to Consider When Evaluating a Child Exposed to Trauma."[33]

What Medical Professionals Can Do About Trauma

Trauma-informed medical professionals *respond* to trauma "by fully integrating knowledge about trauma into policies, procedures, and practices" and also actively seek to resist *re-traumatization*.[2] To *respond* and resist *re-traumatization,* medical professionals should adhere to the SAMHSA 6 key principles of a trauma-informed approach[2] (Box 31.3).

Medical professionals should seek to create a safe and supportive environment in which they can engage, empower, and collaborate with families in response to trauma. This work begins before trauma is even disclosed. Medical professionals can continually create a safe office environment, develop relationships with community resources for trauma, approach parents in an empathetic and collaborative manner, and establish a culture of trauma-informed practices. Cohen, Kelleher, and Mannarino suggest 5 things medical professionals can do to create a trauma-informed practice (Box 31.4).[11] The AAP also has a *Trauma Toolbox for Primary Care* that includes a document, "Addressing Adverse

BOX 31.3

US Substance Abuse and Mental Health Services Administration 6 Key Principles of a Trauma-Informed Approach

1. Safety
2. Trustworthiness and transparency
3. Peer support
4. Collaboration and mutuality
5. Empowerment, voice, and choice
6. Cultural, historical, and gender issues

From US Substance Abuse and Mental Health Services Administration. *SAMHSA's Concept of Trauma and Guidance for a Trauma-Informed Approach.* HHS Publication No. (SMA) 14-4884. Rockville, MD: Substance Abuse and Mental Health Services Administration; 2014. https://store.samhsa.gov/system/files/sma14-4884.pdf. Accessed July 14, 2019.

BOX 31.4
Five Things Medical Professionals Can Do

1. Routinely ask about exposure to potentially traumatic events at office visits.
2. For children who disclose exposure, screen for related functional impairments, including somatic symptoms and emotional and behavioral problems.
3. For children who disclose exposure, provide office-based interventions such as education about the effect of trauma and optimal care for recovery.
4. Monitor children with known trauma exposure to provide early detection of serious psychiatric symptoms and education about the benefits of mental health treatment.
5. For children with significant symptoms, facilitate referrals to appropriate mental health professionals and impress on parents the importance of seeking services for their children.

Derived from Cohen JA, Kelleher KJ, Mannarino AP. Identifying, treating, and referring traumatized children: the role of pediatric providers. *Arch Pediatr Adolesc Med.* 2008;162(5):447–452.

Childhood Experiences and Other Types of Trauma in the Primary Care Setting," which outlines a 4-step process for practices to set up procedures and workflow for the identification and treatment of children with ACEs.[34] What follows in the next sections are specific steps for pediatric practice and decision-making along the same lines as Cohen and colleagues' 5 suggested practices[11] and the AAP 4-step process.[34] These are to establish processes for identifying trauma and assessing traumatic stress, reporting abuse and maltreatment, safety planning, providing education and brief in-office interventions, referring to mental health treatment, managing medications, and following up and monitoring patient progress over time.

Identifying Trauma

The determination as to whether children warrant trauma treatment begins with the identification of potentially traumatic experiences. Inquiring about potentially traumatic experiences at office visits supports early identification of children who have experienced trauma.[11] Traumatic experiences can be detected as part of case finding or as part of a standardized screening process or measure. In some clinical scenarios, the medical professional will be aware that the medical treatment is based directly on or related to a prior traumatic event. Even when new traumatic experiences have occurred, it is always critical for medical professionals to assess for other potentially traumatic events because these are more common among children who have experienced trauma or abuse and a risk factor for acute symptomatology.[35] Cohen, Kelleher, and Mannarino suggest asking a simple question to returning patients at all health supervision visits: "Since the last time I saw you, has anything really scary or upsetting happened to you or your family?"[11] A more thorough history might include asking about children's exposure to intimate partner violence, abuse, neglect, parental substance use, or parental mental health concerns.[16]

Assessing Traumatic Stress

If a child reports exposure to a potentially traumatic event, key to treatment is the assessment of traumatic stress symptoms, because not all children are equally symptomatic. Most traumatic stress screening and assessment tools have been designed for mental health professionals and so might be too lengthy for a typical pediatric practice. These tools might still be considered, however, and include the UCLA Child/Adolescent PTSD Reaction Index (RI),[36] the Child PTSD Symptom Scale,[37] and the Trauma Symptoms Checklist for Children.[38] An abbreviated or brief version of the UCLA PTSD RI per *DSM-5* criteria is currently in preparation for publication. In the meantime, a copy of the *DSM-IV* version of the UCLA PTSD RI, Short Version,[39] is available in Cohen, Kelleher, and Mannarino's article.[11] There is also the Children's Revised Impact of Event Scale and the Pediatric Symptom Checklist, which are listed for trauma in "Mental Health Screening and Assessment Tools for Primary Care" from the AAP *Addressing Mental Health Concerns in Primary Care: A Clinician's Toolkit* (learn more at https://www.aap.org/en-us/advocacy-and-policy/aap-health-initiatives/Mental-Health/Documents/MH_ScreeningChart.pdf). The goal of incorporating a traumatic stress screening tool into the pediatric practice workflow for a child with trauma exposure is to provide meaningful symptom information. The medical professional can then tailor his or her response, including safety considerations, anticipatory guidance, brief in-office interventions, mental health referrals, and plans for follow-up.

Additional assessment information that might be of use in decision-making includes the child's general functioning and environment. Some information about the child's development, strengths, and limitations might already be known to the medical professional or collected in other relevant information forms at the pediatric practice. Of particular interest are details about the child's personal characteristics (eg, age, culture, gender identity, language, developmental ability), medical history, and functioning in the home, family, social, and school environments. Professionals might also want to ask the child or caregiver how the child is functioning since the traumatic event and/or its disclosure. Questions might include, since the trauma, "How is your child doing at home?" "How is your child doing at school?" and "How is your child doing with friends?" Environment and general functioning information might indicate important areas for provider response, including protective factors to promote and risk factors to address.

Mandated Reporting

For children who have been exposed to or experienced trauma, ensuring safety is paramount. Consequently, the first decision is whether a report to state child protective services (CPS) is needed. Mandated reporting largely refers to concerns for child abuse or neglect. However, the definition of *reportable abuse* varies from state to state. The presence of a minor in the event of domestic violence, for example, is considered reportable child maltreatment in some states. Age of consent laws also vary by state. However, all professionals and those providing trauma-informed care are mandated reporters and are obligated to be aware of child abuse reporting laws and requirements in their state. Mandated reporting is a first decision to ensure child safety.

Safety Planning

Returning to a state of safety is important in the treatment and rehabilitation of children exposed to trauma. In addition to mandated reporting, prominent safety considerations that medical professionals should assess and respond to in the course of trauma-informed care include suicidality, self-harm, substance use, other risk-taking behaviors, contact with the alleged offender(s), and unfulfilled basic needs.

Suicidality, in particular, should be assessed for all youth who have been exposed to trauma due to its high comorbidity with trauma as well as its lethality.[40,41] To assess and respond to trauma, medical professionals can follow established practices in their system or directly ask youth or their caregivers probing questions such as, "Have you ever wanted to fall asleep and not wake up?" or "Have you ever wanted or tried to do something to harm yourself?" Some youth will require a full risk assessment, such as by a crisis worker or experienced clinician or, when necessary, in an ED, to determine if urgent and higher levels of care are needed. Other youth will benefit from open communication, safety planning, and monitoring in collaboration with their family and medical professional. Medical professionals providing trauma-informed care assess and address concerns for suicide in youth who have been exposed to trauma. As part of safety planning with patients and their families, there may be specific considerations to make in the event of trauma, such as contact with or exposure to the alleged offender(s) and trauma reminders. Those who have been exposed to trauma can also experience inappropriate guilt and feelings of worthlessness. Medical professionals can have an effect in guiding patients to talk about their strengths and future plans as well as in reassuring them that their guilt is likely misplaced.

Concerns for self-harm, substance use, and other risk-taking behaviors are important to identify and respond to within primary care because they are correlated with suicidality and re-traumatization.[41,42] Medical professionals providing trauma-informed care can be influential in youth behavior change or harm-reduction behaviors. Furthermore, serious and chronic self-harm, substance use, and other risk-taking behaviors are likely indicative of trauma-specific or higher levels of care (eg, specialized, intensive outpatient, day, residential, inpatient treatment). Medical professionals can be pivotal in youth who have been exposed to trauma or who are taking risks accessing appropriate mental health resources.

Ongoing contact with the alleged offender(s) can be a significant stressor and safety concern. At the time of mandated reporting, special consideration might need to be made as to the child's contact with the alleged offender(s), such as when an alleged offender is a caregiver, sibling, or someone with whom the child has daily contact. Medical professionals providing trauma-informed care convey needed child and alleged offender contact information to CPS to inform safety planning. In the event that a child has experienced unsupported allegations of child maltreatment, wherein there was insufficient evidence to support the involvement of CPS, trauma-informed medical professionals can review safety practices and help children and their families access potentially helpful resources (eg, mental health treatment, substance use treatment, food pantries, parenting skills).

Sometimes trauma can upset or alter a child's environment so substantially that it affects their basic needs. A child removed from his or her parents and placed in care, for example, might be unsure of whom to trust and tell if help is needed. A parent affected by domestic violence might not have shelter, food, employment, and health care available without remaining with the abusive partner. A new kinship caregiver might not have all the needed items to care for a child (eg, winter boots and coat, bottles, stroller). Medical professionals providing trauma-informed care discuss safety with children and their caregivers as well as help them to access needed resources and supports in the community.

Providing Education and Anticipatory Guidance

Trauma-informed medical professionals can help children and their families understand trauma, traumatic stress, and available resources. A supportive and informative discussion with the child and his or her caregiver(s) might start with a statement like, "It's really important that you told me you have experienced...and that you're having symptoms like.... Kids exposed to traumatic or upsetting events sometimes have feelings just like yours." This statement praises the child and caregiver(s) for talking about their trauma exposure, a likely vulnerable experience. It also normalizes the child's responses and opens the door to explaining more about trauma, traumatic stress symptoms, and anticipatory guidance. Cohen, Kelleher, and Mannarino suggest that medical professionals can best help children and families who have been exposed to trauma by "[p]roviding education about PTEs [potentially traumatic events] (eg, the common nature of these events, that the pediatrician has seen many other children who have experienced this and recovered, common physical and emotional reactions)"; "[e]ducating families about PTSD or other symptoms children are experiencing"; and "[e]ncouraging families to engage in healthy sleeping and eating patterns, recreation, and exercise and to obtain help from natural support systems (eg, extended family, faith and cultural communities)."[11] Written materials and handouts about trauma and traumatic stress are available from the websites of the AAP (www.aap.org), AACAP (www.aacap.org), and the NCTSN (www.nctsn.org). Specifically, the AAP has designed the *Trauma Toolbox for Primary Care* for medical professionals to incorporate trauma-informed care into practice (visit https://www.aap.org/en-us/advocacy-and-policy/aap-health-initiatives/healthy-foster-care-america/Pages/Trauma-Guide.aspx for more information). This is an excellent source for designing overall processes that identify and respond to trauma in a clinical care setting and includes a number of medical professional– and patient-facing materials.

Delivering Brief, In-Office Intervention

Trauma-informed medical professionals can provide basic information and initial skills for the alleviation of traumatic stress. Decisions as to which symptoms are of highest concern or which skills might be of most interest should be made in collaboration with the child and caregiver(s). However, whenever relevant, basic care needs and disrupted sleep should be addressed first. Medical professionals can follow treatment as usual for child sleep and/or eating concerns, including encouraging routine and caregiver support. Teaching and routinizing relaxation techniques for bedtime might be helpful as well.

Cohen, Kelleher, and Mannarino recommend that in addition to providing education and encouragement to families who have been exposed to trauma, medical professionals can best help by introducing children and parents to simple relaxation techniques such as focused breathing and muscle relaxation.[11] Children and parents can typically identify activities that help them relax, but focused or belly breathing is a technique that travels well and is discrete. There are numerous videos, tools, and phone apps that can assist medical professionals to teach relaxation techniques. Elmo from *Sesame Street* even teaches children to "Belly Breathe" in a song featuring Colbie Caillat and Common (https://www.youtube.com/watch?v=_mZbzDOpylA&t=2s). The National Center for PTSD, within the US Department of Veterans Affairs, has an app and website called PTSD Coach Online that includes learning materials, symptom trackers, coping skills support, and important crisis and mental health resources, including a coping skill guide for focused breathing that may be helpful for adolescents (visit https://www.ptsd.va.gov/apps/ptsdcoachonline/default.htm for more information). A trauma-informed medical professional teaches relaxation techniques to children who have been exposed to trauma and their caregivers and helps them access instructional materials and technology.

Referring to Mental Health Treatment

When traumatic stress symptoms persist after one or a series of abusive or traumatic events, trauma-informed medical professionals respond by explaining that there are effective treatment options and by discussing treatment referrals. Because there is great variability in access to and availability of evidence-based trauma resources, clinics likely need to anticipate that they will be referring families for trauma treatment and identify medical professionals in the area who are competent in delivering evidence-based trauma practices before referral is needed. A primary step when initiating discussions with the family about appropriate treatment includes identifying the type of setting for which the patient's age, symptoms, and functional impairment are most suitable.

In general, if one detects chronic safety issues or global and severe functional impairment, prior to developing an outpatient treatment plan, consideration should be given to whether the patient should be referred to a higher level of care, such as inpatient, residential, day treatment, or intensive outpatient modalities. One should not assume that referral to an outpatient trauma treatment professional will be a successful referral if the child is not stable enough to continue to function in school, home, and social settings with only weekly contact with an outpatient therapist.

Clear indications for a higher level of care include current and severe suicidal and/or self-injurious ideation or behavior; significant substance use; inability to maintain attendance at school due to truancy, missed days, or behaviors at school; and difficulty maintaining a safe and stable home environment based on potentially violent interactions with parents and siblings. Children and adolescents who meet criteria for a substance use disorder, that in and of itself is impairing to the child and resulting in school or family or legal problems, may warrant evaluation by an appropriate substance use facility prior to initiation of trauma treatment.

Not all significant emotional or behavioral reactions that may otherwise impede traditional outpatient trauma treatment will necessitate a higher level of care. One example includes adolescents who experience chronic suicidality and/or self-harm ideation but have been able to maintain some level of safety outside of a hospitalized or more controlled setting. Some of these cases may be adequately addressed within the context of outpatient evidence-based trauma treatment. However, patients with severe and debilitating symptoms may benefit from referral to modalities that directly address suicidal ideation and non-suicidal self-injurious behavior, such as dialectical behavioral therapy. Engaging in dialectical behavioral therapy prior to trauma work can help stabilize an adolescent, decrease the risk for needing higher levels of care such as day treatment or residential treatment, and provide the adolescent with distress tolerance and emotional regulation skills that will directly improve the youth's capacity to address the trauma later in treatment.

In children who meet criteria for outpatient trauma treatment, either initially or after significant safety or behavioral issues have been addressed, there are a number of available options with evidence proving efficacy in the treatment of children who have been exposed to trauma. As a preface, although a variety of treatments are available, many share commonalities and some children respond to some methods better than others. However, at this time, there is a dearth of substantive comparative effectiveness studies and, therefore, it is difficult to know which treatment will be most suitable for which child. In the absence of comparative effectiveness studies, medical professionals are left with meta-analyses that demonstrate the overall effectiveness of evidence-based trauma treatment of children with PTSD and other common sequelae of traumatic experiences such as depression, anxiety, and acting-out behaviors.[43,44] There are also randomized controlled trials that demonstrate effectiveness of evidence-based trauma approaches generally compared to wait-list controls, community care, or a standardized supportive psychotherapy.[43,44]

When deciding on treatment of a child or adolescent, it is best to use shared decision-making methods with patients and their families. When introducing shared decision-making with families, critical points to address include

- Children respond to trauma in different ways, and it is important to understand how a child is responding to the abuse or other traumatic event.
- Although there are many different treatment options, some types of trauma treatment work best for certain types of responses to traumatic events.
- The most appropriate type of trauma treatment of a child is likely dependent on that child's age, duration since the event occurred, type of trauma, and extent of effect.

Evidence-based Treatments of Pediatric Traumatic Stress

Existing research suggests a number of psychological interventions are effective in preventing PTSD and reducing symptoms up to 1 month following the completion of treatment. That being said, research is limited with regard to follow-up with treatment participants and data related to the effectiveness of comparison treatments.[43] While cognitive behavioral therapy shows the best evidence of effectiveness of psychological therapies,[43,44] there are a number of interventions focused on treating children's trauma symptoms that merit more extensive, quality research to gauge their effectiveness. As with any therapeutic intervention, the effectiveness of trauma-specific interventions can be largely dependent on the therapeutic relationship between the child and parent and the therapist.

Examples of common trauma-specific treatments are TF-CBT, PCIT, CFTSI, CPP, and eye-movement desensitization and reprocessing.[11,43,44] There are general components across treatments to be considered in developing a trauma-informed system. Cohen, Kelleher, and Mannarino refer to these components by the acronym DROPS.[11] Common features of evidence-based trauma treatment of children include being **d**evelopmentally and culturally sensitive, **r**esilience based, driven by **o**vercoming avoidance of the trauma experience, **p**arent inclusive, and **s**kills and **s**afety focused. Using written materials and verbal discourse to provide trauma symptom and treatment psychoeducation for children and their caregivers is also an important component of treatment of trauma. This psychoeducation can be provided by the medical professional and therapist.[11,16] To learn more about trauma-informed treatments of children, visit the NCTSN at https://www.nctsn.org.

Trauma-Focused Cognitive Behavioral Therapy

Trauma-focused cognitive behavioral therapy is one of the most well-known interventions for treating trauma symptoms in children and adolescents (approximately 3–18 years old). While TF-CBT was initially designed to treat youth who had been sexually abused, it has now been expanded to treat symptoms associated with a range of traumatic events.[45] Sessions can be one-on-one with the child/adolescent or parent (non-offending in the event of intrafamilial violence), or the child and parent(s) can have conjoint sessions.[46,47]

Trauma-focused cognitive behavioral therapy uses a component approach to treatment. Some of the main components in the TF-CBT process include psychoeducation, parenting skills, relaxation, affective expression and modulation, cognitive coping and processing, and developing a trauma narrative.[46] The components are designed to be flexible with regard to the order of their implementation in the therapeutic setting but always begin with a validated assessment of trauma and behavioral symptoms. While typical length for treatment with TF-CBT in the community is around 20 to 24 weekly sessions, this intervention has been found to be effective at 8 and 16 weeks, depending on the youth.[48] One of the trademark processes in the TF-CBT approach is the development of the *trauma narrative.* The trauma narrative is completed in incremental sessions, whereby the client talks and writes about the events before, during, and after the trauma. A primary goal of the narrative is to "unpair thoughts, reminders, or discussions of the traumatic event from overwhelming negative emotions."[46]

Parent-Child Interaction Therapy

Parent-child interaction therapy is a well-known, evidence-based intervention aimed at increasing positive parenting skills and decreasing problem behaviors in children (approximately 2–8 years old). Parent-child interaction therapy aims to improve parenting skills (including parents who are at high risk for or who previously engaged in physical maltreatment), reduce children's externalizing behaviors, and improve parent-child interactions. It is based on an understanding that negative and coercive interactions between parent and child put parents at a higher risk of maltreating their children.[49] It is suitable for children between 2 and 8 years of age when aiming to change the child's behavior and between 4 and 12 years of age when aiming to change the behavior of a parent who has been physically abusive.[49]

Parent-child interaction therapy seeks to disrupt a maladaptive cycle in the parent-child interaction characterized by negative interactions, overreliance on punishment, and ineffective discipline strategies, which are often followed by aggressive and noncompliant behavior by the children.[49,50] Parent-child interaction therapy is made up of 2 sequential phases, child-directed interaction and parent-directed interaction.[51] On average, the parent-child dyads participate in about 20 sessions, although the number of sessions is largely dependent on parents' ability to master communication and behavior management skills. Parent-child interaction therapy is known for the parent-coaching component, wherein the medical professional observes the parent-child dyads through a 1-way mirror and coaches the parent via a small microphone bud in the caregiver's ear.[51]

Child and Family Traumatic Stress Intervention

Child and family traumatic stress intervention is an early intervention and secondary prevention strategy to prevent the development of PTSD in youth (approximately 7–18 years old) who have experienced one or many traumatic events. This intervention merits further research and is considered a promising intervention to prevent PTSD.[44,52] However, Gillies et al demonstrate that a child's likelihood of being diagnosed with PTSD is reduced if the child receives a psychological therapy such as CFTSI, compared with those who do not.[43]

Child and family traumatic stress intervention is generally initiated within 30 days of exposure to the traumatic event or disclosure of abuse.[52] The intervention consists of 4 to 8 individual and joint sessions between the child and the caregiver. In the case of intrafamilial violence, therapy occurs with the non-offending caregiver.[52]

Child and family traumatic stress intervention targets family support and the development of coping skills. These sessions begin with a psychoeducational session for the caregiver to learn about PTSD and the symptoms associated with experiencing a traumatic event. From here, the medical professional assesses symptoms of PTSD from the caregiver and child's perspectives, compares these responses, and discusses responses to increase the caregiver's awareness of the child's symptoms and the child's communication of his or her symptoms and needs. From here, the medical professional works with the child and caregiver to learn and practice coping mechanisms that address the most salient and impairing symptoms experienced by the child.

Child-Parent Psychotherapy

Child-parent psychotherapy is an evidence-based intervention focused on "nurturing a secure, growth-promoting attachment" between the child and his or her non-offending caregiver.[16] This is a dyadic intervention for very young children (approximately 0–6 years old) along with their caregivers and is primarily based on developing the parent-child relationship.[11,16] The treatment was initially designed for children living in violent homes but has since been expanded to include children exposed to a violent death.[11]

Child-parent psychotherapy typically takes place over the course of 40 to 50 sessions; however, the number of sessions needed rests on advancement of a secure attachment that promotes the child's development and includes an increase in positive interactions between the child and parent. Sessions often take place in an in-home setting. However, CPP can also be effective in a clinical setting, if appropriate.[11,16] Sessions are guided by child-parent interactions, whereby the therapist interprets and directs interactions in more positive and adaptive ways.[16] As a result of CPP, the child and parent can increase their ability to regulate their behaviors and affects, and generally come to better understand each other.[16]

Eye-Movement Desensitization and Reprocessing

Eye-movement desensitization and reprocessing is a promising therapy for the treatment of PTSD in children and adolescents (approximately 3–18 years old).[26,53,54] This therapy, developed by Francine Shapiro in the 1980s, was initially developed to treat adult PTSD but has since been expanded to treat children and adolescents.[53,55]

Eye-movement desensitization and reprocessing comprises 8 phases of treatment: history taking, preparation, assessment, desensitization, installation, body scan, closure, and reassessment.[53] The trademark mechanism incorporated into eye-movement desensitization and reprocessing is the bilateral external stimuli, including the saccadic eye movement (following the therapist's finger from left to right or up and down). This external stimulus has been expanded to include ear tones and tapping the therapist's hand.[54] During the desensitization phase, the client is asked to recall the traumatic memory and any negative associations in combination with the stimuli.[54]

Managing Medications

Trauma-specific therapy models have been shown effective in children with traumatic stress symptoms and should be pursued as the primary, and most often sole, line of treatment.[43,44] There are no US Food and Drug Administration–approved drugs for the treatment of traumatic stress in children.[56] Medications that have demonstrated efficacy for PTSD in adults, such as sertraline, have been studied and found not to be effective in children.[57] Due to lack of evidence, abuse potential, and risk of side effects, there is no clear benefit for the use of benzodiazepines or second-generation antipsychotics in the treatment of pediatric traumatic stress.

Children who have been exposed to trauma are more likely to experience side effects from medications than peers who have not experienced trauma. Trauma-exposed children are more likely to receive psychotropic medications, more likely to receive multiple psychotropic medications at the same time, and more likely to experience side effects from medications than peers who have not experienced trauma.[58–62]

It is possible in some cases for medical professionals to consider short-term use of medications to target specific symptoms in children with traumatic stress. However, it is important to exercise caution. Symptoms common in acute stress may reflect normal post-traumatic hypervigilance and arousal and not warrant pharmacological treatment due to the likely transient nature of the symptoms. One possible area of pharmacological intervention is sleep disturbance, which is common among children who have experienced trauma. Non-pharmacological interventions should be tried first, such as addressing any real or perceived danger at night, returning to previously healthy bedtime routines, practicing relaxation and coping strategies at bedtime, and ensuring that the child is not taking medications (eg, stimulants) or consuming caffeine that may inhibit normal sleep patterns. When non-pharmacological interventions have not improved sleep, over-the-counter medications such as melatonin may be considered. With high levels of traumatic stress or severe sleep disturbances, prazosin may be used at night. Prazosin has been studied and found effective in the treatment of nightmares and other sleep disturbances in adults with PTSD.[63] Preliminary studies have found that use of prazosin in youth with PTSD is tolerated and associated with improvement in sleep,[64] and it has been recommended by the Florida Medicaid Drug Therapy Management Program for Behavioral Health for PTSD-related sleep disturbances in pediatric guidelines.[65] Due to risk of first-dose orthostatic hypotension, prazosin is initiated at 1 mg nightly and can be titrated up by 1 mg every 3 to 7 days until sleep has improved or the patient has side effects such as headaches, dizziness, or anxiety. Most youth who respond to prazosin will respond to a dose between 2 and 5 mg. Benzodiazepines and second-generation antipsychotics should not be used to treat insomnia in pediatric traumatic stress. If initial medication trials do not improve symptoms, psychiatric consultation may be warranted.

Following Up and Monitoring Over Time

Some children who have been exposed to trauma may not initially present with symptoms of traumatic stress; some symptomatic children may not follow through with or complete mental health treatment; and some children may have complex developmental and mental health needs following trauma. The AAP recommends that for trauma, medical professionals adhere to the medical home model.[66] In this framework, medical professionals are critical to helping families navigate service systems by monitoring traumatic stress symptoms, providing ongoing education, and engaging families in appropriate mental health treatment over time.[11]

Conclusion

The beginning of this chapter relayed Delaney's trauma history and detailed some of her subsequent interactions with health care, school, law enforcement, child welfare, and behavioral health professionals. She was sexually abused by her uncle from age 4 to 7 years and experienced nearly a decade of traumatic stress symptoms, functional impairment, and risky behaviors before receiving treatment. Delaney's experience highlights the importance of trauma-informed care and the opportunity medical professionals have to actively recognize and respond to traumatic experiences and traumatic stress in their patients. To reiterate, a trauma-informed medical professional "*realizes* the widespread impact of trauma and understands potential paths for recovery; *recognizes* the signs and symptoms of trauma in clients, families, staff, and others involved with the system; *responds* by fully integrating knowledge about trauma into policies, procedures, and practices; and seeks to actively resist *re-traumatization*."[2]

References

1. Substance Abuse and Mental Health Services Administration. *Trauma-Informed Care in Behavioral Health Services. Treatment Improvement Protocol (TIP) Series 57. HHS Publication No. (SMA) 13–4801*. Rockville, MD: Substance Abuse and Mental Health Services Administration; 2014
2. Substance Abuse and Mental Health Services Administration. *SAMHSA's Concept of Trauma and Guidance for a Trauma-Informed Approach. HHS Publication No. (SMA) 14–4884*. Rockville, MD: Substance Abuse and Mental Health Services Administration; 2014
3. Ko SJ, Ford JD, Kassam-Adams N, et al. Creating trauma-informed systems: child welfare, education, first responders, health care, juvenile justice. *Prof Psychol Res Pr*. 2008;39(4):396–404 https://doi.org/10.1037/0735-7028.39.4.396
4. Flynn AB, Fothergill KE, Wilcox HC, et al. Primary care interventions to prevent or treat traumatic stress in childhood: a systematic review. *Acad Pediatr*. 2015;15(5): 480–492 PMID: 26344717 https://doi.org/10.1016/j.acap.2015.06.012
5. Dubowitz H, Lane WG, Semiatin JN, Magder LS. The SEEK model of pediatric primary care: can child maltreatment be prevented in a low-risk population? *Acad Pediatr*. 2012;12(4):259–268 PMID: 22658954 https://doi.org/10.1016/j.acap.2012.03.005

6. Pediatric Integrated Care Collaborative. Improving the Capacity of Primary Care to Serve Children and Families Experiencing Trauma and Chronic Stress: A Toolkit. Baltimore, MD: Johns Hopkins University Bloomberg School of Public Health Center for Mental Health Services in Pediatric Primary Care; 2015. http://web.jhu.edu/pedmentalhealth/PICC%20Toolkit.pdf. Accessed June 5, 2019
7. Marsac ML, Kassam-Adams N, Hildenbrand AK, et al. Implementing a trauma-informed approach in pediatric health care networks. *JAMA Pediatr*. 2016;170(1):70–77 PMID: 26571032 https://doi.org/10.1001/jamapediatrics.2015.2206
8. Asarnow JR, Rozenman M, Wiblin J, Zeltzer L. Integrated medical-behavioral care compared with usual primary care for child and adolescent behavioral health: a meta-analysis. *JAMA Pediatr*. 2015;169(10):929–937 PMID: 26259143 https://doi.org/10.1001/jamapediatrics.2015.1141
9. Bloom B, Jones LI, Freeman G. Summary health statistics for U.S. children: National Health Interview Survey, 2012. Vital Health Stat. 2013;(258):1–81 PMID: 24784481
10. Lipschitz DS, Rasmusson AM, Anyan W, Cromwell P, Southwick SM. Clinical and functional correlates of posttraumatic stress disorder in urban adolescent girls at a primary care clinic. *J Am Acad Child Adolesc Psychiatry*. 2000;39(9):1104–1111 PMID: 10986806 https://doi.org/10.1097/00004583-200009000-00009
11. Cohen JA, Kelleher KJ, Mannarino AP. Identifying, treating, and referring traumatized children: the role of pediatric providers. *Arch Pediatr Adolesc Med*. 2008;162(5):447–452 PMID: 18458191 https://doi.org/10.1001/archpedi.162.5.447
12. Costello E, Pescosolido B, Angold A, Burns B. A family network-based model of access to child mental health services. *Res Community Ment Health*. 1998;9:165–190
13. Felitti VJ, Anda RF, Nordenberg D, et al. Relationship of childhood abuse and household dysfunction to many of the leading causes of death in adults. The Adverse Childhood Experiences (ACE) Study. *Am J Prev Med*. 1998;14(4):245–258 PMID: 9635069 https://doi.org/10.1016/S0749-3797(98)00017-8
14. National Child Traumatic Stress Network. https://www.nctsn.org. Accessed June 5, 2019
15. Garner AS, Shonkoff JP, Siegel BS, et al; American Academy of Pediatrics Committee on Psychosocial Aspects of Child and Family Health; Committee on Early Childhood, Adoption, and Dependent Care; Section on Developmental and Behavioral Pediatrics. Early childhood adversity, toxic stress, and the role of the pediatrician: translating developmental science into lifelong health. *Pediatrics*. 2012;129(1):e224–e231 PMID: 22201148 https://doi.org/10.1542/peds.2011-2662
16. Sege RD, Amaya-Jackson L; American Academy of Pediatrics Committee on Child Abuse and Neglect and Council on Foster Care, Adoption, and Kinship Care; American Academy of Child and Adolescent Psychiatry Committee on Child Maltreatment and Violence; National Center for Child Traumatic Stress. Clinical considerations related to the behavioral manifestations of child maltreatment. *Pediatrics*. 2017;139(4):e20170100 PMID: 28320870 https://doi.org/10.1542/peds.2017-0100
17. National Child Traumatic Stress Network Core Curriculum on Childhood Trauma Task Force. *The 12 Core Concepts: Concepts for Understanding Traumatic Stress Responses in Children and Families. Core Curriculum on Childhood Trauma.* Los Angeles, CA, and Durham, NC: UCLA-Duke University National Center for Child Traumatic Stress; 2012. https://www.nctsn.org/sites/default/files/resources//the_12_core_concepts_for_understanding_traumatic_stress_responses_in_children_ and_families.pdf. Accessed July 14, 2019
18. Turner HA, Finkelhor D, Ormrod R. Poly-victimization in a national sample of children and youth. *Am J Prev Med*. 2010;38(3):323–330 PMID: 20171535 https://doi.org/10.1016/j.amepre.2009.11.012

19. Finkelhor D, Turner HA, Shattuck A, Hamby SL. Violence, crime, and abuse exposure in a national sample of children and youth: an update. *JAMA Pediatr*. 2013;167(7):614–621 PMID: 23700186 https://doi.org/10.1001/jamapediatrics.2013.42
20. Finkelhor D, Turner HA, Shattuck A, Hamby SL. Prevalence of childhood exposure to violence, crime, and abuse: results from the National Survey of Children's Exposure to Violence. *JAMA Pediatr*. 2015;169(8):746–754 PMID: 26121291 https://doi.org/10.1001/jamapediatrics.2015.0676
21. Saunders BE, Adams ZW. Epidemiology of traumatic experiences in childhood. *Child Adolesc Psychiatr Clin N Am*. 2014;23(2):167–184, vii PMID: 24656575 https://doi.org/10.1016/j.chc.2013.12.003
22. Crouch JL, Hanson RF, Saunders BE, Kilpatrick DG, Resnick HS. Income, race/ethnicity, and exposure to violence in youth: results from the National Survey of Adolescents. *J Community Psychol*. 2000;28(6):625–641 https://doi.org/10.1002/1520-6629(200011)28:6<625::AID-JCOP6>3.0.CO;2-R
23. Hussey JM, Chang JJ, Kotch JB. Child maltreatment in the United States: prevalence, risk factors, and adolescent health consequences. *Pediatrics*. 2006;118(3):933–942 PMID: 16950983 https://doi.org/10.1542/peds.2005-2452
24. Alisic E, Zalta AK, van Wesel F, et al. Rates of post-traumatic stress disorder in trauma-exposed children and adolescents: meta-analysis. *Br J Psychiatry*. 2014;204(5):335–340 PMID: 24785767 https://doi.org/10.1192/bjp.bp.113.131227
25. Cohen JA, Mannarino AP, Perel JM, Staron V. A pilot randomized controlled trial of combined trauma-focused CBT and sertraline for childhood PTSD symptoms. *J Am Acad Child Adolesc Psychiatry*. 2007;46(7):811–819 PMID: 17581445 https://doi.org/10.1097/chi.0b013e3180547105
26. Gillies D, Taylor F, Gray C, O'Brien L, D'Abrew N. Psychological therapies for the treatment of post-traumatic stress disorder in children and adolescents. *Cochrane Database Syst Rev*. 2012;12(December):CD006726 PMID: 23235632 https://doi.org/10.1002/14651858.CD006726.pub2
27. Watts BV, Schnurr PP, Mayo L, Young-Xu Y, Weeks WB, Friedman MJ. Meta-analysis of the efficacy of treatments for posttraumatic stress disorder. *J Clin Psychiatry*. 2013;74(6):e541–e550 PMID: 23842024 https://doi.org/10.4088/JCP.12r08225
28. Bonanno GA, Diminich ED. Annual research review: positive adjustment to adversity—trajectories of minimal-impact resilience and emergent resilience. *J Child Psychol Psychiatry*. 2013;54(4):378–401 PMID: 23215790 https://doi.org/10.1111/jcpp.12021
29. Cicchetti D. Annual research review: resilient functioning in maltreated children—past, present, and future perspectives. *J Child Psychol Psychiatry*. 2013;54(4):402–422 PMID: 22928717 https://doi.org/10.1111/j.1469-7610.2012.02608.x
30. Meyerson DA, Grant KE, Carter JS, Kilmer RP. Posttraumatic growth among children and adolescents: a systematic review. *Clin Psychol Rev*. 2011;31(6):949–964 PMID: 21718663 https://doi.org/10.1016/j.cpr.2011.06.003
31. The Perryman Group. *Suffer the Little Children: An Assessment of the Economic Cost of Maltreatment.* Waco, TX: The Perryman Group; 2014. https://www.perrymangroup.com/publications/report/suffer-the-little-children/. Accessed June 12, 2019
32. American Psychiatric Association. *Diagnostic and Statistical Manual of Mental Disorders.* 5th ed. Washington, DC: American Psychiatric Association; 2013
33. American Academy of Pediatrics. Diagnoses to consider when evaluating a child exposed to trauma. https://www.aap.org/en-us/advocacy-and-policy/aap-health-initiatives/healthy-foster-care-america/Documents/TraumaDiagnosis.pdf. Accessed June 5, 2019

34. American Academy of Pediatrics. Addressing adverse childhood experiences and other types of trauma in the primary care setting. https://www.aap.org/en-us/Documents/ttb_addressing_aces.pdf. Published 2014. Accessed June 5, 2019
35. Goslin MC, Stover CS, Berkowitz S, Marans S. Identifying youth at risk for difficulties following a traumatic event: pre-event factors are associated with acute symptomatology. *J Trauma Stress*. 2013;26(4):475–482 PMID: 23861167 https://doi.org/10.1002/jts.21825
36. Behavioral Health Innovations. UCLA PTSD Reaction Index for DSM-5 (Child/Adolescent)—English. https://www.reactionindex.com/as-uc-ptsd-ri-dsm5-ca.html. Accessed June 5, 2019
37. Foa EB, Asnaani A, Zang Y, Capaldi S, Yeh R. Psychometrics of the Child PTSD Symptom Scale for DSM-5 for trauma-exposed children and adolescents. *J Clin Child Adolesc Psychol*. 2018;47(1):38–46 PMID: 28820616 https://doi.org/10.1080/15374416.2017.1350962
38. Briere J. *Trauma Symptom Checklist for Children (TSCC), Professional Manual*. Odessa, FL: Psychological Assessment Resources; 1996
39. Steinberg AM, Brymer MJ, Decker KB, Pynoos RS. The University of California at Los Angeles Post-traumatic Stress Disorder Reaction Index. *Curr Psychiatry Rep*. 2004;6(2):96–100 PMID: 15038911 https://doi.org/10.1007/s11920-004-0048-2
40. Dube SR, Anda RF, Felitti VJ, Chapman DP, Williamson DF, Giles WH. Childhood abuse, household dysfunction, and the risk of attempted suicide throughout the life span: findings from the Adverse Childhood Experiences Study. *JAMA*. 2001;286(24):3089–3096 PMID: 11754674 https://doi.org/10.1001/jama.286.24.3089
41. Maniglio R. The role of child sexual abuse in the etiology of suicide and non-suicidal self-injury. *Acta Psychiatr Scand*. 2011;124(1):30–41 PMID: 20946202 https://doi.org/10.1111/j.1600-0447.2010.01612.x
42. Jones DJ, Lewis T, Litrownik A, et al. Linking childhood sexual abuse and early adolescent risk behavior: the intervening role of internalizing and externalizing problems. *J Abnorm Child Psychol*. 2013;41(1):139–150 PMID: 22752719 https://doi.org/10.1007/s10802-012-9656-1
43. Gillies D, Maiocchi L, Bhandari AP, Taylor F, Gray C, O'Brien L. Psychological therapies for children and adolescents exposed to trauma. *Cochrane Database Syst Rev*. 2016;10(November):CD012371 PMID: 27726123 https://doi.org/10.1002/14651858.CD012371
44. Leenarts LEW, Diehle J, Doreleijers TAH, Jansma EP, Lindauer RJL. Evidence-based treatments for children with trauma-related psychopathology as a result of childhood maltreatment: a systematic review. *Eur Child Adolesc Psychiatry*. 2013;22(5):269–283 PMID: 23266844 https://doi.org/10.1007/s00787-012-0367-5
45. Child Sexual Abuse Task Force and Research & Practice Core, National Child Traumatic Stress Network. *How to Implement Trauma-Focused Cognitive Behavioral Therapy*. Durham, NC and Los Angeles, CA: National Center for Child Traumatic Stress; 2004. https://www.nctsn.org/resources/how-implement-trauma-focused-cognitive-behavioral-therapy-tf-cbt-implementation-manual Accessed June 12, 2019
46. Cohen A, Mannarino AP, Deblinger E. *Treating Trauma and Traumatic Grief in Children and Adolescents*. New York, NY: The Guilford Press; 2006
47. National Child Traumatic Stress Network. What is child traumatic stress? http://www.nctsnet.org/sites/default/files/assets/pdfs/what_is_child_traumatic_stress_0.pdf. Published 2003. Accessed June 5, 2019
48. Deblinger E, Mannarino AP, Cohen JA, Runyon MK, Steer RA. Trauma-focused cognitive behavioral therapy for children: impact of the trauma narrative and treatment length. *Depress Anxiety*. 2011;28(1):67–75 PMID: 20830695 https://doi.org/10.1002/da.20744
49. The Kauffman Project. *Closing the Quality Chasm in Child Abuse Treatment: Identifying and Disseminating Best Practices*. San Diego, CA: Kauffman Foundation; 2004

50. Thomas R, Abell B, Webb HJ, Avdagic E, Zimmer-Gembeck MJ. Parent-child interaction therapy: a meta-analysis. *Pediatrics*. 2017;140(3):e20170352 PMID: 28860132 https://doi.org/10.1542/peds.2017-0352
51. Thomas R, Zimmer-Gembeck MJ. Parent-child interaction therapy: an evidence-based treatment for child maltreatment. *Child Maltreat*. 2012;17(3):253–266 PMID: 22942167 https://doi.org/10.1177/1077559512459555
52. Berkowitz SJ, Stover CS, Marans SR. The Child and Family Traumatic Stress Intervention: secondary prevention for youth at risk of developing PTSD. *J Child Psychol Psychiatry*. 2011;52(6):676–685 PMID: 20868370 https://doi.org/10.1111/j.1469-7610.2010.02321.x
53. Moreno-Alcázar A, Treen D, Valiente-Gómez A, et al. Efficacy of eye movement desensitization and reprocessing in children and adolescent with post-traumatic stress disorder: a meta-analysis of randomized controlled trials. *Front Psychol*. 2017;8:1750 PMID: 29066991 https://doi.org/10.3389/fpsyg.2017.01750
54. Rodenburg R, Benjamin A, de Roos C, Meijer AM, Stams GJ. Efficacy of EMDR in children: a meta-analysis. *Clin Psychol Rev*. 2009;29(7):599–606 PMID: 19616353 https://doi.org/10.1016/j.cpr.2009.06.008
55. Shapiro F. Efficacy of eye movement desensitization procedure in the treatment of traumatic memories. *J Trauma Stress*. 1989;2(2):199–223 https://doi.org/10.1002/jts.2490020207
56. Keeshin BR, Strawn JR. Psychological and pharmacologic treatment of youth with posttraumatic stress disorder: an evidence-based review. *Child Adolesc Psychiatr Clin N Am*. 2014;23(2):399–411, x PMID: 24656587 https://doi.org/10.1016/j.chc.2013.12.002
57. Robb AS, Cueva JE, Sporn J, Yang R, Vanderburg DG. Sertraline treatment of children and adolescents with posttraumatic stress disorder: a double-blind, placebo-controlled trial. *J Child Adolesc Psychopharmacol*. 2010;20(6):463–471 PMID: 21186964 https://doi.org/10.1089/cap.2009.0115
58. Keeshin BR, Luebbe AM, Strawn JR, Saldaña SN, Wehry AM, DelBello MP. Sexual abuse is associated with obese children and adolescents admitted for psychiatric hospitalization. *J Pediatr*. 2013;163(1):154–9.e1 PMID: 23414663 https://doi.org/10.1016/j.jpeds.2012.12.091
59. Keeshin BR, Strawn JR, Luebbe AM, et al. Hospitalized youth and child abuse: a systematic examination of psychiatric morbidity and clinical severity. *Child Abuse Negl*. 2014;38(1):76–83 PMID: 24041456 https://doi.org/10.1016/j.chiabu.2013.08.013
60. Matone M, Zlotnik S, Miller D, Kreider A, Rubin D, Noonan K. *Psychotropic Medication Use by Pennsylvania Children in Foster Care and Enrolled in Medicaid: An Analysis of Children Ages 3–18 Years*. Philadelphia, PA: PolicyLab at The Children's Hospital of Philadelphia; 2015
61. Raghavan R, Brown DS, Allaire BT, Garfield LD, Ross RE, Snowden LR. Racial/ethnic differences in Medicaid expenditures on psychotropic medications among maltreated children. *Child Abuse Negl*. 2014;38(6):1002–1010 PMID: 24646610 https://doi.org/10.1016/j.chiabu.2014.02.013
62. Singh AB, Bousman CA, Ng CH, Berk M. High impact child abuse may predict risk of elevated suicidality during antidepressant initiation. *Aust N Z J Psychiatry*. 2013;47(12):1191–1195 PMID: 24280998 https://doi.org/10.1177/0004867413510212
63. George KC, Kebejian L, Ruth LJ, Miller CWT, Himelhoch S. Meta-analysis of the efficacy and safety of prazosin versus placebo for the treatment of nightmares and sleep disturbances in adults with posttraumatic stress disorder. *J Trauma Dissociation*. 2016;17(4):494–510 PMID: 26835889 https://doi.org/10.1080/15299732.2016.1141150

64. Keeshin BR, Ding Q, Presson AP, Berkowitz SJ, Strawn JR. Use of prazosin for pediatric PTSD-associated nightmares and sleep disturbances: a retrospective chart review. *Neurol Ther*. 2017;6(2):247–257 PMID: 28755207 https://doi.org/10.1007/s40120-017-0078-4
65. Florida Medicaid Drug Therapy Management Program for Behavioral Health. 2016–2017 Florida Best Practice Psychotherapeutic Medication Guidelines for Children and Adolescents. Tampa, FL: University of South Florida, Florida Medicaid Drug Therapy Management Program; 2017. http://www.medicaidmentalhealth.org/_assets/file/Guidelines/2016%20Florida%20Best%20Practice%20Medication%20Child%20-%20Adolescent%20Guidelines.pdf. Accessed June 5, 2019
66. American Academy of Pediatrics. The medical home approach to identifying and responding to exposure to trauma. https://www.aap.org/en-us/Documents/ttb_medicalhomeapproach.pdf. Published 2014. Accessed June 5, 2019

PART 8

Prevention

CHAPTER 32

Identification of Child Maltreatment

Jill McTavish, PhD
Postdoctoral Fellow
Department of Psychiatry and Behavioural Neurosciences
McMaster University
Hamilton, Ontario, Canada

Harriet MacMillan, CM, MD, MSc, FRCPC, FAAP
Distinguished University Professor
Department of Psychiatry and Behavioural Neurosciences
Department of Pediatrics
Chedoke Health Chair in Child Psychiatry
Offord Centre for Child Studies
McMaster University
McMaster Children's Hospital/Hamilton Health Sciences
Hamilton, Ontario, Canada

Given the high prevalence of child maltreatment[1–4] and the potential deleterious consequences of maltreatment exposure,[5–9] much has been written about recognizing the signs and symptoms of maltreatment and improving detection of children who have experienced abuse and neglect.[10,11] A related issue is consideration of what medical professionals can do to improve identification of those at risk of maltreating children.[12,13] *Screening* and *case finding* are general terms that refer to the identification of a health condition or exposure; this chapter provides an overview of these approaches in relation to child maltreatment, including a summary of the literature evaluating effectiveness of different approaches to identification. Systematic approaches to determine guidelines or guidance for identification of child maltreatment are discussed, including those from the World Health Organization (WHO) and the National Institute for Health and Care Excellence (NICE). Also discussed are examples of alerting features, questions that can be used to move from considering to suspecting maltreatment, and mandatory reporting considerations.

Screening Versus Case Finding

Screening and case finding differ in their approaches to identification in ways that have important implications for patient–medical professional interactions and resources.[14,15] In health care, *screening* is generally defined as the use of tests, examinations, or other procedures "done among apparently well people to identify those at an increased risk of a disease or disorder."[16] It often involves a standardized assessment of patients, regardless of their reason for seeking medical attention.[17] Screening may be applied to an entire population (*mass screening*) or to high-risk groups (*selective screening*).[18] Because child maltreatment is an exposure and not a symptom, disorder, or disease, screening in this population takes on a different meaning: it is typically thought of as identifying children exposed to current or past maltreatment, or those at high risk of being maltreated, using standardized approaches such as questions, checklists, examinations, or other procedures.[13] In recent years, another type of screening has been proposed—adverse childhood experiences (ACEs) screening, or screening children or adults for childhood adversities, including but not limited to types of maltreatment—to assess children and adults' childhood histories.

Alternatively, *case finding* (sometimes referred to as *clinical inquiry*) involves "looking for additional illnesses in those with medical problems."[16] In case finding, the use of questions and other approaches is not applied in the same way to all patients; rather, it depends on the presenting symptoms, direct observations or information provided by colleagues, other history, and, when appropriate, examination of the patient.[19] As such, while screening and case finding are not always mutually exclusive in practice (eg, a medical professional may use case finding following a negative screening result), in this chapter they are considered conceptually different, in that case finding is presented as questioning that takes into account certain indicators and presenting signs and symptoms of the child, as opposed to standardized methods for questioning. The following question may be used as a comparison to illustrate the differences between screening and case finding: "Has anything unsafe happened to you since our last visit?" Mass screening occurs when this question is asked of all presenting children; selective screening occurs when this question is asked of a high-risk group of presenting children (eg, all children who have parents who are struggling with substance use and addiction); and case finding would not use a standard question but would involve the medical professional inquiring about maltreatment in a way that is tailored to how children present with specific alerting features, including signs and symptoms.

Principles of Screening

Key criteria to use when deciding whether or not to screen were published more than 50 years ago by WHO (Box 32.1) and are essential to consider when questioning the utility of screening for child maltreatment.[18] In the interest of space, this discussion focuses on 3 criteria. First, there should be an *accepted intervention* (ideally evidence based) for patients identified as at risk of, or exposed to, child maltreatment. This accepted intervention should be available to any high-risk groups that are identified through screening. Second, there should be a *suitable* test, examination, or procedure; suitability necessitates that the test be sufficiently accurate, ideally as evaluated through randomized controlled trials (RCTs). Third, this test should be *acceptable* to the population. This includes an understanding of potential harms that may arise from screening, where benefits should outweigh harms.

Using just these 3 criteria, it becomes clear why recent systematic reviews and evidence-based guidelines do not recommend screening for child maltreatment.[11,20,21] Although screening for ACEs has not been the subject of a guideline review to date, Finkelhor[22] and others have used similar criteria to identify the lack of evidence to justify screening for ACEs. First, child maltreatment is a complex experience for which limited evidence-based interventions have been evaluated and shown effective.[23] Selection of appropriate interventions requires that children undergo a thorough assessment by a qualified medical professional. For example, trauma-focused cognitive behavioral therapy is an evidence-based intervention for children who have been exposed to sexual abuse,[24] but because the intervention is designed specifically for children with post-traumatic stress disorder symptoms, children must undergo an assessment to determine if this intervention would be helpful. Furthermore, whether or not high-risk groups who are identified by screening would receive the intervention is unclear, because this intervention is not available in all jurisdictions. For example, some research suggests that certain high-risk groups lack access to essential care, such as children in the juvenile justice system with abuse histories,[25] foster children of racial and ethnic minorities,[26] and a significant proportion of children in contact with child welfare services.[27,28]

Second, as will be discussed later in this section, there are no RCTs evaluating screening tests for exposure to maltreatment, and the available diagnostic accuracy studies have serious shortcomings (ie, risk of bias) or the tests are not sufficiently accurate. Third, evidence about the acceptability of these screening tests is sparse. For example, Diderich and colleagues[29] evaluated the acceptability of the Hague protocol, where nurses and doctors in the Netherlands attempted to detect child maltreatment in the emergency department (ED) based on 3 aspects of parental histories: domestic violence, substance use, and suicide attempt or self-harm. The authors suggest that the "majority of parents who agreed to be interviewed were positive and said that they would, if necessary, revisit the ED with the same complaints in the future, suggesting that EDs do not have to fear a decline in the attendance of this specific group of patients."[29] However, the authors note, "It was very difficult to contact the parents by telephone and convince them to take part in the interview,"[29] which may be an indicator of a lack of acceptability for the Hague protocol. More research about the acceptability of screening procedures for children and families is needed before concrete conclusions can be made.

Ideally, screening strategies should be tested through RCTs to evaluate the effect on occurrence or recurrence of maltreatment and child well-being outcomes. For example, systematic reviews of RCTs evaluating screening for women exposed to intimate partner violence (IPV) have indicated that screening does not improve women's mental health,

BOX 32.1

Criteria to Determine the Appropriateness of Implementing a Screening Intervention

1. The condition sought should be an important health problem.
2. There should be an accepted treatment for patients with recognized disease.
3. Facilities for diagnosis and treatment should be available.
4. There should be a recognizable latent or early symptomatic stage.
5. There should be a suitable test or examination.
6. The test should be acceptable to the population.
7. The natural history of the condition, including development from latent to declared disease, should be adequately understood.
8. There should be an agreed policy on whom to treat as patients.
9. The cost of case finding (including diagnosis and treatment of patients diagnosed) should be economically balanced in relation to possible expenditure on medical care as a whole.
10. Case finding should be a continuing process and not a "once and for all" project.

From Wilson JMG, Jungner G. *Principles and Practice of Screening for Disease.* Geneva, Switzerland: World Health Organization; 1968. Public Health Papers No. 34. https://apps.who.int/iris/bitstream/handle/10665/37650/WHO_PHP_34.pdf. Accessed July 14, 2019.

reduce experiences of violence, or increase referrals to support agencies.[30] Comparable studies are not yet available for understanding the effect of screening on children experiencing maltreatment. While there are RCTs[31,32] that evaluate screening as part of an overall intervention, combining screening with other interventions does not allow researchers to isolate the effect of screening on child maltreatment identification or recurrence, as has been done for the IPV screening trials. However, we do know that not all children who are suspected of having been maltreated receive services from child welfare authorities.[33] Even among those receiving services through child welfare, it is unknown whether such services reduce subsequent maltreatment.[34]

While there are no RCTs evaluating the effectiveness of screening for maltreatment, there are several diagnostic accuracy studies. Sensitivity, specificity, positive predictive value, and negative predictive values are common accuracy outcomes that are evaluated in diagnostic studies (Figure 32.1); however, these outcomes are often misinterpreted and may not reflect the effects of the screening test in the population of interest.[35] Instead, rates for true positives, true negatives, false positives, and false negatives may give medical professionals a clearer picture of how many

		Does the index test predict child maltreatment?		
	Total Population	*Yes—positive index test outcome*	*No—negative index test outcome*	**Prevalence of Maltreatment**
Is there a child exposed to child maltreatment present (reference standard)?	*Yes—condition positive*	True positive	False negative (type II error)	**Sensitivity =** # true positive / (sum of condition positive)
	No—condition negative	False positive (type I error)	True negative	**Specificity =** # true negatives / (sum of condition negative)
		Positive predictive value = # true positives / (sum of test outcome positive)	**Negative predictive value =** # true negative / (sum of test outcome negative)	

FIGURE 32.1

Equations for calculating sensitivity, specificity, and positive and negative predictive value.

children will be missed by a screener that should have been caught (false negatives) and how many children who have not been maltreated are falsely identified by the screener (false positives). These numbers have clearer implications, because children who are missed may not receive the services they need and may continue to experience maltreatment and children who are falsely identified may experience an investigation that could be stigmatizing and stressful and, in some cases, may be removed from their home inappropriately.

A diagnostic accuracy study usually involves the following steps: 1) the evaluation of a group of children by the test, examination, or other procedure (hereafter referred to as the *index test*) that is designed to identify children exposed to maltreatment; and 2) the evaluation of this same group of children (or a random subsample) by a reference standard who confirm or deny exposure to maltreatment. The index test and reference standard should be conducted within a short span of one another (eg, within 30 days), so that the situation of the child does not change between tests (if not, bias is introduced). An ideal reference standard (gold standard) is often considered to be an evaluation by a team of child maltreatment experts, although other acceptable reference standards exist, such as child protective services (CPS) assessments and court dispositions. Parent reports of child maltreatment are not considered to be acceptable reference standards due to the potential for false reports and omissions.

There are many ways diagnostic accuracy studies may suffer from poor methodological aspects that affect study quality and the ability to evaluate the accuracy of the results. Factors affecting quality can be evaluated through standardized quality assessment tools, such as Quality Assessment of Diagnostic Accuracy Studies (known as the QUADAS-2).[36] Tools of this type evaluate bias that is introduced into patient selection (eg, did the study avoid inappropriate exclusions?), the index test (eg, were the index test results determined without knowledge of the results of the reference standard?), the reference standard (eg, is the reference standard likely to correctly classify the target condition?), and flow and timing (eg, did all patients receive a reference standard?). For example, verification bias occurs when not every member of the study group is evaluated by the reference standard. This may occur in studies in which the reference standard (eg, a team of child abuse experts) is only called in to verify children who receive positive screening results (and, thus, are already suspected to have experienced maltreatment). In this example, it is likely that some of the children with negative screening results actually experienced maltreatment and had no chance to be evaluated by the child abuse team. Most systematic reviews of identification strategies should employ a quality assessment tool to evaluate potential biases of all included studies.

Evaluation of Screening Tools for Identifying Child Maltreatment

In 2013, Bailhache and colleagues[11] conducted a systematic review of "instruments for identifying abused children during any stage of child maltreatment evolution before their death, and to assess if any might be adapted to screening." While the authors considered 13 studies addressing the identification of physical abuse (7), sexual abuse (4), emotional abuse (1), and multiple forms of maltreatment (1), they concluded that none of the identification strategies were of sufficient quality to use for screening because they were inaccurate, thus missing or overidentifying a significant number of children; they suffered from serious bias that precluded a clear understanding of the study findings; or they identified children too late (ie, when children were already experiencing significant consequences of maltreatment). In 2018, McTavish and colleagues[21] conducted an update of this systematic review and had similar conclusions. This latter review update did, however, identify 2 additional tools that could be considered examples of mass or selective screening tools: the SPUTOVAMO tool and the Escape tool.

The SPUTOVAMO tool is a screening instrument that determines whether there is a suspicion of child maltreatment via a positive answer to 1 or more of 5 questions (Table 32.1). Its use is mandatory in Dutch EDs and out-of-hours primary care locations. One study has evaluated the effectiveness of the SPUTOVAMO tool for identifying physical abuse, sexual abuse, emotional abuse, neglect, and children's exposure to IPV in all children younger than 19 years presenting to out-of-hours primary care locations in Utrecht, Netherlands.[38] This study is an example of a mass screening study. Two other studies used a selective screening approach to evaluate the effectiveness of the SPUTOVAMO tool for identifying exposure to physical abuse or neglect in children younger than 8 years presenting to an ED with a physical injury[37] or children younger than 19 years presenting with burn injuries to a burn center.[39]

The Escape tool is a screening instrument very similar in content and construction to the SPUTOVAMO tool, with 5 or 6 questions that are used to determine whether there is suspicion of child maltreatment, including physical abuse, sexual abuse, emotional abuse, neglect, and children's exposure to IPV (see Table 32.1). Two studies[40,41] have used a selective screening approach to evaluate the use of this tool in ED settings.

While studies evaluating the SPUTOVAMO and Escape tools report good sensitivity and specificity values overall, all but one of the screening studies suffer from serious verification bias, which precludes the ability to trust the findings. For example, only 55 of 18,275 (0.3%) children in one of the studies evaluating the Escape tool[41] were evaluated by the reference standard.

One study evaluating the SPUTOVAMO tool in children younger than 8 years presenting to an ED with a physical injury[37] did not suffer from verification bias, which means one can be more confident in the findings. When using a 2% prevalence of maltreatment (which is approaching the lower end of prevalence in an ED setting[42]), this study indicates that, in this narrow population, the SPUTOVAMO tool misses 0 per 100,000 children suspected of experiencing physical abuse and falsely identifies 13,230 children per 100,000; for neglect, this study suggests that the SPUTOVAMO tool misses 334 per 100,000 children and falsely identifies 13,034 children suspected as having experienced maltreatment.[21] While the study suggests that the SPUTOVAMO tool does not miss children exposed to physical abuse in this population (children <8 years presenting to an ED with a physical injury), there is some evidence to suggest that medical professionals have an easier time identifying suspected physical abuse (especially when a physical sign, such as an injury, is present); conversely, medical professionals have more difficulties identifying less overt forms of

TABLE 32.1
Comparing Questions Included in the SPUTOVAMO and Escape Tools[38,40]

SPUTOVAMO Tool[38]	Escape Tool[40,a]
1. Injury compatible with history and corresponding with age of child?	3. Does the onset of the injury fit with the developmental level of the child?
2. Delay in seeking help without satisfactory explanation?	2. Was seeking medical help unnecessarily delayed?
3. History consistent when repeated?	1. Is the history consistent?
4. Father/mother and child: Appropriate behavior/interaction?	4. Is the behavior of the child, his or her caregivers, and their interaction appropriate?
5. Parents took adequate measures (eg, injury compatible with history and corresponding with age of child)?	5. Are findings of the head-to-toe examination in accordance with the history?
	6. Are there other signals that make you doubt the safety of the child or other family members?

[a] Questions from the Escape tool are rearranged to show their similarity to the SPUTOVAMO tool.

maltreatment, such as neglect, emotional abuse, and children's exposure to IPV.[43] Due to the high number of missed children who are suspected of being neglected and the potential for high numbers of children who are falsely identified by this tool (as well as the limitations in the other screening studies), McTavish and colleagues[21] note that there is still insufficient evidence to warrant screening for child maltreatment. The authors of this SPUTOVAMO study also note that the checklist has a high false-positive rate, does not catch all cases of suspected maltreatment, and should not replace an assessment by a qualified medical professional.[37]

Earlier reviews focused on identification of parents or caregivers at increased risk of committing child maltreatment—specifically child physical abuse or neglect.[12,13] Methods of screening included approaches such as staff- or self-administered questionnaires and standardized interviews. The main problem with these approaches was, again, the high false-positive rate, as well as the lack of evidence-based interventions for those identified as at risk. Among those determined to be at risk of maltreating a child and based on a false-positive rate of approximately 33%, a large number would never go on to commit maltreatment. Labeling caregivers as at risk of maltreating a child can be stigmatizing and stressful, potentially doing more harm than good. Both the US Preventive Services Task Force[13] and the Canadian Task Force on Preventive Health Care[12] noted the lack of screening studies that directly link to health outcomes as well as the limited accuracy of such screening tools. Updated draft recommendations from the US Preventive Services Task Force also suggest the current evidence is "insufficient to assess the balance of benefits and harms of primary care interventions to prevent child maltreatment" and that further research is needed to "determine effective methods for clinicians to identify children at increased risk."[44] Based on these findings, screening for child maltreatment was not recommended by either group. As noted previously, more recent studies about the Hague protocol[45,46] have evaluated the accuracy of identifying children exposed to maltreatment based on parental histories. The authors used a prospective, quasi-experimental pretest/posttest design with a non-randomized control group. Referrals were made for one or more of the following 3 parental histories: 1) IPV, 2) suicidal behavior or other serious psychiatric disorder, and 3) serious substance use. Although the identification rates of child maltreatment increased, there were serious problems in the study design, which diminish confidence in the findings. For example, this study had both verification bias, where only positive screens were evaluated by the reference standard (the number of negative screening results that represented maltreated children was not determined), and incorporation bias, where staff from the Reporting Center for Child Abuse and Neglect (the reference standard) was aware of the results of the index test. As such, there is still insufficient evidence to warrant screening of caregivers.

World Health Organization Recommendations for Identification

The WHO Mental Health Gap Action Programme (mhGAP) was launched in 2008 to facilitate the scaling up of care for mental, neurological, and substance use disorders; the program comprises evidence-based guidelines and practical intervention guides used to assist in the implementation of guideline principles. With no RCTs evaluating identification strategies to assess the effect on child well-being and recurrence and with the questionable effectiveness of available screening tools, recent mhGAP guidance suggests that medical professionals should use a case-finding approach to identify children exposed to maltreatment. This approach requires that medical professionals be "alert to the clinical features associated with child maltreatment and associated risk factors and assess for child maltreatment, without putting the child at increased risk."[20] Attention to minimizing risk requires that certain conditions for safety are met, such as medical professionals who are trained to take histories from children and their caregivers and to provide a safe initial response to disclosures in ways that minimize risk. For example, if a child or caregiver is asked about exposure to IPV without taking into account appropriate need for privacy, this could place the child and other family members at risk. Attending to safety requires a private space to inquire about child maltreatment (and ability to inquire about maltreatment from children without caregivers or others present), an approach to contact CPS according to mandatory reporting legislation, and a strategy for making referrals to support the child and family.

Alerting Features of Maltreatment

Alerting features of possible child maltreatment are signs and symptoms (eg, unexplained marks suggestive of injury on the skin), behavioral and emotional indicators or cues from the child or caregiver (eg, caregiver fails to follow up on the child's treatment), or risk factors (eg, caregiver has substance use difficulties) that prompt a medical professional to consider, suspect, or exclude child maltreatment as a possible explanation for the child's presentation.[47] According to NICE, *suspecting* child maltreatment means that the medical professional has a serious level of concern about the possibility of maltreatment but nothing more definitive. Alternatively, *considering* child maltreatment means that maltreatment may be a possible explanation for the alerting feature and that the medical professional should continue to monitor the child closely. Note that there are different actions for suspecting and considering, which are discussed in the following section.

Inquiring About Maltreatment Through Case Finding

Case finding or clinical inquiry involves asking such questions depending on presenting history and other information that may arise during an assessment. For example, any child being assessed for emotional problems, behavioral problems, or injuries where the cause is unclear should be interviewed alone (when they are an appropriate age and developmental stage to be interviewed) and asked about relationships with caregivers, experiences of discipline, and feelings of safety.[48] Some frontline medical professionals raise concerns about the need to take a history from children alone due to time constraints and lack of resources. The individual history taking from the child does not need to be done by the pediatrician; the important issue is that if one is concerned about a child with these types of problems, a medical professional with sufficient training needs to see a child individually, to ask about these types of exposures.

In many jurisdictions, there is a mandatory reporting obligation for medical professionals when maltreatment is suspected; this is discussed more in the next section. While it is important that a medical professional not conduct an investigation for suspected maltreatment, which is the role of CPS in such jurisdictions (and duplication of investigation efforts may cause the child undue stress), it is also important that the medical professional takes sufficient history from the child about the alerting feature when it is safe and developmentally feasible and appropriate to do so. For example, if a medical professional notices a bruise on a child's head during a visit, it is important to inquire about the lesion in a manner that is safe and developmentally appropriate (eg, "How did you get the bruise on your forehead?"). Other examples of questions that may elicit concerns about maltreatment include

- What things do you worry about?
- What happens in your family when someone gets in trouble?
- Has anyone ever touched you in a way that made you feel uncomfortable or upset?

Questions about maltreatment should be asked in a developmentally appropriate way and should only be asked if the following minimum safety standards are in place:

- The person asking the questions is trained in how to respond to a child's disclosure and familiar with appropriate next steps, including response to the child and to the family.
- Private space is available in the service setting.
- Confidentiality is assured (with limits, considering mandatory reporting obligations).
- Systems for referral are in place.

Training about how to ask about and respond to maltreatment should involve, to some extent, principles related to listening, inquiring about needs and concerns, prioritizing safety, and strategies to support children and families. For example, key principles for listening include using active listening, being empathetic and supportive, and allowing the child to speak without interruption. Although the need for privacy is generally considered for adults, it is often overlooked for children. Asking such questions that could lead to disclosures about maltreatment must involve the use of a private space, and children and caregivers should be asked these questions separately, so as to not put the child at increased risk of harm by asking about exposures in the presence of a caregiver who may be responsible for the maltreatment.

Clinicians who are qualified to inquire about maltreatment should document any responses verbatim and without offering an opinion about the veracity of the information. For example, "While examining child's bruise on lower back, the patient stated, 'That's where Mommy hit me.'" It is important to remember that caregivers may see the report at some point, for example, in legal proceedings. No unnecessary information should be provided (eg, child's general statements about physical appearance of parent, or other nonrelevant information) that may put the child at risk.

When maltreatment is one of many possible explanations for the child's presentation, it is important to look for other potential signs of maltreatment in the child's history, presentation, or interaction with the parent or caregiver.[47] If a medical professional is concerned, but nothing has been identified or disclosed by the child to indicate reason to suspect maltreatment, it may be helpful to consult with a medical professional who has expertise in child development, children's mental health, or child maltreatment. For example, in the case of a child who is running away from home and exhibiting high-risk behaviors but has denied any problems in relationships with caregivers, it would be important to follow up and seek consultation. The urgency of such consultations and follow-up should be based on the severity of the alerting feature (in this case, the high-risk behaviors, including running away).[47]

Mandatory Reporting Considerations

Where mandatory reporting obligations exist, reporters should make an effort to speak to the child and caregiver(s) about the limits of confidentiality, especially when the relationship is ongoing. Doing so before the need to report arises can minimize feelings of betrayal. An example of how to discuss confidentiality follows:

> "I will not tell anyone what you and I talk about without you saying it's all right, unless it has to do with someone's safety." "Do you know what safety means?" (Often the child, depending on the age, can provide an explanation. It is still helpful to clarify what is meant by safety.) "If you, or someone you know, is hurting themselves or being hurt by someone else, then that's a problem with safety."[49]

Children and caregivers who disclose information indicating reason to suspect maltreatment should be informed that a report will be made, although a few exceptions to this responsibility exist, such as if there is a concern that the caregiver may flee with the child. It is also important to inform children and caregivers of possible CPS responses to a report. If the medical professional is unsure if the suspected maltreatment should be reported, consultation with CPS can occur in a confidential manner about the details of the case (without mentioning identifying features of the child or family). Doing so prevents filing of an unnecessary report, which can cause stress to both the medical professional and the child and family. It is also important to remember that a legal duty to report is separate from a moral duty to respond to the child's and family's needs. For example, children who are suspected of having experienced maltreatment should be referred for a comprehensive assessment by a qualified professional.

Conclusion

At this time, there is no evidence to indicate that screening for child maltreatment—either screening children for indicators or screening caregivers for risk factors—leads to reduction in abuse and neglect or improvement in health outcomes for children. Medical professionals should be alert to the clinical features associated with child maltreatment and associated risk factors and ask about exposure to child maltreatment when assessing conditions that may be caused or complicated by maltreatment. Attention must be given to the circumstances of such an inquiry so that the child is not placed at increased risk.

There needs to be an ongoing emphasis on the development of evidence-based interventions for children and families to reduce child maltreatment. Identification should lead to interventions that reduce the risk of recurrence and associated impairment among those who have experienced abuse or neglect and ensure those in need of such interventions have access to them.

References

1. Stoltenborgh M, Bakermans-Kranenburg MJ, van Ijzendoorn MH. The neglect of child neglect: a meta-analytic review of the prevalence of neglect. *Soc Psychiatry Psychiatr Epidemiol*. 2013;48(3):345–355 PMID: 22797133 https://doi.org/10.1007/s00127-012-0549-y
2. Stoltenborgh M, van Ijzendoorn MH, Euser EM, Bakermans-Kranenburg MJ. A global perspective on child sexual abuse: meta-analysis of prevalence around the world. *Child Maltreat*. 2011;16(2):79–101 PMID: 21511741 https://doi.org/10.1177/1077559511403920
3. Stoltenborgh M, Bakermans-Kranenburg MJ, van Ijzendoorn MH, Alink LRA. Cultural-geographical differences in the occurrence of child physical abuse? A meta-analysis of global prevalence. *Int J Psychol*. 2013;48(2):81–94 PMID: 23597008 https://doi.org/10.1080/00207594.2012.697165
4. Finkelhor D, Turner HA, Shattuck A, Hamby SL. Prevalence of childhood exposure to violence, crime, and abuse: results from the National Survey of Children's Exposure to Violence. *JAMA Pediatr*. 2015;169(8):746–754 PMID: 26121291 https://doi.org/10.1001/jamapediatrics.2015.0676
5. Andrews G, Corry J, Slade T, Issakidis C, Swanston H. Child sexual abuse. In: Ezzati M, Lopez AD, Rodgers A, Murray CJ, eds. *Comparative Quantification of Health Risks: Global and Regional Burden of Disease Attributable to Selected Major Risk Factors*. Geneva, Switzerland: World Health Organization; 2004:1851–1940
6. Miller GE, Chen E, Parker KJ. Psychological stress in childhood and susceptibility to the chronic diseases of aging: moving toward a model of behavioral and biological mechanisms. *Psychol Bull*. 2011;137(6):959–997 PMID: 21787044 https://doi.org/10.1037/a0024768
7. McCrory E, De Brito SA, Viding E. The link between child abuse and psychopathology: a review of neurobiological and genetic research. *J R Soc Med*. 2012;105(4):151–156 PMID: 22532655 https://doi.org/10.1258/jrsm.2011.110222
8. Norman RE, Byambaa M, De R, Butchart A, Scott J, Vos T. The long-term health consequences of child physical abuse, emotional abuse, and neglect: a systematic review and meta-analysis. *PLoS Med*. 2012;9(11):e1001349 PMID: 23209385 https://doi.org/10.1371/journal.pmed.1001349
9. Naughton AM, Maguire SA, Mann MK, et al. Emotional, behavioral, and developmental features indicative of neglect or emotional abuse in preschool children: a systematic review. *JAMA Pediatr*. 2013;167(8):769–775 PMID: 23754198 https://doi.org/10.1001/jamapediatrics.2013.192
10. National Institute for Health and Care Excellence. Child maltreatment: when to suspect maltreatment in under 18s. https://www.nice.org.uk/guidance/CG89/chapter/1-Guidance#physical-features. Updated October 2017. Accessed April 4, 2019

11. Bailhache M, Leroy V, Pillet P, Salmi L-R. Is early detection of abused children possible? A systematic review of the diagnostic accuracy of the identification of abused children. *BMC Pediatr*. 2013;13(1):202 PMID: 24314318 https://doi.org/10.1186/1471-2431-13-202
12. MacMillan HL; Canadian Task Force on Preventive Health Care. Preventive health care, 2000 update: prevention of child maltreatment. *CMAJ*. 2000;163(11):1451–1458 PMID: 11192650
13. US Preventive Services Task Force. Screening for family and intimate partner violence: recommendation statement. *Ann Fam Med*. 2004;2(2):156–160 PMID: 15083857 https://doi.org/10.1370/afm.128
14. Dobrow MJ, Hagens V, Chafe R, Sullivan T, Rabeneck L. Consolidated principles for screening based on a systematic review and consensus process. *CMAJ*. 2018;190(14):E422–E429 PMID: 29632037 https://doi.org/10.1503/cmaj.171154
15. Canadian Task Force on Preventive Health Care. Canadian Task Force on Preventive Health Care: Procedure Manual. Ottawa, ON: Canadian Task Force on Preventive Health Care; 2014. https://canadiantaskforce.ca/wp-content/uploads/2016/12/procedural-manual-en_2014_Archived.pdf. Accessed April 4, 2019
16. Grimes DA, Schulz KF. Uses and abuses of screening tests. *Lancet*. 2002;359(9309): 881–884 PMID: 11897304 https://doi.org/10.1016/S0140-6736(02)07948-5
17. Cole TB. Is domestic violence screening helpful? *JAMA*. 2000;284(5):551–553 PMID: 10918685 https://doi.org/10.1001/jama.284.5.551
18. Wilson JMG, Jungner G. *Principles and Practice of Screening for Disease*. Geneva, Switzerland: World Health Organization; 1968. Public Health Papers No. 34. https://apps.who.int/iris/bitstream/handle/10665/37650/WHO_PHP_34.pdf. Accessed April 4, 2019
19. World Health Organization. *Responding to Intimate Partner Violence and Sexual Violence against Women: WHO Clinical and Policy Guidelines*. Geneva, Switzerland: World Health Organization; 2013. https://www.who.int/reproductivehealth/publications/violence/9789241548595/en/. Accessed April 4, 2019
20. World Health Organization. *WHO mhGAP Guideline Update:* Update of the Mental Health Gap Action Programme (MhGAP) Guideline for Mental, Neurological and Substance Use Disorders. Geneva, Switzerland: World Health Organization; 2015. https://apps.who.int/iris/bitstream/10665/204132/1/9789241549417_eng.pdf?ua=1. Accessed April 4, 2019
21. McTavish JR, Gonzalez A, MacGregor JCD, McKee C, Santesso N, MacMillan HL. Identification of child maltreatment: an update of a systematic review. In press
22. Finkelhor D. Screening for adverse childhood experiences (ACEs): cautions and suggestions. *Child Abuse Negl*. 2018;85:174–179 PMID: 28784309
23. Fraser JG, Lloyd S, Murphy R, et al. A comparative effectiveness review of parenting and trauma-focused interventions for children exposed to maltreatment. *J Dev Behav Pediatr*. 2013;34(5):353–368 PMID: 23588113 https://doi.org/10.1097/DBP.0b013e31828a7dfc
24. de Arellano MAR, Lyman DR, Jobe-Shields L, et al. Trauma-focused cognitive-behavioral therapy for children and adolescents: assessing the evidence. *Psychiatr Serv*. 2014;65(5):591–602 PMID: 24638076 https://doi.org/10.1176/appi.ps.201300255
25. Quinn MM, Poirier JM, Garfinkel L. Girls with mental health needs in the juvenile justice system: challenges and inequities confronting a vulnerable population. *Exceptionality*. 2005;13(2):125–139 https://doi.org/10.1207/s15327035ex1302_5
26. Garland AF, Landsverk JA, Lau AS. Racial/ethnic disparities in mental health service use among children in foster care. *Child Youth Serv Rev*. 2003;25(5):491–507 https://doi.org/10.1016/S0190-7409(03)00032-X

27. Raghavan R, Inoue M, Ettner SL, Hamilton BH, Landsverk J. A preliminary analysis of the receipt of mental health services consistent with national standards among children in the child welfare system. *Am J Public Health*. 2010;100(4):742–749 PMID: 19608950 https://doi.org/10.2105/AJPH.2008.151472
28. Burns BJ, Phillips SD, Wagner HR, et al. Mental health need and access to mental health services by youths involved with child welfare: a national survey. *J Am Acad Child Adolesc Psychiatry*. 2004;43(8):960–970 PMID: 15266190 https://doi.org/10.1097/01.chi.0000127590.95585.65
29. Diderich HM, Fekkes M, Dechesne M, Buitendijk SE, Oudesluys-Murphy AM. Detecting child abuse based on parental characteristics: does the Hague Protocol cause parents to avoid the emergency department? *Int Emerg Nurs*. 2015;23(2):203–206 PMID: 25449550 https://doi.org/10.1016/j.ienj.2014.09.004
30. Taft A, O'Doherty L, Hegarty K, Ramsay J, Davidson L, Feder G. Screening women for intimate partner violence in healthcare settings. Cochrane Database Syst Rev. 2013;(4):CD007007 PMID: 23633338
31. Dubowitz H, Feigelman S, Lane W, Kim J. Pediatric primary care to help prevent child maltreatment: the Safe Environment for Every Kid (SEEK) Model. *Pediatrics*. 2009;123(3):858–864 PMID: 19255014 https://doi.org/10.1542/peds.2008-1376
32. Dubowitz H, Lane WG, Semiatin JN, Magder LS, Venepally M, Jans M. The safe environment for every kid model: impact on pediatric primary care professionals. *Pediatrics*. 2011;127(4):e962–e970 PMID: 21444590 https://doi.org/10.1542/peds.2010-1845
33. US Department of Health and Human Services, Administration for Children and Families, Children's Bureau. Child maltreatment. https://www.acf.hhs.gov/programs/cb/research-data-technology/statistics-research/child-maltreatment. Reviewed January 28, 2019. Accessed April 4, 2019
34. Gilbert R, Kemp A, Thoburn J, et al. Recognising and responding to child maltreatment. *Lancet*. 2009;373(9658):167–180 PMID: 19056119 https://doi.org/10.1016/S0140-6736(08)61707-9
35. Mustafa RA, Wiercioch W, Santesso N, et al. Decision-making about healthcare related tests and diagnostic strategies: user testing of GRADE evidence tables. *PLoS One*. 2015;10(10):e0134553 PMID: 26474310 https://doi.org/10.1371/journal.pone.0134553
36. Whiting PF, Rutjes AWS, Westwood ME, et al; QUADAS-2 Group. QUADAS-2: a revised tool for the quality assessment of diagnostic accuracy studies. *Ann Intern Med*. 2011;155(8):529–536 PMID: 22007046 https://doi.org/10.7326/0003-4819-155-8-201110180-00009
37. Sittig JS, Uiterwaal CSPM, Moons KGM, et al. Value of systematic detection of physical child abuse at emergency rooms: a cross-sectional diagnostic accuracy study. *BMJ Open*. 2016;6(3):e010788 PMID: 27006346 https://doi.org/10.1136/bmjopen-2015-010788
38. Schouten MCM, van Stel HF, Verheij TJM, et al. The value of a checklist for child abuse in out-of-hours primary care: to screen or not to screen. *PLoS One*. 2017;12(1):e0165641 PMID: 28045904 https://doi.org/10.1371/journal.pone.0165641
39. Bousema S, Stas HG, van de Merwe MH, et al; Dutch Burn Repository Group, Maasstad Hospital Rotterdam. Epidemiology and screening of intentional burns in children in a Dutch burn centre. *Burns*. 2016;42(6):1287–1294 PMID: 27211360 https://doi.org/10.1016/j.burns.2016.01.009
40. Dinpanah H, Akbarzadeh Pasha A, Sanji M. Potential child abuse screening in emergency department: a diagnostic accuracy study. *Emerg (Tehran)*. 2017;5(1):e8 PMID: 28286815

41. Louwers ECFM, Korfage IJ, Affourtit MJ, et al. Accuracy of a screening instrument to identify potential child abuse in emergency departments. *Child Abuse Negl.* 2014;38(7):1275–1281 PMID: 24325939 https://doi.org/10.1016/j.chiabu.2013.11.005
42. Louwers EC, Affourtit MJ, Moll HA, de Koning HJ, Korfage IJ. Screening for child abuse at emergency departments: a systematic review. *Arch Dis Child.* 2010;95(3):214–218 PMID: 19773222 https://doi.org/10.1136/adc.2008.151654
43. McTavish JR, Kimber M, Devries K, et al. Mandated reporters' experiences with reporting child maltreatment: a meta-synthesis of qualitative studies. *BMJ Open.* 2017;7(10):e013942 PMID: 29042370 https://doi.org/10.1136/bmjopen-2016-013942
44. US Preventive Services Task Force. Draft recommendation statement. Child maltreatment: interventions. https://www.uspreventiveservicestaskforce.org/Page/Document/draft-recommendation-statement/child-maltreatment-primary-care-interventions1. Published May 2018. Accessed April 4, 2019
45. Diderich HM, Fekkes M, Verkerk PH, et al. A new protocol for screening adults presenting with their own medical problems at the emergency department to identify children at high risk for maltreatment. *Child Abuse Negl.* 2013;37(12):1122–1131 PMID: 23768937 https://doi.org/10.1016/j.chiabu.2013.04.005
46. Diderich HM, Dechesne M, Fekkes M, Verkerk PH, Buitendijk SE, Oudesluys-Murphy A-M. What parental characteristics can predict child maltreatment at the emergency department? Considering expansion of the Hague Protocol. *Eur J Emerg Med.* 2015;22(4):279–281 PMID: 24892419 https://doi.org/10.1097/MEJ.0000000000000174
47. National Institute for Health and Care Excellence. *When to Suspect Child Maltreatment.* Manchester, UK: National Institute for Health and Care Excellence; 2009
48. Hibbard R, Barlow J, Macmillan H; American Academy of Pediatrics Committee on Child Abuse and Neglect; American Academy of Child and Adolescent Psychiatry Child Maltreatment and Violence Committee. Psychological maltreatment. *Pediatrics.* 2012;130(2):372–378 PMID: 22848125 https://doi.org/10.1542/peds.2012-1552
49. MacMillan HL, Fleming J, Jamieson E. Psychiatric assessment of children and adolescents. In: Goldbloom R, ed. *Pediatric Clinical Skills.* 4th ed. New York, NY: Churchill Linvingstone; 2010:1–18

CHAPTER 33

Evidence-based Child Abuse and Neglect Prevention Programs

Lisa Spector, MD, FAAP
Professor of Pediatrics
University of Central Florida
Division Chief of Developmental and Behavioral Pediatrics
Nemours Children's Hospital
Orlando, FL

Introduction

Child abuse and neglect is a significant public health issue that can be devastating not only for the children but for parents, siblings, communities, and society as a whole. Prevention of child abuse is the key to reduce childhood exposure to adversity and the accompanying short- and long-term health consequences. The goal is to create neighborhoods and communities where every child has safe, stable, nurturing relationships and environments—where every child can thrive.[1] Yet, prevention of child abuse and neglect is complex and requires a comprehensive approach that addresses factors at all levels of the social ecology—the individual, relational, community, and societal levels.[2]

Child maltreatment is multifactorial; thus, there is no one-size-fits-all child abuse prevention program. While some prevention programs are aimed at the general population (ie, *primary* prevention), others target high-risk groups (ie, *secondary* prevention) or populations that have already engaged in abusive behaviors. Child abuse takes varying forms, which stem from different causes and require different types of treatment and prevention programs. A program that aims to prevent abusive head trauma employs a much different strategy than one to prevent child sexual abuse or neglect. A parent who shakes his or her baby out of frustration requires an entirely different intervention than a person who molests children. Additionally, and unfortunately, prevention efforts require money, and the return on investment takes time. It is the savvy businessperson, government official, or other investor who has the foresight to put forth the money now to reap the benefits of a healthy population and eager workforce with fewer health issues later.

In the past, there was a paucity of data to support prevention programs, but there has been a concerted effort over the past few years to demonstrate the effectiveness of various prevention programs through scientific evidence. There are many venues to obtain information about evidence-based and promising prevention programs. One of the most commonly used is the California Evidence-Based Clearinghouse for Child Welfare (CEBC). The CEBC has a rigorous scientific rating system based on published, peer-reviewed research on each program. Additionally, the Child Welfare Information Gateway connects child welfare and related professionals to comprehensive information and resources to help protect and strengthen families.

This chapter outlines evidenced-based prevention programs aimed specifically at prevention of child maltreatment and provides a resource guide highlighting key components of each program. For a summary of the prevention programs discussed in this chapter, see Table 33.1. Additionally, tangible strategies are provided to assist practitioners in reducing the incidence of child maltreatment in their communities.

The CEBC was a significant resource in formulating the information contained in this chapter. The reader is advised to periodically check https://www.cebc4cw.org for additional information because scientific evidence is continually collected and a program's status may change over time. Level 1 represents the highest level of scientific evidence and is designated as "well-supported by research evidence." To receive a level 1 designation, a program must have at least 2 rigorous, randomized, controlled trials with 1 showing sustained effect of at least 1 year. Level 2 represents "supported by research evidence," and programs must have at least 1 rigorous, randomized, controlled trial with a sustained effect of at least 6 months to receive this designation. Level 3 is "promising research evidence," meaning at least 1 study using some form of control has established the practice's benefit over the control. Level 4 designates "evidence fails to demonstrate effect," and level 5 is a "concerning practice," meaning the program is not recommended for use.

Crying and Abusive Head Trauma (Shaken Baby Syndrome)

Crying is the single most common antecedent event prior to shaking or abusing a baby. Anticipatory guidance addressing newborn and infant crying and, most importantly, the caregiver's ability to cope with the crying is critically important in preventing abuse. Newborn and infantile crying, often referred to as *colic*, begins around 2 weeks of age and continues until

TABLE 33.1
Summary of Prevention Programs[a]

Type of Program	Name of Program	CEBC Rating	Age Group	Participants	Languages	Minimum Provider Qualifications
Home Visiting Program	Nurse-Family Partnership	1—home visiting program for prevention of CAN 1—home visiting program for child well-being 1—primary prevention	0–2 y	Low-income mother	English Spanish	Registered nurse with BS in nursing
	SafeCare	2—home visiting program for prevention of CAN 2—parent training program that addresses CAN 2—secondary prevention	0–5 y	Parents at risk for CAN or who have history of CAN	English Spanish Hebrew French	BS in human services
	Healthy Families America	1—home visiting program for child well-being	0–5 y	Parents at risk for child maltreatment, parental substance abuse, or mental illness	English Spanish	High school diploma or equivalent
	Parents as Teachers	3—prevention of CAN (primary) program 3—home visiting program for child well-being	0–5 y	Families with expectant mothers or parents of children up to kindergarten entry	English Spanish French German Mandarin	High school diploma or GED and 2 y supervised work with young children/ parents
Parent Training Program	The Incredible Years	1—prevention of CAN (secondary) program 1—parent training program that addresses behavior problems in children and adolescents 1—Disruptive behavior treatment (child and adolescent)	0–8 y	Parents, teachers, children	English Spanish French Chinese Dutch Danish Finnish Norwegian Portuguese Russian Swedish	Master's level or equivalent

(continued)

TABLE 33.1 (*continued*)

Type of Program	Name of Program	CEBC Rating	Age Group	Participants	Languages	Minimum Provider Qualifications
Parent Training Program (*continued*)	Triple P	Prevention of CAN (primary) 2—parent training program that addresses CAN 1—parent training program that addresses behavior problems in children and adolescents (only the fourth level [of 5] of the program has the level 1 CEBC designation) 1—disruptive behavior treatment (child and adolescent) (only the fourth level [of 5] of the program has the level 1 CEBC designation)	0–16 y	Parents or caregivers	English Spanish French Arabic Berber Chinese Greek Japanese Malay Portuguese Romanian Swedish Turkish Vietnamese	Post-high school degree in health, education, child care, or social services
	Parent-Child Interaction Therapy	1—parent training program that addresses behavior problems in children and adolescents 1—disruptive behavior treatment (child and adolescent)	2–7 y	Parents or caregivers	English Spanish	Master's degree and licensure as a mental health provider
	Parent Management Training—Oregon Model	1—parent training program that addresses behavior problems in children and adolescents 1—disruptive behavior treatment (child and adolescent)	2–18 y	Parents or caregivers	English Spanish Danish Dutch Icelandic Norwegian	Bachelor's degree with appropriate clinical experience or master's degree in relevant field
	ACT Raising Safe Kids Program	3—prevention of CAN (primary) program	0–10 y	Parents or caregivers	English Spanish Greek Japanese Mandarin Portuguese	Associate degree (bachelor's degree preferred)

(*continued*)

TABLE 33.1 (*continued*)

Type of Program	Name of Program	CEBC Rating	Age Group	Participants	Languages	Minimum Provider Qualifications
Parent Training Program (*continued*)	Family Foundations	2—parent training program that addresses CAN	Birth	Parents or caregivers	English	College education with experience in leading groups and working with families
Primary Care Intervention	Safe Environment for Every Kid	1—prevention of CAN (primary) program 2—prevention of CAN (secondary) program	0–5 y	Parents or caregivers	English Spanish Chinese Vietnamese	Medical professionals in association with master's level mental health professional
Abusive Head Trauma Prevention	Period of PURPLE Crying	1—prevention of CAN (primary) program	0–5 mo	Parents or caregivers	English Spanish Arabic Cantonese French Japanese Korean Portuguese Punjabi Somali Vietnamese	No educational requirements
	Safe Babies New York	1—prevention of CAN (primary) program	0–5 mo	Parents or caregivers	English Spanish	Administration by registered nurse or nurse educator strongly recommended
Child Education Program	Body Safety Training Workbook	3—prevention of CAN (primary) program	3–8 y	Children	English Spanish	Ability to read script; early childhood education (in school setting)
	Who Do You Tell	3—prevention of CAN (primary) program	K–sixth grade	Children	Unknown	Unknown
Staff Volunteer Training Program	Stewards of Children	3—prevention of CAN (primary) program	Volunteers and staff	Youth and adults who work with children	English Spanish Icelandic	Must complete a full-day facilitator workshop

Abbreviations: BS, bachelor of science; CAN, child abuse and neglect; CEBC, California Evidence-Based Clearinghouse for Child Welfare; GED, general equivalency diploma.

[a] Information obtained from CEBC at www.cebc4cw.org.

3 to 4 months of age, with a peak around 2 months of age. Just as successive doses of medications increase the concentration of a drug in the body, the more often the medical professional initiates the conversation about crying, the more it normalizes the behavior and reinforces healthy responses on the part of the caregiver. Ideally, the topic of crying should be broached before the baby is born, again at birth, and then again in each health supervision visit until the child reaches 1 year of age, as well as during high-risk crying times associated with vaccinations and childhood illnesses.

Medical professionals play a critical role in not only normalizing newborn and infant crying and describing methods to soothe the baby (eg, feeding, changing, swaddling) but also providing caregivers strategies to help cope with crying. Caregivers need to know that it is OK to place the unsoothable baby in a safe crib (employing safe sleep practices) for 10 to 15 minutes while caregivers engage in a self-calming activity or just take a break from the crying. This can include a variety of measures, such as calling a friend, family member, or other support; using deep breathing; putting in earphones to dull the crying; watching a calming TV show; listening to calming music; or even stepping just outside the door. Medical professionals can assist families in developing and implementing a strategic plan whereby a caregiver who is struggling with newborn or infant crying can seek assistance in a supportive manner. This may be as simple as having the caregiver call his or her partner, a family member or friend, or even primary care office staff, if available, to help problem solve, provide reassurance, and offer support in a nonjudgmental manner.

There are 2 programs, Period of PURPLE Crying and Safe Babies New York (formerly the Upstate New York Shaken Baby Syndrome Education Program), that address crying in the newborn period in efforts to reduce the incidence of abusive head trauma (formerly shaken baby syndrome). Both programs received the designation of a promising practice through the CEBC (level 3). Both are hospital-based, postnatal interventions for parents of newborns. They share similar goals of normalizing crying, educating about the dangers of shaking, and reducing caregiver frustration around crying.

The Period of PURPLE Crying was developed by the National Center on Shaken Baby Syndrome. The letters in PURPLE describe common properties of crying—namely that crying **p**eaks in 2 months; it is **u**nexpected and **r**esistant to soothing; the baby looks as if he or she is in **p**ain; and crying lasts a **l**ong time and often occurs in the evening hours. The program includes written material and a 17-minute video, which is available on DVD, the internet, and a mobile application. Three points of contact are recommended by the program, the first one being in the first weeks after the baby's birth, the second within the first 3 months, and the third as a public education campaign.

The Safe Babies New York program provides written materials and a video for parents prior to leaving the hospital. One 25-minute contact with a registered nurse is recommended in the program so that caregivers can ask questions and discuss material in the video. Parents/caregivers are asked to sign a commitment statement affirming the receipt of the material. Additional education materials are provided at the first medical professional office visit. In 2014, the program added information about safe sleep in an effort to reduce sleep-related newborn and infant deaths. The program emphasizes the importance of putting babies to sleep on their backs, in a clutter-free environment (ie, no pillows, stuffed animals, crib bumpers, or blankets), and on a firm mattress.

Abusive head trauma is one of the most devastating forms of child abuse, resulting in deleterious outcomes for newborns, infants, and children, including developmental delay, behavioral issues, and death. Additionally, abusive head trauma is associated with high medical costs, as well as an excessive burden on families and society from family court and criminal legal proceedings. While each of the programs described in this section is an effective first step in reducing abusive head trauma in newborns and infants, there is no way to ensure that caregivers read or view the information provided in the hospital. The only way to ensure parents/caregivers receive the information, understand the content, and have a concrete plan to improve coping with crying is for them to have a direct conversation with a knowledgeable medical professional, namely their primary care physician.

Parental Postpartum Depression

Equally important in reducing risk factors for child abuse in the newborn period is assessing for postpartum depression in parents/caregivers. Postpartum depression affects at least 1 in 8 mothers and their babies in the year after childbirth worldwide.[3] Women with depression have been found to have poorer responsiveness to newborn/infant cues[4] and more negative, hostile, or disengaged parenting behaviors.[5] While maternal postpartum depression is becoming more widely recognized and less stigmatized for mothers of newborns, paternal postpartum depression still remains an underrecognized issue for men and other partners. Estimates of the prevalence of paternal postpartum depression in the first 2 postpartum months vary from 4% to 25%.[3] Paternal postpartum depression has high comorbidity with maternal postpartum depression.[6]

The Edinburgh Postnatal Depression Scale (EPDS) has been well validated for women in the United States and non–English-speaking populations in other countries.[7] It has also been widely used in paternal postpartum depression studies. It consists of 10 self-reported items, 8 addressing depressive symptoms (eg, sadness, self-blame) and 2 inquiring about anxiety symptoms (eg, feeling worried or anxious, feeling scared or panicky). Responses are scored 0, 1, 2, or 3 according to severity of the symptom. Postnatal depression is often assessed 6 to 12 weeks after childbirth, but many studies using the EPDS for later postpartum mood evaluation extend to up to 12 months' postpartum. Cutoff scores for depression vary from 9 to 13 points out of a maximum of 30.[6] Other commonly used screening tools with evidence of validity in the puerperium include the Postpartum Depression Screening Scale and the 9-item Patient Health Questionnaire.[3]

The most important aspect of screening for postpartum depression is effective treatment of the caregiver. Fitelson et al published a comprehensive review of treatments of postpartum depression, including psychopharmacological and psychological interventions as well as nonpharmacologic treatments.[3] In summary, psychopharmacological interventions are effective, yet include unknown risks of medications in human milk. Estrogen may be an effective agent for treatment, but data remain limited. Cognitive behavioral therapy, psychodynamic psychotherapy, and other supportive interventions via peer support, health visitor, or partner support have shown benefit over wait-list controls. Data on acupuncture, massage, exercise, and omega-3 fatty acid supplements are limited.

Family Foundations is a series of parenting classes aimed at supporting couples having a baby through recognizing individual adjustment (eg, stress, depression, anxiety) to the new baby and encouraging cooperation, support, and sensitivity between partners. Of the 9 parenting classes, 5 occur before the baby's birth and 4 after the baby's birth. The pre-birth classes focus on promoting communication, how to manage conflict, how to change personal negative storylines, and how to have difficult conversations. The postnatal classes help parents understand the baby's temperament, attachment to the caregiver, dynamics of the parenting team, and appreciation for their partner. Feinberg and Kan demonstrated that parents randomly assigned to Family Foundations displayed significant improvement in distress in parent-child relationship and in maternal depression and anxiety compared with controls who received no treatment.[8]

Home Visiting Programs

Home visiting programs have been providing services to families with young children for many years. They operate under the belief that parents mediate changes for their children.[9] Home visitors provide education and training to parents as well as support and coordination of services. Practitioners vary in their training; some programs use nurses or social workers, while others employ child development specialists, paraprofessionals, or other parents. Common components among programs include education in child health and development, building positive parenting skills, and assistance in accessing social supports and community services. Programs vary with regard to populations served, timing, intensity of visits, and the nature of the home visits.

Children in the birth-to-3-year age group have the highest rate of experiencing child maltreatment and are more likely to die as a result of child maltreatment. In 2014, children 3 years and younger had a child maltreatment rate of 14.8 per 1,000, compared with 10.6 per 1,000 for children aged 4 to 7 years, 7.9 per 1,000 for children aged 8 to 11 years, and 6.9 per 1,000 for children and teens aged 12 to 15 years.[10] According to the 2015 National Child Abuse and Neglect Data System report, an estimated 1,670 children died due to abuse or neglect in the United States that year.[11] Close to three-quarters (74.8%) of the children who died due to child abuse or neglect were younger than 3 years.[11] Nearly three-quarters (72.9%) of child fatalities were attributed to neglect only or a combination of neglect and another maltreatment type, and 43.9% of the children died exclusively from physical abuse or from physical abuse in combination with another maltreatment type.[11]

Prevention efforts geared toward families with infants and toddlers can have a tremendous effect on reducing abuse and neglect as well as reducing death from maltreatment. Home visiting programs appear to be a good fit with regard to prevention of child maltreatment in this age group given the nature of the intervention. However, the research evidence over the years is inconclusive.[12] In 2013, a systematic review to update the US Preventive Services Task Force recommendations found, after review of home visitation programs, that none of the 5 randomized, control trials found differences in the rates of child protective services reports between home-visited children and control children,[13] while 2 trials found a statistically significant decrease in maternal report of use of physical abuse.[13] More recently, a large-scale, mixed-methods study, evaluating the effect of multiple home visiting programs on rates of child abuse–related injury, found that children of parents enrolled in a home visiting program were significantly more likely than controls to experience an abusive episode.[14] However, of the cases describing incidents concerning for abuse and neglect, most involved caregivers other than the client as the perpetrator. Thus, it could be concluded that the effect of home visiting programs can be enhanced through a curriculum that more directly and proactively addresses maltreatment (ie, by helping parents address potential behavior and development concerns with other child care providers, thereby reducing likelihood of abuse, or by promoting use of quality center-based child care) as well as improved access to quality child care options.[14]

One of the most long-standing and commonly recognized home visiting programs is Nurse-Family Partnership, which has the highest rating (level 1) in 2 of the CEBC child abuse prevention categories, home visiting programs for prevention of child abuse and neglect and prevention of child abuse and neglect (primary) programs. The Nurse-Family Partnership enlists registered nurses to provide home visits to first-time, low-income mothers, starting during pregnancy and continuing until the child is 2 years old. The visits are weekly until the infant is 6 weeks old; visits transition at that time to every other week. Olds et al found women visited by nurses were less likely to be perpetrators of child abuse and neglect and had fewer arrests, convictions, and number of days jailed.[15] Subsequent data revealed women visited by nurses experienced less incidences of domestic violence, while children had better language and executive functioning skills and behavioral adaptation during testing.[16]

Healthy Families America is another well-recognized home visiting program. It has a plethora of scientific evidence supporting the program's goal of improving child well-being, including physical health, development, and school readiness, such that it receives a level 1 rating from the CEBC in this area. However, Healthy Families America has yet to have enough scientific evidence to designate it as a home visiting program for prevention of child abuse and neglect (level 4).

Parents as Teachers involves parent educators who provide early childhood parent education. Its 4 goals are increasing parental knowledge of early childhood development, early detection of developmental delays and health issues, preventing maltreatment, and increasing school readiness and success. Visits typically occur every 2 weeks or monthly, depending on family needs, until the child is 5 years old. Parents as Teachers also facilitates parental group gatherings to obtain social support and share experiences. Parents as Teachers is designated by the CEBC as a promising program with regard to primary prevention of child abuse and neglect (level 3).

SafeCare is an in-home parent training program for parents who have abused and/or neglected a child or who are deemed at risk for child maltreatment. The CEBC has ranked it a level 2 program as a parent training program that addresses child abuse and neglect as well as a home visiting program that prevents child abuse and neglect. Caregivers meet with the providers for 1 to 1½ hours a week for 18 to 20 weeks. The curriculum consists of teaching, modeling, role-play, and assessment of targeted skills. Its 3 modules are strategies to improve child-parent interactions, removing home hazards and improving parental supervision, and recognizing and responding to symptoms of illness and injury to reduce medical neglect. Gershater-Molko et al found that families participating in SafeCare who were involved with child protective services had significantly lower rates of re-abuse reporting during the 24-month follow-up period than the control group.[17]

Parent Training Programs

Effective parenting can buffer many adverse childhood events, thereby decreasing toxic stress and improving health.[18] Outside of the newborn period, the toddler's "terrible 2s," which may extend into the preschool years, can be quite challenging for caregivers. As toddlers begin to establish their own identity and attempt to control their environment, caregivers can be at a loss as to how to support their child's growth, yet at the same time set limits and boundaries to protect their child and teach key concepts like sharing. This is a critical time for child development and often a time when caregivers are overly strained and resort to ineffective and harmful discipline techniques. Medical professionals have an essential role in eliciting history about challenges with parenting and providing effective strategies to help teach the child and support the caregiver. *Bring Out the Best in Your Children*[19] is a handout from the American Academy of Pediatrics (AAP) for medical professionals and caregivers describing how to strengthen child-caregiver relationships, set up reward systems, and use time-out effectively. Additionally, the AAP parent-facing website, HealthyChildren.org, provides guidance around discipline strategies for caregivers. Families that require additional support may benefit from a referral to a psychologist, developmental-behavioral pediatrician, or parent training program for more hands-on training in effective behavior management techniques.

There are a multitude of evidence-based parent training programs, including the Incredible Years, Triple P, Parent-Child Interaction Therapy, and Parent Management Training—Oregon Model. Parent training programs are based on common psychological theories such as attachment theory and social learning theory. The focus of these programs is training parents in effective behavior management strategies to reduce child behavior problems, improve child compliance, and, therefore, reduce caregiver stress and the possible sequela of childhood trauma. A variety of formats may be used, ranging from individual therapy with the parent and/or child to group parent treatment or remote training via a book or video. The minimum provider qualifications differ per program.

The Incredible Years provides curricula for parents, teachers, and children that can be used separately or in combination. The Incredible Years parent program can be implemented in an individual or group format. The goals include building positive relationships and attachment, more nurturing and less harsh punishment, and increased social support and problem-solving. The Incredible Years is unique in that it uses a parent-directed approach to skill building in effective behavior management techniques, while also providing rationale for such strategies. The teacher component seeks to increase proactive classroom management skills and strengthen teacher-student partnership. The program is available in multiple languages, and anyone with a master's level of education may be trained to administer the program. Bywater et al[20] demonstrated significant parent-reported improvements in primary measures of child behavior, parent behavior, parental stress, and depression gained initially were maintained at 18 months after baseline. The Incredible Years has the highest rating (level 1) in 2 key CEBC categories, parent training program that addresses behavior problems in children and adolescents and prevention of child abuse and neglect (secondary) program. It is the only parent training program that currently has a level 1 rating in prevention of child maltreatment.

The Triple P Positive Parenting Program is a multitiered system of 5 levels of education and support of caregivers. The lowest level, Universal Triple P, consists of a media campaign about raising healthy children. The next 2 levels, Selected Triple P and Primary Care Triple P, provide brief consultations or seminars to address common childhood issues like toileting and sleeping. Level 4, Standard Triple P, involves individual or group parent training, while the highest level, Enhanced Triple P, involves intense family therapy that targets family stressors and other barriers to standard treatment. Triple P has been shown to lower rates of child maltreatment. This was the result of a study by Prinz et al after 18 counties were randomized to Triple P or service as usual.[21] Treatment counties had 649 service providers trained in Triple P. Pretreatment groups did not differ with regard to substantiated maltreatment. Data collected 12 months after the intervention ceased showed counties receiving Triple P had significantly lower rates of substantiated child maltreatment. Thus, Triple P is listed as a level 2 entity for primary prevention of child abuse and neglect through the CEBC.

Parent-Child Interaction Therapy and Parent Management Training—Oregon Model are 2 equally effective parent behavior management training programs that are well supported by research evidence (CEBC level 1) to address behavior problems in children and adolescents as well as provide treatment of disruptive behavior in children and adolescents. However, neither is listed in the CEBC as supported by research to provide primary or secondary prevention of child abuse and neglect.[22]

The ACT Raising Safe Kids Program is listed as a promising practice (level 3) through the CEBC. ACT is implemented as a 9-session group parent training. It has a universal public health approach addressing use of effective behavior management, child development, discipline methods, medical literacy, parents' anger management, and child aggression. ACT curriculum uses a multimodal education approach through modeling, role-play, constructive activities, and motivational interviewing techniques. The ACT program pairs well with a parent training program that focuses primarily on building effective behavior management skills, like Parent-Child Interactive Therapy, Triple P, the Incredible Years, or Parent Management Training—Oregon Model. Knox et al demonstrated that parent participants in the ACT program reported less spanking and reduced rates of hitting children with objects compared with wait-list controls.[23]

Child Education Programs

While the onus of preventing child sexual abuse does not, and should not, fall onto children, it is essential that children receive education about personal safety as well as reinforcing messages that their body is theirs and they get to decide when, where, and with whom they choose to share their body. This concept is very simply expressed when caregivers do not make a child hug or kiss a family member the child does not want to hug or kiss. Additionally, when a caregiver is tickling a child, if the child says, "Stop," the abrupt cessation of tickling by the caregiver reinforces to the child that the child calls the shots when it comes to sharing his or her body. Medical professionals are in a unique position to educate caregivers about these concepts during health supervision visits in an effort to guide parents in having these potentially difficult conversations with children on a regular basis.

With regard to education about personal safety, the first step is teaching children to use anatomically correct names for their private parts or, at a minimum, labeling their private parts as private. Often caregivers use creative names for private parts, like "pocketbook" or "no-no spot." Vague terms for private parts can impede a child's disclosure of sexual abuse. An unsuspecting teacher may hear the child disclose that someone touched her pocketbook, only to be left thinking that someone took the child's wallet. No-no spot, or similar terms, often ascribe negative connotations to one's genitals, which does not promote a healthy self-image or ownership of one's own private parts.

The next step is helping children understand that private parts are indeed private and that only certain people can look at or touch that area of their body. Concrete examples help children understand this concept; for example, "It is OK when Mom helps you wipe your private area" (for a child working on toilet training); "It is OK if the doctor has to look at your privates as long as Dad is there and says it is OK." A very important follow-up to this instruction is helping children problem solve what to do if someone looks at or touches their private parts in a manner that has not been discussed or in a way that makes the child feel uncomfortable. Children may be advised that they can tell the person "no" or "stop," but most importantly, the child should find a trusted adult to tell about what happened. Children must also be advised that they will not get in trouble for telling and no one will be hurt if the child tells; this may counteract a threatening statement a perpetrator may use to silence the child.

Because children may act out sexually on younger children, it is equally important for medical professionals to assist caregivers in establishing good body boundaries for their children. Children develop a healthy sense of self and also learn body boundaries when they are taught that it is OK for them to touch their own selves in a private setting, when alone in their bedroom or the bathroom, but they are not to touch anyone else's private parts.

There are a multitude of child sexual education programs across the nation, typically administered through local child advocacy centers. The National Children's Advocacy Center website (www.nationalcac.org) is a useful resource to find a local child advocacy center.

Two programs have demonstrated promising research evidence in efforts of primary prevention against child abuse and neglect. The Body Safety Training Workbook consists of 10 lessons administered by teachers or parents. The first 5 lessons address general safety (ie, fire, gun, water, pedestrian, seat belt), while the second set of lessons covers body safety (ie, teaching children the body safety skills of recognizing, resisting, and reporting inappropriate touching). Compared to wait-list control groups, YMCA preschool children receiving the Body Safe Training Workbook

BOX 33.1
Books to Help Parents Talk With Children About Physical and Sexual Abuse

Some Parts are NOT for Sharing by Julie K. Federico
Amazing You! Getting Smart About Your Private Parts by Gail Saltz
Do You Have a Secret? (Let's Talk About It!) by Jennifer Moore-Mallinos
Your Body Belongs to You by Cornelia Maude Spelman
Not in Room 204: Breaking the Silence of Abuse by Shannon Riggs
Some Secrets Should Never Be Kept by Jayneen Sanders
No Secrets Between Us by Rose Morrisroe

demonstrated greater knowledge about sexual abuse and higher levels of personal safety skills, which were maintained 2 months later. Additionally, there was no increase in negative behaviors in the children, nor were the children in the Body Safe Training Workbook group seen as more fearful after participation.[24]

Who Do You Tell is another sexual abuse education program designed in Canada through Calgary Communities Against Sexual Abuse. There are 4 different versions of the program tailored to varying developmental levels: kindergarten, first grade, second grade, and third through sixth grade. Additionally, there is a 1-hour teacher session and a separate parent night, which outlines what will be taught and how to respond to possible disclosures of abuse.

Medical professionals who serve families living in communities with limited resources may be interested in referring parents to watch the Happy Bear Play online video. The 25-minute interactive play for children 4 to 7 years old addresses how to talk about various topics with children, including recognizing welcome and unwelcome touches, practicing resistance skills, and learning to report to a trusted adult. The videos can be found at www.sunflowerhouse.org/happy-bear in English and Spanish. Box 33.1 lists some books to help guide adults in having conversations with their children about body safety and related subjects.

Staff Volunteer Training Programs

Stewards of Children is a 2-hour training that teaches adults who work closely with children in schools, youth-serving agencies, and churches how to prevent, recognize, and respond appropriately to child sexual abuse. The facilitator-led training adheres to the structured DVD content, with intermittent group discussion. The participants receive an interactive workbook to reinforce key concepts and obtain assistance in preparing their personal action plan for protecting children from sexual abuse. Additionally, there is an option for an online format, which requires a score of 80% on the posttest to receive a certificate of completion.

Primary Care Interventions

Safe Environment for Every Kid (SEEK) is the only program that is supported by research evidence as a primary and secondary prevention of child maltreatment. SEEK involves a 15-question screening tool to be administered at regular intervals in the child's first 5 postnatal years. The questionnaire assesses risk factors for abuse, including parental depression and substance use, intimate partner violence, economic hardship, and harsh punishment. Additionally, medical professionals receive training to address positive responses, which incorporates principles of motivational interviewing. SEEK parent handouts are available for all targeted problems as well. Alternatively, medical professionals may elicit support from mental health professionals like social workers to counsel families or assist in finding community resources. After randomization of pediatric practices, Dubowitz et al found that at initial and 12-month assessments, mothers who had participated in SEEK reported less psychological aggression and fewer minor physical assaults than controls.[25]

Conclusion

Prevention of child maltreatment begins with physicians and other medical professionals, whether through advocacy, program development, collaboration with community resources, or consistently integrating conversations about salient topics like crying and personal safety into everyday care and counseling of patients and families.

Providers of health care to children and their families have the knowledge, skills, and tools available to recognize and address many of the common risk factors of child maltreatment, thus reducing its incidence in our communities.

References

1. Fortson BL, Klevens J, Merrick MT, Gilbert LK, Alexander SP. *Preventing Child Abuse and Neglect: A Technical Package for Policy, Norm, and Programmatic Activities*. Atlanta, GA: National Center for Injury Prevention and Control, Centers for Disease Control and Prevention; 2016

2. Centers for Disease Control and Prevention. Child abuse and neglect: prevention strategies. https://www.cdc.gov/violenceprevention/childabuseandneglect/prevention.html. Reviewed February 26, 2019. Accessed July 14, 2019
3. Fitelson E, Kim S, Baker AS, Leight K. Treatment of postpartum depression: clinical, psychological and pharmacological options. *Int J Womens Health*. 2010;3:1–14 PMID: 21339932 https://doi.org/10.2147/IJWH.S6938
4. Murray L, Fiori-Cowley A, Hooper R, Cooper P. The impact of postnatal depression and associated adversity on early mother-infant interactions and later infant outcome. *Child Dev*. 1996;67(5):2512–2526 PMID: 9022253 https://doi.org/10.2307/1131637
5. Lovejoy MC, Graczyk PA, O'Hare E, Neuman G. Maternal depression and parenting behavior: a meta-analytic review. *Clin Psychol Rev*. 2000;20(5):561–592 PMID: 10860167 https://doi.org/10.1016/S0272-7358(98)00100-7
6. Kim P, Swain JE. Sad dads: paternal postpartum depression. *Psychiatry (Edgmont)*. 2007;4(2):35–47 PMID: 20805898
7. Murray D, Cox JL. Screening for depression during pregnancy with the Edinburgh Postnatal Depression Scale (EPDS). *J Reprod Infant Psychol*. 1990;8(2):99–107 https://doi.org/10.1080/02646839008403615
8. Feinberg ME, Kan ML. Establishing family foundations: intervention effects on coparenting, parent/infant well-being, and parent-child relations. *J Fam Psychol*. 2008;22(2):253–263 PMID: 18410212 https://doi.org/10.1037/0893-3200.22.2.253
9. Sweet MA, Appelbaum MI. Is home visiting an effective strategy? A meta-analytic review of home visiting programs for families with young children. *Child Dev*. 2004;75(5):1435–1456 PMID: 15369524 https://doi.org/10.1111/j.1467-8624.2004.00750.x
10. Child Trends. Child maltreatment. https://www.childtrends.org/?indicators=child-maltreatment. Updated 2019. Accessed June 4, 2019
11. Child Welfare Information Gateway. *Child Maltreatment 2015: Summary of Key Findings*. Washington, DC: US Department of Health and Human Services, Children's Bureau; 2017
12. Rubin DM, Curtis ML, Matone M. Child abuse prevention and child home visitation: making sure we get it right. *JAMA Pediatr*. 2014;168(1):5–6 PMID: 24217352 https://doi.org/10.1001/jamapediatrics.2013.3865
13. Selph SS, Bougatsos C, Blazina I, Nelson HD. Behavioral interventions and counseling to prevent child abuse and neglect: a systematic review to update the US Preventive Services Task Force recommendation. *Ann Intern Med*. 2013;158(3):179–190 PMID: 23338775 https://doi.org/10.7326/0003-4819-158-3-201302050-00590
14. Matone M, Kellom K, Griffis H, et al. A mixed methods evaluation of early childhood abuse prevention within evidence-based home visiting programs. *Matern Child Health J*. 2018;22(suppl 1):79–91 PMID: 29855837 https://doi.org/10.1007/s10995-018-2530-1
15. Olds DL, Eckenrode J, Henderson CR Jr, et al. Long-term effects of home visitation on maternal life course and child abuse and neglect. Fifteen-year follow-up of a randomized trial. *JAMA*. 1997;278(8):637–643 PMID: 9272895 https://doi.org/10.1001/jama.1997.03550080047038
16. Olds DL, Robinson J, Pettitt L, et al. Effects of home visits by paraprofessionals and by nurses: age 4 follow-up results of a randomized trial. *Pediatrics*. 2004;114(6):1560–1568 PMID: 15574615 https://doi.org/10.1542/peds.2004-0961
17. Gershater-Molko RM, Lutzker JR, Wesch D. Using recidivism data to evaluate project safecare: teaching bonding, safety, and health care skills to parents. *Child Maltreat*. 2002;7(3):277–285 PMID: 12139194 https://doi.org/10.1177/1077559502007003009

18. O'Connell LK, Davis MM, Bauer NS. Assessing parenting behaviors to improve child outcomes. *Pediatrics*. 2015;135(2):e286–e288 PMID: 25624384 https://doi.org/10.1542/peds.2014-2497
19. American Academy of Pediatrics. *Bring Out the Best in Your Children*. https://www.aap.org/en-us/Documents/ttb_bring_out_best.pdf. Published 2014. Accessed June 4, 2019
20. Bywater T, Hutchings J, Daley D, et al. Long-term effectiveness of a parenting intervention for children at risk of developing conduct disorder. *Br J Psychiatry*. 2009;195(4):318–324 PMID: 19794200 https://doi.org/10.1192/bjp.bp.108.056531
21. Prinz RJ, Sanders MR, Shapiro CJ, Whitaker DJ, Lutzker JR. Population-based prevention of child maltreatment: the U.S. Triple P system population trial. *Prev Sci*. 2009;10(1):1–12 PMID: 19160053 https://doi.org/10.1007/s11121-009-0123-3
22. California Evidence-Based Clearinghouse for Child Welfare. Topic: prevention of child abuse and neglect (secondary) programs. https://www.cebc4cw.org/topic/prevention-of-child-abuse-and-neglect-secondary. Accessed June 4, 2019
23. Knox MS, Burkhart K, Hunter KE. ACT Against Violence Parents Raising Safe Kids Program: effects on maltreatment-related parenting behaviors and beliefs. *J Fam Issues*. 2010;32(1):55–74 https://doi.org/10.1177/0192513X10370112
24. Wurtele SK, Currier LL, Gillispie EI, Franklin CF. The efficacy of a parent implemented program for teaching preschoolers personal safety skills. *Behav Ther*. 1991;22(1):69–83 https://doi.org/10.1016/S0005-7894(05)80245-X
25. Dubowitz H, Lane WG, Semiatin JN, Magder LS. The SEEK model of pediatric primary care: can child maltreatment be prevented in a low-risk population? *Acad Pediatr*. 2012;12(4):259–268 PMID: 22658954 https://doi.org/10.1016/j.acap.2012.03.005

CHAPTER 34

Creating Change Through Advocacy

James G. Pawelski, MS
Director, State Advocacy
American Academy of Pediatrics
Itasca, IL

Advocacy, like medicine, can best be described as an art and a science. As a frontline medical professional, you learn by means of evidence, practice, experience, and shared expertise and apply that knowledge to the clinical evaluation and management of the child who has potentially experienced abuse. Considering the child in the context of his or her family, and the dyad's experience in the social, cultural, educational, spiritual, economic, environmental, and political spheres in which they live, is fundamental to your work.[1]

For decades, we have recognized the need for more than clinical interventions to address the complex issues of child abuse and neglect.[2] Advocating for policy change can support clinical interventions and lead to better outcomes for children.

Prior to 1875 in the United States, efforts to protect children were sporadic and predominantly court based. In 1875, the New York Society for the Prevention of Cruelty to Children became the first organization dedicated to child protection. By 1922, approximately 300 similar nongovernmental child protection groups were formed across the country—many of which were hit hard by the Depression and dissolved. Chicago instituted the world's first juvenile court in 1899, and by 1919, all but 3 states had established similar courts. While their primary focus was on "delinquent children," they were empowered with the ability to adjudicate child abuse and neglect cases. Engagement by community,

---

Portions of this chapter are adapted from American Academy of Pediatrics. *AAP Advocacy Guide*. Elk Grove Village, IL: American Academy of Pediatrics; 2009. https://www.aap.org/en-us/advocacy-and-policy/state-advocacy/Documents/AdvocacyGuide.pdf. Accessed July 14, 2019.

state, and federal government began around 1962 with the publication of *The Battered Child Syndrome* by pediatrician Henry Kempe and his colleagues. This gave rise to the US Congress amending the Social Security Act, emphasizing the role of child protective services in child welfare and requiring states to make child welfare a statewide service. A flurry of state legislation over the subsequent 5 years resulted in every state having a mandated reporting law encompassing professionals such as teachers and physicians. In 1974, the US Congress passed the Child Abuse Prevention and Treatment Act of 1974 (CAPTA), which authorized federal funds to improve the state response to physical abuse, neglect, and sexual abuse, with an emphasis on training, the establishment of multidisciplinary centers, reporting, and investigation.[3]

Since 1974, CAPTA has been amended several times and other important federal laws relating to child abuse and neglect have been enacted. State lawmakers have acted to comply with CAPTA and to enhance the body of public policy reflecting the needs of their states. These system changes, brought about by state and federal policy advances, contribute to better outcomes for children.

Advocacy is the key to building on individual solutions and creating system change—and your expertise and credibility are key credentials for this work.

Advocacy Basics

Broadly defined, *public policy* is the collection of principles, rules, regulations, and laws established through a political process. Public policy influences and can be influenced. Our social environments, principles, and laws are shaped by policy makers with input from advocates. This happens largely at 3 levels of government—municipal/local, state, and federal. Knowing the basics about the structure and function of these levels of government is an important foundation for engaging in advocacy.

Municipal, state, and federal governments have 3 branches—legislative, executive, and judicial. Town and city councils, state legislatures, and Congress are representative groups of elected officials that write, debate, and determine laws for constituents. Executive branches include council chairs, mayors, governors, the president, and the agencies and departments under their jurisdiction. Laws are approved or rejected by executives and implemented by agencies. Budgets are proposed by many government executives, and some have the power to alter what the legislative branch has approved. Municipal, state, and federal courts interpret laws and determine their applicability.

Local Government

Counties and municipalities are the most common forms of local government in the United States, but school districts are also part of this governance structure. Most counties have fiscal authority and exercise power by means of their budgets along with enactment of ordinances. Funding for hospitals, public health and safety programs, and, in some states, services that address child and family welfare often flow from county governments. Municipalities may include cities, towns, and villages. These entities consider proposals, hold public hearings, enact ordinances, and develop budgets—which can all have an effect on child health and well-being.

While there may be differences in the form of these governing bodies and in the processes they use to establish public policy, constituents and advocates often have greater access to these locally elected officials than to those at the state and federal levels.

Some examples of the role that you as a pediatrician could play in community advocacy include

- Partnering with child advocacy organizations in your area
- Informing community leaders, decision makers, and elected officials about issues that are affecting children in your community
- Inviting decision makers to visit your professional setting
- Providing testimony and telling your story at community forums and events and in your local media
- Serving on the board of an organization that supports children's health and well-being or children's interests, such as a school board
- Asking parents, teachers, and other medical professionals in your area to get involved in local abuse and neglect prevention efforts
- Initiating a community project or forming a partnership, alliance, or coalition to address a child protection concern[4(p20)]

State Government

Public policy that affects children's health, in the form of legislation, regulations, and executive decisions, or legal actions, is made almost daily in states across the country.

There are more than 7,300 state legislators across the country who are important players in day-to-day governing. State legislatures are more likely than Congress to enact bills—in some cases, by a substantial margin. States have been described as "laboratories of democracy" and do indeed work to develop innovative solutions to address complex policy challenges. As an advocate, engaging with state legislators is crucial. Many laws related to child protection are enacted at the state level, including determining the definitions of child abuse and neglect, domestic violence, and human trafficking; establishing reporting requirements and immunity provisions; and determining how children should be represented in abuse and neglect proceedings. Some basics to keep in mind when engaging in state advocacy work include

- Although every state legislature is unique, there are some common elements among them.
- Forty-nine states have bicameral, or 2-chamber, legislatures. The "upper" chamber is commonly known as the senate and contains fewer members. The "lower" chamber is known as the house of representatives or the assembly. Nebraska is the only exception; its legislature is unicameral, or one chamber.
- Senate presidents and speakers of the house are the ranking officials in these chambers.
- Committee structures enable legislatures to consider bills by germane subject matter as well as by cost. Committee assignments can sometimes determine the fate of a bill.
- Legislative sessions vary from state to state and year to year. Some state legislative sessions are as short as 30 days; others technically extend over a 2-year period, also known as a *biennium;* and still others meet only during even- or odd-numbered years.
- The governor is the chief executive of a state and is responsible for the administration of the state government. Powers held by governors include approving or vetoing bills passed by the legislature, submitting an annual budget, calling special sessions of the legislature, and overseeing the functions of state agencies.[4(p29)]
- State courts are established and governed by the US Constitution and state laws. Most family law, contract, tort, criminal, and probate cases are heard by state courts; this includes cases related to child abuse and neglect. A "court of last resort," often called a *supreme court,* exists in every state, and in addition to trial courts, many states have intermediate-level appellate courts.
- Figure 34.1 illustrates how a bill becomes a law at the state level.

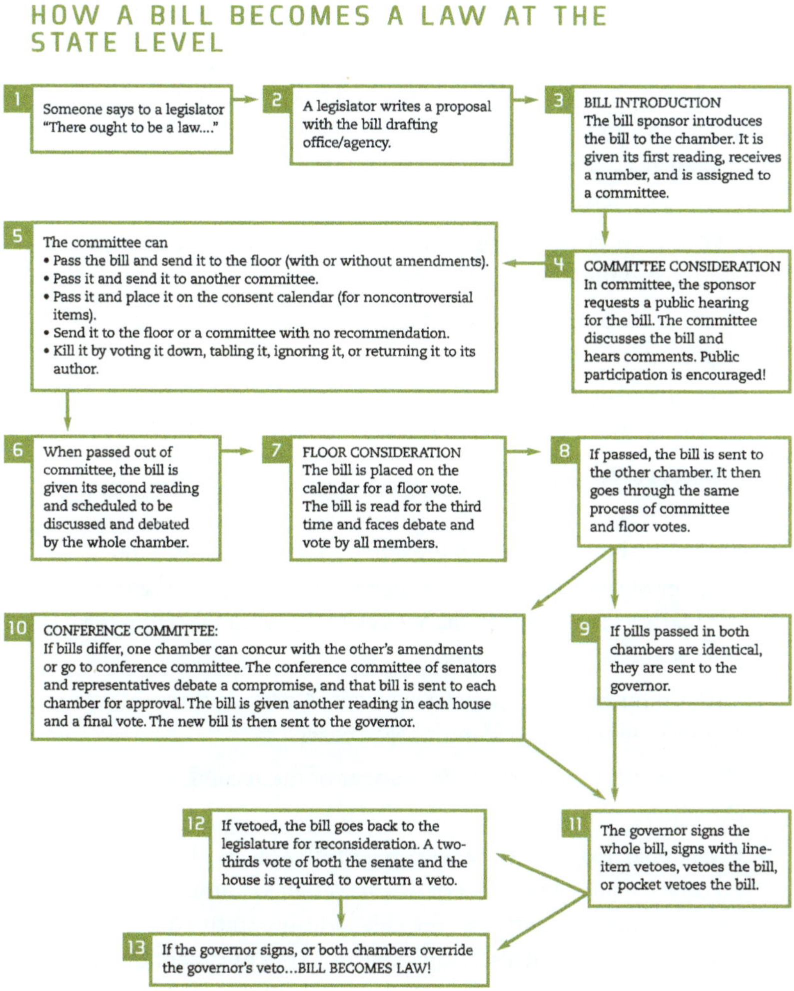

FIGURE 34.1

How a bill becomes a law at the state level.

From American Academy of Pediatrics. *AAP Advocacy Guide*. Elk Grove Village, IL: American Academy of Pediatrics; 2009:47. https://www.aap.org/en-us/advocacy-and-policy/state-advocacy/Documents/AdvocacyGuide.pdf. Accessed July 14, 2019.

Federal Government

The federal government includes 3 coequal branches—legislative, executive, and judicial. The power to enact laws, tax and spend, and confirm or reject presidential appointments is in the hands of the legislative branch, namely the US Congress. The executive branch includes the president, vice president, cabinet, executive departments, independent agencies, and other boards, commissions, and committees.

These individuals and bodies implement and enforce laws. Federal courts and judges, including the US Supreme Court, interpret laws made by the legislative branch and enforced by the executive branch, and determine applicability. These judges and courts, together with the judicial agencies that support their work, comprise the judicial branch. The following fundamentals will help with your federal advocacy:

- Like most state legislatures, the US Congress has 2 chambers, the Senate and the House of Representatives.
- There are 100 US senators and 435 members of the US House of Representatives.
- Each chamber has its own leadership, its own committee structure, and its own set of rules.
- Senators serve 6-year terms and representatives serve 2-year terms.
- Each state has 2 senators representing the entire state. The number of representatives for each state depends on the state's population. This number changes every 10 years following the census and reapportionment.
- Each Congress has 2 one-year sessions. A new Congress always begins in January of odd-numbered years.
- National elections occur in November of the second session of a Congress.
- Each department of the federal government is headed by a secretary who is a member of the president's cabinet. A cabinet secretary not only serves as the chief administrative officer for that department but also as an advisor to the president on the policies and programs related to her or his department.[4(p30)]
- There are 3 main levels in the federal court system. The district courts act as the trial courts; the circuit courts are the first level of appeal; and the Supreme Court is the final level of appeal in the federal system and takes judicial precedence over all other courts in the country.
- Figure 34.2 illustrates how a bill becomes a law at the federal level.

Getting Started

There is no right or wrong way to get involved in advocacy. Your interest, experience, and expertise in seeking policy solutions that support your work to care for children who have experienced neglect and abuse is a solid

HOW A BILL BECOMES A LAW AT THE FEDERAL LEVEL

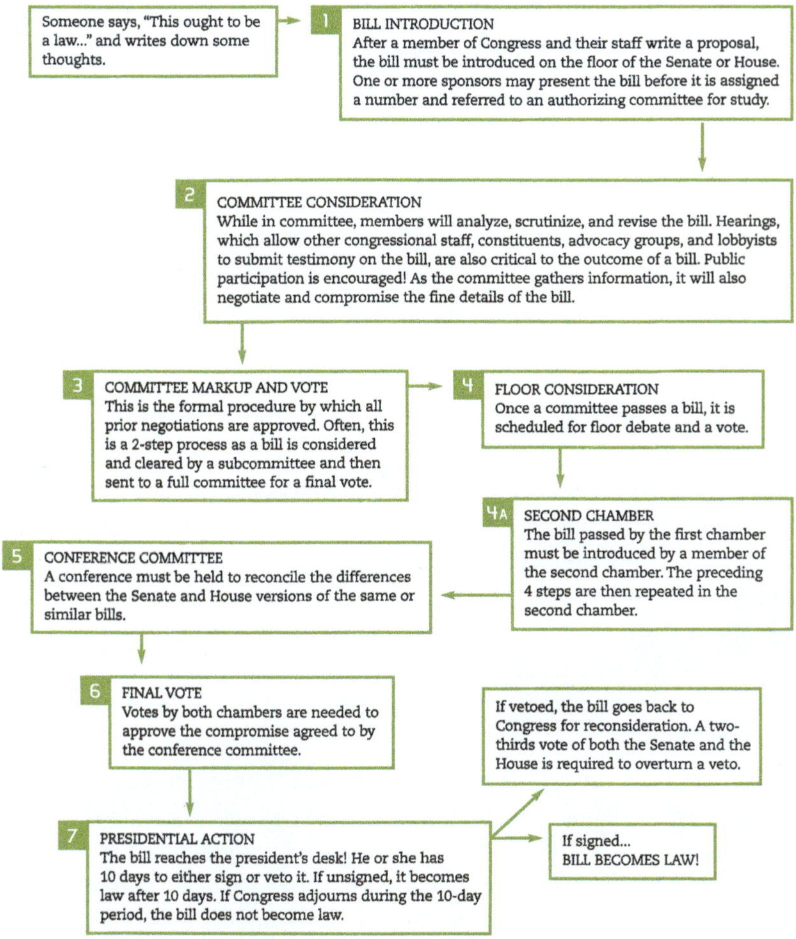

FIGURE 34.2

How a bill becomes a law at the federal level.

From American Academy of Pediatrics. *AAP Advocacy Guide*. Elk Grove Village, IL: American Academy of Pediatrics; 2009:51. https://www.aap.org/en-us/advocacy-and-policy/state-advocacy/Documents/AdvocacyGuide.pdf. Accessed July 14, 2019.

foundation on which to build. There are several factors, though, that may influence your decisions, including

- *Time.* Depending on your schedule, workload, and other constraints, you may determine that you are better suited for one type of advocacy or that your engagement will be most effective if focused on a combination of efforts. Some activities will be long-term, such as relationship building. Others require immediate attention, such as when a crucial bill is being considered by lawmakers.

- *Opportunity.* Your own experiences, trending policy issues, media stories, and, sometimes, the need to push back against proposals that will further harm children present numerous possibilities for engagement. Assessing such opportunities in the context of your time are key steps in your path to acting.
- *Need.* Is your issue being played out on the local, state, or national scene? In the courts or in the media? Can you spend time in your state capitol testifying? Can you call you member of Congress? Can you engage in awareness raising via social media? Fine-tuning your advocacy actions to each opportunity and its timing demands creates a formula for successful engagement.[4(p33–34)]

Once you have assessed your time, the opportunities, and the need, you will likely find that the issue you want to act on to create tangible change will require some realistic goal setting. Consider the following simple steps as you approach your goal:

- *Be realistic.* Make sure your goal is attainable. Consider focusing on no more than 3 goals. This will allow you to channel your energy and reduce the risk of spreading yourself too thin.
- *Think incrementally.* Advocacy is a bit like training for a marathon. Long-term goals may be bold and aggressive, but shorter-term benchmarks that will allow you to assess and celebrate your progress along the way are vital to your progress. For example, if your long-term goal is to introduce legislation to ensure that state and local agencies improve communication and information sharing about at-risk children, an example of a shorter-term goal could be that you have initiated conversations with an interested decision maker.
- *Think broadly.* Success comes in many forms. It may begin by raising awareness of your issues, then increasing the number of people engaged in supporting it, followed by identifying decision makers who understand the need for policy change. A win may be a letter to the editor focusing on your issue published in your newspaper or organizing a related social media campaign.[4(p57)]

Taking Action

The ties between advocacy and protecting children from abuse and neglect are inextricable. Once you know that you can create change and learn the basics of how it can be accomplished, you can get started by assessing key factors that will influence your goals. Then, it is time to act. You will find that advocacy is doable and does not always require a lot of time.

Consider the following ways that you can effectively incorporate advocacy into your already busy schedule:

In Less Than 1 Hour Per Month

- Vote. Decisions about child protection and well-being are make at the local, state, and federal levels. Every election is important. Children cannot vote, but you can be their voice.
- Call, email, or write a letter to your decision makers on behalf of a child protection issue that is important to you.
- Contribute to an advocacy organization or campaign that focuses on children's health, safety, and well-being.
- Provide information in your professional setting on community resources to which you can refer patients.
- Sign up for 1 or 2 email lists that focus on key policy issues.
- Patronize businesses that donate a percentage of their profits to child protection causes and services.

In About 1 Hour Per Month

- Cultivate long-term relationships with a public official or other decision maker in your community.
- Write a letter to the editor of your local newspaper.
- Talk to other professionals and parents that you encounter about the advocacy issues you care about. Encourage them to get involved as well.
- Submit an article on an advocacy issue you care about to a professional or community group's newsletter or website.
- Invite a decision maker to your workplace or a community site to experience what is happening.
- Attend community forums and events sponsored by decision makers or children's safety groups in your area.

In More Than 1 Hour Per Month

- Testify before your town or city council or the state legislature. Participate in a community forum.
- Set up an advocacy booth or display in your professional setting that explains the issue you care about and gives people information and resources for getting involved.
- Serve as a spokesperson for a local issue or community-based organization.
- Volunteer as a board member of a child protection organization working on advocacy in your community.
- Apply for community advocacy grants.
- Become a member or chairperson of your professional association's advocacy committee.[4(p25)]

Sustaining Your Efforts

When it comes to advocating on behalf of children's health and well-being, advocacy work can involve many wins along the way, and they should be celebrated to sustain your efforts. Ongoing work and long-term relationships with elected officials or community leaders are important to ensure that change occurs. Keep the following tips in mind as you continue your advocacy journey:

- *Be patient.* Relationships with elected officials take time to develop. Be patient and remember that each interaction you have with your decision makers gives you a chance to build a stronger relationship and ultimately bring about change in the issues you care about.
- *Choose issues that you are passionate about.* Having a personal connection to the issue you are working on provides you with ongoing motivation to stay involved.
- *Set realistic time frames and identify milestones along the way.* By marking important interim steps, you can track your progress along the way. Milestones could include attracting a bipartisan cosponsor, a hearing being held, a vote being taken (even if you do not win), or an important community leader expressing support.
- *Celebrate often.* Consider each interaction you have with your decision makers a step forward in creating meaningful change for children and child protection professionals.

- *Evaluate your effort.* Take time to assess what is going well and where plans must be changed. Incorporate what you are learning along the way and reassess your goals as needed.[4(p60)]

You Can Make a Difference

As a medical professional caring for vulnerable children, your stories make the issue of children's safety, health, and well-being real in a way that fact sheets or statistics alone cannot. You put a human face on an advocacy issue. By nature of your profession, education, and training, people in your community respect and trust you. When you speak on behalf of an issue, you bring credibility to the issue. Because you instill trust and are credible, you can easily inspire others to get involved in children's health issues. Others in your community will be influenced by what you have to say and will want to become part of your efforts. The same skills you use every day to establish trust, develop relationships, and provide solutions can be applied in your advocacy work. Advocacy allows you to dig deeper into your interests and touches on why you became involved in child protection. Through advocacy, you can channel your passion into meaningful and lasting change.

Most importantly, many of the children you care for do not have the power to advocate for themselves and cannot vote. They need you to tell their story. Through advocacy, you can help ensure that decision makers do not just say children's safety, health, and well-being is a crucial issue but that they actually act on the issue too. You can be the voice children need.[4(p24)]

References

1. American Academy of Pediatrics Council on Community Pediatrics. Community pediatrics: navigating the intersection of medicine, public health, and social determinants of children's health. *Pediatrics*. 2013;131(3):623–628 https://doi.org/10.1542/peds.2012-3933
2. Nazarian LF. A look at the private practice of the future. *Pediatrics*. 1995;96(4 Pt 2):812–816 PMID: 7567362
3. John EB. Myers, A short history of child protection in America. *Fam Law* Q. 2008;42(3):449–457
4. American Academy of Pediatrics. *AAP Advocacy Guide*. Elk Grove Village, IL: American Academy of Pediatrics; 2009. https://www.aap.org/en-us/advocacy-and-policy/state-advocacy/Documents/AdvocacyGuide.pdf. Accessed April 4, 2019

Index

F

N

O

S